INTRODUCTORY MEDICAL ~ SURGICAL NURSING

Jeanne C. Scherer, R.N., M.S.
Assistant Director and
Medical-Surgical Coordinator
Sisters of Charity Hospital
School of Nursing, Buffalo, N.Y.

INTRODUCTORY MEDICAL ~ SURGICAL NURSING

Second Edition

17 92

J. B. Lippincott Company
Philadelphia
NEW YORK SAN JOSE TORONTO

Distributed in Great Britain by
Blackwell Scientific Publications
London Oxford Edinburgh

ISBN 0-397-54200-3

Library of Congress Catalog Card Number 76-57782

Printed in the United States of America

2 4 6 8 9 7 5 3 1

Library of Congress Cataloging in Publication Data

Scherer, Jeanne C.
Introductory medical-surgical nursing.

First ed. (1972) by D. W. Smith and C. P. H. Germain, published under title: Nursing of adults.
Includes bibliographies and index.
1. Nursing. 2. Surgical nursing. I. Title.
[DNLM: 1. Nursing. 2. Surgical nursing.
WY100 S326n]
RT41.S579 1977 610.73 76-57782
ISBN 0-397-54200-3

PREFACE

This text is designed for the student studying medical-surgical nursing for the first time. It offers a complete and thorough coverage of medical-surgical nursing for the beginning student or the practitioner requiring an up-to-date review of the field.

Each chapter is prefaced with objectives that are student and instructor oriented. The student may view the objectives as a guide to the learning experience; the instructor may use the objectives as goals of a particular unit in a program of studies.

Tables have been added to clarify and emphasize the nursing management of major disorders. This tabular material serves as an easy reference and study guide to essential points.

The emphasis of the book is on clinical practice with pathophysiological and psychosocial aspects serving as background for the teaching of nursing management of patients with medical-surgical disorders. Material on patient education, particularly discharge teaching, has been included where appropriate.

A summary of general pharmacological and nutritional considerations has been included at the end of appropriate chapters to succinctly emphasize the important points in nursing management. A glossary of medical terms and an appendix of common laboratory values are included for easy reference.

A separate workbook has been designed for use with this textbook. All questions contained in the *Student Work Manual for Introductory Medical-Surgical Nursing* have been taken directly from this textbook.

There were many individuals involved in the production of this book. The general format and the establishment of guidelines came from David T. Miller, managing editor of the nursing department at J. B. Lippincott Company. To Mary Dennesaites Morgan I owe special recognition for her encouragement, guidance, ideas, and editorial assistance. The thoughtful attention of copy editors Joyce Mkitarian, Val Rementer, and Elaine Terranova is especially appreciated. Dorothy W. Smith and Carol Hanley Germain, the authors of *Nursing of Adults,* on which this book is based, allowed some of their original material to be retained in this text.

The photographs taken by Mr. Dennis Atkinson demonstrate professional capability in capturing what the author had in mind. The assistance of Paul S. Milley, M.D., attending pathologist, and H. A. Revollo, M.D., attending pathologist, both of Sisters of Charity Hospital is appreciated. Mrs. Agnes O'Shea, Director of Public Relations at the same hospital was an invaluable assistance in arranging some of the photographic sessions.

The cooperation and assistance extended by the nursing staff at Sisters of Charity Hospital of Buffalo and De Graff Memorial Hospital of North Tonawanda, New York provided the author and photographer with the situations which complement the textbook material.

Special recognition must go to those wonderful people called patients who consented to be a part of this textbook, and to the students of the class of 1977 at Sisters of Charity Hospital School of Nursing to whom this textbook is respectfully dedicated.

Jeanne C. Scherer

CONTENTS

UNIT FOUR
Disorders of cognitive, sensory, or pyschomotor function

UNIT FIVE
Threats to adequate respiration

UNIT SIX
Insults to cardiovascular integrity

INTRODUCTORY MEDICAL ~ SURGICAL NURSING

UNIT ONE

Concepts basic to the care of patients

- Care of adults throughout the life cycle
- Nurse-patient relationships
- Fundamental processes of health and illness
- The interaction of body and mind
- The patient in pain
- Dependence on and abuse of alcohol, drugs, and tobacco
- Care of the dying patient
- Nursing in emergencies
- The surgical patient

CHAPTER 1

Care of adults throughout the life cycle

On completion of this chapter the student will:

- **Identify physical and mental commonalities and differences at various levels of human development.**
- **Discuss the implications of physical and mental changes for the development of an individual nursing care plan.**
- **Describe and compare specific physical changes in the aging process and the effects these changes may have on the nursing management of the patient.**
- **Discuss the physical and emotional effects of the aging process.**
- **Describe and discuss the special needs and problems relative to the young, middle-aged, and elderly.**
- **Discuss the current problems of the senior citizen.**

The developmental process

Growth, decline, change and development: all are parts of the dynamic thing we call living. The changes that people experience over a lifetime are often described as *aging*. The aging process occurs at different rates in different individuals.

Just as the age at which menstruation begins may vary, the time of the changes that come later in life can vary. One person may be mentally alert, vigorous, and active at 80, while another, aged and infirm at 60. For purposes of discussion, young adulthood is that period when the individual is establishing himself, roughly between the ages of 18 and 35. Middle life, from about 35 to 65, the established years, is the period when a person has found his place and is enlarging it and making it more secure. Sixty-five has become a common designation for the beginning of old age, since pension and retirement plans normally start at this age; physiological and mental aging, of course, may begin earlier or later.

It is important to understand the developmental pattern of the adult so that normal changes are not confused with the changes of disease. Some changes are obvious and familiar to all. For example, hair gradually turns gray as age advances and reflexes become slowed. Contrast the speed of a 17-year-old on crutches with the movement of an 80-year-old getting out of bed for the first time after surgery. If the nurse knows what to expect from patients on the basis of development and aging, a plan of care may become more effective and patient teaching more realistic.

Developmental tasks of adults in our culture

The baby under 2 has to learn to walk. One of the 6-year-old's tasks is to learn to read, and the adolescent is expected to establish relationships with the opposite sex that are different from those of childhood. In our society one of the responsibilities of the young adult is to establish a home and career. In middle life there is increasing community responsibility, whereas the elderly lend to others the wisdom gathered through a lifetime.

Every stage of development has its own tasks—hurdles to be surmounted, things to be learned, changes to be accomplished. Developmental tasks are achieved most readily at certain ages; failure to accomplish these at one time may make their later realization difficult.

There is a progression in the scope of developmental tasks as the individual grows from childhood to adulthood. For example, in adjusting to his own body, it is the young child's task to learn what is part of the physical self and what is not (his toy is not, but his toes are) and to develop skill in using his body for walking, holding a spoon, dressing, running, and other activities. It is the adolescent's task to make a socially satisfactory adjustment to the maturing changes that his body undergoes, and to accept and utilize these changes. It is an adult's task to maintain a healthful physical regimen in spite of the pressures of his life and to learn what new motor skills are needed in his work, home, or recreational activities; and it is the task of the older adult to adapt his living to diminished strength and agility.

Developmental tasks are culturally determined. Whereas in our culture young people are expected to become independent of their parents, in some societies young adults marry but continue to live in the parental household and to obey their parents' wishes. Although our society places great emphasis on working, making money, and getting ahead, some people place a major value on enjoying each moment of life as it is lived. In planning health care, account must be taken of such differences. Clinic appointments may be broken if the individual believes more in today than in tomorrow. If he feels ill on the day of his appointment, he will come; if he feels well, he may go fishing instead.

There is, and probably should be, wide variation in the degree to which adults achieve various tasks. One may be a loving husband and father but a poor provider. Another may earn a very large salary but spend little time with his family. The fact that individuals progress in such different ways is a gain for society. Discussing developmental tasks of adults does not imply that every individual should conform to a mold labeled "The Perfect Adult."

Oversimplification of the concept of developmental tasks is to be avoided. Adjustments must be made over and over, as each period of life, or each change in the environment, makes new demands. For example, fear of being alone, experienced early in life, may seem to be solved during middle life by close relationships with a growing family, only to reappear in later life when family and friends die or move away. Rather than viewing developmental tasks as achieved or not achieved, it is more accurate to recognize that people of all ages are in the process of realizing them and that the degree of success with each task may vary markedly at different periods of life.

Some intangibles

While the more tangible accomplishments of establishing a home and earning a living are easier to observe, the search for meaning, for identity, and for lasting values involves tasks which determine the quality of the patient's life and relationships. The degree to which one performs these tasks may influence his response to illness.

Whether the individual is successfully dealing with these inner tasks is likely to become evident in times of stress such as during illness or bereavement. Some people are aided by a strong religious faith. Illness, aging, and the loss of loved ones bring fundamental questions to the fore, such as, "What is the purpose of my life?" or "Now that I am old and cannot work, what use am I?" Patients sometimes voice these thoughts to the nurse when given an opportunity; however, many patients do not ask these questions directly, but may imply them by their attitudes and reactions. The nurse sees people under circumstances which tend to reveal inner strength, or a lack of it. Just as it is important to accept patients whose values and beliefs are different from one's own, it is also important to accept the patient's progress, as far as achievement of various life tasks is concerned. The patient who has been primarily concerned with surface events may continue to focus on them during illness. The nurse should respect this attitude and not seek to change it. However, if the patient shows that he wishes to discuss some of his concerns about the meaning of life, or about his illness, the nurse can help by listening, and showing sympathy. Some patients mobilize themselves after illness and misfortune; others, seemingly no worse off, do not. The inner strength which an individual has may not be known, even to him, until it is tested by an ordeal. This inner strength is related to ability and willingness to withstand the pain and anxiety involved in facing some of the fundamental issues of one's life, and to accept help from others when it is needed. The patients to whom you can be of most genuine and lasting service are those who can accept your help and use it to strengthen their own forces in their struggle with illness or disability.

How can the nurse answer such questions as, "Why must I suffer so much pain?" or "Why did my husband have to die so young?" The nurse is not in a position to provide the answers—especially not for another person whose values and experiences may be quite different from her own. The nurse can listen to the patient and convey concern for him as he puts these questions to himself.

Illness is quite naturally regarded as a misfortune. For some, going through illness opens up new opportunities to explore the meaning and values of life; for these patients it can be an opportunity for personal growth. Because the nurse cares for people during crises, such as illness and bereavement, it often becomes necessary to support and help patients during these experiences.

Coping with illness is part of living. Few escape it. How illness is dealt with depends on how the person has learned to handle stress, on the severity of the condition, and on the support afforded by the environment, of which the nurse may be a significant part.

The young adult

The young adult is usually physically more resilient than the older person. Two days after an appendectomy he may be able to carry out activities which a middle-aged patient who had the same operation must postpone for a week. The young person often has an emotional resilience, too, enabling him to mobilize energy quickly after a shock or a loss. This does not necessarily mean that he has dealt adequately with the experience inwardly. He may at a later time need to go back and reexamine the experience, and its meaning to him.

The young person's resilience is enhanced by the supports which society offers him. Our society invests heavily in the young; they are, after all, its future. The young person is also more likely to have intact family relationships than is an elderly person. Often the young adult's ties with his parents are still strong, and in addition, he may have founded a young family of his own.

Because many young people have other sources for support and assistance, the nurse may fail to notice the ways in which young patients require help. Visits from friends and family may seem to imply that the young adult has many meaningful relationships with others and that he is receiving much support. However, this is not necessarily so. The relationships may be superficial, leaving the patient very much alone. In any case, personal relationships do not take the place of the professional helping role of the nurse and other members of the staff. The nurse must not assume that the young patient (or a person of any age) who is surrounded by cards, flowers, and candy does not need attention to his physical or emotional needs.

The patient's resilience may be another factor which deters the nurse from recognizing his need for a supportive listener. Nevertheless, it is important to help the patient to assimilate painful experiences. Too often, family and friends discourage the patient from talking about the experience. They may be eager to forget an event which is also painful for them. Because the nurse listens, the patient is helped to review what has happened and to confront some of his feelings about his illness during his stay in the hospital. Such nursing intervention may or may not help a patient deal with the experience and move on to new opportunities.

The hospital is an environment where authority and rigid adherence to a routine are much in evidence, and where patients usually have little voice in making the rules. If the young adult is hospitalized for more than a brief period, the rigidity of rules and authority is likely to become especially irritating. He may find various ways to express his dissatisfaction such as turning up the volume of the radio or television, disregarding the doctor's orders, and so forth. To whatever extent possible, it is important to include the young patient in the decision-making process, while making a special effort to interpret hospital rules to him. Even if rules cannot be changed, they will be less likely to cause anxiety to the patient who understands their purpose. For instance, enforcing the rule limiting visitors to two at a time per patient makes it impossible for a young man to entertain a group of friends. He may find his disappointment softened, however, by realizing the impracticality of allowing each patient as many visitors as he wishes. Even if the young patient does not concede this point, he will have received the interest and concern of the nurse who, instead of officiously quoting the rules, took time to explain them.

Relationships with physicians and nurses can also reveal to the young person that basic human questions affect people of all ages. While one's perspectives on these questions differ with age, sharing of views can lead each person to deeper understanding. The physician and nurse can provide experience with rational authority. Previously, the young patient may have viewed authority as essentially arbitrary and negative—inciting his antagonism. However, professional people, by the nature of their work, have many opportunities to emphasize the rational aspects of authority. The physician recommends bed rest, not in order to impose his will on the patient or to restrict his freedom, but because the patient's condition requires it. The nurse firmly encourages the postoperative patient to walk, not out of a wish to inflict pain but because walking will help him to recover. Emphasizing the reasons behind the staff's actions and decisions, and avoiding arbitrary use of authority, may help the young person appreciate authority and discipline. These qualities are not necessarily negative and restrictive, but can also be positive forces enabling those with special knowledge and skill to exercise them for the benefit of others.

What of the nurse's own reactions to working with young adults? For the nurse who is in this age group there may be a particular tendency to identify with the patient; this may be a problem if the patient has a terminal illness, such as leukemia. Caring for a fatally ill young person is a stark reminder of the unpredictability of each person's life span. Working with young adults may make it especially difficult for a young nurse to keep professional and social roles differentiated. The older nurse may carry over to the patient previously experienced conflicts with adolescent children. For nurses of all ages, the challenge in caring for a young adult lies in helping the patient move forward with the developmental tasks of his age period to the extent his illness allows, as well as in providing appropriate care.

Physical changes

Following the rapid changes of puberty, physical growth ceases between 18 and 20. Thereafter a slow and barely perceptible decline in many physical abilities begins. At about 20, the body and general appearance no longer change quickly.

Visual Accommodation. The ability of the eye to adjust to near and far vision is one of the reliable physiological indicators of age. Children can see an object clearly when it is held almost at the tip of their noses. Even before puberty this ability begins to diminish gradually, and continues to decline during most of adult life.

Changes in Hearing. These also occur throughout life. Loss of ability to hear high tones begins in childhood. Hearing is most acute at about the age of 14; thereafter it declines gradually. It is established that persons exposed to loud noise, both industrial and environmental as well as loud music, over prolonged periods, often develop a hearing loss. Those working in an area where noise is unavoidable should take steps to prevent hearing loss. A protective device, resembling earmuffs or stereo headphones, is almost always supplied by the safety division of an industrial organization. Those exposed to loud music should seriously consider the consequences of such exposure. As a rule, hearing loss is gradual and often irreversible and may go unnoticed until a severe loss has occurred.

Position Sense and Speed of Reaction. These reach their peak between the ages of 20 and 30. Some youths tend to be too sure of their fast reaction time and push their luck beyond their ability to respond. You will meet as patients some of the luckier young men and women whose accidents did not prove fatal.

Developmental tasks

A task of young adults in our culture is to work toward independence and self-esteem. One aspect of achieving independence is to gradually differentiate oneself from one's parents. This process involves developing values and making decisions. An aspect of developing self-esteem is learning respect for one's own competence. This, in turn, results in respect for others and their competence; it also furnishes a basis for finding a place as a productive member of society.

Young adults are expected to become independent of their parents, gradually developing a different type of relationship with them, one in which the young person begins to accept the consequences of his own actions. Such a development does not take place suddenly; indeed, it has its beginnings when the child is encouraged to make decisions of his own. Young people whose parents have helped them gradually to assume more independence usually find this transition period easier than those whose parents continue to exert very strict control through late adolescence.

As part of his independence from his parents, the young adult is expected to learn a trade or a profession and begin to support himself. In our technologically advanced society, learning a profession usually entails extended schooling and prolongs economic dependence on parents well beyond the point at which physical maturity has been reached.

Young adults are expected to make decisions, stick to them and take the consequences. The adult should be able to face reality and differentiate between it and fantasy. Progress in this task, as in others, is achieved gradually throughout childhood and adolescence. Its accomplishment is of major importance in helping the young adult to sort out his own strengths and weaknesses and to set realistic goals for himself.

Implications for nursing

Most people have been taught through their childhood years to control expressions of strong emotion. Before surgery, the child may plainly express his fear, giving those who care for him a chance to reassure and comfort him. The young adult may be no less frightened but may show fear in less obvious ways. He too requires reassurance, but sometimes it is harder to recognize his need.

Because they are involved in achieving independence from their parents, many young people have difficulty accepting their parents' suggestions, even when these suggestions could prove useful. The nurse can be especially helpful to these patients by allowing them opportunities to express their ideas and to ask questions about matters that interest or concern them, and by conveying respect for them as individuals. Members of the health professions can offer help and suggestions that might be rejected if parents offered them. Counseling in matters of personal health, such as the hygiene of menstruation or care of the skin in acne, is an example of the kind of problem for which young people may seek the nurse's help. Recognizing the young person's struggle for independence, the wise nurse carefully avoids a patronizing air; instead, she provides sound information that the young person may consider in coming to his own decisions.

Some adolescents may be placed on adult hospital units. Other hospitals have adolescent units with policies that provide opportunities for socialization, music, and snacks. On adult wards, noncritically ill adolescents and young adults often benefit when they are assigned beds near each other, because they have similar interests.

The adolescent or young adult who is still developing a concept of his physical self and working through his feelings about sex often finds illness frightening. Illness and surgery may mean that his ideal picture of a beautiful body cannot be his. Surgery on or near genitals can greatly intensify the fear of castration. Embarrassment—so easily brought on—is conscious, but the underlying basis for it may be subconscious. Providing maximum protection against unnecessary exposure and fully explaining what is going to happen before a procedure is started, and why it is done, lessen some of the anxiety. The very fact that the nurse shows interest can convey to the patient that the hospital staff is concerned with his welfare, understands his feelings, and respects his right to privacy.

Because he is not yet sure of his own strengths, the young person may worry about the impression he makes on others. The hard job of working out how much dependence he can accept without interfering with his struggle for independence can make the patient irritable. He may retort angrily when he does not mean to. An angry response from the nurse, although understandable, compels the patient to prolong his anger to save face. Youth is a period of intense testing—of oneself and one's abilities, of the endurance of one's body, of one's influence on others.

Being sick and in a hospital removes from the individual the opportunity to test himself in his usual environment. It is an interruption that few welcome.

Growth as well as activity has high energy requirements, so the caloric needs of those who have not attained their full growth are higher than those for older persons engaging in the same amount of activity. Young patients may require a diet higher in calories, larger food portions, or between-meal snacks.

At any age, success in coping with difficult problems can increase an individual's confidence in himself and his skill in dealing with similar situations in the future. Pain, fear, loneliness, and anger reappear many times in the lives of most people. The young person who is helped to combat them during a personal crisis, such as illness, is girded for future encounters.

Creating a Positive Environment. The young patient with a chronic disease or a permanent disability is in danger of missing the challenges and the learning opportunities appropriate to his age. The nurse might search for ways to change the patient's environment so that he has experiences that are more typical of his culture. Are there courses that the homebound or hospitalized adolescent can take? Is there a party he can attend? Can transportation be provided to a church group? When parents, adolescents, and nurses put their heads together and community resources are investigated, ways can often be found to provide the handicapped young person with the experiences he needs.

Working with Parents. In addition to working with the young adult, the nurse has a role in working with his parents. Particularly when illness strikes, parents can be helped greatly by explanations and reassurances from the nurse. Even though they share a home, communication between family members may be inadequate. This is often the case between an adolescent and his parents.

In the tension and the conflicting demands of everyday life, many people experience twinges of regret and self-reproach for not having been, on one occasion or another, more perceptive of another's needs, or more generous in giving of their time and attention. When sudden illness occurs, such feelings sometimes surge to the fore and may be expressed as, "Is this partly my fault? Is there something I should have done to prevent it?" The wise nurse will allow the family or friends to discuss the matter but will avoid any comment which implies blame. After the sudden shock of the illness and after the patient has received initial treatment, the nurse can assist the family to recognize ways in which they can help to prevent, or detect promptly, similar problems in the future.

It is important to help the adolescent to deal with his illness, whether temporary or permanent, and to avoid unnecessary threats to his health in the future. All this requires knowledge and understanding on the part of the patient. He will be better able to meet his health needs in the future if he has some understanding of the reactions of his own body in health and in illness. Understanding one's own illness is never purely an intellectual undertaking; it is a combined intellectual and emotional process that includes accepting what has happened and planning what to do about it.

The adult in middle life

Middle life is the period when dependence on others is least acceptable—to the patient, his close associates, and to those who care for him. The middle years are usually characterized by productivity, self-satisfaction, and responsibility toward others. A change from independence and productivity toward dependence and curtailment of productivity may constitute a major crisis for this age group. To become partially or totally dependent on others, even for short periods of time, is often difficult for the patient who is accustomed to independence in his thinking and actions.

Physical changes

Strength. Change occurs continuously but so gradually that it is often not noticed. Nevertheless, a particular event can bring the change suddenly into sharp focus. For example, a man of 55 is driving along the parkway and has a flat tire. Through good luck and good management it has been years since he has had a flat. He begins the job of jacking up the car. All goes well until it is time to lift the spare tire into place. It is just too heavy. He realizes with a start that he is not as strong as he used to be. This fact is emphasized painfully when a lad of 20 stops to help him. With a cheery, "Stand aside, sir," the younger man easily places the tire in position. The loss of strength which seemed to make its appearance in this man's 50s had actually been going on for two or three decades but had gone relatively unnoticed until an unusual event demanded the physical prowess that he no longer possessed. However, some of the loss of strength may be attributed to disuse atrophy, suggesting that regular exercise over a lifetime contributes to well-being. The middle-aged laborer may note less loss of strength than the middle-aged man who has spent most of his time at his desk.

HEIGHT AND WEIGHT. These show continuous increase until about age 20. Height tends to remain constant until old age, when posture and settling of bones cause a slight decline. In contrast, weight continues to increase until about 60. Commonly there is a lessening of exercise and slowing of metabolism without a corresponding decrease in caloric intake. If an individual has reached optimum weight during young adulthood, it is undesirable for him to continue to gain weight as he grows older. However, it is often difficult for him to stay slim.

During middle life there is a gradual slowing of metabolism and reaction time, as well as a gradual decline in visual and auditory perception. During this period early signs of aging make their appearance. Sometimes these early and obvious changes are traumatic for the individual in a youth-worshiping culture. This attitude is reflected in the American preoccupation with cosmetics and youthful clothes. Bernard Shaw once said that while the 30s are the old age of youth, the 40s are the youth of old age.

PACE. During middle life, the individual gradually modifies his pace. This modification by no means indicates "sitting back," for these are usually the busiest years of life. However, there is a subtle change in the tempo of living, such as walking up steps instead of racing up two at a time, and shifting participation in sports from the most strenuous and competitive to those somewhat less demanding. During active adult life many of the extremes of physical strength are not required, and their gradual loss is scarcely noticed.

Subtle but important cultural influences, as well as physical changes, cause a slow shift in activity at various ages, so that the older person often no longer seeks more strenuous activities. Society shifts its expectations of what pursuits are considered appropriate for various age groups. These shifts are not always consistent with desirable health practices.

There has been increasing recognition of the ill effects of lack of exercise, particularly during middle and later life. Lack of regular exercise may contribute to obesity, lessened efficiency of the circulatory and respiratory systems, and decreased muscle tone and strength. Rather than gradually slipping into a routine of too little exercise, persons in middle and later life should undertake regular activities that provide exercise as well as enjoyment. Exercise that is suitable, and possible, varies over the life span and from person to person. Brisk walking, swimming, gardening, and bicycling have been suggested as activities that can be engaged in by older persons who are in good health. Social pressures exert an influence, perhaps not wholly desirable, on the kind of exercise older people feel free to undertake. Emphasis on conformity and on youthful glamor in sports attire discourage some older people from activities such as swimming and bicycling. Cost must be considered, as well as availability.

The middle-aged person who has neglected physical activity and who decides to begin a program of exercise should first see his physician for a physical examination. It is not unheard of for a middle-aged, sedentary person who decides to exercise in order to prevent myocardial infarction, to suffer just this occurrence during an ill-considered burst of exercise for which he has not gradually prepared himself.

Physical examinations in the middle years emphasize the detection of illnesses most commonly found in this age group—heart and blood vessel disease, cancer, and diabetes.

MENOPAUSE. Menopause usually occurs between the ages of 45 and 55, but may vary considerably. Puberty is marked by rapid growth, maturation of reproductive organs, and the development of secondary sex characteristics in response to the stimulation of sex hormones. Menopause, on the other hand, is characterized by shrinkage of reproductive organs due to the gradual reduction in sex hormones. Gradually, ovulation and menstruation cease.

This period of life is probably more difficult for women than for men. There is no physiological climacteric or "change of life" among men, as there is among women, but, rather, a gradual decrease of sexual vigor. However, a proud new father at the age of 70 is by no means unknown. The fact that menopause usually coincides with the growing independence of children causes profound changes in many women's responsibilities and activities, while men may continue to be very much absorbed in their careers during middle life. Contrary to popular belief, marked diminution in sexual response does not necessary accompany menopause.

VISUAL ACCOMMODATION. Loss of visual accommodation, called *presbyopia,* which interferes with reading, sewing, and other close work usually starts between ages 40 and 50. The individual holds reading matter farther and farther from his eyes in order to see it clearly. This adjustment of position, known as the "tromboning effect," has given rise to many jokes about needing longer arms for reading. The individual achieves artificial accommodation by using reading glasses for close work or by wearing lenses especially ground to provide for accommodation (bifocals, trifocals). Gradual decline in visual acuity also occurs; significant changes usually do not appear until about the age of 40. More light is needed for such activities as reading and sewing.

Changes in Hearing. Hearing gradually diminishes with age, and some people, particularly in later middle life, find that the decrease is sufficient to interfere with their communication with others. Loss of hearing which occurs as a result of aging is called *presbycusis*.

By speaking slowly and clearly, the nurse can improve communication with the hearing-impaired patient. If the patient has been fitted with a hearing aid he may have to be reminded to wear it when communicating with hospital personnel. The nurse should face the patient while speaking so that he can note lip movement and facial expression.

Developmental tasks

In middle life the person is at the period in which society is making the greatest demands on him. He is responsible not only for himself but also for the care of his children and often, his aging parents. It is at this time that the individual acquires most of his material possessions. Maximum earning power may be reached during this period.

Adjusting to Independence of Children. Often it is difficult for middle-aged parents to accept their children's growing independence. The necessary changes in attitude may be especially difficult for the mother whose entire life has been devoted to her children and her home. The fact that women are living longer and are in better health than ever before means that those who have children are still active and vigorous when their children are grown. Keeping house is usually not sufficiently challenging to women during later middle life. The menopause often coincides with these events. The woman's total reaction may be a feeling of despair and uselessness. In contrast, the man with a family is usually still very much involved in his work and career; therefore, he may find it less difficult to accept his children's growing independence.

Women who have been employed may view the independence of their children differently from those who have remained at home. For these women, employment may provide involvement and a challenge during their children's transition from dependence to independence, as well as mental and emotional diversion.

Adjusting to Dependence of the Aged. The increasing dependence of the aged also presents strains on persons in middle life, not only financially, but also socially and emotionally. Apartments and homes tend to be small in modern urban society. They were planned to accommodate only the family of parents and children. Most people in our society prefer separate dwellings for each nuclear family. Some families manage very well, however, with a three-generation household. When families live together for economic reasons, even though they would prefer to live separately, strains and conflicts often result.

Because more people are living to an advanced age when the likelihood of physical and mental infirmity increases, their grown children may become increasingly involved in care of aged parents. The needs of the parents, which become more pressing as time passes, revive the old problem of independence from parents. This time the problem is set in a new context, since now it is the child who is stronger and the parents who are weaker; the child who is richer, and the parents who are poorer. The person in middle life may experience difficulty in meeting the needs of both growing children and aged parents.

It may become necessary to consider placing an aged parent in a public or private nursing home. At this time the nurse can be of assistance in helping the family choose one where standards are high: where the menus are well planned, where there is enough well-qualified staff, where the building is safe, and where there are opportunities for rehabilitation. Care in a geriatric setting need not mean severing close family ties or a termination of responsibility and participation in the care of one's parents. Grown children often feel guilty about placing their parents in an institution, even though it does not seem feasible for them to take the parent into their own homes. Their guilt often leads them to express anger and dissatisfaction toward the home and the care given. The reluctance that people often have in acknowledging the declining abilities of their parents presents problems in setting realistic rehabilitation goals. Understanding the purposes of the various treatments, such as exercises, helps to lessen the tendency of the grown children to view the facility and its staff with dissatisfaction.

Foster-home care may be provided by a couple or a widow who enjoys the company of older people and who has a large house. The advantages to the older person include living in a home environment without having responsibility for its upkeep; and the possible strain of different generations of the same family living together is prevented. The older person brings income to the family who is boarding him; in some instances the state finances the foster care. Foster homes, like institutions, can be poor or excellent. Much depends on the personalities of the people providing the care.

Observing the aging of one's parents is, for many people, a difficult experience. Changes that tend to occur with very advanced age—such as forgetfulness, loss of physical strength, and diminution of vision and hearing—may be very distressing. For a few people the experience of watching their parents age is so painful, particularly if the aging process is complicated by illness or marked impairment of function, that they find ways to withdraw from it. They may avoid visiting the parent or giving assistance that seems within their ability to provide.

Certain guidelines can be helpful in such situations. Remember that people vary in their ability to cope with stressful situations. Blaming the son or daughter for what appears to be neglect of his parents is usually ineffective in helping him to assume more responsibility. This approach may, in fact, make the son or daughter even more likely to avoid the situation, whereas an attitude of acceptance may help the grown child to become better able to assist his parents.

Regardless of the attitude of the grown children, the nurse can be most helpful if she recognizes that the decision concerning future care of the older person rests with the parent and the children. She should not attempt to impose personal views on others, but help them to find their own solutions.

THE SINGLE PERSON. For a variety of reasons, many people remain single. Individual, creative, or sometimes religious fulfillment may be served best by remaining single. The single person may be lonely, as might anyone, but he or she may have a full life of varied and rich relationships. Many who remain unmarried develop a certain self-reliance that serves them well in later life because they tend to plan ahead and provide for the time when loneliness, lack of interest, and too much free time are a torment to many others.

TIME. Some interesting changes occur in the way the person in middle life views time. Time not only seems to be shorter, but it *is* shorter. A person who feels himself to be in the wrong job and would like to enter another is aware that soon there will be no time left to make such a major change. The woman who has no children may feel that it will soon be too late to have any. Just as it is inevitable that children will grow up, it is also inevitable that parents will die in due course, probably during this period of a person's life. The changes in his own body also remind him that time has not stood still.

SATISFACTIONS OF MIDDLE AGE. Just as young adulthood has its satisfactions as well as its stresses, so is middle life a mixture of the two. At this period the person has a chance to reap the harvest of his early struggle to establish a home and earn a living.

The person in middle life perceives his own assets, and can utilize them for the good of his family, the community, and society, as well as for his own self-development. He can harness his energies to the accomplishment of goals that are significant and worthwhile. With a channeling and focusing of his energies may come additional time for enjoyment.

Middle life makes an individual increasingly aware of choices. Some of the choices he has made himself; others have been made by circumstances. If the direction of one's life is recognized as essentially consistent with one's values, middle life can be richly satisfying.

Of course, as at any period in life, not everything will always go well. The person may never achieve success at home or at work. Nevertheless, it is during middle life that most people (if they are going to do so at all) bring their dreams and abilities to fulfillment.

IMPLICATIONS FOR NURSING

A major problem confronting the individual who becomes ill during middle life is change from independence and productivity to dependence and curtailment of productivity. These changes also create problems at other age periods, but their impact is particularly severe during middle life.

In what ways may the nurse assist the patient with this problem—or at least avoid adding to it? One way is to avoid adopting stereotyped expectations concerning the patient's response to illness, but instead be observant of his individual way of reacting. For example, there is a widespread expectation among nurses that the mother who becomes ill is more concerned about her children's welfare than her own, and that the father-provider who becomes ill is more worried about his family's welfare and support than he is about his own recovery. It seems likely that to some extent such statements reflect the expectations of nurses, rather than necessarily the reactions of patients. Some patients do respond to illness with greater concern for others than for themselves. However, a common response to illness, at any age, is increased concern for, and preoccupation with, one's own welfare, and diminished capacity to be concerned about the needs of others.

Just as it is important to avoid burdening the patient with stereotyped expectations of his behavior and attitudes toward others, it is also important to support his remaining independence and ability to make decisions and to participate in planning his own care. Because the shift from independence to dependence is already a problem, it is particularly important to use nursing approaches which foster the degree of independence of which the patient is capable.

For example, a man who is recovering from myocardial infarction must rest. He must stay in bed and allow the nurse to bathe him. Frequently these patients express anger at curtailment of their activities and, particularly, at having decisions made for them. Many patients who suffer myocardial infarction are active, hard-driving people who are very much involved in their work. Suddenly, with the onset of infarction, the patient is reduced to the helpless physical dependence of an infant. If a patient expresses anger over the abrupt curtailment of his independence, one of the things a nurse can do is consider with him the areas where he can make decisions, such as selecting food choices from a special diet menu.

A great variety of illnesses usually associated with emotional stress, such as asthma, peptic ulcer, and colitis, are common during this time of life. Recognition of this period as one in which the individual's responsibilities and stresses are numerous may help the nurse to care for patients whose illness is greatly affected by emotional strain.

The modern independent small family consisting of parents and children encounters extra problems when illness strikes. If the mother becomes ill, no one is there to take over the housework and care of the children. Employing someone to do this work is often difficult and unsatisfactory, even if the family can afford it.

It is sometimes hard for those working with the hospitalized patient to recall that he is part of a family. It is so easy for nurses to sympathize only with the patient, since it is his need that they see, and to view his family in a supporting role. You may hear a nurse say at morning report, "And poor old Mr. Jones—his children hardly ever come to see him. It's a shame." It is easy to sympathize with Mr. Jones and disapprove of the children who fail to visit him at a time when he needs them most. But the situation affecting Mr. Jones's children may be completely unknown to the nurse. It is possible that Mr. Jones's son has a sick wife at home, and it is all he can do to go to work and care for his wife and children. Parent-child relationships during middle and later life are an outgrowth of those developed throughout the years, and the situation may involve complex emotional and social factors. Usually, the members of the patient's family are doing the best they can within the limitations of the emotional, social, and economic pressures placed upon them.

For many people during middle life there is a quickening of interest in their own thoughts and inner experiences. No longer as concerned and absorbed in establishing a place for themselves in work, community, and family life, they begin to turn inward to greater consideration of their own values, life style, and relationships with others. Illness can spark this process by posing some profound questions concerning the meaning of life and death, as well as by providing a respite from usual activities, thus affording time for reflection. The nurse can help the patient by listening if he wishes to discuss some of these concerns.

The experience of illness can provide an opportunity for personal growth. It allows the patient to confront fundamental issues of life and to deepen his understanding and the quality of his relationships. The nurse must recognize this opportunity and support the patient in his experience.

The older adult

Associated with physiological changes of aging is an increased susceptibility to illness, and slowness to recover from it. In our society many of the aged are disadvantaged also in relation to family ties, income, housing, and opportunities to perform useful and respected work.

The care of the aged is the responsibility not only of their children but of society as a whole. The view that families alone are responsible for care of the aged has brought some results which are tragic for individuals and, in the long run, for society. For instance, a couple in their late 50s may be continuing to support one or two aged parents in a nursing home, at a time of life when they should be saving money for their own rapidly approaching retirement. When their retirement does come, they may be obliged to seek assistance through public welfare.

It is essential for nurses to understand these problems and to recognize that they may significantly affect the lives of several members of a family, rather than just the aged. It is also important for nurses to recognize their role in helping families make their own decisions in these matters, rather than making the decisions for them, or subtly influencing them about what course of action to take. The nurse who is quick to recommend a nursing home, and the nurse who subtly implies that placing a relative in a nursing home is tantamount to abandonment, are both imposing their own values on others, rather than helping the elderly person and his family to consider alternatives and to decide what is best for them.

The assumption is sometimes made that later life is synonymous with incapacity. One often hears an achievement of an older person received with astonishment: "Imagine, at *his* age!" Such responses actually reveal condescension, and an expectation that the significant part of life is over, once one has passed middle age. But is it really? And even more important, does it *have* to be, or do our expectations sometimes make it so? The news that an elderly man and woman plan to marry is often greeted with amusement, as though somehow the individuals are expected to have outlived their human need for closeness and companionship. Such views by the young are presumptuous, and can undermine the confidence and resilience of many older people who sense that they are not seriously expected to seek new experiences, whether in work or in personal relationships. The process of aging brings many doubts and uncertainties of ability to support oneself financially, or to find companionship and useful work. *Attitudes of younger people, including those in the health professions, are especially important.* We can convey that we see nothing odd or humorous about an older person's desire to work, or to remarry, and particularly, that we are not overcome by surprise that significant achievements can occur in later life. Instead of "Why, at your age?" we can convey "Well, why not?"

The aged experience many losses—personal relationships, income, health, agility, and opportunities to learn new things and to continue employment. However, it is necessary to view the losses not in the context of the values and goals of youth and middle life, but in *the context of later life*. Thus, a decrease in physical strength or agility is expected at this time of life and should be viewed not as a loss but as an expected change. The stark reality of physical decline must be viewed from the perspective of the older person's life, and not just in terms of measurements of the loss of youthful vigor and physiological efficiency.

We hear a great deal too about the older person's lessened concern with daily events, and increased preoccupation with his own thoughts. An increased concern with assessing one's life and accomplishments, and one's relationships with others and with work occurs for many people during middle age, and continues into later life. The older person often shows greater selectivity of involvement with certain people and with those aspects of his work which have most meaning and value for him. Whether or not this change constitutes loss depends upon one's values. In a society in which "busy-ness" and involvement with many individuals and groups is highly valued, and where little recognition is given to the importance of developing personal inner resources, these changes with age may be viewed as loss. However, if a high value is placed on development of the inner life, these changes with age can be viewed as manifestations of personal maturation.

Physical changes

The elderly seek medical care more frequently than younger people because of the higher incidence of certain health problems among older age groups. For example, the highest incidence of impaired vision and hearing occurs among older people. During later life certain prominent causes of illness and death, such as cancer, cerebrovascular accidents, and heart disease, also reach their peak. Knowledge of normal physiological changes which occur with aging can help the nurse to plan for care of elderly patients, and to assist patients and their families to cope with the aging process.

Nutrition. There is a tendency for people to lose weight during old age, and nutritional deficiency is often a serious problem. This may be related to the lack of dentures, to boredom at eating alone, or to lack of money. Chronic constipation may be a problem. Diet planning for the geriatric patient should limit calories to match lessened energy output, but also maintain weight unless the patient is obese. Yet well-seasoned foods should be included because the sense of taste dulls with age. The older person continues to need a well-balanced diet that includes fresh fruit and vegetables, milk, eggs, and meat. He should have enough fluid and roughage to encourage normal bowel function. Many older people find that a light supper (perhaps of soup or cereal, bread, and fruit) is sufficient for them at the end of the day when they are tired. Their heavier meal comes, then, at midday. Serving unrecognizable pureed or ground foods insults the taste and the sensibilities of some elderly people; their intake increases when foods are offered in other ways, such as stews. The elderly patient may need help with his meals. Appetite may increase, however, when food is served in a way that enables him to help himself as much as possible. The patient who cannot feed himself an entire meal may be able to feed himself a small part of it, provided that meat is cut, containers (milk, juice) are open, and hot beverages have been poured.

Position Sense and Speed of Reaction. These show gradual decline until the age of about 70, when the decline becomes rapid. The decline of these two faculties, together with diminished vision, is frequently a cause of accidents.

Diminished agility, position sense, vision, and hearing make older pedestrians prone to injury. Older people should be discouraged from walking unaccompanied at night. If they must walk alone after dark, encourage them to use the best-lighted streets, and to be alert to traffic.

Falling is a common cause of injury to the elderly and is usually due to diminished agility, vision, and position sense.

The susceptibility of older people to falls and fractures (their bones are more brittle and break more readily) should affect the planning of homes and apartments. Because of the increasing proportion of older people in the population, it is advisable to have basic safety factors included in all housing and not to confine safety devices to units designed especially for the elderly.

Skin. Gradual changes in the skin and in the body's ability to adjust to heat and cold occur with age. The skin becomes drier and prone to wrinkling. In old age it may become thin, flaky, and susceptible to irritation. The hair, also, becomes drier, thinner, and gray. Nails, particularly toenails, often become thickened and brittle as a result of poorer circulation to the extremities.

During later middle life and old age the body gradually loses some of its ability to adjust to extremes of temperature. It is harder for an old person to keep warm in cold weather because his metabolism is slower, and he lacks physical vigor for the strenuous exercise that would help him to keep warm. In hot weather, the older person does not dissipate heat as efficiently as a younger one, because his cutaneous vessels may not dilate as much and his sweating mechanism may not function as effectively as it formerly did. Today there are many welcome aids for keeping older people comfortable in very hot weather and in cold weather. Modern heating that provides uniform warmth in the entire house is another boon. Air conditioning has made summers more comfortable for everyone.

The nurse can help by making adjustments to keep older people more comfortable, remembering that they tolerate temperature changes poorly. If an older patient shares a room with younger people, fewer problems in regulating temperature may occur if the older patient is placed farthest from the window and is offered an extra blanket.

Teeth. Since considerable individual differences exist in the resistance of teeth to decay, some people lose their teeth as they grow old despite good dental care. Others have almost all their own teeth. The older person who needs dentures should be encouraged to obtain them, since his appearance and nutrition will benefit.

Other Physical Changes. Other important physical changes include a considerable decrease in cardiac output. Since cardiac output affects nutrition to all parts of the body, this change is of great significance. Vital capacity (the amount of air that can be expelled after taking a deep breath) also diminishes markedly with age.

The aged individual has diminished ability to maintain homeostasis during stress; he has less "reserve" with which to deal with exertion, infection, and fatigue.

Physiological response to exercise also changes with age. The circulatory system cannot respond as efficiently to the demands of exercise, and the heart and blood vessels cannot supply the increased demands of the muscles for blood.

Developmental tasks

Sometimes it is assumed that there is one accepted pattern of aging. In our society continued active involvement in work and family affairs tends to be admired; therefore, those who adapt to aging in this way are especially likely to be considered successful. Others, however, adapt successfully by withdrawing somewhat from activities and relationships, and investing more time and energy in solitary pursuits, such as gardening, reading, and reflection (Fig. 1-1).

Behavior considered maladaptive at one period in life may be an asset at another period. For example, a person who was regarded in youth as somewhat distant in his relationships may in later life seem to cope particularly well with situations in which he is alone a great deal. Conditions which for other older persons might spell intolerable loneliness may, for this person, constitute welcome relief from the pressures of maintaining close personal relationships.

Life does not cease making demands when the responsibilities of middle life have passed. In fact, some of the most difficult problems are reserved for the last part of life. Negative attitudes in our culture toward aging play no small part in aggravating the problems and decreasing the satisfactions of later life.

Coping with Dependence. Many problems of aging revolve around dependence. People who live long enough become, to some extent, dependent on others for companionship and often for financial support and physical care. Change from independence to dependence is usually gradual unless, for example, a sudden illness renders a previously self-sufficient person dependent.

Many older persons find dependence on others difficult to accept, even though they may recognize the necessity for it. Some of the elderly deny the need for any help, sometimes jeopardizing their own safety. Others readily become very dependent. Such older people tend to hang on to others, sometimes causing friction within the family as the demands for assurance exceed the capacities of others to meet them. Similar problems are observed in nursing homes in relationships between patients and nurses. In such instances the nurse should recognize the patient's needs for dependence, and gradually help him to become more self-reliant. Ignoring the older person can cause him to redouble his efforts to gain the nurse's attention and support with a resultant increase of friction in the relationship. On the other hand, if the nurse shows interest and concern for the patient, the patient often begins to show interest in his progress, initially to please the nurse, and as a way of establishing a relationship with her, but later because he himself, with help, has grown more self-reliant.

Economic Concerns. One of the tasks of later life involves adjustment to decreased income. Many factors are responsible for the economic plight of the aged. Compulsory retirement is an important cause. Older people who are willing and able to work, often find themselves at age 65 without any work to do and with a vastly decreased income. Physical decline plays a part, too. Sometimes the individual's working life is terminated by an illness from which he never fully recovers. The fact that more people are reaching old age means that the economic problems of this age group are multiplied many times.

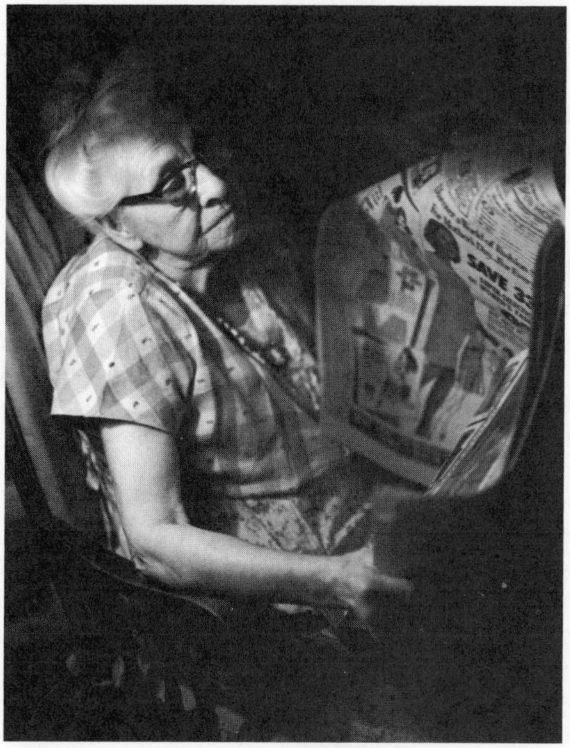

figure 1-1. Many older adults remain active even into the late years, gardening, reading, and enjoying other hobbies. (Photograph—D. Atkinson)

The reluctance of employers to hire older workers shows that the attitudes of society have played a part in the problem. There have been tendencies to emphasize the liabilities of age and to fail to recognize the assets which older workers possess. Studies have shown repeatedly that in some ways this stereotype is not accurate, and that other elements have been magnified beyond their true proportions. It is true, certainly, that the time needed for recovery from accidents or illness tends to increase with age. On the other hand, older workers tend to be careful, accurate, and dependable, although they are also likely to be slower than younger people and to have greater difficulty in adapting to change.

Older people particularly need money to help them to overcome or to compensate for some of the infirmities of age. Medical expenses increase with age, and the older person is in need of services to carry out tasks now physically beyond him.

The enactment of federal legislation (Medicare) providing health benefits to the aged has been an important advance in helping the elderly to meet the costs of health care. This program of federal assistance has also indirectly eased the burden on families of elderly people, which often bore the entire cost of medical care.

Lack of money is not the only problem caused by retirement. Idleness, boredom, and loneliness often result, since work has absorbed so large a portion of most people's time and interest and has provided many contacts with other people. Because the ability to earn his way has been removed, a person may suffer a loss of self-esteem.

Use of Time. The problem of how to spend time looms large because there often is so much free time. During his working life, leisure after a day's work may have been highly prized because it was limited. Too much leisure may lead to feelings of futility and uselessness. Much has been written about the value of hobbies and interests in later life. However, older people tend not to develop new interests but to continue those they already have. There is an amazing continuity in interests throughout each individual's life. The interests developed throughout childhood and early adulthood tend to remain those of the later years.

When emphasis is placed on the development of hobbies during early and middle life, in later years these activities will be available to cushion the problem of having too much spare time. Older women who have been housewives encounter less of a transition in this respect than do their husbands, whose retirement from work is often abrupt. The older woman continues her accustomed housekeeping duties, while her husband may feel out of place when he is at home all day.

Hobbies, however, do not provide most people with a wholly satisfactory solution to problems related to increased leisure. Most individuals in our society have been taught that work is a necessity, and that performing productive work is important in giving meaning to life. Hobbies are sometimes trivial; they may be merely measures to pass the time, rather than to use time productively. The elderly person requires opportunities for meaningful, productive work and relationships—opportunities that are often lacking in clubs for the aged. The eager response of some older people to opportunities to serve, such as helping disadvantaged children learn to read, underscores the need of older persons to occupy their time usefully and productively.

Coping with Loneliness. The problem of loneliness is acute for most older people. In addition to lack of contact with co-workers on the job, separations occur among families and friends. Inevitably, one spouse dies first. Grown children often live at a considerable distance. Regardless of physical distance, the emotional and social distance between generations may be hard to bridge. The very old person outlives most of his contemporaries, and difficulties in travel make it hard for him to see old friends or to make new ones. Those who have developed interests and activities that they can enjoy alone are in a better position to cope with the problems of loneliness than those who have rarely undertaken any project or diversion by themselves. Being able to tolerate and to enjoy periods of being alone is an important asset at any age, but is particularly important during later life.

The older person who has the capacity and energy to develop new relationships has an asset in dealing with loneliness. Some older persons seek situations, such as retirement villages, where they will have greater opportunities to meet people and form new friendships.

Securing Adequate Housing. Finding living accommodations is difficult for many older people from the standpoints of both money and companionship. Lack of money often forces older people to find cheaper and less desirable accommodations. Usually, the new dwelling is smaller, and reduction in living space makes it necessary for the older person to part with many treasured objects accumulated over a lifetime. Older people sustain so many losses that they tend to cling to their possessions, sometimes hoarding objects that appear to others to be of little value.

Objects with which the individual must part may remind him of past accomplishments and relationships and, therefore, be especially comforting to him. It is important that the elderly person be permitted to keep as many of his treasured possessions as possible, since they provide him with a link to his past and a comfortable feeling of "belonging here, among these things." Because being surrounded by familiar possessions is so large an environmental support, it is important to increase facilities for home care of the aged, and also to be as flexible as possible in permitting the older person to take some possessions with him if it becomes necessary for him to reside in an institution.

Some small communities are being established for older people which combine a chance to live in apartments or small homes with such conveniences as an infirmary, shopping service, and recreational facilities. Not surprisingly, the greatest need exists among those least able to pay for ideal retirement living. Some communities are establishing recreational and guidance centers for older people. Some centers serve a hot meal at noon, thus providing a place where older people who live in furnished rooms, with cooking facilities that are limited or nonexistent, may enjoy recreation and companionship as well as a good meal.

Retirement communities and separate, smaller retirement neighborhoods made up of several housing developments for older persons have, despite their advantages, the disadvantage of limiting contacts between older people and younger people. Different age groups seem to need this contact, and separate housing developments for the aged seriously limit such interaction. In response to the increase in the number of older people, many more nursing homes and homes for the aged have been established. Some of these are excellent, but others fall below adequate standards.

Implications for nursing

Attitudes. Care of the elderly evokes varied reactions. For some nurses, it can be an unpleasant reminder that they too will grow old and die. Working with elderly patients may remind the nurse of troubling aspects of a relationship with aging parents. Sometimes the physical appearance of the aged is distasteful to nurses. These reactions may lead to an avoidance of elderly patients.

On the other hand, the nurse may idealize the elderly person, perhaps in response to family teachings that older people are wise, and have earned a place of honor and respect. The nurse who has idealized the aged, viewing them as benevolent and kindly, and generously sharing their wisdom with the young, may also do an injustice to her elderly patients, by expecting them to exemplify her ideal. Thus, nurses who have a very negative or a very positive stereotype of aging may both fail to take account of an individual patient's strengths and weaknesses.

One's views of aging can be made more realistic, perhaps, by remembering that the aged are a disadvantaged group in our society. They are disadvantaged in relation to income, employment, housing, health, and companionship—some of the important ways in which most of the aged do not share equally with those who are younger. While disadvantaged people may become more patient, tolerant, and generous, in many instances the reverse is true. They may become selfish, resentful, and demanding. The latter characteristics are sometimes attributed to age, whereas such characteristics, when observed, may actually reflect the individual's deprivations, more than his chronologic age. In addition, some people simply are more pleasant to be with than others—a fact which is true during every period of life.

Teaching the Older Patient. Suppose that a 67-year-old woman has just discovered that she has congestive heart failure. The doctor has recommended rest, a low sodium diet, digitalis, and a diuretic. This woman has many new things to learn. Perhaps the most important of these will be the fact that she *can* learn. Older people themselves often have the false notion that ability to learn ceases at some point during life. Encouraging self-confidence in older people is the first big step in helping them to learn.

When teaching the older patient, the nurse must convey to him the belief that he *can* learn. It is necessary to proceed more slowly than with younger patients, and to give them the extra time they need to think about and respond to new ideas. Speak slowly and distinctly to help the individual compensate not only for slowed reaction time but also for the probable hearing deficit. If you use visual aids, such as graphs or pictures, allow the person extra time to study them, and be sure he is wearing his glasses (if necessary) and that he has a good light. Use visual materials which are large enough to be seen easily, and which are clear and uncluttered.

Find out about the patient's past experience and relate new material to it. Because older people have accumulated a vast store of experience, helping them to draw on it aids learning. In teaching, the first step involves finding out what the patient already knows. This is determined by asking questions and listening to what the patient says. Learning is an important means of compensating for losses. Being able to master new knowledge and skill is important to self-esteem. Consider the blow which may come to the pride of a man in his late 60s who observes that the nurse is teaching his daughter how to administer his insulin injection without first evaluating whether he can learn this himself. Many times older people are unnecessarily denied the opportunity to learn new skills, thereby making it all the more difficult for them to

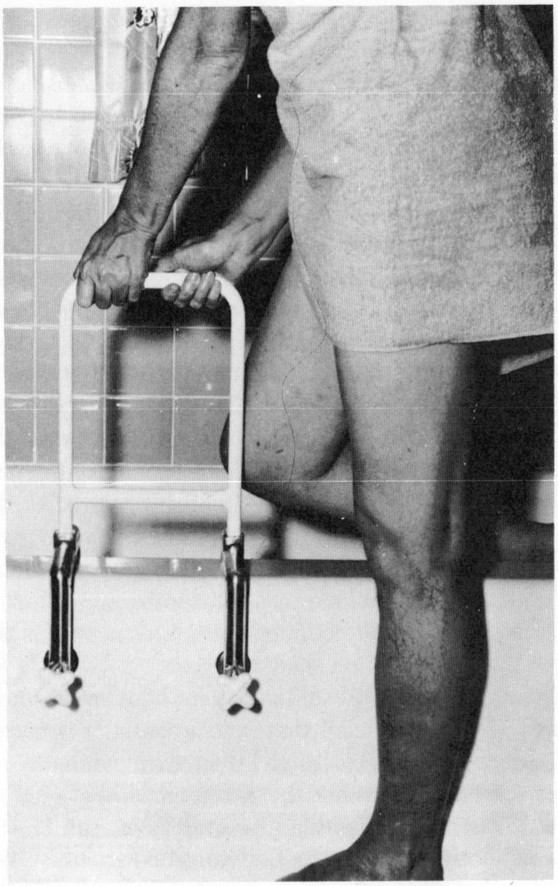

figure 1-2. An attachable grab bar for bathtubs helps to prevent falls. (Bollen Products, Cleveland, Ohio)

compensate for illness and disability, and to continue their productive roles at work and in family life.

Physical Care. Perhaps the older person's need to adjust to increasing physical limitations is the problem most familiar to nurses. Older people need gradually increasing amounts of help with self-care as their own ability to care for themselves diminishes. The thoughtful nurse will plan for this need, and she will help the patient's family to do so.

Many older people do not receive the kind of physical care they should. Sometimes it seems especially hard for others to carry out these measures. For instance, in the home the nurse may find that an elderly woman living with a married daughter has very poor habits of personal hygiene. Her hair may be dirty and her clothing soiled, while the home, her daughter, and the grandchildren seem to be shining with cleanliness. As the nurse begins to talk with the daughter about her mother's care, the daughter may say, "Mother doesn't seem to notice things like that any more, and I try to let her do as she wants to." Or the daughter may say that it is hard for her to remind her own mother about personal cleanliness and to offer help.

Neglecting the physical needs of the aged is quite common in hospitals, too. It is not unusual for a nurse to say, "I can do these things for a baby. I expect him to be helpless. But with an old person—." To most people, the elderly lack the appealing quality in their helplessness that infants possess; they do not seem cute or attractive. Perhaps they are not expected to be helpless, either. Nevertheless, if people live long enough, there comes a time when they need assistance with personal hygiene. Recognition of this necessity can help the nurse to plan for and to give this care and to teach family members to do so. Very old people become forgetful and unmindful of details, but it is not kind to allow them to have poor hygiene. Old people may have severe scalp irritations, excoriated skin, and pressure sores which cause discomfort and pain.

The prevention of physical discomfort is not the only reason for emphasizing the physical care of older people. Another is to help them maintain dignity and self-respect. Contrast the demeanor of the neglected old person with that of one whose snow-white hair is neatly coiffed, whose skin is clean and healthy, and whose dress is attractive. To augment this concept of self-respect, the nurse should make it a rule to call each patient by name. To address an older person by his own name, rather than as "Pop" or some other patronizing nickname, helps him maintain his dignity and identity. The older person should be encouraged to care for himself as much as possible as long as he is able. Many devices are available to encourage self-help (Fig. 1-2).

Because circulation to the extremities is often poor, care of the feet and the toenails is important. Lessened circulation may result in injuries or infections healing poorly and even becoming gangrenous. Because the skin on the legs and the feet is usually very dry, cream or lotion should be used after bathing. Thickened, brittle nails should be trimmed carefully, a little at a time. Soften the nails first by soaking the patient's feet in warm water. Very thick nails that have been neglected may need the attention of a podiatrist. If the feet are cold, bedsocks and extra blankets are a help. Hot-water bottles and electric heating pads should be used cautiously because of the danger of burns. The combination of diminished sensation and lessened circulation makes this danger more acute in the aged.

Alcohol should not be used as a back lotion, since it is drying, and the skin of older people tends to be dry and scaly. Instead, cream, an emollient, or lanolin lotion should be used. Frequent hot baths also tend to be drying. Instead of a daily tub, patients may have a partial bath on alternate days. All the soap must be rinsed off the skin, since dried soap on the skin can be irritating. Friction from clothing and bedding should be minimized. For example, sleeves on the patient's gown should be drawn over elbows to decrease irritation caused by rubbing against the sheets.

Bath oil may also be helpful in overcoming dry skin; when it is used, particular care must be taken to avoid the patient's slipping in the tub. A rubber mat is essential in a tub made slippery by the bath oil.

A stall shower is desirable since it avoids the need to step over the side of a tub, and then lower oneself into the tub. If the patient is weak and unsteady on his feet, a chair may be placed under the shower, making it possible for him to bathe while seated. The shower provides the most thorough rinsing of soap from the skin, thus helping to minimize skin irritations so common in the elderly. Whatever method of bathing is used, particular care must be taken to insure privacy, since many older people are especially distressed when they cannot maintain their usual standards of personal modesty.

Dentures require regular cleaning and brushing. If removed, they should be stored in an opaque covered jar. Instruct the patient not to roll them in tissues, as they can be easily thrown away or lost this way. If you are helping the patient to clean his dentures, put them in a small basin and take them to the sink to clean them. Avoid holding them directly over the sink—they are easily dropped and broken.

Older women sometimes have problems with slight incontinence of urine when they are coughing or sneezing (stress incontinence) or with vaginal discharge. Late in life the vaginal mucous membrane becomes thin and subject to infection. The nurse or a family member may notice that this problem exists; the doctor should be consulted. He may recommend, among other treatments, a cleansing douche. Help the patient to keep clean through perineal care and use of disposable pads, if necessary.

Increased facial hair may be distressing to elderly women. It may be removed by careful cutting or shaving or by the use of a depilatory. A physician's order is needed for the two latter methods of removing facial hair. Older men may need help with shaving. Tactful reminders and provision of enough clean clothing will help the patient to maintain his appearance. A predictable routine for changing clothing is helpful; for example, place clean clothes on the patient's bed for him to wear when he has finished bathing.

Elimination may pose particular problems in the elderly. Frequency of urination is not uncommon. Many older men have hypertrophy of the prostate. Older women often have relaxation of perineal structures with less efficient emptying of the bladder. Symptoms of frequent urination should be noted carefully and reported to the doctor. Care must be taken to prevent falls when the patient gets up during the night. Making sure the call light is nearby or leaving the bedpan or urinal within easy reach may limit the need for getting out of bed during the night. Some older people are constipated; this is likely to be especially troublesome to those who cannot get up and move around. Helping the patient to maintain adequate dietary and fluid intake and to have a regular time for evacuation may be the remedy. Sometimes enemas, mild cathartics, or stool softeners, are ordered by the doctor.

Being confined to bed has other adverse effects on older people. Older people expand their chests less fully because of loss of elasticity of structures that increase and decrease the size of the thoracic cavity. Confinement to bed accentuates this problem and often leads to development of hypostatic pneumonia. (See p. 267 for further discussion of hypostatic pneumonia.) Decubitus ulcers are common among the aged because of the lessened ability of the skin and subcutaneous tissues to tolerate pressure. Circulation tends to be lessened with age; confinement to bed often aggravates this tendency. Diminished circulation to the brain may cause disorientation. Muscle tone is readily lost during bed rest. Extreme weakness often results and is difficult to overcome.

In view of these complications, doctors usually permit elderly patients out of bed as soon as possible. The patient should be encouraged to take a few steps with help and gradually to increase activities. When you know that the patient will be allowed up shortly, ask his family to bring his clothes, particularly his shoes.

Time. The older patient is slower in his movements and responses than a younger one. Attempts to make him hurry often result in confusion, irritation, and accidents. It is wise to plan nursing care so that he has more time for his activities. For instance, since

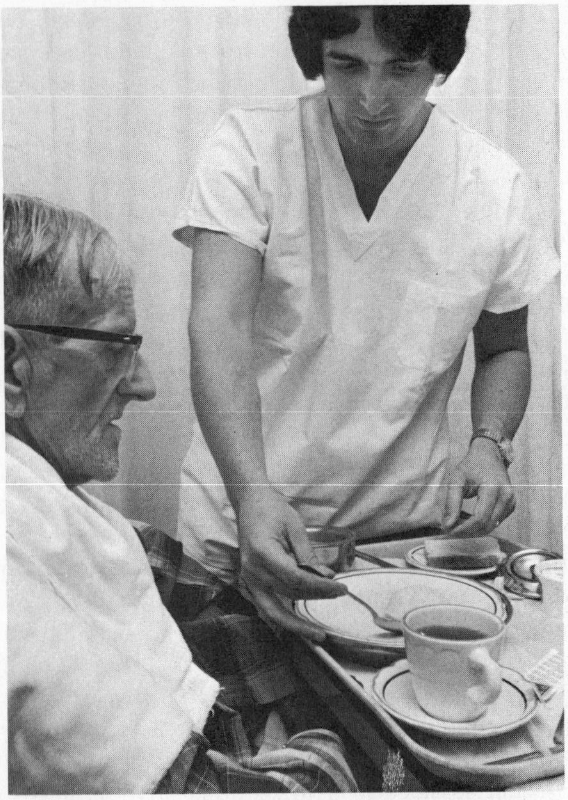

figure 1-3. The nurse should serve the older patient his tray first and collect it last. Food containers should be opened and eating utensils accessible. (Photograph—D. Atkinson)

he eats slowly, serve him his tray first and collect it last (Fig. 1-3). The thoughtful nurse will prepare everything the patient needs for self-care and then let him proceed at his own pace to complete those aspects of care that he can tend to himself. Explanations of tests and treatments should be made slowly and, if necessary, repeated.

Even comparatively minor illnesses or injuries can have serious consequences for the older person, because they can tip the already precarious balance from independence to dependence. Often, the older individual unnecessarily gives up some of his usual activities, because others (and sometimes the patient himself) are too quick to assume that he will never be able to resume these activities.

Hospital Care. Recognizing that the older person is likely to have greater difficulty adapting to a hospital environment, the nurse can make his adaptation easier and less hazardous for him. High beds are a potential danger, since the older person may misjudge the distance to the floor and fall as he is getting up. Hi-lo beds, which are adjustable, permit the ambulatory patient to get out of bed easily. If high beds are used, have a sturdy footstool in place. If an electric bed is used, the patient will need instruction in operating the controls. The bed should be left in the low position except when direct nursing care is administered. It is wise to leave a dim light in the older patient's room during the night so that he can more readily orient himself to his surroundings as he awakens, and avoid falling if he gets up. It may be helpful to leave the door to the hall partially open for this reason also. The use of side rails should be explained to the patient; the call light should be readily available when the side rails are raised.

The elderly usually require less sleep which may present a problem when a hospital room is shared with others. Keeping the patient awake and interested during the day may help him sleep better at night. Barbiturates often cause confusion and restlessness in aged patients. Whenever possible, it is preferable to encourage sleep by relying on general nursing measures rather than on drugs.

Even without the use of drugs, nighttime confusion and disorientation are common among the elderly, particularly when an older person is moved away from his familiar surroundings to a hospital or nursing home. These episodes of confusion, which are especially likely to occur at night, are disturbing to the patient and to others, and are hazardous to the patient's safety. Unfortunately, mismanagement of this problem is very common, leading to the patient's becoming more confused and disturbed. Initial reactions to the patient may be to *control* him and to lessen the noise he makes by such measures as scolding him and quickly closing the door of his room so that other patients are not awakened. Sometimes restraints, such as a Posey belt, are quickly applied before other measures are tried. These actions quite predictably increase the patient's agitation and he becomes more anxious and confused; at this point orders for sedation may be sought. Sedatives and hypnotics, even when used in low doses, can result in wakefulness, excitement, and confusion in elderly patients. Sometimes the use of restraints and sedatives can be avoided and the patient calmed by other measures.

The elderly patient should be checked frequently during the night, especially if he is noisy or appears to waken frequently. Touching and talking to him, or adjusting his pillow or blanket might be all that is needed to calm him; on the other hand, being near or touching the patient may aggravate his confusion.

The nurse should try to determine what is causing the confusion and then attempt to reduce or eliminate it. Some patients will remain noisy and confused despite all efforts, but others are trying to communicate something without being able to state the problem—the need to use a urinal, the discomfort of constipation, being too hot or too cold, fear, and loneliness. The nurse may determine what is wrong by observing those clues and hints which the patient reveals.

Measures to help the patient maintain his contact with reality are, of course, necessary at any time, and to some extent prevent episodes of acute confusion. Elderly, confused patients may benefit from a mode of therapy called "reality orientation" (Table 1-1).

The nurse who speaks slowly and distinctly, and who presents one suggestion or request at a time, rather than a rapid barrage of instructions, is facilitating the older person's ability to respond, and showing she expects that he can do so. There is no quicker way for an older person to lose ability to care for himself than to be in a situation where he is treated as though this capacity has already been lost. The older person senses that he is no longer considered capable of managing such tasks as storing his dentures safely in the jar on his stand, or cleaning them himself; he gives over these self-care functions, which would help him maintain some privacy, independence, and contact with reality. A vicious circle may ensue, in which the staff grow more impatient with the elderly person's detachment, less inclined to talk with him and encourage his participation, and he in turn turns more and more to his inner world of fantasy. Meaningful relationships are an important measure in helping the patient to maintain contact with reality; the relationship with the nurse can be significant. It is, however, difficult to bridge the gap between generations.

The difficulty is increased if the nurse considers certain topics "taboo." For instance, some nurses believe that the aged should not talk about the past but, instead, must be engaged in conversation solely about present and future events. For many elderly persons, however, daily events are relatively insignificant compared with events in the past. Is it any wonder that a retired archeologist may sometimes prefer to reminisce about his explorations in far-off lands, rather than sticking to conversation about card parties held in the nursing home? One need of the aged involves assessing past events, achievements, and losses, and integrating these life experiences. If we recognize that the older person has something valuable to contribute at home, at work, and in his community, we can feel proud to have a part in helping him to maintain his health and continue to make his unique contribution as long as possible.

Table 1-1.
Reality orientation

Beginning
The date is prominently displayed on a sheet of paper placed in the patient's line of vision or on a blackboard situated in the solarium or dayroom —"Today is Sunday, June 19, 1977."
Each time a nurse or nurse assistant enters the room or gives bedside care (bath, medications, linen change) identification is made—"Hello, Mrs. Green, I'm Mrs. Wilson, your nurse." This is repeated until the patient can identify the nurse by name.
The time of day is stated—"Mrs. Green, it's 2 o'clock and time for your pill."
Progressive
The patient is given portions of current newspapers or magazines, starting with one or two pages or pictures and increasing gradually.
A large clock on the wall is used for orientation to time, and a large calendar for day and date (a calendar that shows one page per day is preferred). Personnel should draw patients' attention to both.
Current events are discussed: changes in the weather, major elections, sports events, and other things of interest to a particular patient. Discussions should become more detailed as orientation increases.
Happenings in the patient's life are compared from day to day.
Television and radio are used to provide news, weather reports, and entertainment. A routine of daily programs provides continuity and encourages recall of recent events.
Social interaction with other patients is encouraged, as are hobbies, cards, and group and individual projects.

General nutritional considerations

Early years

- Eating habits may be irregular:
  The patient may not be hungry when the meal is served.

The patient may desire snacks which may not be available because of dietary restrictions.

- Food preferences may lean toward "empty" calories rather than a well-balanced diet. The patient may need to be taught good eating habits.
- Fad dieting may result in various dietary deficiencies.
- Certain deficiencies, such as a vitamin C (ascorbic acid) deficiency, may interfere with the healing process.
- Caloric needs are greater, therefore larger portions and the addition of snacks may be needed to meet the patient's caloric requirements.
- Eating habits may be established. The patient may find it difficult to adjust to hospital food and/or special diets.
- The patient may need counseling on nutrition from the dietitian or nurse.

MIDDLE YEARS

- Food patterns and eating habits are definitely established, making it difficult for some patients to accept special diets or dietary restrictions.
- The overweight middle-aged adult may have tried fad diets, with uncertain results.

LATE YEARS

- The eating habits of the elderly may be determined by such factors as a limited income, inadequate cooking facilities, and poor dentition.
- A dietary deficiency may complicate medical or surgical problems.
- The general physical condition of the patient may affect digestion and absorption of food.
- Food preferences may be hard to change, making special diets or regulation of food intake difficult.

General pharmacological considerations

- All patients taking drugs after discharge from the hospital will have to be cautioned on the use of any drug—prescription or nonprescription—unless ordered by the physician. Interactions of various drugs may have serious results.
- Patients should thoroughly understand drug use: quantity of the drug (number of capsules or tablets, amount of liquid), the time it is to be taken (for example, 10 AM and 2 PM), and any instruction relating to a specific drug.
- Sedatives and hypnotics, even in low doses, can result in wakefulness, excitement, and confusion in *any* patient, and particularly, the elderly.

Bibliography

BURNSIDE, I. M.: *Psychosocial Nursing: Care of the Aged.* New York, McGraw-Hill, 1973.

———: Touching is talking, Part 5. Am. J. Nurs. 73:2060-3, December, 1973.

CAHALL, J. B. et al: Considerate care of the elderly. Nurs. '75, 5:38, September, 1975.

DOLAN, M. B.: Shelly was angry. So was the staff. Nurs. '74, 4:86, January, 1974.

EARHART, M.: Beverly—dealing with a difficult adolescent patient. J. Pract. Nurs. 24:24, January, 1974.

FUCHS, L.: Talking to the elderly. Nurs. Care 8:16-7, March, 1975.

GREENBERG, B.: Reaction time in the elderly, Part 3. Am. J. Nurs. 73:2056, December, 1973.

HAYTER, J.: Biologic changes of aging. Nurs. Forum 13:289, No. 3, 1974.

KIMMEL, D. C.: *Adulthood and Aging: An Interdisciplinary, Developmental View.* New York, Wiley, 1974.

LORE, A.: Adolescents: people not problems. Am. J. Nurs. 73:1233, July, 1973.

OREMLANK, E. K. et al: How to care for the "between-ager." Nurs. '74, 4:42, November, 1974.

PENETAR, M. P.: *Education and the Family.* Buffalo, Boncroft Books, 1971.

SCARBROUGH, D. R.: Reality orientation: a new approach to an old problem. Nurs. '74, 4:12, November, 1974.

SCHWAB, M.: Caring for the aged, Part 1. Am. J. Nurs. 73:2049, December, 1973.

STAFFORD, S.: Trivia, illusions and quirks—what they can tell you about your patients. Nurs. '75, 5:6, September, 1975.

STEVENS, C. B.: Breaking through cobwebs of confusion in the elderly. Nurs. '75, 4:41, August, 1974.

———: *Special Needs of Long-Term Patients.* Philadelphia, Lippincott, 1974.

UJHELY, G. B.: The environment of the elderly. Nurs. Clin. N. Am. 7:281, June, 1972.
July, 1975.

VINCENT, P.: The sick role in patient care. Am. J. Nurs. 75:1172,

WEFFORD, W.: Closing the communications gap. Nurs. Times 71:114, January 26, 1975.

CHAPTER—2

On completion of this chapter the student will:

- Describe and discuss the essential components of, and guidelines for, nurse-patient relationships.
- Discuss the anxiety of patient and nurse and its relevance to their relationship.
- Discuss frustration, anxiety, anger, conflict, and grief and how the nurse may work with the patient experiencing these emotions.
- Understand how to provide emotional support to the patient undergoing tests and treatments.
- Discuss the implications of sustained nurse-patient relationships.
- Understand the problems involved in giving nursing care to the patient who is physically unattractive.
- List the essentials of teaching the self-care patient undergoing diagnostic tests.
- Discuss the problems encountered with the patient who refuses treatment.
- Evaluate interventions and relationships of the patient's family in the clinical area.

Nurse-patient relationships

There are some basic guidelines for adapting general knowledge of nurse-patient relationships to the particular requirements of medical-surgical patients:

- In most instances the medical-surgical patient has sought care for some physical condition; this condition may, of course, be aggravated by emotional stress, or may even be caused by it. Keeping in mind that the patient's attention is usually on his physical condition, and that he is not primarily concerned with solving personal problems, will help set the tone for the nurse-patient relationship. The nurse's ability to give emotional support will be enhanced by recognition of the patient's view of why he is seeking treatment.
- In caring for medical-surgical patients, the nurse must be able to consider both the physical care of the patient and his emotional reactions to illness and treatment. Often it is possible to combine these two aspects of care. *Listening* is a very important part of nursing care; what the patient says may give clues to physical and mental states.
- The manner in which physical care is administered is important. Touch should be gentle, not rough.
- Frightening and painful procedures are common on medical-surgical units. Although at first the nurse is a stranger to the patient, the stress of experiences such as undergoing surgery can lead the patient to rely on the nurse more quickly and more fully for emotional support than if he were not faced with these experiences.
- Medical-surgical patients are likely to be more outwardly poised than pediatric, geriatric, or psychiatric patients. One of the challenges in working with this group will involve helping them maintain poise in stressful circumstances (when the patient shows that to do so is important to him), but also encouraging expression of personal feelings.
- There is enormous variety among medical-surgical patients in terms of age, diagnosis, degree of illness, and other factors. Some patients will be completely helpless; others will seem able to care for themselves. The approach to each patient should be different.

The following points will help review some basic guidelines for nurse-patient relationships applicable in any setting:

- Be yourself. You can borrow techniques from someone you admire, but do not try to imitate someone else. Sick people are perceptive, anxious, and suspicious, even if they do not show it. If they feel the nurse is sincere they will be more trusting.
- Small points of care are important to the sick. Reactions to something as personal as illness are not always logical and rational. The big fact of recovering may be lost in the little annoyance of being served cold coffee. But if the patient *feels* your interest in him, your concern for his welfare and comfort, he is less likely to become angry.
- Size up the situation between your patient and yourself. Do not rush in with too many busy activities at once, unless they are of vital necessity to the patient. Learn to get the "feel" of your patient. What is his general condition? What is he expressing? Is he in pain? Does he seem to be resigned or apprehensive?
- Besides giving the expert technical care that you will gradually learn to give, there are several ways in which you can help your patient by the relationship you establish with him. One is to help him gather as many facts as possible about his situation so that he can make reasonable decisions. Another is to teach him new skills with which he can help himself to live with or to recover from his illness. And, particularly important, you can support him as he goes through the various stages of illness and recovery.
- If the patient asks no questions and discusses none of his feelings with you, do not pry; but do not assume either that he understands all, or that he has perceived nothing of what is going on around him. If it appears that he wants to know, explain treatments and tell him what to expect, so that he can use the information to orient himself to his new surroundings. But do not urge discussion on the unwilling patient.
- Such trivial reassuring clichés as, "Don't worry" and "Everything will be all right" mean the same thing to a patient as, "I don't want to hear about your troubles." If your patient says that he is worried or does not feel well, he has opened the door to expression of his feelings. If the nurse unperceptively pushes aside his remark by saying something like

"Everything will be fine," she shuts the door, thus avoiding involvement but leaving the patient to cope with his feelings alone.

- Accept every patient as an adult who perhaps for the present must be cared for physically as a baby. *Never talk down to a patient.* Avoid the use of patronizing expressions, particularly the "we" which is notorious in the nursing profession.
- At the same time, be generous with gentle ministrations. A patient needs to feel that someone cares about him.
- Never smother a patient with the kind of attention that retards his ability to do as much for himself as he can.
- When a patient is angry, let him be. He may not be angry with you, even though it is you he is scolding. Although crankiness is hard on others, it is often better for the patient than swallowing his anger and getting indigestion, or worse, from it. However, this depends on the patient and on the situation. Some people are more comfortable when helped to preserve their aplomb. To perceive these differences is a difficult but important part of nursing.

Some basic concepts

Terms such as anger and anxiety are commonplace. Most of us have become so accustomed to these words that we sometimes use them too loosely. What is the difference between fear and anxiety? In the following section there is a discussion of the following terms: anxiety, frustration and anger, conflict, and grief.

Anxiety

Anxiety is different from fear. The person who is afraid usually can identify the cause of his fear. His knees may tremble after a narrow escape from an auto crash; trembling and a pounding heart are natural reactions to danger. In anxiety, the external circumstance is identified less clearly. Often the patient feels uneasy, or he has a general feeling of impending unpleasantness or disaster but is unable to explain why he feels this way. The patient is usually not aware of the underlying cause of his anxiety, although he may be aware of situations which precipitate it. Because he is unable to identify the cause of his anxiety, he frequently feels helpless and overwhelmed.

Anxiety has been defined in various ways: as an energy, and as an emotional response without a specific object; as a response to a threat to one's self-respect and to the respect in which one is held by others. There are many facets to the concept of anxiety; these are but a few. Threats to survival, whether physical survival or survival as an integrated personality, elicit profound anxiety. You will observe anxiety among patients who have emphysema and coronary artery disease, for example.

The levels of anxiety vary from mild to panic level. In mild anxiety, the individual's ability to observe is heightened; this ability is reduced in moderate and severe anxiety, when the individual tends to focus on details. In mild anxiety the individual's ability to perceive relationships between events is enhanced; as anxiety becomes more severe, he progressively loses this ability. Ability to learn is thus enhanced by mild anxiety, but is impaired in moderate and severe anxiety. In panic level anxiety the individual may describe feelings of "disintegrating" or "being swept away." It is important to realize that, whatever the individual's physical capacities, he is helpless while in this state, and requires assistance to reduce the anxiety to more manageable levels. Staying with him is one measure which is useful. Listening to him is another. He may speak of one detail, and this in distorted fashion. As the nurse listens, and as the patient becomes somewhat less anxious, he begins to "put together" in a more coherent way what he is trying to communicate, thus enabling the nurse to respond.

We know that when a person is very anxious, he cannot see all aspects of a problem. He tends to see and to magnify only a single detail or a few details, and sometimes he makes the wrong connections. An anxious person often becomes confused and unable to follow directions or the explanation given to him about a treatment.

Avoid cutting off patients when they begin to talk. Although verbalizing does not in itself relieve anxiety, it can be the beginning of understanding. The problem will never be solved until it is understood. Letting a patient talk opens the way to understanding and dealing with problems. Sometimes a patient can recognize the need for further, more expert help.

There are times when the matter should not be pursued. For example, when the nurse's skills are not adequate for the amount of help the patient seems to need, or when other factors, such as the patient's physical condition, make further discussion of anxiety-producing material unwise, it should be postponed. A patient who has just suffered myocardial infarction may, as he speaks of his recent close encounter with death, experience an increased pulse rate and restlessness. In such circumstances the wise nurse will not encourage the patient to explore the problem further, but will suggest he save further discussion until later. In such a situation, administration of a "p.r.n." order for sedation may also be appropriate, in order to alleviate physiological manifestations of anxiety which are particularly hazardous to a patient who has experienced recent myocardial infarction.

There are other times when it is not helpful to encourage a patient to look more closely at his problems. In these instances, instead of an approach which conveys, "Tell me more about it," measures can be used that support the patient in other ways and help him through the crisis. When a patient has a life-threatening physical need and is also terrified, attention must be given first to the physical need; psychological needs can be considered after the emergency is over. When a patient is in pain, the pain should be relieved, if possible, before consideration is given to how he reacts to it. Attention to physical needs is one way of communicating support to the patient. Ignoring physical needs, even such simple ones as giving fresh water or lowering the bed to a more comfortable position, is a way of telling the patient that no one cares and of increasing his anxiety. Words should not be used when action is more appropriate.

Some patients prefer not to discuss their emotional problems with the nurse, and the nurse should respect a wish for privacy. The nurse's need to help should be tempered by an understanding of what will bring relief to the particular patient. Some patients find it most helpful for the nurse to give support in nonverbal ways; others are benefited if they are encouraged to talk about how they feel.

Sometimes, because the patient's anxiety is so great, he bursts out with a flow of emotion-laden personal concerns even when the nurse's contact with him has been relatively brief. The patient may later worry about revealing so much of his personal life. Stay with him and listen supportively during his period of distress, but avoid questioning him or encouraging him at this time to go on. When the patient is calmer and has had a chance to think over what has been said, he will be better able to assess what topics (if any) he wants to pursue.

Dealing with personal anxiety

What are some of the things that can be done when you become anxious? If you can, leave the situation for a moment to think it through. However, there are times when you cannot leave; for instance, when there is bleeding present. Try to concentrate on some concrete, helpful thing you can do. Hold a compress in place, empty the emesis basin, or take the patient's pulse. These actions give you time to think what to do next.

Merely learning to recognize when you are anxious often will keep you from being helpless in the grip of anxiety. When you know you are anxious—except in an emergency—stop! Think the situation through. Find help; do not race blindly ahead with what you are doing. At such times the patient gets the wrong medication, or the side rail is left down, so that he falls out of bed. Every person who deals with helpless people has the responsibility to stop work when he is unable to function. Extreme anxiety can keep one from functioning and cause hazardous behavior; so can physical illness or excessive loss of sleep. None of these "excuses" is accepted legally if a patient is harmed.

Knowledge and competence are an insurance against anxiety. If you do not know the proper procedure so well that it is almost automatic, you may become anxious when you find yourself fumbling. Do you know what to do if a patient has a convulsion, if he faints, if he bleeds? Are you skilled in handling oxygen? When you need it in a hurry, will you be able to remember which handle does what? Can your hands manage the suction tubing so well that you can keep your eyes on the patient if he starts to choke? Do you know the locations of the fire extinguishers in the area—and how to operate them?

On the other hand, do not expect too much of yourself. As you learn new things, you will have moments of insecurity. Just as the patient who is anxious concentrates on smaller and smaller details, you, too, will find that your ability to perceive the whole situation narrows with anxiety and grows with the increase of knowledge and capability. The first time you gave an enema you probably concentrated so hard on the tubing that you may not have remembered to see whether or not the patient was comfortable. As you become more professional, you can extend your attentions to include the patient.

Frustration and anger

What happens in frustration? A person sets a goal, but some barrier prevents its fulfillment. The result is frustration, which is made up of feelings of helplessness and anger. The amount of frustration one feels is dependent on how important the goal was, what similar past experiences the person has had, and how he handles feelings of helplessness and anger. A patient who fails to walk well on his new artificial leg will be frustrated, especially if his job depends on his ability to walk well. We do not always know what goals another has set for himself. Therefore, we cannot assume that the failure that does not frustate one person will not frustrate another. One patient may be thrilled to find that he can walk around his bed; another may be dismayed to find that he will be barred from entering an athletic contest. Frustration ends in anger. People can become very angry and not know it. The anger may be too painful to face; it may interfere with the picture the person has formed of himself. Anger becomes subconscious when a person has to hide from himself the fact that he is angry. Unknown anger that is still present as energy is harder to handle. The trouble with feelings and reactions of which one is not aware is that they complicate and obscure the situation, making a rational solution to the problem difficult to achieve.

Patients have many reasons for being angry. Merely being sick is frustrating. To be sick and in the hospital is bad enough, but worse yet, one has to pay for it! Restriction of activity, such as that imposed by an illness or disability, is frustrating. Being unable to control the most ordinary daily routines, such as getting a hot cup of coffee, brushing one's teeth, or urinating, is frustrating. The confinement to a room makes smaller details more and more important.

Some things the patient expresses anger about can be remedied; for instance, try to see that he receives hot coffee if cold coffee upsets him. Many of the main causes of anger, however, cannot be remedied. If the patient must remain in traction for 6 weeks, and therefore misses a long-awaited trip, there is nothing he or anyone else can do about changing the situation. In addition to giving your patient opportunities to express his anger, help him to find activities to use up the excess energy mobilized by anger. Physical activity is especially beneficial. The patient with a lower limb in traction can still exercise his arms; these exercises can be useful not only in preparing him for crutch walking, but also in using some of the pent-up energy engendered by anger, thus helping him to relax.

Conflict

The medical-surgical patient is often confronted with making decisions which have far-reaching consequences, and often he is expected to arrive at his decision promptly. Such situations set the stage for conflict—the patient feels torn between opposing goals. It is not uncommon for patients to have to choose "the lesser of two evils"; sometimes neither alternative is really desirable, and the question revolves around which choice has the most assets. Often the situation is complicated by the fact that no one can predict the outcome of a particular treatment or surgery. Nevertheless, the patient must reach a decision. The nurse can act as a sounding board while the patient expresses the conflict and considers the alternatives.

When a patient is in conflict, it is important to help him get the necessary information to help him in decision making. It is also important not to try to make the decision for him.

Grief

Grief is an intense sadness. It is an emotional state, a reaction to severe loss. Normally, appropriate responses are crying, withdrawal, depression, and lack of appetite. Further responses that may be seen are anger, feelings of emptiness, and despair.

The intensity of grief usually depends on the cause: the greater the loss the more intense the grief.

The patient grieves for what is important to him, and for those he loves, regardless of the appropriateness of his reactions. Physicians and nurses often have mental yardsticks which they use to measure the appropriateness of patients' reactions, and which often blind them to what an experience means to the patient. Losses have very personal meanings to the individual who experiences them. The patient's reaction is also affected by the magnitude of other serious losses in his life, how well he has recovered from them, and his personal resources and assets. For the elderly lady who has outlived all of her relatives and close friends, the death of a beloved pet during her hospitalization may be overwhelming, while for a patient with family and friends and a challenging career, the loss of a pet, although painful, may not constitute a major loss. Likewise, one patient may seem withdrawn and apathetic for months following removal of a gangrenous toe, while another patient may, a few weeks following amputation of his leg, begin learning to use his artificial limb, and start making plans to return to work.

Brief nurse-patient relationships

What are some measures which help the nurse to develop a supportive relationship with a patient during a brief period? (Some of these points are also

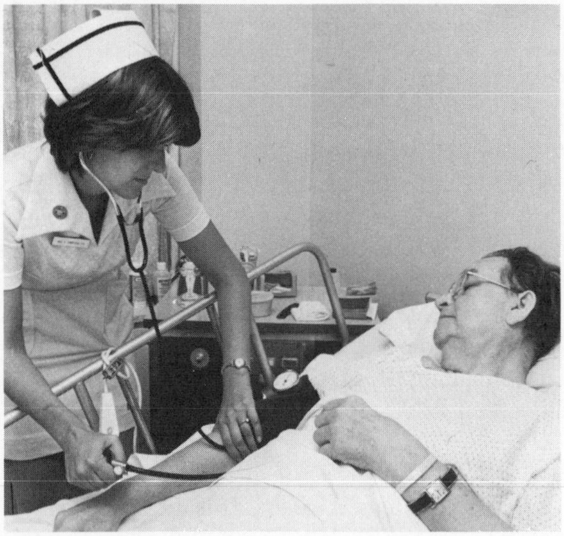

figure 2-1. Even routine nursing procedures and diagnostic tests can produce stress in the patient. (Photograph —D. Atkinson)

applicable to caring for patients during diagnostic and therapeutic procedures; see below.)

- Concentrate on what the patient is going through. Avoid social clichés which are not only meaningless but often offensive in such situations, because they imply denial of the stressful experience the patient is facing. At such times the patient needs to focus his energy on the situation at hand; he should not be expected to divert some of it into an effort to be sociable.
- Diverting the patient's attention toward some concrete action or observation is different from merely expecting him to socialize. The patient recognizes this difference by the context of the relationship which the nurse establishes with him. One nurse talked on and on to a patient undergoing initial treatment in the emergency room. She asked where he lived, how many children he had, what kind of work he did—all in the tone one would use when making a new acquaintance. Another nurse was helping care for a woman who had been in an automobile accident. When this nurse saw that the physician was about to perform a painful procedure, such as cleaning the wound or suturing, she said to the patient, "Now look at me, and squeeze my hand hard. It's going to hurt for a minute." Sometimes a patient is helped by being asked to count aloud, thus giving him something specific to concentrate on when he is anxious and in pain. The essential ingredient in all these situations is the patient's feeling of support and encouragement from the nurse.
- Establish some physical contact and eye contact with the patient. Occasionally, your patient will show that he does not welcome physical contact, in which case it should be kept to a minimum. Gently placing your hand on the patient's shoulder may be more appropriate and more effective in some instances than verbal reassurance.
- Have equipment handy, neat, and in good condition. You cannot concentrate on the patient if you are frantically hunting for a sterile syringe of the proper size. Also, remember that an environment which is orderly and clean can increase the patient's confidence in his care.
- Perform technical skills with as much confidence and dexterity as possible. If some of them are new, practice away from the patient until you gain proficiency.
- Be alert to the patient's physiological as well as his emotional reactions. Are his lips becoming cyanotic? Did his pulse rate increase?
- It may seem difficult to concentrate on a variety of factors simultaneously—the patient's pulse, skin color, respirations. With experience, many of these observations become automatic. You don't have to tell yourself, "Check the pulse; observe skin color." You will just *do* these things, and as you become more quickly responsive to various indices of the patient's condition, you will find that you are more alert to danger signals in the patient's physiological and emotional state.

Supporting the patient during tests and treatments

Usually the nurse has primary responsibility for providing emotional support and observing the patient's response during various procedures, such as paracentesis or liver biopsy. However routine such procedures may seem to professional staff, they usually represent stressful experiences for the patient (Fig. 2-1).

Collaborating with the physician

The physician, nurse, and patient are typically the three persons involved during care, although, of course, additional personnel may be required for more complex procedures such as renal dialysis. The primary focus of each of the three is different; the interaction among them is important. The physician concentrates on the procedure, although this does not mean that he ignores the patient. Nevertheless, the main focus of his attention must be on performing the procedure. The patient's role involves getting through a painful, humiliating, frightening, or sometimes simply tedious experience with the best grace possible. The nurse functions in two roles, which may be complementary or antagonistic to each other, depending upon how the situation is handled. The nurse must support the patient, both physically and emotionally, as well as assist the physician, obtain necessary equipment, and so on. The patient's confidence is increased if nurse and physician are collaborating and genuinely appear to respect each other. One very obvious (but frequently ignored) aspect of this collaboration involves avoiding any conversation between physician and nurse during the procedure, which does not pertain to the patient's immediate care. It is not uncommon for doctors and nurses to use social conversation to ease the tension of a situation, or even to use the time to catch up on sharing information and plans about other patients' care. Such conversations are to be avoided.

Make it a practice to begin a procedure (especially if you have not worked with the physician before) by asking the physician whether anything additional, or different, is needed. This step will help avoid tension during the procedure. Particularly if the procedure proves difficult (such as a lumbar puncture, in which the spinal fluid is difficult to obtain), a minor problem with equipment may assume major proportions as physician and nurse vent their tension and frustration over the situation.

Concentrating on the patient's reactions

Often the nurse has a tendency to concentrate on assisting the physician, rather than combining this role with support of the patient. What may be some reasons for this? It is frequently disquieting to observe another person's response to a painful procedure. Sometimes, the nurse has not personally experienced the procedure, and may exaggerate the discomfort the patient is actually experiencing, and withdraw from him on the basis of an erroneous perception of what he is going through. To see another person lose composure is disquieting, because the potential for similar behavior lies within all of us. The nurse is likely to be more vulnerable to anxiety as a result of these factors than is the physician, since his attention is centered on performing the procedure.

Routinization of the procedure is another problem that is more acute for the nurse than for the doctor. Unless the nurse concentrates on the patient's reaction, the assisting role can become quite routine, particularly if one repeatedly helps with the same tests. For example, there is little difference from one patient to another in the preparation of equipment for "routine" pelvic examination. While the physician has some variety by focusing on possible pathology (Is the cervix eroded? Are there tumors?), the preparation and cleaning up of equipment can be almost identical from one patient to another. In order to avoid falling into a highly routinized approach, it is essential for the nurse to concentrate on the patient's reaction. Each patient will respond somewhat differently and require a slightly different approach.

Failure to provide emotional support during the stess of diagnostic tests and treatments may leave some patients angry and critical of this aspect of their care; others, for whom emotional support is crucial, are lost to treatment, or suffer serious emotional disorders precipitated by their illness and its treatment. (Of course, not all such reactions can be prevented, even by the most skillful support from the nurse and physician.) If, by support and encouragement, you enable a patient to keep on with a series of painful procedures until he has had an opportunity to benefit from them, is this not just as important as performing the procedure?

Sustained nurse-patient relationships

Working with long-term patients provides many satisfactions; it also poses some problems. While you have the satisfaction of seeing some patients improve, others for various reasons will remain unchanged, or may even get sicker. The nurse will be called upon to continue working with the patient and family during extended periods often marked by exacerbations and remissions of the illness.

Maintaining a professional role with the patient presents additional challenges. Because you have known him for a long time, it may be difficult for you to differentiate between a professional role and a social role. There is also greater likelihood, because of your familiarity with family problems, of becoming a protagonist for one family member or another, rather than helping the family to assess problems and deal with them.

Long-term patients in the general hospital often get "lost in the shuffle." The acutely ill surgical patient, for example, or the accident victim may claim the staff's time and attention in a way that an elderly man with chronic congestive heart failure may not. As you work in the general hospital, be alert to the special requirements of long-term patients. Are there activities in which they can participate, such as use of a library, playing cards, and so on? Is there a place where the patient can eat his meals out of bed, with others, if he is able?

When working with these patients, avoid reminding them that others are sicker and require more of your time. The long-term patient typically has significant problems in adapting to the restrictions imposed by his illness. Listening to these patients and their families, and helping them take stock of their situation is an important part of your role.

The care of long-term patients highlights the importance of faithfully carrying out necessary care every day, even though there is no quick improvement. Sometimes there is no improvement at all, and one realizes that treatment is serving only to hold ground which might otherwise be lost, rather than to provide improvement. The very sameness of the care, day by day, can be discouraging to both nurse and patient. Almost anyone can perceive the drama of bringing a patient out of anaphylactic shock, but not every nurse is attuned to helping an emphysema patient do his breathing exercises daily, and to feeling joy when the patient blows out one more candle today than he did yesterday.

The relationship which the nurse has with the long-term patient is especially important since many of these patients have few ties with their families and friends. Because other significant relationships are so often lacking, what the nurse provides as a listener and as one who is concerned about the patient's welfare can be especially important. Nurses can show their interest and support of patients by attending to the daily matters which help the patient acquire greater freedom and mastery of the situation. They can also aid him to use the abilities which he has, and assist him to keep in touch with those people who are important to him. Wheeling the patient to the phone booth and helping him get the necessary change to call his family can be just as significant an aspect of nursing, particularly for this group of patients, as giving back rubs or providing adequate fluid intake.

Patient behavior

The facial expression assumed by a patient is not necessarily a good indication of what is happening inside him. Cheerfulness can be a mask behind which lurk fears and anger of a most urgent nature. The need of the quiet person to talk may be great, and it may be hard for him to express himself. On the other hand, a patient may attempt to please the staff by not complaining, not even telling the nurse he has pain or discomfort. This behavior may mask his condition, resulting in a more serious condition.

Other patients, by their behavior, may make it hard for nurses to accept them. For instance, some grown-up patients act like uninhibited children. They demand more service than anyone could give. They cry. They are stubborn, not doing what was ordered by the physician. They do not act as persons of their age usually do. Such patients sometimes cause anxiety in the nurse, because they do not meet her expectations. However, the nurse should remember that the patient who seems to be willful and obstinate may be trying to maintain his integrity and his will to fight. The patient who gives in to every demand may have given up.

Some adults may be ashamed of their behavior if it becomes childish when they are sick and forced to depend on the care of others; they may cry and complain more easily. If a patient is embarrassed by his behavior, the nurse can point out to him the temporary nature of his dependence. Nurses see people *in extremis,* with their defenses badly shaken. A matter-of-fact, "This is not unusual" acceptance of the situation may help to convey to the patient recognition of the temporary nature of the circumstance and a subtle tone of support. When people are temporarily shorn of their usual poise and self-control, the nurse can help them to maintain their dignity.

It is important to assess the patient's capacity for control at a given time and also to consider some possible reasons for his behavior. While it is not only useless, but also possibly harmful, to demand that a patient show greater control than is possible for him, it is important to establish a plan of care which enables the patient to maintain the self-control which he can muster. For example, a patient with multiple sclerosis had tremors of his hands; each time he tried to take a sip of water, he spilled it on the bed, and then burst into tears of frustration. The nurse, noting the difficulty, placed the water glass, half full, on the overbed table close to the patient, and put a flexible straw in the glass. The patient could draw the table toward him when he wanted to drink and sip the water without having to handle the glass. A patient who is incontinent at night may be able to avoid soiling himself if the urinal is left where he can reach it.

In working with patients who have a variety of illnesses—many of which have no ready cure, and some of which have none—there is a great temptation for the nurse to adopt a manner which implies to the patient that there is no cause for concern. One nurse said to an elderly lady who had just learned that she had cataracts developing in both eyes, "You have nothing to worry about." Such an attitude, in effect, denies the patient any opportunity for help with the very real worries of how to get along with impaired vision (for example, if he depends on his car for his livelihood); how to deal with the possibility of blindness; how to defray the expense of surgery; and how to meet the other direct and indirect effects of the operation. It has been said that the only really minor operation is the one someone else is having. Doctors and nurses sometimes have a tendency to speak of diseases as more amenable to care and cure than is actually the case, leaving the patient and family to find out the truth for themselves and to deal with their plight unaided. Dismissing the problems of patients with the statement, "Don't worry," is probably a self-protective mechanism for health personnel; they should remember that it is good practice to allow patients and families to voice their misgivings.

The nurse's feelings

The nurse may avoid a patient for reasons other than personal behavior. He may speak a different language, or his customs may be so strange that the nurse feels that there is no common meeting ground for communication. Many of us have a tendency to avoid the unfamiliar, because it usually provokes more anxiety than the familiar. We may be uncertain what to do or say. Because we do not know what to expect next, we feel uneasy. Yet there is a certain sense of adventure in exploring the unknown. What are the thoughts and the feelings of a person different from us in background or age? As the unknown unfolds, we find that we have grown, and that our own perspectives have been enriched.

Not all cultures view cleanliness in the same way. Most Europeans do not consider themselves clean without frequent cleansing of the rectal and genital regions, especially after a bowel movement. There are people in other groups who do not believe in a daily bath. If a patient enters the hospital with nits clinging to the shafts of his hair and black lines under his fingernails, will his condition color your feelings about him as a person? If your answer is "Yes" (and it may well be), try to draw a distinction between a person's standards of hygiene and the person as an individual.

You may become attached to some patients. You have cared for them a long time. They like you, and you like them. They are *your* patients. You may be unwilling to relinquish them to their families or to death. Although you should not be afraid to like your patients, emotional involvement with a patient does not mean the same thing as emotional involvement with a friend or a family member. Relations with patients are more temporary. You are maintaining a tacitly understood relationship based on service. Usually, you do not call your patient by his first name; you do not display your personal life to him; you are not coy. You can be warm and express your interest in a different fashion. You show a patient that you like him by taking him as he is, by perceiving his needs and meeting them promptly. The tender touch at just the right moment, the word of encouragement when he is feeling low will bring satisfaction to both of you. The more you understand what comforting the patient means to you, the more free you will be to do it well.

Guarding against suicide

The depressed patient bears watching; he may be thinking of suicide. Signs of depression are: lack of enthusiasm, prolonged insomnia, listlessness, reluctance to speak, neglect of appearance, withdrawal, lack of interest in anything, and feelings of worthlessness. It may be difficult to get the patient to say anything. Suicide in the nonpsychotic patient is often an attempt to escape from an overwhelming situation, which frequently is the loss of love. Hostility is often a factor, too. Anger at self, the wish to hurt those close to him who have hurt him—usually such influencing factors are unrecognized by the patient. In some instances it is possible to avert suicide if the patient thinks that one person in the world will listen to him and is concerned for him. That one person can be a nurse. The background leading to suicide is a long, complicated web of events and feelings. The nurse is expected to recognize depression and protect the patient by reporting her observations promptly to the doctor. Obvious hazards, such as a razor in the patient's stand, can be removed quietly.

If a patient threatens suicide, pay attention to him. He may mean it. Do not leave the patient alone. Communicate with the doctor. Alert the rest of the nursing staff. Chart your observations. Where pain, incurable disease, crippling disability, and impending death are present—as they may be on any general hospital floor—suicide, like fire, is an ever-present possibility.

Patients' complaints

Some patients continually complain about pains and aches or the service of the hospital. These patients are often disliked, particularly by the nursing staff. Perhaps complaints about what little can be done leave the nurses feeling helpless. What is it that lies at the root of the patient's bitterness and continual complaints? Has anyone tried to find out? Is this the only way the patient can get any attention? In the course of this patient's day, does he have any warm human contact? Any opportunity for a feeling of accomplishment or satisfaction? A patient, because he is a patient, is cut off from his family and friends, his work, and his home. His habitual sources of satisfaction are usually not available in the hospital, where his sore toe and his elevated leukocyte count may receive attention while he himself is starved for human contact.

Patients who voice many complaints are sometimes labeled as chronic complainers, those who are never satisfied, or uncooperative individuals. This form of labeling reveals a lack of perception and understanding on the part of the speaker. Perhaps nurses label patients as a way of putting distance between themselves and the patients who make them anxious. The subconscious reasoning may be that a patient who is labeled as uncooperative is so unworthy that nurses are excused for avoiding him. By stereotyping and labeling a patient, the nurse will in a sense dismiss him. Stereotyping can be done by a whole group, with disastrous effects on the patient. The night nurse reports to the day staff, "He's uncooperative," and sets up the climate and expectations. Once a patient is labeled as uncooperative, he probably will not disappoint anyone. He will be uncooperative.

Who are the "good" patients? Many nurses think that submissive patients are "good," and by bestowing approval on the quiet ones they force patients to hide their feelings. Often the behavior expected of patients is made evident to them subtly but very clearly. "Mrs. Glenn is a wonderful patient, Doctor. She's always smiling." Therefore, Mrs. Glenn must go on smiling, "even if it kills her." Her ulcer may grow bigger, but she is smiling.

Some patients do not complain because they are at the mercy of the nurse. They dare not antagonize her, or the doctor, or the orderly. A patient lying in bed, sick and in pain, depends on the hospital staff. He is in a vulnerable position, and the danger of being ignored—psychologically and physically—is a real one. A patient may be afraid to complain, no matter how miserable he feels, because he may observe that the more cranky patients are left thirsty and in wet beds. But fear of expressing one's feelings is not a stepping stone to health.

The patient who is physically unattractive

Our culture places heavy emphasis upon cleanliness, pleasant odors, and attractive appearance. The patient who has had radical head and neck surgery for removal of cancer and has not had plastic surgery is badly disfigured; the patient with infected skin lesions has an unpleasant odor; patients with a staphylococcal infection can transmit the condition to others.

The nurse is bound to be affected by unpleasant sights and odors, but must learn to accept these situations. Odors can often be controlled, but disfigurement due to radical surgery may or may not be corrected by cosmetic surgery. The nurse must be aware of her outward reactions, such as facial expressions, when giving care. What is most important is that *no* negative feelings or emotions be conveyed to the patient.

It may be helpful to ask someone else (such as your teacher) to observe unobtrusively as you give care to the patient, and to evaluate afterward your interaction with the patient. Sometimes you will be unaware of how your facial expression or gestures come across to another person, and a candid impression from someone else can alert you to trouble spots, as well as help you become aware of your strengths. Another important barometer of your approach is the reaction of the patient. Of course, if he shows embarrassment or withdrawal, it may be due entirely to his own reaction to his situation; it may also, however, be an indicator that he perceives that you do not accept him. Accepting the patient definitely does not mean accepting disarray of the surroundings and inattention to the patient's personal hygiene.

The "self-care" patient

A good many medical-surgical patients are described as "self-care." Some are on general units; others are on separate units designed especially for them. These patients present no less of a challenge than the more physically helpless patients in the establishment of the nurse-patient relationship, but the challenges are somewhat different.

Among the "self-care" patients are many who are undergoing diagnostic tests. Frequently the patient has a good deal of free time; in fact, some patients describe the experience as one of interminable waiting: waiting to go to scheduled appointments, waiting for test results. Frequently the waiting is accompanied by anxiety. Until a diagnosis is made, the patient has no concrete "enemy" to grapple with. Instead, he may have many vague fears about what may be wrong and a general feeling of powerlessness.

One important aspect of care of these patients involves explaining diagnostic tests. The patient should know what will be involved—for example, fasting from food or fluids, the need for radiologic examinations, having blood drawn, saving urine samples. He should also be informed of the time of the test, how long it will take, where it will be performed, and how he will get there (cart, wheelchair). Depending on the type of test, some or all of the information may be given by the nurse. It is the initial responsibility of the physician to provide the patient with information about what tests are needed and why, and to interpret the test results to him. The nurse should talk with the physician so that she knows what explanations the patient has received. Within this framework, the nurse reviews and clarifies information with the patient. If a patient is scheduled for some test or procedure about which he seems to know nothing, bring this to the physician's attention.

Patients need opportunities, too, to review with the nurse the results of their tests, the diagnosis the doctor has made, and the treatment which he has prescribed. Often, after the physician has given the patient the information, the patient wants a chance to talk about it again—to review what was said, to clarify terms, and the like. If the patient needs an operation it may be necessary to refer his questions to the physician. The patient may have forgotten, or become confused about, what the doctor told him. Opportunity to discuss this again with the physician is helpful to the patient once the first shock of the diagnosis has diminished. If the situation is very threatening to the patient, he will require repeated opportunities to talk with the nurse and physician in order to prepare himself for treatment.

The patient who is unconscious

Some nurses find it very difficult to care for a patient who cannot respond in some way; others may find it a relief not to have to relate verbally to the patient. The nurse must try to avoid, on the one hand, treating the patient as though he were an object, rather than a person, and on the other hand, feeling overwhelmed by the seriousness of his condition. When caring for these patients try to think of concrete, individual nursing needs which you observe, and plan ways to meet them. Is the skin on the patient's sacrum redder? How can you position him to promote good body alignment and prevent pressure sores? Has he shown any sign of returning consciousness—the flicker of an eyelid? Concentrating on such practical and individualized observations will help you to avoid being overwhelmed by the gravity of the patient's condition and also, to avoid thinking of him as an object.

Care of an unconscious adult, particularly if he is heavy, is best undertaken by two nurses working together. The physical and emotional burdens for the nurses are made lighter when they are shared. Each can encourage the other and trade information on how best to give mouth care, prevent obstruction of catheters, and so on. However, it is essential to keep in mind that the patient may hear you, even though he cannot respond, therefore, make it a rule never to say anything in your patient's presence which you do not want him to hear, even though he *appears* to be unconscious, he may still be able to hear.

The patient who refuses treatment

A teacher, lawyer, salesman, or whatever, is, upon admission to the hospital, expected to "take orders" unquestioningly. A host of indignities surround him. No matter how necessary these may be from the standpoint of running the hospital, they can upset the patient. The abrupt change from being in charge of his own affairs to following the directions of others is difficult for many patients. Anxiety over the diagnosis and its implications plays a part in a patient's refusal to follow treatment. He may refuse treatment because he cannot acknowledge that he could be sick enough to need it. When a patient refuses treatment, he places the nurse in a difficult position. The nurse is expected to see that prescribed treatment is carried out, whether this involves taking medication, staying in bed, or keeping within a prescribed diet. Frequently the nurse assumes more responsibility than can be handled, and the frustration which results may get in the way of effectively dealing with the patient. It should be remembered that it is the nurse's responsibility to see that the patient stays in bed or follows his diet. It is the patient's responsibility to follow his treatment and, except in unusual circumstances when unable to make his own decisions, it is basically a matter for the patient to decide if he will accept treatment, once he has acquired the necessary facts. It is also the physician's responsibility to see that his patient has necessary information concerning the treatment, and encouragement to follow it. Keeping these factors in mind will help you maintain perspective concerning your role and your responsibility. By concentrating on what your responsibility really is, and recognizing the limits of your authority, you will be less likely to feel overwhelmed by the situation, and more able to concentrate on what you can do to help the patient. For example, suppose you are informed during morning report that a coronary patient refuses to stay in bed, and that it is your job to see that he does. The entire responsibility for seeing that he remains in bed does not rest on your shoulders, nor will it be "all your fault" if he keels over during one of his trips to the bathroom. You do, however, have a responsibility to do all in your power to help the patient follow his treatment. With your responsibility cut down to more manageable size, how will you approach the patient?

Start by thinking of his situation. What may be some reasons for his not staying in bed? Did his physician explain the need for bed rest fully, and did the patient understand the explanation? Is his call bell answered promptly, or does he feel that he must choose between wetting the bed and getting up to go to the bathroom? Does the thought that he has had a coronary make him so anxious that he does everything possible to deny his illness? These are possibilities. How can you find out what is troubling the patient?

If you scold him, he is likely to "tune you out." So, instead, try to give him care, and then gently ask him what makes it so difficult for him to stay in bed. Listen carefully to what he says, and avoid cutting him off. The most important reason may not be mentioned until some of the lesser ones have been expressed. Avoid giving the patient a lecture on the pathophysiology of myocardial infarction, and of the possibility of dire consequences if the order for bed rest is not followed. Most patients are already only too well aware of the seriousness of heart attacks. Emphasizing this is likely to frighten the patient further, and make him more prone to deny his condition.

As you listen to the patient, keep attuned not only to underlying fears which he may express, but also to his recounting of daily annoyances. Often these patients, in their frustration and anger at being suddenly stopped in the midst of a busy life by a serious illness, comment about cold coffee, unemptied urinals, and so on. Let the patient know that you will do what you can to remedy these problems. When the patient senses your concern about his daily frustrations and notices that you are interested in seeing what can be done about them, he may be more likely to confide other concerns to you.

The nurse is often asked to enforce rules concerning treatment of diabetics. Here again, it is essential that you examine your role and responsibilities. Suppose, for instance, that when you are assigned to care for a diabetic patient you are told, "Watch him. He sneaks food from other patients' trays." What is your role here? Can you, in light of your other patients' requirements, watch this one so closely that you are sure he does not help himself to extra food? Probably not. It is the patient's responsibility to follow his diet, and it is your job to help him do so, by finding out what the difficulty is, and helping him to deal with it. But you cannot force him to follow a diet against his will.

One crucial consideration, when working with a patient who refuses his treatment, is acknowledgment that the patient has the right to do so (except under unusual circumstances which concern legal aspects of nursing). The nurse who recognizes this will make a more realistic assessment of the patient's role and of her own. It is then the nurse's job to help the patient make the best possible decisions for his own welfare, rather than to place herself in the false position of deciding for him what he may and may not do.

Families

Nurses have specialized knowledge and skills that help patients to recover. But a loved one can make contributions to the peace of mind and the comfort of a patient that, because of the closeness of the relationship, has effects which surpass any professional skill.

When it is appropriate, capitalize on what the family can do for the patient; do not exclude them. Help the family to encourage the patient in what he must learn. Is he walking better? A word of praise from a loved one may mean more to the patient than the applause of the entire hospital staff. Is a patient worried about his new diet? Let his wife show him how she will fit it into their daily lives. Perhaps Mr. Cole will eat better if his wife brings some food from home. With permission of the doctor and the physical therapist, encourage the family to participate in the rehabilitation program in speech and exercises.

It may not be easy for a daughter to sit passively by while others care for her mother. The illness alone makes her uneasy, and her inactivity may make her feel even more powerless. Action is a good antidote for this kind of feeling. Instead of allowing her to feel left out, suggest that her mother might be cheered by the evening paper, or ask her to encourage the patient to drink beverages if she needs fluids.

Family feelings of guilt about illness are common and usually unfounded. A son might think, "If I had spent more time home, Father would not have had this heart attack." A wife may think, "If I had gone on that trip with John, he wouldn't have been in this car accident." The irrationality of these thoughts does not lessen their sting. Being able to participate in the care of the patient may help the family to alleviate feelings of guilt. The nurse should provide opportunities for the family to talk about the experience, if they wish.

Visitors should be made to feel welcome. They are the patient's contact with his usual life. Show them how to cheer the patient without tiring him. Is the visitor standing at the bedside, awkwardly clutching his coat? Draw up a chair for him; show him where to hang his coat.

Several other challenges must be considered when working with patients' families, particularly in long-term illness. (Although the terms "relative" and "family" are used here, they signify those persons closest to the patient. For some patients this is a close friend.) It is easy for nurses to view family members only in their role of helping the patient and to disregard their other responsibilities. In an acute illness, it is common for relatives to discontinue other responsibilities temporarily in order to help the patient. If illness continues, however, the patient's family must begin to resume other obligations. In talking with the patient's relatives, try to consider the situation which they face. One aspect of it, to be sure, is the patient's illness. However, do not close off other topics of conversation, if the family member wishes to introduce them. As you listen to some of his other concerns, such as the fact that one of his children has cerebral palsy, or that he belongs to a union that is now on strike, you will gain greater appreciation of his situation and you will have less tendency to consider him solely in the role of the patient's helper.

Society sets certain standards concerning responsibility when a family member is ill. Perhaps nowhere are these standards so forcefully upheld as in health care institutions. At morning reports and team conferences, one frequently hears negative comments about patients' families: the family does not take the patient home; they do not visit, and so on. This criticism is understandable; health personnel must rely on families to assume their role in helping the patient. When families do not meet these expectations, not only does the patient lack the support and encouragement that he needs, but also the work of physicians and nurses is made more difficult. Remember that not all families can meet your expectations in helping the patient, for a variety of reasons, many of which may remain unknown to you. As you work with the patient's family, be alert to their attitudes and to their resources for helping the patient. This approach will enable you to aid them in using the resources they have available. What questions do they have about the patient's care? What community resources may be of help to them?

Evaluate your own intervention with family members. Do you, without meaning to, encourage family members to alter their usual relationships with the patient? Suppose you are teaching the patient's wife how to irrigate and dress his colostomy. In your emphasis on the procedure, and your zeal to help her perform it correctly, are you losing sight of the fact that you and she are beginning to talk as though she were another nurse rather than the patient's wife? The family member, particularly if he or she is well informed about medical and nursing matters, may have a tendency to substitute a highly "clinical" approach for the personal relationship with the patient if the illness poses problems affecting this relationship. For instance, although the patient's wife may spend a great deal of time at the hospital, most of it may be focused on concern for her husband's diet, his dressing, the condition of the skin around the stoma, and so on. This approach may indicate a failure to deal with the implications of the husband's illness for their personal relationship. The patient is often acutely aware that his role has suddenly shifted exclusively to that of patient in his wife's eyes. Although a relative's reluctance to learn to care for the patient is usually quickly noted, an overly "clinical" approach may not attract attention, since it fits in with the staff's expectations. If you notice that a relative is beginning to speak of the patient's care almost as though she were the "assistant nurse," perhaps you can spend some time talking with her—other than the time you have allotted to teaching her procedures. By showing interest in her, and in her concerns, rather than just in her ability to carry out her husband's care, you may make it possible for her to talk over some of her personal reactions with you. No matter how well informed a patient's wife may be about her husband's condition, she is still his wife, and not another nurse.

Keep in mind that illness, such as cancer or heart disease, in a family member is a powerful force in mobilizing the anxiety of relatives. They may show their anxiety in various ways: by withdrawing, by becoming too "clinical," by talking about the patient rather than to him, or by blaming the family's difficulties on the patient's illness. The more you can recognize the part anxiety plays in such reactions, the better able you will be to help the family care for the patient.

The transition from hospital to home can be a stressful experience for the patient and his family. Often it is possible for the patient to reestablish his ties with family and friends when he returns home. Sometimes it is not, and the patient must recognize that his place in the lives of others, to which he was so eager to return, no longer exists, and that he must begin all over again to develop new relationships. As you work with patients who are making the transition from hospital to home, your appreciation of these factors will help you to assist the patient's family to assess the situation realistically.

Bibliography

Amacher, N. J.: Touch is a way of caring. Am. J. Nurs. 73:852, May, 1973.

Anderson, L. et al: *Nutrition in Nursing.* Philadelphia, Lippincott, 1972.

Crary, W. G. et al: Depression. Am. J. Nurs. 73:472, March, 1973.

Dodge, J. S.: What patients should be told: patient's and nurse's beliefs. Am. J. Nurs. 72:1852, October, 1972.

Kelly, Sister P.: Diagnostic tests: what should we tell the patient? Nurs. '74, 4:15, December, 1974.

Novak, B. J. et al: From the patient's point of view. Nurs. Care 8:28, June, 1975.

Quint, J. C.: *The Nurse and the Dying Patient.* New York, Macmillan, 1967.

Robinson, L.: The demanding patient, Part 1. Nurs. '73, 3:20, January, 1973.

Rogers, J. et al: Nurses can help the bereaved. Canad. Nurs. 71:16, June, 1975.

Scherer, J. C.: *Introductory Clinical Pharmacology.* Philadelphia, Lippincott, 1975.

Schoenberg, B., ed.: *Loss and Grief: Management in Medical Practice.* New York, Columbia University Press, 1970.

Starr, B. D. and Goldstein, H. S.: *Human Development and Behavior: Psychology in Nursing.* New York, Springer, 1975.

Wolff, I. S.: Acceptance. Am. J. Nurs. 72:1412, August, 1972.

CHAPTER—3

Fundamental processes of health and illness

On completion of this chapter the student will:

- **Discuss the basic concepts of stress in regard to illness and health.**
- **Discuss the role of the nurse in dealing with stress and clinical situations producing stress.**
- **Define and use correctly the disease terminology in this chapter.**
- **Describe the basic principles of water and electrolyte regulation and the normal function of body fluids.**
- **Describe the principles and purpose of intravenous therapy.**
- **Discuss the basic principles of: the major internal body defenses, the inflammatory response, tissue repair, and body responses to infection.**
- **List some of the more common causes of allergy and describe the common forms of treatment for an allergy.**
- **List the signs of anaphylactic shock and the emergency treatment for it.**

Nursing, as a health profession, helps people to reach and maintain optimal health. It is also concerned with preventing disease and caring for those who are ill.

Health and illness are relative states. Constantly in flux, they depend on the satisfaction of biological, psychological, and sociological needs and the individual's ability to make suitable adaptations to internal and environmental stresses as they arise.

Homeostasis

Homeostasis is the term used to describe the state of the body when it is in a dynamic state of equilibrium. The word dynamic is used because in order to maintain this equilibrium, the body is constantly at work to balance the components of the internal environment: endocrine secretions, water, electrolytes, proteins, vitamins, minerals, and oxygen. The body must obtain the materials needed and convert or eliminate what is superfluous. Thus, pathology can arise from deprivation such as vitamin deficiency, or from excess such as too many sodium ions. Endocrine disturbances can arise when one has too little of a hormone or too much.

Concept of stress

Another derivative from the concept of homeostasis is the concept of stress. Stress, according to Engel (1953), can be "any influence, whether it arises from the internal environment or from the external environment, which interferes with the satisfaction of basic needs or which disturbs or threatens to disturb the stable equilibrium."

In Selye's theory (1956), stress is a specific physiological condition manifested by a general adaptation syndrome. Whether a stressor is biological, such as surgical trauma or bacterial toxins; psychological, such as worry, fear, rage; or sociological, such as a new job or increased family responsibilities, the same nonspecific general adaptation syndrome results if the stressor is excessive, ill-timed, or too sudden in onset.

The general adaptation syndrome consists of three stages: the alarm reaction, the stage of resistance, and the stage of exhaustion or death. Most stressors evoke the first two stages of response. An individual goes through these defensive stages a great many times during life. They are purposeful homeostatic reactions.

The general response to a stressor is accomplished through the coordinated efforts of the endocrine and nervous systems. Acting through the nerves, stressors produce norepinephrine and acetylcholine in nerve endings; and a few nerve filaments go directly to the adrenal medulla. Also, through the endocrine system, stressors stimulate the pituitary to secrete ACTH, which in turn acts on the adrenal cortex to produce predominantly anti-inflammatory glucocorticoids, namely cortisone and cortisol. Glucocorticoids tend to be inhibitory and catabolic.

The adrenal is also stimulated to produce proinflammatory corticoids or mineralocorticoids, namely aldosterone and desoxycorticosterone. Mineralocorticoids tend to be stimulative and anabolic.

Selye found that imbalances between these two types of hormones as well as an excess of ACTH can be responsible for disease by affecting certain "target organs." These include the thymus and lymphatic system; joints and connective tissue; blood vessels; the liver, kidney, pancreas, and gastrointestinal tract.

The adaptive hormones of the pituitary-adrenal system appear to be necessary to maintain life during the alarm reaction of the general adaptation syndrome, when large tissue regions are under stress. The body then gains the time necessary for the development of specific local adaptive phenomena in the directly affected region.

During the stage of resistance the directly affected region can cope with its local task without the help of adaptive hormones.

At times, when the body uses one organ system repeatedly to cope with a threatening situation, disease can result from its disproportionate excessive development, or from its eventual breakdown due to wear and tear. Specifically, Selye uses the term "diseases of adaptation" to refer to maladies resulting from the excess, deficiency, or improper mixture of adaptive hormones.

Stress is obviously not an entirely negative concept. Inherent in each individual's growth and development are markedly stressful situations which, if mastered, give zest and fullness to life. In the oyster the pearl is produced in response to a stressor. One needs stress to live. Each stage of development has its stressful tasks to be learned and mastered which ready one for the next stage of development.

The person who subjects himself to the stress of physical conditioning involved in a daily two-mile run gradually increases the efficiency of his cardiovascular system. This is beneficial stress, denied to the person who limits his exercise to changing the channels on his television set.

Trying something for the first time, whether it be a new job, a new skill, or a new role in life, is often a stressful experience. But as one perseveres and ability and confidence increase, the apprehension diminishes and life is enriched because of the continuing effort to learn and grow.

Biologically, the individual's mode of adaptive responses is limited by genetic endowment as well as by morphology and physiochemical structure. Psychological adaptation also depends on genetic endowment plus one's relationships with significant others, and one's beliefs. Though individuals have greater latitude sociologically for new adaptive modes, inertia and cultural tradition may impede the development of new coping mechanisms, particularly if they contradict old values.

The body, with its marvelous capacity for coping with large variations in the assaults of various stressors, sometimes reaches a point when quantitative excesses cannot be compensated for and symptoms result. Symptoms represent the evidence of damage or the defense reaction to excessive stress. Though symptoms have been categorized classically as mental or physical, each disease process involves all tissues of the body, directly or indirectly, and in varying degrees.

Though symptoms may indeed reflect an organic disturbance, cellular pathology need not have initiated the symptom complex. Disease is usually the result of multiple factors. A female diabetic patient, well controlled with diet and insulin, may be looked upon as being in a state of equilibrium. But the social and psychological stressors of her husband's sudden death may be sufficient to provoke acute symptomatic illness. Organic disorders are concomitants in the complex of biological, psychological, and social patterns of adaptation, and illness should be looked upon as a breakdown in total living. Good treatment, then, emphasizes the function of the individual in all his dimensions.

Nursing and stress

How does nursing fit into this more comprehensive view of health and illness? Examining some of its dimensions, nursing care involves:

1. Preventing, modifying, reducing, or removing stressors.

Nurses can anticipate the adaptive tasks facing an individual through a knowledge of the developmental needs and tasks facing him at his particular stage in the life cycle. The prevention of illness at crisis points in life is enhanced when individuals are prepared for new adaptive tasks. Nurses can assist in the maintenance of homeostasis by participation in programs of health education. Participating in immunization programs, encouraging routine Pap smears, or speaking to members of a Golden Age Club on the prevention of falls are other ways.

In the hospital, the nurse who cares for the patient with an acute myocardial infarction monitors the electrocardiogram continuously to detect the added stressor of dangerous cardiac arrhythmias to keep them from interfering with the heart's effective function and healing.

2. Supporting the adaptive processes utilized by the patient in his attempt to establish a new state of equilibrium.

During the illness, support of the patient's natural defenses and adaptive processes can be accomplished while working with the physician and other members of the health team. Management of the internal environment through such activities as the control of pain with drugs, the administration of fluids and electrolytes or antibiotics and other medications offers specific help.

Understanding the mental mechanisms patients use to cope with threats to their integrity enables the nurse to be supportive. Non-judgmentally listening to him as he confronts his weaknesses, identifies his strengths, and attempts to reassess the direction of his life relieves the patient of the burden of carrying this load internally. The nurse who listens supportively may help the patient to deal with an amputation although she cannot prevent the amputation. Nor can she solve the patient's problems for him. She can assist him to identify what the problems are and where she and the other available resources can be of assistance.

Management of the external environment is often necessary to promote rest, a major treatment for many illnesses. Nursing activities which promote rest include arranging for a comfortable room temperature, providing a cotton blanket instead of a woolen one for the allergic patient, noise control, provision for a pleasant, appropriately cheerful environment, and spacing nursing activities for the benefit of the patient rather than for the convenience of hospital departments.

The nurse's good judgment regarding the number of visitors and the length of visitation assists the patient in his attempt to regain equilibrium. The elderly lady might greatly benefit by having the rules relaxed and her daughter near at hand most of the time whereas the active businessman might need to be protected from the over-solicitude of his office associates.

3. Recognizing that applying stressors is a necessary part of the treatment process and that, in moderation, stress is necessary for life.

There are optimum stress tolerance levels. These need to be accurately assessed so that patients are guided to use their adaptation energy at a rate and in a direction appropriate to the capacity of their minds and bodies.

The patient in shock has the capacity for only essential physical activity so that his metabolic demands are minimized.

The nurse who encourages the postoperative cholecystectomy patient to cough up secretions introduces another stressor, but minimizes its effect by splinting the incisional area. Stress is also minimized by teaching the patient to cough properly preoperatively when he is apt to be more comfortable. Letting the patient know what is expected of him, commending his often heroic efforts, and giving him pain medication as warranted after he has performed his task are ways of supporting the patient through this stressful experience. Introducing minimal stress through coughing and deep-breathing exercises prevents the major stress resulting from atelectasis and hypostatic pneumonia.

Though bed rest is a treatment designed to reduce stress in many illnesses, it can be hazardous in itself. The nurse who uses good judgment in encouraging deep breathing and in turning and properly positioning the patient on bed rest prevents more stressful complications. Providing the usually active business executive on enforced bed rest with diversional material of his preference reduces his discomfort and promotes his adaptation.

When the nurse attempts to teach a diabetic patient how to inject himself with insulin, she indeed may introduce a stressor. His normal emotional response may result in trembling, pallor, or profuse diaphoresis.

Thus, the diabetic should learn self-care after he has some control of symptoms and he is not in severe disequilibrium. The judgment that comes from knowledge and experience enables the nurse to determine how much stress is appropriate for the individual patient, when to apply it, and when to lessen or remove it.

Disease terminology

The word *acute* can be misleading to patients and their families. It does not necessarily refer to the seriousness of disease; rather it describes the rapid nature of the onset and the progress. In contrast, the term *chronic* describes the lengthy, sometimes endless persistence of a condition without much change for the better.

The seriousness of the problem is graded as *severe, moderate,* or *mild.* A stage of the disease may be described as *early, late,* or *terminal. Terminal* usually means a stage preceding death.

A disease may be described also as *primary* or *secondary.* A *primary* condition is assumed to have developed independently of any other. A subsequent disorder that developes as a result of an original illness is called *secondary.* To illustrate, a patient sustains multiple injuries in an automobile accident with one of the injuries a compound fracture of the femur. Because part of the bone punctured the skin, bacterial contamination of the wound occurred with a subsequent infection of the bone (osteomyelitis). The fracture is a primary condition; the osteomyelitis developed as a result of the injury and therefore is a secondary condition.

Morbidity means sickness. It usually is expressed as a rate in relation to population. If 39 people are ill in a population of 1,000, the morbidity rate is 39 per 1,000. *Mortality* means death. If 25 people die in a population of 1,000, the mortality rate is 25 per 1,000.

Hereditary Conditions. Heredity can be an etiological (causal) factor. From the moment of conception the destiny of thousands of traits is decided. Some of these inherited traits can impair the function of the body, and the individual is born with hereditary disease or a tendency to develop it. Hemophilia and color blindness are disorders transmitted by the genes from parent to child. Many hereditary diseases are carried in the genes as recessive traits and are not manifested in every generation.

Congenital Defects and Diseases. Although they are often confused with hereditary conditions, congenital diseases are not necessarily the same. Although congenital disease is present at the time of birth, it is not always transmitted by the genes. It can result from some unfavorable event or unfortunate environmental condition experienced by the fetus during the period of pregnancy. For example, drugs and radiation can affect the developing fetus. The mother can transmit an infection of her own, such as syphilis, to the fetus, and as a result, the child is born with congenital syphilis. An illness of the mother, such as German measles, may impair normal development of the fetus, and the resulting defects would be termed *congenital.*

The etiology of the congenital defect may be unknown. Until it is known, it is difficult to take steps to prevent it. The cause of congenital heart disease is obscure in most instances. The congenital irregularity may be a serious threat to life, as when a baby is born missing a vital organ; or disfiguring, as in polydactylism (more than the usual number of fingers or toes); or it may be so slight as to escape notice completely.

Few, if any, people are born perfect. The flaw may be tiny, a mole or the deviation of a minor blood vessel; or the defect may be important to appearance or health. Most people find deformities difficult to accept. Through the ages such persons as dwarfs have been objects of morbid curiosity, social ostracism, and fear of ill omen; the present is not entirely free of this attitude. Those with obvious major deformities face the constant reminder of their imperfection, their "wrongness." The experienced nurse can come across the grossly deformed person and show no surprise, shock, or curiosity, but, instead, an acceptance of the patient as a fellow human being.

TRAUMA. The term *trauma,* meaning injury, applies to both physical wounds, such as those a person suffers in an automobile accident, and to psychic wounds, such as those suffered in the loss of a loved one.

DEFICIENCY DISEASES. Disorders resulting from the lack of dietary substances required by cells for their normal function and maintenance are deficiency diseases. Some specific deficiencies can produce clear-cut disorders; for instance, lack of vitamin C causes scurvy —historically, the disorder that affected seamen on long voyages. It was found that citrus fruit, commonly limes or lime juice, prevented the disease, and the world had a treatment for scurvy long before its etiology was understood.

DIETARY EXCESSES. The body is harmed not only by the deficit of materials that it requires but also by excess. Too many calories produce obesity, and overdoses of certain vitamin and mineral preparations can be harmful.

HYPOXIA. Hypoxia (insufficient oxygen) produces dramatic effects, for all body cells require an adequate uninterrupted supply of oxygen. Mental impairment quickly follows hypoxia and anoxia (lack of oxygen). The brain is very sensitive to an inadequate supply of oxygen. Irreversible damage to the brain can occur if this organ is deprived of oxygen for more than five to seven minutes.

It is possible for specific areas of the body to be deprived of oxygen while other areas receive a sufficient supply. Reduction of the blood supply to a local area is called ischemia. Thus, if a patient has a narrowing of the coronary arteries, a reduction in blood flowing through these arteries results. The myocardium (heart muscle) is therefore receiving less oxygen and becomes ischemic.

Ischemia may damage nerves irreparably, and even less sensitive tissue, like muscle, can undergo damage. If the ischemia is relieved and has not been too severe or prolonged, healing may occur in time. However, serious and long-continued ischemia can cause necrosis (death) of the involved tissues. Decomposition of the necrotic tissue begins, and gradually the area darkens to purple and eventually to black. This massive death of tissue is called *gangrene.*

When an area of tissue is deprived of blood supply long enough to become necrotic, the affected tissue is described as an area of *infarction.*

NEOPLASMS. This term refers to the new formation of abnormal tissue. Such growths are called *tumors.* A *benign tumor* is one usually similar to the tissue in which it originates, and it is covered by a capsule of fibrous tissue. It may have little activity except local growth, or it may carry on the processes characteristic of the tissue from which it started. Benign tumors of endocrine glands can produce the hormone of the gland. A type of benign tumor of the pancreas is capable of making insulin. Benign tumors typically stay within their capsules and do not spread to other sites.

A benign tumor may cause trouble for several reasons. In certain locations it is disfiguring. In other cases it grows to occupy too much space and crowds the normal structures so that they cannot function properly. A hormone-producing tumor may function outside of the organized body commands, secreting the hormone in excess or at inappropriate times.

Once located, benign tumors usually can be excised and will not grow again. However, while benign tumors usually are considered less dangerous than cancer, they can prove just as deadly. A benign tumor in the brain or the spinal cord that grows in an inoperable site can be fatal.

Malignant tumors (collectively called *cancers*) grow

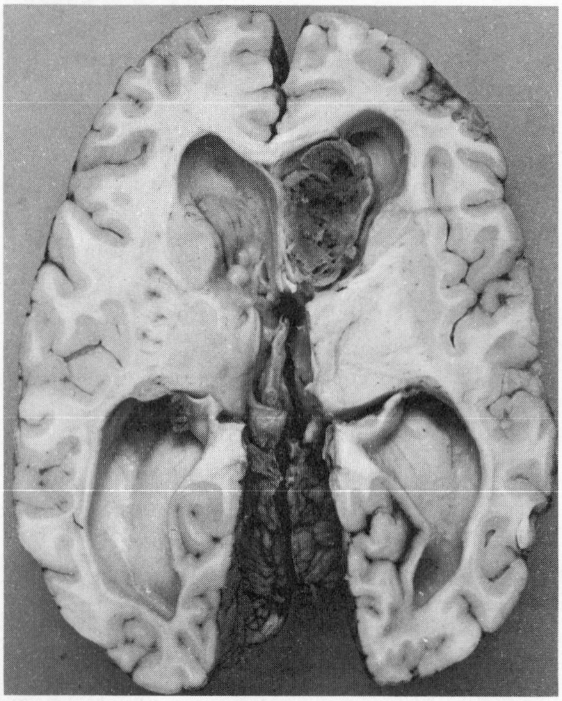

figure 3-1. Tumor (ependymoma) of the lateral ventricle of the brain. (Courtesy of K. L. Terplan, M.D. Photograph—D. Atkinson)

and act in total disregard of body order (Fig. 3-1). Their cells may differ considerably from the tissue of their origin. They tend to spread (metastasize) to other parts of the body. To track down all the metastatic "seeds" of a malignant tumor may be impossible. The malignant tumor can invade, crowd, and weaken normal structures. Some cancers arising from endocrine glands may secrete hormones and produce additional disorder. The capacity of cancer for causing destruction and pain is so great and the control of many of the malignant neoplasms is so difficult that cancer is one of the most dreaded of all diseases. For further discussion of cancer, see Chapter 10.

Infection. Organisms classified as protozoa, yeasts, molds, bacteria, rickettsiae and viruses, can harm human cells by growing within them or producing *toxins.*

Infection is invasion of the body by an organism that produces harm (called a *pathogenic organism* or *pathogen*). Each organism must live in an environment suited to its needs, and not all tissue sites appeal to it. For example, the bacillus that causes typhoid fever thrives in lymphoid tissue. The organism of tetanus cannot survive in oxygen; hence, to multiply and produce the toxins of its serious disease it needs to live deep in a wound. Viruses live inside cells and may be very selective as to the kind of cell they will inhabit; for instance, the polio virus inhabits the anterior horn cells of the spinal cord.

Because we do not live in a sterile environment, we are constantly bombarded by organisms, but we are not always sick. Becoming infected depends on several factors: (1) the number of invading organisms, (2) how virulent they are, and (3) the resistance of the host.

As a rule, foreign material, dead or alive, is tolerated poorly by the tissues. Whether infecting organisms consume nutrients needed by the cells, invade them and disturb their structure or activity, or in some other unknown way offend the tissue, they do produce injury and death of body cells. The group of organisms finds food in the host, adapting its enzymes to the chemical compounds in the host. This is the incubation period, and during it the host is usually unaware of the organisms and may be symptomless. The organisms thrive on the food, and they multiply. Ultimately, the host may become ill.

Idiopathic (Unknown) Etiology. Though they are being extensively studied, cancer, diabetes and rheumatoid arthritis are diseases of unknown origin. The effects of aging are apparent, but *why* these changes take place is not clear. There are many other disorders of obscure etiology. For some of them there is a satisfactory treatment. As a general rule, cure must await knowledge of cause, but this is not always true.

Water and electrolyte regulation

Normal functioning of the body fluids

Approximately 75 pounds of a human body that weighs 125 pounds is made up of water. Much as appearance may belie it, approximately 60 percent of the adult human body is water. Body water is kept within the cells (*cellular* or *intracellular*), between the cells (*interstitial*), and in the bloodstream (*intravascular*). The interstitial and intravascular spaces are called, somewhat misleadingly, the *extracellular* (outside the cells) *compartment.*

Every one of the countless number of cells that make up an inch of skin, muscle, or any tissue is a tiny pond of fluid, held together by the cellular membrane. Around these skin cells is the bath of interstitial fluid. Within each cell is constant chemical activity, as well as constant interchange with the interstitial fluid.

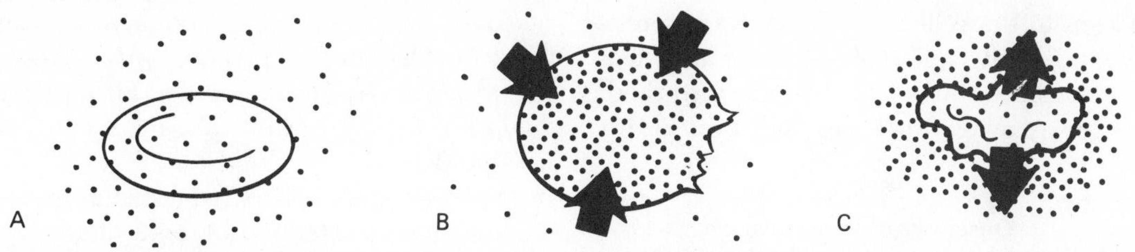

figure 3-2. Concentration of particles in cells in relation to surrounding fluid. (A) Isosmotic: the number of particles within the cell and in the fluid surrounding the cell are approximately equal. Water passes across the cell wall in both directions. (B) Hypo-osmotic: the number of particles in the fluid outside the cell is less than the number inside the cell. Water flows into the cell until the concentration is equal on both sides of the wall, or until the cell bursts. (C) Hyperosmotic: the number of particles in the fluid outside the cell is greater than the number inside the cell. The cell becomes dehydrated as the water leaves it.

Electrolytes are in the water of both the cellular and the extracellular spaces. These electrolytes include such ions as potassium, magnesium, sodium, phosphate, sulfate, calcium, chloride, bicarbonate, protein, and organic acids such as carbonic acid and the amino acids. There is a striking difference between the extracellular and the cellular fluids in terms of the concentration of ions. The sodium, calcium, and chloride ion concentrations are many times higher in the extracellular fluid. In contrast, potassium, magnesium, and phosphate concentrations are many times higher cellularly than extracellularly. These differences are responsible for electrical potentials that develop across the cell membrane and perhaps also for the degree of permeability of the membrane. An incorrect concentration of these ions on both sides of a membrane will affect the transmission of impulses across nerve fibers.

Most cell membranes are apparently completely permeable to water, and the total exchange is enormous. The net exchange of water is governed by the osmotic pressure changes in the two compartments. *Osmotic pressure* (power to draw water) is exerted by concentrated solutions on one side of a semipermeable membrane drawing water from dilute solutions on the other side. Osmosis takes place whenever a concentration gradient exists across a semipermeable membrane. If the concentration is higher within the cell, water will be drawn through the membrane into the cell from the interstitial space until the concentration of particles in the fluid is the same on both sides of the membrane. If the concentration is higher in the interstitial space, water will be pulled from the cell. By means of osmosis the system tends to achieve a situation of uniform osmotic pressure (Fig. 3-2).

Ordinarily, a healthy person consumes more water and electrolytes than the body needs. Water is in everything he eats. Water is formed also within the body during the metabolic processes. Fluid requirements vary, depending on the size of the person, his activity, and conditions in the external environment that affect fluid loss, like temperature. Normal daily fluid requirements for an adult range from 1,500 to 3,000 ml.

Water and electrolytes normally leave the body by way of skin, lungs, kidneys, and bowel. *Insensible fluid loss* is that which is lost through skin and lungs, and is not measurable except by the use of special equipment. Perspiring is the primary cause of insensible loss, but water is exhaled also from the lungs as vapor. The largest amount of fluid is excreted by the kidneys, and a relatively small amount is lost in feces. The tubules of the kidneys select and return to the general circulation electrolytes needed by the body. Those ions not needed by the body are excreted in the urine.

The kidneys remove approximately 180 liters of fluid from the bloodstream each day. All but about 1 to 1½ liters are reabsorbed into the blood. This 1 to 1½ liters passes into the renal pelvis in the form of urine. The kidney also makes a continuous adjustment in ion selection according to the needs of cells. Thus, if an individual increases his salt intake and has an excess of sodium and chloride ions, the healthy kidney will adjust by excreting excess sodium and chloride.

The total daily urinary output for the average adult is usually under 2 liters, and total fluid output ranges from 1,850 to 3,600 ml. To keep the body in good condition, the amount of fluid lost each day should be balanced approximately by the amount taken in.

The normal functioning of the body depends on the maintenance of constant conditions within the body's internal environment. Body fluids carry nutrients and oxygen to the cells and remove waste products from them. Relative quantities of water and electrolytes must not be disturbed; if they are disturbed, severe symptoms, damage to tissues, and even death may result.

Observations and nursing management

Do you see the pitting edema on the ankle of a patient with cardiac disease? The clear fluid in a blister? The sweat on the forehead of a patient in pain? The mucoid return at the bottom of a gastric suction bottle? Vomitus in the basin? Diarrheal stool in the bedpan? There are valuable electrolytes in each, as important to the patient as his blood.

Careful observation of fluid intake and output is important in the early detection of water and electrolyte imbalance. The amount of vomitus should be measured and charted, and the amount of perspiration should be noted and described as accurately as possible. Since water and electrolytes are lost through the abnormal drainage that is part of therapy, such as aspiration of secretions of the gastrointestinal tract, it is essential to measure the contents of all drainage bottles accurately. Note by measurement the amount of blood or other drainage coming from a wound or a body orifice, or, if this observation is impossible, estimate the amount as accurately as possible. Although accurate tabulations of intake and output are singularly rare in hospital practice, *this phase of nursing, on which the doctor may judge his replacement therapy, is of the greatest importance to the patient* (Table 3-1).

Daily weight is often requested as an aid in determining loss or retention of body fluids. One liter of water weighs 2.2 pounds. Always weigh the patient at the same time of day, in the same amount of clothing, and on the same scale. If there is a marked change in the patient's weight, notify the doctor.

Unless contraindicated by a physician's order, it is important to encourage fluid intake by those patients who do not take in an adequate amount of fluid or who need extra fluids because of excessive fluid loss. For example, the patient with diarrhea, an elevated temperature, and diaphoresis is most probably losing more fluid than he is taking in. Because he is ill, he may need encouragement to take extra fluids.

If the amount is to be in any way unusual, this will be specified by the doctor—for example, "encourage fluids to 2,000 ml." or "restrict fluids to 750 ml./day." Taking fluids helps to regulate water and electrolytes and reduces the need for prolonged intravenous therapy, thereby canceling some discomforts. Patients usually tolerate fluids best when they are given frequently in small amounts. Whenever the patient's preferences for certain fluids do not conflict with the doctor's orders, giving him the fluids that he likes will increase his intake. Some postoperative patients can retain carbonated beverages, like ginger ale, better than plain water.

Table 3-1.
Intake and output: important points to remember

Intake includes all fluids plus those foods that are liquid at room temperature (gelatin, ice cream, ice chips).

Output includes urine as well as vomitus, diarrhea, drainage, and blood.

A physician's order is not needed for measurement of intake and output.

Remind the ambulatory patient that all urine must be measured; therefore a urinal or bedpan must be used and the urine is not to be discarded until it is measured.

The intake and output record should include the amount and the time of day fluid is taken in or excreted.

The intake and output record is checked and totaled at the end of each shift.

Intravenous therapy

Parenteral Replacement Therapy. Some of the solutions commonly used for parenteral replacement therapy are the following:

- Glucose in water, given in 5 percent or 10 percent solutions, supplies carbohydrate in a readily usable form.
- Isotonic solution of sodium chloride (sodium chloride 0.9% solution).
- Plasma expanders, such as dextran, can be used as substitutes for whole blood and plasma to maintain the volume of circulating blood and to treat shock. Dextran contains an unusually large sugar molecule. Because of these large particles it increases the amount of circulating fluid in the bloodstream by pulling

tissue fluid into the blood vessels. The volume of circulating fluid is expanded, thus lessening shock due to too little fluid in the vascular system. The use of plasma expanders is especially applicable when adequate supplies of whole blood and plasma cannot be quickly obtained.

- Whole blood is used to supply red cells and plasma. Plasma (blood minus red blood cells) alone may be given when additional red blood cells are not needed. Because plasma can be stored for long periods, and whole blood cannot, plasma is more readily available in emergencies.
- Electrolyte solutions contain many of the electrolytes found in the cellular and extracellular spaces. These solutions are chosen for replacement therapy on the basis of the patient's needs for electrolytes and water.
- Amino acid solutions also may be given intravenously. Their use is especially important in conditions involving prolonged malnutrition. Amigen is one preparation containing amino acids for intravenous use. It should be administered slowly so as not to produce symptoms such as nausea and a feeling of warmth.

Although the procedure for intravenous therapy can be reviewed readily in texts on the fundamentals of nursing, several points are especially important and should not be overlooked:

- The rate of administration is usually expressed as number of drops per minute. The usual rate of flow is 40 to 60 drops per minute, depending on the number of drops per milliliter delivered by a specific type of intravenous administration set. The maintenance of a proper speed of infusion (or the number of drops per minute) is the responsibility of the nurse. A pharmacology text should be consulted for the methods of calculating the amount of fluid infused during a specified time interval.
- The physician may request more rapid administration if the patient is severely dehydrated, or he may ask for slower administration with a microdrip set in elderly persons, those with cardiovascular disease, or for solutions containing potent drugs.
- Explain to the patient the basic reasons for administering intravenous fluids—that is, the provision of fluid and sugar or other nutrients when the patient is unable to take these on his own.
- Promptly after the absorption of the solution in the bottle, the intravenous infusion should be discontinued, or more solution should be added as ordered. Allowing the solution to run out and the blood to clot in the needle closes the vein, with the result that the needle must be reinserted, causing the patient needless pain.

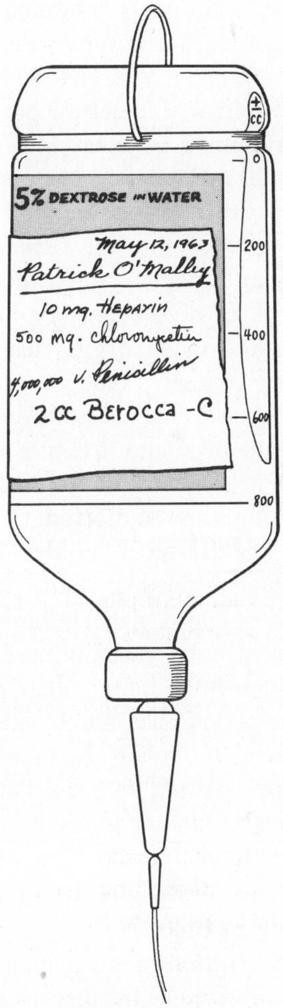

figure 3-3. The label on an infusion bottle should include the name of the patient, the date of preparation, and every ingredient in the bottle. The patient's label is taped on the bottle so that it does not cover the name of the solution.

■ In some hospitals nurses are asked to add medications to intravenous solutions when the solution is being prepared for administration. Always indicate what is added by labeling the bottle clearly (Fig. 3-3).

■ Never administer medication by injecting it into the tubing after the intravenous infusion has been started, unless such administration has been specifically ordered, and unless the administration of intravenous medications is considered part of the nurse's function in that hospital. Injecting medication into the tubing gives the patient a more concentrated dose than does adding medication to the bottle.

■ Unless there is a specific, written order to the contrary, solutions containing potassium should not run into a patient's vein at a rate faster than 40 mEq. every 4 to 6 hours for fear of too rapid rise in serum potassium and cardiac arrhythmias. In emergencies, the maximum rate is 40 mEq. every 2 hours.

■ Watch the site of injection carefully for infiltration of solution into the tissue, evidenced by swelling and blanching of the skin. This observation is always necessary and is especially important when drugs that can cause sloughing of tissues, such as levarterenol (Levophed) are being administered.

■ If a needle is used and it enters an arm vein at a joint or in the back of the hand, the arm or the hand should be supported. Use a wooden splint or a special metal holder. If the arm does not have excessive hair, fastening it loosely to the board with adhesive tape or Velcro straps at both ends and near the needle will sometimes hold better than gauze bandage. If the patient has much hair it can be shaved off over the area to be taped. Whether gauze or tape is used, be sure that it is snug enough to hold but not so tight that it compresses the blood vessels. Venous catheters allow more flexibility and are tolerated for longer periods of time.

■ The administration of intravenous infusions should not interfere with nursing care. If the arm is supported carefully in the correct position, the patient can be turned without dislodging the needle or intracath. Keep the arm well splinted and the tubing loose while turning the patient.

■ Blood transfusion reactions may occur during or after the administration of blood that has been incorrectly typed and cross-matched or given to the wrong patient. A reaction may also be seen if there has been bacterial contamination of the blood or the transfusion set or if the patient has an allergic reaction to the donor blood. Allergic reactions are seen when blood donors are not carefully screened. For instance, the donor may not admit to taking a particular drug. If a person has been taking penicillin, denies taking the drug and then donates blood, the penicillin will be present in the donated blood. If the patient receiving the blood is allergic to penicillin, he may have an allergic reaction during or after the transfusion. The patient should be observed for chills, fever, dyspnea, cyanosis, and sudden sharp pain in the lumbar region. If any of these symptoms appear, stop the transfusion and seek additional direction from the physician. If it is decided that the transfusion is not responsible for the symptoms, it can be restarted. However, if the blood is at fault, permitting additional blood to enter the patient's body while seeking advice may cause serious and even fatal consequences. Careful checking of labels on the blood to be administered is of crucial importance.

■ Be careful! Plain distilled, sterile water is *never* given intravenously. It is hypo-osmotic and will destroy the patient's red blood cells. Some head nurses keep the supply of sterile distilled water separate from the supply of intravenous fluid bottles to prevent its accidental use.

Body defenses

Sources of body protection

The body maintains many reserves. When a blood vessel fails, often the body can replace its function with the development of other vessels to the stricken part (collateral circulation). Oxygen cannot be stockpiled, but the body does have a supply of minerals, vitamins, food, and fluid beyond immediate requirements. There is a reserve capacity for many vital functions of the body. For example, there is more lung tissue than is normally required. There are two kidneys, although one could provide satisfactory renal function. There is reserve liver function, and dual organs of sight and hearing.

Hyperplasia. This extra growth of normal tissue

is a mysterious body asset resulting in *hypertrophy* (enlargement). We do not always know how the body commands this extra growth, but it occurs in certain tissues in time of extra need. If one kidney is removed, the remaining kidney may enlarge, increasing the amount of available kidney function. Other examples in endocrine glands, muscles, heart, and lymphatic tissue are common.

At times hyperplasia can occur when no apparent need for it exists. There may be hyperplasia in the thyroid gland, with secretion in such excess that it is toxic to the body.

THE AUTONOMIC NERVOUS SYSTEM. Another source of body protection is the organized provision for *adjustment* through the autonomic nervous system. Orders through the autonomic nervous system regulate sweating, alter the size of the pupils of the eyes, speed and slow heartbeat, and direct many other adjustments in the body that are beyond voluntary control. Moment to moment, whether human beings are awake or asleep, the autonomic nervous system is making adjustments in response to the ever-changing environment around and inside them.

PROVISIONS AGAINST HAZARDS. Externally, the skin shell, with its superficial layer of dead cells, is a relatively impermeable covering. As long as it remains intact, it is the major protection of the body from invasion by organisms. The outer layer of the skin prevents soaps, lotions, perfumes, and other chemical irritants from coming in contact with living cells.

Openings into the body also have their protection. Hydrochloric acid in the stomach creates an environment in which bacteria do not thrive. The reflexes of blinking and sneezing guard the eyes and the respiratory tract. Secretions in these areas have antimicrobial activity. The unprescribed use of washes, gargles, douches, and irrigations often do not offer as much protection as the natural material they wash away. Body openings have a rich blood supply and abundant lymphatic tissue to serve the cells of the area, if they are invaded by organisms.

The hard bony skull is protection for the delicate tissues of the brain. The rib cage is protection for the thoracic organs. A whole series of defensive barriers protects the lungs from infection by organisms of the air and the teeming bacterial population of the nose and the throat, through which every breath passes. Tears and mucus wash away particles of dust and microorganisms. Tiny cilia beat against foreign matter to hasten its exit from the body.

MAJOR INTERNAL DEFENSES. These are the highly organized reactions called forth when the body is threatened. These reactions can originate in the endocrine glands, through their chemical messengers, the *hormones*. For example, in times of sudden, urgent distress everyone has experienced the sensations of a large dose of epinephrine (Adrenalin). When the sympathetic division of the autonomic nervous system orders this hormone released from the adrenal medulla, it enters the bloodstream and produces a massive body-wide reaction. The alert state of the body produced by epinephrine has been described as preparation for "fight or flight."

A second hormonal reaction can occur when the pituitary gland orders the adrenal cortex to discharge its adrenal cortical steroid. Hydrocortisone constitutes a major part of the substance released. Blood pressure, water and electrolyte regulation, the membranes covering cells, and the metabolism of glucose are only a few of the structures and the mechanisms affected. Particularly during periods of prolonged stress, the hormonal activity of the adrenal cortex provides a key to the widespread reaction that defends the body. Hormones also regulate many processes to maintain a normal cellular environment. The hormones help to avoid the harm that could follow those occasions when excess fluid, sugar, or salt ingestion otherwise would radically upset the normal environment of the cells.

THE INFLAMMATORY RESPONSE

A wound is a break in the continuity of tissue, caused by physical means, such as a cut or burn. How does the body handle the localized problem of injury or necrosis, in which some special attention is required that is not routine for the rest of the body? First, the injured area must be able to signal its distress. There must be provision for the removal of dead cells, and some kind of replacement to fill in the defect left behind.

Inflammation is the body's response to damage of cells. Regardless of the cause, whether it is a cut, a burn, a bruise, or a pinch, the reaction is similar. The signal that starts the reaction may be the release from dead or injured cells of some of their internal substances, such as histamine. These substances have a profound effect on the capillaries. The capillaries dilate widely and thus bring greatly increased amounts of blood to the area. If the action takes place in the skin or in tissues close under it, the redness produced by this flushing is visible. This site is warm to touch, because it has a greater supply of blood than the tissue around it.

Not only do the capillaries dilate, but the "mesh" of their walls also is opened. Normally, capillaries are permeable to the passage of water and electrolytes, but in this situation they permit extra fluid and some protein of the plasma to escape. This extra fluid in the tissue spaces results in swelling, along with discomfort and a throbbing sensation. Often the swelling is sufficient to stimulate the receptors for pain. The blood vessel changes are responsible for the *cardinal symptoms of inflammation: swelling, pain, redness, and heat.*

Among the substances released by the injured cells is one which attracts leukocytes. They pass through the capillary walls into the damaged tissues. When there is extensive tissue damage, with consequently great release of the substance that attracts leukocytes, this material may be absorbed and may circulate in the blood. It appears to stimulate the production of more white blood cells. A blood count taken at this time will demonstrate an increase in the white cells (leukocytosis) beyond normal.

Fever often accompanies inflammation. How inflammation influences the temperature-regulating center is not clear. Possibly a substance absorbed from the injured cells is the signal that stimulates this response.

These effects of inflammation might prove to be beneficial. The protein escaping into the damaged tissue tends to gel and impede movement of materials within the site. Swelling and pain encourage the individual to keep the injured part at rest, which prevents activity from dispersing the contents of the injured area. Bacteria or an offensive substance, such as a foreign chemical, could create additional harm if distributed beyond the local tissue.

Inflammation attracts attention. The patient feels

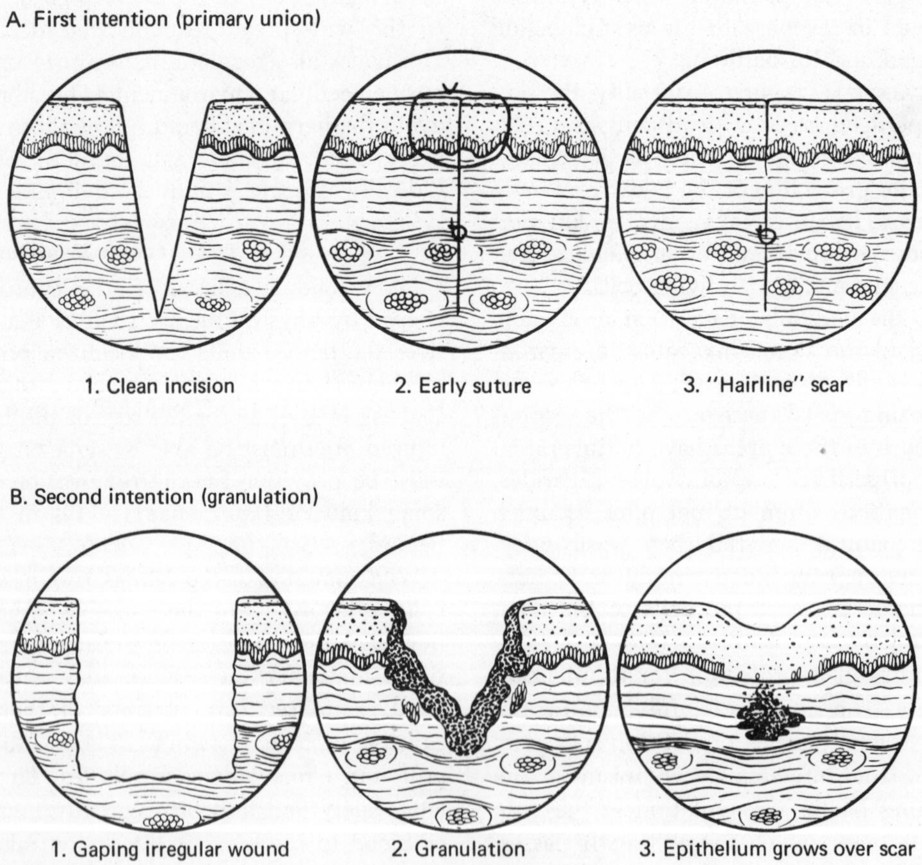

figure 3-4. First and second intention wound healing. (Rhoads, J. E., et al: *Surgery—Principles and Practice,* ed. 4. Philadelphia, Lippincott)

its effects, and the doctor relies on its features to help locate and identify the place and the type of body injury. By watching the sequence of symptoms it is possible to decide whether the body is overcoming its problem successfully or needs help to master it.

At times it is desirable to combat inflammation by countering the vascular dilatation. For example, cold compresses may be prescribed for a sprained ankle, because there is no apparent benefit from the painful swelling, and no microorganism needs to be isolated. The removal of necrotic tissue still takes place, although at a slower pace because of the vasoconstriction induced by the cold. Sometimes the doctor prescribes cold compresses for the first 24 hours to impede swelling, and then warmth to increase blood supply and to hasten the removal of waste.

Tissue repair

As damaged tissue is being cleared of its debris, the signal for repair is given. One of two types of repair may follow: replacement with tissue identical with that destroyed or replacement with scar tissue.

When there is a break in tissue the cells bordering this area begin to multiply and fill in the defect. However, if the defect is large, the ability to reestablish identical cells is diminished or lost. To encourage repair with normal or near-normal structures, the sides of identical tissue are brought together. In the case of an operation, the surgeon lines up each of the surfaces of tissue he cut through. The sutures hold the tissues firmly in this position and allow the patient reasonable freedom of movement without worry that the wound edges will shift. Healing occurs, using normal cells and some scar tissue to fill in the defect. This is ideal healing or "healing by first intention."

The edges of a traumatic wound may be so far apart that they cannot be pulled together satisfactorily; sometimes the products of infection separate the tissue surfaces. The open skin is a way of escape for dead cells and other debris that must be removed from the area before regrowth can be complete. In such cases, packing may be used to keep the wound open and methods to promote drainage, such as irrigation, may be ordered. Scar tisssue is allowed to fill the defect from the bottom. This is called "healing by secondary intention." In "third intention healing," a large gaping wound is filled in with granulation tissue (Fig. 3-4).

The scar mass is formed by cells called *fibroblasts*. These cells locate through the protein gel and start to extend little fibrils or threads from the cell body. As

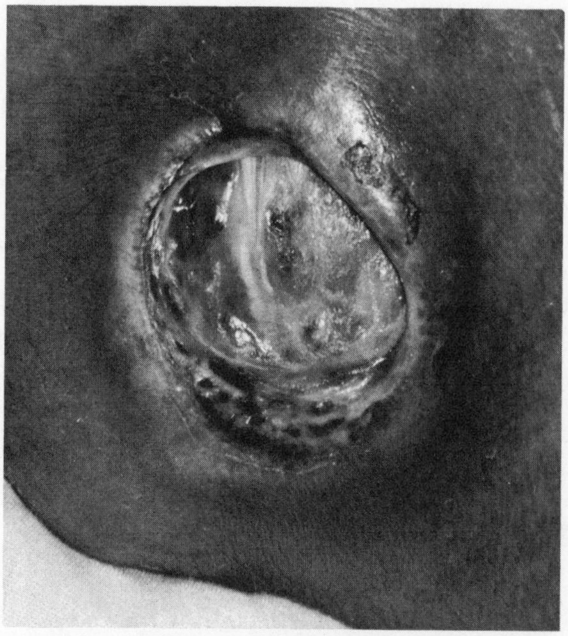

figure 3-5. A decubitus ulcer showing third intention healing with the wound filled with granulation tissue. (Photograph—D. Atkinson)

the threads weave and intertwine, a network is formed from side to side. To nourish the working cells in this area, otherwise deprived of circulation, capillaries from normal tissue bud out and crisscross the defect. They give a pink or bright red appearance, and at this stage the tissue being formed is called *granulation tissue* (Fig. 3-5).

Granulation tissue is delicate and very vascular. Great gentleness should be used when changing dressings to avoid damaging newly forming tissues, as well as to spare the patient any unnecessary discomfort. Packing or gauze that adheres to the tissues should be moistened with sterile saline before removal, to avoid pulling the delicate tissues apart.

When the union of tissues is satisfactory, a signal stops further work by the fibroblasts. In the weeks to follow, fibrils tend to harden and contract. The drawing tight of the network of tough fibrils can cause deformity. The pull of a contracted scar is strong enough to tilt the head or keep an entire limb in a contorted position. This problem is one reason for attempting care that allows healing with minimum scar formation.

The scar is as strong at three weeks as it ever will be, but it continues to change for a long time. With contraction, the scar squeezes out the capillaries that once richly infiltrated its network. It begins to blanch, and over months and years it becomes colorless.

Blood flow is the key to healing. Healing is poor where there is normally a poor supply of blood. The anterior portion of the lower leg is such a site, and injuries there heal slowly. Because adipose tissue has poor vascularity, it heals slowly. The surgeon knows extra care and time will be required for healing in an obese person where pads of fat have been joined together within the wound. Circulation must never be impaired by carelessness. Tight garments or dressings on or above a wound should be loosened. When there is a leg wound, the patient must be encouraged to move from an unfavorable position, such as crossed legs. Excessive tension or pulling on wound edges can delay healing. Be alert for any signs of impaired circulation, such as swelling, coldness, absence of pulse, pallor, or mottling, and report them. In applying a dressing, particularly to an extremity, make certain that it is not tight enough to impair circulation.

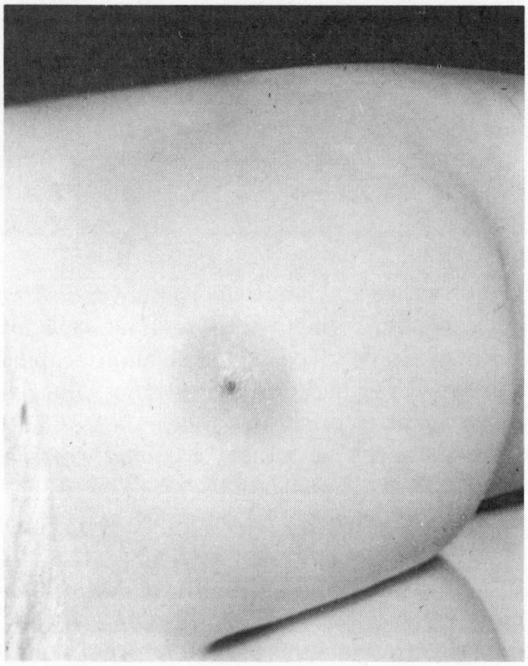

figure 3-6. This painful abscess followed an intramuscular injection. Note the swelling and the redness. (Medichrome—Clay-Adams, Inc., New York, N.Y.)

Body responses to infection

Inflammation

The inflammatory defense in infection is usually greater than that in which no pathogen is involved. The patient with an injured area of heart muscle due to a coronary occlusion will have an inflammatory response: a slight fever and a slight leukocytosis; whereas in infection, the leukocytosis is usually pronounced. Infection also influences the kinds of white blood cells that will appear. In viral disease the response may not be characteristic, or there may be little response. However, in many bacterial infections rapid changes occur that demonstrate how the body is handling the infection. When a doctor suspects that a patient may have an appendicitis attack, he can have a white blood cell count taken every few hours. If there is a growing inflammation and infection, the white cells increase in number.

An infection that has not spread is said to be *localized.* A white, thick exudate of dead cell debris develops inside an outer shell. This material is pus, and a pocket of pus is called an *abscess* (Fig. 3-6). A furuncle (boil) is an abscess of the subcutaneous layers of skin. Around its edges the fight between leukocytes and bacteria continues and adds to the pus accumulation. The pressure of the pocket of pus causes pain.

Infections caused by some organisms localize more readily than others. The streptococcus, for example, can produce materials that tend to break down the confining protein gel of the inflammatory exudate, enabling it to spread in the tissues and to invade lymphatic channels. Wide tissue inflammation without pus is characteristic of its infection (Fig. 3-7).

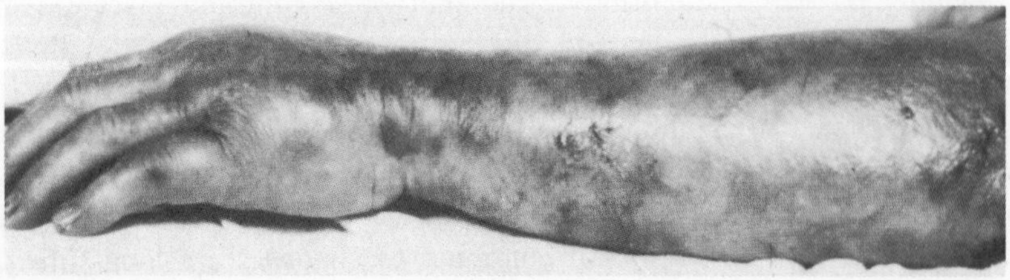

figure 3-7. Streptococcal infection of hand and arm. There is no localization. (Rhoads, J. E., et al: *Surgery—Principles and Practice,* ed. 4. Philadelphia, Lippincott)

The infection caused by the staphylococcus tends to become walled off. The organism can multiply rapidly inside the walls, but has less chance to extend into surrounding structures.

Appearing at frequent intervals throughout the body, the nodes of the lymphatic system are a defense against infection (Fig. 3-8); sometimes they become infected themselves. Inflammation of the lymph glands is called *lymphadenitis.* The swelling in the lymph gland at the node produces a tender, firm lump—a signal that organisms have reached this point. If the organisms are sufficiently numerous and virulent, they may resist destructive forces in the lymph channels and pass through node after node. Eventually, the lymph glands drain into the veins, and bacteria are deposited in the bloodstream. When infective organisms circulate in the blood, the condition is called *septicemia.* Although organs such as the lung, spleen, and liver are rich in lymphatic tissue traps, septicemia threatens by blood-borne delivery every tissue in the body in which the organism might find suitable living conditions. Once in the blood, the organisms may spread thoughout the body to infect many tissues.

Fever is a cardinal sign of infection. It is almost always present when there is septicemia. The temperature may increase as the infection grows. A very sudden high fever is not uncommon in infection. The superficial blood vessels constrict to avoid loss of warmth from the blood. Sweating stops, and circulation is diverted to the deepest, most protected blood vessels. The patient feels cold. Muscles begin to contract in uncontrollable shivering and shaking. Heat is being produced by the activity of the chill. Suddenly the patient feels extremely hot. Sweating and vasodilation occur. Fever at this time can be dangerously high. It tends to subside gradually over a period of hours, but in some patients the new excessive temperature level remains relatively unchanged hour after hour.

A chill often signals that the body is responding to microorganisms that have entered the bloodstream. At this time the physician may order a blood culture, in an effort to identify the organisms.

A severe chill is both uncomfortable and frightening for the patient. The chattering of his teeth and the shaking of his body—movement that he cannot control—may be so violent that the whole bed shakes. This will stop only after his skin is warmed. He may need several blankets over him. Bath blankets placed next to his skin will help. Antipyretic-analgesic drugs such as aspirin are useful for reducing temperature and making the febrile patient more comfortable.

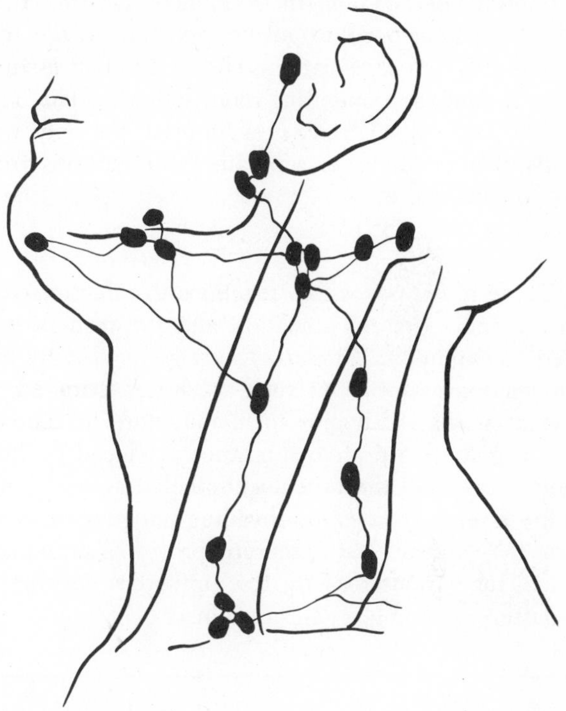

figure 3-8. Lymph nodes of the neck help to prevent spread of infection from a primary site in the head or neck to the rest of the body.

As soon as the chill is over, some of the covers should be removed. Sudden extremes of temperature should be avoided, but too much covering could increase the patient's temperature. Since a chill is a result of peripheral blood vessel constriction, it is not infrequent for a patient to have a fever of 103°F. and complain of feeling cold. The patient's temperature, pulse, and respiratory rate should be checked hourly, or as ordered by the physician. The patient may be drenched in perspiration as the temperature begins to drop. To prevent too rapid cooling and to lessen discomfort, replace his gown with a dry one and change any damp bed linen.

Hospitals present a problem in terms of infection due to the high population of pathogens from patients whose infections release billions of organisms. These pathogens become resident organisms on the skin and the mucous membranes of hospital personnel, and also survive on hospital floors and equipment. When numbers of available virulent organisms come in contact with many vulnerable hosts, such as the patients debilitated by other diseases or those with wounds, infection can become common. Many organisms, especially staphylococci, have developed resistance to certain antibiotics. Because of these known hazards, rules have been developed to govern practices in the hospital—rules about isolation, changing of dressings, housekeeping, and operating room activities. The basis for all these rules is that, in a hospital, the only way to avoid infection is to separate the organisms from the potential hosts.

Immunity

There are two possible reactions to infection—the basic response of inflammation and the response related to immunity. When the body is invaded by foreign material (antigens) such as viruses, bacteria, or foreign protein, it begins to manufacture antibodies. An antibody is a protein substance produced by lymphoid tissue and the reticuloendothelial system. Antibodies attempt to destroy invading antigens; in some cases they are successful, thereby providing immunity. When, for various reasons, the antibodies are unable to destroy invading organisms, illness occurs.

There are three types of immunity, (1) *actively acquired immunity,* (2) *artificially acquired immunity,* and (3) *passive immunity* (Fig. 3-9). Actively acquired immunity is immunity to a specific disease because of a previous infection by the same microorganism. An example of this is immunity to chicken pox after having had the disease. Artificially acquired immunity is created when an antigen that has been killed or attenuated (weakened) is injected into the body. The body cannot distinguish between a dead or weakened antigen and a virulent one and will manufacture antibodies in the presence of antigens in any of these forms. Therefore, the weakened or killed antigen can be used to provide immunity without infecting the patient with the disease. An example of this type of immunity is the use of the Salk vaccine to immunize children and adults against poliomyelitis.

The third type of immunity—passive immunity—uses antibodies produced by another organism, either animal or human. This type of immunity is short lived but is used when antibodies are needed *immediately.*

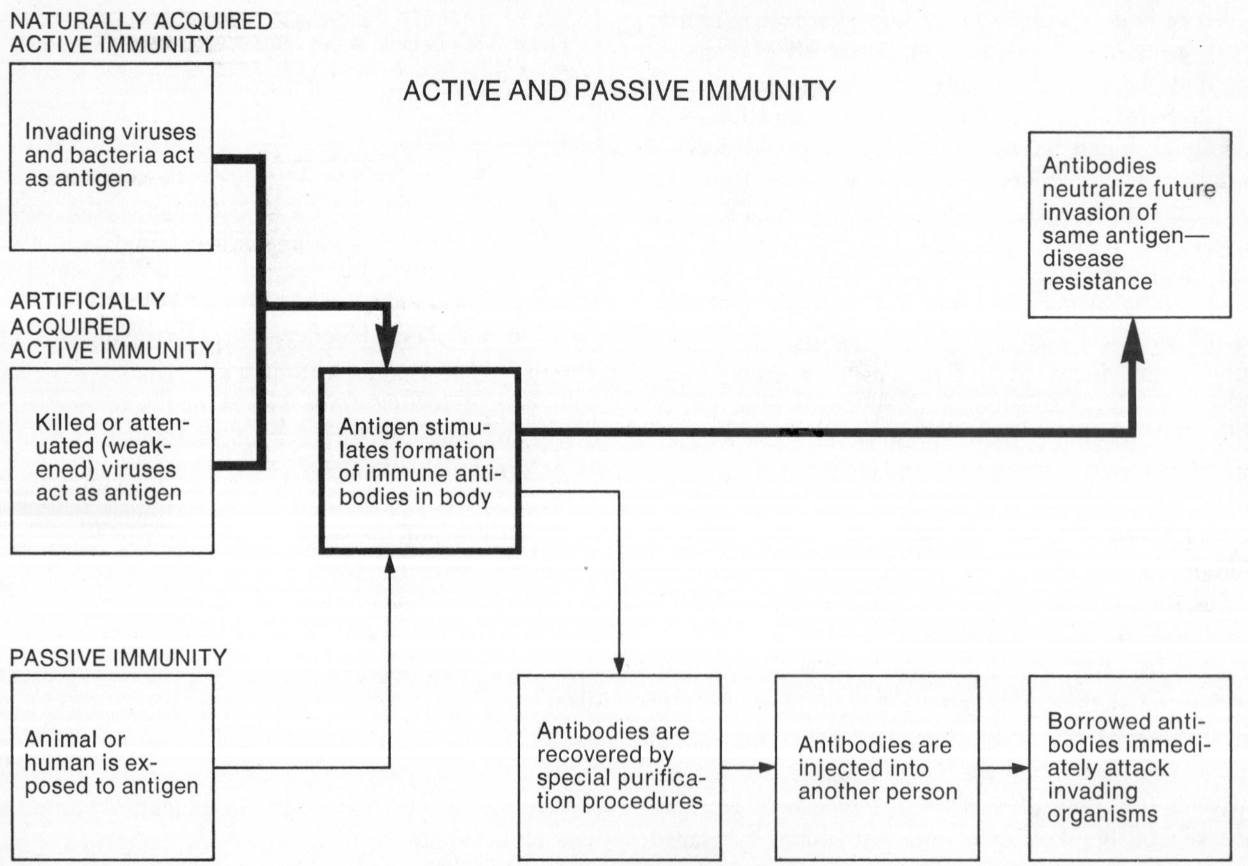

figure 3-9. Active and passive immunity.

The development of an artificially acquired active immunity takes several weeks to several months.

Passive immunity most always involves the injection of *antitoxins,* formed in the body after exposure to a *toxin.* A toxin is a substance produced by a particular strain of bacteria, as for example the bacteria causing tetanus. Like antigens, toxins also stimulate lymphoid tissue and the reticuloendothelial system to produce antitoxins. If a patient were to develop tetanus, the physician would administer tetanus *antitoxin,* thus using antibodies formed by another organism. The immunity is immediate. If the physician wishes to create an artificially acquired immunity to tetanus, an injection of tetanus toxoid is used. A *toxoid* is a weakened toxin and is capable of stimulating the body to produce antitoxin.

Allergy

To most people, allergy is synonymous with hay fever, asthma, and hives. In its most general sense, allergy refers to a state of *altered* immunologic reactivity whereby the body is injured in the course of its immune response against an agent "recognized" as something foreign to the body. It has been estimated that approximately 10 percent of the population has a tendency to develop clinically significant allergies. Sensitivity to certain substances appears to be quite common.

Allergy can occur at any age, and in the same individual the pattern of allergic response often varies over the years. A person may suddenly show an allergic reaction to a substance with which he has had contact for years. On the other hand, allergic responses to one agent may disappear gradually, to be replaced by sensitivity to another substance. Why these changes occur is not clear. As in many other conditions, fatigue, emotional stress, and the presence of infections contribute to the development of allergic reactions in susceptible persons.

Substances commonly causing allergy

Allergens may be classified as those that are inhaled or ingested and those that come in contact with the skin. Here are some common examples:

Inhalants	Ingestants	Contactants
Dust	Eggs	Wool
Feathers	Seafood	Nylon
Animal danders	Nuts	Dye (such as hair dye, shoe dye)
Pollens	Chocolate	Cosmetics

Drug allergy is common and can be caused by almost any drug. Certain drugs, such as penicillin, are especially likely to cause allergic reactions. An allergic response to drugs is a different phenomenon from toxicity due to overdosage; even a minute amount of a drug to which the patient is sensitive can cause symptoms. Such commonly used and relatively safe drugs as aspirin can produce severe allergic response. Sometimes in giving a new drug to an allergic patient, small doses are given initially to determine the patient's reaction, or an antihistamine is administered simultaneously. Allergic reactions to drugs may be immediate, or they may be delayed for several hours or days. A variety of common allergic responses may occur, although some drugs are noted for causing a particular type of reaction, such as the rash that follows the administration of penicillin.

If a patient says, "Is that aspirin? I'm allergic to it," take his word for it. Withhold the drug (whatever it may be) and check with the doctor. Never assume that a small dose will not matter, or that the patient is mistaken. You are the one who administers many potent drugs—often drugs that the patient has never received before. Be alert for any symptoms that may indicate allergy, and report them promptly.

When preparing medications, you can minimize your own contact with drugs by working neatly, avoiding spilling, and washing your hands afterward. Never out of curiosity taste the drugs that you are administering. These simple measures will help avoid the possibility of allergies developing due to contact with drugs during work.

Diagnosis

The diagnosis of allergy may be the simplest and the most clear-cut matter, or it may tax the resources of the most astute physician and require a high degree of assistance from the patient, his family, and the nurse. A patient may develop typical symptoms of allergic rhinitis only when ragweed is pollenating, leading the doctor to suspect immediately that ragweed is the offender and to perform a skin test to confirm this diagnosis. The cause-and-effect relationship may be so clear that the patient himself may affirm, "I can't eat strawberries. They give me hives." On the other hand, a patient may have symptoms throughout the year without any apparent relationship to the substances that he eats or inhales. Sometimes by very careful observation and skillful interviewing the doctor may discover clues that previously had passed unnoticed. For instance, the patient or a family member may recall that symptoms became more noticeable after visiting friends who had a dog. Such a clue is followed with skin tests for sensitivity to animal dander and further observation of the relationship between allergic symptoms and contact with dogs. The diagnosis is complicated by the fact that the patient may be allergic to several things, and that his tendency to develop symptoms varies with the degree of fatigue or emotional stress and with the presence of infection. Symptoms may not occur each time the patient is in contact with the allergen.

Skin Tests. There are two methods of skin testing, the scratch test and the intradermal injection. The physician decides if either or both methods will be used. The scratch test involves making a scratch on the skin and applying the test antigen to the scratch. This lessens the danger of a severe reaction in a highly sensitive individual. There have been reports of sudden anaphylactic reactions from intradermal injection of penicillin in persons suspected of penicillin allergy. If the scratch test is negative, tiny amounts of the suspected antigen are injected intradermally. After about 20 minutes the physician inspects the site of the injection. If the area has a wheal, surrounded by erythema, a positive reaction to the antigen has occurred. Extracts of various substances such as pollens, animal danders, and food may be injected intradermally or applied to a scratch on the skin. Sometimes, even though the patient has had a positive skin test, he encounters no symptoms when he is in contact with the substance; or, despite a negative skin test, all the evidence seems to point to a particular substance. Most skin testing is performed in the physician's office.

The Nurse's Role. The nurse can help with diagnosis by being alert to the possible relationship between the patient's symptoms, his contact with substances in the environment, and his physical and emotional state at the time the symptoms appear or grow worse. These observations must be made unobtrusively and then reported. Avoid constant reminders or suggestions like, "Maybe it's those flowers—we'll have to get rid of them." Continued reminders of possible allergens may make the patient feel that his environment is filled with lurking danger and cause him to fear contact with things that may have nothing to do with his symptoms.

The nurse may be asked to assist with skin tests. In addition to assembling and preparing equipment for the doctor to use (syringes and needles, extracts of various antigens), the nurse should observe the patient during the interval between the injections and the reading of the test. During this period of approximately 20 minutes, the patient may note the development of itchy wheals, indicating a positive skin reaction to the substance injected at that site. Assure the patient that the wheals and the itching will subside soon, just as mosquito bites do, and advise him not to scratch them.

Observe the patient very carefully for any sudden sneezing, difficulty in breathing, pallor, faintness or sweating that might indicate a severe generalized allergic reaction. If you notice any such symptoms, the physician is to be notified immediately.

Treatment

Avoidance of the Allergen. When possible, of course, allergens are to be avoided. However, avoiding strawberries is a relatively simple matter, but it is not easy to completely avoid dust. Once the physician has determined which substances are causing difficulty, instructions are given regarding modification of living habits. For example, if the patient is allergic to feathers, he will need to eliminate all pillows and comforters filled with feathers and to substitute those filled with foam rubber or a variety of synthetic fabrics. The patient should be given a list of allergens to be avoided and may need an explanation of how to avoid them.

By reading the labels he can find out the ingredients in commercially prepared foods and the material used to stuff pillows. When a person who has food allergies eats out, he should avoid mixtures, confining himself instead to plain foods of known composition.

When avoidance is not possible as, for example, when the patient is allergic to pollen, and he must continue to live and work where the pollen is troublesome during certain seasons, he may be treated by desensitization or antihistamines.

Desensitization. Administering tiny doses of the antigen subcutaneously and gradually increasing the dose results in desensitization. In this way the patient slowly develops increased tolerance for the substance and fewer symptoms. Sometimes symptoms can be relieved completely.

Desensitization is usually started before the season begins, if the patient's allergy is seasonal, and it may be continued throughout the season. If symptoms persist throughout the year, often the case when such substances as house dust are involved, treatment must be continued during the entire year. Generally, the time between injections varies.

While many patients are helped by desensitization, it is a prolonged and usually a costly treatment and is not effective with some types of allergy.

The same precautions required during skin testing are necessary during desensitization. The patient is observed with special care when treatment is first begun, and whenever the dose of antigen is increased. Syringes containing doses are so finely calibrated that 1/10 or even 1/20 ml. can be measured accurately. Under no circumstances should the patient leave the clinic or the doctor's office before 20 minutes have elapsed. Severe reactions are most likely to occur during this period. The patient is instructed to place ice on the site of injection, to take an antihistamine, and to call his doctor, if he notes an increase in symptoms after he returns home.

Drug Therapy. The rationale for use of drugs is their ability to interrupt the inflammatory cycle and antagonize the effects of released histamine.

Antihistamines are given to provide symptomatic relief. It is believed that their effectiveness is due to inhibiting the action of histamine within the body. While they give temporary relief, they do not decrease the patient's hypersensitivity, and symptoms recur when the drugs are discontinued. Antihistamines are especially useful in relieving symptoms of short duration, such as hay fever, which occurs for a few weeks in the fall, or allergic reactions to drugs. Therapy with antihistamines may be combined with desensitization in long-term management of allergy.

Overuse of antihistamines can worsen the situation in asthmatics by drying secretions and increasing the difficulty with which they are removed. Antihistamines cause drowsiness. Occasionally, dryness of the mouth and dizziness also are noted. Since many different preparations are available, if one preparation causes marked side effects, the doctor usually prescribes a different one. It is important that medication used during the day does not make the patient sleepy, particularly if he drives a car or performs other activities requiring alertness. A number of these preparations are available in tablets having prolonged action. Thus, instead of taking the drug every 4 hours, once every 8 to 12 hours may suffice.

Adrenergic Agents such as epinephrine and isoproterenol (Isuprel) are used principally for their ability to dilate the smooth muscles of the bronchi. This drug action is especially useful in the treatment of asthma. They also reduce congestion of bronchial mucosa and constrict small blood vessels in the skin.

Corticosteroids may be given to relieve the symptoms. Usually these drugs are given only during a brief period when symptoms are very severe. Therapy is then continued with other measures, such as desensitization.

Anaphylactic shock

Anaphylactic shock is a term used to describe a sudden, severe allergic reaction. The blood pressure falls sharply, the pulse is rapid and weak or may be imperceptible, the skin becomes pale and diaphoretic, and consciousness is lost. The exact mechanism of anaphylactic shock is not fully understood. It is believed that the sudden liberation of large amounts of histamine causes heavy loss of plasma from the bloodstream. Capillary damage permits plasma to flow out through the walls of the blood vessels, thus suddenly diminishing the volume of circulating blood. An insufficient volume of blood is returned to the heart; the heart cannot pump enough blood to maintain adequate circulation. As in any case of shock regardless of the cause, the patient may die quickly due to insufficiency of the blood supply to the vital organs, such as heart and brain.

Prompt treatment is essential to avoid irreversible shock—the condition in which damage to the tissues from lack of blood makes it impossible for the patient to respond to treatment. The doctor immediately gives treatment to increase the circulating blood volume, to restore normal blood pressure, and to combat hypoxia.

- It may be necessary to perform a tracheotomy if laryngeal edema interferes with breathing.
- Epinephrine may be lifesaving. Small amounts are given intravenously.
- Antihistamines may be administered intravenously or intramuscularly.
- Intravenous solutions such as plasma or balanced electrolyte solutions may be administered.
- Drugs such as levarterenol (Levophed), which raise blood pressure (vasopressors), may be added to the intravenous infusion.
- Oxygen may be given to help compensate for the poor oxygenation of tissues that occurs when adequate circulation is not maintained.
- Corticosteroids and antihistamines may be administered to combat the allergic response.

Treatment and observation do not stop when the patient recovers from shock. Although use of intravenous solutions and vasopressors is limited usually to the treatment of sudden acute symptoms, corticosteroids and antihistamines will probably be continued for several days or longer to avoid further symptoms. The patient is observed carefully for any evidence of further allergic reactions.

Summary

The homeostatic processes by which the body protects and defends itself are constantly in use, and most of the time they are impressively successful. Their activity is noticeable only when they are severely challenged. If the defenses are weakened, inhibited, or destroyed, the body can be an easy victim of unfavorable influences that it could normally be expected to counteract without difficulty.

When the patient's adaptive responses, time, or therapy falter, one complication can follow another. Then the struggle between health and illness is on full force, and attention to nursing details can make a vast difference to the patient.

General nutritional considerations

- Patients receiving IV therapy should know why they may not be permitted any fluids or foods by mouth (NPO). It is also important that they know the nature of the IV and its purpose.
- If permitted, the patient on NPO may be given ice chips when his mouth is dry.
- If patient intake and output is to be recorded, the patient and/or family or friends with the patient should be informed.
- A complete food allergy history is necessary as this may give clues to potential drug allergies.

General pharmacological considerations

- Electrolytes such as sodium (Na), potassium (K), and calcium (Ca) may be given as drugs for replacement of lost electrolytes.
- The dosage of electrolytes must be carefully measured and given only as directed by the physician, since these drugs are potentially dangerous.
- It is possible to be allergic to *any* drug. A thorough allergy history is important, for it may uncover hidden allergies.
- Drugs used in the treatment of anaphylactic shock are potent. The use of these preparations requires extreme accuracy in measurement and administration.

Bibliography

Baker, B.: Immunology, Part 1. Nurs. Care 7:11, September, 1974.

Carey, L. C.: Pathophysiology of shock. AORN J. 18:311, August, 1973.

Derbes, V. J.: Rashes: Recognition and management. Nurs. '73, 3:44, March, 1973.

Engel, G.: Homeostasis, behavioral adjustment and the concept of health and disease, in R. Grinker, ed., *Midcentury Psychiatry.* Springfield, Thomas, 1953.

Grant, M. M. and Kudo, W. M.: Assessing a patient's hydration status. Am. J. Nurs. 75:1306, August, 1975.

Guyton, A.: *Textbook of Medical Physiology,* ed. 4. Philadelphia, Saunders, 1971.

Lee, C. A. et al: What to do when acid-base problems hang in the balance. Nurs. '75, 75:32, July, 1975.

MacBryde, C. M.: *Signs and Symptoms,* ed. 5. Philadelphia, Lippincott, 1970.

Metheny, N. M. and Snively, W. D.: *Nurses' Handbook of Fluid Balance,* ed. 2. Philadelphia, Lippincott, 1974.

Rodman, M. J. and Smith, D. W.: *Clinical Pharmacology in Nursing.* Philadelphia, Lippincott, 1974.

Safran, C.: Those summer allergies. Today's Health 51:18, July, 1973.

Saylor, D. E.: The disoriented patient . . . reorienting reactions. J. Prac. Nurs. 23:24, January, 1973.

Scherer, J. C.: *Introductory Clinical Pharmacology.* Philadelphia, Lippincott, 1975.

Selye, H.: *The Stress of Life.* New York, McGraw-Hill, 1956.

TeWinkle, M. B.: Immunization and communicable disease. J. Prac. Nurs. 24:22, March, 1974.

CHAPTER—4

The interaction of body and mind

On completion of this chapter the student will:

- **Discuss the concepts, treatment, and nursing management of the patient with a psychosomatic illness.**
- **Discuss the problems that may be encountered when giving nursing care to the patient with a psychosomatic illness.**
- **Define the terminology used in describing various types of deliria.**
- **Describe and discuss the nursing management of the delirious patient.**

The concept of psychosomatic illness

Psycho, refers to mind, and *soma,* to body. Psychosomatic illness is the occurrence of bodily symptoms which are psychological or emotional in origin.

Mind and body are not separate; one affects and is affected by the other. Who has not experienced some physical manifestation of emotional stress? Such experiences as a headache after a quarrel and urinary frequency or diarrhea before an examination are not uncommon, and for most people they are of a transitory nature. The symptoms disappear and are forgotten after the crisis has passed. No treatment may be needed, or the patient may use simple remedies to relieve the discomfort. One person may find that a leisurely walk is the best cure for a headache; another may take aspirin.

Certain conditions have been considered classic examples of psychosomatic illness: peptic ulcer, eczema, colitis, and asthma. Personality profiles have been developed to describe the typical characteristics of persons who develop such illnesses. Another point of view is that human beings are more complex and varied in their responses than such profiles would indicate, and that the type of illness a patient develops in relation to stress varies with many additional factors, such as heredity and environment. Much remains to be learned about the relationship between stress and physical illness.

Physical symptoms, such as palpitation, tachycardia, sweating, or disturbance of sleep, which reflect anxiety, may occur over a prolonged period. The symptoms may seem mysterious and threatening, because the patient is unaware of their cause. The patient whose heart beats more rapidly and forcefully as a manifestation of anxiety may report this symptom to his doctor, believing that something is wrong with his heart. Often the patient is not aware that he is anxious. He knows only that his heart keeps pounding for no apparent reason.

Almost any symptom can have its origin in emotional stress. Some patients almost invariably have the same symptom when they become anxious. One may have diarrhea, another asthma, and a third may develop hives or eczema. Some people develop two or several different symptoms; often the symptoms are experienced in an alternating fashion.

The development of bodily symptoms is only one manifestation of anxiety. It may show up also in symptoms that are primarily mental, such as the inability to concentrate or to remember. Such symptoms, too, vary in degree. Many people occasionally experience symptoms like moodiness or depression. When such symptoms are severe or long-lasting, they interfere with the functioning of the individual in daily life and with his relationships with others.

Sometimes a person subconsciously develops an illness as a way of handling a desperate need, such as the need for affection. The only real cure is to satisfy the primary desire. An example is a woman who has pain in her heart, not because of organic heart disease, but because the symptom is a way of gaining, if only temporarily, the love and the attention for which she longs. Her husband cannot leave her when she is so sick; her children are concerned. Her pain is just as severe as if it had a physical cause.

The reality of psychosomatic illness

Is the patient with psychosomatic illness really sick, or does he merely imagine he is sick? Many people, including the families of patients and members of the health professions, believe that physical illness which is influenced by emotional stress is less real, or wholly imaginary. Acknowledging the reality of the patient's illness is important; it is the first step in helping him.

Patients with psychosomatic illness are likely to be neglected. The same staff who give excellent care to other patients, not uncommonly ignore them. Some possible reasons for the stigma may include the use of the term *psycho* as a prefix. Perhaps this conveys the idea that such patients are mentally ill, and therefore have no physical illness. Perhaps they are considered weaklings. One hears comments like, "He could snap out of it if he wanted to." Prejudice against these patients may be due to a belief that they are feigning illness in an attempt to get attention or favors.

A patient with psychosomatic illness may be confused with a malingerer, one who deliberately shams illness in order to achieve some secondary gain, such as financial compensation or excuse from work. Pretending illness is considered an unhealthy and unsatisfactory solution to the problems of life. Often it adds to the patient's difficulties, as he makes elaborate attempts to avoid detection. A malingerer can be helped sometimes to find other ways of coping with difficulties. The essential difference between psychosomatic illness and malingering is that the malingerer feigns symptoms. It is a conscious process and he is aware that he is pretending to be sick. The patient with psychosomatic illness develops symptoms as a manifestation of largely unconscious psychic conflicts. The symptoms are real.

Condemnation of the patient with psychosomatic illness can persist despite intellectual understanding of theories about its causes. The patient can sense immediately whether those who care for him are trying to help him, or whether they are belittling him. It is important to understand that:

- The patient with psychosomatic illness is really sick. He is not pretending or imagining his symptoms.
- The idea that he can "snap out of it" at will is no more true than it is of those with diseases like pneumonia, whose need for care is readily acknowledged.

Treatment of psychosomatic illness

The first step in helping the patient is to accept and acknowledge his illness. The cause of symptoms must be found, and measures to relieve them and to prevent recurrence must be taken. Thorough examinations are essential. Although the physician may suspect that the illness is due to emotional rather than physical causes, he must search carefully for any evidence of physical disease. It is not unknown for an illness considered psychosomatic to be later diagnosed as cancer or some other disease. The thorough search for physical causes of the symptoms helps to gain the patient's confidence. He knows that his condition and welfare are being taken seriously. If no organic basis for his complaints is found, he usually will find this news easier to accept when he knows he has had a thorough examination.

Finding no physical cause for the disorder points the way to understanding the patient's condition. What is the cause? Is it emotional stress? If so, what kind? What are the problems which are upsetting the patient?

Sometimes, by talking with the patient the physician can learn about the emotional difficulties he is experiencing and can help him to see the possible relationship between his symptoms and emotional stress. Until the patient himself begins to see this relationship, the relief of symptoms is transitory and random. When he begins to understand the cause-and-effect relationship, he may begin to find other ways of handling his emotional problems. Almost any example is an oversimplification, because there are many diverse and subtle aspects to each situation. Perhaps the patient will be helped by learning to express anger, as well as by avoiding situations that make him angry.

Sometimes the patient's physician recommends the services of a psychiatrist. The two physicians may work together closely in helping the patient, one concentrating largely on the emotional causes and the other on the relief of physical symptoms. Some hospitals have separate units for the care of psychosomatic patients, where emphasis is placed on both emotional and physical components of the illness.

The patient's physical discomfort should not be ignored. While the emotional factors responsible for his illness are being studied, he needs to feel that others are concerned about his symptoms, and that he will be helped to be more comfortable. The patient's symptoms indicate the type of treatment that may provide relief. Sometimes sedatives or tranquilizers are prescribed to lessen the patient's anxiety, thus helping to relieve his physical symptoms. However, these drugs do not provide a substitute for the patient's understanding of the relationship between his symptoms and stress situations. Sometimes psychotherapy is carried on individually; sometimes, in groups. One of its objectives is to help the patient become aware of the deep-rooted and often unconscious causes of his anxiety.

There is no easy cure for psychosomatic illness. Discovering the causes of the patient's illness and helping him to understand and to find more satisfactory ways to cope with his problems are challenges to all who work with him. Frequently, the process takes many years. Some patients are unable to accept the idea that their symptoms originate in emotional conflicts; therefore, they cannot begin to move toward identification of their emotional problems. These patients may continue to be treated symptomatically by such measures as diet and medication. At some future time it may be possible for them to recognize a relationship between their physical symptoms and their emotional conflicts.

Nursing management

Nursing management of the patient with psychosomatic illness requires tact, insight, and judgment. The patient needs someone to listen to him, to be concerned about his symptoms, and to respect him. Prying or attempting to force on the patient an acceptance of the relationship between his symptoms and his emotional problems can make him more anxious. Such efforts may result in intensification of his physical symptoms and resistance to any later suggestion by the physician that he have psychotherapy.

The nurse may make observations that point to a relationship between the patient's physical symptoms and other events in his life. It is important to make these observations. Do symptoms come and go, leaving the patient free of discomfort for part of the day, or do they persist most of the day and night? What kinds of things tend to relieve the symptoms? Medication? Diversion?

It is also important to know how to act on your observations. For instance, the nurse may note that an asthmatic patient almost always has an attack after his mother visits him. Recognizing that this sequence may be an important clue, the nurse should discuss this observation fully with the patient's physician. Through such collaboration the nurse can share in helping the patient, increase her understanding of his emotional needs, and receive guidance from the physician on how to proceed with this aspect of the patient's care. For one thing, she can listen carefully to the patient. Perhaps he will begin talking about his mother, or, equally significant, he may carefully avoid any mention of her. This information, too, can be shared with the physician and may prove to be very useful in planning the patient's treatment. The nurse's observations thus form a basis not only for her own intervention, but also for collaboration with others who care for the patient.

Observing such a relationship between the patient's symptoms and events in his life is a clue that the patient may experience considerable anxiety in relation to these aspects of his life.

The nurse gradually develops a relationship with the patient; she can listen with greater sensitivity to his concerns, and often she can find opportunities, during this process, to help the patient see connections between his symptoms and his reactions to daily experiences. In this process the patient himself often begins to see a relationship between the bodily symptoms he is experiencing and the emotion which he is describing.

The delirious patient

Delirium is a state of disorientation and confusion caused by interference with the metabolic processes of the neurons of the brain. The condition tends to be temporary and reversible. Delirium usually subsides when its cause has been removed.

The delirious patient is disoriented as to time and place and may have illusions and hallucinations. An *illusion* is an inaccurate interpretation of stimuli within the environment. The patient may think that his sister is calling him, when actually the nurse is calling him. *Hallucinations* are subjective sensory experiences that occur without stimulation from the environment. The patient may hear a voice when no one is calling.

The delirius patient is restless and confused. He has defects in memory and judgment. He often behaves impulsively and acts on incorrect interpretations of his environment. For instance, he may believe that a window is a door and attempt to escape through it. Often delirium develops suddenly; it can subside equally quickly. A patient may seem well oriented at bedtime but be delirious an hour later, with symptoms usually worse at night.

Nursing care of the delirious patient involves protecting him and others from harm and helping him (as far as possible) to minimize disorientation and confusion. The basic cause (drug intoxication, fever, alcoholism) is treated medically.

- Keep sensory stimuli to a minimum. The room should be quiet. Avoid unnecessary conversation. Be specific and repetitive in conversation. For example, repeating, "You're in the hospital, and I am your nurse," can help the patient to orient himself to his environment. Keep explanations brief and simple, such as "Here is your soup" or "I'm going to wash your back." Try not to reflect the patient's restlessness and agitation. Feelings can be contagious. Speaking quietly and slowly may help to lessen the patient's apprehension.
- Keep the patient's room softly lighted during the night. Soft light will help to prevent the increased disorientation that usually occurs when the patient is left in a darkened room, and it will contribute to his safety by enabling others to observe him.
- Protect the patient from harm. Most hospitals require a doctor's order before restraints can be used. If your delirious patient has such an order, be sure that the restraints in *no way impair circulation,* and that they give the patient as much movement as is compatible with safety. Many people, delirious or not, react to physical restraints with anger; the delirious patient may be made more excited by them. Remove the restraints whenever there is adequate supervision so that the patient can move about. If he has been pulling against them, his skin may be reddened—or worse, cut. Help him to sit up as much as possible, if he is permitted to sit up.
- The delirious patient usually is incapable of feeding himself. Feed him slowly and allow him to assist, if he is able. Encourage fluid intake, unless the doctor has left orders to limit fluids.

- Side rails can help to keep the patient in bed. Explain their purpose, so that he will not consider them a confining cage from which he must escape. A patient who is physically strong enough can climb over side rails.
- Having someone remain with the patient, assuring him that he is being cared for, can help greatly to lessen his agitation and to prevent him from hurting himself. Perhaps a family member can stay with the patient, if shortage of staff makes it impossible for nursing personnel to do so.
- Keep objects capable of causing harm away from the patient. For instance, a paper drinking straw should be used instead of a glass one and a paper cup instead of a water glass. Cigarettes and matches should not be left within reach.
- Remember that the patient cannot control his behavior. Scolding is both inappropriate and ineffective.

Delirious patients require a great deal of nursing care. Their unpredictable behavior often interferes with the goals of those caring for them. As far as possible, modify the environment and the plan of care to help prevent incidents that can upset the patient and those around him.

General nutritional considerations

- Patients under stress may tend to lose their appetites; it is important to provide them with simple, attractive, nutritious foods and liquids.
- If a patient is placed on psychotropic medications, the nurse should read the package insert accompaning the medication, check drug information in text references, and/or check with the hospital pharmacist for any dietary considerations affecting the specific drug. For example, some psychotropic medications should not be given with a diet which includes cheese, chocolate, alcohol, or caffeine.

General pharmacological considerations

- A complete current medication history should be obtained for each patient. Many people under stress take over-the-counter drugs, stimulants, and tranquilizers which they may not mention unless asked.
- Some patients under stress increase their consumption of alcohol.
- Disorientation and confusion may be an adverse side effect of medications; appropriate action to withdraw or reduce the dosage must be taken promptly.

Bibliography

Barnard, M. U. et al: Psychosocial failure to thrive. Nursing assessment and intervention. Nurs. Clin. North Am. 8:557, September, 1973.

Berni, R. and Fordyce, W. E.: *Behavior Modification and the Nursing Process.* St. Louis, Mosby, 1973.

Burnside, I. M., ed.: *Psychosocial Nursing Care of the Aged.* New York, McGraw-Hill, 1973.

Carlson, C. E.: *Behavioral Concepts and Nursing Intervention.* Philadelphia, Lippincott, 1970.

Fann, W. E. and Goshen, C. E.: *The Language of Mental Health.* St. Louis, Mosby, 1973.

Halberstam, M.: Can you make yourself sick? Today's Health 50:24, December, 1972.

Kneisl, C. R. and Ames, S. A.: *Mental Health Concepts in Medical-Surgical Nursing: A Workbook.* St. Louis, Mosby, 1974.

Kyes, J. J. and Hoffling, C. K.: *Basic Psychiatric Concepts in Nursing,* ed. 3. Philadelphia, Lippincott, 1974.

Mastrovito, R. C.: Psychogenic pain. Part 8. Am. J. Nurs. 74:514, March, 1974.

Robinson, L.: *Liaison Nursing: Psychological Approach to Patient Care.* Philadelphia, Davis, 1974.

Rosenbaum, V.: How to handle psychological regression in patients. Nurs. Care 75:20, July, 1975.

Starr, B. D. and Goldstein, H. S.: *Human Development and Behavior.* New York, Springer, 1975.

Stevens, C. B.: *Special Needs of Long-Term Patients.* Philadelphia, Lippincott, 1974.

CHAPTER—5

The patient in pain

On completion of this chapter the student will:

- **Discuss the reasons that patients may react differently to pain.**
- **State the factors that can influence the degree of pain.**
- **Describe ways to evaluate the degree of pain.**
- **List nursing measures that may be employed in the management of pain.**

Pain may be described as a disagreeable sensation which results from a potentially harmful stimulus. What may be mild pain for one person can be moderate or even severe pain for another. There is no method the nurse can use to determine the actual amount of pain experienced. The only information the nurse has is what comes from the patient—an expression, a statement, an emotional reaction. If the patient says he has pain—*he has pain!*

Not everyone reacts to pain in the same manner, nor does everyone experience it in a like way. The patient who cries when he is in pain is *no different* than the patient bearing

Table 5-1.
Evaluation of pain

INITIAL EVALUATION

Location

Description of the pain:
Sharp, dull, knife-like, throbbing, squeezing, radiating, intermittent, steady, severe, mild, bearable, superficial.

Relation to circumstance:
What (if anything) brought on the pain? Does anything relieve the pain (change of position, walking, etc.)?

Onset:
Sudden, gradual.

FOLLOW-UP OF NURSING MANAGEMENT

Was the pain relieved by an analgesic?
Were nursing measures used? Were they successful?

severe pain in silence. For each, pain is a very real and a very private sensation.

Many factors influence the individual's interpretation of pain. Physical activity may increase pain or may make an individual temporarily forget about it. Anticipation can heighten the response to pain, for example, the patient watching the nurse prepare an injection may anticipate pain. Response to pain may also be learned; as is the case with the child who imitates his parents' reaction to pain. On the other hand, parents may suggest to their children what they believe is the correct response to pain. A son may be reminded that "men don't cry if they have pain," or a daughter encouraged to miss school if she does not feel well.

Pain experienced in the past may influence a present or future response to pain. This is an important point to remember during preoperative preparations of the patient who has had previous surgery. The pain or discomfort experienced at that time may influence his response to pain during the postoperative period.

Response to pain or discomfort may be culturally influenced. In one culture or ethnic group, pain may evoke a highly charged emotional response in either or both sexes; in another, pain is met with stoical silence. Of course, emotional reactions to pain are by no means consistent for all members of any particular group, and the nurse must avoid stereotyped opinions when evaluating the patient who is in pain.

Implications for nursing

Any patient who has pain deserves *immediate* attention. Before nursing measures are instituted, the patient must be quickly and accurately evaluated (Table 5-1). The exact location of the pain is important. The patient who has had abdominal surgery but complains of pain in his incision *and* his leg will require examination by a physician. Pain in the incision is to be expected, but leg pain may be a complication of surgery. If the patient is not asked *where* the pain is, a potentially serious condition may go unnoticed.

Description of the pain is patient-oriented; in other words, it gives the patient's "view." An exact description may, in some instances, aid in diagnosis. Pain changing from dull to sharp, pain in the chest that is now radiating down the arm, intermittent pain that becomes a steady pain—all these could indicate a specific disease, problem, or change in the patient's condition. In turn, such a change may prompt the physician to institute a new medical or surgical treatment, order diagnostic studies, or prescribe additional medication. Noting whether a specific situation or activity brought on the pain may clarify the diagnosis or indicate a need for additional therapeutic measures.

It is also important to know what, if anything, relieves the pain. For example, the patient who has abdominal pain may notice that food relieves the pain.

Table 5-2 lists nursing measures that may relieve pain. These procedures can be instituted for any patient with pain or discomfort, whether mild, moderate, or severe. They will not be effective for all patients.

Analgesics should be administered *promptly* (Fig. 5-1). Making a patient wait creates anxiety, and anxiety increases pain. It is also true that if an analgesic is not administered promptly and pain is allowed to reach maximum intensity, the analgesic will not be as effective as when it is given promptly. Nurses sometimes tend to become hardened to demands for analgesics, and the patient may be labeled a "clock-watcher" or a "baby about pain."

Sometimes pain can be lessened if the patient assumes a more comfortable position. Moving a shoulder, changing the position of a leg, or raising the head of the bed are some measures that may be of value. Such measures should not replace the administration of an analgesic; rather, they should be carried out *in addition to* the administration of these drugs.

Pain can be intensified by *additional* discomforts.

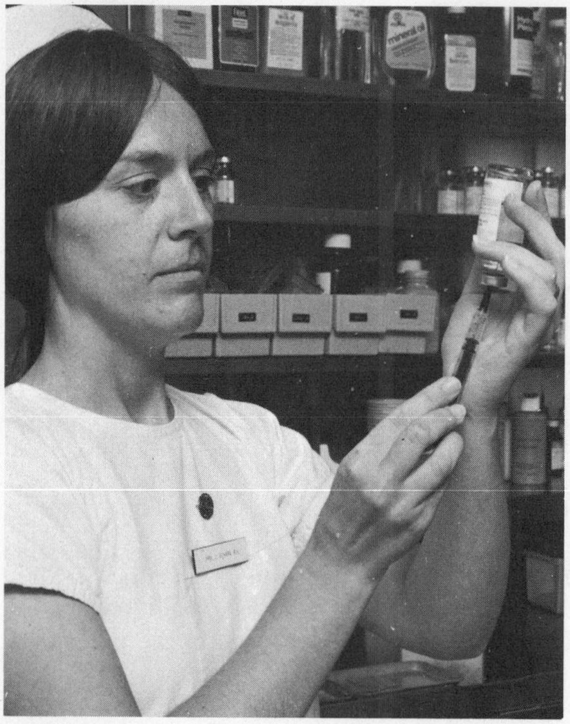

figure 5-1. When the patient has pain, analgesics should be prepared and administered promptly. (Photograph—D. Atkinson)

An example is the patient with pain in a surgical incision *and* back pain from lying in one position for an extended period of time. Noise may also decrease the ability to tolerate pain and in many instances aggravates the pain. It is important to speak softly when talking to a patient (a harsh, shrill, high-pitched voice can be extremely annoying) and perform activities quietly; this may aid in reducing those stimuli that aggravate pain.

While narcotic and non-narcotic analgesics reduce pain during the postoperative period, nursing measures may be used to further reduce discomfort. Support of the incision while the patient is coughing and deep breathing takes the strain off the incision and reduces the pulling or tearing sensation often felt during these movements. The patient should be shown how to use a pillow for support and encouraged to use the pillow when coughing. Chest tubes, urethral catheters, and suprapubic tubes may also be used and these should be checked for excessive tension; tubes should normally have some slack. In addition, uncomfortable positions, rigid restraint of the arms during administration of intravenous fluids, wrinkles or lumps in the bedding, drafts, and so on add discomfort. Extra effort and ingenuity go a long way toward relieving these problems.

Those with constant or severe pain for a long period may need to talk about their pain. Sometimes just talking will help ease some of the emotional impact of the experience. Nurses may feel that unless they are actively doing something, they are not helping patients. This is not so. Listening is an art, and being an attentive and interested listener can sometimes be as valuable as medications and treatment. Note also that *no one task* stands alone as the accepted method in the management of pain.

The effects of pain

Sudden severe pain can cause shock; if the patient is already in shock, pain can deepen the condition. It is obvious, then, that severe pain must be relieved as soon as possible. Such pain can also increase restlessness, which may be undesirable in patients with severe injuries or cardiac problems. Another conse-

Table 5-2.
Nursing management of the patient with pain

Administer analgesics promptly. Note whether the medication relieves pain.
Create a position of comfort for the patient.
Provide distraction or diversion: television, radio, the companionship of other patients.
If the pain is caused by pressure on one or more parts of the body, attempt to relieve the pressure. Change the patient's position frequently.
Reduce or eliminate noise and disturbances.
Be gentle in giving care.
Reduce as much as possible excessive and unnecessary activities during morning care, turning, feeding, changing bed linen, and so on.
Ice (chips, collar, packs) can relieve certain types of pain. A physician's order for them is usually needed.
Moist heat may relieve muscle pain and stiffness. It usually requires a physician's order.
Surgical patients need support for the incision when they are coughing, turning, and doing deep-breathing exercises.

quence of prolonged pain is loss of appetite, which can also be serious. The patient needs a nutritional, well-balanced diet as diet is often an important part of treatment. In addition, administration of narcotic analgesics to relieve pain can decrease the appetite. It may be necessary for the nurse and the dietician to discuss this problem with the patient, choosing his favorite foods. Small servings and between-meal feedings may be needed to supply an adequate and nutritional diet. Pain affects the mind as well as the body. Constant pain wears down the ability to tolerate any pain or discomfort. This in turn can have a variety of effects, both mental and physical. The need for analgesics may increase, the patient may become exhausted, or depression may occur.

Surgical measures for the relief of pain

There are times when pain cannot be controlled by analgesic medications and good nursing management. When this occurs it is termed *intractable pain* and the surgeon may decide to perform a neurosurgical procedure to provide relief. Neurosurgical procedures for the relief of pain are:

- *posterior rhizotomy*—a sectioning of the posterior nerve root just before it enters the spinal cord. Posterior spinal nerves are sensory, thus sectioning prevents sensory impulses from entering the spinal cord and going up to the brain. This results in a *permanent* loss of sensation in the area supplied by the nerve sectioned. More than one nerve may be sectioned to produce the desired results. Some patients, especially the terminally ill, may be unable to tolerate this major surgery. A chemical rhizotomy (using chemicals to destroy the nerve) is an alternative and often gives the same result.
- *cordotomy*—an interruption of pain pathways in the spinal cord. Like a rhizotomy, this is major surgery. Sensory nerve tracts in the spinal column are destroyed, thus preventing sensory nerve impulses from going to the brain. Loss of sensation in this case is also permanent.
- *percutaneous cervical cordotomy*—basically the same as a cordotomy, carrying less surgical risk and often better tolerated by the terminally ill. Using x-ray as a guide, a needle is inserted through the skin (percutaneous) in the area of the neck (cervical) near the mastoid bone. Pain pathways are interrupted by movement of the needle. This procedure is performed under local anesthesia.

Nursing management

A laminectomy must first be performed on the patient who has a rhizotomy or cordotomy. This procedure is necessary in order to expose the operative area. Care during the postoperative period is standard for any laminectomy (see Chapter 17). Initially, the patient is likely to complain of pain in the operative site; he may state that there is no relief from the pain for which the surgery was performed. He should be assured that it takes several days before relief is noted. In reality, the patient has no sensation of pain in the areas supplied by the sectioned spinal nerves or spinal tracts. Possibly, the brain has "learned" that this is a painful area, and the sensation of pain may remain for several days or longer, even though there are no sensory impulses reaching the brain. Other patients may notice relief almost immediately.

Nursing observations include checking for sensory and motor integrity. The physician may request sensory evaluation by use of a (sterile) pin. The area is pricked by the pin; the patient is then asked if he feels anything and the type of sensation is noted. The nurse's fingertip should be used several times, instead of the pin, to confirm the validity of the patient's response. The patient should be asked to move all four extremities (motor loss is abnormal) as a check for motor ability. Any change in motor ability must be reported at once. The bed is usually kept flat and the patient log-rolled every 2 hours.

Discharge teaching

Since sensation is lost in those areas supplied by the sectioned nerves, the patient and his family must be cautioned against the use of excessive heat or cold on these tissues. Precautions include the use of heating pads, ice, and exposure to the sun. The area should be inspected daily for injury; the patient would not be able to feel it if an injury occurred.

Other measures to relieve pain

Investigation is constantly being directed toward finding alternative methods of relieving pain. Electrical stimulation is currently being used to treat some forms of chronic pain. Three methods may be employed: (1) the transcutaneous method, (2) the percutaneous method, and (3) the dorsal column stimulator. The transcutaneous method uses electricity, delivered by electrodes placed on the skin. In the percutaneous method, a wire is inserted into or near a major nerve. The dorsal column stimulator (DCS) requires surgical implantation of an electrode over the dorsal column of the spinal cord. All these methods use electrical current provided by a portable battery. Studies show that the use of a mild electrical current relieves pain, enabling some patients to decrease their need for analgesics.

Acupuncture, although not accepted by all medical personnel, has provided relief for some patients. Needles are inserted at selected sites and twirled, or vibrated, by means of an electrical current. How acupuncture works is not completely understood.

Meditation techniques, such as yoga and transcendental meditation, are being used to control certain types of pain. Meditation should only be attempted with medical approval and should not be used to replace conventional medical treatment. Successes attributed to meditation apparently depend on the individual's ability to use the proper technique in meditating. Meditation should be learned from reliable teachers.

General nutritional considerations

- Efforts should be made to determine which foods the patient in pain particularly likes and can tolerate.
- Painful procedures should be timed so that the patient is at maximum comfort at mealtime.
- Small servings and between-meal feedings may be particularly helpful.

General pharmacological considerations

- Administering medication before pain reaches maximum intensity will be more effective.
- Time pain-relieving medication so as to permit maximum patient cooperation in care such as turning, walking, and coughing.
- Observe the patient for untoward side effects, especially depressed respirations.

Bibliography

Brunner, L. and Suddarth, D. S.: *The Lippincott Manual of Nursing Practice.* Philadelphia, Lippincott, 1974.

Carini, E. and Owens, G.: *Neurological and Neurosurgical Nursing.* St. Louis, Mosby, 1973.

Copp, L. A.: The Spectrum of Suffering. Am. J. Nurs. 74:491, March, 1974.

Drakontides, A. B.: Drugs used to treat pain. Am. J. Nurs. 74:508, March, 1974.

Gaumer, W. R.: Electrical stimulation in chronic pain. Am. J. Nurs. 74:504, March, 1974.

Goloskov, J. and Leroy, P.: Use of the dorsal column stimulator. Am. J. Nurs. 74:506, March, 1974.

Isler, C.; New approach to intractable pain. RN 75:17, January, 1975.

Johnson, J. E. and Rice, V. H.: Sensory and distress components of pain. Nurs. Res. 23:203, May-June, 1974.

LeMaitre, G. and Finnegan, J.: *The Patient in Surgery: A Guide for Nurses.* Philadelphia, Saunders, 1975.

Mastrovito, R. C.: Psychogenic pain. Am. J. Nurs. 74:514, March, 1974.

McCaffery, M.: *Nursing Management of the Patient with Pain.* Philadelphia, Lippincott, 1972.

———: Intelligent approach to intractable pain. Nurs. '73, 3:26, November, 1973.

McLachlan, E.: Recognizing pain. Am. J. Nurs. 74:496, March, 1974.

Rodman, M. J. and Smith, D. W.: *Clinical Pharmacology in Nursing.* Philadelphia, Lippincott, 1974.

Scherer, J. C.: *Introductory Clinical Pharmacology.* Philadelphia, Lippincott, 1975.

Siegle, D. S.: The gate control theory. Am. J. Nurs. 74:498, March, 1974.

CHAPTER—6

Dependence on and abuse of alcohol, drugs, and tobacco

On completion of this chapter the student will:

- **Define commonly used terms associated with drug use and abuse.**
- **Describe some of the common methods of treating drug dependence.**
- **Describe methods of drug rehabilitation.**
- **Discuss some of the sociological effects of drug abuse.**
- **List some of the common signs of drug withdrawal.**
- **Discuss some of the harmful physical effects of drug abuse.**

Repeated consumption of some drugs leads to dependence—a complex interaction between physical craving and psychological longing. Most habit-forming drugs are harmful when taken in excess over long periods of time. They can compel enslavement that overrules the better judgment of the user, and they may ruin his health.

In 1957 the World Health Organization Expert Committee on Addiction-Producing Drugs defined drug addiction and drug habituation:

DRUG ADDICTION

Drug addiction is a state of periodic or chronic intoxication produced by the repeated consumption of a drug (natural or synthetic). Its characteristics include:

1. An overpowering desire or need (compulsion) to continue taking the drug and to obtain it by any means;
2. A tendency to increase the dose;
3. A psychic (psychological) and generally a physical dependence on the effects of the drug;
4. Detrimental effect on the individual and on society.

DRUG HABITUATION

Drug habituation (habit) is a condition resulting from the repeated consumption of a drug. Its characteristics include:

1. A desire (but not a compulsion) to continue taking the drug for the sense of improved well-being which it engenders;
2. Little or no tendency to increase the dose;
3. Some degree of psychic dependence on the effect of the drug, but absence of physical dependence and hence of an abstinence syndrome;
4. Detrimental effect, if any, primarily on the individual.

When the topic of drug dependence is discussed, there is a tendency to think first of narcotics. Alcohol frequently is not regarded as a drug but as a beverage. However, alcohol has potent pharmacological effects, and dependence on alcohol is common. Dependence on smoking is in still a different category. Recent emphasis on the harmful effects of smoking has led many smokers to try to stop the habit. Many have found the process difficult; some have found it impossible. The report of the Advisory Committee to the Surgeon General of the United States Public Health Service states that "habituation" is the correct term to apply to cigarette smoking.

Characteristics of dependence

In varying degrees, according to the agent and the individual, dependence on alcohol and drugs includes a strong need to continue taking the agent, ambivalence toward it, and withdrawal symptoms when it is withheld.

ONSET OF DEPENDENCE. Drug dependence takes time to develop. The length of time varies with the drug or drugs used and the individual using the drug. There is no clear-cut point at which the person who drinks changes from a social drinker to an alcoholic who can no longer control his drinking, or heroin will become more important to the drug user than family or job. By the time the person realizes that he is dependent, he has changed. He has lost control over the habit before he knows that he has. It may take ten years for alcoholism to develop fully, and several more years before it is identified as a problem by the patient. However, dependence on narcotics may occur within a few weeks.

TOLERANCE. Tolerance buildup is a major problem in drug dependence. When tolerance develops, the dose that was previously effective no longer gives relief, and an increased dose is necessary to obtain the original effect. For example, as the dependence progresses, the alcoholic can indulge in heavy drinking without getting drunk, and the person dependent on drugs requires higher and higher doses. Although tolerance to these substances can increase, it is limited, and can be exceeded, in which case, poisoning results.

WITHDRAWAL SYMPTOMS. If a strong psychological and physiological dependence on the substance is established, the patient suffers psychological and physical symptoms when the drug is abruptly discontinued.

Incidence and economics

Dependence on alcohol and drugs is a persistent social problem. Of particular concern is the incidence of drug abuse among the very young. There appears to be an increase in the use of alcohol among teenagers and young adults, with some becoming alcoholics before their twenty-first birthday.

Drug dependence is a major health and economic problem. Alcoholism is responsible for loss of time from work and for inefficiency at work, and it is unusual for the person dependent on narcotics to be able to work in a regular job. In addition, the care of both types of patients in general and mental hospitals and penal institutions is costly to the community.

Drug dependence is as expensive to the individual as to society. The person dependent on illegal drugs is placed in an impossible financial position. He depends on the pushers who sell them, and has no recourse if the price is exorbitant, if he does not have the money, or if the drug he buys is diluted. Many soon find themselves without funds, and turn to theft, prostitution, and other illegal activities to support their drug habit. The alcoholic often misses work and may ultimately lose his job because of excessive absenteeism and/or poor work performance.

Treatment

Treatment comprises two phases. Initially, it is aimed at alleviating the physical symptoms caused by withdrawal of the drug and giving psychological aid to help overcome the acute sense of loss that the patient suffers. Even after physiological adjustments have been made to reduce physical craving, the psychological craving remains and requires continued, long-term consideration. Treatment and nursing care that ignore the long-term rehabilitative aspects of a therapeutic program are doomed to fail. Unless the patient solves some of the underlying emotional and social problems which led to dependence, there is great likelihood that he will relapse after the first phase of treatment.

Overcoming physical dependence on drugs is sometimes the beginning, but it is never the end of the patient's struggle to overcome his drug dependence. He may be offered individual or group psychotherapy, community-based follow-up clinics, or he may join special groups such as Alcoholics Anonymous (AA).

Facilities for treatment of the person dependent on narcotics are not as widespread as those for the alcoholic, but are increasing as more attention is being paid to these health problems. Sometimes community resources exist, but the patient is unaware of them. Helping patients to find facilities as well as helping communities to develop them are a part of creative nursing that can make the difference between health and disease.

Alcoholism

Many efforts have been made to differentiate excessive drinking and alcoholism, but as yet there are no wholly-agreed-on criteria.

Etiology

There may be a physiological as well as a psychological basis for alcoholism. Although there is no agreement among authorities on alcoholism, it would seem that many theories, whether physiological, psychological, or socioeconomic may have some merit.

Personal problems often lead to excessive drinking as drinking is one way to relieve anxiety and escape from problems that seem insurmountable. Alcohol is commonly used as a means of expressing hostility. Frequently, the rage and the frustration are turned inward on the alcoholic himself. Self-destructive tendencies are common. Often alcoholics feel such hopelessness that they see little point in taking ordinary measures to protect themselves against illness, exposure, and accidents. The high incidence of pneumonia and tuberculosis among alcoholics is related closely to personal neglect. Suicide is a particular problem among alcoholics. It has been stated that low self-esteem and conflicts over dependence are important factors in the causation of alcoholism.

Incidence

Only a small percentage of alcoholics live in the skid-row sections of our cities; they come from all occupational and social groups—rich or poor, executives or laborers—and they are scattered throughout the community from elementary schools to homes for the elderly.

Despite the manifold problems associated with alcoholism, many alcoholics have an amazing ability to maintain themselves in the community. They manage to continue to work and, sometimes, to conceal their disability from all but their families and closest friends. Often the condition continues with varying degrees of severity for a large part of the individual's life.

Women as well as men become alcoholics, although they are less well accepted than are men alcoholics. However, because women tend to confine their drinking to their own homes, sometimes the mistaken assumption is formed that alcoholism is largely a man's disease. Although the effects of a woman's drinking are less noted in public places, the effect of a woman alcoholic on her family is devastating.

Because many alcoholics try to hide their condition, it is especially important to show sensitivity when dealing with them. Illness and accidents associated with drinking are occasions when alcoholism comes to the attention of nurses and physicians, and are opportunities for the patient to acknowledge his problem and to seek help. Unfortunately, the alcoholic is often rebuffed by health professionals, and the opportunity to assist the patient to acknowledge and deal with his drinking is lost.

Physiology

Alcohol is absorbed directly from the stomach and small intestine into the bloodstream, without digestion. The rate of absorption of alcohol is slowed by the presence of food in the stomach. When alcohol is taken on an empty stomach, its effects are felt quickly, and reach a peak in about 20 minutes.

Alcohol is a central nervous system depressant. The highest intellectual functions, such as judgment, are the first to be impaired, and the vital physiological functions such as breathing, which are under control of the brain stem, are the last to be affected. Thus, the inebriated individual may lose his life due to an error in judgment while driving, although the same level of alcohol intoxication would not jeopardize his vital physiological functions such as respiration.

Alcohol is not a stimulant, although many people regard it as such because an inebriated person may feel or act stimulated due to lessening of inhibitions.

The effects of alcohol on the central nervous system are related to the levels of alcohol in the blood and brain tissue. When alcohol enters the capillaries it diffuses into all body tissues. The tissues which have the best blood supply have a particularly rapid accumulation of alcohol. For example, the level of alcohol concentration in the brain quickly comes into balance with that of the blood. Later, alcohol is taken up by tissues with lesser blood supply, thus drawing some alcohol away from the brain. However, the most important factor in reducing brain levels of alcohol is oxidation of alcohol by the patient's body.

Between 90 to 95 percent of alcohol is metabolized to carbon dioxide and water. Most of the rest is excreted unchanged in the breath and urine. The first steps in metabolic breakdown of alcohol occur in the liver. Later, metabolism of alcohol occurs in all cells of the body, where the acetate derived from alcohol is fed into the cellular system for obtaining energy from food.

Energy is produced in the process of oxidation of alcohol to carbon dioxide and water, and in this sense alcohol is a food. Alcohol produces 7 calories for every gram oxidized. However, alcohol does not contain essential nutrients such as vitamins and amino acids. Therefore, although the individual who uses alcohol as a significant source of calories may maintain or even gain weight, he frequently suffers malnutrition because he relies substantially on alcohol, rather than on nutritive foods, for his caloric intake. The prevalence of malnutrition among alcoholics is believed to be a factor in causing cirrhosis of the liver. However, there is also evidence that prolonged excessive consumption of alcohol has, in itself, adverse effects upon the liver and leads to fibrosis and to fatty infiltration which gradually impair the functioning of the liver.

Alcohol also affects other parts of the body. It can irritate the mucosa of the mouth, the throat, and the stomach leading to hoarseness and gastritis.

Symptoms

Drinking patterns vary widely. Some alcoholics maintain themselves most of the time in a state of intoxication that dulls their reactions to personal problems, interferes with judgment and human relationships, but permits them to perform some routine tasks. Others alternate periods of sobriety with drinking sprees, when they continue drinking until they are unconscious. The alcoholic may stick to one drinking pattern, or he may vary the pattern at different periods of his life; no one pattern invariably characterizes his behavior. However, the alcoholic often feels the need to drink regularly during the day, and often drinks alone. Others who are developing the condition drink heavily in the evening but abstain during the workday. Later the individual usually finds that he must also drink during working hours.

Usually the alcoholic does not talk about drinking, although he may say that he is not feeling well. He often becomes terrified of his condition, but is afraid to admit to others (or even to himself) that anything is wrong.

Hangovers increase in severity; nausea, vomiting, weakness and headache are the typical symptoms. The patient misses work more and more frequently, and he has blackouts (amnesia). He sneaks drinks and gulps them as fast as he can.

The patient's disease has serious repercussions in the rest of his life. His employer notices increased absence from work and lessened efficiency when the patient is at work. Most of Monday may be spent at the water cooler or in the rest room while the alcoholic tries to pull himself together.

The alcoholic tells himself that he can stop drinking any time he wants to. This statement is true. He can and does stop drinking—sometimes for months. He stops long enough to convince himself that he can stop; but he goes back to it, sure that he has the problem under control. His ability to have lapses in his drinking proves to him that he is not dependent. Unfortunately, the "proof" is not true; he *is* dependent on alcohol.

Often the alcoholic becomes so overwhelmed with guilt over the effects of his drinking on both himself and his family that he drinks increasingly, thus establishing a vicious circle.

Some alcoholics may have brief episodes of a mental disorder called *delirium tremens* or the DT's. The onset of delirium tremens is sudden, although before it an alcoholic is often restless, anxious, and sleepless. DT's are especially likely to occur when the individual cannot maintain his usual high alcohol intake. Gastrointestinal disturbance, hospitalization, or imprisonment are examples of circumstances which may precipitate delirium tremens because the person is temporarily unable to drink alcoholic beverages. The alcoholic admitted to the hospital for reasons other than alcoholism usually tries to hide the drinking problem. Some may try to bring a supply of alcohol with them. Others, such as the acute surgical patient, will of necessity be deprived of oral fluids—including alcohol. Such patients usually develop signs of DT's in two to three days.

Characteristics of DT's are hallucinations and tremors that may shake the whole body. The patient sees—and less frequently hears—things that are not there. Most commonly he sees fast-moving animals of grotesque shapes and colors. Some patients see small people running over the floor or climbing on the chair. Restless, violent, unceasing activity that may take the form of running from the animals accompanies DT's. The activity is so great that it may lead to death from heart failure or exhaustion, especially if the patient is malnourished.

The patient experiencing DT's is in the throes of extreme anxiety. He knows who he is, but he may misidentify other people or identify objects incorrectly. He may understand that he is having hallucinations, but this realization does not make the animals go away. He perspires, and therefore dehydration and electrolyte imbalance are further increased. Respiration, pulse, blood pressure, and, often, temperature are elevated. If DT's come when the body has an added strain, such as pneumonia, the body's resistance to alcohol poisoning is decreased.

Effects on the family

Alcoholism has widespread and often long-range effects on the family. Although the problems differ, the general effects are loss of income if the alcoholic is the wage-earner, tension between the alcoholic and the spouse, separation or divorce, strained relationships with the children, and social stigma.

Because alcoholism is socially unacceptable, the family usually makes every effort to conceal the problem from others. They are thus cut off from the kind of help and support they might receive if the condition were more acceptable.

Problems in family relationships are often compounded by the way in which alcohol affects the alcoholic's behavior. For example, his gross neglect of the usual standards of dress and of personal cleanliness and his angry outbursts during intoxication tend to lower the alcoholic's self-esteem as well as the esteem of others.

Perhaps the most difficult aspect of all for the family is the fact that the alcoholic cannot be treated successfully until *he* seeks treatment. The family may find many community resources for treatment, but they are useless to the alcoholic unless he himself decides to use them. One of the commonest errors of the family is to attempt to arrange for treatment when the alcoholic does not accept it. Success in treatment of alcoholism rests on the alcoholic's desire for help, not on his family's wish (or desperate need) that he be helped.

Often the alcoholic does not seek help until he has hit bottom—perhaps he has lost his job and alienated his family. Experiences like waking up in a jail or a hospital with no recollection of how he got there may shock the person into being able to admit the need for help and into beginning to seek it.

Treatment

The patient brought to the hospital with acute alcoholic poisoning is highly agitated, and may have or will soon develop DT's. Blustering, noisy behavior may be part of a defense against feelings of utter helplessness and fear. The nurse must protect the patient from injury. If he perceives that he is being chased by animals, he may run, and an open window may look like a welcome escape from his pursuers. Physical restraints are avoided whenever possible, because they often aggravate the condition by making the patient feel fettered and more helpless. Closing and locking the window and placing side rails on the bed are examples of measures that can help to protect the patient. The presence of a nurse or a nursing assistant who is calm, firm, and watchful helps to protect the patient from injury as well as lessening extreme agitation.

Drug therapy for acute alcohol poisoning includes:

- Vitamins, especially the vitamin B group. Alcoholics usually suffer from vitamin deficiency; vitamin B deficiency may be so severe that the patient develops pellagra.
- Paraldehyde, which may be used as sedation during periods of acute agitation.
- Tranquilizers, which are widely used to lessen the patient's restlessness and agitation.

Phenothiazine-type tranquilizers must be administered cautiously because they potentiate the depressant and hypotensive effects of alcohol. Tranquilizers may be used to control withdrawal symptoms, such as nervousness and tremulousness, when the patient is being helped to abstain from alcohol. Continued use of these drugs presents hazards as alcoholics are likely to become dependent on tranquilizers and sedatives, such as phenobarbital. Medical supervision of drug therapy is essential for alcoholics, who readily transfer their dependence on alcohol to other agents.

Intravenous fluids and electrolytes may be given until anorexia, nausea, and vomiting are controlled sufficiently to permit an adequate intake of oral fluids. Encouragement of a nutritious diet is essential as soon as the patient is able to tolerate oral fluids and food.

After the acute phase has passed, the patient requires long-term treatment. Disulfiram (Antabuse) is a drug sometimes used as an adjunct to other kinds of therapy for chronic alcoholism. The drug causes no apparent effects when given alone, but the ingestion of even small amounts of alcohol by a patient taking disulfiram causes severe nausea, vomiting, and diarrhea. Hypotension, which may become severe, may also accompany gastrointestinal symptoms. The patient must consent to the use of disulfiram and be fully aware of the symptoms he will experience if he takes a drink.

The alcoholic is particularly perceptive of the attitudes of others toward him. Because of unfortunate past experience, he often expects to be treated with scorn and condescension, and he may be ready to defend himself in a demanding, restless manner. Such behavior may be a cover for feelings of helplessness, anxiety, and self-loathing. By kindness, patience, and tact the nurse can show him that she considers him a worthwhile individual. By her actions and words she can convey to him that she regards him as a sick person who needs treatment, that her relationship with him is based on helping him toward recovery, and that she believes recovery is possible. The nurse should try not to lecture the patient about anything, even Alcoholics Anonymous. Instead, she should emphasize acceptance of him as he is and give him opportunities to talk about his situation and his feelings. The nurse should let the patient say what he wishes, but avoid prying and giving advice. It is not likely that she can give him advice that he has not heard already many times.

Rehabilitation

Some hospitals have carefully planned programs of follow-up care for their alcoholic patients. The patients may come back to the hospital one evening a week for group discussions shared with other alcoholics. The hospital dietitian may lead a discussion on planning an adequate diet, and a member of Alcoholics Anonymous may talk with the group about the work of that organization. Others who may be invited to participate in this type of discussion are physicians, clergymen, nurses, and social workers.

Psychotherapy may help the patient to gain greater insight into the emotional problems that have led to dependence on alcohol. Psychotherapy may be carried out individually or in groups.

Alcoholics Anonymous (AA) is an organization composed of and run by alcoholics who by helping each other find that they themselves have been helped. The organization has been notably successful. Often it has helped people who have failed to be helped by other means.

The philosophy of AA is disarmingly simple. It is expressed in a prayer its members use, "God grant me the serenity to accept the things I cannot change, courage to change the things I can, and the wisdom to know the difference."

Abuse of other drugs, such as amphetamines, LSD, marihuana

Drug abuse and dependence are problems of vastly increasing importance, because of the effects of these substances on the individual and society. The problem of drug use is highly charged emotionally, making it especially necessary for nurses and other health professionals to be aware of their own emotional reactions to drug use, and to try to avoid having their personal views interfere with ability to work with patients who have this problem.

Some characteristics of drug users and abusers

There appears to be no one reason why an individual uses drugs. Different kinds of people use drugs for different reasons; thus, there is no stereotype of "the drug addict." It is essential to consider the differences among drugs (there is considerable difference between occasionally smoking marihuana and becoming dependent on heroin) as well as among drug users, with regard to personality, motivation to use drugs, and patterns of drug use.

Low self-esteem may be a personality characteristic in some who misuse and become dependent on drugs. The drug experience temporarily conveys a feeling of competence, power, and excitement which increases the individual's sense of worth while he is experiencing the effect of the drug. Drugs are also a way of withdrawing from problems, of making problems seem insignificant, and, therefore, not worth solving. Persons who use drugs often do so as a form of protest and an expression of anger against others. Drug use may also be a form of escape, a substitute for affection, or a search for meaning or values. The individual may or may not know why he uses drugs.

Although drug use occurs in all age groups, it is particularly prevalent among young people. The drug experience may be a way of life, a way of relieving loneliness, or a way of belonging to a group. Often, a person will begin to use drugs because of curiosity or peer pressure.

Although it was previously assumed that drug abuse was primarily a problem of persons who are economically, socially, and educationally disadvantaged, it has become clear in recent years that the problem exists, and is sometimes especially common, among the socially, economically, and educationally advantaged. Despite obvious advantages, these young people are sometimes seriously lacking in parental love and concern, and in opportunities for meaningful and satisfying relationships with adults.

Relevance to nursing

As the nurse becomes more involved with the community, the problems of drug abuse increase significantly in nursing practice. The student nurse has a particular stake in this matter. She may experience a feeling of interest in and loyalty to the youth-culture which encourages use of drugs, while at the same time, an identification with and loyalty to a profession which seeks to limit use of potent and hazardous drugs without medical advice, and whose members, regardless of age, tend to be viewed as authorities on matters affecting health.

The consequences of being known as a drug abuser can be very serious for members of the health professions, such as nurses, physicians, and pharmacists, whose work requires a high degree of responsibility in adherence to laws concerning use of drugs. Their work also provides easy access to certain types of drugs commonly used in therapy, such as sedatives, tranquilizers, and narcotics. Thus, the nurse and other health professionals may be faced with the problems of defining personal feelings toward drug abuse and considering the consequences of drug use or abuse upon a future career.

Drugs subject to abuse

Amphetamines. Amphetamines (or "speed") are central nervous system stimulants. They increase the individual's sense of alertness and wakefulness, and they also alter mood. Misuse of amphetamines varies from brief and relatively infrequent use of moderate amounts of these drugs in order to postpone fatigue, to drug abuse by "speed freaks" who take massive doses, seeking extended periods of euphoria and wakefulness until they "crash" or come down off a "high." After using amphetamines to produce an unnatural wakefulness and alertness, the individual often experiences a "let-down" characterized by physical and mental exhaustion.

Serious consequences of amphetamine abuse are exhaustion, marked nervousness, weight loss, and, in some instances, psychosis. Misuse of amphetamines also leads to drug dependence. Death from an overdose of amphetamines may occur in the chronic user, especially when the drug is used intravenously.

LSD (lysergic acid diethylamide) is a drug which produces mental states said to be similar to those observed in some psychoses. For this reason LSD is often called a psychotomimetic drug (a drug which mimics psychosis). The drug causes visual hallucinations and illusions, as well as mood changes. The results are highly variable and individual, from one person to another, and in the same person, when the drug is taken under varying circumstances.

Medical evidence indicates that self-medication with LSD constitutes a serious form of drug abuse, even though the drug is not addictive in the sense that narcotics are. Among the reasons for this belief are:

- LSD has precipitated prolonged psychotic reactions and suicide attempts.
- Persons who are experiencing an LSD "trip" can seriously hurt themselves or kill themselves, because they may believe they are invulnerable to hazards, such as falling from heights, or being struck by cars.
- A sense of extreme terror sometimes occurs as a result of using LSD. This result is variable and unpredictable, and is referred to as a "bad trip."

Marihuana is derived from the cannabis plant, is popularly referred to as "pot," and is usually inhaled by smoking. Considerable controversy exists concerning the harmfulness of marihuana, but it is generally believed to be one of the least harmful of the frequently abused drugs. Its use does not lead to physical dependence and tolerance. The effects of smoking marihuana are variously described as subtly pleasurable changes in mood, perception, and consciousness, a feeling of bodily lightness, and sometimes hallucinations. The use of marihuana does not necessarily lead to experimentation with other more harmful substances.

Barbiturates, Nonbarbiturate Sedative-Hypnotics, and Minor Tranquilizers. These drugs, called "downers" by drug abusers lead to sedation and somnolence. The barbiturates and minor tranquilizers are dangerous when misused by persons who seek to control their nervousness by self-medication with these agents.

Because of the frequency with which sedatives and minor tranquilizers are prescribed to help control anxiety, many persons who misuse these drugs have been introduced to them through a physician's prescription. Particularly dangerous is the use of amphetamines and barbiturates in combination, and combinations of alcohol with barbiturates or with other sedatives, hypnotics, and the minor tranquilizers, such as diazepam (Librium). Because alcohol potentiates the depressant and hypotensive effects of these sedative drugs, this combination can be especially hazardous, and could lead to coma and death.

Use of barbiturates and similar sedatives, hypnotics, and tranquilizers can lead to serious physical dependence and to withdrawal symptoms when the drugs are abruptly discontinued. Withdrawal symptoms are characterized by nervousness, extreme restlessness, and insomnia. Prolonged insomnia and agitation sometimes lead to hallucinations or to a full-blown psychosis. Muscular tremors and even convulsions may also occur. Withdrawal of barbiturates in persons dependent on them must be *undertaken gradually, under close medical supervision.* Physical dependence on minor tranquilizers can also occur. This is manifested by an abstinence syndrome when the tranquilizer is abruptly withdrawn. Its signs and symptoms are similar to those for withdrawal of barbiturate: nervousness, tremors, hallucinations, delirium, and convulsions.

Potent Narcotic Analgesics. Heroin (diacetylmorphine) is a potent and illegal narcotic which produces an intense euphoria or "high." Tolerance and physical dependence occur rapidly, thus making heroin one of the most potentially dangerous of the illegal drugs. Intravenous self-administration of heroin can lead to serious infections such as septicemia and hepatitis. Since the drug is usually administered by this route, many addicts develop either or both of these problems.

The consistent administration of a powerful narcotic can allow pain from another disease to go unrecognized and, therefore, untreated. Whenever an addict requires treatment for any disease, it is essential that physicians and nurses know that he is an addict. Addicts usually require larger doses of premedication and anesthesia for surgery. Because he is engaged in an illegal activity, an addict often will hide the fact that he is addicted; yet this information is important to the anesthesiologist. The observation of constricted pupils, which may mean that the patient is addicted to morphine, would be a most valuable observation to make. Because the addict's technique may not be sterile, he may develop complications like local infections or hepatitis from the use of unsterile syringes and needles.

Signs of drug withdrawal

Withdrawal sickness, a self-limiting but extremely uncomfortable illness, occurs when addicts do not take the narcotic to which they are addicted. The symptoms of withdrawal from narcotics begin to become severe approximately 24 hours after the last dose, and they reach their peak in 36 to 72 hours, after which they taper off. The individual feels sick and becomes apprehensive. His eyes tear, his nose becomes congested, and he usually experiences repeated yawning. In addition, he perspires profusely and feels hot and cold flashes. "Goose bumps" (pilomotor response) are raised on his skin. He may also feel anxious and restless and have an intense craving for the drug. Temperature, blood pressure, and pulse are elevated. Vomiting, diarrhea, anorexia, headache, muscular aching and twitching, and severe abdominal cramps follow. Coma and collapse are possible.

It is important to differentiate between *physical* withdrawal and psychological dependence. Physical withdrawal symptoms are of a few days' duration, but psychological dependence and the craving for the euphoria produced by the drug can last for years, even when the patient is prevented from obtaining the drug during that prolonged period. This emphasizes the need to focus on helping the addict deal with his psychological craving which can, after several months in a hospital, lead him to seek narcotics upon his release.

Treatment

People dependent on heroin and other opiates may be weaned from these drugs with the aid of methadone. This drug is itself addicting, but its use seems justified in some circumstances. When used as an adjunct to the gradual withdrawal of opiates, its main advantage is that it keeps the patient comfortable without producing a euphoric "high." Eventually, when dosage of the opiate has been gradually reduced and finally eliminated, the physician must also withdraw the methadone. Fortunately, this is usually accomplished with only relatively mild discomfort, as physical dependence on this drug is not as powerful as dependence upon heroin.

Methadone has been used in still another way to aid in the long-term rehabilitation of narcotic addicts. In this so-called methadone maintenance therapy, methadone is not withdrawn, but is instead administered for a prolonged period of time. It is claimed that patients taking methadone are unable to experience the characteristic euphoria produced by heroin. Similarly, patients taking methadone in doses that reduce or eliminate the craving for heroin are able to carry on activities requiring mental alertness and motor coordination. Thus, former heroin addicts can hold jobs, go to school, and perform the activities expected of them.

As a result of reports of successful rehabilitation programs based upon the adjunctive use of methadone, clinics have been set up in some large cities where addicts are treated with a combination of methadone, counseling, and assistance with finding and keeping jobs and homes.

When methadone is used to aid in withdrawal of opiates, symptoms of lassitude, nausea, vomiting, dizziness, sweating, anorexia, and insomnia still may occur and last for weeks, but the most acute symptoms of withdrawal illness are largely avoided.

Psychotherapy is an important aspect of treatment. Treatment involves not only breaking the pattern of addiction to a narcotic, but, even more difficult, treatment of the underlying personality disorder and dealing with the complex web of social problems that accompany the addiction.

Other methods of treatment include the use of narcotic antagonists such as naloxone (Narcone) and group therapies much like Alcoholics Anonymous.

Prevention

Dependence on drugs by a person with severe, long-term pain is a tragedy. Use of narcotics to relieve the pain of such conditions as arthritis and peripheral vascular disease usually is avoided for this reason. Some patients, for example, those who require relief from severe pain due to terminal cancer, cannot obtain relief by any other therapy. If dependence on narcotics occurs in these instances, it is viewed as an unavoidable complication during treatment of an acutely painful terminal illness. In most hospitals, narcotics must be reordered by the physician at frequent intervals (e.g., every 48 hours), thus bringing to the attention of the physician the question of whether the patient should continue to receive the drug. If the nurse observes that a patient seems to be relying on narcotics, she should consult the physician. Above all, she should never use narcotics ordered by the physician for the relief of pain merely to quiet a patient who is making difficult demands on the staff. Instead, she should consider the reason for the patient's behavior, and in consultation with the physician develop a plan for dealing with the patient's discomfort. Any person who regularly receives narcotics for whatever reason can become dependent. Dependence is *not* limited, as is commonly supposed, to those who are socially and educationally disadvantaged.

Physicians, nurses and pharmacists have a special responsibility in prevention and early detection of drug dependence, because they are the ones who handle narcotics as part of their work. Destroying disposable syringes and needles before discarding them to prevent their possible use later by addicts is an example of something nurses can do to help to combat the problem. Keeping the medicine closet locked is another. Those whose work involves handling narcotics are especially vulnerable to dependence. Honest recognition of this possibility has helped many professional people to avoid the pitfall of taking unprescribed drugs with the idea that it will be all right "just this once."

Smoking

Any discussion of habituation and dependence syndromes would be incomplete without attention to the problem of habituated tobacco smokers. It has become increasingly apparent that the undesirable effects of smoking constitute a real health hazard to the large segment of the population who are heavy smokers. Consequently, the problem of tobacco habituation is a rightful concern for all health professionals.

Lung cancer

There is an increased risk of developing lung cancer related to the number of cigarettes smoked per day and the duration of smoking. Pipe and cigar smokers, who usually do not inhale, develop cancer of the lung more frequently than nonsmokers, but less frequently than cigarette smokers. Pipe smokers are especially prone to cancer of the mouth.

Physical effects of tobacco

Cigarette smoking causes breathlessness, both at rest and on exertion, decreased pulmonary function, and a chronic productive cough. Paralysis of the cilia caused by smoking prevents the clearing away of foreign particles, such as those found in tobacco smoke, which are then deposited on the epithelium. In addition, pathology seen in chronic bronchitis can be caused by smoking. Smoking has not been as clearly identified as a cause of emphysema, but the rupture of alveolar septa and the fibrosis caused by smoking seem to be related to this disease. And, it is known that the death rate from emphysema, like that from bronchitis, is higher in the smoker than in the nonsmoker. The symptoms of bronchitis and emphysema tend to be progressive, especially in smokers, and may result in respiratory crippling to the extent that the patient is unable to work or even to walk because he cannot breathe adequately.

Effects of Withdrawal. When a smoker stops smoking, he may experience such physical symptoms as constipation, irritability, a slowing of the pulse, hunger, and weight gain. Some individuals will experience a variety of symptoms; others few or none. The craving may be so urgent that the person engages in some remarkable mental gymnastics as to why he should have a cigarette immediately. As a result, he often takes one in spite of his resolve not to do so. This process is hard to believe unless one experiences it. Although the craving may disappear after a few days or months, it may persist for years.

Decreasing the number of cigarettes smoked a day may be the most satisfactory solution for some people. However, many soon find themselves smoking the same number of cigarettes as before. The longing is kept alive.

Some people report that they feel wonderful after giving up smoking; there is no morning cough, food tastes better, they have more energy, and there is the thrill of accomplishing a difficult task. Others find the depression, irritability and craving not worth the compensations.

Assisting the Patient. The attitudes of those in contact with the person who is attempting to become an ex-smoker are of prime importance. Although the nurse may be in a position to inform the patient about the dangers of smoking, fear techniques and preaching are known to fail. Authoritatively telling people to stop smoking because cigarettes are harmful may be like daring them to continue. Such an approach may instill fear but not change the habit.

The nurse may be asked to give suggestions on how to stop smoking. There is no method that will help all individuals, but antismoking clinics and hypnosis have helped some. Others find serious reasons for stopping and will do so themselves by either stopping suddenly or by slowly decreasing the number of cigarettes smoked per day.

With all patients the nurse's approach should be supportive. She should be especially careful not to push the person who reacts to stopping smoking with increased anxiety. Instead, she should encourage the patient to seek further help, and assist him to do so, if he wishes, by providing him with names of resources where individual and group counseling are available. In this way the patient can receive expert assistance with personal problems which may be affecting not only his problem with smoking, but other aspects of his life as well.

General nutritional considerations

- The alcoholic patient may have a vitamin and nutritional deficiency and a well-balanced diet is usually ordered.
- The nurse should encourage the alcoholic patient to eat. Small and frequent feedings may be better tolerated than three regular meals.
- Patients going through medically supervised drug withdrawal may require additional dietary supplements and between-meal feedings.
- The meal trays of the alcoholic or drug dependent patient should be checked after each meal as these patients have a tendency to eat poorly. Any evidence of reduced dietary intake should be reported to the physician.

General pharmacological considerations

- It is essential that the alcoholic patient receive vitamin therapy.
- Paraldehyde, which may be used as sedation during periods of acute agitation, may be given orally, either undiluted or diluted in juice, or by the intramuscular route.
- Because of postural hypotension, alcoholics receiving phenothiazine-type drugs, for example chlorpromazine (Thorazine), should be warned against rising rapidly from a lying or sitting position.

- Disulfiram (Antabuse) may be given to the alcoholic as part of a rehabilitation program. The patient should be fully aware of the symptoms he will experience if he drinks alcohol while taking the drug (i.e., severe nausea, vomiting, and diarrhea).
- Patients receiving tranquilizers or barbiturates should be warned about the use of alcohol while taking these drugs. The combination of alcohol and tranquilizers or barbiturates can be hazardous and could lead to coma and death.
- Patients receiving *methadone* as part of a narcotics rehabilitation program should have this noted on the front of their chart and on the patient Kardex. Being a narcotic, methadone can potentiate the action of certain drugs —most notably narcotics, tranquilizers, barbiturates, and anesthetics.
- Patients receiving methadone will usually require lower doses of drugs such as tranquilizers, barbiturates, and so on when it is necessary to administer these agents.

Bibliography

Boyson, M. A.: Helping the alcoholic cope with sobriety. RN 75:37, July, 1975.

Dever, Sister M. Charles et al: Methadone maintenance treatment at Sisters of Charity. Buffalo, New York. Hosp. Prog. 55:32, February, 1974.

Elaine, B. et al: Helping the nurse who misuses drugs. Am. J. Nurs. 74:1665, September, 1974.

Funston, F. D.: Detoxification: An alternative in transition. Canad. Nurs. 69:27, November, 1973.

Gay, G.: Treatment of acute drug reactions and overdose in a free clinic. Nurs. Dig. 3:32, November-December, 1975.

Guthrie, H. A.: *Introductory Nutrition,* ed. 3. St. Louis, Mosby, 1975.

Krepick, D. S. et al: Heroin addiction: A treatable disease, Nurs. Clin. North Am. 8:41, May, 1973.

Lewis, L. W.: The hidden alcoholic: A nursing dilemma. Nurs. '75, 5:20, July, 1975.

Mitchell, H. S. et al: *Nutrition in Health and Disease,* ed. 16. Philadelphia, Lippincott, 1976.

Morgan, A. J. and Moreno, J.: *The Practice of Mental Health Nursing.* Philadelphia, Lippincott, 1973.

———: Attitudes toward addiction. Am. J. Nurs. 73:497, March, 1973.

Mueller, J. F.: Treatment for the alcoholic: Cursing or nursing? Am. J. Nurs. 74:245, February, 1974.

Newman, R. G.: Methadone maintenance treatment. J. Prac. Nurs. 24:22, October, 1974.

Odom, C.: The enigma of drug abuse. J. Prac. Nurs. 24:19, September, 1974.

Pillari, G. and Naries, J.: Physical effects of heroin addiction. Am. J. Nurs. 73:2105, December, 1973.

Ray, O. and Leith, N. J.: *Drugs, Society and Human Behavior.* St. Louis, Mosby, 1972.

Razzell, M.: No thanks, I've quit smoking. Canad. Nurs. 71:23, September, 1975.

Rodman, M. J. and Smith, D. W.: *Clinical Pharmacology in Nursing.* Philadelphia, Lippincott, 1974.

Scherer, J. C.: *Introductory Clinical Pharmacology.* Philadelphia, Lippincott, 1975.

CHAPTER—7

Care of the dying patient

On completion of this chapter the student will:

- **Recognize some of the problems of the dying patient.**
- **Describe the important aspects of nursing care of the dying patient.**
- **Discuss the needs of the family of the dying patient.**
- **Begin to formulate personal ideas about death and the dying process.**

There are many indications that death has become a taboo subject in our society, much as sex was a taboo topic in the Victorian era. Euphemisms are widely used in place of the word "death," and great effort and expense are often employed to prepare and to show the body of the deceased in a way which makes it appear that death has not occurred at all.

Many people have little contact with death occurring naturally in the home. Frequently death occurs among awesome equipment and busy physicians and nurses dedicated to saving lives, to whom the death of a patient may signify their failure as healers. Seldom, in the hospital environment, is death viewed and discussed as a natural and universal experience. The role of health workers in supporting the patient and his loved ones during this experience is often de-emphasized in the stress on details of therapy which, though necessary and important, do not in themselves convey human caring. Nurses have opportunity to be involved with patients and families at the time of death —an opportunity which can enable them to help others during one of life's crucial experiences, as well as to grow personally in their understanding and acceptance of death as a part of life.

Attitudes of falseness and denial interfere with provision of supportive care for the patient and family. The patient whose illness is terminal is often dealt with by evasion and a false and superficial cheerfulness which he is usually quick to detect. Family members who realize that death of a loved one is near frequently have little opportunity to discuss their feelings with nurses and physicians. Avoidance of the dying patient and his family is common, and serves to protect staff from confronting their own anxieties about death and their own feelings when one of their patients has a terminal illness. Although death can occur in any clinical setting, it is most frequent on medical-surgical units and in geriatric services.

Many persons have their first experience with death in a highly charged emotional situation with the death of a parent or close relative.

Of primary concern is the consideration of one's personal view of death and the recognition that many patients and their families come to this experience quite unprepared to deal with it. The person whose only experience with death has been a visit to a funeral parlor, where someone has explained, "See, he is not dead; he is sleeping," is not well prepared for the reality of the change which occurs with the cessation of breathing and sudden stillness, as the patient crosses the threshold between life and death.

The development of one's philosophy and religious beliefs concerning death and of one's ability to accept the reality of death is a lifelong task to be dealt with again and again as life makes new demands and presents new challenges. The individual who thought he understood his views on death may find that he has hardly begun this process when confronted by a sudden death. For the nurse, as for all people, considering death is a process of personal growth which can occur over a lifetime. Persons in the health professions are among those who have opportunity, by care of patients and their families at the time of death, to enhance their own personal growth in the process. The nurse's ability to help patients and their families at the time of death is based upon understanding and inner growth. It is through understanding, humility, recognition and acceptance of death as part of life that the nurse ministers to dying patients and to their families. Emphasis is upon recognizing what this experience means to the patient and to those close to him, helping them to express their thoughts and feelings, and supporting them as they go through the stages of the experience.

Elizabeth Kübler-Ross defines the five stages prior to death as denial, anger, bargaining, depression, and acceptance. These stages apply to those patients who are aware that they have a terminal illness.

The individual first denies that the illness is terminal. He may believe that the x-rays are in error or the laboratory tests were mixed up with those of another patient. Sometimes the patient goes through elaborate mental gymnastics to prove to himself that this illness is not happening to him.

The second stage is one of anger—or, "Why me?" The anger may be directed toward others: doctors, nurses, family, other patients.

The third stage is an attempt to postpone death by bargaining. Usually these bargains are secretly made with God, with the patient promising to do something if death is postponed.

The fourth or depression stage is the patient's first realization of the truth of the situation. During this stage he may have a sense of great loss which may have many facets. He may mourn the loss of money, a change in body image, or the loss of employment.

The fifth or last stage is one of acceptance. In this stage the patient appears detached, is tired and weak, and may sleep often. He may wish to be left alone.

Patients may not follow these stages in an orderly manner and may even be in several stages at once. It may also be difficult to recognize all of these stages, especially if the patient is in more than one and has mixed symptoms or characteristics of several.

One consideration is especially important in working with dying patients. Often the nurse avoids talking with these patients in any but a very superficial way, out of uncertainty about how to respond when the patient asks, "Am I going to die?" Tension increases when the nurse (usually unrealistically) views herself as the only one to whom the patient can turn for help in dealing with his illness. Often the patient gradually recognizes clues in the behavior of others toward him that indicate that his illness is terminal. Thus the view of the patient as thoroughly unaware and seeking a disclosure from the nurse is often incorrect, and it greatly interferes with the nurse's relationship with the dying patient. When patients are given the opportunity, they often bring up awareness of their own approaching death by a remark about plans for providing for their children, leaving gifts for their families, and so on. Such comments, when they reflect the patient's realistic assessment of his situation, should be accepted rather than refuted by such replies as, "You shouldn't talk like that." Sometimes no verbal reply is necessary, as the feeling of acceptance of what has been said is expressed nonverbally in the way that the nurse conveys caring.

Three important aspects of nursing care of dying patients are: (1) supporting the patient as he begins to consider his approaching death; (2) fostering communication with the patient so that he does not face this experience in increasing isolation from others; and (3) talking with family members and with others who care for the patient about the patient and plans for his care.

The patient requires thoughtful attention to his physical comfort: position change, sips of fluids if he is able to tolerate them, a quiet restful environment. Primarily, he needs consideration as a human being, in all the varied ways that this can be demonstrated through thoughtful care. He requires particularly to be protected from routine, impersonal care typified by large numbers of health workers arriving to carry out, impersonally, the taking of his temperature, the provision of a water pitcher, or a check on the liter flow of oxygen being administered to him.

It is important to spend time with the dying patient over and beyond that required for physical care and treatments. The patient may bring up his concerns during his bath and treatments. Because of the tendency for dying patients to become isolated from others, it is particularly important to provide additional time when the primary objective is listening and supporting them as they come close to the time of their death.

It is important to be sensitive to the patient's spiritual concerns and to help him obtain the religious counseling and rites which he wishes. If the patient is too ill to express his wishes, the family should be consulted concerning spiritual care.

The patient can grow and mature as a person when he approaches death. The patient's philosophical and religious views may mature; he may develop a broader view of his life as part of the cosmos, and his death as a natural event in the ebb and flow of life. He may experience a tenderness and closeness toward family and friends which he has not felt before. On the other hand, the patient may become progressively disengaged from others as death approaches. If so, his family, particularly, will need help in understanding this change. Often the patient has a particular need for familiar and treasured possessions. It is especially important to keep the possessions the patient shows he values near him.

Families of dying patients particularly need the support a nurse can give. Often their own process of grieving begins when they learn that the patient's illness is terminal. Some family members begin to withdraw emotionally from the patient at this time because they find the experience too painful. Others draw closer, realizing the shortness of the time left with the loved one. The family's feelings do not conform necessarily to others' idealized views of what these feelings should be. For instance, the family may feel anger that the patient is about to leave them. The more the family member can express his feelings to an understanding listener, the better, because it helps the family member to recognize the emotion, and to consider whether it is one which would be beneficial to share with his dying relative. He can thus avoid burdening the patient and he can free himself to relate as constructively as possible to the dying patient. However, the possible harm from direct expression of feelings between relatives and the dying person is often overestimated. Family members may be so cautioned against showing any but cheerful feelings that they assume an air of false cheerfulness when visiting the patient. The patient senses the "mask" and feels isolated from the persons to whom he turns for closeness. When the family member finally can no longer keep up the pretense, but shows grief, both the relative and the patient often experience relief at the honest communication between them. Of course this does not mean that it is helpful for the family to burden the patient again and again with their grief or with their refusal to let him go when death is near. However, one big problem among family members of dying patients in our culture seems to lie in the inability to communicate frankly with the dying person—to express feelings and accept his expression of feelings. The regret at tenderness unexpressed, and thereafter unable to be expressed, is among the most poignant problems of grieving relatives. The nurse who can accept direct, straightforward communication from families can help them be more direct with the patient, thereby assisting them to have this enriching experience.

Perhaps nowhere is the stereotyped expectation of what the family *should* do, and how they *should* react, so strong as it is toward relatives of dying patients. The family may have their opportunity to experience this significant event in their lives impaired by the expectations of others about how they should react. The nurse needs to notice how the patient's relatives respond and what they seem to want and need.

One patient's husband may want to stay with his dying wife most of the day, sitting quietly with her. To argue with this man that he should "get more rest" may be useless and irritating both to him and to the nurse. Instead, it would be more helpful to provide him with an easy chair, encourage him to visit the coffee shop for nourishment, and help him to feel comfortable and accepted as he does what he shows he wants to do: remain with his wife. On the other hand, for the husband who shows that short visits are best for him or may be all that is possible for him in light of responsibilities to others and to his work, it is important to help the husband and wife to have these short visits free of other interruptions, e.g., by making a special effort not to schedule treatments during the husband's visit and avoiding conveying any attitude of, "It's about time you came," or, "Where have you been?" Some family members will openly express their grief—and it is helpful if they can do so to the nurse, in a private room away from the patient. Others seem to need a "stiff upper lip" in order to cope with the experience. In either case it is important to respect the way the relative is dealing with the situation.

It is important for the family to have a room where they can go to have privacy to talk with other relatives, to cry, and to rest. Facilities are extremely limited in this regard, and often family members are seen standing for long periods in the corridor (while one or two relatives remain with the patient). Every effort should be made to find a place where the family can have some privacy and can be seated comfortably. Frequent visits can be made if they show they wish this contact. Just sitting with the family for a short time and expressing concern for their comfort and welfare and listening to some of their concerns can bring comfort. The family frequently worry about how much the patient is suffering. It is helpful to explain that, as life ebbs, so usually does awareness of pain and discomfort. Thus, as the patient's death draws near, he may seem "detached," very often he slips into unconsciousness. It is then that the family's suffering is likely to be acute, although the patient's is lessened.

Helping the family to express their emotions and, as much as possible, to understand what is occurring can help them recover from grief after the patient's death. The nurse has many opportunities to assist the family to deal with the reality of death.

When death has occurred, it is usual for the relatives to leave the hospital at once. However, some may wish to remain for a time with the body of the deceased, and it is important to provide them a period of privacy before postmortem care is given. Particularly if only one relative is present at the time of death, it is important to offer to stay with the relative for a while before he leaves the hospital. If the relative seems very distraught, it is wise to telephone another family member to come and be with him or call the hospital chaplain.

General nutritional considerations

- Dietary considerations will vary depending on the cause and nature of the patient's illness.
- If the patient has abandoned hope, he may have little or no appetite. He will have to be encouraged to eat by the provision of a selection of his favorite foods, mealtime companions, and attractive preparation.
- Sound nutrition should be encouraged as an aid to helping the patient feel as well and as strong as possible, for as long as possible.
- See Chapter 5, "The Patient in Pain."

General pharmacological considerations

- Control of pain is often a great challenge. See Chapter 5, "The Patient in Pain."
- Fears of the patient and staff regarding the possibility of the patient's building a tolerance to pain-relief medications should be discussed.

Bibliography

Davis, B. A.: Until death ensues. Nurs. Clin. North Am. 7:303-309, June, 1972.

Freidman, M.: *The Story of Josh.* New York, Ballantine Books, 1974.

Kobrzycki, P.: Dying with dignity at home. Am. J. Nurs. 75:1312-3, August, 1975.

Kübler-Ross, E.: *Death: The Final Stage of Growth.* Englewood Cliffs, N.J., Prentice-Hall, 1975.

———: *On Death and Dying.* New York, Macmillan, 1969.

———: *Questions and Answers on Death and Dying.* New York, Macmillan, 1974.

Lacasse, C. M.: A dying adolescent. Am. J. Nurs. 75:433-4, March, 1975.

Myers, S.: Effects of death on the living. J. Prac. Nurs. 25:31+, January, 1975.

O'Brien, M.: *The Care of the Elderly Person: A Guide for the Licensed Practical Nurse,* ed. 2. St. Louis, Mosby, 1975.

Quint, J. C.: *The Nurse and the Dying Patient.* New York, Macmillan, 1967.

Rinear, E. E.: Helping the survivors of expected death. Nurs. '75, 5:60-5, March, 1975.

Schoenberg, B. et al, eds.: *Psychosocial Aspects of Terminal Care.* New York, Columbia University Press, 1972.

Walker, M.: The last hour before death. Am. J. Nurs. 73: 1592-93, December, 1973.

CHAPTER—8

Nursing in emergencies

On completion of this chapter the student will:

- **List and discuss general principles of first aid for major and minor emergencies.**
- **Understand the rationale for nursing measures in specific first aid situations.**
- **Discuss principles of emergency nursing measures in the hospital setting.**
- **Function as a member of the health team in emergency situations.**

General principles of first aid

First aid is not the amateur practice of medicine; it is a series of measures designed to keep the patient alive and prevent further damage until definitive medical treatment can be initiated.

Some important general principles of first aid, adaptable to particular situations, follow:

- Establish an airway and adequate respiration.

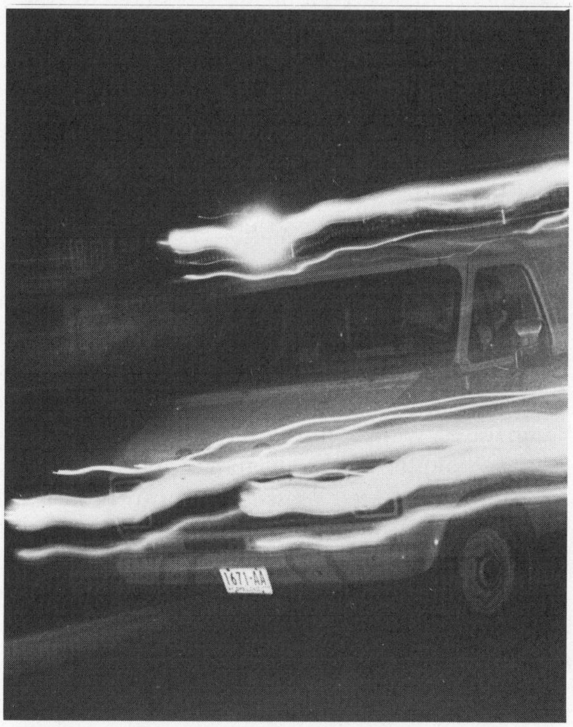

figure 8-1. Every emergency is traumatic, requiring calmness on the part of all involved, until the patient is brought to the hospital. (Photograph—D. Atkinson)

- Stop bleeding, especially from an artery.
- Do not move the patient unless he is further endangered by remaining where he is. A minor injury can become a major one when the patient is moved incorrectly. The rule is to keep the patient lying flat until he is seen by a doctor, or until a plan to move him has been evolved on the basis of the nature and the extent of his injuries. If the patient *must* be moved immediately, handle him as little and as gently as possible, especially where he is injured and try to keep his body as straight as possible. Do not jackknife him. Get enough help—for the patient's sake and your own. Sometimes in an emergency people forget others are around, and try single-handedly to move a heavy person.
- Search for injuries systematically. Carry out this search as soon as possible after stopping the patient's bleeding and establishing respiration. Start at the head and work down to the toes. A wound that is tiny or hidden by clothing may still be very dangerous, for instance, a small puncture wound in the chest that penetrates to the pleura. An abdominal wound or hidden bleeding could also be present. Nothing is lost by caution, and an injury actually may be more serious than it looks.
- Think of the underlying anatomy and physiology. For example, if the patient has a hole in his chest that sucks in air with every breath, it is a sign that the wound extends to his pleural cavity. When his rib cage expands, he is pulling air into the pleural space through the wound. The immediate first aid measure is to close that wound to prevent further collapse of the lung. Use a pressure dressing or, if one is not available, the palm of your hand.
- Prevent chilling. Almost all emergency conditions entail some degree of shock, so chilling should be avoided. Do not make the patient too warm. Excessive heat can increase shock.
- Do not give the patient anything to drink or eat until the full extent of his injuries has been determined by a physician. Never give an unconscious person anything to drink. No injured person should ever be given alcohol. Alcohol acts as a vasodilator, so that heat loss from the body is increased, thus increasing shock. Vasodilation also increases bleeding.
- Stay with the patient until a doctor arrives, unless there are a number of casualties, and you must leave one to attend another.
- Further injury is prevented by transporting the patient flat. The nurse should take command, so that untrained persons do not unintentionally harm the patient.
- Report the symptoms that were noted and the treatment, if any, that was given. It may be necessary to put these observations in writing.
- Communicate calmness. Every emergency is traumatic but the calmness of those caring for him gives the patient a sense of security (Fig. 8-1). Fear and confusion can be minimized by a calm but firm manner.
- Apply to psychological emergencies the same principles as to any other emergency nursing situation: prevent further injury and seek medical care. Anyone who has attempted suicide requires medical attention. The person who is acutely confused, disoriented, or disturbed also needs help. Stay with the patient. If he has a distorted impression of reality, do not argue. Talk to the patient and allow him to talk to you.

First aid in various emergencies

Hemorrhage

It is important to look for bleeding, and stop it quickly. Most people can tolerate the loss of a pint of blood, but losing a quart or more leads to shock. A patient can hemorrhage to death in less than one minute from a large artery that is severed, but most bleeding can be stopped by pressure and elevation. To control bleeding:

- Apply direct continuous pressure to the wound, which will usually stop the hemorrhage. If you do not have a sterile bandage to place over the wound, use a clean handkerchief or a piece of cloth. Lacking these, use your bare hand.
- Apply pressure on a major artery leading to the wound. Press the artery against the bone (Figs. 8-2 and 8-3).
- Elevate the part.

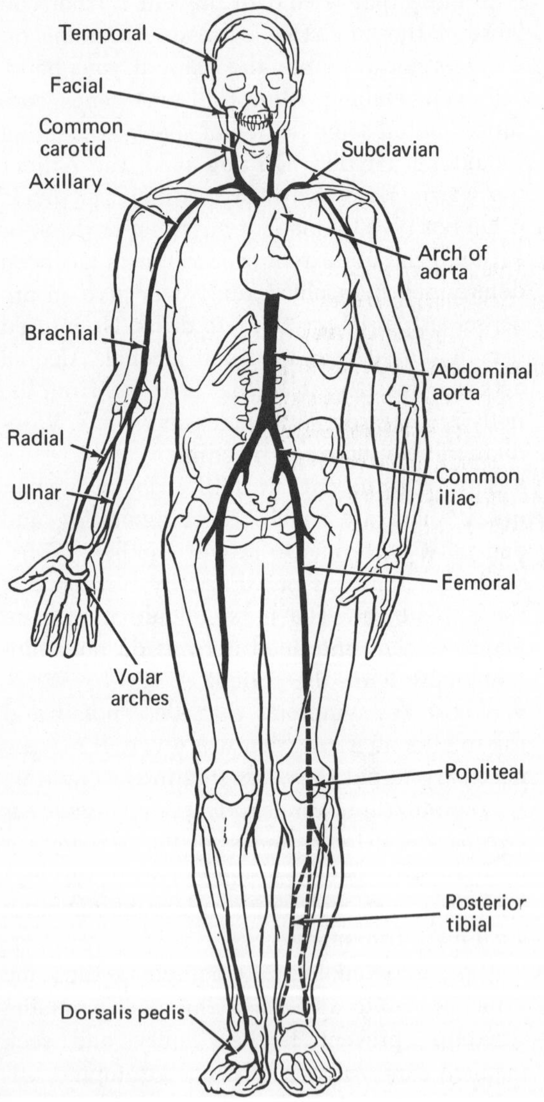

figure 8-2. Arteries that may be palpated (except the aorta and the common iliac) and compressed. The dotted line on the left leg indicates that the arteries travel along the back of the leg.

If bleeding cannot be controlled by the application of pressure and elevation of the part, a tourniquet may be necessary. An extremity that is mangled, crushed, or amputated will require a tourniquet to stop bleeding. A tourniquet of the inflatable (pneumatic) type is preferable. A blood pressure cuff can be used as a tourniquet; the cuff is inflated to a level above the patient's systolic blood pressure. If the blood pressure is not obtainable, the cuff is inflated until bleeding stops. An inflatable tourniquet should not be removed except by a physician.

Cessation of respiration

This condition may be due to drowning, electric shock, carbon monoxide or other gaseous poisoning, or to disease. Treatment must be begun at once.

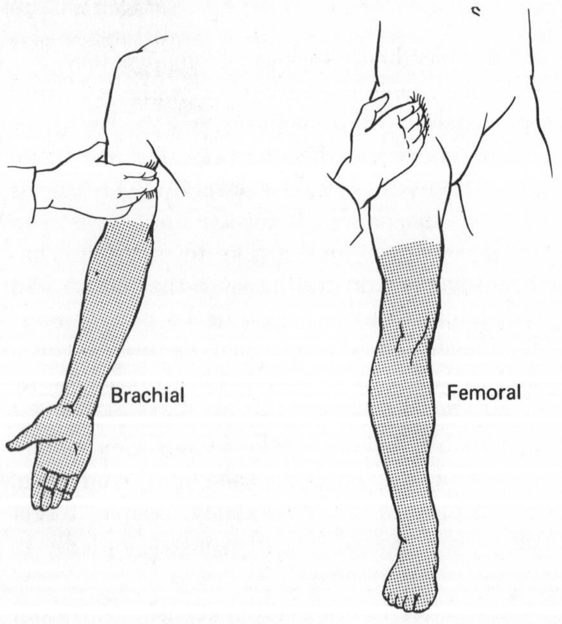

figure 8-3. Methods of occluding the brachial and femoral arteries to control bleeding from injuries in the shaded areas. Pressure is applied to artery and bone behind it.

Mouth-to-mouth breathing is the most effective method of resuscitation. Properly performed, it can maintain in good physiological condition a patient who is not breathing for himself. Speed in initiating the procedure is important. The procedure follows:

- First, clear the airway. An obstruction in the mouth, the trachea, or the bronchi will prevent ventilation of the lungs. Wipe the inside of the patient's mouth with a handkerchief. If it is necessary, turn him on his side and sharply slap his back. This procedure may dislodge an obstruction in a bronchus.
- Make sure the tongue does not obstruct the airway.
- Hold the patient's nose, so that the air you blow into his mouth does not escape.
- Take a breath, and blow into the patient's mouth until you see the chest rise. Listen for the rush of expired air while you take your next breath. Watch for relaxation of the chest wall.
- Reinflate the patient's lungs as soon as his expiration is complete. Repeat this procedure 12 times a minute. Make the breaths deep enough to inflate the patient's lungs. Continue until the patient breathes for himself or until he is declared dead by a physician. When the patient does start to breathe for himself, watch him continuously for at least 1 hour.

Many people recoil from this close physical contact, if the patient looks especially unhealthy or unkempt. If you wish to place a thin cloth between your mouth and the patient's, do so. It will not impede ventilation. If a double-ended plastic airway is available, it can increase the efficiency of artificial respiration considerably.

Shock

Keep the patient lying flat with his feet 8 to 12 inches higher than his head (unless there is dyspnea in this position), and as still and quiet as possible. He should be warm, yet not hot. Excessive heat results in vasodilation, which can increase shock. Do not give anything by mouth to an unconscious patient, to one with a head injury or an abdominal wound, or to any patient who will receive medical attention within 2 hours. If a long interval is anticipated, and the patient is not vomiting, start him on sips of water.

Electric shock

A severe electric shock results in cardiac arrest from ventricular fibrillation. The only definitive treatment for this is defibrillation. If a defibrillator is not immediately available, cardiopulmonary resusciation is administered while the patient is being transported to the nearest hospital. When removing the patient from the electrical contact, it is most important that the rescuer avoid touching him; rather, use an object that will not conduct electrical current—wood or plastic—to push or pull the patient away. If a live wire is involved, it can be moved away from the patient with a nonconductive object.

Wounds

Unless a sterile bandage is available, most wounds should be left uncovered and exposed to the air until they have been treated by a physician. Wounds should not be washed or treated with an antiseptic until a physician has examined the patient.

Snakebite

Persons bitten by snakes native to the United States usually recover, but snakebite may also be fatal. In all likelihood, the victim will be extremely apprehensive. It is most important to identify the snake, as treatment may include the administration of antivenin. If the individual saw the snake, it is important to ascertain from him the color of the snake, and the shape of its head.

First aid is directed toward keeping the venom from entering the bloodstream and thus spreading to other areas of the body. This can be accomplished by keeping the patient quiet, immobilizing the affected part, applying a tourniquet *above* and *below* the area of the bite, and, possibly, applying cold. If available, antivenin is administered. The value of incision and suction to remove snake venom is questionable.

Animal bites

Bites from any warm-blooded animal must be regarded as potential rabies threats. Such wounds should be washed and debrided if necessary and tetanus immunization given to the victim. If a person is bitten by an animal that may have rabies, the rabies vaccine is given if (1) the animal is found and appears rabid or develops rabies after it has been impounded, or (2) the animal itself cannot be found but the type of animal is known to carry rabies, for example bats, skunks, or raccoons.

Poisoning

Food poisoning can be caused when food is contaminated with such organisms as *Staphylococcus aureus, Clostridium botulinum,* and *Clostridium perfringens.* Toxins produced by these organisms cause the illness. Food serves as a vehicle that transfers pathogenic organisms (such as *Salmonella*) from a contaminated source to the victim.

Food poisoning may be of nonmicrobial origin, in cases of contamination by insecticides for example. Naturally toxic plants, such as various strains of mushrooms, some berries, and some wild plants, may be ingested through accident or ignorance.

Clostridium botulinum produces a neurotoxin that may cause nausea and vomiting, headache, lassitude, double vision, muscular incoordination and inability to talk, swallow or breathe. This organism, an anaerobe, is found most often in foods that have been improperly canned at home.

Botulinus toxin is destroyed by heat just below the boiling point; therefore, food which has been boiled in the previous few hours is considered safe. However, the *spores* of botulinus are not killed by boiling, even for hours. Therefore, food which is boiled and then kept in closed containers for several days can be lethal. Botulism can also be acquired from improperly cured sausage and fish. Ordinarily, this bacterium does not grow in a highly acid medium, so most fruit preserves are quite safe. Any can which is swollen or seems to contain gas should be discarded unopened. Foods suspected of being contaminated should not be tasted. There have been deaths from a single taste. Smoking, salting, marinating, and drying food do not necessarily kill the spores of *Clostridium botulinum.*

Botulism is treated with antitoxin, a positive-pressure respirator, and intravenous therapy. Early treatment is important; the mortality rate is about 65 percent. Death is often due to respiratory failure.

Staphylococci grow in food, especially creamed food that has not been sufficiently refrigerated. Symptoms may include weakness, diarrhea, nausea, vomiting, and abdominal cramps that develop a few hours after ingesting the contaminated food and last for a day or two. Death is rare. Food poisoning may not be recognized until the food is absorbed and the patient has symptoms, usually diarrhea and vomiting. The patient should be kept quiet, and medical help obtained as quickly as possible. Parenteral fluids and sedation may be given. To help prevent food poisoning, nurses should teach the importance of cleanliness in food preparation, and of prompt and adequate cooking and refrigeration. In preparation for a picnic, for example, it should be stressed that the arrangements must include refrigeration. Sometimes food such as potato salad is prepared in large quantity and left out of the refrigerator for hours before it is consumed because of lack of room on the shelves. This is a dangerous practice.

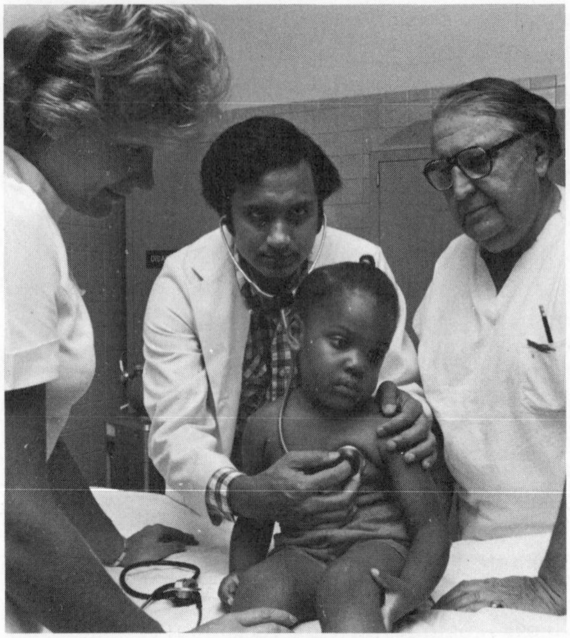

figure 8-4. Children frequently ingest drugs and chemicals found in and around the home and should be treated as soon as possible. (Photograph—D. Atkinson)

Drug poisoning may result from an accidental or intentional overdose of drugs or the ingestion of poisonous chemicals. Treatment of drug poisoning will depend on the type of drug(s) or chemicals ingested, the amount or dose, the route (oral or intravenous), the length of time since ingestion or injection (if known), and the patient's present condition (Fig. 8-4). It is extremely important to determine the drug or chemical involved and the amount, as correct treatment or administration of an antidote often depend on drug identification. Burns on the mouth suggest that a corrosive acid or alkali has been swallowed. If the container is not found immediately, the poison may be diluted by giving the patient (if he is conscious) as much water as possible. Rapid action is important.

Induce vomiting unless the poison is ammonia, or a strong acid or alkali (which would reburn the tissues of the mouth and esophagus as the chemical is brought up), or any petroleum product, such as gasoline, lighter fluid, or kerosene. Vomiting is not induced in these instances because of the danger of aspiration. Vomiting should not be induced if the patient is already comatose or convulsing. If the patient complains of severe pain or a burning sensation in his mouth and throat, vomiting should not be induced.

It is necessary to smell the breath for fumes. If you see no burns and smell no fumes, vomiting may be induced. Putting one's finger down the patient's throat to induce vomiting is less preferable than the administration of syrup of ipecac, a drug that does not require a prescription and should be in all households with small children. Every precaution must be taken to avoid aspiration.

Most cities have poison information centers with a 24-hour telephone answering service. If a child or adult has ingested a drug or chemical, the poison center can provide information regarding emergency treatment and the antidote to be used. If the container is found, it should be saved; if not, a specimen of the patient's vomitus or a urine specimen should be saved for the doctor. The observation of vital signs and the prevention of chilling are important first aid measures. The patient should be transported to the hospital as quickly as possible.

POISONING BY GAS. When gas poisoning is suspected, the patient must be removed from the area of the fumes. If he is overcome at home, it is necessary to open the window immediately and remove the patient from the room. If he is not breathing, mouth-to-mouth resuscitation is started. There is no other first aid measure. The patient should be hospitalized as rapidly as possible. The ambulance or an emergency squad may have resuscitating and oxygen equipment.

EXPOSURE TO TEMPERATURE EXTREMES

HEATSTROKE (SUNSTROKE). In this disorder, the body's normal responses to increasing temperature are not functioning. The patient feels dizzy, weak and nauseated; he may have a headache, but there is no perspiration. The skin is red, hot, and dry to the touch. There may be convulsions or collapse. The immediate first aid measure is to cool the patient. He must be removed from the direct sunlight, and immediately cooled with wet, cold towels applied to the entire body. If he is conscious, he may have cool drinks. If ice is available, it can be put in packs and placed on forehead, axillae, and on the body and legs. Cold water can be poured on the patient, or he can be fanned or put into a cool tub. Temperature should be taken frequently, and cooling continued until his temperature is down to about 101°F. Sustained high fever will result in brain damage. These patients need hospitalization even if they respond to first aid measures. The patient may have a lifelong problem with heat regulation after an episode of heatstroke, possibly necessitating a move to a cooler climate or the regulation of his life so that he is not exposed to heat for long periods of time.

HEAT EXHAUSTION. This disorder is characterized by circulatory disturbances brought about by an excessive loss of salt and water due to prolonged sweating. The patient feels dizzy and faint, and he may have headache, muscle cramps, and nausea. In contrast with heatstroke, the skin is pale and damp. Uncorrected, the condition leads to collapse, but it is usually possible to rouse the patient.

Heat exhaustion is treated like shock, except that it is necessary to cool the patient. Water with a teaspoon of table salt in each glass is given. To relieve muscle cramps, firm pressure against the muscle with the flat of the hand is applied. Heat exhaustion often can be prevented by taking adequate salt and water during a time of excessive exposure to heat and by observing such common sense precautions as avoiding strenuous exertion and wearing suitable clothing.

At times, patients may have a combination of heatstroke and heat exhaustion, and the physical signs may not be as distinct as descriptions suggest.

FROSTBITE. Severe cold causes injury to tissues; frostbite is a degree of cold injury. There is extreme vasoconstriction and thrombosis, as well as direct injury to the walls of the blood vessels and the cells. Exudate escapes from the damaged vessel walls, resulting in edema. There is ischemia of the tissues, and the skin blanches. The frostbitten part becomes numb and stiff. As it warms, it turns a bright pink and blisters.

Experience in World War II and the Korean War showed that the previously common practice of slowly warming a frostbitten part causes more tissue damage than rapid warming. Bathe the affected part in comfortably warm water for 10 minutes. Be sure the temperature of the water is comfortable for the patient. Let him test it; water that may feel warm to normal skin may feel hot to frostbitten skin. After bathing, the skin should be blotted dry, and a dry sterile dressing applied, using sterile gauze to separate skin surfaces. The part requires elevation. Snow or cold water should not be applied to the affected areas. If legs or feet are involved, the patient should not walk.

Debridement and grafting may be necessary if blistering has occurred. Because deep circulation is less affected than is superficial circulation, this surgical treatment usually is effective.

The degree of injury varies in severity. In mild cases, recovery is complete. In severe cases, amputation may be necessary. Patients who have been severely frostbitten may, for years afterward, experience numbness and tingling when the affected area is exposed to cold. Such patients are advised to protect this area in the future from injury or exposure to cold.

Prevention of frostbite includes:

- Avoiding skin contact with the CO_2 in fire extinguishers.
- Avoiding constricting clothing, such as shoes and socks that are too tight, or the use of circular garters in cold weather—these further impair blood supply.
- Keeping the entire body as warm and dry as possible when in extreme cold.
- Teaching persons likely to be affected, such as soldiers, to exercise legs, feet, arms, and fingers if they are in a situation likely to cause frostbite.
- Teaching persons vulnerable to frostbite to observe each other's skin for the development of yellow-white patches (on the ear lobe, for example) and to heed such sensations as pricking or pain, which may herald frostbite.

First aid in minor emergencies

Fainting. A momentary deficiency in cerebral oxygenation causes fainting. It can be distinguished from other forms of unconsciousness by its temporary nature. Usually, the patient regains consciousness as soon as he has attained a horizontal position.

If a person feels faint, he should lie flat, without a pillow. Tight clothing around the neck and the waist should be loosened and falling prevented when possible, since the injury sustained by the fall may be far more serious than the faint. If the patient cannot lie down, he may sit down and put his head between his knees. A physician should examine the patient to determine the cause of the fainting.

Sunburn. A first-degree burn may be soothed by cool compresses. To avoid further trauma to his skin, the patient must be handled gently. Blisters should be dressed with sterile gauze and not punctured. If the burn is extensive, it requires medical aid.

Bites and Stings. *Ticks.* The tick may be killed with a few drops of turpentine, or a hot needle may be used to make it release its hold. Then, with tweezers, it can very gently be removed from the skin. Crushing the tick could transmit to the patient virulent pathogenic microorganisms which some ticks carry. Excessive force in trying to remove a tick must be avoided. The area should be scrubbed with soap and water afterward.

Bees, Wasps, Hornets. The stinger should be removed with a sterile needle or tweezers (only honey bees shed their stinger). An icebag or a paste made of baking soda will reduce the swelling and the itching. If the person is allergic to the sting of that insect, it may be fatal. Any symptoms of allergy after a sting demand immediate medical attention.

Poisonous Spiders, Tarantulas, and Scorpions. Death of a healthy adult from spider bite or scorpion sting is rare, but the symptoms can be extremely painful. Deaths have occurred in children and in adults in a weakened condition. The best known toxic spider is the black widow which secretes a neurotoxin. This spider is a shiny black color with a red to orange hourglass on its ventral surface. A less well-known spider is at least as dangerous. The brown recluse spider originally was reported in Missouri but seems to have spread throughout the continental United States. It is somewhat smaller than the black widow, and ranges from light tan to dark brown in color. It has a banjo-shaped spot on its *dorsal* surface. The brown recluse is a shy animal and is usually hidden from view. It bites when it feels trapped. Unfortunately, it sometimes lives in old clothing or shoes kept in a garage or basement. When a person tries to put these garments on, the spider, presumably in self-defense, bites. The initial bite is seldom painful and often is unnoticed. The toxin, however, contains an extremely potent digestive enzyme, and after a few hours, it destroys a large amount of tissue, leaving an open wound which may not heal for many months. Secondary infections can ensue. For this reason, a report of spider bite must be taken seriously, even if there is no pain, and no initial evidence of toxicity. If possible, the spider should be identified. If this cannot be done, any person bitten by a spider of unknown species should be referred to a physician for immediate observation and definitive management. A spider bite should not be incised by a first aid worker. For temporary relief, cold applications to the bitten area are helpful, but freezing of tissues must be avoided. There are specific medical treatments for black widow spider bites, including the intravenous injection of calcium gluconate and the use of an antivenin. At present, there is no antivenin available for brown recluse spider venom.

Emergency nursing in the hospital

Some large hospitals have emergency departments in which patients stay during the first hours or days of an acute disorder.

When the emergency is over, the patients are transferred to regular hospital units, where treatment is continued.

Following are some principles of emergency nursing in the hospital. They apply to any nursing situation:

- Recognize an emergency. Know enough about each patient to recognize when an illness has become serious. Know the diagnosis of each patient and learn what the danger signs are. An important part of good emergency nursing involves recognizing danger and knowing when to call the doctor.
- Apply first aid. The nurse may be the first person to see a patient in an emergency. Whether the patient is hospitalized or comes into the nurse's care from the street, the principles of first aid apply. Establish priorities of care. Highest priorities are severe hemorrhage, acute respiratory difficulty, shock, severe chest pain, multiple injuries, high fever, and coma.
- Adjust your pace to the rapidly changing situation. The nurse must move fast to aid respiration, stop the bleeding, and call the doctor. Her report to the doctor must be as accurate as it is prompt.
- The nurse is often first to greet the patient and his family, and must not, in haste, neglect a kind word of encouragement. The right word at the right moment, the touch on the arm, the chair offered, the assurance that the doctor is on his way, the deft application of a dry sterile dressing—all can help to make the patient and his family feel that he will be cared for at the time when he desparately needs help.
- Support the patient in every way possible. Call for the priest, minister, or rabbi if the patient wishes. Providing dramatic treatment and concentrated care often helps to allay anxiety. On the other hand, the extent of the patient's injuries should be explained realistically by the physician. The patient should be allowed to discuss what happened and his reactions to it; ignoring him does not help him to assimilate the traumatic experience. The nurse should be especially observant for symptoms which seem in excess of the injury, or for denial of the injury, and report these observations to the doctor.
- Remember the legal implications of the situation. The patient's valuables should be collected carefully and sent home with a relative or deposited in the hospital safe. Handle all clothing with care, even if it is bloody or dirty. A patient who sees the nurse handle his clothing as if it were repugnant to her may feel himself rejected. If the clothing must be cut, cut along a seam, when it is possible. The nurse may work with the police to help to establish the identity of an unaccompanied, helpless person. If the patient is unable to sign a consent for surgery, his family must be located.
- Be alert to your function in relation to others on the health team. An acute emergency demands smoothness, with each member of the team contributing his share of efficiency. The nurse should anticipate the information that the doctor will want.
- Be sure that supplies are ready for use. Such emergency equipment as oxygen or a cardiac pacemaker are of no value unless they are available when needed. It is every nurse's responsibility to know where the emergency supplies and equipment are, and how to use them.
- Be clear and complete in regard to follow-up care. Because patients and their families tend to be anxious, instructions are easily confused or forgotten. When possible, instructions should be written as well as given verbally.

Emergency nursing requires judgment, timing, alertness and knowledge. There is no substitute for knowing the basic principles of physiology, sterile technique, and first aid so well that under pressure one can function without hesitation. A nurse should not expect to manage first emergencies as well as later ones. It is possible to learn from each of them.

General pharmacological considerations

- Nurses should be familiar with the use, action, side effects, and precautions of drugs used in emergency situations.
- Drugs used to treat shock are potent vasopressors requiring a determination of the patient's blood pressure every 3 to 5 minutes and adjustment of the rate of drug administration (as drops per minute) according to blood pressure.
- When tetanus immunization is necessary, the nurse should only administer tetanus *toxoid*. Tetanus toxin-antitoxin should be administered by a physician.
- Accidental drug ingestion is a relatively common occurrence, especially among children. Patient discharge teaching should include instructions regarding safekeeping of drugs.
- It is important to locate the drug or chemical container in cases of accidental poisoning in order to identify the material and possibly the amount ingested.
- Syrup of ipecac is available in a 1-ounce size without a prescription and should be kept in all households with young children. The directions for administration are clearly printed on the label. For children over 1 year, give one-half the container (15 ml.). Parents should be advised to contact the local poison control center before giving this or any drug.

Bibliography

COSGRIFF, J. H. and ANDERSON, D. L.: *The Practice of Emergency Nursing.* Philadelphia, Lippincott, 1975.

DIAMOND, E. F.: Emergency care of acute poisonings. RN 36:OR/ED 8, June, 1973.

Emergency Care and Transportation of the Sick and Injured. Chicago, American Academy of Orthopedic Surgeons, 1971.

JELENKO, C.: Emergency treatment of small deep burns. Hosp. Med. 11:92, January, 1975.

MILLER, R. H. et al, eds.: *Textbook of Basic Emergency Medicine.* St. Louis, Mosby, 1975.

MITTY, W. F. et al: Treating shock in the emergency department. RN 36:OR/ED 1, August, 1973.

ROYCE, J. A.: Shock: Emergency nursing implications. Nurs. Clin. North Am. 8:377, September, 1973.

SCHULBERG, H. C.: Picking up the pieces—intervening in disaster situations. Nurs. Dig. 3:50, July/August, 1975.

SCHWARTZ, A. R.: Culture—positive. Emer. Med. 7:227, April, 1975.

STEELE, J. H.: Salmonellosis: A growing threat. Consultant, 13:166, March, 1973.

STEPHENSON, H. E.: *Immediate Care of the Acutely Ill and Injured.* St. Louis, Mosby, 1974.

TAYLOR, A.: Botulism and its control. Am. J. Nurs. 73:1380, August, 1973.

The deadly mushroom. Newsweek 81:48, January 15, 1973.

Those critical first minutes. RN 35:46, June, 1972.

When the shock is electric. Emer. Med. 5:88, June, 1973.

CHAPTER 9

The surgical patient

On completion of this chapter the student will:

- Discuss and list routine preparation of the patient going to surgery.
- Describe the influence of thorough preoperative teaching on the postoperative recovery rate.
- List the routine nursing tasks performed during the immediate postoperative recovery period.
- Describe the postoperative management of the patient with pain.
- Discuss the importance of oral fluids and diet in the postoperative period.
- Give the rationale for frequent coughing, deep breathing, and leg exercises in the immediate postoperative period.
- Explain the importance of early postoperative ambulation in the prevention of postoperative complications.
- Recognize and list overt, major complications that may occur during the postoperative period.

The immediate preoperative preparation of the patient almost always takes place on the nursing unit. A preoperative check-

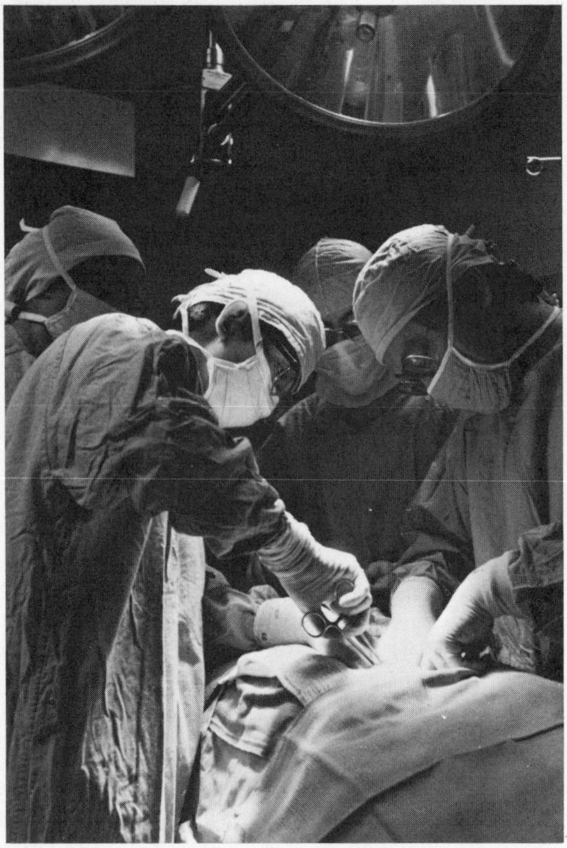

figure 9-1. The patient who consents to surgery is completely dependent on the abilities of the surgical team. (Photograph—D. Atkinson)

list is usually used to ensure completion of observations and nursing tasks. Typical items include making sure that the operative consent has been signed and that the patient has voided. When these details have been carried out with careful attention and due consideration for the patient and his family, the nurse and the assistant from surgery help the patient onto the stretcher for safe transportation to the surgical suite.

The patient who consents to have surgery, particularly surgery that requires taking a general anesthetic, renders himself completely dependent on the knowledge, skill, and integrity of those who care for him (Fig. 9-1). In accepting this trust, members of the surgical team have an obligation to make the patient's welfare their first consideration during this period.

Preoperative apprehension

What fears may the surgical patient have? Consider the woman who is to have surgery of the breast. Fear of the diagnosis probably looms large. Today most women recognize that a lump in the breast may be cancerous, and they know that the diagnosis will be determined during surgery and the subsequent examination of tissue. Even though a prosthesis may be worn that keeps others from realizing she has had surgery, the patient will experience a change in body image. She may be very concerned about her husband's reaction to her changed appearance. The possibility of cancer—and of major surgery—may arouse fears of pain and death. The thought of being unconscious and unable to know or in any way control what is happening is disquieting. Fear of unrelieved pain after surgery is often a source of apprehension.

Patients who are extremely frightened respond poorly to surgery; they seem to be particularly prone to complications like cardiac arrest and irreversible shock. Unless the operation is an emergency, many surgeons defer surgery if the patient is very frightened. If the patient has been extremely fearful before surgery, he may show unusual behavior afterward, perhaps not recognizing changes in his body that have resulted from surgery, or withdrawing from others and seeming very depressed. Be alert for symptoms of unusual emotional reaction during the preoperative period and report them promptly.

Preoperative preparation

With the exception of emergency surgery, preparation for surgery should begin 1 to 2 days before it has been scheduled. A clear, careful explanation by the surgeon is most important as the patient should understand the reason for surgery and the results to be expected. When the team knows what information the doctor has given, nurses are in a better position to help the patient to understand any points that are not clear or to clear up any misconceptions he or his family may have.

After the doctor has discussed the surgery with the patient, the nurse explains the plan for preoperative and postoperative nursing care and ways in which the patient can participate in his care. For example, the nurse explains the purpose of deep-breathing exercises, turning from side to side, and range-of-motion (ROM) exercises. This is followed by a demonstration of these exercises or movements. If possible, the patient should practice these maneuvers before surgery.

Preoperative explanations

Before surgery the patient is usually alert and sometimes free of pain. During the immediate postoperative period he is drowsy from medication and anesthesia, and often he has pain. Pain and sleepiness interfere with learning. Thus it is preferable to teach patients during the preoperative period. Repetition and review will be necessary postoperatively, but the patient will be better able to participate, because he knows what to expect. The patient is probably anxious, and anxiety may interfere with learning. For this reason, the nurse learns to recognize defenses, such as denial or forgetting, and plans her explanations in accordance with the patient's readiness and ability to receive instructions. Planned use of simple, factual explanations that are adjusted to the patient's ability and need is an essential part of the nursing care plan. A patient who is helped to understand what he can do to help himself is prepared to cooperate with the health team.

The patient who enters the hospital for emergency surgery must be prepared as quickly as possible. There is not a great deal of time for reassurance and explanation. Even though explanations must be brief, they should be given if the patient is aware enough to understand them. As soon as emergency measures have been carried out, it is especially important to spend time talking with the family, helping them to understand what has happened. When the patient recovers sufficiently, extra thought and attention should be given to helping him to understand the illness or the accident that has overtaken him.

Religious faith is a source of strength and courage for many patients. Opportunities for contact with the patient's clergyman for the sacraments of his denomination are especially important during a crisis like an impending operation. Every effort should be made to help the patient to maintain his religious ties, either through the services of the patient's own clergyman or through the hospital chaplain.

The patient's family

Family members need to understand what measures are necessary to prepare the patient for surgery, so that they can participate intelligently in his care and provide him with further explanation and encouragement. Sometimes the patient can better accept the necessity for surgery if it is explained further to him by a relative whom he loves and trusts. Many family members want to be near the patient and to help in any possible way to prepare him for surgery. Their presence helps the patient to feel less alone and assures him of his family's concern and interest.

The nurse who believes that family members have a right to be with the patient, and that their presence can be helpful, will reveal this attitude in her manner toward the family. On the other hand, if she believes that the family is in the way or likely to upset the patient, she will behave in a way that is conducive to this very occurrence.

Preoperative medication

Tranquilizers such as chlordiazepoxide (Librium) or sedatives such as phenobarbital may be given several days prior to surgery to relieve apprehension. The evening before surgery a hypnotic drug such as secobarbital (Seconal) may be given. About 30 to 60 minutes before the patient goes to the operating room, a preoperative medication is administered. This medication may consist of one, two, or three drugs: a narcotic or a sedative, an antiemetic, and a drug to decrease the secretions of the respiratory tract. Examples of these drugs are meperidine (Demerol), a narcotic; or secobarbital (Seconal), a hypnotic/sedative; perphenazine (Trilafon), an antiemetic which also has some sedative properties, especially when administered with a narcotic; and atropine, a cholinergic blocking agent which will dry secretions of the nose, mouth, throat and bronchi. The preoperative medication is usually ordered by the anesthesiologist, with the choice of drugs based on the patient, the surgery, and the type of anesthetic to be used.

The patient should have an explanation of the effects that will be experienced after the preoperative medication is administered. He should also be instructed to remain in bed; the side rails should be raised and the call light placed within easy reach. He should be told not to smoke after the medication has been given but if the patient feels he must smoke one last cigarette just before surgery, someone should stay with him while he is smoking.

Physical preparation and hospital procedures

Preoperative preparation may extend over a period of several days or weeks, and it may include many tests, x-ray studies and laboratory procedures, as well as education of the patient and the family. The nurse plays an important part in explaining the necessity for preoperative tests and in carrying out the preparation for these tests.

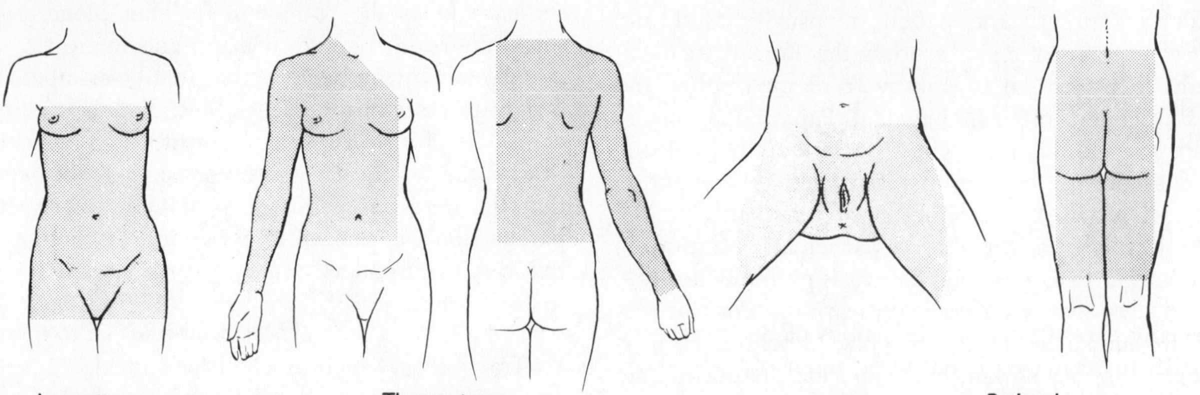

figure 9-2. These diagrams indicate areas of skin prepared before laparotomy, thoracotomy, and surgery in the perineal area. Note the extensiveness of the skin preparation in each of these examples. The procedure of each hospital varies somewhat in the designation of the areas to be prepared.

A medical history is taken and a physical examination performed prior to surgery. In addition, laboratory tests such as urinalysis, complete blood count (CBC), hemoglobin, and hematocrit are usually ordered. These studies are carried out to discover any pre-existing disease that might alter the patient's response to surgery or his recovery from it. For instance, urinalysis may suggest the presence of diabetes mellitus or chronic nephritis. In many hospitals a routine chest x-ray is taken to make certain that the patient has no unsuspected pulmonary disease, such as tuberculosis. If unsuspected disease is discovered, the operation may be delayed while measures to treat or to control the conditions are instituted.

Often surgery must be undertaken despite the presence of other illnesses. A patient with multiple sclerosis may require surgery for a broken leg, or a patient with heart disease may have to have his appendix removed. These long-term illnesses affect plans for medical and nursing care. The surgeon often consults the patient's medical doctor concerning the management of the coexisting disease. For instance, the patient with heart disease may require daily doses of digitalis, as well as a low sodium diet. The patient with multiple sclerosis may need considerably more assistance with activities of daily living than would most surgical patients. A diabetic patient needs special treatment before, during, and after surgery. These needs have to be considered in planning nursing care.

Immediate preoperative care

Immediate preparation for surgery usually starts the afternoon before surgery.

Skin Preparation. The purpose of skin preparation is to make the skin as free of microorganisms as possible, thus decreasing the possibility of the entrance during surgery of bacteria into the wound from the skin surface.

Most hospitals have manuals describing specifically the areas of the skin to be prepared for certain types of surgery and the procedure to be used. Figure 9-2 shows areas of the body customarily prepared for common types of surgery. Before commencing any skin preparation, it is well to look up the procedure and the area to be prepared in the hospital manual. If there is doubt, the doctor should be consulted. It is very important to have the skin preparation meticulously complete before surgery, because last-minute additional preparation, along with the tension generated among the staff by the necessity for this procedure, is very upsetting to the patient and may shake his confidence in those caring for him.

Although the procedure for skin preparation varies in different hospitals, cleanliness of the skin and the removal of hair from its surface without injury or irritation are fundamental. The skin cannot be made completely sterile, but the number of microorganisms on it can be substantially reduced. Hair is shaved because microorganisms readily cling to it and to prevent it from entering the wound, where it acts as a foreign body to prevent healing. Plain soap and water are sometimes used for cleansing the skin. Solutions effective in decreasing the number of microorganisms on the skin are now very widely used.

Before starting the procedure explain briefly what you are going to do and why it is being done. Drape and screen the patient to prevent unnecessary exposure. In most hospitals a male nurse or nursing assistant takes care of the skin preparation for male patients. Preparation for orthopedic surgery must be especially careful, because infections of bone are very difficult to manage, even with intensive antibiotic therapy.

Elimination. Before certain types of surgery it is particularly important that the bladder be empty. Distention of the bladder makes lower abdominal surgery more difficult and increases the possibility that the bladder may be injured during the operation. For this reason some surgeons ask that the patient be catheterized, and a catheter be left in place. If the patient is not to be catheterized, make certain that he voids just before surgery. Even in operations far removed from the region of the bladder, the patient will be more comfortable and at ease if he has voided just before going to the operating room. Too often the patient is given the bedpan or the urinal hastily, with little attention to position or to privacy, when the stretcher arrives to take him to the operating room. Under these circumstances many patients become tense, are unable to void, or void in insufficient quantity. Plan the patient's care in such a way that there is time for the important details of positioning and privacy, without obvious haste or impatience. If the patient has had a thorough explanation of the *pre*operative period, he will most likely have voided upon waking and before the preoperative medication is administered. The bed patient should be given the urinal or bedpan about an hour before surgery.

Enemas may be ordered before surgery to clean out the lower bowel. The act of straining to have a bowel movement is painful after any abdominal operation. If fecal matter is left in the bowel preoperatively, it may become hard and even impacted before the patient is able to bear down painlessly enough to evacuate. In addition, an enema is particularly important when surgery is performed on the bowel.

Sometimes, enemas are ordered for patients whose surgery involves distant organs. For instance, enemas often are ordered before eye surgery, so that the patient will be spared the strain and the exertion of moving his bowels in the immediate postoperative period; this exertion might cause hemorrhage in the operative area.

General anesthesia produces muscular relaxation; having the bowel empty prevents the possibility of involuntary bowel movement during or immediately after the operation. The patient's comfort and peace of mind are enhanced if he has moved his bowels before going to the operating room. Small-quantity commercially prepared enemas are usually used for preoperative preparations. Most patients find them more comfortable and less tiring than the large-quantity enemas.

Food and Fluids. The doctor will leave specific directions concerning the length of time during which food and fluids are to be omitted preoperatively. Usually, midnight preceding surgery is specified as the time for terminating food and fluids. Before this time the patient should be encouraged to eat and drink in order to maintain fluid and electrolyte regulation and to provide nutrients necessary for wound healing. Protein and ascorbic acid (vitamin C) are especially important in promoting wound healing. Except in emergencies, a patient whose nutrition is poor usually has surgery deferred until deficiencies of food, fluids or electrolytes can be corrected. Parenteral administration may be necessary if the patient is unable to take a sufficient amount of oral fluids.

Care of Valuables. Attention is given to the care of valuables on admission. Sometimes, despite these measures, the nurse finds that the patient has valuable jewelry or documents with him on the morning of the operation. It is the policy in most hospitals that valuables be placed in the hospital safe before the patient goes to surgery. It is important to always chart what has been done with valuables (such as depositing them in the safe). You may not be working when the patient asks for them, but if you have written the information on the patient's chart, another nurse can locate them readily.

Nails and Hair. Details of personal grooming, such as trimming the nails and shaving, should be completed before surgery. Women are asked to remove bobby pins or any metal or plastic objects in the hair as these might cause injury if the patient is restless during or immediately after surgery. A special cap covering the hair is usually placed on the patient's head, either in the operating room or just before the patient leaves his room.

Attire. The patient is given a clean hospital

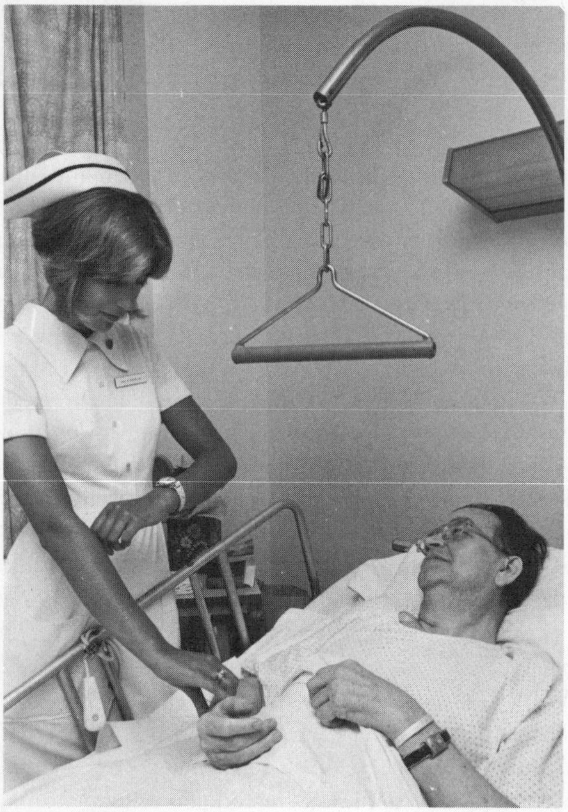

figure 9-3. The blood pressure of the surgical patient is taken prior to the administration of narcotics. (Photograph —D. Atkinson)

gown; personal clothing is not worn in the operating room.

PROSTHESES. In most hospitals the patient is asked to remove dentures, so that they will not become dislodged and cause respiratory obstruction during the administration of anesthesia. However, some anesthetists prefer that well-fitting dentures be left in to preserve the contours of the face. Acquaint yourself with the policy at your hospital. If dentures are to be removed, the patient should be tactfully asked if he has any. If he does, he should be given an opaque denture jar; then, unless he needs help, he can be left alone for a few minutes while he removes and cleans them and places them in the jar. In most hospitals the denture jar is left in the patient's bedside stand until he returns to the ward. Other prostheses, such as eyes or limbs, must be removed before surgery.

MOUTH CARE. All patients should have thorough mouth care before surgery; a clean mouth makes them more comfortable and prevents the aspiration of particles of food that may be left in the mouth. Chewing gum is not permitted, since it, too, could be aspirated.

MAKEUP AND JEWELRY. Because the anesthetist carefully watches the color of face, lips and nailbeds for cyanosis during surgery, patients are asked to remove their makeup. Jewelry should be removed for safekeeping; a valuable ring might slip off the finger of an unconscious patient and be lost. If the patient is reluctant to remove a wedding band, it may be tied to the wrist with a piece of gauze; the gauze is slipped under the ring, then looped around the finger and wrist. Care should be taken to avoid tying it tightly enough to impair circulation.

TRANSPORTATION OF THE PATIENT TO THE OPERATING ROOM

When it is time for the patient to go to the operating room, he is placed on a stretcher and covered with cotton blankets. All necessary information should be recorded on the chart before the patient leaves his room: medications, T.P.R., voiding, disposition of valuables and dentures, and pertinent observations concerning the patient's condition. The chart and x-ray films are taken to the operating room with the patient. The blood pressure is taken and recorded by the nurse before the patient goes to the operating room; it is helpful to have a record of the patient's preoperative blood pressure so that it can be compared with blood pressure readings during surgery. The blood pressure should be taken before narcotics are administered, since they may lower the blood pressure (Fig. 9-3). Always check the patient's identification bracelet before taking him to the operating room to be sure the right patient is being taken for surgery.

CHECKLIST FOR PREOPERATIVE CARE

Here are a few hints on organizing preoperative care. Some hospitals put a checklist or reminder sheet on the front of the chart of each preoperative patient.

A. General goals for the whole preoperative period
   1. Emotional support
   2. Instruction
   3. Spiritual needs; visit from clergyman
   4. Planning with family; teaching family
B. The afternoon before surgery
   1. Check preoperative orders carefully; note orders for enemas, catheterization, medications, and any other procedures that are to be carried out preoperatively

2. Have patient sign consent
3. Prepare skin of operative area
4. Safeguard valuables
5. Give sedative, if ordered, to promote sleep
6. Withhold food and fluids as ordered (usually after midnight)
7. Make certain that all specimens requested have been collected (urine, blood)

C. The morning of surgery
1. Take and record, T.P.R., B.P.
2. Assist the patient with personal hygiene as necessary
3. Help the patient to dress for the operating room
4. Remove prostheses (including dentures, if it is hospital policy that they be removed)
5. Administer preoperative narcotic, as ordered
6. Have patient void
7. Leave patient resting in bed, with call bell handy
8. Make certain that all charting is complete

These measures cannot and should not always be carried out in this order. *The needs of each individual patient are more important than any routine.*

The postoperative phase

Postoperative nursing care involves intensive nursing designed to:

- Prevent and detect complications
- Protect the patient from injury during this period of helplessness
- Relieve discomfort, pain
- Help the patient to regain independence

Factors such as age of patient, nutritional status, or disease conditions requiring more intensive therapy will affect the duration of the postoperative period. The kind of surgery will have a bearing on how long the patient will require continuous surveillance beyond the immediate postanesthetic period.

During the immediate postoperative period, the patient is in the recovery room or an intensive care unit. These are rooms specially designed for the care of the patient requiring close observation and prompt care in the event of a sudden complication. Patients going to the intensive care unit are sent there because the doctor anticipates a more prolonged stay (over 24 hours) while patients in the recovery room usually stay just long enough to recover from the anesthetic.

Postanesthesia recovery

The recovery room (P.A.R. or R.R.) usually has accommodations for a group of patients to be under the continual surveillance of highly skilled personnel. Equipment is available for immediate use in case of need. Recordings of vital signs are made at frequent intervals and the progress of recovery from the anesthetic is charted on the patient's bedside record.

As a general rule, the endotracheal tube is removed by the anesthesiologist before the patient leaves the surgical suite. A complication which can arise during this critical time is laryngospasm. The natural respiratory response to noxious gases is a forced expiratory grunt as the thoracic and abdominal muscles tense into a protective shield. Too light a plane of anesthesia allows this protective reflex to narrow the laryngeal space, resulting in high-pitched inspiratory stridor, or a "crowing" sound. This condition requires that the patient be assisted with respiration manually, along with being supplied a slightly higher oxygen content than ordinary air. An oropharyngeal airway is inserted to prevent the tongue from obstructing the air passage during this phase of the patient's recovery from anesthesia. This airway is left in position until the patient begins to regain consciousness, giving evidence of the return of the swallowing and cough reflexes. Even then, the patient is so positioned that vomitus or secretions will not be aspirated into the tracheobronchial passages. If necessary, suction is used to promptly remove vomitus and secretions so that the patient will not aspirate them.

When the patient is fully reacted and there is no evidence of complications, he is prepared to return to the nursing unit. The length of time varies, but an average duration of the postanesthetic period may range from ½ hour to 2 or more hours. If the surgery is of such a nature that intensive nursing care is required, the patient may be sent to the intensive care unit. In this unit, similar measures are taken as in the recovery room to foresee and prevent critical complications.

The chief responsibilities of the nurse during the *immediate* postoperative recovery period are (1) to assure a patent airway, (2) to help maintain adequate circulation, (3) to prevent and/or treat shock, and (4) to attend to proper positioning and the function of drains, tubes and intravenous infusions.

Positioning the patient is an important measure in preventing interference with circulation; normal body alignment should be maintained. Precautions are taken to prevent displacement of the infusion needle because maintenance of the infusion is important to adequate circulatory function.

Nursing care and observation are important after spinal anesthesia, although the fact that the patient does not lose consciousness simplifies some aspects of postoperative care. Even though the patient is conscious, it is important to remember that he usually has had medications that make him sleepy. Side rails should be in place and the call bell handy.

At first the patient's lower extremities will feel numb and heavy. Even though an explanation of this feeling was made before surgery, it is important for the nurse to repeat the explanation that numbness is usual and will subside in a short time. Many patients become apprehensive because of this symptom, and fear that the anesthesia has resulted in paralysis of their legs.

The patient usually is kept flat in bed for 6 to 12 hours after the surgery. Unless the doctor has ordered otherwise, he may be turned from side to side. As the anesthesia wears off, he will begin to have sensation in the anesthetized parts. Often he describes this as "pins and needles." He also will begin to experience pain in the operated area; analgesics usually are ordered to relieve the pain. Those patients who develop headache may have to remain flat for a longer period. There has been so much discussion about "spinal headache" that patients sometimes think it an inevitable sequel to spinal anesthesia. Remember not to contribute to this impression by the power of suggestion. A statement like "I'll keep your bed flat so you can doze" is preferable to "I'll keep the bed flat so you won't get a headache."

Postsurgical shock due to blood loss, fluid shifts, and neurogenic factors is usually mild and amenable to therapy. Intravenous fluids are regulated to prevent overhydration but are specified in amount and rate of flow to treat dehydration. The kind and specific amount of intake for fluids and blood depends on the patient's requirements and the kind of surgery performed. The rate of flow is carefully determined at the start and checked frequently to keep the flow at the number of drops per minute ordered by the physician. Medication for pain relief or sedation is ordered by the surgeon. The recovery room nurse exercises judgment in administering the first postoperative medication. Judgments in this matter are based on knowledge of the drugs used for anesthesia and their effect on the action of drugs used for pain relief. The physician is guided by these considerations when ordering analgesics for postoperative patients. The pattern of the vital signs gives the nurse a clue to the degree of shock and the value of judiciously administered sedation for control of the autonomic nervous system, which regulates many of the reflex mechanisms involved in shock.

The number and kind of drains and tubes vary with the surgical procedure. The nurse determines the adequacy of drainage so that when drains are not functioning properly, measures may be instituted to correct the malfunction. In order to prevent further complications and delayed healing, indwelling drains must be kept in proper position and in working order. Catheters and tubes must be checked to prevent kinking or clogging that interferes with adequate drainage of urine or bile. Calm, patient and, if necessary, repeated explanations will be required to help the patient understand the purpose of these drains and tubes. This is much more difficult to do in the postoperative period if adequate explanation has not been included in the preoperative instruction.

Intravenous fluids are usually administered throughout the operation and into the recovery phase until the patient's blood pressure is stabilized. This is a routine precaution that is desirable in the event of sudden reaction which might precipitate shock. Maintenance of adequate circulation is essential for prompt treatment of vascular collapse even in a mild form. If the surgical procedure is a major one, fluids are needed to maintain nutritional status until the patient is able to resume oral nourishment.

Postoperative nursing management

THE MANAGEMENT OF PAIN

Because a certain amount of pain is expected after surgery, the doctor will leave orders for analgesics so that the patient will be as comfortable as possible. The most severe pain occurs during the first 48 hours. Pain arouses varying degrees of anxiety in different people. Some take it in stride; others greatly fear it, and their tenseness and fear increase the pain. Intense pain can also cause shock.

It is the responsibility of the nurse to evaluate the need of the patient for the narcotic. Usually the medication, such as morphine or meperidine (Demerol), can be repeated at 3- to 4-hour intervals. In no aspect of nursing is sound judgment more vital than in the administration of narcotics to postoperative patients. What at first appears a simple procedure (he has pain; you give the drug) is really a complex one.

Here are some factors that must be considered before administering the narcotic:

- Narcotics are not without side effects. For example, morphine as well as other narcotics may depress respirations; meperidine (Demerol) can cause hypotension.
- Consider the timing of narcotics in relation to getting the patient out of bed. It is sometimes unwise to get a patient up shortly after he has had a narcotic, because he is more likely to feel dizzy and faint. However, the timing of narcotics in relation to ambulation is a matter requiring astute judgment. Some patients require medication for the relief of pain before they can tolerate the additional discomfort entailed in getting up. In such instances it is usually wise to allow the patient to rest in bed for about an hour after administering the medicine to permit some relaxation, and then, when assisting him out of bed, perhaps to have the assistance of a second person in case the patient should become faint or dizzy.
- If narcotics are continued for prolonged periods, the danger of addiction arises. However, their use during the early postoperative period usually does not cause addiction.
- Have nursing measures been tried to relieve the pain? Sometimes pain in the operative site is intensified because the patient has minor physical discomforts. Along with the administration of a narcotic, the nurse should try simple comfort measures such as a change of position, use of a small pillow for support for the back or shoulders, or massaging areas subject to pressure such as the elbows and hips. These nursing actions may also enhance the effect of the narcotic. A comfortable patient can rest and receive the full benefit of the medication without being disturbed for nursing routines.
- Never give a narcotic to a patient whose blood pressure is low and unstable without first consulting the physician. If shock is imminent, administration of a narcotic can precipitate it.
- Usually it is advisable to wait until the patient has reacted fully from anesthesia before giving a narcotic. While he may mumble about pain, he often is not fully aware of it until he opens his eyes and knows where he is. The patient's condition and recovery from anesthesia can be evaluated more accurately if the medication is withheld until he has reacted.
- The purpose of the medication is to relieve pain, not to render the patient stuporous. Oversedation makes it impossible for the patient to practice such preventive measures as deep breathing and coughing.
- Morphine depresses respirations. Withhold it and consult the doctor if the patient's respirations are fewer than 12 per minute.
- Narcotics and sedatives should be given with special caution to older people, because they have a tendency to become restless and disoriented as a result of the medication.
- When giving medicine for the relief of pain, take advantage of its psychological as well as its physiological effect. All medicines convey some psychological meaning, along with their physiological action. For example, do not rush in and give an intramuscular injection of meperidine, saying only, "Turn over." The patient may also be receiving penicillin or neostigmine (Prostigmin) as part of his therapy, and he may think that nothing has been done to relieve his pain. You might say, "I'm going to give you some medicine to lessen the pain. In a few minutes you'll find it will be much less severe. Maybe you can doze off for a while."
- Give the medication promptly when it is required. Minutes seem like hours to patients who are in severe pain.
- Determine whether the pain is incisional pain, for which the narcotic is ordered, or whether it stems from another source. It is not enough to know that the patient has pain. Find out *where* the pain is. If he had abdominal surgery and the pain is in his chest, do not give the narcotic. Call the doctor instead, so that he can determine the cause of the pain.
- Most patients do not require frequent administration of narcotics after the third postoperative day. At this time the physician may

either decrease the dose of the drug or increase the time interval between injections, e.g., from q4h to q6h. Another alternative is to order a less potent analgesic. There is no set time limit with regard to how long after surgery narcotics will be needed, as much depends on the type and extent of surgery and the patient. If the patient continues to complain of pain after the dose, the drug, or the time interval has been changed, the physician should be notified. Perhaps a complication like wound infection is developing. Or perhaps the patient is beginning to rely on the drug to relieve worry and anxiety rather than pain. This tendency should be noted early, because it can lead to addiction.

Exercises in the early postoperative period also can increase the patient's pain. Assisting the postoperative patient to carry out measures to forestall complications and discomforts requires a great deal of tact, patience, and skill. It is all very well to say that the patient must turn, cough, and take deep breaths. Persuading him to do these thing when they cause him considerable apprehension and pain is not so easy.

Oral fluids and diet

Regardless of how much intravenous fluid the patient is receiving, nothing soothes his parched, dry mouth and throat like cool liquids that he can swallow.

Table 9-1.
Schedule for postoperative exercises

Time	Nursing Action
12 noon	narcotic analgesic administered
12:45 1:45 2:45	deep-breathing and coughing exercises
4:30	narcotic analgesic administered
5:30 6:30 7:15	deep-breathing and coughing exercises
8:45	narcotic analgesic administered

The deep-breathing and coughing exercises were performed 6 times during the 8-hour period, and were planned according to the analgesic effects of the narcotic.

Patients usually ask for water almost as soon as they begin to complain of pain in the incision. Several important points must be considered, though, before the patient is given fluids by mouth:

- Check to make sure that the doctor's order indicates that fluids may be given postoperatively. Sometimes the order reads, "Food and fluid as tolerated." At other times it may say, "Nothing by mouth."

  If the patient is not allowed oral fluids, rinsing his mouth and placing a cool, wet cloth or some ice chips against his lips will help to relieve the feeling of dryness.
- Make certain that the patient has recovered sufficiently from anesthesia to be able to swallow. Ask him to try swallowing without drinking anything. If he can, give him a small sip of water.
- Give only a few sips at a time. Fluids should be introduced slowly and given in small amounts; otherwise vomiting may occur. Give fluids through a straw rather than directly from the glass, so that the patient does not have to sit up. If the patient vomits, assure him matter-of-factly that he will be able to retain fluids later. Offer him mouthwash to help to get rid of the taste of anesthetics and of vomitus, and make sure that he is kept dry and clean. Try not to make him feel that the vomiting was a great calamity, or that it is likely to continue for a long time.

Coughing, deep-breathing, and leg exercises

Coughing and deep breathing help remove secretions from the lungs and bronchi. Usually ordered every 1 to 2 hours, these exercises are essential if postoperative respiratory complications are to be prevented. Coughing will usually place a strain on an incision, especially if the surgery was in the chest or abdomen. Using a pillow or the hand to give support to the incision may eliminate some of the discomfort experienced when the patient is coughing. Also of value is the administration of a narcotic followed in 45 minutes to 1 hour by deep breathing and coughing exercises. The nurse can time these exercises during the early postoperative period as shown in Table 9-1.

Intermittent positive pressure breathing (IPPB) may be ordered two to six times per day. This procedure delivers air or oxygen into the lungs and removes carbon dioxide. It may also be used to administer medications, by the aerosol method, into the lungs. IPPB is particularly effective for those who cannot or will not deep breathe after surgery. Pain associated with coughing that usually follows the procedure may cause a patient to be uncooperative and to refuse the treatment. It then becomes essential that the nurse *stress* the importance of the procedure and try to gain the patient's cooperation.

Leg exercises are usually ordered for the surgical patient in an effort to prevent the formation of a thrombus. Unless the physician leaves orders to the contrary, postoperative patients should begin to move their legs as soon as consciousness returns. These exercises are not complicated; they can be taught readily by the nurse during the preoperative period and then reviewed with the patient postoperatively. Instruct the patient to move his toes and feet, alternately flexing and extending them. Then have him flex and extend his legs by bending his knees and then straightening his legs. These exercises should be repeated regularly. It is much more effective to advise the patient, "Exercise each leg the way I have shown you 10 times every hour," than to say, "Move your legs as much as you can." Remind the patient to exercise each time that you check vital signs. If he is still sleepy from anesthesia, he cannot be expected to remember to do exercises.

Early ambulation

The term *early ambulation* is widely used to describe one aspect of postoperative treatment. *Ambulation* means walking. The patient is helped to walk about early in his postoperative period.

Help the patient to a sitting position at the side of the bed. If dizziness is *more than* momentary, help him to lie down again. If the height of the bed can be adjusted, place it in the lowest position possible. If this type of bed is not available, use a footstool. While you support the patient firmly, let him step to the floor and take one or two steps to a chair.

Exercise and erect posture help the patient to breathe more deeply, and the change of position helps to prevent congestion of the lungs with fluid. Walking stimulates circulation in the lower extremities, thus lessening the problem of venous stasis. Erect posture and exercise also help to overcome problems of urinary retention, constipation, and distention. Early ambulation helps patients to regain their appetites, and greater activity during the day helps them to sleep better at night. Several important points are:

- Early ambulation is a therapeutic measure. Its primary purpose is to prevent complications.
- Ambulation means walking, not sitting. Frequently the treatment is misunderstood to mean just getting out of bed, and the patient is assisted to a chair in the morning, where he sits until evening! Prolonged sitting, by putting pressure on the legs, may predispose a patient to thrombophlebitis. The patient should sit for short periods, take frequent short walks, and alternate these with resting in bed.
- Walking soon after surgery often causes the patient pain and apprehension. He needs a great deal of explanation about the purpose of the treatment, so that he does not consider it merely a lack of attention or concern for his comfort.
- Special equipment, like catheters and infusion bottles, need not restrict the patient to bed. However, their management does require some ingenuity, so that the treatment may be continued safely and effectively while the patient is out of bed.
- Having plenty of assistance will add greatly to the patient's confidence, as well as ensure his safety. Don't hesitate to ask another nurse to help, particularly if it is the patient's first time out of bed, or if the patient is aged.
- Early ambulation helps the patient to feel less helpless, and it tells him that he is recovering quickly and satisfactorily from his operation. One of the dangers of early ambulation is this same confidence. Because patients look more self-sufficient, they themselves may be misled into taking on too much activity too soon.

Visitors

The patient's relatives usually feel less worried when they are kept informed of the patient's condition, given opportunities to express their interest and concern, and allowed to participate, when possible, in the patient's care.

Seeing the patient, if only for a few moments, often does a great deal to assure a relative that the patient really is all right—that he actually has come through the operation. Careful explanation of what to expect (for example, that the patient is drowsy or confused, or that he is receiving intravenous fluids) is essential in lessening apprehension. A brief visit from a relative just after surgery often assures the patient that his family is there, and that they are concerned about him.

It is important to keep family members informed of the patient's condition and of the time that he returns to his own room. Some hospitals provide a visitors' lounge adjacent to the area of the operating room and the recovery room. Opportunities for contact with the staff are fostered by such an arrangement because of its convenience to all concerned. If the surgeons and the nurses know that family members are nearby, they can more easily stop to speak to them. The provision of such areas for the family conveys concern for them as well as for the patient. Such an arrangement is in marked contrast with the still prevalent practice of providing no particular place for the families of patients to wait during the surgery and recovery period. Especially in multiple-bed rooms the presence of the family over an extended period can be disturbing to the other patients.

It is sometimes possible and desirable to allow a responsible member of the family to sit quietly beside the patient during the early postoperative period. Having a member of the family near is especially helpful if the patient is aged or extremely apprehensive, or if he is unable to speak English.

Possible postoperative complications

The first 24 hours after the surgery require alert attention to prevent the possible occurrence of four important complications of the immediate postoperative period: hemorrhage, shock, hypoxia, and vomiting. The patient may have been moved from the recovery room so that each member of the nursing team must be alert to the signs of change that result from or point to these complications.

Hemorrhage

Hemorrhage can be internal or external. If a large amount of blood is lost, there will be signs of shock: fall in blood pressure, weak and rapid pulse, pallor, increased respiratory rate, restlessness, and cool moist skin. The amount of blood lost need not be great enough to produce symptoms of shock in order to cause serious complications. For example, after thyroidectomy, a small amount of blood seeping from a capillary may be sufficient to compress the trachea, resulting in respiratory difficulty.

Dressings must be inspected regularly for any sign of bleeding. Also the bedding and the dressing under the patient are inspected, because blood may pool under the patient's body and be more evident under him than on his dressing. In such an eventuality it may be necessary for the patient to be taken back to the operating room for ligation of bleeding vessels. Blood transfusions may be ordered to replace the blood lost.

When reporting bleeding, always note the color of the blood. Bright red blood signifies fresh bleeding. Dark, brownish blood indicates that the bleeding is not fresh. When the patient is first transferred to your care, it is important to find out whether drains have been inserted and what type of drainage is expected. If you know that a drain is in place, you will not be surprised when brownish-red drainage appears on a dressing. Dressings that become soiled may be reinforced, but they never should be changed except at the direction of the surgeon. If drainage is to be expected, the patient should be told that the drainage is a normal consequence of the surgery and does not indicate any complications.

The color and the amount of any drainage should be reported accurately on the patient's chart.

Shock

The loss of fluids and electrolytes, trauma (both physical and psychological), anesthetics, and preoperative medications may all play a part in precipitating shock. The symptoms include pallor, fall in blood pressure, rapid, weak pulse, restlessness, and cold, moist skin. Narcotics should never be administered to a patient in shock or to one in whom shock seems imminent, unless the patient's condition has been evaluated by the doctor and he expressly orders that the medication be given. Narcotics given to a patient in shock may not be absorbed, due to the decreased volume of the circulating blood. As the patient recovers from shock and the circulation improves, several doses of the narcotic may be absorbed at once, resulting in an overdose. Narcotics may precipitate shock in patients in whom this complication is imminent.

The patient in shock should be kept flat unless the physician orders otherwise. Some physicians advocate elevation of the legs to enhance the flow of venous blood to the heart.

Patients in shock are placed with their heads lower than their feet. Patients who have had brain surgery or spinal anesthesia should be kept flat; for these patients the foot of the bed should not be elevated. (The spinal anesthetic might travel upward and paralyze the diaphragm; placing the head lower than the rest of the body following brain surgery may increase cerebral edema.)

The treatment of shock includes the administration of whole blood, other parenteral fluids, such as plasma expanders, and drugs that help to raise blood pressure. Medications are usually administered intravenously to patients who are in shock.

Hypoxia

Hypoxia may complicate postoperative recovery. Sometimes anesthetics and preoperative medications depress respirations, thus interfering with oxygenation of the blood. Because mucus may block tracheal or bronchial passages and interfere with breathing, the amount of oxygen entering the lungs may be lowered. Oxygen and suction equipment always should be ready for emergency use, and the patient should be watched carefully for cyanosis and dyspnea. If breathing is obstructed because the tongue has fallen back and obstructed the nasopharynx, the lower jaw is pulled forward and an oropharyngeal airway inserted (Fig. 9-4). This type of obstruction can also be relieved by turning the patient on his side.

Other factors, such as residual effect or overdose of drugs, pain, poor positioning causing pressure, a pooling of secretions in the lungs, or an obstructed airway also predispose to hypoxia. Restlessness, crowing or grunting, respiratory efforts, perspiration, bounding pulse, and rising blood pressure should arouse suspicion of embarrassed respiration.

When indicated, positive pressure ventilation is applied by the use of a mechanical respirator. Any one of several types may be used. Many hospitals have the advantage of inhalation therapy services. Personnel in these services are specially trained to take care of the equipment and to assist with this important aspect of care.

Vomiting

If vomiting is severe or prolonged, oral feedings are discontinued temporarily, the patient is fed intravenously, and a nasogastric tube is inserted and connected to suction. Most patients can begin to take food and fluids a few hours after surgery, unless it has involved the gastrointestinal tract. The nurse's own attitude is important. Never suggest to the patient that he will vomit after surgery. The skillful nurse keeps an emesis basin nearby but not prominently displayed during the postoperative period.

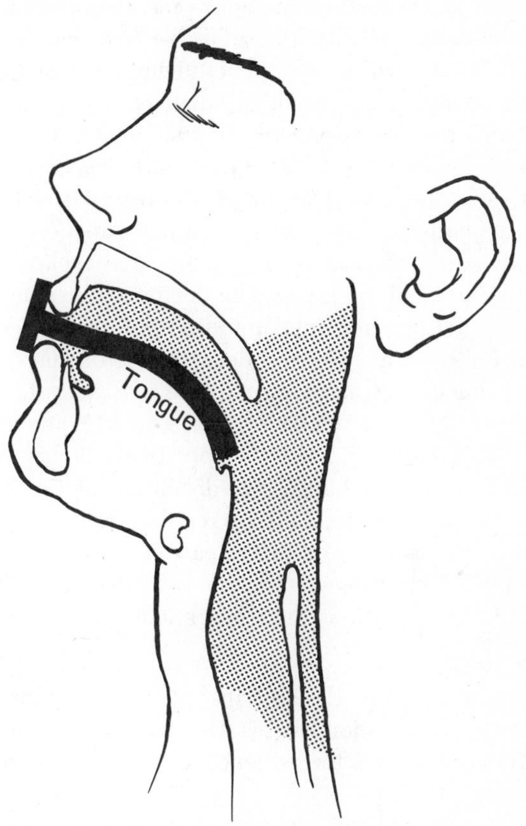

figure 9-4. An oropharyngeal airway in place. Note how the airway prevents the tongue of the unconscious patient from blocking the air passages. As long as the airway is unobstructed and in place, there is a free route for air between the pharynx and the outside.

Urinary retention

Patients who have had abdominal surgery, particularly if it has been in the lower abdominal and pelvic regions, often have difficulty voiding after surgery. Operative trauma in the region near the bladder may temporarily decrease the patient's sensation of needing to void. The fear of pain also causes tenseness and difficulty in voiding. The discomfort and the lack of privacy associated with using the bedpan may play a part. Position is very important. Many women cannot void lying down, but they can void if allowed to sit up. Men often have difficulty voiding when recumbent, but they can void normally if permitted to use the urinal while standing at the bedside.

Those patients having major surgery on or near the bladder almost always have a retention catheter inserted. If a catheter was not inserted, it should be remembered that any surgery—major or minor—on any area of the body can cause difficulty in voiding. Catheterization entails the risk of bladder infection; it should be avoided when simple nursing measures, plus a little patience, can result in adequate voiding.

It is important to record the time and the amount of each voiding for 1 or 2 days after surgery (the length of time that this part of the record should be kept depends on how quickly normal function is resumed). No order is necessary for this record, and usually none will be given. The doctor will expect you to know the patient's intake and output and to record them. Follow any specific orders the doctor may leave concerning the measuring of intake and output.

If the patient is unable to void, 8 to 12 hours is the usual time that is allowed postoperatively before catheterization is considered. Overdistention of the bladder must be avoided, as it makes the patient restless and uncomfortable, and in the case of abdominal surgery puts extra pressure on the operative site. There are several indications that the patient needs to void:

- Restlessness
- Distention of the area just above the pubis. Careful palpation of this area causes discomfort and makes the patient feel that he has to void
- Large intake of oral or parenteral fluid, with no unusual loss of fluid, such as that from prolonged vomiting or profuse sweating

Distention

Abdominal distention results from the accumulation of gas (flatus) in the intestines. It is caused by a failure of the intestines to propel gas through the intestinal tract by peristalsis, and it is aggravated by the tendency of some patients to swallow large quantities of air, especially when they are frightened or in pain. The handling of the intestines during surgery may cause postoperative distention, because the trauma of handling temporarily inhibits normal peristalsis. Contributing factors are immobility following surgery, interruption of the diet necessitated by surgery, and anesthetics and drugs given during or after surgery.

Sometimes, if the symptoms are mild, they can be relieved by nursing measures. If the patient is permitted out of bed, help him to walk about and to go to the toilet. Sometimes walking, plus some privacy in the bathroom, will help expel the gas. Encourage him to eat as normally as possible within the limits specified by the doctor's orders.

If the patient's discomfort is severe, or if it is not relieved promptly by nursing measures, the doctor should be notified. Usually he orders one or several of the following measures:

- Insertion of a rectal tube to dilate the anal sphincter and to release the gas that may have accumulated in the rectum. The tube is inserted as if giving an enema. The bedding, in case some fecal matter is expelled with the flatus, is protected by covering the end of the tube with an absorbent disposable pad. The best results are achieved by leaving the rectal tube in place for about 20 minutes, removing and cleaning it, and then inserting it an hour or so later. The constant presence of the tube both day and night makes the patient uncomfortable and messy, and using it continuously can render it ineffective.
- Use of neostigmine (Prostigmin) intramuscularly to stimulate peristalsis, thus helping the patient to expel gas. The usual dose is 1 ml. of a 1:1,000 or a 1:2,000 solution.

A very serious condition called *paralytic ileus* sometimes occurs. The patient has paralysis of the intestines and thus absence of peristalsis.

Acute gastric dilatation, a condition in which the stomach becomes distended with fluids that do not pass normally through the gastrointestinal tract, is another complication similar to that of paralytic ileus. The patient frequently may regurgitate small amounts of liquid, his abdomen appears distended, and, as the condition progresses, he may develop symptoms of shock. Acute gastric dilatation is treated by passing a nasogastric tube to the patient's stomach, applying suction, and removing the gas and fluid. Some surgeons use suction of the gastrointestinal tract routinely to prevent paralytic ileus and acute gastric dilatation.

Pneumonia and atelectasis

Pneumonia may result from failure to expand the lungs sufficiently, from accumulation of fluid in the lungs, which is favored by lying quietly in one position, and from failure to cough up mucus. Patients with chronic respiratory diseases such as bronchitis and elderly patients whose breathing has become more shallow are especially susceptible to postoperative pulmonary complications. Pneumonia of this type is sometimes called *hypostatic* or *postoperative pneumonia.* It occurs because the condition of the patient's lungs favors infection (any fluid which stagnates in the body tends to become a culture medium for bacteria) rather than because the patient has been exposed to virulent organisms, such as those that often cause pneumonia in healthy people. Because conditions in the patient's own respiratory system offer so little resistance to infection, it may be set up by organisms normally harbored in his mouth and throat, organisms that usually are not harmful.

The symptoms of pneumonia include fever, cough, expectoration of purulent or blood-streaked sputum, dyspnea and malaise. Treatment involves the use of antibiotics, such as penicillin. If a mucus plug should obstruct a bronchial passageway, causing the part of the lung served by that portion of the bronchial tree to fail to expand normally, this condition is called *atelectasis.* (Since unconsciousness and immobility are important predisposing factors, these complications can also develop in nonsurgical patients.)

The nurse should help the postoperative patient maintain conditions in his respiratory tract that help to avoid pneumonia and atelectasis. Specifically, nursing tasks include:

- Suctioning mucus from his nose and mouth while the patient is unconscious.
- Having the patient rid his respiratory tract of mucus by taking deep breaths, coughing, and expectorating mucus.
- Helping him to change his position frequently.

Thrombophlebitis

When patients lie still for long periods without moving their legs, particularly if there is pressure on their legs from a tight strap or a pillow roll under the knee, venous circulation may be impaired. Blood may flow sluggishly through the veins (venous stasis). This condition predisposes a patient to the development of inflammation, with consequent formation of clots within the veins, a condition called *thrombophlebitis.* There is another condition in which clots form, but in which inflammation is minimal or absent. This is called *phlebothrombosis.* These conditions occur most frequently in the legs. Inflammation helps the clots to adhere to the walls of the veins; therefore, thrombophlebitis is considered to be less dangerous than phlebothrombosis.

Clots that do not stick to the wall of the vein but travel in the bloodstream are called *emboli.* By lodging in a distant blood vessel they may obstruct circulation to a vital organ, such as a lung, and cause severe symptoms and even death.

The nurse may help to prevent thrombophlebitis by avoiding prolonged pressure on the patient's legs which might impair circulation and by encouraging leg exercises.

Unless specifically ordered by the surgeon, the use of pillows under the knees or calves is to be avoided. Use of elastic stockings or elastic bandages is considered of value in preventing thrombophlebitis and phlebothrombosis. If elastic bandages are used, they should be removed and reapplied *every 6 to 8 hours.* Elastic stockings should be removed and reapplied once or twice a day (Fig. 9-5, p. 104).

Wound infection

The postoperative patient must be observed carefully for symptoms of wound infection. The first symptom may be increasing pain in the incision. (In normal recovery, pain in the incision decreases.) Other symptoms of wound infection include localized heat, redness, swelling, and purulent exudate. Systemic symptoms of infection include fever, chills, headache, and anorexia.

If there is drainage from the incision, culture and sensitivity studies may be ordered. It may be necessary to place the patient in isolation to prevent the spread of the infection to other patients. The treatment of wound infections involves local and parenteral use of antibiotics, measures to drain pus, if any, and maintenance of the patient's resistance through rest and nutritious diet.

Wound disruption

Dehiscence means the separation of wound edges without the protrusion of organs. *Evisceration* means the separation of wound edges with the protrusion of organs. These complications are most likely to occur between the sixth and the eighth postoperative days, when the sutures hold the wound less firmly, and the wound itself may not yet be strong enough to hold the edges together. Predisposing factors include those that interfere with normal healing, such as malnutrition (particularly insufficient protein and vitamin C), defective suturing, or unusual strain on the wound from severe coughing, sneezing, retching, or hiccuping.

The patient may say that he has a sensation of something "giving way." Pinkish drainage may appear suddenly on the dressing. If you suspect wound disruption has occurred, the patient should be placed at complete rest in a position that puts the least strain on

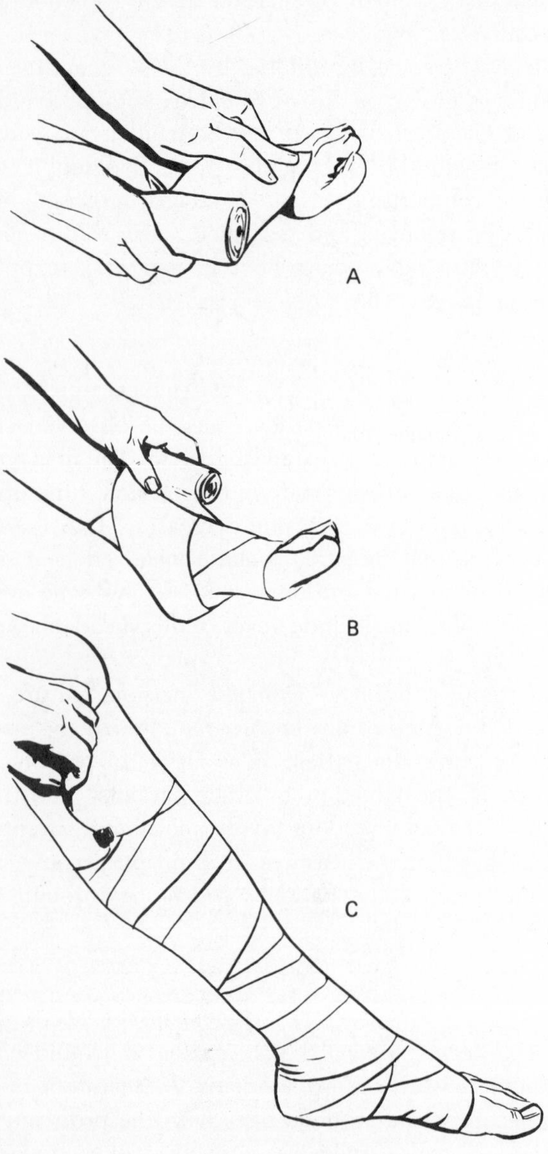

figure 9-5. Steps in applying an elastic bandage. (A) Use 4-inch bandages, starting as close to toes as possible to assure maximal venous return. (B) Anchor bandage around ankle, completely covering heel. (C) Overlap one-half to two-thirds of bandage. Continue wrapping to knee or thigh. Use additional bandages as needed. Secure with fasteners.

the operative area. If evisceration has occurred, place sterile dressings moistened with sterile normal saline over the protruding organs. Report the symptoms immediately. Emotional support and reassurance are as necessary as in any other emergency.

General nutritional considerations

- Food and fluid requirements may be provided by the intravenous route until the patient is able to take oral feedings.
- Anesthesia decreases peristalsis, therefore food and fluids are not given orally until peristalsis returns.
- Depending on the surgery, the physician usually orders a progressive diet: clear liquid diet, full liquid diet, soft diet, regular or house diet.
- Some patients may progress from a liquid to a house diet.
- Vitamins B and C are often added to intravenous feedings as these vitamins aid wound healing.
- Vitamins B and C are water soluble vitamins and are not stored in the body and therefore are given daily.
- Before discharge from the hospital, some surgical patients may require special instructions regarding dietary intake and limitations.

General pharmacological considerations

- Some patients experience acute anxiety before surgery and the physician may prescribe a tranquilizer or sedative during the preoperative period. The nurse should notify the physician if the medication does not appear to be effective.
- The evening before surgery a hypnotic drug may be ordered to ensure rest. The results of the medication should be documented on the patient's chart.
- Medications administered 30 to 45 minutes prior to surgery may include narcotics, sedatives, antiemetics, and a drug to dry respiratory tract secretions.
- Explanation to patients of the effects of the preoperative medication depend on the drug(s) administered but usually include: (1) the drowsiness that will occur and the extreme dryness of the mouth, nose, and throat; and (2) the importance of remaining in bed after the injection has been given.
- Narcotic analgesics should be administered as ordered and as needed. The patient should

not be made to wait for relief of pain providing the established time limit has passed.

- Narcotic analgesics should *not* be administered to a patient in shock or if shock appears imminent without first checking with the physician.
- Morphine and other opiates depress respirations; therefore the respiratory rate is counted *before* these drugs are administered and the medication withheld if the respiratory rate is 10 to 12 or below.

Bibliography

BAKER, B. H.: Medical bacteriology: The "WBC" and "diff." Nurs. Care 6:25, August, 1973.

BALLINGER, W. F. et al.: *Alexander's Care of the Patient in Surgery,* ed. 5. St. Louis, Mosby, 1973.

BILLARS, K. S.: You have pain? I think this will help. Am. J. Nurs. 70:2143, October, 1970.

CODD, J. et al.: Postoperative pulmonary complications. Nurs. Clin. North Am. 10:5, March, 1975.

COLLART, M. E. and BRENNEMAN, J. K.: Preventing postoperative atelectasis. Am. J. Nurs. 71:1982, October, 1971.

CONDON, R. E. and NYHUS, L. M.: *Manual of Surgical Therapeutics,* ed. 2. Boston, Little, Brown, 1975.

DODGE, J. S.: What patients should be told; Patients' and nurses' beliefs. Am. J. Nurs. 72:1852, October, 1972.

HARDY, J. D., ed.: *Rhoads' Textbook of Surgery: Principles and Practice,* ed. 5. Philadelphia, Lippincott, 1976.

HEASTER, P.: Isolation isn't just a technique. J. Prac. Nurs. 75:28, June, 1975.

LAIRD, M.: Techniques for teaching pre- and postoperative patients. Am. J. Nurs. 8:1338, August, 1975.

LEMAITRE, G. and FINNEGAN, J.: *The Patient in Surgery: A Guide for Nurses.* Philadelphia, Saunders, 1975.

METHENY, N. A.: Water and electrolyte balance in the postoperative patient. Nurs. Clin. North Am. 10:49, March, 1975.

RODMAN, M. J. and SMITH, D. W.: *Clinical Pharmacology in Nursing.* Philadelphia, Lippincott, 1974.

SCHERER, J. C.: *Introductory Clinical Pharmacology.* Philadelphia, Lippincott, 1975.

WILLACKER, J.: Bowel sounds. Am. J. Nurs. 73:2100, December, 1973.

WILSON, J. L., ed.: *Handbook of Surgery,* ed. 5. Los Altos, Lange, 1973.

Wound suction—better drainage with fewer problems (pictorial). Nurs. '75, 5:52, October, 1975.

UNIT TWO
Oncologic nursing

- **Care of the patient with cancer**
- **Nursing management in radiotherapy**

CHAPTER—10

Care of the patient with cancer

On completion of this chapter the student will:

- Be able to name the seven warning signs of cancer.
- Discuss some of the factors or situations that may predispose an individual to cancer.
- Discuss the importance of a routine physical examination in the detection of cancer.
- Differentiate and describe malignant and benign tumors.
- Discuss the various methods of diagnosis and treatment of cancer.
- Assess and discuss personal feelings regarding patients with cancer, especially the terminally ill or those with disfiguring surgeries.
- Discuss the emotional impact associated with the diagnosis of cancer.
- Discuss the personal and family problems that may occur when the patient is told he has cancer.
- Discuss the problems involved when the question arises, "should the patient be told he has cancer?"
- Specify ways to help the patient with cancer maintain dignity throughout treatment of his disease.

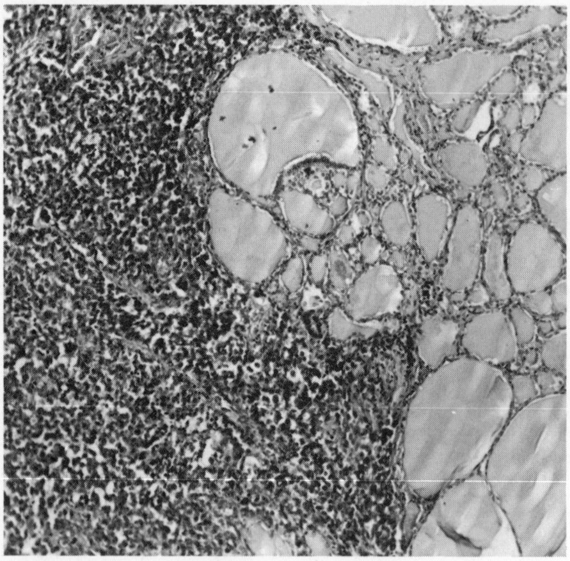

figure 10-1. A microscopic section of thyroid tissue showing normal thyroid cells (*right*) and malignant anaplastic metastatic melanoma (*left*). (Courtesy P. S. Milley, M.D. Photograph—D. Atkinson)

Table 10-1.
Classification of tumor cells

Origin	Malignant	Benign
Skin	squamous cell carcinoma	papilloma
	malignant melanoma	nevus (mole)
Epithelium	adenocarcinoma	adenoma
Muscle	myosarcoma	myoma
Connective Tissue		
fibrous tissue	fibrosarcoma	fibroma
adipose (fatty) tissue	liposarcoma	lipoma
cartilage	chondrosarcoma	chondroma
bone	osteosarcoma	osteoma
Nerve Tissue	neurogenic sarcoma	neuroma
	neuroblastoma	ganglioneuroma
	glioblastoma	glioma
Bone Marrow	multiple myeloma	—
	leukemia	—

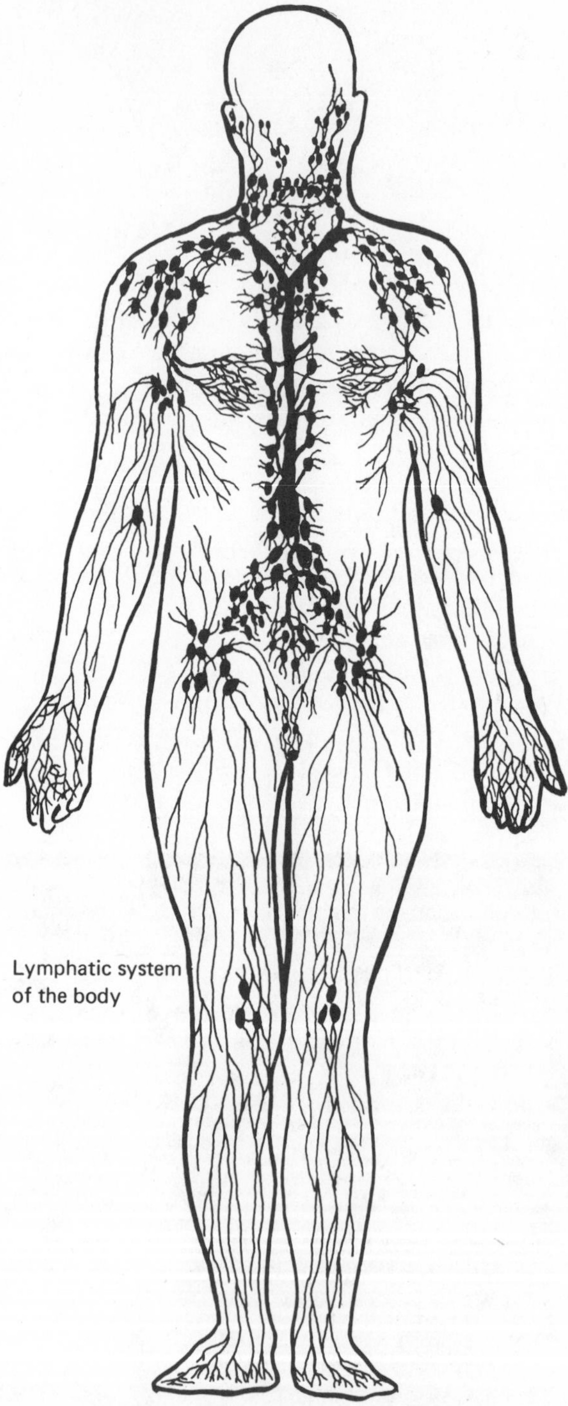

figure 10-2. One route by which malignant cells can spread to other areas of the body is the lymphatic system. Cancer cells can also be carried by the blood.

Pathology and epidemiology

Body cells sometimes undergo changes in their structure and appearance, begin to multiply, and then give rise to a colony of cancer cells (Fig. 10-1). These cells may arise in any part of the body, at any time, and from any cell that can proliferate. They multiply rapidly, invading and destroying surrounding normal tissues by causing pressure and competing with normal cells for nutrients and oxygen. Cancer cells, though changed in appearance, usually retain enough resemblance to the tissues from which they arose to be recognized, if found, in any other part of the body. For example, if a tumor from the neck shows malignant cells arising from breast tissues, it is known to have spread from the breast. Sometimes the secondary tumor is found even before the primary tumor has been discovered.

Although all forms of malignant growth may be referred to as cancer, more specific terms are used to describe particular types of cells that have undergone malignant transformation.

In order to name tumors some knowledge of embryology is necessary. Malignant tumors may arise from any or all three embryonal tissues. When a tumor contains all three embryonal components it is referred to as a teratoma.

The embryonal tissues are as follows:

- Ectoderm—outer layer of the embryo—which produces the skin and the nervous system.
- Mesoderm—middle layer of the embryo—which produces bones, cartilage, muscle, fat, blood, and all other connective tissues.
- Endoderm—inner layer of the embryo—which produces the linings of the gastrointestinal tract, respiratory system, spleen, liver, etc.

It is customary to name tumors after the types of tissues from which they arise. Some examples of names of tumors which relate to types of tissue are given in Table 10-1.

Malignant tumors differ from benign tumors in several ways (Table 10-2). Benign tumors are usually encapsulated while malignant tumors tend to infiltrate surrounding tissues and even metastasize. Cancer is known to spread to the lymph nodes that drain the tumor area. For this reason a lymph node dissection is often performed in addition to wide excision of the tumor (Fig. 10-2).

Cancer can spread by:

- Direct extension to adjacent tissues.
- Extension from lymph vessels into the tissues which lie alongside lymphatic vessels.
- Being carried in the stream of lymph or blood, often to distant sites (embolism).
- Diffusion within a body cavity.

The area in which malignant cells first arise is called the primary site. The regions of the body to which cancer cells are spread are termed secondary or metastatic sites. The metastasis phenomenon is one of

Table 10-2.
Characteristics of malignant and benign tumors

Malignant	Benign
1. Grow rapidly	1. Grow slowly
2. Rarely enclosed in a capsule (encapsulated)	2. Almost always enclosed in a capsule
3. Infiltrate surrounding tissues	3. Do not infiltrate surrounding tissues
4. Spread from original site by metastasis	4. Remain localized
5. May recur after removed	5. Usually no recurrence after removal
6. Harmful to host	6. Usually not harmful to host
7. Prognosis depends on the type and location of the tumor, speed of diagnosis, presence or absence of metastasis	7. Prognosis almost always good*

* The exception may be the presence of a benign tumor causing compression of a vital organ, for example, a benign brain tumor.

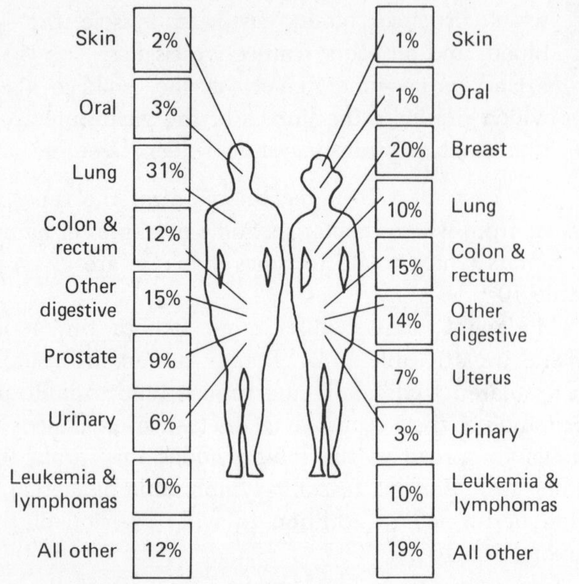

figure 10-3. Cancer deaths by site and sex. (The American Cancer Society: Cancer Facts and Figures, 1974)

the most discouraging characteristics of cancer as even one malignant cell can start a metastatic lesion in a distant part of the body. Today, these metastases are treated aggressively and, as a result, there are now more long-term survivors. The importance of good follow-up care with an interval history and physical examination must be emphasized to the patient and his family.

Benign tumors remain at the original site of their development. They may grow larger, but their rate of growth is slower than that of malignant tumors. Benign tumors usually do not cause death unless their location impairs the function of a vital organ. On the other hand, malignant tumors grow rapidly and unless they are completely removed before metastasis has occurred they are likely to spread.

Etiology

So far the cause of cancer has not been determined. Early detection is stressed but not enough emphasis is being placed upon the prevention of cancer which in some instances is possible.

Cancer is a category of diseases which are characterized by the spread of malignant cells. There is question about whether one cause or a combination of causes is responsible for the development of cancer. Research relating the incidence of cancer to possible causative factors is being carried out.

Environmental and social factors strongly influence the incidence of some types of cancer (Fig. 10-3). Skin cancers, the most common, are often induced by prolonged exposure to sunlight. Fortunately, such cancers are easy to detect and are highly curable. Physical agents such as x-rays and gamma radiations are well established causes of squamous cell and bone sarcomas. Chemicals have been known to produce skin cancers in industrial workers. The inhalation of cigarette smoke over a period of many years has been implicated as a major cause of lung, pharyngeal, oral, and laryngeal cancers.

Some factors are thought to predispose the individual to cancer. Leukoplakia of the mouth or genitals, for instance, may remain benign or undergo malignant change, and should be removed when feasible.

It is thought that cancer occurs only when a certain combination of factors favors its development. These factors may include heredity, hormonal state, and exposure to carcinogens. In addition to efforts to find the causes of cancer, attempts are being made to understand factors that affect host resistance in the hope that susceptibility to the development of cancer can be decreased.

Symptoms

Cancer is an insidious disease that tends to develop slowly and with few or no early symptoms. Every effort must be made to discover it in its earliest stage, which facilitates complete removal and a good prognosis.

Everyone should be familiar with the seven warning signals of cancer listed by the American Cancer Society.

- A sore that does not heal
- A lump or thickening in the breast or elsewhere
- Unusual bleeding or discharge
- Any change in a wart or mole
- Persistent indigestion or difficulty in swallowing
- Persistent hoarseness or cough
- Any change in normal bowel habits.

Diagnosis of cancer

The diagnosis of cancer begins with the recognition that the disease may assume many forms and guises. Sometimes the symptoms are so obvious that the patient proclaims the diagnosis himself. At other times the doctor's suspicion is aroused by an apparently minor condition that does not respond to therapy.

A complete regular physical examination is the first weapon in the struggle to discover cancer in its early stages. Every physician's and dentist's office, clinic, and industrial clinic should be a cancer detection center. With effective teamwork the doctor, dentist, nurse, laboratory technician, and others, can make the cancer detection examination a simple, routine, and, sometimes, lifesaving procedure.

Cancer is diagnosed by a combination of methods: (1) a thorough patient history and physical examination, and (2) by special diagnostic studies. A careful history will define the patient's complaints and, on occasion, reveal enough positive findings for the physician to suspect a malignant process. The physical examination may reveal a suspicious growth or the presence of enlarged lymph nodes that may be indicative of metastasis; or it may prove negative. Special diagnostic tests include x-ray examinations, biopsy of the tumor, blood or bone marrow samples, urine specimens, smears, and bronchial washings. The types of tests ordered will depend on the (probable) location of the tumor. In many instances the biopsy is the definitive examination; it nearly always provides differentiation between malignant and nonmalignant (benign) tumor cells. There are times when the pathologist (a specialist in identifying tissue changes) is unable to determine if a section of biopsied tissue is malignant or benign; that is, the cells are "questionable." Depending on the location of the tumor and other factors, the surgeon must decide the extent of surgery.

The patient's reaction to diagnosis

Once a diagnosis of cancer has been confirmed, either by positive studies or biopsy, the question arises: should the patient be told? The woman who has had a breast removed will know, soon after waking from anesthesia, that her breast was removed and the lump must have been malignant. The man who has had a bone marrow aspiration for possible leukemia usually does not know he has cancer immediately after the study was done—he has not experienced any physical change as did the woman with breast cancer.

There are many views as to whether the patient should be told. Most physicians and nurses feel that the patient should know his diagnosis. There are exceptions of course; some patients cannot emotionally accept the diagnosis and others may be too ill to understand. The physician may discuss the problem with the family and the family, for any number of reasons, may ask him not to reveal the diagnosis to the patient. At this time the physician may present the family with the pros and cons of their decision. They should understand that it is often very hard to keep the diagnosis from the patient for an indefinite period of time. If radiation treatments or chemotherapy are the chosen methods of treatment, either in conjunction with or instead of surgery, the patient will probably realize that he has cancer. Nurses must respect the decision of the family or the physician in withholding information, regardless of their own feelings in the matter. Such a decision has usually required much thought and consideration.

Even though research has made notable advancement, the word "cancer" still has a tremendous emotional impact. When the diagnosis is first known, most patients respond with shock, disbelief, fear, anguish, and worry. Their whole world has changed. These feelings may last indefinitely. Eventually, however, many patients decide to face the problem, do all they can to recover, and try to live a normal life. Others may never recover emotionally, and this has been known to affect their physical progress. Sometimes acceptance of the diagnosis and a positive outlook can be fostered by the family, the physician, and the nurse. *How* the patient is told of his disease *is* important. The physician and nurse who show sincere interest and concern may help the patient through this traumatic period.

Treatment

There are three basic methods employed in the treatment of cancer: (1) surgery, (2) radiotherapy, and (3) chemotherapy. These methods may be used alone or in combination; no one is superior to the others, nor will any one method necessarily give better results.

Surgery

Surgery may range from a simple removal of the tumor to extensive surgical excision, which includes removal of the tumor and adjacent structures such as bone, organs, and lymph glands. What and how much is removed depends on the surgeon's judgment. The surgeon will base his decision on the findings of the pathologist, the physical condition of the patient, the results that may be expected, and other factors which vary according to the particular situation. Thus, a lump in the breast may prove to be malignant, requiring removal of the breast. Biopsy of adjacent tissue may show infiltration of cancer cells and the

Table 10-3.
Antineoplastic agents

GENERIC NAME	TRADE NAME	USE
ALKYLATING AGENTS		
busulfan	Myleran	chronic myelocytic leukemia
chlorambucil	Leukeran	chronic lymphocytic leukemia, Hodgkin's disease, other malignant lymphomas
cyclophosphamide	Cytoxan	malignant lymphomas, multiple myeloma, neuroblastoma, ovarian cancer, chronic leukemias
mechlorethamine	Mustargen	Hodgkin's disease, lymphosarcomas, tumors of the breast, ovary, nasopharynx, stomach, uterus, kidney, myelocytic and lymphocytic leukemia
melphalan	Alkeran	multiple myeloma
thiotepa	—	advanced carcinoma of breast, ovary, lung, chronic granulocytic and lymphocytic leukemia, Hodgkin's disease
triethylenemelamine	TEM	Hodgkin's disease, chronic lymphocytic and myelogenous leukemia, lymphosarcoma
uracil mustard	—	chronic lymphocytic and granulocytic leukemia, Hodgkin's disease, lymphosarcoma
ANTIMETABOLITES		
cytarabine	Cytosar	acute leukemias of adults and children, solid tumors, lymphomas, Hodgkin's disease
floxuridine	FUDR	intra-arterial infusions in the palliative management of tumors
fluorouracil	5-FU	palliative treatment of solid tumors not amendable to surgery or radiation
hydroxyurea	Hydrea	melanoma, chronic myelocytic leukemia
mercaptopurine	6-MP Purinethol	acute leukemia
methotrexate	—	choriocarcinoma, palliative treatment of acute leukemia, intra-arterial infusion of solid tumors
procarbazine	Matulane	Hodgkin's disease, treatment of solid tumors
thioguanine	—	acute leukemia, chronic myelocytic leukemia
NATURAL PRODUCTS		
bleomycin	Blenoxane	malignant lymphomas, squamous cell carcinomas, choriocarcinoma, intra-arterially in treatment of otorhinolaryngeal tumors, intrapleurally in the prevention of pleural fluid
dactinomycin	Cosmegen	malignant melanoma, some lymphomas, Wilm's tumor
doxorubicin	Adriamycin	acute lymphoblastic and myeloblastic leukemia, osteogenic sarcoma, ovarian, breast and thyroid carcinoma
mithramycin	Mithracin	malignant testicular tumors
vinblastine	Velban	Hodgkin's disease, other malignant lymphomas, carcinoma of the breast
vincristine	Oncovin	acute leukemia

Modified from Scherer, J. C.: *Introductory Clinical Pharmacology*. Philadelphia, Lippincott, 1975.

surgeon may then perform more extensive surgery, removing lymph nodes in the axilla. Another patient, with the same type of cancer and metastasis may have less extensive surgery because of age or other contributing factors.

An extensive operation may be followed by reconstructive or plastic surgery to cosmetically or functionally correct defects caused by the original surgery. For example, a patient with cancer of the face with removal of part of the nose and cheek may have surgery at a later date to improve the appearance. Or a patient with a colostomy may require revision of the stoma (the opening on the abdomen) to release adhesions and thereby improve function of the colostomy. Not all patients are candidates for reconstructive surgery, especially if tumor growth was not halted or their physical condition is poor and they are unable to tolerate further surgery.

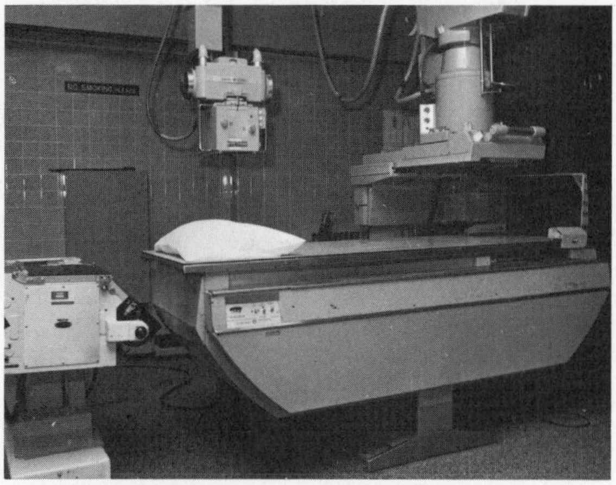

figure 10-4. Superficial and deep x-ray therapy is one method of treating cancer. (Photograph—D. Atkinson)

Radiotherapy

Radiotherapy, or radiation therapy, is the treatment of cancer using x-ray (Fig. 10-4) or radioactive isotopes. *Radiation* is the emission or giving off of rays; *radioactivity* is the ability of a substance to emit alpha, beta, and gamma rays. A concentration of radiation is harmful to living cells, including cancer cells.

Chemotherapy

Chemotherapy, or the use of drugs, is a third method of treating cancer (Table 10-3). Generally, antineoplastic drugs can be divided into (1) alkylating agents, (2) antimetabolites, (3) natural products, (4) hormones and hormonelike agents, and (5) miscellaneous agents. Many of these drugs affect cells that divide at a rapid rate; this includes tumor cells *as well as* some normal body cells such as bone marrow, lymph tissue, and the epithelial cells that line the gastrointestinal tract. Most antineoplastic agents are capable of causing moderate to severe side effects.

Antineoplastic drugs may be given by oral, intramuscular, or intravenous routes. There are specialized methods for delivery of a maximum dose of a drug to an isolated part of the body—the tumor—with minimal amounts reaching other body tissues. This technique is called perfusion and there are various types. Intra-arterial perfusion is the introduction of an antineoplastic drug, under pressure, into an artery that supplies the tumor or organ containing the tumor. Isolated perfusion (Fig. 10-5) is the introduction of an antineoplastic drug to a tumor area after the blood supply is isolated from the rest of the circulation. The

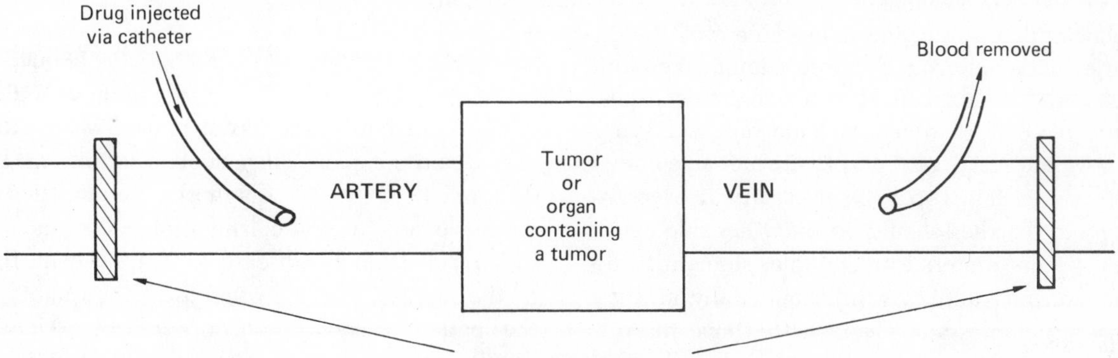

figure 10-5. A schematic representation of the technique of isolated perfusion. The artery and vein leading to and from the tumor are temporarily isolated and the antineoplastic drug is delivered directly to the tumor.

Table 10-4.
Nursing management of the patient receiving chemotherapy

Consult references for the side effects and toxic effects of the drugs administered.

Inspect the oral mucosa daily, using a lightly padded tongue blade and flashlight. Any reddened areas or white spots should be reported. Check lips, especially at the corners, for cracks or open sores.

Give good oral care:

- allow frequent rinses with warm water
- apply a mixture of glycerine and lemon to the lips, if dry; use a mouth wash recommended by the physician if severe oral inflammation occurs.

If stomatitis is apparent, see that the patient has a soft, bland diet.

Encourage nutritional and fluid intake:

- frequent sips of water
- frequent, small feedings of high caloric food.

Report early signs of infection (fever, sore throat, chills), nausea, vomiting, diarrhea.

Change the patient's position frequently.

drug is injected into the isolated artery, it flows through the tumor, and the returning venous blood containing the drug is removed. Surgery may or may not be required for this procedure.

Drugs used in the treatment of cancer have a wide variety of side effects and patients receiving chemotherapy by any route often experience them. Appropriate references should be consulted with regard to the side effects of each agent.

In chemotherapy, nursing management of the patient varies with the drug, the dose administered, and the route used (Table 10-4). Some patients experience little discomfort; others, a wide range of symptoms. Gastrointestinal side effects are not uncommon and intravenous fluids may be necessary if excessive vomiting and diarrhea should occur. Other side effects that may be encountered are fatigue, stomatitis, alopecia, leukopenia, and easy bruising. Many of these drugs have a depressant effect on the bone marrow, thus inhibiting the manufacture of red and white blood cells and platelets. In some instances a profound decrease in these blood components may occur, resulting in anemia, a tendency toward bleeding, and a low white blood cell count. The anemia and bleeding tendencies may be treated with blood transfusions (whole blood, packed cells, or platelets). A decrease in white blood cells decreases resistance to infection, in some cases, the white blood cell count dropping so low that even a minor infection could have a lethal effect. These patients are placed in reverse isolation, with the patient protected from contact with microorganisms. Some hospitals use special isolation rooms (germ free unit, "Life island," laminar air flow room) for those undergoing intensive chemotherapy or who develop seriously low white blood cell counts.

Certain hormones slow the growth of malignant cells by providing a less favorable environment for their growth. For example, men with disseminated prostatic cancer may have symptomatic improvement when the effects of male hormones are counteracted. This counteraction is achieved by the administration of estrogens or by removal of the testes (bilateral orchiectomy).

Corticosteroids are used in the treatment of some forms of acute and chronic leukemia and lymphomas. These drugs have the ability to depress the bone marrow, especially the manufacture of white blood cells. By a mechanism not fully understood, they provide symptomatic relief and for a time the patient looks and feels better. Corticosteroids also reduce elevated serum calcium levels seen in cancers that have metastasized to the bone.

Supportive Therapy. In addition to chemotherapy, surgery, and radiation therapy, the treatment of cancer also includes supportive therapies such as special diets or blood transfusions. There may also be a need for drugs such as analgesics, electrolytes, vitamins, and intravenous fluids.

Nursing the patient with cancer

The nursing needs of the patient with cancer are varied and complex. They depend on his and his family's reactions to the diagnosis, the location of the cancer, consequent impairment of body functions that may result from the disease or its treatment, the stage of the disease, and the prognosis. The quality of care the patient receives not only reflects scientific advances in drug therapy, surgery, and radiotherapy, as well as the availability of equipment; it also reflects the attitudes towards cancer of those who take care of the patient. Most patients with cancer are extremely sensitive and can detect any insecurity or distaste on the part of the nurse. Each staff member's actions and attitudes are important and affect the patient's response to others on the health team. Two guidelines can help the nurse in communicating with the patient, and with other members of the health care team:

- The patient's questions and concerns must not be avoided. He should be allowed to express them without being interrupted or having the subject changed. When a patient has a question the nurse should decide whether it is one which can, and should be, answered. The patient can be helped to find the answer, or referred to the appropriate person with whom to discuss it. For instance explanation of the diagnosis and plan of therapy is the responsibility of the physician.
- It is important to be clear about what others, particularly the physician, have explained to the patient. Ideally such matters should be discussed regularly among all staff. It is unwise to work with any patient without knowing the framework of explanation given to him by the physician. With the cancer patient it is especially necessary that communication be kept open among all who care for the patient. Sensitivity and judgment are required in determining what to tell the patient, in order to promote his comfort and well-being.

Helping the patient maintain dignity is important. Perhaps in no other disease is there such a threat to "wholeness" as exists in cancer. The disease itself and the treatment are often destructive of tissue, and sometimes disfiguring. Some patients who know they have cancer state that they fear the pain or disfigurement or any other specific aspect of the illness not so much as they fear possible overall loss of self-control and dignity during the final stages of the illness. The nurse must not lose sight of this important concern of her patients. The process of physical care is often demanding: tubes to keep patent, skin care, and many other tasks which can tax the resources of the nursing staff. Every effort should be directed towards helping the patient maintain his self-respect. Care in draping during treatments, strict attention to cleanliness, and allowing him to participate in planning his care as long as he is able to do so are all measures to help him maintain his dignity. It is essential for the nurse to aid the patient and his family in recognizing that a diagnosis of cancer is not synonymous with death, to help them make use of available treatment, and to establish a regimen which encourages as full a return to usual activities as possible. The patient who is physically able to continue working is encouraged to do so, as well as to continue his usual home life and recreation. Family members can be helped by professional staff to realize that the patient will benefit (as will those in close association with him) if he is encouraged to live as full a life as possible. Patients who have cancer and who nevertheless continue most of their usual activities have many realistic concerns. The nurse can help by listening, clarifying, and assisting the patient and family to find their own solutions.

More patients are now being cured of cancer, and these patients, too, require assistance from health professionals. Usually it is not certain at the outset whether or not the patient has been cured. A patient with cervical cancer may undergo hysterectomy, and the physician believes all malignant tissue has been removed. Nevertheless, it is of the utmost importance that the patient return regularly to the clinic or to the physician's office for periodic examinations, so that any new evidence of the disease can be promptly detected and treated. Many patients, having been through the ordeal of the diagnosis of cancer and treatments with surgery or radiation, want nothing so much as to forget the experience. A visit to the clinic or physician not only reminds them of the experience, but brings with it suspense and dread concerning what may be found at follow-up examinations. Nurses, especially nurses in public health and industrial settings, can help by encouraging and supporting the patient, by showing understanding and acceptance of the patient's feelings, and also by stressing the necessity for, and the advantages to the patient, of follow-up care. In time, when no new evidence of cancer is found, the patient usually relaxes more, as each favorable report brings greater feelings of security that he is, in fact, cured.

If the patient's disease becomes widespread, certain nursing considerations become especially important. The patient may conjure up dreaded fantasies of agonizing pain and mutilation. Too often his opening and sometimes fumbling comments and questions to express these concerns are met by avoidance or by an overly jolly approach which denies the seriousness of his situation. It is important to consider what the patient says, to assist him in expressing his fears, and to discuss them with him. In doing so, some of the vague, enormous, and very threatening fears can be lessened and made more manageable. The patient who has opportunity to express fear that the pain may later become unbearable can consider, with the nurse and doctor, what is available to relieve his pain, and can receive reassurance from them that they will not desert him—that they will be there, and help him remain as comfortable as possible. It has been observed repeatedly that patients who receive emotional support from the nursing staff and who are in an atmosphere which fosters dignity, self-care to the extent possible, recreation, and companionship, experience less pain. It may help patients to speak of their fear of death, of separation from loved ones, of loss of control, and of mutilation.

It is especially important to observe patients with metastatic cancer for complications. Bleeding or even serious hemorrhage may occur if a blood vessel is eroded by malignant tissue. Infection, manifested by such symptoms as fever and chills, may occur since the tissues undergoing malignant change are vulnerable to infection. Pathologic fractures may result if the patient has metastases to bone. In addition, complications may occur as a result of physical inactivity: thrombophlebitis is an example. Vigilant nursing care is required to prevent complications when possible, and to detect their occurrence promptly.

Prevention and control

EDUCATING THE PUBLIC. Education has encouraged the awareness of warning signals and the willingness to seek diagnosis and treatment. Women are realizing the need to seek early treatment for breast tumor or abnormal vaginal bleeding. Some people have become so fearful of cancer that every symptom, however minor or transient, causes near panic. Such reactions do not indicate less need for public education. On the contrary, this points to the extreme fear that people have of cancer and the need for better information on the ways by which cancer can be controlled and cured. These reactions emphasize the importance of teaching in a manner that does not provoke needless alarm. Patients who refuse to go to doctors or clinics are not necessarily uninterested or even uninformed. People who are very frightened may react with seeming apathy. Their fear of cancer may be so great that they are unable to face examination and the possible discovery that they have cancer.

Besides teaching the seven warning signals of cancer and advising early diagnosis and treatment, nurses can encourage people to avoid practices believed to favor the development of cancer—smoking, excessive exposure to sunlight, and contact with certain types of chemicals. What is most important in public education is promoting the importance of a periodic physical examination. Statistics have proved that early detection of most cancers increases the chances of curing the disease.

General nutritional considerations

- Patients with stomatitis due to the side effects of antineoplastic drugs should be given a soft, bland diet.
- Intake of food and fluids should be encouraged. Many patients develop anorexia due to radiotherapy, chemotherapy, or the course of their disease.
- Some patients may require frequent small feedings rather than three standard meals.
- Adequate fluid intake is necessary to prevent dehydration and electrolyte imbalance. This is especially important in patients with frequent episodes of vomiting.
- Patients who develop diarrhea due to radiotherapy or chemotherapy usually require a bland or low-residue diet.

General pharmacological considerations

- Drugs used in the treatment of cancer—antineoplastic agents—are potentially toxic drugs.
- Nurses should be thoroughly familiar with side effects and toxicity of the antineoplastic agents administered. The dose or length of treatment depends in some cases on the patient's response to this method of therapy.
- Many antineoplastic drugs have a profound effect on the bone marrow. Patients should be observed for signs of bone marrow depression, namely (1) infection: fever, sore throat, chills and (2) bleeding: evidenced by oozing from venipuncture or parenteral drug injection sites, bleeding from the gums, or signs of blood in the urine or stools.
- Intravenous or intra-arterial administration of antineoplastic agents may lead to thrombo-

phlebitis. Sites should be inspected daily for tenderness, pain, swelling, or induration above or below site of use.

- Nausea, vomiting, and diarrhea may be observed during administration of many antineoplastic agents. These side effects must be reported immediately, since dehydration and electrolyte imbalance often occur rapidly. Antiemetic or antidiarrheal drugs or intravenous fluid and electrolyte replacement may be needed.
- Physical side effects such as alopecia and skin pigmentation may be distressing to the patient. A wig, or use of cosmetics to cover mild cases of skin discoloration should be encouraged.
- Patients referred to outpatient clinics for further drug therapy must be encouraged to keep clinic appointments. Therapeutic drug results are often based on specific time intervals between drug administration.
- Patients referred to outpatient clinics should be encouraged to report any and all unusual symptoms or effects experienced at the time of each clinic visit.

Bibliography

American Cancer Society: *A Cancer Source Book for Nurses.* New York, American Cancer Society, 1975.

Bell, M. et al: Care of the patient for cordotomy. J. Neurosurg. Nurs. 5:27, July, 1973.

Bouchard, R. and Owens, N. F.: *Nursing Care of the Cancer Patient.* St. Louis, Mosby, 1972.

Bruya, M. A. and Madiera, N. P.: Stomatitis after chemotherapy. Am. J. Nurs. 75:1349, August, 1975.

Buehler, J. A.: What contributes to hope in the cancer patient, Part 6. Am. J. Nurs. 75:1353, August, 1975.

Copen, P.: The terminal cancer patient. Nurs. Care, 6:27, May, 1973.

Davison, R. L.: Cancer and the nurses' social role. Nurs. Times, 69:601, May 10, 1973.

Herbst, S. F.: A new approach to parenteral drug administration . . . Anderson Hospital, Houston, Texas (pictorial), Part 3. Am. J. Nurs. 75:1345, August, 1975.

Hoffman, E.: "Don't give up on me." Am. J. Nurs. 71:60, January, 1971.

Leitch, W. H.: Review your knowledge of brain tumors. AORN J. 17:71, February, 1973.

Lerner, R. A. et al: The human lymphocyte as an experimental animal. Sci. Am. 228:82, June, 1973.

Lord, E. A.: My crisis with cancer. Am. J. Nurs. 74:647, April, 1974.

Lund, D.: *Eric.* Philadelphia, Lippincott, 1974.

Parsell, D. and Tagliareni, E. M.: Cancer patients help each other. Am. J. Nurs. 74:650, April, 1974.

Pohutsky, L. C. et al: Cancer update. Computerized axial tomography of the brain: A new diagnostic tool (pictorial). Am. J. Nurs. 75:1341, August, 1975.

Robinson, C. H.: *Normal and Therapeutic Nutrition,* ed. 14. New York, Macmillan, 1972.

Rodman, M. J.: Anticancer chemotherapy, Part 1. RN 35:45, February, 1972.

———: Anticancer chemotherapy, Part 2. RN 35:61, March, 1972.

Rothschild, M. A.: Nuclear medicine—new procedures for diagnosing disease. Nurs. Care, 8:25, September, 1975.

Scherer, J. C.: *Introductory Clinical Pharmacology.* Philadelphia, Lippincott, 1975.

Sometime soon I will be dead of cancer. Med. Insight, 5:22, May, 1973.

Storlie, F.: Gloria. Am. J. Nurs. 75:1188, July, 1975.

Taif, B.: Nutritional considerations in radiation and chemotherapy. J. Prac. Nurs. 25:16, May, 1975.

Williams, S. R.: *Nutrition and Diet Therapy: A Learning Guide for Students,* ed. 2. St. Louis, Mosby, 1973.

CHAPTER—11

Nursing management in radiotherapy

On completion of this chapter the student will:

- **Describe the various types of radiotherapies employed in the treatment of cancer.**
- **Discuss nursing management of patients receiving internal and external radiotherapy.**
- **Recognize and describe the hazards of overexposure to radiation.**
- **Identify and discuss the safety principles of time, distance, and shielding.**
- **Recognize and list the side effects that may be seen during and after internal and external radiotherapy.**

The term radiotherapy refers to the therapeutic application of ionizing radiation from x-ray machines (Fig. 11-1) or radioactive materials. Radiotherapy deals mainly, but not exclusively, with the treatment of cancer. The aim of radiotherapy is an orderly destruction of malignant, rapidly dividing cells, while leaving the rest of the body well or able to recover and capable of eliminating the killed cancer cells. This destruction is

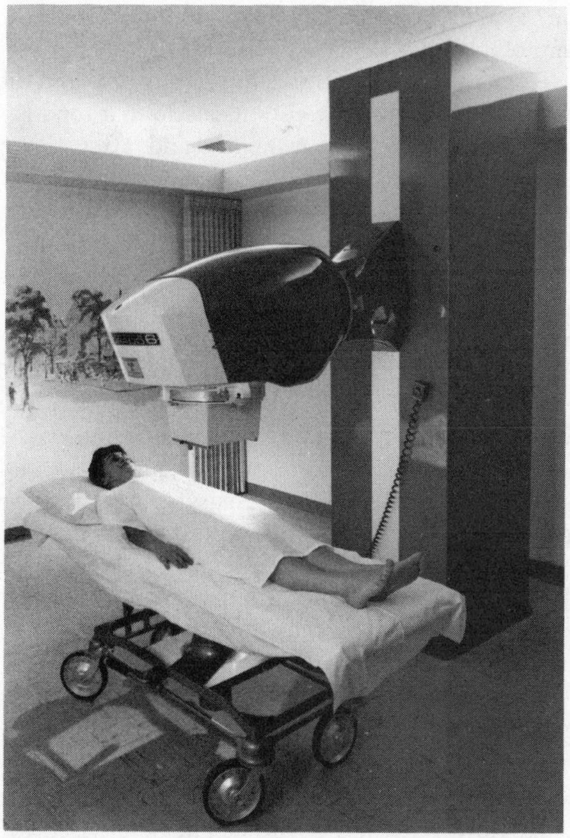

figure 11-1. A vertical teletherapy unit. The radioactive source is Cobalt^{60}. (Atomic Energy of Canada, Ottawa, Canada)

accomplished by x-rays or radioactive materials. When the malignancy is far advanced, radiotherapy is used palliatively to cause a remission of symptoms so that the patient will be more comfortable. Radioisotopes are used for both diagnostic and therapeutic procedures.

That radiation is invisible and inaudible makes it seem menacing, and it is difficult for some patients to understand. Diagnostic tests and treatments often involve the use of large machines that are, for the patient, strange to behold. Because radiotherapy is used for the treatment of cancer more often than for any other condition, and because most patients know this, radiotherapy itself suggests a serious condition.

An adequate knowledge of radiation is necessary not only for the safety and protection of personnel, but also for countering superstition, misconception, and fear of radiation. A more realistic attitude toward clinical uses of radiation is necessary if we are to be truly successful in the management of patients receiving radiotherapy. Uncertainty or confusion on the part of hospital personnel will only increase the patient's fears and damage his morale.

Radiation deserves the same respect as is given to other modalities of therapy for cancer. As noted in Chapter 10, radiotherapy is one of three accepted forms of treatment for cancer and allied diseases. These methods are used singly or in combination. The choice is left to the judgment of the physician. It must always be remembered that it is the patient rather than the cancer which is being treated. All available means must be used to support the patient while he is receiving radiotherapy for his disease.

Clinical application of radiotherapy

Radiotherapy is an exacting science. Its administration is as meticulous and often as tedious as that of surgery or chemotherapy. The application can be as extensive as that of an operative procedure. Major and minor surgical procedures are often performed for the express purpose of treatment with radioisotopes. Like surgery, radiotherapy can result in painful and unpleasant complications.

The patient's basic needs for information must be met. Silence or vague answers can be more disturbing to him than the truth. It is well to use the exact terms the therapist has used to explain the effects of treatment ("melting" or "shrinking" of the tumor). This should be noted on the nursing care plan. Lay terminology is best understood by most patients. Technical terms may add to the patient's fears. Most patients tolerate therapy and bear some discomfort if they are given simple explanations. Discussion of the side effects of therapy should be minimized until they are imminent or actually occur.

When preparing the patient for radiotherapy and assisting him during the period of therapy, it is important not only to explain the treatment to him, but also to listen to his views, doubts, and concerns about the treatment.

Sensitivity of Tissues to Radiation. Rapidly dividing cells are more sensitive to radiation than those which divide slowly. However, radiosensitivity does not imply curability of cancer. For example, the lymph nodes in Hodgkin's disease, a lymphoma, are quite radiosensitive, and radiotherapy is the treatment of choice, but the disease itself is a progressive one. Great strides have been made in the treatment of the lymphomas with the newer supervoltage machines so that the malignancy is held in check for longer periods of time. On the other hand, a basal cell cancer, usually of the face, is quite radiosensitive and the cure rate by radiotherapy is usually very good.

INDIVIDUAL REACTIONS. Individual differences may alter the patient's response to therapy. Infection or ischemia may decrease the radiosensitivity, and poor response is evident more often among the cachectic than in well-nourished patients. On entering tissues, radiation produces ionization of atoms with chemical alteration of tissue proteins. Ionization is facilitated by the large amounts of water and oxygen present in the tissues. The maintenance of good hydration of the patient receiving radiotherapy is an important nursing responsibility. When the oxygen-carrying ability of the blood is impaired as a result of anemia, there is a reduced response to radiotherapy. Therefore, it is important to maintain the patient's hemoglobin at near normal levels.

External radiotherapy

Most patients know that they are receiving x-ray therapy for cancer. The physician discusses the diagnosis with the patient and his family. In some instances, a young or frightened patient is not told that he has cancer; a term such as "cyst," "ulcer," or "inflammation" is used to describe the disease. It is important that all members of the health team be aware of the explanation given the patient and his family. The nurse is perhaps of greatest help when she listens and allows the patient to express his feelings. By quiet acceptance of his emotional state, nursing personnel can help him accept therapy and come to terms with his illness. Many social and psychological problems can be resolved once the diagnosis and its implications are openly or tacitly accepted. For the patient with incurable disease, the palliation achieved may permit normal or near normal activities for a long period of time. The nursing management of the patient receiving external radiotherapy is given in Table 11-1.

RADIATION REACTIONS. A systemic effect, radiation sickness, is sometimes experienced by patients undergoing radiotherapy. The amount of radiation sickness depends upon the site, dose, and size of area treated. For example, a patient undergoing therapy for a small basal cell cancer of the face will not be expected to experience radiation sickness; while patients who have larger areas of the body treated may experience radiation sickness. The symptoms may include weakness, nausea, vomiting, diaphoresis, and sometimes chills. The symptoms are handled prophylactically and symptomatically.

To avoid nausea and vomiting, the nurse and dietitian should plan the patient's meals so that food is not served at least one hour before and after therapy. Some therapists may decide to order an antiemetic to be given one-half hour before therapy. Rushing the patient should also be avoided, and diagnostic tests should not be scheduled immediately before or following therapy. Emphasis upon emotional support and a program including necessary rest and pleasant diversion often obviate the problem of nausea. If radiation reactions should become severe, the therapist may halt treatments to give the body a chance to recover. The reason for this should be explained to the patient and his family to avoid misunderstandings, feelings of discouragement, and setback. It should be explained that deviations from the original plan of therapy are not unusual. Normal activities are encouraged as much as possible. Rest periods should be provided after therapy, as some patients tire easily.

With better radiation techniques and patient management, many side effects have been reduced or nearly eliminated. It is unwise to burden the patient by telling him of side effects which may or may not occur. However, the patient should be advised to report any discomforts he experiences to the staff. When the patient reports symptoms, such as itching or burning, it is essential to take his statements seriously and to see that the appropriate member of the health team receives the information about the patient's symptoms. The patient should know that the skin in the treated area may become reddened, and that this

Table 11-1.
Nursing management of a patient receiving external radiotherapy

The course of therapy is explained to the patient by the physician, preferably with the nurse present.
Patients should be observed for radiation reactions which may occur during or after therapy: nausea, vomiting, diarrhea, anemia, signs of infection, loss of hair, fatigue, anorexia, weakness. Any evidence of symptoms should be reported at once.
Skin markings are *not* to be washed off or removed by any other means.

is a normal reaction to therapy. The term "burn" should never be used as it may connote overtreatment or carelessness.

The patient is instructed to keep the radiated skin clean and dry, and to avoid unprescribed ointments or creams. The radiated skin should be protected against extremes of heat or cold. Heat pads, ultraviolet light, diathermy, whirlpool, sauna or steam baths, and direct sunlight must be avoided. Careful bathing is advised and soap and friction over the treated skin must be avoided. The skin markings must *not* be washed off as they are used as guides by the radiologist and technicians. These marks are necessary for the setting and adjusting of the x-ray machine over the area to be radiated, before each treatment. Loose clothing is advised to avoid irritation.

Intense itching is sometimes experienced. A steroid-type cream or aerosol spray is sometimes prescribed for relief. Cornstarch may be prescribed for use over radiated areas where two skin surfaces are in contact, for example, axillary and groin areas, and areas under the breasts, provided there is no breakdown of the skin.

If the scalp is being irradiated, shampoos, tinting, and permanent waving should be avoided. Upon completion of therapy, the therapist may recommend a mild baby shampoo. Partial, temporary hair loss is seen, with regrowth usually occurring in from 4 to 6 months. A wig is recommended to restore appearance and morale.

Patients receiving radiotherapy may develop varying degrees of bone marrow depression. Periodic complete blood counts, weekly or more often, and occasional whole blood, packed cells, or platelet transfusions are necessary as a decrease in the white cell count lessens the patient's ability to fight infections. Visitors and hospital personnel with colds or other infections should not be in close contact with radiotherapy patients. If the reduction in white cells (leukopenia) is severe, the therapist may temporarily halt treatments and perhaps put the patient on reverse isolation precautions.

FLUIDS AND DIET. Most patients tolerate a well-balanced diet. Because large amounts of tumor are being lysed during therapy, it is important to maintain effective kidney function to avoid uric acid crystalluria and possible kidney shutdown. Good hydration and maintenance of dilute urine are measures used to prevent this rare complication. The patient should take up to 3,000 ml. of fluid daily. If the fluid intake is inadequate, the therapist may wish to order a supplementary intravenous infusion to make up the deficit. Accurate intake and output records are essential. Most patients who are able like to do this themselves once they have been taught. Unless the patient has been on a special diet for some medical reason, a regular diet is usually recommended. Allopurinol is sometimes prescribed when the uric acid level in the blood is high.

FOLLOW-UP CARE. The patient is encouraged to live as normal a life as possible. The help of the patient's family is often enlisted toward that end. When the family is offered the opportunity to express their own misgivings and questions to the staff, they are better able to offer assistance and support to the patient. The patient is referred to the social worker for assistance with such matters as housing, transportation, and family problems. In some instances homemaker or housekeeping services may also be necessary.

It is important for the nurse in all clinical settings to be alert to the need for continuity of care and to initiate referral to other nurses when necessary. For example, if the patient is treated initially in the hospital and subsequently as an outpatient, referral to a community health nurse may be indicated. Side effects from therapy can occur after the course of treatment has terminated. The therapist will, therefore, prepare the patient for this possibility and stress the importance of returning to the clinic if he experiences any discomfort, so that medication and treatment can be prescribed if necessary.

Internal radiotherapy

All persons involved in the care of patients receiving radioisotopes must recognize the necessity for limitations to radiation exposure. The degree of possible hazard depends upon the type and amount of radioactive material used for treatment.

Generally, no special precautions are required when patients receive small amounts of radioactive material for diagnostic studies. If any precautions are necessary, they are specified by the radiologist. There is usually no hazard to personnel or visitors. Patients receiving moderate or large amounts may present a hazard unless simple precautions wirtten by the radiation safety officer are carried out.

The safety principles of time, distance, and shielding (where applicable) must always be borne in mind.

TIME refers to the length of exposure. The less time spent in the vicinity of a radioactive substance the less the radiation received. Nurses should plan carefully so that less time will actually be spent at the bedside. The nurse must learn to work quickly and efficiently. Careful psychological preparation helps the patient to accept the limited amount of nursing time.

DISTANCE refers to the distance from the radioactive source. The patient's bed assignment and degree of isolation are determined by the radiation safety officer after monitoring the patient. The inverse square law applies to radiation exposure. The rate of exposure varies inversely as the square of the distance from the source (patient). A nurse standing 4 feet away from the source of radiation receives 25 percent as much radiation as she would if she were standing 2 feet away from the source (patient) (Fig. 11-2).

SHIELDING refers to the use of any type of material to lessen the amount of radiation reaching an area. The material usually used is lead, but other materials have the capability of shielding. Examples include the concrete walls usually found in radiotherapy and diagnostic radiology departments. Lead-lined gloves, leaded aprons, and drapes are also examples of shielding.

Since radiation produces no immediate symptoms, one can receive radiation injury without being aware of it. The National Committee on Radiation Protection publishes guides for radiation safety for all hospitals, clinics, and laboratories engaged in the handling of x-rays and radioactive materials. The effects of long and short exposures must be taken into account. The latent period between the exposure and the accumulated biological effect is often long, and great care is taken to protect occupationally exposed workers from radiation injury which can accumulate over the years.

Despite precautions, absolute protection for all personnel is not possible, and those who work in this field must deal with the risk involved. Radiation risks are very small, and scientists have made great progress in reducing radiation exposure to the barest minimum. However, all women who are pregnant (whether staff or visitors) should avoid any exposure to radiotherapy.

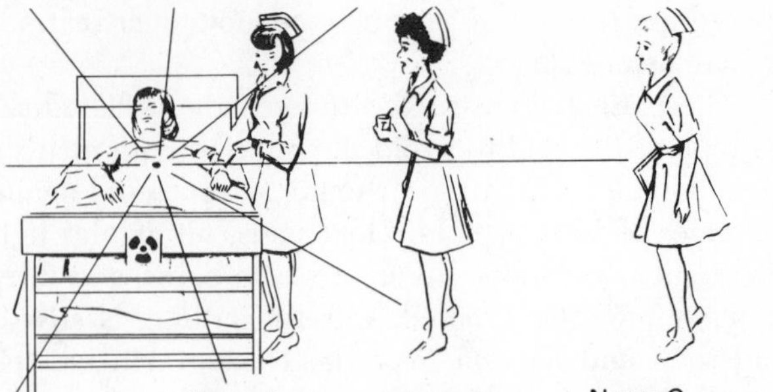

figure 11-2. Examples of distance. Nurse B (4 feet away) receives approximately 25 percent of the radiation received by Nurse A (2 feet away), and Nurse C (8 feet away) receives approximately 25 percent of the radiation received by Nurse B.

RADIOISOTOPES

In certain instances, it may be more advantageous to use radioactive sources within the tumor itself (interstitial), rather than using a distant source (external radiotherapy). This method has the advantage of delivering the highest dose within the tumor, with a rapid fall off of dose in the surrounding tissues. Radioisotopes may also be administered orally or intravenously for systemic effect, placed in solid tumors inside the body or into body cavities for local effect, or applied topically for local lesions using various kinds of applicators.

NURSING MANAGEMENT OF THE PATIENT RECEIVING INTERNAL RADIOTHERAPY

Nursing care will depend on the method of administration, and the type and dosage of radioactive substance used. The radiation safety officer or the radiologist will specify the necessary safety precautions.

Before therapy is begun, the physician or clinical nurse specialist must explain the procedure to the patient and his family. Specific treatment, if necessary, such as the insertion of an indwelling catheter, should also be explained. Follow-up explanations, as needed, are given by all nurses caring for the patient.

If an applicator is used to hold the radioactive source, it may be inserted into the patient in the operating room or in the patient's room. The radioactive substance may be inserted along with the applicator, or it may be introduced after the applicator has been put in place (the afterloading technique). Nursing management of the patient receiving internal radiation therapy is given in Table 11-2.

The patient's chart will list specific orders for treatment and the precautions that are to be taken during treatment. A notation will be made regarding the type and dosage of radioactive substance, the time and area of insertion, the type of applicator used, and the time the material is to be removed. The chart may also give the name of the individual to be notified if an emergency occurs, for example, the dislodging of a radium applicator inserted into the vagina. If any orders are unclear, the nurse should contact the radiologist.

Table 11-2.
Nursing management of the patient receiving internal radiotherapy

Three important aspects of exposure to radiation must be remembered:

TIME: Spend as little time as possible in the room. Organize all needed materials, such as linens, before entering the room, and work quickly but carefully, avoiding unnecessary steps and activities.

DISTANCE: When possible, stand in the doorway of the room to communicate with the patient. Only approach the bed when giving nursing care.

SHIELDING: If increasing the length of exposure is absolutely necessary, contact the radiation safety officer about the advisability of wearing a lead apron. Room walls act as shields, protecting those in the hallway.

Check the patient's chart for special precautions, such as the saving of urine, disposing of linen, wearing of gowns or gloves. Some hospitals have these precautions listed in a hospital procedure manual.

Attach a radiation sign to the door (if the door is kept closed) or to corridor wall next to the doorway of the room.

Generally, if an applicator has been inserted into a body cavity, the patient should stay in bed. For some types of applicator insertion and other types of radiotherapy ambulation may be allowed, but the patient must stay in his room.

If an applicator becomes dislodged, pick it up with long-handled tongs and place it in the shielded lead container. The tongs and container are usually left in the room during treatment. Call the radiologist or the radiation safety officer immediately. NEVER TOUCH THE APPLICATOR WITH THE BARE HANDS!

Patients receiving internal radiation may experience varying degrees of gastrointestinal disturbances during or after the period of treatment.

In preparing the private room prior to treatment, the nurse must check to see if essential items are available: paper tissues, paper bags, water glass, straws, and so on. Furnishing these items *before* the treatment reduces exposure of nursing personnel once treatment has begun. The patient should have adequate reading material or other forms of diversion. (These items will not become radioactive unless directly contaminated with a radioactive material.) Some hospitals use a special room for radiotherapy, which accommodates more than one patient. The beds are kept a specific distance apart for the safety of other patients.

All personnel and workers in the area should be made aware of radiotherapy, even though a radiation sign is posted on the wall (Fig. 11-3). This is especially important for cleaning and maintenance personnel who may not be aware of the signs even though they are posted in a prominent place. Visitors for other patients may inquire about the radiation signs and should be assured that neither they nor the patients are in danger.

Radioactive iodine (^{131}I) is used for the treatment of thyroid cancer, thyroid metastases, and some types of hyperthyroidism. For therapy, radioactive iodine is administered orally in liquid form as a clear, colorless, tasteless preparation. The patient will need to fast, because food delays the obsorption of the isotope. The precautions specified by the radiation safety officer must be strictly observed.

Radiogold (^{198}Au) is used to retard the accumulation of malignant effusions in body cavities. Also, this isotope is sometimes injected interstitially (liquid form) directly into an unresectable tumor, or interstitially in stainless steel seeds as a permanent implant. Small amounts of this isotope are eliminated in the urine, while most of it remains in the injected area. Contamination may easily be seen by the appearance of a pink or red stain on the dressing, gown, or bedding.

With intracavity use, radiogold produces irradiation of the lining of the cavity. It will reduce or suspend tumor activity and will deliver a lethal dose to tumor cells. The radiotherapist will use and remove his own equipment, usually sterile disposable paracentesis or thoracentesis sets. When the isotope is used in body cavities, the position of the patient must be rotated every 15 minutes for at least 2 hours. This will assure equal distribution of the isotope throughout the cavity. Sometimes the polyethylene tubes used for administering the isotopes are clamped and left in place to facilitate further treatment at a later date.

Radiophosphorus (^{32}P) concentrates in the nuclei of cells where it forms an important constituent of their chemical structure, nucleic acid. The nuclei of rapidly proliferating cells tend to have more nuclear material than normal cells, so they concentrate the

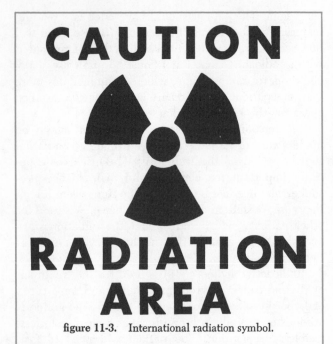

figure 11-3. International radiation symbol.

radiophosphorus. Temporary isolation is not necessary because the patient's own body serves as an effective shield. Contamination can easily be seen by the appearance of a blue stain on the dressing, gown, or bed linen. Contaminated items must be handled carefully. The nurse must wear disposable gloves and use waterproof containers. Contaminated items are removed for proper disposition by radiation safety personnel after monitoring. Radiophosphorus may be administered orally or intravenously for the treatment of chronic leukemia or polycythemia vera. The isotope tends to deposit in bones and in the cells of the reticuloendothelial system. Some of the isotope is excreted in the urine and stool in the first few days. The patient should flush the toilet three times and should wash his hands thoroughly. As with radiogold and all radioisotopes, the patient's chart should contain the appropriate information.

General nutritional considerations

- To avoid nausea during treatment, the patient should *not* be served meals one hour before or after a treatment has been given.
- If the patient is experiencing nausea *during* the days or weeks required for external radiotherapy, he may find food more palatable and acceptable if served in small amounts.
- A well-balanced diet is important *during* radiotherapy.
- Fluid intake should be increased with fluids offered frequently and in small amounts. If nausea is present, fluids should be given to the patient after he experiences relief of the nausea.

General pharmacological considerations

- Nausea is a common side effect of radiotherapy and antiemetics may be needed to control nausea and vomiting.
- Drugs may be ordered for other side effects that may occur during radiotherapy: aspirin for fever, antibiotics for infection, various ointments and creams for the skin over the radiated area.
- When creams or ointments are ordered for the skin over the area radiated, these products are to be applied exactly as ordered, for example, sparingly, or liberally.

Bibliography

American Cancer Society: *A Cancer Source Book for Nurses.* New York, American Cancer Society, 1975.

Arena, V.: Radiation accidents: What you need to know about them. RN 36:42, September, 1973.

Bouchard, R. and Owens, N. F.: *Nursing Care of the Cancer Patient*, ed. 2. St. Louis, Mosby, 1972.

FDA establishes protection standards. AORN J. 17:55, February, 1973.

Gribbons, C. A. et al: Treatment for advanced breast carcinoma. Am. J. Nurs. 72:678, April, 1972.

Hendrickson, F. R. et al.: Radiotherapy treatment for cancer: Guidelines for nursing care. J. Prac. Nurs. 22:18, February, 1972.

Isler, C.: Radiation therapy. The nurse and the patient, Part 2. RN 34:48, March, 1971.

Prosnitz, L. R.: Radiation therapy. Treatment for malignant disease, Part 1. RN 34:42, March, 1971.

Sutton, M.: Radiotherapy—treatment for cancer by x-rays. Health 7:42, Winter, 1970-71.

Taif, B.: Nutritional considerations in radiation and chemotherapy. J. Prac. Nurs. 25:16, May, 1975.

Turnbull, F.: Pain and suffering in cancer. Canad. Nurs. 67:28, August, 1971.

UNIT THREE

Disturbances of body supportive structures and locomotion

- The patient with a fracture
- The patient with a disease of the bones and joints
- The patient with an amputation

CHAPTER—12

The patient with a fracture

On completion of this chapter the student will:

- List the symptoms of a fracture.
- Describe and discuss the principles of first aid for the individual with a fracture.
- Identify the types of reduction of a fracture.
- List the problems and complications that may follow the application of a cast.
- Give basic cast care instructions to the patient discharged from the emergency department after the application of a plaster cast or an immobilizing dressing.
- State the basic principles of traction.
- Give basic nursing care to a patient in traction.

Types of fractures

A fracture is a break in the continuity of a bone. A simple classification of fractures follows:

- *Open* (compound)—the bone breaks through the skin. Because there is an open wound, the danger of infection is greatly increased.
- *Closed* (simple)—any fracture that is not open is a closed fracture.
- *Displaced*—the bone ends are separated at the fracture line.
- *Greenstick*—the bone bends and splits, but it does not break clear through. This kind of fracture occurs primarily in children.
- *Complete*—the fracture line goes all the way through the bone.
- *Comminuted*—the bone is splintered into many small fragments at the fracture site, with the bone ends separated and usually misaligned.
- *Impacted*—one portion of the bone is driven into another.
- *Complicated*—a fracture with injury to the surrounding tissues, such as blood vessels, nerves, muscles, tendons, joints, or internal organs.
- *Pathologic* (spontaneous)—the bone breaks without sufficient trauma to crack a normal bone. This kind of fracture occurs in such conditions as osteoporosis (porous bones), cancer, certain instances of malnutrition, Cushing's syndrome, and as a complication of cortisone and ACTH therapy.

The pathology of fracture and the physiology of bone repair

For 10 to 40 minutes after the fracture the muscles surrounding the bone are flaccid. Then they go into spasm, and when they do, they cause increased deformity and additional interference with the vascular and the lymphatic circulations. Traction at this later stage is accomplished only with difficulty. The application and the maintenance of traction immediately after a fracture avoids the later complication of spastic muscles.

When there are bone fragments as a result of fracture, the local periosteum and surrounding blood vessels are torn. The tissue surrounding the fracture shows inflammation with swelling due to hemorrhage and edema. The blood in the area clots, and a fibrin network forms between bone ends. This changes into granulation tissue. The osteoblasts, proliferating in the clot, increase the secretion of an enzyme that restores the alkaline pH, and the result is the deposition of calcium in the callus and the formation of true bone. At the stage of the consolidation of the clot (6 to 10 days after the injury) the healing mass is called a *callus.* The callus holds the ends of the bone together, but it cannot endure strain.

Interference with the removal of the debris will interefere with the healing process. Nonunion of the fracture—a permanent break in the continuity of the bone—may result. Nursing measures that promote adequate circulation in the affected part foster deposition of calcium and healing of the bone. This is one reason that elevation of the affected limb, which helps to reduce edema, is so important. Because early mobilization of the patient encourages favorable nitrogen balance and counters poor circulation, many patients with a fractured hip are treated with pin fixation instead of traction.

Bone repair is a local process. About a year of healing must take place before bone regains its former structural strength, becoming well consolidated and remolded, and possessing fat and marrow cells.

Incidence

Most accidents occur in the home and on the highways. Slippery wet tubs, scatter rugs, highly polished floors, and activities involving a precarious balance, such as standing on a rickety chair to hang a curtain—all can be hazardous. The incidence of fractures is greater among persons who have predisposing conditions, such as osteoporosis and cancer which affects bone. Poor coordination, diminished vision and hearing, the frequency of dizziness and faintness, and general feebleness make falls and resultant fractures a common problem among the aged. Other high-risk groups include patients with diseases affecting locomotion, such as arthritis, Parkinson's disease, and multiple sclerosis. The fact that bone breakage in older persons is more frequent across the neck of the femur is attributed partially to atrophy of bone.

Symptoms

- *Pain*—one of the most consistent symptoms of a broken bone is pain. It may be severe, and it is increased by attempts to move the part and by pressure over the fracture.
- *Loss of function*—skeletal muscular function is dependent on an intact bone.
- *Deformity*—a break may cause an extremity to bend backwards or to assume another unusual shape.
- *False motion*—unnatural motion occurs at the site of the fracture.
- *Edema*—swelling usually is greatest directly over the fracture.
- *Spasm*—muscles near fractures involuntarily

contract. Spasm, which accounts for some of the pain, may result in the shortening of a limb when a long bone is involved.

If the sharp bone fragments tear through sufficient surrounding soft tissue, there will be bleeding and black and blue discoloration of the area. If a nerve is damaged, there may be paralysis.

First aid

BLEEDING. Blood can be lost in both open and closed fractures, with the greatest amount usually lost from an open (compound) fracture. Control of bleeding is often difficult. Initially, direct pressure should be applied to the bleeding wound with sterile dressings and a pressure bandage. If the bleeding is extensive or it is believed that there may be many bone splinters around or near a major artery, the application of a tourniquet is warranted.

EVALUATION. It is safe to assume that a fracture has occurred if the limb is misshapen, if the patient states that he has heard the bone snap, or if there is a loss of function. Overcaution is never misplaced. It is better to splint a sprain than not to splint a fracture.

"SPLINT THEM WHERE THEY LIE" is the motto. The ragged edge of a broken bone can do great damage to the soft tissues around it. Fragments of bone can cut through periosteum, fascia, muscle, nerves, blood-vessel walls and even skin. The protrusion of a fragment of bone through skin is very dangerous, since dirt or perhaps bits of clothing may be introduced into an otherwise clean wound. Pulling a patient to the side of the road and lifting him into a car without supporting the fracture can create an open fracture from a closed one. It is better to stop hemorrhage, treat shock, and immobilize the fracture before the patient is moved.

SPLINTING. Before the patient is moved, the affected limb or part must be immobilized (Fig. 12-1).

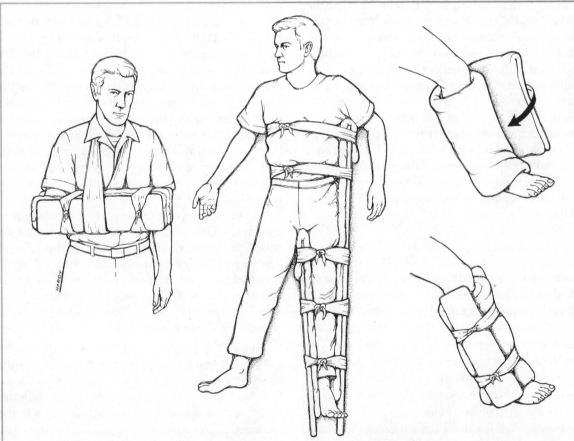

figure 12-1. Splinting techniques using padded boards and circular conforming gauze bandage. Patients with a suspected forearm fracture should be immobilized using splints and a simple sling. A lower extremity may be immobilized using longer padded-board splints and circular conforming gauze. The ankle can be splinted by wrapping it in a towel (to keep pressure off bony prominences) and using supporting, lightly padded splints exteriorly, maintained in position by circumferential conforming gauze.

Immobilization prevents further damage to surrounding tissues and structures and reduces pain and discomfort. To splint an extremity, padded wood, inflatable plastic splints, or metal splints such as the Thomas ring-traction splint may be used. If possible, the splint should be applied so that it includes the joints above and below the fracture site. For example, if the tibia is broken, include both the ankle and the knee in the splint. Be sure to pad the appliance, so that the soft tissues are protected. Remember that the arm and the leg bones are especially close to the skin, and that extreme gentleness is needed in handling a fractured limb to prevent a simple fracture from tearing the skin and becoming a compound fracture. Tie the splint in place securely but not so tightly that circulation is impaired.

The inside fold of a clean handkerchief may be placed over the wound. If the bone disappears into the wound, surely carrying some dirt back with it, write a note that the bone has broken through the skin, and pin the note to the clothing of the patient. When he gets to the hospital, the doctors then will know that deep, thorough cleansing will be necessary.

Infection is a prime concern in an open fracture. For this reason early débridement of the wound in the operating room is considered essential. Excision of necrotic and severely traumatized tissue, plus careful cleansing and flushing out of the wound, helps to remove the contaminated foreign materials, thus decreasing the likelihood of infection. Osteomyelitis can be a complication of open fractures. In compound fractures the incidence of delayed union and nonunion tends to be increased, especially if infection occurs.

Hospital treatment of fractures

If the patient arrives with a splint, do not remove it. X-ray films are taken before any treatment is given. If the fracture was not splinted outside the hospital, a splint is usually applied to immobilize the part while the patient goes to the x-ray department and waits for the x-ray films to be developed and read. Keep the injured part elevated to minimize edema. The doctor usually orders medication for pain. Immobilization of the part also helps to reduce pain.

In removing clothing, help the patient to keep the injured part as motionless as possible. For example, to remove a jacket when the left arm is broken, have the patient remove his arm from the right sleeve first, freeing the jacket, so that it can be slipped off his left arm without moving that arm. On occasion it may be necessary to cut clothing away. When it is possible, cut along the seam, making sure that no threads fall into any open wound.

When a patient is admitted to the hospital with multiple injuries, the doctor decides which problems are to be given prior attention. Bleeding and shock will be first on the list. Vital signs should be checked every 15 to 30 minutes and the patient observed for any general physical changes.

The aim of treatment is to help the body reestablish functional continuity of the bone. One aspect of treatment does pose a dilemma: the fragments will not heal unless they are immobilized; at the same time, it is necessary to treat the limb in such a fashion that circulation is maintained and muscles will not atrophy. Early, active use of nearby muscle groups is one of the most effective ways to encourage adequate circulation. The solution to this problem is active use of the injured part without disturbance of the injured bone.

Types of reduction

The method of treatment selected by the doctor for a fracture depends on many factors: the first aid given, the location and the severity of the break, and the age and overall physical condition of the patient. First, the doctor *reduces the fracture* (replaces the parts in their normal position) by manipulation of the fragments. He takes the broken limb in his hand and, by gentle manipulation, redirects it to its normal position. This kind of reduction is a *closed reduction.* Then he immobilizes the part by bandage, cast, traction, or internal fixation.

In an *open reduction,* which is performed in the operating room, the bone is exposed and realigned under the direct vision of the orthopedist. The operation usually is performed under general or spinal anesthesia. A cast is applied, and x-rays taken while the patient is still anesthetized so that any needed correction can be made. This method is used frequently for dealing with soft tissue, such as nerves or blood vessels, caught between the ends of the broken pieces of bone; for wide separation of the fragments; for comminuted fractures; for fractures of the patella and other joints; for open fractures when débridement of the wound is necessary; and for internal fixation of fractures.

Skin Preparation for Open Reduction. Because osteomyelitis (infection of bone) is difficult to cure and may result in the patient's being permanently crippled, careful attention is paid to the preparation of the skin before any orthopedic surgery. In an emergency, shaving and cleaning the skin may be done in the operating room. When there is time, preparation usually begins the day before the surgery. The skin is shaved and scrubbed with a cleansing agent and an antiseptic applied. The area then may be wrapped in a sterile covering, which is removed the next day, when scrubbing and application of an antiseptic are repeated. A new sterile covering may be put on and left in place until the operation. In some hospitals the scrubbed area is left open.

Cast application

Other fractures, such as those of long bones in which there is no impaction, are immobilized by casts (Fig. 12-2). Casts hold the bone in place while it heals, and permit early ambulation when a leg is broken. The patient may be given a narcotic before the cast is applied, or general anesthesia may be used. Sometimes a local block is performed, such as infiltrating the brachial plexus with procaine when reduction of a fracture of the arm is to be undertaken.

The doctor positions the patient as he wishes the part to be immobilized. An assistant holds the arm or leg exactly in place. Casts that include joints are usually applied with the joints flexed to lessen stiffness. A break in the lumbodorsal spine is corrected by allowing the patient to assume a position of hyperextension and immobilizing him in that position in a cast.

During the application of a cast the nurse should assist the physician by obtaining needed materials. The patient will most likely be frightened as well as experiencing discomfort and/or pain due to the injury. Each step of the cast application should be explained: application of sheet wadding and stockinette, the wet plaster bandage, and the warm sensation that occurs while the cast is setting. The nurse must also provide emotional support, as anticipation and fear increase anxiety, which may interfere with the patient's ability to cooperate while the cast is being applied.

After the fragments of bone have been manipulated into place and the cast has been applied, a second x-ray film is taken, so that bone alignment can be checked. Whenever a cast is removed or applied, an x-ray picture is taken.

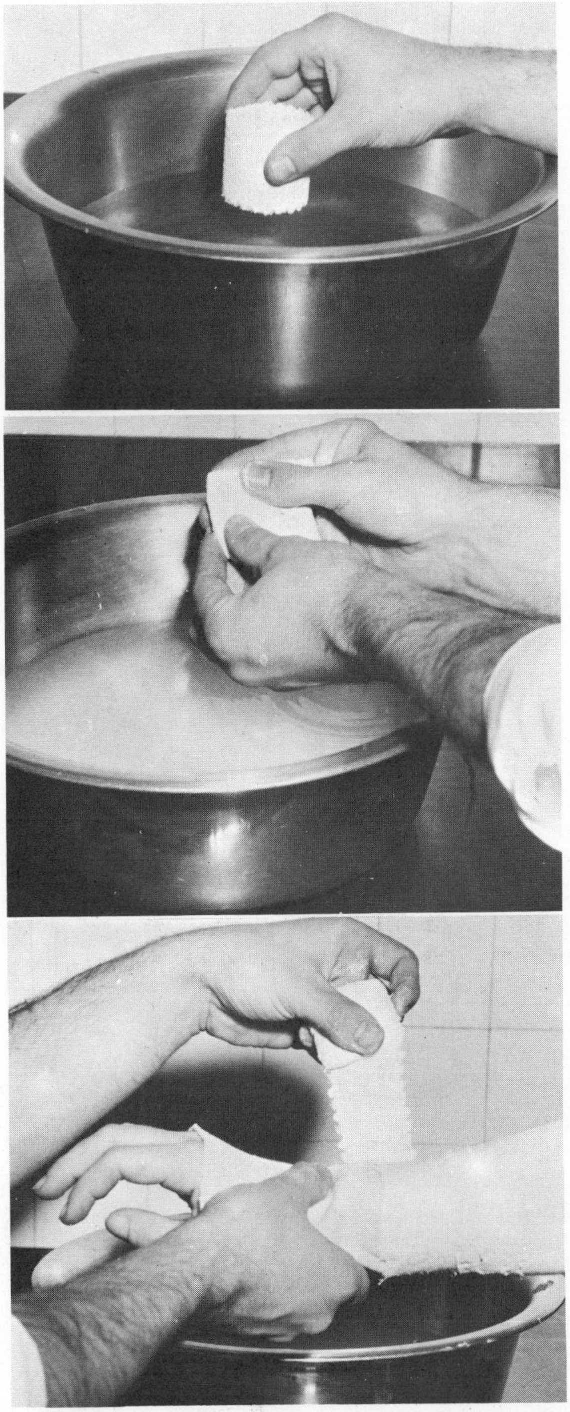

figure 12-2. Applying a cast. (*Top*) The roll is soaked in an upright position. (*Center*) The water is pressed out evenly and gently. (*Bottom*) The part is supported in the proper position during the bandaging.

Drying and finishing the cast

There are various types of cast materials, some setting in a few minutes, others taking up to 24 hours to become completely dry. During the drying period the cast needs protection. A thumbprint on the cast, while

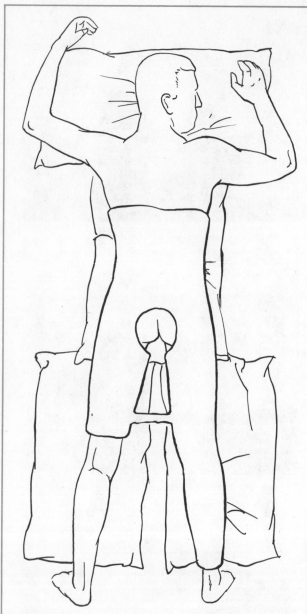

figure 12-3. The wet spica cast is supported on pillows until it dries. When the patient lies on his abdomen, his feet are positioned over the edges of the pillows, which are so placed that they support the patient in good body alignment.

it is drying, can leave an indentation that later may cause a pressure sore on the patient's skin. The cast should be supported with the palm of the hand rather than the fingertips. No draft ever should be allowed to fall directly on a patient in a wet cast.

The cast itself must be left uncovered so that water can evaporate from it. Many doctors prefer natural evaporation, but some ask the nurse to use cast dryers to speed the drying. Intense heat should never be used. Not only is there danger of burning the patient, but the heat will dry the outside of the cast and leave the inside wet, so that later it may become moldy. Intense heat can also crack the plaster.

The damp cast never should be placed on a hard bed, where it automatically will flatten over bony prominences, later causing damage to the soft tissue between the cast and the bone. Instead, place the cast on a pillow or a series of pillows covered with plastic to protect the pillow from the dampness of the cast. The pillow prevents flattening of the cast and elevates the part.

A spica (body) cast is supported on pillows until it is dry along its entire length (Fig. 12-3). After several hours, the patient is turned as directed by the doctor to allow the undersurface of the cast to dry. The damp cast is handled with a flat hand; the fingertips are kept away to avoid indenting it. A spica cast is never lifted by the foot or the ankle; rather, the hand is slipped under the patient's buttocks.

After 48 hours, when the cast is thoroughly dry, it can lie on a hard surface. Although casts are durable, they do break. A particularly active patient may need to be told of this possibility.

EDGES. After a cast is dry, the rough edges will require finishing. Rough edges can be temporarily covered with a gauze dressing which is anchored in place with adhesive tape to prevent the dressing from slipping down inside the cast. If the cast is lined with a stockinette, this is pulled over the edge and taped to the cast. Some doctors secure the stockinette over the edge of the cast with plaster (Fig. 12-4).

SPICA CASTS need special attention to the finishing of the area near the buttocks. If there is not enough room for defecation, tell the doctor, so that he can enlarge the space. To protect the cast from getting wet and soiled, the nurse can fit some waterproof material around the edge and tape it to the cast. A consistently damp cast will become moldy and very malodorous.

Whenever the patient is turned, the buttocks should be inspected, and any pieces of plaster that may have accumulated brushed away. You will note that the buttocks are creased where the cast has pressed against the skin; these creases are lines of potential skin breakdown. The physician should be consulted concerning any local medication that may be applied. Sometimes he recommends rubbing the involved area with skin cream or oil or painting it with tincture of benzoin.

Nursing management of the patient in a cast

Elevation of the limb

While the patient wearing a cast is in bed, the injured limb should be kept elevated to prevent edema. Pillows may be used to elevate the limb, or the physician may order a special sling to provide greater elevation of the affected part.

Nursing observations

General observations of a patient with a cast are given in Table 12-1. It should be noted that these observations are *extremely* important, as serious complications have resulted when casts have become too tight. Look at all edges of the cast—top and bottom—for any place where the edge cuts into the skin. Although this possibility is more likely to occur during the first 24 hours, it can happen at any time. In cases of pressure against the skin where there is no edema, the doctor may split the cast and loosely pad the area with cotton. If there is edema around the edge of the cast, the doctor must be notified at once. If edema causes pressure, the doctor may bivalve the entire cast to release the pressure.

Color is another useful index of pressure. The skin showing at the ends of the cast should be the same color as that of the rest of the body; it should not be white or cyanotic. Be sure that you see 5 fingers or 5 toes. The little toe has a tendency to get lost and to be compressed inside a cast that covers most of the lower leg. Teach the patient to move his fingers or his toes at the end of a cast periodically. Look to see that they move freely. One of the benefits of motion is that it helps to reduce edema in a nearby area.

The *blanching sign* is a useful color index. The nail of the great toe or of the thumb is compressed briefly and then released. The blood should rush back into it as quickly as it does in your own thumb.

Make sure that the fingers and toes at the end of the cast are as warm as those on the other side of the body. If they are not, notify the doctor at once—day or night. Compression of blood vessels and nerves by a cast can cause irreparable damage. The diminished supply of oxygen and food to the tissues may cause their death. Volkmann's contracture apparently results from pressure, perhaps on the radial artery. The etiology is not entirely clear, but compression of vital structures in the arm plays a large role. The hand is swollen and blue, and the radial pulse diminished or absent.

Sometimes the only indication that tissues inside the cast are undergoing necrosis is the odor emitted. The patient may not complain of any pain or discomfort *beneath* the cast because loss of sensation may develop in a pressure sore. When the pressure sore becomes necrotic, infection almost always results.

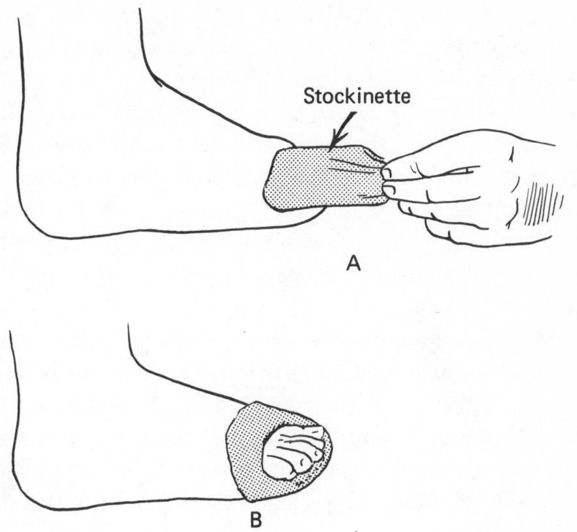

figure 12-4. The edges of this cast are made smooth by pulling out the stockinette (A) and fastening it to the outside of the cast (B).

Table 12-1.
Nursing observations of a patient with a cast

Check all cast edges for smoothness, once the cast is dry.
Check the extremities for *any* change in skin color and temperature.
Note any drainage: color, amount, or increase in amount.
Check the cast for any unusual odor.
Carefully investigate *any* complaints the patient may have.
Check the pulse in the extremity, if possible. Report absence of a pulse *immediately*.
Check for movement or lack of movement in the extremity.

Note: The above observations should be made at least 2 to 3 times per day.

Although some pain at the fracture line is expected the first few days, continued pain means that something is wrong. If the patient complains of any pain or discomfort above, below, or underneath the cast the complaint should be thoroughly investigated before an analgesic is administered. The compression of a nerve or a blood vessel can lead to permanent damage and crippling.

Cast Windows. A window cut in a cast over the area of discomfort will permit visualization of that area of the skin.

Some doctors have a window cut over the radial pulse in an arm cast for the express purpose of feeling the pulse. The purpose is not to check on the patient's general condition so much as to check the circulation of the affected arm. The window can be observed for edema that may puff the flesh through the opening.

If a cast is put on a patient after an open reduction, and there is bleeding from the wound, it may take longer for the blood to seep through the plaster than it would to pass through an ordinary bandage. If the nurse sees a red spot, it should be circled with a pencil or ballpoint pen, the time noted, and the physician notified. If the red spot enlarges beyond the penciled boundaries, the bleeding is continuing.

The patient may return from the operating room with a drain inserted inside the cast. In 24 hours the drain may be removed through a window.

Moving the patient

Most patients in casts become amazingly adept at locomotion in a very short time, but in the beginning, turning in a spica cast is frightening. Perhaps the worst aspect is that the patient feels helpless. He is encased in plaster, unable to help himself if he falls—a possibility that seldom escapes the attention of patients.

The first day or two, while the cast is still damp and the patient is unsure of himself, two people should help him turn, one standing at each side of the bed. Since the damp cast should not be placed directly on the bed, the covered pillows are laid in position to receive the cast while the patient is at one side.

To turn a patient in a body cast, have the patient move to one side of the bed. You stand on the other side of the bed. If you are turning him alone, be sure that he does not move so far to the opposite side of the bed that he falls out. The affected leg is the one that swings up and over. Before turning, the patient should put his arm on the unaffected side over his head, to get it out of the way. Remove the head pillows. With one hand on the patient's shoulder and the other on his hip, using good body mechanics so that you do not hurt your own back, turn the patient toward you. Do not pull on the abduction bar to turn the patient. It is more fragile than it looks. If the patient was lying on his back, he is now prone. Do not leave him with his toes digging into the bed. You can have the patient move down so that his toes hang free over the edge of the mattress, or you can elevate the cast, making sure that support all along its length leaves his toes hanging free over the end of the pillow. Each time after turning the patient, look at the exposed skin along the cast edges to see whether the new position is exerting excessive pressure.

To place a patient in a spica cast on a bedpan, pad the space just behind the pan, and elevate the head of the bed slightly to keep the fluid from running up the patient's back. Support the legs with pillows to avoid strain on the cast. Sometimes the head of the bed is elevated on blocks. The nurse cleans the patient after he has used the bedpan, if he cannot reach far enough to clean himself.

Itching

The very old patient or the very young patient may push any kind of object into his cast. Coins, knitting needles, spoons, etc., may disappear inside. The pain of pressure may pass off in a few days as the wound becomes anesthetized. But a hot spot may develop on the cast over the trouble area, and perhaps a stain will appear.

Itching, especially during hot weather, can cause great discomfort. Nothing should be inserted down into the cast as injury to the skin or underlying structures can result in an infection. If itching is severe, the physician should be consulted.

Exercise

It may be necessary to set up a routine of daily exercises using the unaffected limbs. For example, the patient with a fracture of the left leg should exercise the right leg and possibly the arms. For those whose activities are limited by the type or size of cast, coughing and deep-breathing exercises are necessary to prevent atelectasis and pneumonia.

Psychological problems

The physical discomfort of a cast, especially a body cast, can cause serious psychological problems. A full body spica can reduce a grown man to the helplessness of a baby. He cannot go to the faucet to get a drink of water; he cannot go to the bathroom by himself. The prevention of the elementary impulse of motion is one of the most unendurable of constraints. Although most patients are grateful for the care they receive, it is natural, normal, and healthy for them to resent the restrictions imposed by the cast. Many orthopedic patients who are in a state of sustained anger are not necessarily aware of why they feel that way. The anger is not directed purposely at the nurse, but the nurse may be the only person around on whom the patient can vent his feelings.

The nurse helps the patient to dispel some of his anger by not becoming upset when an orthopedic patient shows anger, by encouraging as much self-sufficiency and motion (good antidotes to helplessness) as allowed, and by listening to the patient without becoming defensive.

ENCOURAGING SELF-HELP. Implements for the care of the patient should be arranged so that he can do as much for himself as possible. Even in a spica cast, a patient can wash the upper parts of his body. The food tray can be placed on a table or stand at the same level as that of the mattress so that he can feed himself. If he cannot pour his coffee or cut his meat, perform these services for him. A wooden prop may be used to support the patient on his side while he eats, or he may eat while lying prone. A bag placed at the head of the bed can hold toilet articles. An electric razor and portable mirror will make it possible for most male patients to shave themselves. Keep the patient's water pitcher, reading material, and urinal within easy reach, so that he can help himself without needing to ask for aid. Whatever helps the patient to feel adequate instead of helpless benefits him psychologically. Remember, too, that exercise with a purpose is a better morale builder than exercise for its own sake, which can be a bore. Exercise which the patient can undertake with others and projects he can do in a group are helpful in providing companionship as well as exercise. Patients who are in private rooms require particular thought, since they lack opportunity for group activities. Sometimes patients in private rooms can be moved to a dayroom for exercise sessions or other forms of diversion.

EXPLANATIONS. The doctor may show the patient his x-ray films, which are not only interesting to him, but also enable him actually to visualize the fracture. Explaining what to expect, the length of time that he probably will spend in the cast, what he will be able to do, and what limitations he will have helps the patient to know what to expect, and, therefore, lessens fear of the unknown. For example, if a man knows about how long his cast will be on, and about how much limitation of motion he will have, he can make plans for returning to his job. If he has no idea about the outcome of his treatment, he may worry unnecessarily about a permanent loss of income or other things that may never happen. To be crippled is a fearful thought. Most people are afraid of the possibility, and a fracture can create deep-seated anxiety.

LATER CARE

If the patient is kept in the hospital only overnight or not at all, he and his family must be taught to care for his cast. Because the patient is likely to be excited from his accident, it takes a skillful teacher to reach him so that he fully understands and remembers the

Table 12-2.
Instructions for home care—patients with plaster casts

1. Go to bed as soon as you get home. Stay in bed for the next 24 hours. You may get up to go to the bathroom.
2. While you are in bed, keep the injured arm or leg elevated on a pillow. (Protect the pillow with plastic material as long as the cast is damp.) The hand or the foot should be the highest part of the body.
3. Whenever you get out of bed, keep the injured arm in a sling. If your leg is injured, and you sit for longer than 15 minutes, elevate your leg on a chair or stool.
4. Move your fingers (arm cast) or toes (leg cast) for several minutes every half-hour.
5. If the cast feels tight, exercise the fingers or the toes and elevate the limb. If the tightness is not relieved, come to the hospital (emergency entrance). Immediately (day or night) report to the hospital or your doctor if you notice any of the following:

   Numbness of fingers or toes
   Swelling of fingers or toes
   Blueness of fingers or toes
   Severe pain in the limb

   A crack or break in your cast (if noticed at night, wait until morning to report to the hospital)

important points. If the hospital does not have a printed form of instructions for patients with plaster casts, the nurse should write out just what he should do: elevate the part; watch for coldness, numbness, blueness, swelling; return to the doctor the next day; do not allow the cast to get wet, etc.

Table 12-2 is an example of a printed instruction sheet that gives directions for home care.

When the patient with an arm fracture gets out of bed, the arm that has been elevated on a pole or a pillow still has to be kept raised, with a sling used to support it (Fig. 12-5). It is important to remember that the sling supports the entire arm, including the wrist. If the wrist is allowed to drop over the edge of the sling, the fingers can become edematous, circulation impaired, and nerves compressed. A permanent deformity could result. Make sure that the knot does not rest exactly at the back of the neck, or it will hit the cervical vertebra with each step that the patient takes. To prevent edema of the fingers, the sling should be adjusted so that the fingers are higher than the elbow. Advise the patient to exercise the shoulder that bears the weight of the sling and the cast. If the elbow is outside the cast, it, too, should be exercised.

Removal of Cast. Casts are removed by a mechanical cast cutter. Although cast cutters are noisy and frightening, the patient should be assured that the machine will not cut him.

When the cast is removed, continued support to the limb is necessary. An elastic bandage may be put on a leg; the arm may be kept in a sling.

The patient will have pains, aches, and stiffness, and the limb will feel surprisingly light without the cast. The skin will look mottled, and it may be covered with a yellow crust composed of exudate, oil, and dead skin. It may take a few days to remove this crust, but there is no hurry. Olive oil and warm baths will soften it.

Exercise. After removal of a cast the patient's muscles will be weak. Graded active exercise, directed by the doctor or the physical therapist, should help the extremity to regain its normal strength and motion. Resistive exercises that are beyond the patient's capacity result in further limitation of motion. Exercises should be active, not passive, and progressively graded so that muscles and joints are coaxed rather than forced into full range and strength of motion.

Bivalve Cast. If a cast is put on an extremity before edema has developed fully, compression of the tissues will result, because there will be no room for expansion inside a cast. To avoid this possibility, the doctor may apply the cast and, as soon as it is dry, split it along both sides. The cast sides then are refitted on the patient's limb and bandaged in place. This kind of cast is called a bivalve cast. It may also be used for a patient who is being weaned from a cast, when a very sharp x-ray film is needed, or in the treatment of such conditions as arthritis, in which the method is a convenient one for splinting the part intermittently. A bivalve cast should be removed daily, unless the doctor orders otherwise. Note any pressure areas on the skin. While the patient is out of the cast, his skin can be washed, rubbed, oiled or powdered, and the exercises ordered by the doctor can be given. Be careful not to pinch the skin when you reapply the cast.

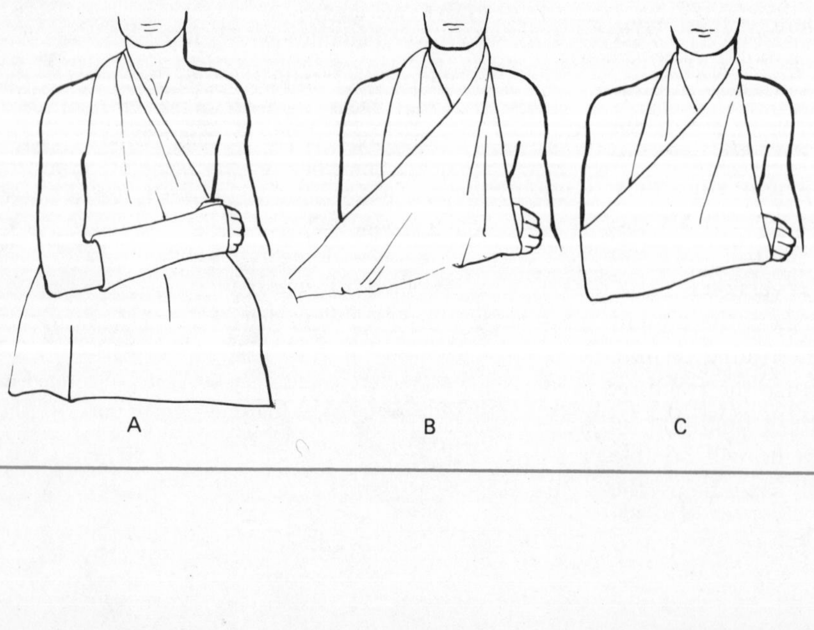

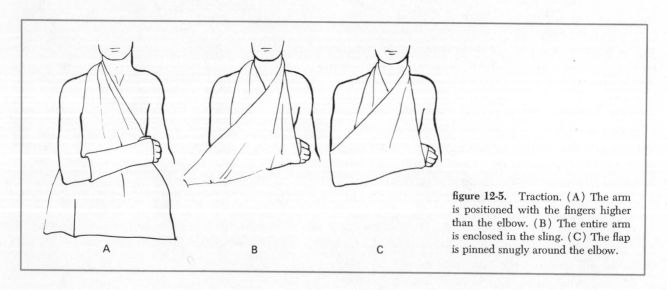

figure 12-5. Traction. (A) The arm is positioned with the fingers higher than the elbow. (B) The entire arm is enclosed in the sling. (C) The flap is pinned snugly around the elbow.

The patient in traction

Various types of traction can be used to maintain alignment and immobilization. The two most common types are *skin traction* and *skeletal traction.* Skin traction utilizes pull on tapes or traction strips attached to the skin, usually by elastic bandages (Fig. 12-6). Skeletal traction uses a wire (Kirschner) or pin (Steinmann) inserted in the bone, with pull (traction) applied to the pin or wire.

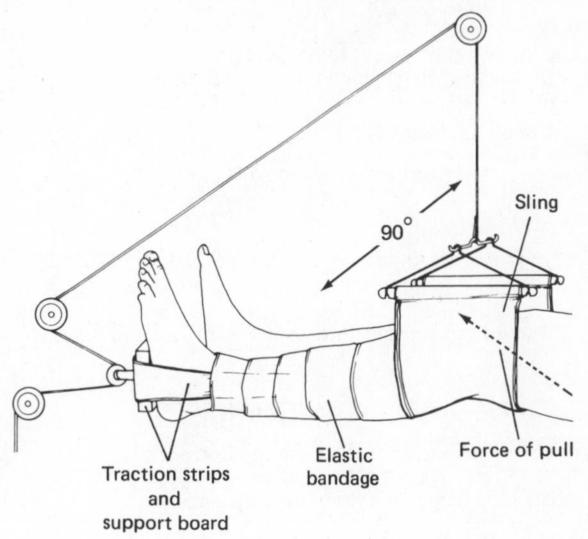

figure 12-6. Russell traction, a form of skin traction, which may be used for fractures of the hip and femur.

Explanations. The array of bars, ropes, and pulleys may frighten the patient at first. Most fracture patients come to the hospital on an emergency basis, and may be in traction before they have had time to recover from the shock of their experience. At first, simple and direct explanations should be given to the patient. Most important of all, he should be assured that his needs will be taken care of. Be sure that his call bell or light is within reach, that he knows how to use it, and that it is answered quickly. Concerned nursing care will soon minimize his feeling that he is helplessly anchored in one place with no one to hand him a urinal or blanket.

It is important for the nurse and the doctor to correct later any misconceptions that the patient may have as to the purpose of the equipment, the approximate length of time that he will be in it, the pains and the aches to be expected, and the probable outcome.

Placing the Patient in Traction. The mattress on the traction bed should be firm and level. A patient in traction should never lie on a lumpy or a soft mattress. A bed board may be used under the mattress. The doctor places the patient in traction.

The patient may remain in traction for many weeks, making nursing care a *very important* part of the return to optimum function. As traction is used to realign and immobilize the fractured bone, it is imperative that correct principles of traction—that is, traction and countertraction, or two forces pulling away from a center—are maintained (Fig. 12-7). Weights must hang free, ropes and pulleys must be free from interference, and splints and slings must be suspended without interference. Depending on the type and location of the fracture and the type of traction used, the patient may or may not be allowed certain movements—e.g., turning, lifting the hips, having the head of the bed raised. The amount of movement allowed will be ordered by the physician, but the nurse should never hesitate to ask when there is a question of how much movement is permissible.

Buck's extension is a simpler traction that may be used to align bone fragments temporarily while the patient awaits internal fixation. Foam rubber strips, moleskin tape, and then an elastic bandage are applied to the skin of the leg; traction is accomplished with a single pulley.

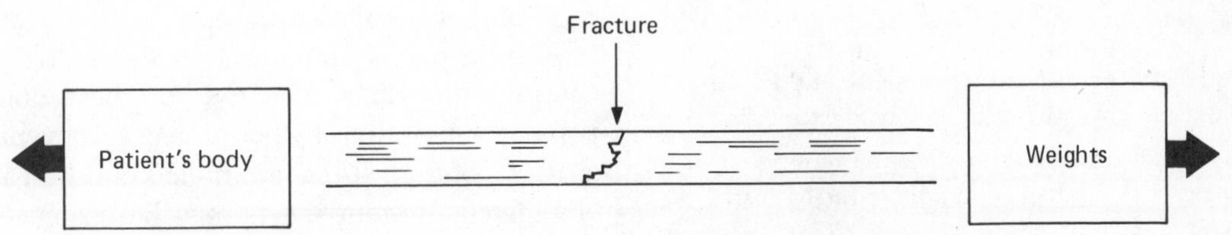

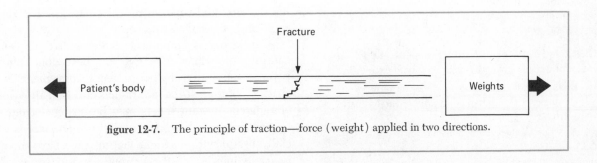

figure 12-7. The principle of traction—force (weight) applied in two directions.

Table 12-3.
Nursing management of the patient in traction

Check traction alignment:

- Weights, splints, and slings should hang free;
- The body should be in alignment with the force of traction;
- The head of the bed is raised only to the prescribed height.

Encourage motion and exercise in the *unaffected* limbs.

Use a footboard to prevent footdrop.

Use a trochanter roll for the unaffected leg(s).

Encourage participation in daily care.

Have the patient do deep-breathing exercises every 1 to 2 hours while awake.

When giving care, use gentle movements and avoid excessive jarring of the bed.

Give frequent skin care, with particular attention to bony prominences.

Check for early signs of decubitus formation: blanched skin, reddened areas, pain or discomfort over pressure points.

Keep bottom sheets taut and free of wrinkles.

Use sheepskin pads, foam rubber supports, or an alternating pressure mattress at the first sign of skin breakdown (elderly patients may need these measures from the beginning).

Be alert to signs of infection at sites of pin or wire insertion and operative site (if surgery was performed).

Push fluids unless specifically contraindicated by a physician's order.

Keep all items within reach: bedside stand, call light, personal effects, etc.

Make sure that traction is continuous and that weights are *never* released unless so ordered by the physician.

Check for signs of circulatory impairment in all extremities but especially in the affected extremity:

- Blanching or discoloration of the extremity;
- Coolness of skin when compared to the opposite extremity;
- Absence of peripheral pulse(s).

Nursing management of the patient in traction

The patient in traction is more or less immobile in that he is confined to bed. This, then, prompts the institution of special points of nursing care to prevent the complications that arise from immobilization: skin breakdown, pneumonia and other respiratory disorders, infection, footdrop, muscle atrophy, and so on. The principles of nursing management are given in Table 12-3.

Check frequently to see that the patient's hand or foot is warm and of normal color. Sensation should be normal when the foot or the hand is touched. There should be no numbness or tingling.

See to it that all the ropes are in their grooves. During movement a rope can jump its track. When it does, it no longer moves. A frayed cord should be replaced before it breaks. Make sure that the patient's footpiece does not touch the pulleys at the foot of the bed. There is no traction when it touches the pulleys. If suspension traction is working properly, the patient's leg will rise when he lifts his hips. If his leg does not rise, check to make sure that the traction rope is in the grooves of the pulley, and that the weights are hanging free. If the leg still does not rise, inform the doctor. He may wish to adjust the traction.

Check to see that the patient's elbows are not becoming sore from rubbing the sheet. Long-sleeved gowns may help to protect them. After the patient's bath, apply lanolin, followed by tincture of benzoin. Teach the patient to use the overhead trapeze to lift himself in bed; he should not push up with his elbows.

To prevent atrophy, exercises are encouraged. The physical therapist will direct the patient in those exercises performed on the affected extremity; the nurse must encourage use of the unaffected extremities. This can be done, in part, by having patients assist in their own care as often and as much as possible. Range-of-motion (ROM) exercises may be ordered. The nurse or the physical therapist is responsible for performing these exercises on those incapable of self-exercise and for showing and supervising the exercises of those not requiring physical assistance.

Gentleness is important, as excessive movement causes pain. Linen changes are best done by two people, especially if the patient's movement is restricted. Bottom sheets are pulled taut and all wrinkles eliminated. Bottom sheets may be changed from side to side or top to bottom. The latter maneuver is especially useful with accident victims who have incurred multiple injuries of the extremities and trunk. With this method, the bottom linen is removed by starting at the head of the bed and pulling the sheet down under the patient; at the same time clean bedding is positioned and follows the soiled linen to the foot of the bed. The reverse direction, that is, changing linen from bottom to top, can also be used.

A fracture pan (or orthopedic pan) rather than a regular bedpan is usually preferred as it eliminates elevation of the hips. A kidney (emesis) basin may be used for female patients if urination is difficult on a fracture pan. Stool softeners may be necessary as confinement to bed and the use of a bedpan encourage constipation.

Back care may offer a challenge, especially when movement is limited. Firm, downward pressure on the mattress near the part to be massaged will give room for the nurse's hand. Keeping the skin soft and smooth is important as decubitus formation is a frequent complication, especially in the thin or elderly patient. Special attention should be given to the sacral area—a common early site of skin breakdown—which is not easily inspected when the patient cannot turn from side to side. Lambswool padding or an alternating pressure mattress may prevent decubitus ulcers, but should not be used in place of good skin care!

If the patient complains of chilliness in the suspended arm or leg, and it is certain that there is no impairment of circulation, a small cover (flannel sheet or light blanket) may be placed over the extremity. The covering should be light, and should not interfere with the slings, splints, or ropes of the traction.

Intake and output should be measured for the first several postoperative days and continued if fluid intake is low. Fluids must be encouraged as an increase in fluid intake reduces the chance of kidney stone formation—a complication of prolonged bed rest and limited fluid intake. Fluids should be readily available by placement of the bedside stand close to the bed.

Diversion therapy, often neglected by busy nursing personnel, is important for any patient confined for a long period of time. An occupational therapist can offer suggestions or plan therapy that is tailored to the patient's needs and preferences. Diversional therapy helps the mind and the body, the mind by creating interest and the body by encouraging movement and

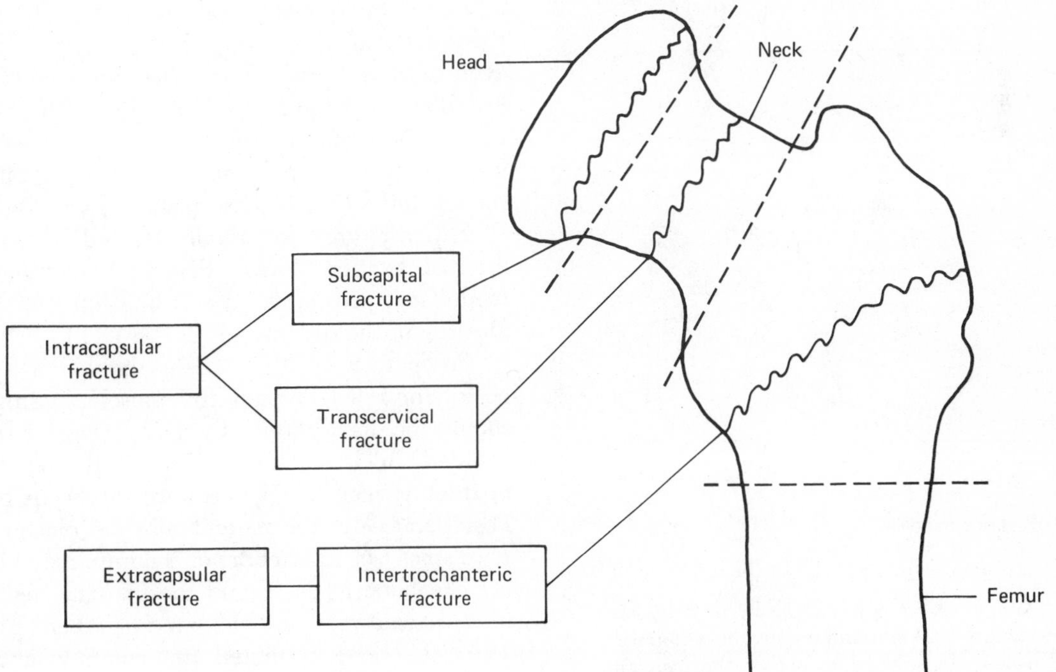

figure 12-8. Types of fractures of the femur.

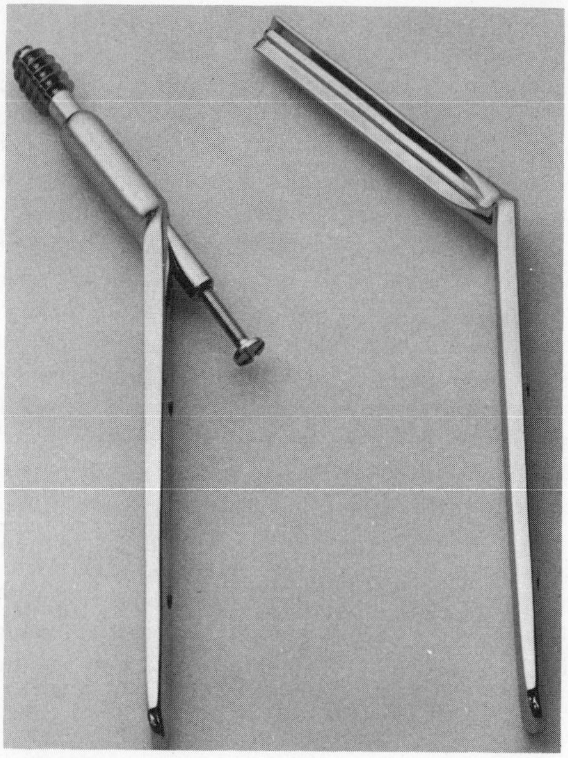

figure 12-9. The Richard adjustable hip screw (*left*) and the Jewett nail (*right*). Both are used to repair intertrochanteric fractures. (Photograph—D. Atkinson)

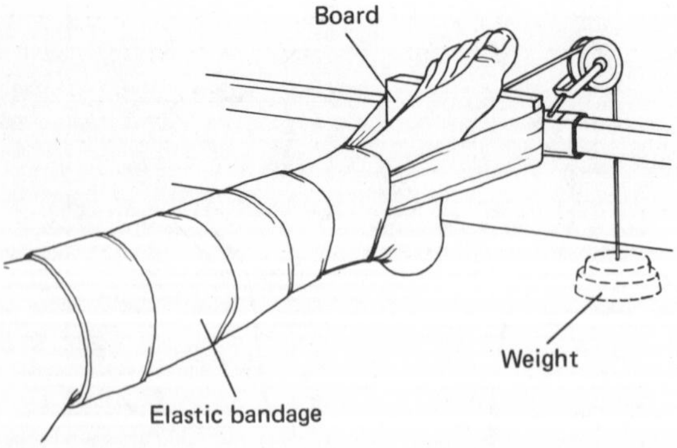

figure 12-10. Buck's extension may be used for hip fractures until internal fixation (surgery) is performed. An Ace bandage is applied to anchor the moleskin straps applied to the skin (dotted lines). The strips may be applied in various ways, one of which is illustrated above.

use of muscles. If an occupational therapist is not available, the nurse can try to provide diversion through the use of reading materials, television, painting, sewing, etc.

Removal from traction

When a patient is removed from skin traction, the adhesive tape is first soaked with ether or acetone. Then a swab moistened with ether or acetone is used to help loosen the tape from the skin. The leg is washed and oiled. Find out from the physician how much movement of the affected part the patient is allowed, and make certain that the patient understands what movement is permitted. If the limb has been in any type of traction for a considerable time, it will at first feel stiff, and there may also be some atrophy of muscles, making the limb look thinner than the other. Explain to the patient that the feeling of stiffness will disappear as he becomes able to exercise, and that the muscles will gradually grow firm and strong again as he uses the leg.

The patient with a fractured hip

Hip fractures are not uncommon in the elderly and may also occur in anyone who has had a serious injury or fall. Because of osteoporosis, the bones of the elderly are fragile and brittle; fracture may occur even after a minor injury. The types of hip fracture are shown in Fig. 12-8, p. 139. Signs of hip fracture are: (1) pain in the affected area, (2) shortening of the leg, and (3) external rotation (a turning outward) of the leg and foot. Diagnosis is made by x-ray.

Hip fractures are usually treated by means of an internal fixation device, that is, a nail or an intramedullary prosthesis, depending on the type and location of the fracture (Fig. 12-9).

Preoperatively, the patient should be given analgesics for relief of pain and muscle spasms. The leg should be handled gently and excessive movement avoided. Buck's extension (Fig. 12-10) or other forms of traction may be applied until surgery is performed. Postoperatively, the patient may be placed in a cast (hip spica) or in traction, or the limb may be left free.

The bone heals around the metallic device, which in the meantime holds the bone together (Fig. 12-11). Thus the bone is united immediately, and patients can be mobilized much earlier than with treatment by traction. Plates, bands, screws, and pins may be removed after the bone has healed, or may be left permanently in place.

Another device to produce internal fixation is the intramedullary rod, which is inserted in long bones. It may be used when, for example, the patient has had a pathologic fracture. Such a patient is likely to suffer additional pathologic fractures. The patient usually is placed in traction after this procedure and may bear weight in about three weeks.

BONE GRAFTS. Sometimes cancellous bone (the reticular tissue of bone) is packed around the fracture line to stimulate bone growth. Heterogenous bone (bone from another species), homogenous bone (bone from the same species but another person), or autogenous bone (bone from the body of the patient) may be used. Autogenous bone, which may be taken from the tibia or the iliac bone, seems to be accepted best by the body. The grafted bone eventually is replaced by the growth of new bone.

COMPLICATIONS. Blood vessels run close to the neck of the femur. When the bone fragments produced by the fracture divide these vessels, the neck and head of the femur suffer a loss of blood supply, which may cause avascular necrosis (also called aseptic necrosis). Dead bone, which looks like live bone on an x-ray film, will unite with the live part of the femur and may even support the weight of the patient for some months following an internal fixation, but then it collapses. The incidence of nonunion is also attributed to divided arterial blood supply. Aseptic necrosis and secondary arthritic changes in the joint may occur.

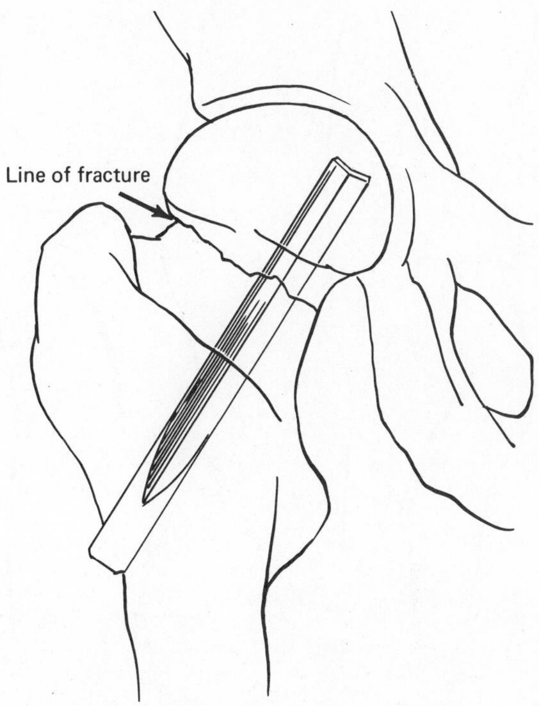

figure 12-11. A Smith-Petersen nail through the fractured neck of a femur.

POSTOPERATIVE NURSING MANAGEMENT

Because these patients usually are elderly and have suffered two major physical insults (the trauma of the fracture and the surgery), alert, supportive nursing care and careful judgment are especially important to their life and comfort. Hemorrhage is an immediate postoperative concern. So is postoperative pain, which may be severe. Narcotics should be administered judiciously and with consideration of the dangers of disorientation and depression of respiration. The postoperative exercises of deep breathing and moving the unaffected extremities are often even more of a trial for the older patient, who might not have been agile when well. Yet the complications resulting from not participating in these exercises are life-threatening.

When there is a surgical wound in which a large skin flap covers a dead space, the patient may come from the operating room with a drain that may be connected to a low suction drainage device, such as the Hemovac; the drain may be left in place for 1 or 2 days to prevent the collection of fluid in the space.

When a bone is nailed, there is no need for a cast. Postoperatively, the doctor will order to which side the patient may be turned. If it is toward the affected leg, the bed provides a comfortable splint and reduces the pain of movement. Place a pillow lengthwise between the patient's legs before turning him. Turn the patient all at once, keeping the fractured leg in a straight line with the trunk. If the patient may be turned to his unaffected side, use one pillow lengthwise under his upper leg and another behind his back.

Depending on the condition of the patient, possibly on the day after the operation, exercises prescribed by the doctor are started by the physical therapist. The role of the nurse is to encourage the patient, to make the exercises as pleasant as possible, and to see that they are done at least 4 times a day. The nurse reminds the patient to avoid external rotation while he is in bed by "toeing in."

After pinning for internal fixation some patients are placed in traction for 1 or 2 days to help to relieve muscle spasm. Then they are helped out of bed, sometimes to ambulate without weight bearing on the

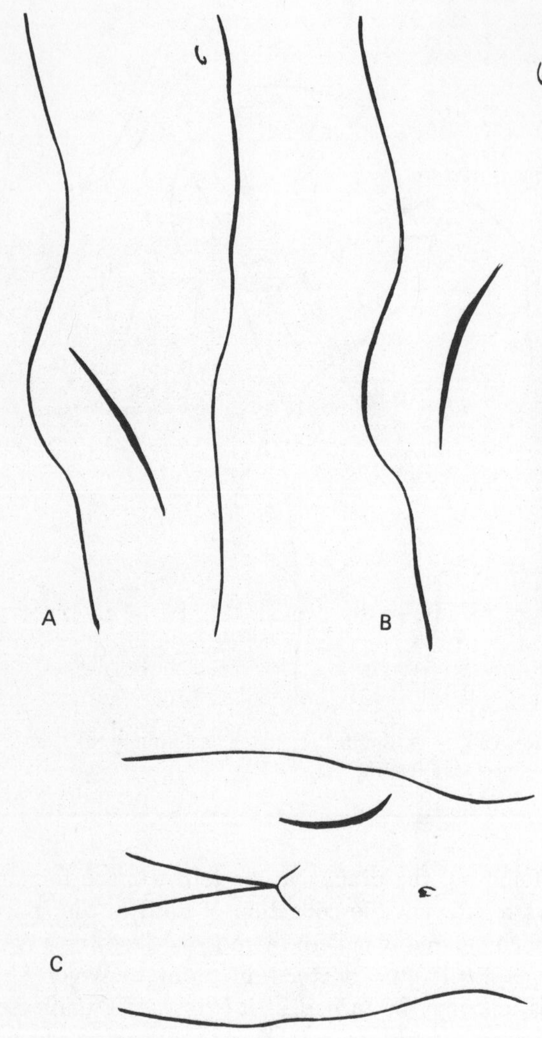

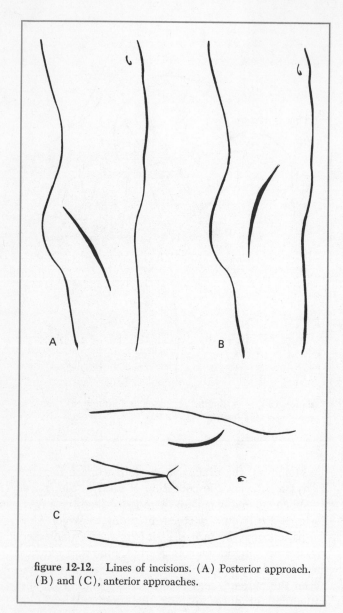

figure 12-12. Lines of incisions. (A) Posterior approach. (B) and (C), anterior approaches.

affected leg and sometimes just to use a wheelchair. Weight bearing on the operative side is avoided until evidence of healing is seen on x-ray film.

After the insertion of a prosthesis, the position of the patient is determined by the line of the incision in the capsule (Fig. 12-12). The objective is to prevent strain on the incision that would result in pushing the prosthesis through it. When the surgical approach has been posterior, the patient is kept relatively flat in bed, with the operative leg somewhat abducted and in external rotation (here is an exception to the rule). When the incision is anterior, the leg is kept in internal rotation, and the patient may sit up. He is helped out of bed on the first postoperative day and is encouraged to walk with weight bearing as soon as the soft tissues have healed. X-ray films are taken about every 3 months the first year.

When there is necrosis of the femur after a pinning, the patient will have pain and muscle spasm, and he will limp. Early recognition is important, because further weight bearing will cause crumbling of the bone. Depending on the age, condition, and degree of disability of the patient, reoperation for the insertion of a prosthesis may be considered.

Total Hip Replacement. Total hip replacement may be indicated in those patients with severe arthritic degeneration of the hip, disabling pain, and severe limitation of movement in the hip joint. In this surgery, the head of the femur and the acetabulum, a ball-and-socket joint, are replaced with metals and plastics.

Postoperative management of the patient with a total hip replacement will vary and often depends on the degree of bone damage, the age of the patient, the variances in the surgical procedure, and the surgeon's preference. Most surgeons write detailed postoperative orders.

Following surgery, the patient may be placed in Buck's traction, or a splint which insures abduction of the operative leg may be applied. Depending on the surgeon's orders the patient *may* or *may not* be allowed to turn on his side. If turning is allowed, pillows are placed between the legs before the patient is turned on his side. The leg *must* be kept in an abducted position at all times, or else the prosthetic femoral head may dislocate from the acetabulum. If dislocation occurs, repeat surgery may be necessary.

Exercise of the operative limb may begin on the day after surgery, starting with foot and ankle motion. As this movement will be painful, exercises are best done ½ to 1 hour after the administration of an analgesic. The patient may begin active movement of the knee, hip, and ankle by the third to fifth postoperative day. This movement may be done with the help of a physical therapist or by using a knee sling attachment to the bed frame. Ambulation usually begins approximately 1 week after surgery.

Crutch walking

The physical therapist measures the patient for crutches. It is important that they be the proper height, so that as the patient learns to walk he can hold himself erect and experience as little strain as possible. A principle of any rehabilitative measure is that it should produce the most natural situation possible. Crutches that fit properly allow the patient to walk more naturally than do ill-fitting ones.

In preparation for walking with the aid of crutches, the patient may be taught the following exercises to strengthen his arm and shoulder muscles: to lie on his abdomen and do push-ups, to lift sandbags up while he is lying on his back, and to sit up with both palms on the mattress and to push up until his buttocks clear the bed. In crutch walking the weight is carried on the hands, not the axillae. Branches of the brachial plexus run through the axilla; the patient who leans on his crutches may damage these nerves, so that paralysis of his arm results. This condition, known as *crutch palsy,* has been known to develop after only 4 hours of leaning on crutches without the use of handgrips.

For a day or two the patient stands before he walks. Parallel bars may be used before he tries the crutches. Standing gives him the feel of being upright with crutches. He is taught the tripod position, with the crutches ahead of him and to the side. He leans forward slightly from the ankles—not from the neck, waist, or hips. A mirror helps the patient to obtain and maintain good position. The patient with a pinned hip does not touch his affected leg to the floor. Shoes should fit well and have nonslip soles and heels. The patient is taught by diagram and demonstration before he actually tries his crutches (Fig. 12-13).

Ordinarily, the physical therapist teaches crutch walking. (If there is no physical therapist, the teaching is carried out by the nurse.) The nurse should work with the physical therapist and know what he has taught the patient. When crutches are used for the first time, precautions must be taken to ensure the patient's safety. Ambulation should be with the assistance of one or two nursing personnel. All objects must be removed from the area and the floor clean and dry. If the patient has been using crutches for some time, the patient should be taught to inspect the crutch tips for wear. If the rubber shows signs of wear, the tip should be discarded and a new one used.

Other fractures

FRACTURE OF THE SPINE. The patient with a fracture of the spine is usually placed in a position of hyperextension, a position that best reestablishes the normal position of the spinal column and exerts the least pressure on the spinal cord. Continuous hyperextension may be accomplished by a cast or by immobilizing the body with head traction and sand-

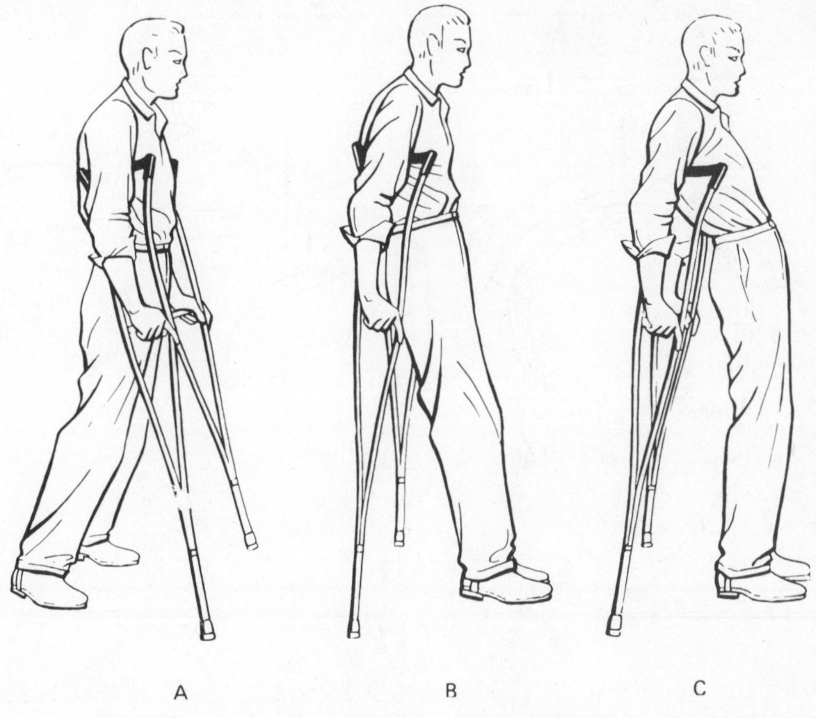

figure 12-13. A man with paraplegia using the swing-through gait. (A) He puts the crutches well in front of him. (B) The swing through. (C) The position in which he lands. He next puts the crutches in position (A).

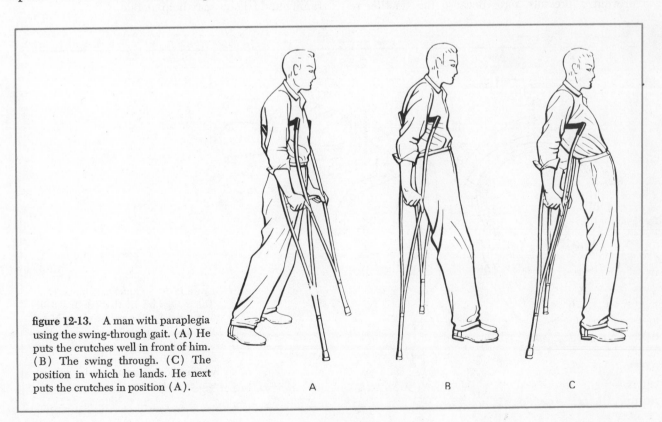

bags over a Gatch bed. Traction may be accomplished by making small burr holes in the skull into the outer layers of the parietal bones on each side and inserting tongs, such as Crutchfield tongs, which then are connected with a pulley and weights (Fig. 12-14). Sandbags may be placed at the shoulders to help to keep the patient down in bed, or the head of the bed may be raised for countertraction. The patient may turn from side to side only if a doctor gives an order. The patient must be turned without bending his spine. If the patient may be turned, a Stryker or a Foster frame facilitates care. When head traction is used, the head of the patient is placed at the foot of the bed.

If, as may rarely be the case, the patient is not allowed to turn, his body may be held still by sandbags at his sides, or a drawsheet may be placed over his abdomen. As the patient may have to lie still in the same position for as long as 6 weeks, the care of the skin is of the utmost importance. Back care is given by compressing the mattress with one hand and slipping the other hand under the back of the patient. All of the back cannot be washed and rubbed at one time, but no area should be neglected. Beware of the development of decubitus ulcers at the back of the head. The patient is not allowed to have a pillow, but a thin piece of foam rubber under his head may help to prevent a pressure sore. Because the traction relieves pain, patients often are more comfortable in tongs than they appear to be. However, the family may need to be assured that the tongs grip only the bones of the head, and that there is no danger of puncturing the patient's brain. Signs of infection around the burr holes should be watched for.

Sometimes traction is accomplished by leather or webbed straps on the head and under the chin. These can cause considerable skin irritation. Thin strips of foam rubber between the skin and the strap may help. Traction may be released momentarily for skin care only if the head is supported in the same position with the other hand, and only if the physician allows it. A doctor's order is required for release from traction long enough for a barber to shave a male patient. Be especially careful that there is no jerk when traction is reapplied.

A patient in the position of hyperextension may have difficulty swallowing and should be fed slowly. A suction machine should be kept nearby in case he needs it. The suction machine should be checked to be sure it is functioning properly *before* the patient is fed.

The position is a tiresome one. There is little for the patient to look at, and his body grows weary from lying still. A radio, television, and visits from family and friends may help morale.

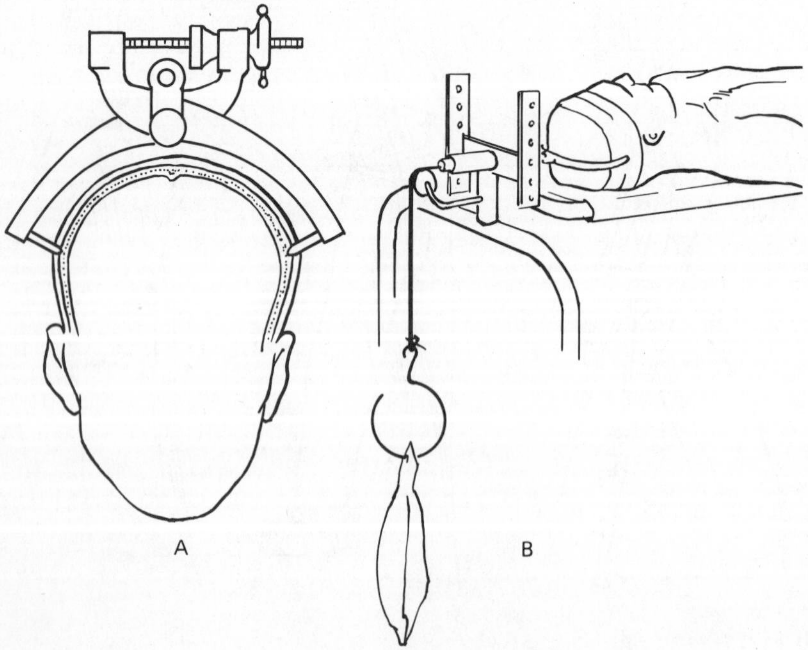

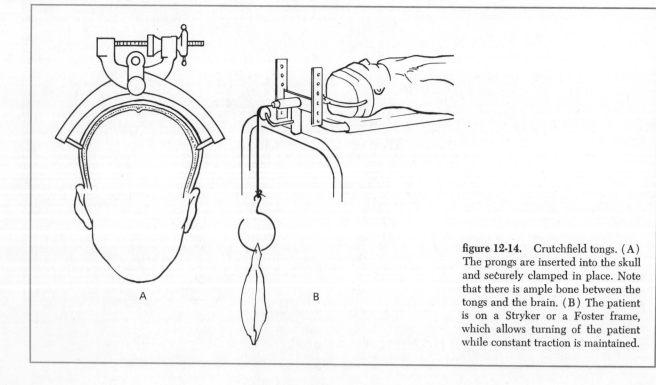

figure 12-14. Crutchfield tongs. (A) The prongs are inserted into the skull and securely clamped in place. Note that there is ample bone between the tongs and the brain. (B) The patient is on a Stryker or a Foster frame, which allows turning of the patient while constant traction is maintained.

Massages of the parts of the body on which he lies and range-of-motion exercises for his limbs help to maintain muscle tone. Patients who are in casts and traction are particularly susceptible to hypostatic pneumonia. Deep-breathing exercises, blowing into a bottle of water through a straw, or IPPB treatments should be carried out 4 to 6 times per day.

If a patient has a fracture of a cervical vertebra, he may graduate to a neck brace. Since he cannot look down with this brace on, he has to be careful not to trip when he walks.

FRACTURE OF THE MANDIBLE. Fractures of the mandible are treated frequently with wires that splint the lower jaw to the upper jaw. The nurse should be familiar with the wire loops that can be unhooked, and she should keep a pair of scissors strapped to the head of the bed for use in case the patient vomits. Because the patient cannot chew, the diet is liquid or, at best, semiliquid, and he may be fed through a straw. The patient's mouth should be cleansed thoroughly after each meal and every 2 hours. The cheeks are retracted with a tongue depressor, and a flashlight is used to see into the mouth. These fractures usually are compound. Complications include primary hemorrhage, asphyxia, and infection, which may lead to osteomyelitis.

FRACTURE OF THE CLAVICLE. A fractured clavicle may be immobilized by a figure-of-8 bandage. When a fractured clavicle is immobilized with plaster, the cast is usually placed over padding applied in a figure-of-8 design. Felt is placed in the axilla to protect the axillary vessels and nerves. Initially, the patient may be uncomfortable. Pressure against the axilla can be relieved by abducting the arm or resting the elbows on the arms of a chair or table. The patient should be encouraged to use his arms as naturally as possible. Motion will help to prevent "frozen shoulder."

FRACTURED RIBS. Broken ribs are uncomfortable, since they must move when a person breathes. Often they are strapped for support, and they usually heal without trouble. They are treated with adhesive strapping, which crosses the midline to the unaffected side, front and back, and is applied as the patient exhales. The skin is first shaved and the nipple area is padded to facilitate removal of the tape.

Dislocations and sprains

Dislocations occur when the articular surfaces of a joint are no longer in contact. In adults they are caused by trauma or, less frequently, by disease of the joint. The symptoms are pain, malposition leading to an abnormal axis of the dependent bone, and loss of the function of the joint. Treatment consists of manipulation of the joint until the parts are again in normal position, followed by immobilization by Ace bandage, cast, or splint for several weeks to allow the joint capsule and surrounding ligaments to heal.

Manipulation never should be attempted by anyone except a physician, who usually makes an x-ray examination first and may anesthetize the patient for the procedure. Amateur attempts at reduction may further injure the capsule of the joint and surrounding structures, and sometimes cause fractures or hemorrhage.

If the patient must be transported to the hospital, the affected joint should be splinted. After the reduction of the dislocation the nurse watches for compression resulting from tight bandages or a tight cast.

Sprains are injuries to the ligaments surrounding a joint. They are accompanied by pain, swelling, and loss of motion. They may become ecchymotic because of the rupture of the nearby blood vessels. An x-ray film may be taken to differentiate a sprain from a fracture. Treatment consists of elevation of the part and application of an elastic bandage.

General nutritional considerations

- A diet high in proteins, vitamins, and minerals may be ordered for the patient immobilized for a long period of time.
- Calcium is needed for the repair of bone. A diet high in calcium and restricted in foods that inhibit the absorption of calcium (such as fats, certain breakfast cereals) may be ordered.
- Phosphorus is also needed for the repair of bone and is usually present in adequate amounts in the average diet.
- Many patients develop anorexia during a prolonged period of immobilization and may require small frequent feedings to provide an adequate dietary intake.
- Fluids should be forced to prevent formation of kidney stones, one of the hazards of immobility. Additional fluids can be supplied between meals in the form of milk shakes, gelatin, and other foods, as well as water.

General pharmacological considerations

- Stool softeners such as dioctyl calcium sulfosuccinate (Surfak) may be necessary to prevent constipation in the patient immobilized for a long period of time.
- Vitamin and mineral supplements may be ordered for patients immobilized in traction, especially if dietary intake is poor.
- Patients receiving calcium as a mineral supplement will also require additional vitamin D as an adequate amount of this vitamin must be present for calcium to be absorbed from the gut wall.
- If osteomyelitis should occur, antibiotic therapy is instituted. The patient may require systemic antibiotics for a long period of time. The nurse should be aware of the possibility of the development of drug-resistant microorganisms. If this should occur, the patient will develop symptoms of a recurrence of the osteomyelitis.

Bibliography

Anderson, L. et al: *Nutrition in Nursing.* Philadelphia, Lippincott, 1972.

Barrett, A. M.: Improving nutrition for the elderly. Nurs. Care 75:28, July, 1975.

Brown, S.: Easing the burden of traction and casts. RN 75:36, February, 1975.

Brunner, N. A.: *Orthopedic Nursing, A Programmed Approach.* St. Louis, Mosby, 1970.

Committee on Injuries, American Academy of Orthopaedic Surgeons: *Emergency Care and Transportation of the Sick and Injured.* Menasha, Wisconsin, George Banta Co. Inc., 1971.

Cosgriff, J. H. and Anderson, D. L.: *The Practice of Emergency Nursing.* Philadelphia, Lippincott, 1975.

Eyre, M. K.: Total hip replacement. Am. J. Nurs. 71:1384, July, 1971.

Gartland, J. J.: *Practical Orthopaedics,* ed. 2. Philadelphia, Saunders, 1972.

Guthrie, H. A.: *Introductory Nutrition,* ed. 3. St. Louis, Mosby, 1975.

Hogberg, A.: Preventing orthopedic complications. RN 75:34, March, 1975.

Larson, C. B. and Gould, M.: *Orthopedic Nursing,* ed. 7. St. Louis, Mosby, 1970.

Law, J.: The fat embolism syndrome. Nurs. Clin. North Am. 8:191, March, 1973.

Meltzer, W., ed.: *Orthopedics.* New York, Harper and Row, 1971.

Miller, M. and Sachs, M.: *About Bedsores: What You Need to Know to Help Prevent and Treat Them.* Philadelphia, Lippincott, 1974.

Rhomas, B. J.: Total knee, new surgical miracle. RN 73:25, September, 1973.

Rodman, M. J. and Smith, D. W.: *Clinical Pharmacology in Nursing.* Philadelphia, Lippincott, 1974.

Townly, C. and Hill, L.: Total knee replacement. Am. J. Nurs. 74:1612, September, 1974.

Twedt, B.: Control of pain in orthopedic patients. RN 75:39, April, 1975.

Webb, K. J.: Early assessment of orthopedic injuries. Am. J. Nurs. 74:1048, June, 1974.

CHAPTER—13

The patient with a disease of the bones and joints

On completion of this chapter the student will:

- Describe the more common symptoms and modalities of treatment of the patient with a disease of the bones and joints.
- Discuss the social, economic, mental, and physical problems of the patient with rheumatoid arthritis and the problems encountered during rehabilitation.
- Give postoperative care to the patient with corrective or reconstructive hip and knee surgery.
- Discuss the use of physical devices for preventing deformities and skin breakdown in the orthopedic patient immobilized for long periods of time.
- Recognize and list the side effects of drugs usually used in the treatment of diseases of the bones and joints.
- Educate the patient regarding the importance of drug and nutrition therapy in the treatment of disorders of the bones and joints.

Arthritis

Arthritis means inflammation of a joint. The disease has been known throughout human history, as evidence of arthritis has

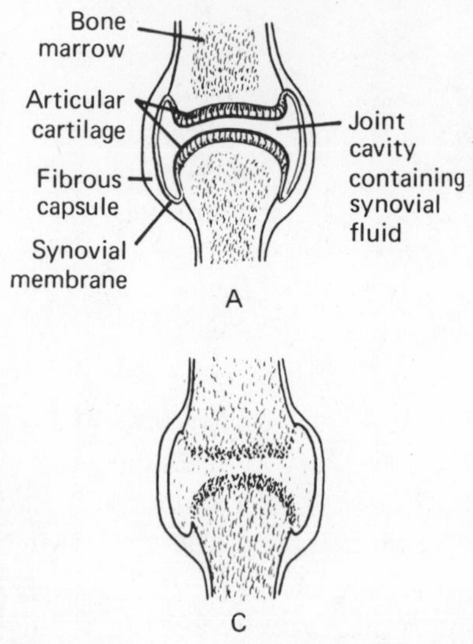

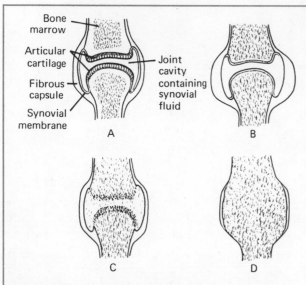

figure 13-1. Pathologic changes in rheumatoid arthritis. (A) Normal ball-and-socket joint. (B) Same joint, showing progression of pannus formation, destruction of cartilage and acute inflammation. (C) Inflammation subsided; fibrous ankylosis. (D) Bony ankylosis; the joint is immobile.

been found in Egyptian mummies, and clear descriptions of the disease go back almost as far as the written word.

There are many forms of arthritis. The term is applied usually to diseases in which the major symptom involves joints. The etiology and the relationships of the various forms of arthritis are subject to various interpretations. It has been suggested that rheumatoid arthritis is a collagen disease. Considerable medical attention has been focused on attempts to understand the pathology, the cause, and the interrelationships of the collagen diseases, including rheumatic fever, systemic lupus erythematosus, periarteritis nodosa, and rheumatoid arthritis. Because the cause (or causes) of rheumatoid arthritis remains unknown, the way in which the condition is classified varies widely in the literature.

Types of arthritis

The following is a partial classification of the complex disease entities usually included in the term *arthritis*:

- Infectious arthritis
- Traumatic arthritis
- Polyarthritis of unknown etiology (example, rheumatoid arthritis)
- Degenerative joint disease (example, osteoarthritis)
- Arthritis associated with biochemical or endocrine abnormalities (example, gout)
- Tumor
- Allergy and drug reaction

Infectious arthritis

Infectious arthritis is caused by a specific microorganism. For example, in untreated tuberculosis, the tubercle bacillus may proceed to invade the joints. Staphylococci or streptococci may infect a joint, as may many other microorganisms. Usually only one joint is involved, which shows the usual signs of infection: warmth, redness, pain, and swelling. Joints normally are sterile, and the products of bacterial growth are harmful to the lining of the joint. In an effort to dilute these harmful products, fluid is poured into the joint cavity. This fluid accounts for some of the pain and much of the swelling. After the infectious organism has been identified (a culture may be taken from aspiration of the fluid in the joint), the arthritis is treated with a drug to which that organism is sensitive. In the case of bacterial infection, the antibiotics are administered systemically, and sometimes injected directly into the joint. The use of antibiotics has made infectious arthritis relatively uncommon.

Traumatic arthritis

Arthritis due to direct trauma may be caused by a sudden twist, a direct blow to the joint, or a multitude of small insults. In this category fall such disorders as arthritis of the feet of ballet dancers.

Rheumatoid arthritis

Along with degenerative joint disease, rheumatoid arthritis is one of the major causes of arthritic disability in adults. Rheumatoid arthritis is an inflammatory disease of connective tissue, characterized by chronicity, remissions, and exacerbations. Constitutional symptoms and joint changes, which may become permanent deformities, are part of the disease (Fig. 13-1).

Incidence

Rheumatoid arthritis is found throughout the world. This crippling disease strikes during the most productive years of adulthood, usually in the 20 to 40 age group. Three times as many women as men are affected.

Pathology

Rheumatoid arthritis is a systemic disorder; its nature is not fully understood, and its etiology is unknown. However, the local effect in the joint can be described. Some of this effect is due to the disease itself and some to the body's reactions against it. For example, the replacement of damaged tissue by fibrosis is a defense mechanism of the body. However, scars due to fibrosis can lead to crippling contractures.

Synovitis, inflammation of the synovial membrane surrounding a joint, the earliest pathological change, causes congestion and edema. Pathophysiological changes follow, leading to the formation of a tissue which adheres to the opposite joint surface, inhibiting motion. This is the stage of *fibrous ankylosis* (abnormal immobility of a joint).

When the restricting band of tissue becomes calcified, as it may, the stage of *osseous ankylosis* has arrived, and the joint no longer exists. This process from nonspecific synovitis to complete ossification of the joint may take years, and it may proceed at different rates in different joints in the same patient.

Some patients develop subcutaneous nodules. These appear over pressure points, such as the elbow or the base of the spine. Though usually painless, they may be quite painful if continuous pressure is put on them, as in a chair-bound patient with nodules at the base of the spine.

Muscles become weak and atrophy, partially from disuse. Because of connective-tissue changes and neurovascular changes, the extremities often have a smooth, glossy appearance, and they may be cold and clammy.

Etiology

Although the causes of rheumatoid arthritis have not yet been discovered, it is probable that one or more factors trigger the onset of the disease.

Children of arthritic parents have a greater tendency to develop the disease than those whose ancestors have no such history. Heredity may be a factor, but the evidence pointing to this theory could be explained also by environmental factors.

Symptoms

In most patients the onset is insidious. Over a period of time patients notice that a joint or two is stiff when they wake up in the morning. There are twinges of momentary discomfort in a finger or two. Slowly some joints, usually the fingers, become moderately sore, red, and swollen. Over a period of weeks, other joints become involved. Swelling and pain come and go. In the meantime the patients find that they tire easily. They lose weight, and may develop a fever and malaise. Tolerance for any kind of stress is lessened, and temperature changes are tolerated poorly. Although the diet may be adequate in iron, patients characteristically have a persistent anemia because of the effect of this chronic disease on the blood-forming organs.

As the disease progresses, the muscle wasting around affected joints accentuates the appearance of swelling. The proximal finger joints swell the most, and as deformity develops, the fingers point toward the lateral aspect of the hand (Fig. 13-2). Extremities

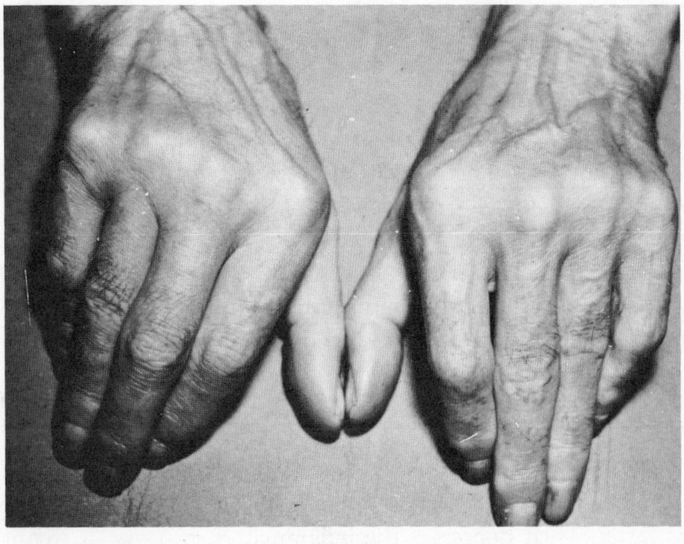

figure 13-2. Appearance typical of arthritic hands. The joints become sore, swollen and deformed. (Medichrome—Clay-Adams, Inc., New York, N.Y.)

become cold, moist, and mauve-colored. Patients in this stage of the disease have considerable pain at rest, and especially on motion.

The symptoms may vanish suddenly for no apparent reason. Inflammation leaves joints that were sore and red; the patient is not stiff, he has no fever, and his pain is gone. However, the symptoms almost invariably return after the patient has had a symptom-free period. Inflammation causes more joint damage, followed by another remission. The pattern of remissions and exacerbations continues for years.

Without treatment—and sometimes with it—the joint may be totally destroyed. As the synovial space is replaced with bony growth, motion is lost. When the joint becomes immobile, the pain of the inflammation is lessened, but there still is discomfort because of contractures and immobility. One of the aims of treatment is to decrease the inflammation of the joint before it has become one bone.

Treatment

Although the cause of rheumatoid arthritis remains unknown, and the disease cannot be cured, much can be done to lessen its damage. Early treatment before the onset of fibrous or bony ankylosis gives the best results. Treatment is designed to make the patient more comfortable, to prevent or to correct deformities, and to maintain or to restore function of the affected parts of the musculoskeletal system.

Optimal health conditions should be maintained, since supporting the resistance of the body to the inflammation is one of the few truly therapeutic steps that medicine has to offer. Rest, both systemic and local, is balanced carefully with exercise. Even during an acute phase of the illness, some movement of the affected parts is usually prescribed to help lessen the possibility of bony ankylosis, muscle wasting, osteoporosis, and the debilitating effects of prolonged rest. Deep breathing and prescribed exercises, graded to the condition of the patient, strengthen general body tone and keep specific muscle groups from atrophy. The patient should be encouraged to eat an optimum diet, even though he may have little appetite. Unless there are other medical complications, such as diabetes or hypertension, this diet need not be modified from that of a normal individual.

Drug therapy

Drug therapy in rheumatoid arthritis is not curative, but it helps the patient to feel less pain, and, in some instances, it depresses the inflammatory process. Because of the long-term nature of this disease, relief of pain by the use of narcotics is avoided.

The Salicylates. Aspirin (acetylsalicylic acid) is the major drug in the group. In early rheumatoid arthritis, it seems to have an anti-inflammatory action and to afford specific relief of joint pain. In chronic rheumatoid arthritis, the relief appears less dramatic, but it still is present, and probably it is more related to the general analgesic properties of aspirin than to any specific action. The manner in which this common drug works still is not fully understood.

Large doses of aspirin, which may help the inflammatory process to subside, also may give rise to salicylism: headache, tinnitus, nausea, vomiting, and increased pulse and respiratory rate. Another serious problem with prolonged use of aspirin is erosion of the stomach lining, leading to multiple small spots of bleeding. Patients on high doses of aspirin should be instructed to watch their stools for evidence of gastrointestinal bleeding (black, tarry stool). The patient may note easy bruising, as large doses of aspirin affect the clotting mechanism of the blood. Aspirin cannot be used in patients with ulcers, history of ulcers, or bleeding disorders.

Milk and crackers taken before the drug may help to prevent gastric distress. If the patient experiences distress that seems to be related to his aspirin intake, the physician should be notified. Some patients decrease the dose or omit the tablets entirely without consulting the physician, and yet control of the symptoms depends on a high, sustained blood level of the drug. If the patient is experiencing toxic side effects, the physician should be notified. The patient should be instructed *not* to substitute buffered aspirin or enteric-coated aspirin for regular aspirin unless the physician approves the change.

Other Drugs. Phenylbutazone (Butazolidin) and oxyphenbutazone (Tandearil) are pyrazolone derivatives with analgesic and anti-inflammatory activity. Because both drugs can cause serious side effects, particularly to the bone marrow and kidneys, patients must be under close medical supervision while taking them. Ibuprofen (Motrin) is a newer preparation used in the treatment of rheumatoid arthritis. Like aspirin, Motrin has anti-inflammatory, analgesic, and antipyretic activity. The most common side effect is gastrointestinal disturbance.

Gold salts, such as aurothioglucose (Solganal) and sodium thiomalate (Myochrysine), produce less dramatic results in treatment as there may be 2 or 3 months between the start of gold therapy and the therapeutic results of decreased inflammation and pain. The time lapse may be very discouraging to the patient. Therapy with gold is not always effective. The use of gold can result in serious side effects, including jaundice, blood dyscrasias, hepatitis, hematuria, toxic nephritis, and severe gastrointestinal upsets. The patient is observed carefully with blood counts and urinalysis, and is questioned about skin manifestations, in order to detect early the more severe toxic effects. Gold salts are given intramuscularly.

Corticosteroids. Corticosteroids do not cure arthritis, but they give the patient prompt relief from pain and stiffness. Both physical and mental well-being are improved. However, the long-term use of a corticosteroid may result in side effects that are more disabling than the disease being treated. Close supervision by the physician of the dosage is imperative.

Nursing management

During an early acute phase of rheumatoid arthritis, the patient feels both ill and frightened. If he is febrile, he may be kept in bed, and every effort is made to reduce his pain. A cradle or a footboard keeps the bedcovers from pressing tender feet into abnormal positions, such as outward rotation.

A patient at the early stage of rheumatoid arthritis—or any chronic disease, for that matter—needs accurate information about the probable course of the disease, so that he can plan for the future. As rheumatoid arthritis progresses slowly in about 80 percent of the cases, the immediate way of life of a patient need not change drastically. If he understands the disease process, there are things he can do at the very early stages that will help to prevent present fatigue and later deformity.

He will need to learn about the pathology of the joint changes, so that he will understand why he must both exercise and rest, and that the disease has spontaneous remissions. He should be told what does *not* cure arthritis, so that he can avoid spending money on worthless "treatments."

Exercise. Appropriate exercise has three objectives: (1) to preserve or to increase the function of the joint by preventing ankylosis, (2) to maintain muscle tone, and (3) to improve the strength and coordination. Disuse of a joint leads to stiffness, which leads to more disuse. The patient with deformities tends to avoid the use of deformed joints or to move in ways that increase the deformities.

Relative amounts of rest and exercise are planned carefully for each individual patient. Reparative processes are favored by rest, but prolonged immobilization may lead to ankylosis. Some exercises may be done while the patient is lying down; thus he avoids the extra work of overcoming the pull of gravity. The joint needs protection against overuse, wobbling, and partial dislocations. If it is possible, after heat and perhaps light massage, each joint should be exercised several times a day.

Only gentle stretching is permissible. Excessive activity to the point of pain or fatigue, vigorous exercise of an inflamed part, or movement that increases joint instability and abnormal deviation and dislocation can cause further damage. Active exercise is more therapeutic for the muscles than passive movement.

Many hospitals and community health agencies have physical therapists who will be responsible for teaching the patient his exercises, applying heat, massage, and perhaps whirlpool baths or contrast baths to limbs. Where there is no physical therapist, the nurse has the responsibility for teaching the exercises. Some rules for exercises are:

1. The number and the duration of the rest and exercise periods change as the patient's condition changes. These are determined by the physician and governed by how the patient feels. The exact nature of the exercises is prescribed by the physician.
2. Exercises can seem a tiresome chore, and they may be uncomfortable. Discomfort during or immediately after an exercise should be expected. However, exercise that causes excessive pain should be decreased.
3. Affected joints should go through their prescribed exercises several times a day.
4. Several short periods of 5 to 10 minutes are better than fewer, longer ones of 20 to 30 minutes.
5. As the tolerance of the patient improves, the number of exercise periods can be increased.

Rest. To maintain motion, the arthritic joint needs rest as well as exercise. Because joints limited in motion tend to take the form of flexion, which leads to contractures, the resting position of the joints should be the position of greatest possible extension without actual pain. Therefore, the frequent, necessary rest periods are not as comfortable for the patient as they might be if the line of least resistance were followed. The proper position for rest is flat on the back on a well-supported bed.

HEAT. Heat is more of a comfort than a curative measure. Because it improves circulation and relieves muscle spasm and pain, it allows the part better rest and easier exercise. Heat can be applied dry or wet. Dry heat sometimes is applied by a heating pad, a paraffin bath, or an infrared bulb. The ordinary heating pad is not as effective as other measures. Infrared heat penetrates deeper than the level of the skin. Even superficial heat affects deeper-level blood vessels by reflex action.

Many arthritic patients prefer wet heat, claiming that it penetrates better. Wet heat can be applied in the form of baths, either local or tub, or by the use of specially insulated heating pads that can be used with moisture. *No* heating pad should be used with or near moisture unless of the type clearly identified as insulated and usable with moisture. Heat in any form should be applied for 20 to 30 minutes. The application of pure lanolin or other lotions may help to counter the drying effects of this treatment.

EQUIPMENT. Various mechanical aids have been devised to help the disabled in the performance of day-to-day tasks. Rare is the arthritic for whom a mechanism cannot be fashioned that helps him to feed himself, to comb his own hair, to select his own programs on the television set, and to cope with more complex and specialized problems. Some mechanical aids are currently on the market; others can be custom-built, very often of improvised materials, if a little ingenuity is employed. A device should be lightweight and as simple as possible. If the patient finds the device inconvenient or does not like it for any reason, he will not use it.

Not every action of the arthritic should be governed by a gadget. Indeed, his life will be simpler if he has to take care of only a few appliances; but if a device can give a patient the independence of necessary self-help, he should be encouraged to use it.

Braces, bivalve casts, or splints applied to joints that are painful and in spasm help to prevent dislocations and deformity and to keep the rest of the joints mobile. Splints have three basic functions: (1) immobilization for local rest during an active phase of the disease; (2) to correct deformities, such as a long brace with a turnbuckle across the back of the knee to help place that joint in extension; and (3) to help overcome weakness.

If poor posture is imposing an abnormal strain on weight-bearing joints, the patient may be fitted with a corset that improves posture. The splint or brace must fit well, be neither constricting nor loose, be lightweight, and maintain the joint in a good functional position. The nurse should observe for friction on the skin. Adequate padding and good skin care protect the skin. Rough edges that might tear the skin of the patient should be checked. Once a week the leather parts should be saddle-soaped, and the metal joints should be oiled.

The bed should be flat and firm with only one small pillow. A bed board that fits should be placed under the mattress and firmly attached, so that when the patient moves near the edge, he is not in danger of tipping the bed board over. The height of the bed should be level with that of the wheelchair, if the patient moves back and forth between the two.

REHABILITATION. Rehabilitation is an important aspect in the management of patients with rheumatoid arthritis. Both the patient and the family must be given facts about the disease, the limitations of the patient, the need for certain changes in life style, and rehabilitation exercises. The prime focus of rehabilitation is making the patient as independent as possible for as long as possible. The patient's disability must be evaluated, and a plan of care developed that will enable the patient to remain independent. For example, the housewife with severe deformity of the fingers will need extensive reevaluation of her daily activities. Vacuuming the rug or making the bed which once may have been easily accomplished are now nearly impossible for her to do. A lighter, smaller vacuum cleaner or fitted contour sheets may help her to perform these activities. Some activities may have to be either discontinued or performed with help from family members or friends. Thus, the husband may have to move furniture, but the patient still may be able to dust. One very important point to be considered is the expense of some of the alterations of life style. A dishwasher may be an easy alternative to washing dishes, but for some this may be impractical or financially impossible. The nurse must remember that suggestions should be within the financial capabilities of the family.

CORRECTIVE SURGERY. The use of surgery to overcome or prevent deformity is becoming an increasingly important aspect of early treatment. Previously surgery was resorted to only late in the disease after extensive damage had occurred. Synovectomy (removal of the diseased lining) performed early is being extensively investigated as a means of preventing destructive changes in affected joints, particularly those of the hands, feet, and knees. When muscle spasm is causing progressive deformity, tendons may be transplanted to change the direction of pull to a corrected one. An artificial angling of the bone through surgical fracture (osteotomy) may improve the utility of a deformed limb.

Table 13-1.
Postoperative management of the patient with an arthroplasty

HIP ARTHROPLASTY

The leg *must* be maintained in a position of *abduction.*

Balanced suspension traction is used for approximately 3 weeks.

A pillow is placed between the knees to prevent accidental adduction.

A trochanter roll is used for the unoperated leg to prevent external rotation.

Isometric exercises are instituted.

Deep-breathing exercises are performed hourly for the first 1 to 2 days postoperatively, then every 2 to 3 hours while awake.

The head of the bed is kept flat until orders are written to raise the head of the bed. Increase in height should be gradual.

Blood pressure, pulse, respirations are taken every 1 to 2 hours for the first 24 hours, then every 4 hours. Nursing judgment or the physician's orders may alter the frequency of these measurements.

Temperature is taken every 4 hours for 5 or more days.

The dressing is checked for drainage, and reinforced if necessary.

Voiding and intake and output are checked.

The color and temperature of the extremity are checked and any changes reported immediately.

KNEE ARTHROPLASTY

The leg is elevated to prevent edema.

Vital signs and temperature are checked as above.

Voiding and intake and output are checked.

The color and temperature of the extremity are checked and any changes reported immediately.

Leg exercises, which usually begin the first or second postoperative day, are supervised.

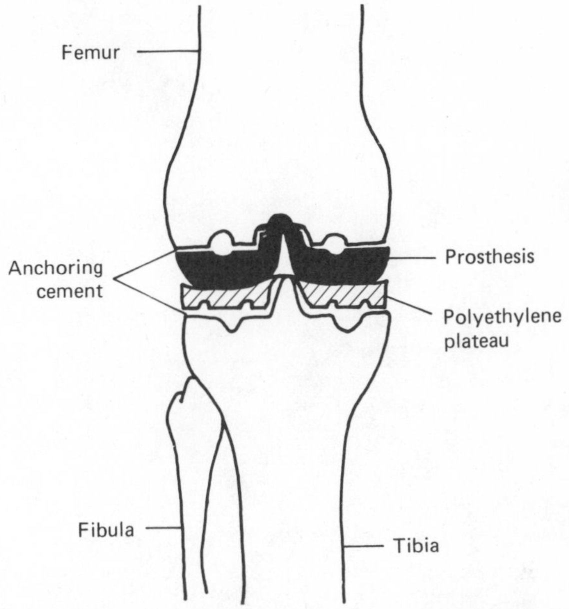

figure 13-3. A total knee replacement showing the insertion of the prosthesis and the polyethylene plateau. The prosthesis allows for full movement of the knee.

Arthroplasty, the fashioning of a new joint with artificial material, may be resorted to. When all hope of salvaging a joint is gone, but it is still painful and troublesome to the patient, an arthrodesis (fusion of the joint surfaces) may be performed, eliminating the joint but relieving the pain. Nursing management of a patient with an arthroplasty is given in Table 13-1. In some instances, nursing care will vary; use of pillows and trochanter rolls and the institution of isometric exercises should be prescribed by the physician.

Recently, newer surgical procedures have been devised for total hip and knee replacements (Figs. 13-3, 13-4). In some cases, these procedures have given better results than the knee or hip arthroplasty. In general, care of the patient is the same as that for an arthroplasty; however, different types of traction and postoperative exercises may be used. In addition, turning may or may not be allowed and the patient's position in bed may be varied. As there are various techniques of total hip replacement, the physician's orders are usually detailed (see Chapter 12). If there is *any* question about the meaning of an order or what can or cannot be done, the nurse should consult the surgeon before instituting any nursing task.

Infection and thrombophlebitis are two serious complications of orthopedic surgeries. The patient's

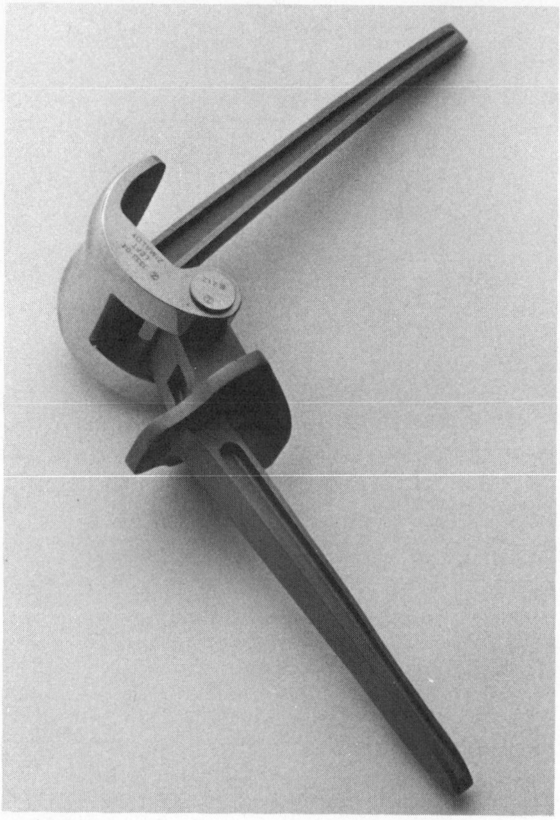

figure 13-4. The Guépar-type total knee prosthesis. (Photograph—D. Atkinson)

temperature should be monitored every 4 hours during the immediate postoperative period—approximately 5 days. Laminar airflow rooms have reduced the incidence of postoperative infections. Any signs of thrombophlebitis—elevated temperature, calf tenderness, pain, warmth, or redness in an extremity—must be reported immediately as there is always the danger of a pulmonary embolus. Fat emboli are common complications when there is a fracture of or surgery on the long bones, for example, the femur. The symptoms of a fat embolus, for example, petechial hemorrhages on the skin of the chest, are the same as those for an embolus due to a blood clot. Fat emboli usually occur earlier in the postoperative period than emboli due to a blood clot.

Patient education

Emotional factors play a great part in the management of the patient with rheumatoid arthritis. There are two factors to be considered: (1) the crippling aspects of a disease with an uncertain and precarious future, and (2) the emotional toll extracted by pain, discomfort, and physical limitations. These factors may make teaching the patient difficult, especially when he is in the advanced stages of the disease. The points to be stressed in teaching are:

- The importance of consistent medical supervision, even though the patient may feel good and have relief from pain and stiffness.
- The medications prescribed by the physician are important and should *not* be omitted, even if the patient feels better.
- Other drugs or treatments should not be used unless approved by the physician, for example, switching from plain aspirin to a buffered variety. A change should not be undertaken even though both products are, in essence, aspirin. The buffered aspirin contains an alkali and in high doses can cause electrolyte imbalances.
- The physician's advice regarding rest and exercise should be followed Both are important; too much or too little of either can be harmful.
- The side effects of the prescribed medication(s) should be included in the discharge teaching.

Some arthritic patients have deformities that are far advanced, and the nurse may find these patients seemingly beyond rehabilitation. Sometimes the disease is overpowering; treatment was not begun in time, or was inadequate. Perhaps present methods of treatment were not available when the illness started.

Whatever the condition of the patient, the nurse should concentrate on making the most of his remaining capabilities. The best way to begin is to look for little things that hold promise of improving the situation.

Ankylosing spondylitis

Ankylosing spondylitis, or Marie-Strümpell disease, is a chronic inflammatory disease of the joints of the spine usually beginning in the sacroiliac. If the disease progresses, rigidity and fixation (ankylosis) of the spine result. Diagnosis is made by x-ray examination. Treatment is similar to that for rheumatoid arthritis (see pp. 148-153). Adequate bed rest, a firm mattress with a bed board, exercise, and improved posture are advised. Salicylates or phenylbutazone may be prescribed; in addition, deep radiotherapy has been used for those who do not respond to more conservative treatment.

Degenerative joint disease (osteoarthritis)

This type of arthritis is a disease of the joints characterized by a slow and a steady progression of destructive changes. Unlike rheumatoid arthritis, degenerative joint disease has no remissions and no systemic symptoms, such as malaise and fever.

Incidence and etiology

This is a wear-and-tear disease that may start as early as the middle 30's, but it is mainly an affliction of later middle life and old age. Repeated trauma may lead to degenerative changes. Obese people, whose joints must bear heavy weight, are more likely to develop early symptoms than lean people. It has been suggested that osteoarthritis is more common in people who use muscular effort as a way of coping with anxiety and aggression. Men and women appear to be affected equally.

Pathology

Osteoarthritis is a reflection of generalized aging. The cartilage that covers the bone edge becomes thin and ragged, and no longer springs back into shape after normal use. Finally, the bone end is bare.

The synovial membrane, which at first is normal, becomes thickened. The fibrous tissue around the joint ossifies. These changes, which occur slowly, give the patient pain and limited motion of the joint. Ankylosis does not occur.

Symptoms

Osteoarthritis is a progressive disease. Early symptoms are stiffness—usually at night or in the morning—and pain which may be noted after exercise. Later, symptoms are more prominent: marked joint enlargement, pronounced stiffness, and pain after exercise. Diagnosis is made on the basis of the patient's symptoms and examination of the affected joints. X-ray studies also demonstrate joint changes.

Many older patients who are admitted for other medical or surgical disorders may also have osteoarthritis; this fact should be considered, along with the primary reason for hospital admission, when planning and implementing patient care. These patients may have morning or evening stiffness, which may cause them to move slowly and, in some cases, with great difficulty. The self-care and partial-care patients should be allowed to complete morning care at their own rate. Young nurses, especially, may become impatient by the seemingly long time these patients may take for morning care. It should be remembered that many of them experience quite a bit of pain and discomfort early in the morning. Ambulatory patients should be encouraged to wear their own shoes rather than slippers, especially if they have special orthopedic-type shoes. Shoes permit better foot and leg support and lessen discomfort.

Treatment

Proper local rest of the affected joints is more important than total body rest. Short periods of moderate exercise are helpful. Exercises should never be a strain to the patient. Normally repeated five to six times a day, they should be regulated by the feeling of the joint. Postural defects that add to the strain on a joint theoretically should be corrected; but since posture is the result of the habit of a lifetime, it probably will not be changed after middle age. Heat to the part is a comfort to the patient. If massage is used, it must be done gently to avoid further damage. Obese patients should lose weight. Anything that helps to relieve strain on the sore joints helps the patient. Support may be given with strapping, belts, braces, canes, or crutches. In some instances, the patient may gain relief while in traction.

Aspirin affords relief from pain. Narcotics are to be avoided. Corticosteroids may be injected into areas of inflammation during an acute stage. Daily traction and swimming may be prescribed.

Because both osteoarthritis and rheumatoid arthritis are called "arthritis," and patients may know that rheumatoid arthritis causes deformity, those with osteoarthritis may worry that their disease also will result in deformity; but osteoarthritis does not have the crippling effect of rheumatoid arthritis.

Gout

Gout is a metabolic disorder in which the body is unable to properly metabolize purines, which are end products of the digestion of certain proteins. This inability results in an accumulation of uric acid in the bloodstream (hyperuricemia). Deposits of urate (a salt of uric acid) crystals occur in body tissues, chiefly in and around joints, causing local inflammation and irritation.

Symptoms

An attack of gout is characterized by a sudden onset of acute pain and tenderness in a joint. The skin turns red, the part swells, and is warm. Fever is usually present. The attack may subside in 1 to 2 weeks, but moderate swelling and tenderness may persist beyond that time. There is usually a symptom-free period followed by another attack, which may occur at any time.

Diagnosis is made by examination of the affected joint, a thorough patient history, serum uric acid levels (which may or may not be elevated), finding of uric acid crystals in synovial fluid obtained by aspiration of the affected joint, x-ray examination, and the finding of tophi—subcutaneous deposits of uric acid crystals (Fig. 13-5). Tophi are usually found on the outer ear (pinna) and at affected joints. Administration of colchicine gives dramatic relief during an acute attack and may be used to distinguish gout from other forms of acute arthritis.

Treatment

Although gout cannot be cured in the sense of removing the basic metabolic difficulty of constant or recurrent hyperuricemia, the attacks usually can be controlled to the point that they no longer occur. The regimen must be individualized for each patient and changed from time to time in response to the changes in the course of the disease. For treatment to succeed, the patient must understand the nature of gout, have self-discipline, and conscientiously maintain contact with his physician.

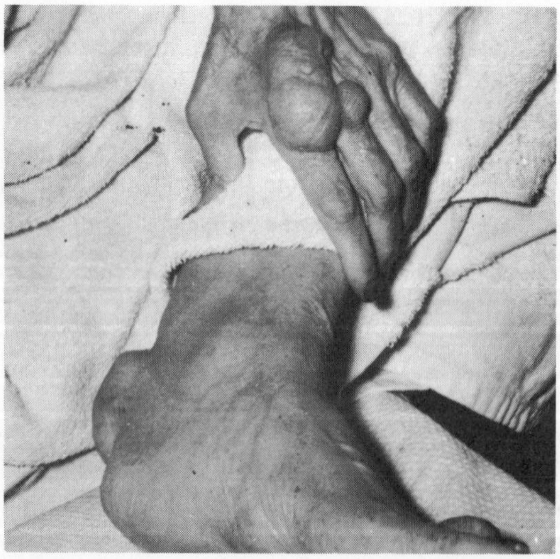

figure 13-5. Gouty tophi. (Vakil, R. J., and Golwalla, A.: *Clinical Diagnosis*, Bombay, Asia Pub. House)

The aim of treatment is to decrease the amount of sodium urate in the extracellular fluid, so that chalky deposits do not form. This is attempted in two major ways: (1) by decreasing the amount of purine ingested, and (2) by using uricosuric drugs, which promote the renal excretion of urates by inhibiting tubular reabsorption of urates. The excess uric acid in the body of a patient with gout is derived from a process of internal biosynthesis; consequently, except for severe tophaceous gout, there is less emphasis on strict diet restriction than on uricosuric drugs. The majority of patients are not placed on a rigid diet, although they are instructed not to eat foods high in purine. The reaction to food and alcoholic drinks is extremely individual.

The prescribed diet is adequate in proteins—with concentration on low-purine proteins—low in fat, and rich in carbohydrates. Large fluid intake and no alcohol usually are recommended. High-purine foods to be avoided include liver, kidneys, brains, anchovies, sardines, herring, smelts, bacon, goose, haddock, mackerel, mutton, salmon, turkey and veal, yeast, beer, meat broth, and leguminous vegetables, such as beans.

Low-purine or purine-free foods usually allowed include chocolate, coffee, tea, fruit juices, fruits, breads, cereal and spaghetti, eggs, gelatine, milk, nuts, pies (except mincemeat), sugar, and other than leguminous vegetables.

When instructing a patient with gout about diet, the nurse avoids any implication that he is "bad" if he goes off his diet, although she points out that the nature of the chemical disorders will cause pain if he takes food that markedly increases the urates in his body. Formerly dietary management was considered most important in gout control and rigidly prescribed. However, since the effect of dietary control on urate levels is relatively small, a much more lenient attitude has been taken.

Drugs. Because of the urgent nature of the pain, narcotics may be justified. However, they are rarely used, because drugs specific for gout are available. Acute attacks of gout are treated with colchicine, given hourly until the pain subsides or nausea, vomiting, intestinal cramping, and diarrhea develop. When one or more of these symptoms occur, the drug is temporarily stopped. Other drugs that may be used are oxyphenbutazone (Tandearil), allopurinol (Zyloprin), probenecid (Benemid), sulfinpyrazone (Anturane), and phenylbutazone (Butazolidin). Analgesics may be ordered until the drugs specific for gout have taken effect. Treatment is also aimed at preventing future attacks and permanent joint damage. Increased fluid intake is also recommended to reduce the possibility of urate stone formation in the kidney, and, if the patient is obese, a weight-reduction diet is planned to reduce strain on the involved joints.

Nursing management

Nursing management during an acute attack involves keeping the patient as comfortable as possible. During an attack a bed cradle is placed over the affected joint to protect it from bedding, breezes, and bumps. This is one bed that never should be jarred. A sign "Don't Bump the Bed" may remind auxiliary personnel and visitors to be careful. Either warm or cold compresses may be ordered and applied very gently. Elevation of the joint may make the patient more comfortable. Only after the pain and the redness have disappeared is the joint to be exercised. Then early ambulation is necessary to ensure good joint function.

An explanation regarding the hourly administration of colchicine should include the necessity of giving the drug until gastrointestinal symptoms develop or the pain is relieved. This can be the starting point in discharge teaching because it involves the patient in the management of his disease, the purpose of medication, and how the medication is administered. Knowing *what* to expect and *why* the gastrointestinal symptoms may have to be tolerated for a short time reduces anxiety and lets the patient know that interest is being taken in him and his problem.

Other treatment of advanced gout includes surgery to remove large tophaceous masses. Surgery may also be employed in an attempt to correct crippling deformities that may result when treatment is delayed, and to fuse unstable joints to increase their function.

Bone tumors

Bone tumors may be malignant or benign. Malignant tumors may be primary, that is, originating in the bone, or secondary, originating elsewhere in the body and traveling to the bone (metastasized). Primary malignant tumors are called *sarcomas* (e.g., osteogenic sarcoma, Ewing's sarcoma, and chrondrosarcoma), are highly malignant, and metastasize early, usually to the lungs. Symptoms of malignant tumors of the bone are persistent pain, swelling, and difficulty in moving the involved extremity. Diagnosis is made by x-ray examination and an open or closed biopsy of the tumor. The serum alkaline phosphatase may be elevated.

Treatment of primary malignant bone tumors involves surgical removal of the tumor by amputation of the extremity or by wide local resection. Radiotherapy and chemotherapy may be used in addition to surgery. These latter two measures rarely cure primary tumors but may slow tumor growth and help to relieve pain. Chemotherapy after surgery may destroy tumor cells that have escaped from the original tumor site.

Metastatic bone tumors are usually found in the pelvis, spine, and ribs. These tumors are not operable but may be controlled (but not cured) with radiation, antineoplastic drugs, or hormone therapy.

Benign tumors are removed by curettage (scraping) or by local excision.

Nursing management will depend on the type of tumor. The patient with a benign tumor will require normal postoperative care. The affected part is usually placed in a splint, or heavy dressings may be applied to immobilize the part. The patient with a malignant tumor will have the same *physical* care as the patient with an amputation who is confronted with an alteration of body image. In addition, he may have been informed of the diagnosis and possibly the prognosis. This requires exceptional nursing care as the prognosis of bone cancer is relatively poor. Depending on the type of tumor, statistics quote a 15 to 50 percent 5 year survival rate. Thus, the nurse may have to help the patient cope with fears and anxieties accompanying this type of diagnosis and surgery. While false hope should never be given, the patient should understand that the physician and nursing personnel will do all they can to keep him comfortable.

Discharge planning will vary, depending on the extent of the surgery, the patient, and whether metastasis has occurred. To plan effective discharge teaching the nurse must first consult with the physician to find out what special teaching is required. The patient may need special planning, and a referral to a social service agency, community health nurse, or a community agency is often required to meet a specific need. The family may have to be shown how to apply

Table 13-2.
Nursing management of the patient with osteomyelitis

Isolation techniques should be instituted if drainage is present.
A deodorizer is used if the drainage has an unpleasant odor.
Pillows, trochanter rolls, sandbags, and so on should be used to support and keep the unaffected extremity in proper alignment.
The affected side should be kept in proper alignment if a splint has not been applied. This may be difficult because of severe pain.
The affected parts are handled gently and with great care.
Sheepskin boots or pads, or sponge rubber should be used to protect elbows and heels.
A footboard is used to prevent footdrop.
An alternating pressure mattress is used if there is early evidence of decubitus ulcer formation.
Fluids are encouraged, intake and output are measured.
A good dietary intake is important. A high-protein, high-vitamin diet is essential to healing.
Signs of recurrent infection should be looked for: chills, fever, rapid pulse, pain, redness, tenderness.

dressings as well as how to assist with the prosthesis, if one can be used.

Osteomyelitis

Osteomyelitis is an infection of the bone, most commonly caused by the organism *Staphylococcus aureus. Acute* osteomyelitis is most aften caused by bacteria reaching the bone by way of the bloodstream. *Acute localized* osteomyelitis is most often caused by direct contamination of the bone due to trauma, for example, penetrating wounds or compound fractures. Occasionally, surgical contamination or direct extension of bacteria from an infected area adjacent to the bone can cause osteomyelitis.

Symptoms occur suddenly; high fever, chills, rapid pulse, tenderness, and/or pain over the affected area, redness, and swelling. Laboratory tests usually show a rise in the leukocyte count, an elevated erythrocyte sedimentation rate (ESR), and possibly a positive blood culture. Diagnosis may be made by x-ray examination; however, x-ray evidence may not be apparent during the early stages of infection. Diagnosis is almost always made by the symptoms presented.

TREATMENT. There are three weapons to combat osteomyelitis: (1) the patient's own defenses, aided by rest and good nutrition; (2) antibiotics; and (3) surgical drainage of the pus that forms. In the early stage of treatment the antibiotic may be given by continuous drip infusion. Some physicians make a series of drill holes in the bone to evacuate pus and to relieve the pressure. Antibiotics are put directly into the wound, and a catheter may be left in place for periodic irrigation or continuous drip of antibiotic solution. The wound is kept open for drainage, and the extremity positioned so that the mouth of the wound is down, utilizing the help of gravity in draining the pus. Sometimes a closed irrigation and drainage system is used, with a low-pressure pump providing intermittent suction that allows the wound to fill periodically. The affected part may be immobilized with plaster, such as a half cast. The patient may be placed in isolation until the infection is controlled.

NURSING MANAGEMENT. Table 13-2 summarizes nursing management of the patient with osteomyelitis. The nurse must be especially mindful of the patient's pain. Movement causes great distress to the patient; yet he cannot lie continuously in one position. When turning the patient, movement should be smooth, careful, and unhurried. The part is well supported over its entire length and perhaps splinted with a pillow. A firm pillow held in place with sandbags keeps the affected part still. Immobilization of the part, which is a comfort to the patient while slightest movement is agony, can be accomplished by a cast, a brace, or the judicious placement of sandbags. It is extremely important that the patient's bed is placed where it is least likely to be jarred.

The nurse, aware that the infection can spread to other bones, informs the physician immediately if swelling, redness or pain elsewhere over a bone develops. Pathologic fractures (fractures that occur without severe trauma) may occur. These are singularly difficult to recognize, because the pain of osteomyelitis is so great that the pain of the fracture is masked.

COMPLICATIONS. The diseased bone may lengthen

as bone growth is stimulated, or it may shorten because of the destruction of the epiphyseal plate. Another complication of osteomyelitis may be the result of the nurse's negligence. If the application of dressings become too routine over a period of months, she may become careless with her aseptic technique, and fresh organisms may be introduced into the wound.

Perhaps the most discouraging complication of all is the tendency of osteomyelitis to become chronic. The sinus from the bone to the outside may drain for years. The inactivity of the part, the muscle spasm, and the despair of the patient take their toll. The patient with chronic osteomyelitis frequently is wasted, weak, and burdened with a deformed extremity. Sometimes amputation is necessary. Fortunately, antibiotic therapy has lessened the incidence of chronicity and heightened the chances of recovery.

General nutritional considerations

- Patients with arthritic deformities of the hands, arms, and shoulders may need assistance in cutting their food and opening cartons or covers on the hospital tray.
- Severely arthritic patients may require a soft diet if they are learning to use special feeding devices.
- Arthritic patients should be cautioned against fad diets or food claims that cure arthritis. No special dietary changes should be undertaken without approval of the physician.
- Occasionally, patients with gout may need to restrict their intake of foods high in purine, for example, liver, kidney, and meat extracts.
- Overweight patients with osteoarthritis should be encouraged to lose weight and may need a reduction diet prescribed by the physician and tailored to their needs.
- Patients with osteomyelitis may require a high-calorie, high-protein diet as an aid in repair of diseased bone.

General pharmacological considerations

- Arthritic patients should be warned about drugs, health foods, and certain food substances available in drug form and promoted as "cures" for arthritis.
- Patients taking large doses of salicylates should be told the (1) signs of gastrointestinal bleeding (black, tarry stools), (2) signs of salicylism, and (3) possibility of easy bruising and other bleeding tendencies.
- The signs of salicylism include: headache, nausea, vomiting, tinnitus, increased pulse and respiratory rate, fever, mental confusion, drowsiness.
- Large doses of salicylates can interfere with the clotting mechanism of the blood. Patients taking these drugs are instructed to inform their physicians and dentists of this fact.
- Patients with gout will need detailed instructions concerning their medical regimen with regard to the drug(s) to be taken and the importance of increasing their fluid intake to reduce the possibility of urate stone formation in the urinary tract.
- Salicylates do not require a prescription; therefore, patients taking these drugs for arthritis on advice of their physicians must be warned about substituting the various types of aspirin and aspirin-related products unless the change has been approved by their physicians.
- Patients with diseases of the bones and joints should be cautioned against discontinuing their drugs if and when they begin to feel improved.

Bibliography

About gout: Emergency Med. 5:180, January, 1973.

Brunner, L. and Suddarth, D. et al: *Lippincott Manual of Nursing Practice.* Philadelphia, Lippincott, 1974.

Driscoll, P. W.: Rheumatoid arthritis; understanding it more fully. Nurs. '75, 5:27, December, 1975.

Ehrilich, G., ed.: *Total Management of the Arthritic Patient.* Philadelphia, Lippincott, 1973.

Goldenberg, D. L. et al: Arthritis: a differential guide (pictorial). Hosp. Med. 10:68, February, 1974.

Gumpel, J. M.: Ankylosing spondylitis (pictorial). Nurs. Times 70:1308, August 22, 1974.

Haslock, L. et al: Gout (pictorial). Nurs. Mirror 140:49, January 23, 1975.

Lamb, C., ed.: RA therapy: three-step therapy for rheumatoid arthritis. Patient Care 8:21, May 15, 1974.

———: What does high uric acid mean? Patient Care 8:164, August 1, 1974.

Larson, C. B. and Gould, M.: *Orthopedic Nursing,* ed. 8. St. Louis, Mosby, 1974.

LORBER, A.: Gold therapy in rheumatoid arthritis: improving results. Consultant 14:95, November, 1974.

MACRAE, I.: Arthritis: its nature and management. Nurs. Clin. North Am. 8:643, December, 1973.

MASON, M. and CURRY, H. L. F., ed.: *An Introduction to Clinical Rheumatology*, ed. 2. Philadelphia, Lippincott, 1975.

MCCAFFERY, M.: *Nursing Management of the Patient with Pain.* Philadelphia, Lippincott, 1972.

PITORAK, E. F.: Rheumatoid arthritis: living with it more comfortably. Nurs. '75 5:33, December, 1975.

ROBINSON, C. H.: *Normal and Therapeutic Nutrition,* ed. 14. New York, Macmillan, 1972.

RODMAN, M. J. and SMITH, D. W.: *Clinical Pharmacology in Nursing.* Philadelphia, Lippincott, 1974.

SOIKA, C. V.: Combatting osteoporosis. Am. J. Nurs. 73:1193, July, 1973.

STAUDT, A. R.: Femur replacement . . . Memorial Sloan-Kettering Cancer Center (pictorial) Part 4. Am. J. Nurs. 1346, August, 1975.

THOMAS, B. J.: Recognizing and treating arthritis in the young. RN, 37:64, September, 1974.

WALLACH, J.: *Interpretation of Diagnostic Tests,* ed. 2. Boston, Little, Brown, 1974.

WILLIAMS, S. R.: *Nutrition and Diet Therapy,* ed. 2. St. Louis, Mosby, 1973.

CHAPTER—14

The patient with an amputation

On completion of this chapter the student will:

- **Discuss the physical, social, economic, and psychological problems encountered by an individual with an amputation.**
- **Describe the basic nursing care of the patient with an amputation.**
- **Discuss the important aspects of the rehabilitation of the patient with an upper or lower extremity amputation.**
- **Discuss the elements of emotional support and understanding needed by the patient undergoing amputation of an extremity.**

Usually, the loss of a limb is psychologically damaging. An amputation can make a patient feel that he is less acceptable than others, can lessen his self-esteem, and can affect his self-image. The patient can be expected to experience grief over his loss and, depending on his adjustment, work through the various stages of the grieving process. The nurse helps by assessing the stage of grief the patient is in and providing appropriate support.

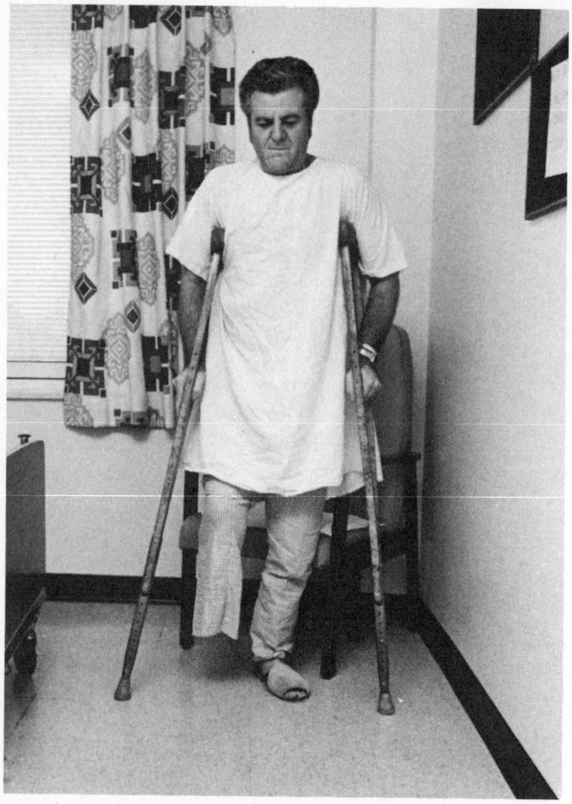

figure 14-1. The response to an amputation is highly individual. This patient ambulated on crutches soon after surgery and showed determination in his rehabilitation. (Photograph—D. Atkinson)

Not only does the loss of a limb mean that the person may consider himself to be no longer whole, but it may also create difficult practical problems. Depending on the situation, the patient will face the possibility of loss of locomotion, lifelong invalidism, a change in home-making practices, and perhaps the loss of a job.

Even if the mechanics of rehabilitation can be accomplished perfectly, the loss of a limb may cause such anxiety and grief that the patient is unable to use a prosthesis. A young healthy person who loses a leg in an automobile accident, often is able to make the necessary physical adjustments, so that after only a relatively short time he can continue a full, active, and productive life. On the other hand, the young college athlete or cheerleader who has had an amputation due to cancer of the bone has overwhelming adjustments to make. While the entire response to amputation is highly individual, it is affected by such factors as age, reasons for amputation, prognosis regarding underlying condition, and the patient's emotional state and developmental level (Fig. 14-1).

As opposed to the younger person, the older person requiring an amputation is more likely to have widespread concomitant disease that may be disabling in itself. There may be generalized weakness, poor vision, or cardiovascular disease. Changing lifelong habits requires stamina, courage, patience, help, and a certain degree of health. Yet some elderly patients, especially those who are supported emotionally by loved ones, do very well in adjusting to great changes in their lives.

The physician may decide that it is better for family members to learn of an impending amputation before the patient does, so that they will have time to adjust to the idea and can help the patient when he learns about it.

If the amputation is necessitated by trauma, and the patient is brought to the operating room directly from the ambulance or the emergency room, the psychological adjustment is even more difficult. That morning the patient rose from sleep with an intact body. He thought, perhaps, that a usual day lay ahead of him. That night he will be minus a leg.

An amputation is irrevocable, carrying a deep sense of loss, even for the patient who has had severe pain in the limb. The patient who awakens from anesthesia to find a limb amputated needs people around him who can help to cushion the emotional impact by their acceptance of his feelings and their faith in his ability to eventually cope with the problems.

Etiology

The causes of amputation are (1) accidental and extensive violence to extremities, (2) death of tissues from peripheral vascular insufficiency or from peripheral vasospastic diseases such as Buerger's disease and Raynaud's disease, (3) malignant tumors, (4) longstanding infections of bone and other tissue which prohibit restoration of function, (5) thermal injuries, due to both heat and cold, (6) a useless, deformed limb which is a hindrance to the patient, (7) conditions which may endanger the life of the patient, such as vascular accidents and gas bacillus infections.

Nursing management

The successful management of amputees requires cooperative teamwork among physicians, nurses, therapists, and prosthetists. Although amputation involves loss of a significant body part with all this entails for the patient, it can also be viewed as reconstructive surgery. A functioning organ, the amputation stump, is left, providing the opportunity for the patient to use one of the modern prostheses from which he can gain the greatest degree of functional performance.

Preoperative phase

Psychological Preparation. When amputation is inevitable, the physician discusses with the family, and ultimately with the patient, the extent of physical disability, the psychological, esthetic, social, and vocational implications, and the realistic possibilities for prosthetic restoration. He promptly attempts to reduce anxieties and misunderstandings because radical surgery constitutes a severe threat to most people. Although the patient is still faced with a crisis, this approach establishes the groundwork for assisting the patient to accept and to adjust to the realities of the situation. Not all amputees can benefit from a prosthesis, and the surgeon is careful not to make casual promises to soothe a patient prior to surgery.

Patients vary in their reactions to the impending loss of a limb. These reactions are based upon such variables as age, the educational, intellectual, economic, and emotional status of the individual, what the loss of the part means to him, and how he has dealt with previous losses. In general, a gradual state of depression and a degree of hopelessness are common. Those with diabetes, for example, may be angry because despite the extra care they gave their legs and their dietary deprivation, they still must lose a limb.

The amount of grief is thought to be proportional to the symbolic significance of the part and the resultant degree of disability and deformity. It is recommended that the physician, in his preoperative explanation, emphasize the necessity for the amputation without criticizing the patient for his reservations and recognize the anger the patient may feel about the threat to his body integrity. This helps clear the way for the expression of grief as well as the patient's concern about the disposition of the amputated part. The patient usually wants the separated part of himself treated with respect, which includes decent burial of the part. The nurse discusses with the physician what was told to the patient and the patient's response, and gives the patient the opportunity to further express his thoughts and feelings.

The nurse can help the patient and family by accepting their reaction of shock and grief at the news and by letting the patient and his family talk about their feelings. Before the operation, she can help them to learn how others have managed with one arm or one leg, how the patient can help himself (by diet and exercises), and what to expect during the postoperative period. She can resist the temptation to make preoperative promises that cannot come true when attempting to aid the patient to accept the thought of an amputation.

Although it has been stated frequently that nurses should encourage patients by showing enthusiasm and optimism themselves, patients do not necessarily share this attitude. Sometimes this results in the patient perceiving the subtle message that he is expected to smile bravely and undertake his rehabilitation exercises with enthusiasm. This he may do as a facade to smooth relationships with the staff. He meets their need for an eager, smiling patient, rather than his own needs. Although it is important for the nurse to feel and show confidence in the patient's ability, a forced cheeriness may not be the best way to do this. It is usually preferable that she listen while the patient discusses his concerns, realizing that he is likely to express grief and anger. If possible, the nurse can have an amputee who has coped successfully with his handicap visit the patient.

Many of the serious psychological problems resulting from the thought of amputation are lessened by recently improved surgical procedures, making it possible for amputees to ambulate almost immediately after surgery. Despite immediate postsurgical fitting and early amputation, the patient cannot be hurried through his stages of grieving, and each patient needs support to proceed at his own pace to fully integrate the experience.

Most physicians assure a patient who will lose one limb and has three remaining normally functional limbs that he will derive practical function from the use of a prosthesis. This applies to almost all lower extremity amputees and most upper extremity amputees, regardless of age. The great majority of amputations in the lower extremity are performed on patients over age 60. Unfortunately, it is in this older age group that coexisting debilitating and degenerative diseases exist, many of which are disabling in themselves. The nurse must be careful not to become overenthusiastic about how much function will be regained after the amputation, since in the older age group, the quality of performance with prostheses falls far short of the normal, both for upper and lower extremity amputations. Some patients are unable to

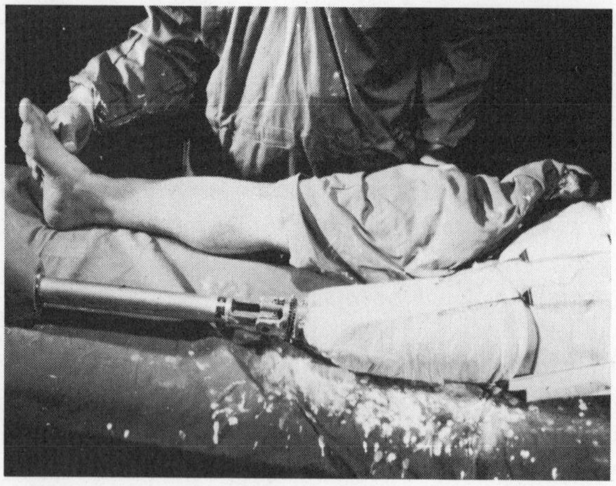

figure 14-2. Above-knee rigid dressing and immediate fitting in the operating room. (Institute of Rehabilitation Medicine, New York University Medical Center, New York, N.Y.)

accept amputation. Unfortunately, many of these do not receive sufficient help for their emotional requirements. One task of the nurse is to continually support patients who initially cannot accept amputation. Later they may begin to progress toward acceptance, especially if they have family and friends as well as nurses and physicians who don't give up on them.

PHANTOM LIMB. The surgeon may inform the patient of the phenomenon of phantom-limb sensation. This is the patient's sensation of the presence of the amputated limb. It is a normal, frequently occurring physiologic response following amputation surgery.

On the other hand, phantom-limb pain is the presence of pain or other abnormal sensations such as burning, tingling, throbbing, or itching in the amputated extremity. If the phantom is painful, it can be an extremely serious problem with regard to the emotional status of the patient and his ability to use a prosthesis. The sensation of a phantom limb should be explained to the patient as a normal phenomenon

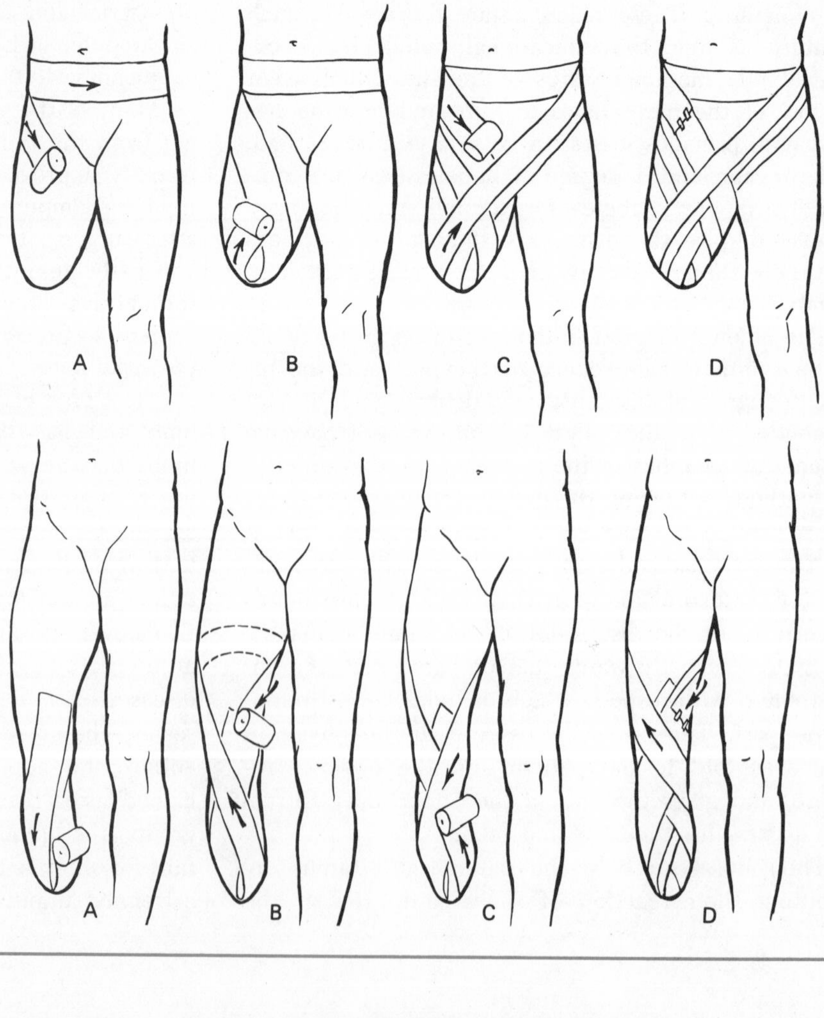

figure 14-3. In bandaging a stump of the upper leg, the bandage is anchored at the waist. Apply the bandage while the patient is standing on his unaffected leg. A crisscross (rather than a circular) pattern is followed around the leg, starting at the stump end. Each loop overlaps the previous one by at least half its width. The same principles apply to bandaging a stump of the lower leg. Note that anchoring is accomplished without a circular turn around the leg.

so that he will not be disturbed by his awareness of the amputated part. After a patient learns to use a prosthesis, although he still is aware of the phantom, he usually learns to ignore its presence. The patient may merely feel that the foot or the hand is still there. He should be encouraged to talk about the sensation. He may be embarrassed, or he may fear that he is losing his mind or that the staff will think that he is emotionally disturbed. The experience of phantom limb as a usual occurrence after amputation consists of somesthetic and kinesthetic sensations which feel as real as those in the opposite limb or as in the limb before amputation. Amputation phantoms can persist for months or decades, or can come and go.

Physical Preparation. If the operation is not an emergency, there is time to prepare the patient for some of the things he will be required to do after amputation. A good diet, including plenty of fluids, helps the patient to withstand the shock of the operation. If the patient's condition permits, he is prepared for postoperative exercises by starting them preoperatively. The patient can do pushups while he is lying prone. In anticipation of crutch walking, he can push down on the bed with his hands while he is in the sitting position. The patient practices until he can lift his buttocks off the bed. The three unaffected limbs are put through the normal range of motion. If the patient is old, ill, or weak, care is taken not to tire him. An exercise done two or three times a day is better than one done ten times all at once. An overhead bar and trapeze should be put on the bed.

Surgical phase

Amputation can be performed at any level in the lower extremity. There are preferred levels above and below the knee to facilitate fitting with available prostheses. A stump that is too long or too short creates fitting problems and discomfort. Over 90 percent of amputations in the lower extremity are at the standard above- or below-knee levels. The ideal level above the knee is in the middle third of the thigh, the longest preferred stump being to within 4 inches of the knee. The standard below-knee level of choice is in the middle third of the leg, but not lower than the musculocutaneous junction of the calf muscles. Hemipelvectomy and hip disarticulations are relatively infrequent and are performed almost exclusively for malignant tumors. Knee disarticulations, disarticulation at the ankle joint (Syme's amputation), and partial foot amputations are occasionally performed.

When the surgeon decides that amputation is inevitable, the first decision he makes is the level of amputation. Although he has a number of tests available, including arteriography, the final decision can be made only by observing the vascularity of the tissues on the operating table.

In the upper extremity the principle followed is to save all possible length and tissue with the exception of partial hand amputations. An amputation through any part of the hand that does not leave functioning elements is obstructive to the use of a prosthesis. In such cases, amputation is generally by disarticulation through the wrist or just proximal to the wrist.

In the lower extremity, unless there is unequivocal evidence that the knee cannot be saved, an attempt is made to amputate below the knee. Amputation above the knee is disabling. Since function is achieved in relationship to agility, older people do not do as well with an amputation above the knee, although the majority of them can be fitted with a prosthesis.

With modern techniques and the use of a rigid plaster dressing (cast) applied at the time of surgery (Fig. 14-2), many of the borderline cases who were previously considered to be candidates for above-knee amputation, particularly diabetics with gangrene of the toes, can survive with below-knee amputations in greater proportion than was previously recognized.

If the rigid dressing is not used at the time of surgery, the amputation stump must be shaped and conditioned by bandaging with elastic bandages or by using elastic stump shrinking socks or both (Fig. 14-3). With the use of the rigid dressing and immediate or early ambulation, the entire preprosthetic management period is altered, since the most efficient way of conditioning, shrinking, and shaping the amputation stump is by using it. Even when immediate ambulation is not anticipated, the use of the cast considerably lessens the former lengthy period of stump conditioning for prosthesis fitting.

Other Amputations. Hemipelvectomy, interscapulothoracic amputation, and translumbar amputation (hemicorporectomy) are radical procedures used in specialized centers when the patient has a bone or soft tissue malignancy. The nursing care is complex and depends on the patient's disturbance in self-image, loss of function, and involvement of other organ systems. Special prostheses are required for some return of function.

Amputation of an upper extremity

The arms are highly specialized in function. Loss of an arm or any part of an arm—especially the dominant arm (i.e., the right arm in right-handed individ-

Table 14-1.
Postoperative nursing management of the patient with an amputation

No Prosthesis Fitted at the Time of Surgery	Prosthesis Fitted at the Time of or Immediately after Surgery
Bed boards and/or a firm mattress must be in place before the patient returns from the operating room.	The stump must remain in the plaster cast.
Skin traction apparatus is affixed to the bed if a *guillotine, or open amputation* (i.e., no skin covering the stump) is performed. The physician usually orders the equipment to be put on the bed before surgery.	If the cast becomes dislodged from the stump, the stump is wrapped immediately with an elastic bandage and the physician called.
Any overhead frame with a trapeze may be added to the bed to aid in moving the patient.	If dressings covering the operative area also become dislodged, sterile nonadhesive dressings (such as Telfa pads) are placed over the incision before the elastic bandage is applied. Several rolls of elastic bandages and sterile nonadhesive dressings are kept at the bedside and in plain view.
To prevent edema, elevation of the stump on pillows, or elevation of the foot of the bed for the first 24 hours after surgery may be necessary.	A suspension harness, fitted around the waist, is attached to the cast to keep it secure and in place. The harness is slightly tightened when the patient is ambulatory and slightly loosened when the patient is in bed.
A footboard is used to support the unoperated extremity.	A drain covered with a small dressing may be inserted in the incision and protrude through the end of the cast. The color and amount of drainage (if any) is noted and recorded on the patient's chart.
Isolation technique is usually necessary if control of infection was the reason for amputation.	
The stump is checked for drainage, and the color and amount recorded on the patient's chart.	
A plastic-backed drainage pad is placed beneath or on top of the stump to reduce linen changes due to drainage.	
A tourniquet must be kept in *plain sight*. If gross hemorrhage occurs, the tourniquet is applied and the physician called immediately.	
Range-of-motion exercises are begun as soon as movement is tolerated.	

uals)—often requires great physical and emotional adjustment during the preoperative as well as the postoperative period.

Postoperatively, a soft dressing anchored with an elastic bandage is usually applied to the stump. In some cases, a prosthesis is attached immediately after surgery. It may be necessary to elevate the stump on a pillow and to start exercises as soon as movement of the stump is tolerated. Exercises may have been started during the preoperative period, depending on the emotional acceptance of the patient. Hematoma and infection are complications and any excessive drainage or signs of infection must be reported immediately.

Long-range planning requires teamwork. Each team member—physician, nurse, therapists, and prosthetist—has an important role in rehabilitation of the patient. It should be noted that not ALL upper extremity amputees can be fitted with or learn how to use a prosthesis. Some find it difficult to accept the "hook" type extremity and prefer no prosthesis. This may be especially true if the nondominant limb was amputated. Vocational and psychiatric counseling is often needed, especially for the younger patient.

Amputation of a lower extremity

Amputation of a lower extremity is more common than upper extremity amputation. This amputation may or may not be an emergency procedure and requires preparation of the patient, if there is time. Because a lower limb prosthesis is sometimes less conspicuous and has a more natural appearance than an upper limb prosthesis, it may be accepted more readily.

Postoperative care may vary, depending on the type of amputation and whether the prosthetic device was fitted at the time of surgery or later. Postoperative management of a patient with an amputation of an upper or lower extremity is given in Table 14-1.

Postoperative phase

Lower Extremity. When the patient is returned to the unit and the immediate postoperative reaction is past, the nurse plays an important role in making observations regarding the status of the amputation stump. Some oozing will take place and stain the rigid plaster dressing. The stain is marked with a pencil and observed periodically, to determine whether or not excessive bleeding is taking place. If such bleeding occurs, the physician should be notified immediately. When a rigid dressing is not applied, the same principle is used in observing the compressive dressing with the elastic bandages.

There is the possibility of hemorrhage in an amputation stump when a rigid plaster dressing is not applied. A tourniquet should be kept in view in the event that massive bleeding is evident.

In a closed or flap amputation, skin flaps cover the bone end. In an open or guillotine amputation, the end of the stump is open, with no skin covering the stump. Open amputations are usually performed in the presence of infection. Skin traction is applied and the infected area allowed to drain.

The traction must be continuous. The surgeon may arrange the traction so that the patient can turn over in bed and even get up in a wheelchair with a specially designed traction board without interrupting the pull of the weights. If the patient is incontinent, waterproof material is secured around the outside of the bandage to prevent soiling of the wound.

If the wound is infected, reoperation or perhaps amputation at a higher level may be performed after the infection is cleared and the patient's condition is improved. Sometimes the stump is allowed to heal without revision (re-amputation). Sometimes revision is done. For instance, a guillotine operation may be revised later to provide a stump suitable for the prosthesis.

Closed amputations are usually covered with pressure dressings. Drains may or may not be inserted in the incision. The stump may be elevated on a pillow for the first 24 hours, thus preventing edema of the stump. Many physicians prefer elevation of the foot of the bed as stump elevation promotes contracture of the remaining leg muscles. A bed board and/or a firm mattress provides firm support under the hips, thus preventing flexion and contraction of the hip joint. While some drainage is usually considered normal, hemorrhage is a complication of amputations. Oozing around the incision may be seen and the dressing is reinforced as needed. Plastic-backed drainage pads can be placed under the stump. If drainage is near the top, a smaller pad may be placed between the stump and the top sheet. This protects the linen, reduces linen changes, and also prevents unsightly drainage from staining the top sheet. Stains, odors, and the sight of blood are upsetting to the patient and his visitors. If a top sheet directly over the stump is uncomfortable, a drainage pad is laid lightly over the stump and the top sheet secured around the groin and the unoperated side.

Exercises are encouraged during the early postoperative period. Usually physical therapy is started early, with the physical therapist instructing the patient in the type of exercises to be performed. The patient should be encouraged to use the trapeze to assist movement in bed.

Bed positioning of the patient is important. With the rigid dressing there is no danger of the development of flexion contractures of the stump. When the rigid dressing is not used, bed positioning to prevent contractures is quite important. The nurse may assist in the prevention of contractures by:

- Assisting and teaching the patient to roll from side to side and in the prone position in order to create extension for the amputation stump. Know what the physician and physical therapist permit. Because the patient may experience a great deal of pain in the immediate postoperative period, a good time for placing him prone is about a half-hour after he has received medication for pain. Then he will be more comfortable and better able to move.

  While he is lying on his abdomen, the patient may be instructed to adduct the stump so that it presses against his other leg. His toes should extend over the end of the mattress so that they are not pressed down into the mattress. When the patient lies on his unaffected side, he may be taught to flex gently and to extend his stump. When a patient with a BK (below-knee) amputation is in the supine position, and a pillow has been placed momentarily under his knee on the operative side, he can flex gently and extend his knee. He is taught to pull himself up in bed by using his arms and the trapeze rather than pushing with his heel, which may become sore.

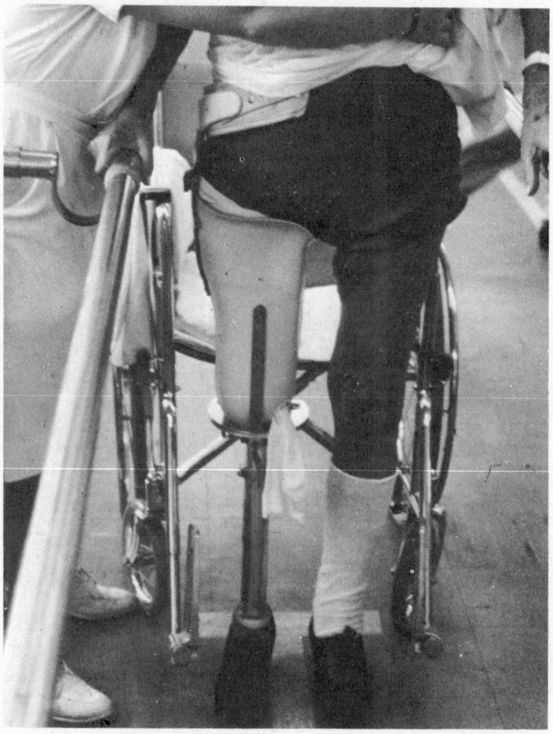

figure 14-4. Temporary, removable above-knee socket and walking pylon. (Institute of Rehabilitation Medicine, New York University Medical Center, New York, N.Y.)

- Being sure that the patient is lying on a firm mattress. A sagging mattress can cause a flexion contracture.
- Working with the physical therapist so that a program of exercises to prevent contractures is implemented for the patient who progresses to the point where he is up in a wheelchair most of the day. For example, to prevent hip flexion contracture, the patient can be taught to suspend his stump over the edge of the bed and go through the full range of joint motion before he gets up and when he returns to bed. Attention is paid to the remaining limb as well as to the stump. Good muscle tone is maintained by range-of-motion exercises, with the patient doing the work. Footdrop is avoided by ankle exercises and the use of a footboard.

Temporary Prosthesis. Immediate fitting of a temporary prosthesis in the operating room is intended to get the patient up as soon as possible. Thus, the patient with a rigid plaster dressing may be allowed to sit on the edge of the bed and dangle his unaffected leg on the day of surgery. If he has the stamina the first or second postoperative day, he may be permitted to stand and regain his sense of balance. Touching down on the floor with the improvised prosthesis and weight bearing of about 10 percent of body weight is permitted.

The patient can progress to walking with crutches or a walkerette or in parallel bars 1, 2, or 3 days after the amputation with a high degree of safety if the rigid dressing is properly applied. He is not permitted to put full weight on the amputation stump until 6 weeks after amputation. The reason is that the skin may heal in 2 weeks, but the deep tissues take at least 6 weeks for maturity of the scars to withstand the forces of full weight bearing.

The patient with a temporary leg prosthesis may be ambulatory several days after surgery. A pylon with a foot and ankle attachment is fitted to the cast (Fig. 14-4), and the patient allowed to stand with a limited amount of weight placed on the amputated extremity as the stump begins to heal and edema disappears. Later, a second cast may be fitted. Ultimately, a conventional prosthesis (Fig. 14-5) is fitted.

The nurse works with the physical therapist by positioning the patient properly in bed, by encouraging exercises, and by supervising him as he attempts to stand, transfer weight, and maintain balance.

Whenever the patient returns from the physical therapy department, the nurse should question him with regard to shortness of breath, the presence of pain, his response to exertion, and how he feels when walking with a prosthesis.

After removal of the sutures, the patient is fitted with a temporary prosthesis with which he walks until his stump is in condition to tolerate a permanent prosthesis. Under these conditions, it is possible for the patient to leave the hospital ambulatory on two legs about a month after surgery, if the scar is healed and all other conditions are satisfactory.

The attitude of family members, especially of the spouse, will have a great bearing on how the patient accepts surgery and cooperates in his postoperative care and rehabilitation.

Upper Extremity. A similar approach is used in amputations in the upper extremity. The surgical objective here is to create a gently tapering stump with muscular padding over the end. The upper extremity amputation stump moves within the socket more and is subject to more variations in friction than the lower extremity stump. For this reason *the myoplastic closure* and loose approximation of the skin flaps is essential. The myoplastic form of amputation consists of sewing opposing muscles to each other and down to the bone

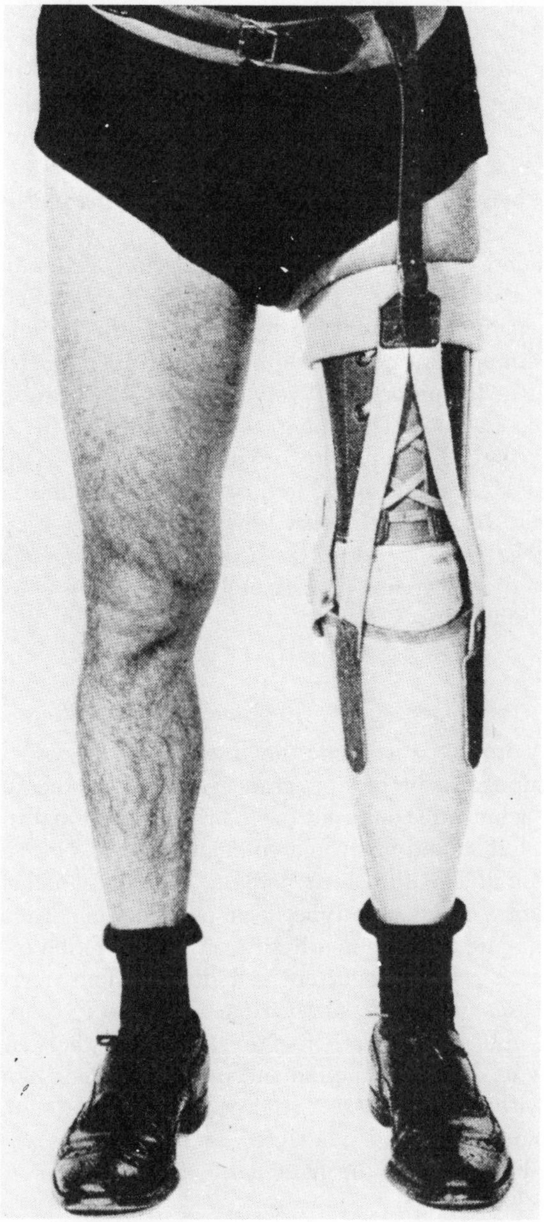

figure 14-5. Conventional below-knee wood socket with knee joints and laced thigh corset. (Institute of Rehabilitation Medicine, New York University Medical Center, New York, N.Y.)

from which they originate, thus allowing the muscles to contract isometrically. Tight skin across a subcutaneous cut bone end is the primary cause of the pain in an upper extremity amputation at any level.

Most patients with upper extremity amputations can be measured for a prosthesis shortly after the surgical scar has healed. It is necessary to maintain a full range of motion in the remaining joints and build up strength in the muscles by the time the prosthesis is finally delivered. This is accomplished by passive exercises and encouraging the patient to perform active exercises within his tolerance. The application of a rigid dressing can simplify the postoperative care of the upper extremity amputee, but it is seldom used. The reason is that most upper extremity amputations are performed following extensive trauma or infection and the greatest length is being preserved. In emergencies, the application of a rigid dressing adds to the risk since frequent inspection of the part is necessary. The dressing of an upper extremity stump usually consists of a thin strip of non-adherent material such as silk or petrolatum gauze, covered with fluffy gauze and kept in place with a gently compressive bandage. This bandage is not designed for shrinkage, but simply for external support to hold the dressing on and to some extent control posttraumatic and surgical edema.

During the healing period, the patient may become ambulatory and is made aware of the importance of good posture. In amputations above the elbow and higher, there is a tendency for the trunk to tilt away from the side of the amputation and for the head to tilt toward it. Eventual foreshortening of the shoulder girdle can result in scoliosis (curvature of the spine). This is of greater importance, of course, in growing children. For this reason, deep breathing, bilateral adduction and abduction exercises for the scapulae, and shoulder shrugging should be practiced several times daily. The nurse gives the patient support and supervision as necessary and is guided by the therapist.

Only when there is no longer the possibility of infection and the scar is well on the way to healing is shrinking bandaging done. The elastic bandage is applied in the same manner as for lower extremity stumps. Compression proximally is achieved by spirals and doubling back the bandage to avoid circular constriction. Upper extremity stumps do not need massive shrinkage over a long period as do those of the lower extremity. They will not be subjected to the great forces of body weight support even while using a prosthesis, and usually stabilize in about 6 months.

A person who loses his dominant hand has the choice of learning to do everything (write, light a match, count change, eat, and so on) with his other hand or of learning to use a prosthesis. Since the loss of a hand is a devastating disability, one that makes a difference to the patient almost every minute of the day, early restoration of the sense of purposeful use is important and can be accomplished by placing a temporary cuff over the stump and fitting it with a clip or clamp which can hold a pencil, piece of chalk, or a spoon. The patient can then have the satisfaction of practicing writing on paper or a blackboard and attempting to feed himself as training procedures.

The nurse can play a very important part of this preprosthetic-training program in association with the occupational therapist. With persistence and support, the painful phantom is eliminated by purposeful use of a functional prosthesis, whether the upper or the lower extremity is involved.

Complications that may occur late in the postoperative course include chronic osteomyelitis (following persistent infection) and, rarely, a burning pain (causalgia), the etiology of which is not known. Pain may also be caused by a stump neuroma, which is formed when the cut ends of nerves become entangled in the healing scar. A neuroma may be treated with injections of procaine, or reamputation may be necessary.

Caring for the Stump. The type of surgery performed influences the length of time for stump conditioning, shrinking, and shaping. However, there are some general principles to be observed.

To help the stump shrink and shape properly for the wearing of a prosthesis, two or three elastic bandages may be sewn together and applied to the stump. The physician generally determines the method for applying the bandages. The stump is usually bandaged first with an over-and-under motion and then with a spiral motion (Fig. 14-3). All parts of the wrapped limb should be equally compressed. If the proximal part of the stump is compressed more tightly than the rest of the limb, edema will result in the end of the stump (bulbous edema). When a bandage is applied to an above-knee amputation, the spirals arc continued as high as possible to avoid a roll of flesh above the bandage. The bandage is changed at least twice during the day and before the patient retires for the night, at which time the underlying skin is inspected. In the summer especially, when the patient perspires profusely, the stump is washed each time the bandage is changed, and talc applied. If the skin is dry, petrolatum or cold cream may be used.

If the patient will have to bandage his stump at home, he and a member of his family should be taught how to apply the bandage and how to care for the stump. He should also be taught to wash the bandages between wearings, to rinse them well and to lay them flat to dry, since hanging tends to decrease the elasticity. When the bandages are dry, they should be rolled without stretching. If the patient uses a leather shrinker, he should be cautioned to use it with the same precautions that he would use with elastic bandages, giving special attention to cleanliness, frequent changes, prevention of tightness on the top, and skin irritation. It is safer to use safety pins instead of clasps to secure the end of the bandage.

The nurse should check to make sure that the patient is applying the elastic bandage or any other device for shrinkage with even pressure from the tip of the stump on up the limb. The patient and the nurse should look for shrinkage without pockets of flabbiness. The patient should return to his physician if the stump becomes uneven.

Successful ambulation depends on maintaining both the stump and the prosthesis in good condition. The patient should learn to protect both. Trauma to the stump may necessitate a return to the wheelchair or even to surgery, and repair of the prosthesis is an added expense. The stump is protected also by good daily care. It should be inspected for skin irritation, bathed, aired and powdered twice a day. Stump socks should be washed every day. When they tear or stretch, they should be discarded; the roughness of a darn or the crease of a stretched sock may cause a decubitus ulcer.

Training with prosthesis

A prosthesis is not designed to replace the lost part, its functions, or its appearance. Therefore, the function achieved should not be compared to normal function, but should be evaluated against the patient's best potential. The amputee's potential depends upon such variables as his age, type of amputation, condition of the amputation stump, physical status, condition of the remaining leg, concurrent debilitating illness, visual motor coordination, motivation, acceptance, cooperation, and insight. Patients vary greatly in their capability of deriving function and in their learning capacity with their prosthesis; the period allotted for their training varies and is affected by such factors as the speed with which the patient learns and his potential for rehabilitation.

For some a prosthesis signifies tragedy; to them it is a constant reminder of inadequacy. For others a prosthesis is an expensive, sometimes troublesome piece of machinery that nevertheless enables them to walk. If mental depression prevents its use, it is equally important to relieve the depression and to concentrate on ambulation. For some, alleviation of despair is a more important consideration than the mode of getting from one place to another.

The purpose of a lower extremity prosthesis is to provide weight support and comfort as well as the capacity to ambulate with safety, with or without mechanical aids. The process is begun by teaching the patient to apply the prosthesis properly without assistance. His training starts with standing and weight shifting to get the feel of weight support and balance, between parallel bars. He is then taught heel and toe balance and rocking and hip hiking to get the prosthesis off the ground. Early steps begin by advancing the prosthesis first and bringing up the other leg to the standing position. With practice, alternate steps and increasing weight bearing are progressively accomplished. Initially crutches, the walkerette, or canes are used until the patient has sufficient confidence and stability to discard them. It takes about 2 weeks of daily training to determine what any individual patient's best function will be. Daily practice for about 2 months thereafter usually permits the patient to achieve a satisfactory level of function. Learning to walk correctly takes time and practice. The patient may learn this skill in a physician's office, a rehabilitation center, or a hospital clinic.

Any discomfort caused by the prosthesis should be corrected as soon as possible. The nurse is in a position to discuss the progress with the patient and to examine the stump. Any observations relating to fit, comfort, or general physical stress should be reported to the physician, the physical therapist, or the prosthetist.

Upper extremity amputees are trained by occupational therapists and assisted by the nurse. The training consists of teaching the patient to apply and operate the prosthesis. He is taught procedures to bend and lock the elbow and proper use of the harness. He is given very small increasingly difficult operations to perform with the terminal device, whether it is the hook or the hand. All of the operations of the elbow and terminal devices are controlled by the shoulder on the amputated side.

TEAMWORK. One of the most important advances is the concept of the teamwork approach in the rehabilitation of the amputee. The nurse has more personal contact with the amputee than any other member of the team. The nurse is in a position to encourage and to help him become motivated, and to keep his wounds clean, and gain his confidence and participation.

Rehabilitation is not an all-or-nothing proposition. It does mean assessing strengths and liabilities and helping the patient to make the most of what he has. It is equally vital that the physician, the nurse, the physical therapist, the family, and the patient be realistic about what is expected. The nurse can also help the patient realize that he has assets as well as problems. When people are discouraged, they sometimes fail to see that they have strengths with which to work. The nurse who can help a patient to see both sides of the ledger will be better able to help him to become self-directing.

General nutritional considerations

- The deep feelings of loss and depression which follow an amputation can result in loss of appetite. The patient will need to be encouraged to eat and snacks should be provided.
- Concomitant diseases, which have sometimes led to the necessity of amputation (e.g., diabetes), may influence the diet selection.
- Rehabilitative efforts for the patient with an amputation of the arm include use of the prosthesis while eating and the selection of foods and utensils which the patient can easily manage.
- If the amputation is not an emergency procedure, attention should be given to a nutritious diet preoperatively.

General pharmacological considerations

- Patients with concomitant illness such as vascular disorders should be observed carefully for possible pre- and postoperative reactions to sedatives.
- Patients receiving medications for an underlying illness may require dosage changes or discontinuation of the medication prior to anesthesia (e.g., insulin or anticoagulants).

Bibliography

BALLINGER, W. F., TREYBAL, J. C., and VOSE, A. B.: *Alexander's Care of the Patient in Surgery*, ed. 5. St. Louis, Mosby, 1972.

BOSANKO, L. A.: Immediate postoperative prosthesis. Am. J. Nurs. 71:280, February, 1971.

BRUNNER, L. and SUDDARTH, D. S.: *Lippincott Manual of Nursing Practice*. Philadelphia, Lippincott, 1974.

FOLSOM, F. *Extracation and Casualty Handling*. Philadelphia, Lippincott, 1975.

JEGLIJEWSKI, J. M.: Target: outside world. Am. J. Nurs. 73:1024, June, 1973.

JORDAN, H. S. and CYPRES, R. M.: All around care for the leg amputee. Nurs. '74, 4:51, April, 1974.

LARSON, C. B. and GOULD, M.: *Orthopedic Nursing*, ed. 7. St. Louis, Mosby, 1970.

LEMAITRE, G. and FINNEGAN, J.: *The Patient in Surgery: A Guide for Nurses*. Philadelphia, Saunders, 1975.

Manual of Orthopaedic Surgery. Chicago, American Orthopaedic Association, 1972.

UNIT FOUR

Disorders of cognitive, sensory, or psychomotor function

- The patient with neurological disturbance
- The patient with cerebrovascular disease
- The patient with spinal cord impairment
- The patient with visual and hearing impairment

CHAPTER—15

The patient with neurological disturbance

On completion of this chapter the student will:

- Collect materials necessary for and assist with the neurological examination.
- State the rationale for the various tests used in the diagnosis of neurological diseases and disorders.
- Prepare a nursing care plan for a patient having (1) a lumbar puncture and (2) contrast studies.
- List the points for assessment of the level of consciousness of the patient with a neurological disease or disorder.
- Prepare a nursing care plan for a patient with a neurological disease or disorder.
- Describe the nursing management of patients with chronic neurological diseases such as parkinsonism or multiple sclerosis.
- Describe the various forms of epilepsy, listing the prominent symptoms of each.
- List general seizure precautions and describe the nursing actions taken when a patient has a seizure.

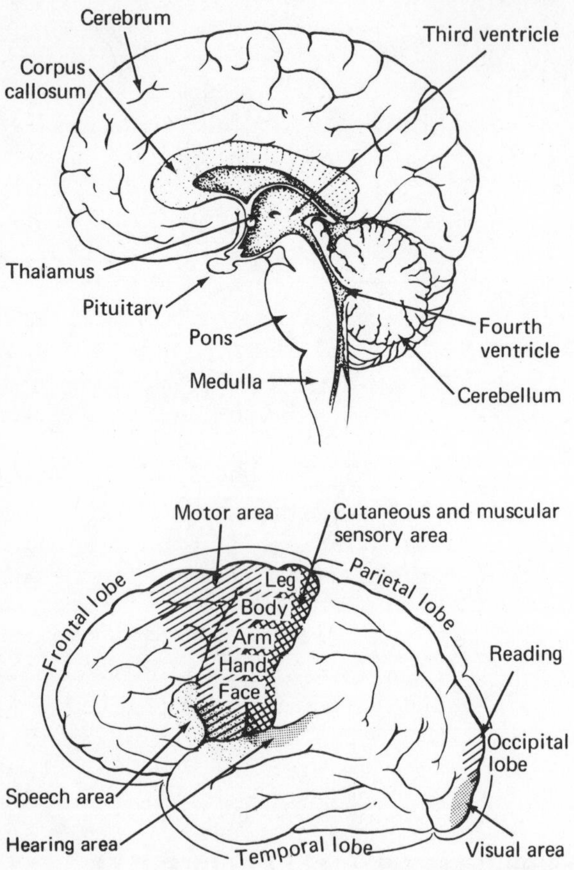

figure 15-1. (*Top*) Major structures of the brain. (*Bottom*) Diagrammatic representation of approximate areas of the brain that control various functions.

Table 15-1.
Equipment used during the neurological examination

Flashlight	Stethoscope
Ophthalmoscope	Sphygmomanometer
Tongue depressors	Percussion hammer
Cotton-tipped applicators	Tape measure
Pins (or sterile needles)	Cotton balls
Tuning fork	
Empty test tubes (which later are filled with hot or cold water)	

NOTE: not all of the above may be needed for a neurological examination. In some instances, additional equipment may be required.

Nursing care for patients with nervous system disorders challenges the nurse's observational powers and bedside skills. The patient may be extremely ill, demonstrate physical signs (such as tremors or weakness) and personality changes that require detailed observation, thoughts for the safety of the patient, and highly skilled hands to make the patient more comfortable. Neurological lesions that change physical function or the ability to think and to communicate are especially distressing to both the patient and his family. The patient who cannot think clearly, or who must learn to feed himself again, or who is in deep coma for weeks requires both psychological understanding and such thorough attention to nursing details that visitors leave the bedside with the comforting thought that the patient is receiving the best possible care. The nurse should be alert for early opportunities to help the patient to become self-sufficient. Throughout the hospital stay of the patient the nurse makes the detailed observations that may be of diagnostic importance, such as where the convulsion started, the slight drag to the left leg, the transient nystagmus.

Neurological examination

A neurological examination is performed to identify and, in some instances, to locate disorders of the nervous system (Fig. 15-1). The physician, and sometimes the nurse, looks for normal and abnormal responses to certain tests. The nurse may also be responsible for preparing the patient for the examination and for collecting the equipment needed. As the neurologist may have conducted part of this examination in an office or clinic prior to the patient's admission, the nurse should first ask what equipment will be required (Table 15-1).

In addition to examination of the senses and reflexes, there may also be tests for muscle coordination, abnormal gaits (walking), and abnormal movements such as tremors and muscle spasms. The patient may be asked to walk while he is observed for abnormal movements or a peculiarity of gait. Various tests may include climbing a small set of stairs and walking, then turning abruptly and walking "heel to toe," similar to walking a straight line for a sobriety test. Another test, the Romberg, has the patient stand with feet close together and eyes closed. If swaying is noted and there is a tendency to fall, this is considered a positive Romberg, indicating a problem with equilibrium. When this test is performed the nurse should stand fairly close to the patient, in case a loss of balance occurs.

Additional testing may include questioning the patient and the performance of mental tasks. In some instances these may appear to be relatively simple mental maneuvers. Asking a middle-aged adult to count backwards from one hundred or holding up three fingers might seem to ridicule the patient's intelligence; it does not. Those who have diseases or disorders of the nervous system may have difficulty with the easiest tasks or may be unable to answer simple questions. *At no time must the nurse display any outward emotion during this part of the examination.*

Other tests may include the finger to nose test with the eyes closed, writing words, and identifying common objects. Much depends on the original complaints and, possibly, the findings of diagnostic tests.

Diagnostic evaluation

Most hospitals require that a patient sign a statement of consent for diagnostic tests. Hospital procedures and equipment vary. The nurse should check the hospital procedure book before assisting with any of these tests.

Lumbar puncture

Cerebrospinal fluid surrounds the brain and the spinal cord. By acting as a cushion, it protects them and helps to maintain a relatively constant intracranial pressure.

A lumbar puncture (LP or spinal tap) is performed to obtain samples of cerebrospinal fluid for laboratory examination and to measure spinal fluid pressure. A lumbar puncture may also be performed to inject a drug (intrathecal injection) such as an antibiotic, to administer a spinal anesthetic, to withdraw spinal fluid for the relief of intracranial pressure, or to inject air, gas, or dye for a neurological diagnostic procedure. In health, cerebrospinal fluid (CSF) is clear and colorless, with a pressure of 80 to 180 mm. of H_2O; a pressure over 200 mm. of H_2O is considered abnormal.

Changes in cerebrospinal fluid occur in many neurological disorders. For example, meningitis (inflammation of the membranes that surround the brain and the spinal cord) causes a marked increase in the number of leukocytes in the cerebrospinal fluid, making it appear cloudy or even purulent. Often in a cerebral hemorrhage blood will be present in the spinal fluid, causing it to contain many red blood cells and to appear reddish. Cerebrospinal fluid pressure is increased when intracranial pressure is increased, whether the cause be an abscess, a blood clot, a tumor, or any lesion that takes up space.

Bacteriological tests on specimens of spinal fluid may reveal the presence of pathogenic organisms, such as the tubercle bacillus. Serological tests for syphilis may also be performed on spinal fluid.

Glucose will be decreased in bacterial meningitis. Protein is usually elevated when there is a spinal cord tumor or a brain abscess. Special analyses of the cerebrospinal fluid proteins (electrophoresis, immunophoresis) are frequently helpful in multiple sclerosis and other diseases.

Strict aseptic technique is required during the procedure. The equipment normally needed is a lumbar puncture tray, sterile gloves, a local anesthetic, and skin antiseptic. The hospital procedure manual should be consulted for the exact materials needed; it is also necessary to consult the physician regarding his preference for a local anesthetic and skin antiseptic. These materials should be brought to the patient's room immediately prior to the procedure. Leaving the equipment in the room, even for a short time, can create undue and unnecessary anxiety in the patient.

An initial explanation of the procedure is best given by the physician, but the nurse can describe the body position to be assumed. During the procedure, the patient is placed in a lateral recumbent position with the back 3 to 4 inches from the edge of the bed, the knees drawn up, and the head bent downward. Keeping the patient in a tightly curled position increases the space between the vertebrae, easing the entrance of the spinal needle. The top shoulder is kept as straight as possible and not allowed to rotate forward. The elderly or arthritic patient may have some difficulty with this position.

On occasion a *cisternal puncture* is performed to remove spinal fluid instead of a lumbar puncture. The back of the neck is shaved, the skin washed with an antiseptic, and a needle inserted just below the occipital bone of the skull. The patient lies on his side, with a small firm pillow or sandbag placed under the side of the head, and the head flexed forward.

If the pressure of the cerebrospinal fluid is measured, the nurse may be required to hold the manometer while a reading is obtained. It is necessary to hold the very top of the manometer in order to avoid a break in sterile technique. If a Queckenstedt test is done, the nurse may be asked to apply pressure to the jugular veins which are located on the side of the neck. This test is performed to determine spinal fluid pressure changes when the jugular veins are compressed; a sluggish rise or no rise when the veins are compressed may indicate an obstruction in the circu-

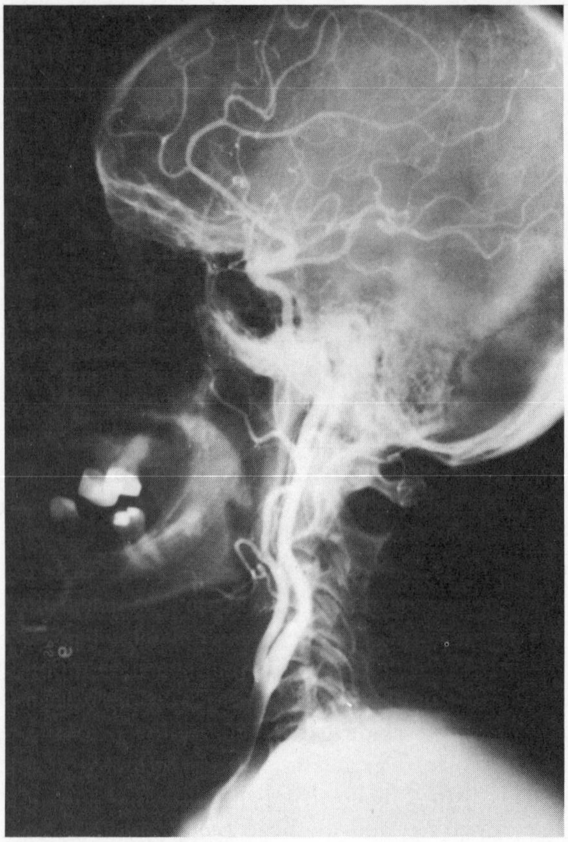

figure 15-2. A normal cerebral arteriogram. (Courtesy H. Revollo, M.D. Photograph—D. Atkinson)

Table 15-2.
Nursing management of the patient after a lumbar puncture

Complete bed rest is required for 8 to 24 hours or as ordered by the physician.

The bed should be kept flat for 6 or more hours. A pillow may or may not be allowed.

Analgesics may be ordered for headache and a force fluid regimen prescribed to assist in the replacement of cerebrospinal fluid.

Vital signs should be taken immediately after the procedure and hourly for 4 to 6 hours, if necessary.

If nausea, vomiting, or pain in the back of the legs occurs, this must be reported to the physician.

lation pathways of the spinal fluid. Since there are several minor variations of this procedure, specific instructions from the physician may be needed.

At the end of the procedure, samples of cerebrospinal fluid are usually sent to the laboratory. It is essential that the test tubes containing the specimens be properly labeled and that request slips clearly identify the patient and the tests desired. Loss or breakage might necessitate a repeat of an uncomfortable procedure. Caution is also exercised during the procedure by providing a firm container for holding spinal fluid samples.

Care of the patient after a lumbar puncture is discussed in Table 15-2. Some patients experience a "spinal" headache which is thought to be due to the removal of spinal fluid. Applying an ice bag to the head, keeping the room dark and quiet, and administering analgesics usually relieves some of the discomfort. If no pillow is allowed, a small towel covered with a pillowcase will provide some support for the head and take the strain off the neck muscles. A quiet, understanding manner before, during, and after the procedure may also lessen postprocedure discomfort.

Contrast studies

Cerebral angiography (Fig. 15-2), *ventriculography* (Fig. 15-3), *pneumoencephalography* (PEG), and *myelography* are contrast studies; that is, radiopaque dye or air is injected for visualization of cerebral or spinal structures.

A cerebral angiogram (also called cerebral arteriogram) is a diagnostic study that may detect distortion of cerebral arteries and veins indicating an aneurysm, tumor, or other vascular abnormality. A radiopaque dye is injected into the right and/or left arteries of the neck (carotids), or the brachial artery. A rapid sequence of x-ray films is taken as the dye circulates through the cerebral arteries and veins.

It is essential that the patient be given a full explanation of the procedure, especially if it is performed under a local anesthetic, when patient cooperation is necessary. If the physician has failed to give an adequate explanation and the patient or his family persist in asking questions, the nurse should call the physician for clarification. Preparation of the patient includes an explanation of the procedure (preferably by the physician) and fasting from fluid and food for 6 to 8 or more hours.

This procedure may be performed under general or local anesthesia. If local anesthesia is used, the patient will experience discomfort and pain during the procedure. Some of the discomfort is due to the positioning and anchoring of the head with tape. Administration of a local anesthetic is followed by the insertion of needles into the carotid arteries, causing discomfort and a feeling of tightness in the throat. Following injection of a radiopaque dye under pressure, there will be a warm, flushed feeling followed by a severe burning sensation lasting about 10 seconds. The simultaneous clicking or chattering sound is the rapid movement of x-ray film beneath the patient's head.

An angiogram is not without danger; death has been known to occur during or after the procedure. Table 15-3 describes nursing management after the procedure. It should be noted that care will vary according to the patient's condition prior to the procedure and the specific orders of the physician.

The patient may experience difficulty in swallowing and talking for a few hours after the procedure but any severe difficulty in swallowing or breathing must be reported at once. Any change in the level of consciousness or numbness or paralysis in the face or extremities must also be reported immediately. The ice collar should be checked periodically and refilled as necessary. If the brachial artery (in the arm) is used as an injection site, careful attention is given to the pulse of the arm. Absence, or a change in the quality of the pulse, or redness, swelling or edema of the arm must be reported immediately.

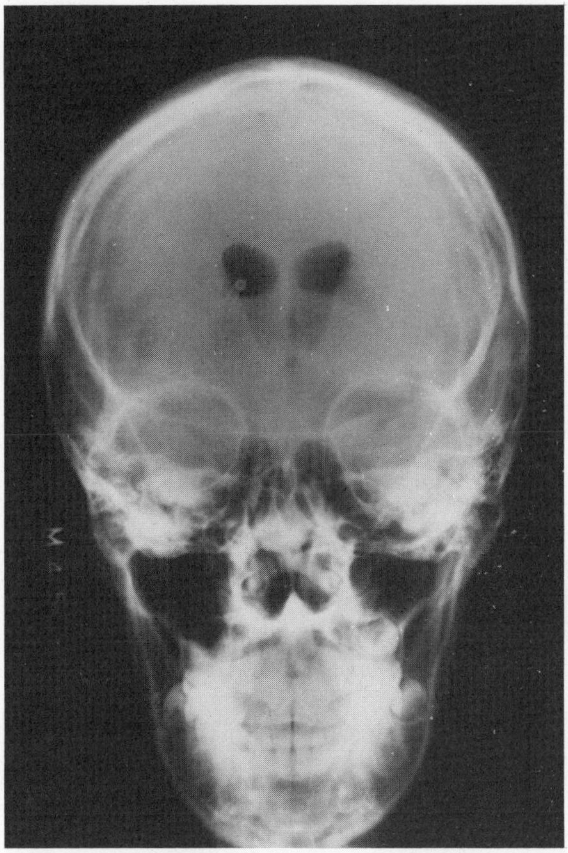

figure 15-3. Normal ventriculogram. (Courtesy H. Revollo, M.D. Photograph—D. Atkinson)

Table 15-3.
Nursing management of the patient after a cerebral angiogram

The head of the bed should remain flat or slightly elevated, depending on the physician's orders regarding height.

An ice collar or cold pack should be applied to the neck to prevent subcutaneous swelling and edema, and relieve discomfort (if the carotid artery is the site of the injection). This is usually a written order.

Vital signs should be checked every ½ hour until the patient is stable or as ordered by the physician.

Puncture sites should be inspected for swelling and formation of a hematoma every hour.

A tracheostomy set should be available.

Oral fluids are usually withheld for several hours. Sips of ice water or ice chips may be allowed.

Patients allergic to iodine cannot receive radiopaque dye material containing iodine. Even though proper precautions, such as skin testing and an allergy history are taken, sensitivity to iodine can occur. This phenomena may be manifested by a sudden onset of anaphylactic shock: severe hypotension, weak rapid or imperceptable pulse, a sudden change in the level of consciousness, and profuse diaphoresis. This is an emergency situation requiring cardiopulmonary resuscitation (CPR) and other emergency measures.

Pneumoencephalogram (PEG)

A pneumoencephalogram is an air contrast study performed when there is a suspected abnormality such as a brain tumor. The patient may be given a local or general anesthetic. Cerebrospinal fluid is removed by means of a lumbar puncture, followed by an injection of air or gas. If only a small amount of spinal fluid is removed this is called a *fractional* pneumoencephalogram. After injection of air or gas, a series of x-ray films are taken.

The preparation of the patient for pneumoencephalography is similar to that of a preoperative patient. The patient must give written permission for the procedure. An enema may be ordered the evening before. A sedative is usually ordered the night before, and often is repeated the morning of the procedure. Ordinarily, an injection of atropine and Demerol or other premedication is administered ½ to 1 hour before the pneumoencephalogram is begun.

Other aspects of preoperative care that are applicable to patients being prepared for pneumoencephalography include:

- Attention to personal cleanliness
- Removal of dentures
- Noting and recording vital signs on the patient's chart
- Omission of food and fluids for 6 hours before the procedure

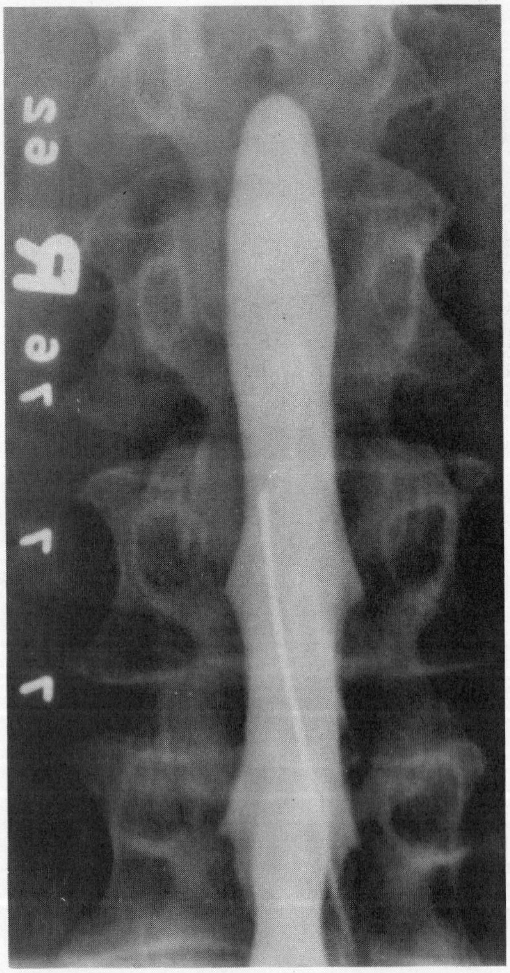

figure 15-4. A normal myelogram. (Courtesy H. Revollo, M.D. Photograph—D. Atkinson)

Patients usually experience a severe headache after pneumoencephalography. Some have nausea, vomiting, and fever; they may also have shock, convulsions, respiratory distress, or symptoms of increased intracranial pressure. The patient may hear a splashing noise when he turns his head. This reaction is due to the presence of air in the ventricles. The symptoms gradually subside over a period of about two days, as the air is absorbed gradually, and cerebrospinal fluid is produced to replace that which was removed during the test.

After a pneumoencephalogram, the patient is placed flat in bed, at complete rest. The movement of his head tends to increase the severity of the symptoms. Application of an ice cap to the head, codeine, and aspirin may be ordered. The patient should be fed, bathed, and given assistance when he turns. Fluids are encouraged in order to increase production of cerebrospinal fluid. Level of consciousness, state of pupils, pulse, respiration, and blood pressure are observed and recorded frequently, on the basis of the doctor's order. Usually, these observations are made every 15 minutes or every half-hour at first. On the second or third day after the test, the patient is usually assisted to get up. He should sit up first and then slowly assume a standing position. If he experiences headache, he may be placed on bed rest for another day.

A serious complication in patients with brain tumors is a shift of the tumor, caused by the injection of air. In its new position the tumor may encroach on brain centers vital to the patient's life. Emergency surgery to remove the tumor may be necessary. Tumor shift may be evidenced by a change in vital signs, or level of consciousness, or the development of such neurological symptoms as paralysis, altered sensation in a part, or a dilated, poorly reactive, or nonreactive pupil on one side. Symptoms will depend on the area of the brain affected by the tumor. The physician should be notified immediately if any new neurological symptoms appear, or if there is intensification of preexisting symptoms.

Ventriculography

The procedure for ventriculography is similar to that for pneumoencephalography, except that the air is injected into the ventricles of the brain through burr holes made in the skull. Ventriculography is used when pneumoencephalography is not possible. For example, obstruction of the spinal canal may make it necessary to secure a ventriculogram rather than a pneumoencephalogram. In this case, the air injected during a lumbar puncture could not rise to the ventricles if the spinal canal were blocked, so the air is injected into the ventricles. Ventricular puncture is the procedure preferred by many neurosurgeons when increased intracranial pressure is known or suspected, because lumbar puncture may permit shifts of brain tissue downward through the foramen magnum from loss of fluid below.

Hair that covers the area where the burr holes are to be made must be shaved before the ventriculography is performed. Other preparation is similar to that for pneumoencephalography. Ventriculography is performed in the operating room under local or general anesthesia.

The care of the patient after ventriculography is also similar to that after pneumoencephalography. However, the patient is less likely to suffer from a headache, because there is less chance that air will enter the subarachnoid space. Sterile brain cannulas in a sterile test tube should be taped to the head of the bed. If there is a sudden increase in pressure after the ventricular puncture, the physician may need to do an immediate tap.

Myelography

A lumbar puncture is performed in myelography, and a radiopaque substance is injected through the spinal needle into the spinal canal (Fig. 15-4). X-ray films are then taken to demonstrate abnormalities of the spinal canal, such as tumors or a ruptured intervertebral disc. When the roentgenograms have been taken, the dye is removed via the spinal needle to prevent irritation of the meninges by the dye. Movement of the spinal needle is necessary in order to remove the dye. This manipulation of the needle sometimes causes pain, due to the contact of the needle with the nerve roots. If the patient is told just before this procedure that some pain is commonly felt, and that it does not indicate any untoward response to the procedure, it will be easier for him to tolerate the discomfort. Afterward the patient rests flat in bed for a few hours. He should be watched for signs of meningeal irritation (stiffness of the neck and pain when an attempt is made to bend the head forward).

Other diagnostic studies

Electroencephalography

The electroencephalogram is a record of the electrical impulses generated by the brain. Electrodes are placed on the patient's scalp, and the graph is recorded by a machine called an *electroencephalograph*. Usually, the patient is taken to another room, where a technician carries out the test. The procedure is not painful, and it does not cause after effects. The patient is instructed to sit comfortably in a chair, or to lie on a bed or a stretcher, and to relax while the machine makes the recording. The test is run for varying lengths of time (½ to 2 hours). It is important to explain the test to the patient before it is begun, so that he will not fear that the wires and the machine will give him a shock. The patient follows his usual activities after the test. No special care or observation is necessary. If the doctor approves, a shampoo may be given after the test to remove the conducting jelly from the patient's hair. If a shampoo is contraindicated, the patient's hair can be gently and briskly rubbed with a towel and combed until the jelly is removed.

Brain scan

A brain scan may be ordered if an abnormality of the brain is suspected. The brain scan may identify brain tumors, hematomas in or around the brain, fluid accumulation in the area surrounding the brain, cerebral abscess, cerebral infarction and displacement of the ventricles. A radioactive material such as technetium^{99m} per technate is injected prior to the procedure. Depending on the type of scanner used, this procedure can take as long as 1 hour or as little as a few minutes. It may be necessary for some patients to return for follow-up scans at 24-, 48-, or 72-hour intervals. The procedure is not painful.

Levels of consciousness

The following classification of *levels of consciousness* (LOC) applies to altered consciousness from any cause, including increased intracranial pressure; cerebral vascular accident; edema; effect of a drug, such as alcohol; anesthesia; fever; and disorders of brain physiology that may be brought about by such deviations as hypoxia and hypoglycemia. At times it may be difficult to differentiate between the levels of consciousness. Some patients may show characteristics of two or more levels.

Consciousness. The patient responds immediately, fully, and appropriately to visual, auditory, and other stimulation.

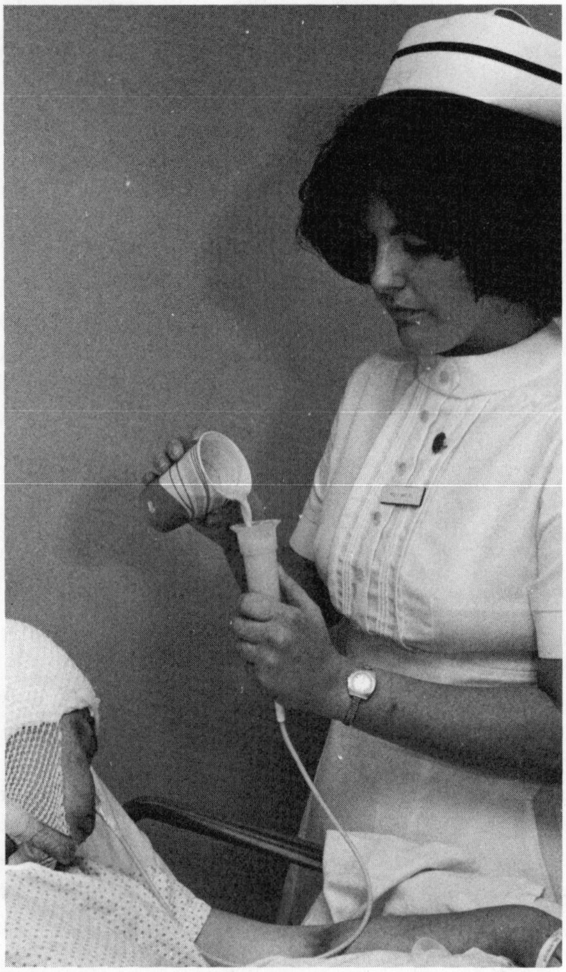

figure 15-5. The unconscious patient will need feeding by nasogastric tube or other methods to meet nutritional requirements. (Photograph—D. Atkinson)

Somnolence or Lethargy. The patient is drowsy or sleepy at inappropriate times. He can be aroused but will fall asleep. He also may answer questions but the answers may be delayed or inappropriate. The speech may be incoherent. He may respond to verbal commands but the response will be slow. There is usually a response to painful stimuli.

Stupor. The patient can be aroused only by vigorous and continuing stimulation, usually by manipulation or perhaps by strong auditory or visual stimuli. Such stimulation may arouse him enough to answer simple questions with one or two words, or his response may be only restless motor activity or purposeful behavior directed toward avoiding further stimulation.

Semicoma. The patient is unresponsive except to superficial, relatively mild painful stimuli to which he makes some purposeful avoiding motor response. Spontaneous motion is uncommon, but the patient may groan or mutter.

Coma. He is unresponsive to all but very painful stimuli to which he may make fragmentary, delayed reflex withdrawal or, in deeper stages, may lose all responsiveness. There is no spontaneous movement and respirations may be irregular.

Nursing management of the neurological patient

Maintenance of an Adequate Airway. Some patients may have an inadequate exchange of air. There are several nursing measures that may increase the amount of air inspired with each breath. When he is lying on the side or back, the patient's head can be *slightly* hyperextended. Keeping the head of the bed slightly elevated lessens the pressure of abdominal organs on his diaphragm. Coughing and deep breathing, unless contraindicated by the physician's order, clears the respiratory tract of pooled secretions. It should be noted that coughing may be contraindicated in patients with increased intracranial pressure, therefore the nurse would not encourage this maneuver in any patient suspected of having this condition. IPPB (intermittent positive pressure breathing) may be ordered for those with respiratory problems. Suctioning may be necessary if the patient is unable to raise secretions. The nurse suctions the patient as frequently as necessary, being careful not to traumatize the tissues. If the tip of the catheter is pushed roughly against the tissues of the nose or the throat, or if suctioning pressure is applied directly to a tissue, the injured membrane may become edematous, bleed, or produce even more mucus. Suction should be applied only when the catheter is withdrawn and never when it is inserted. Oxygen by nasal catheter may be ordered.

Nutrition. Meeting the patient's nutritional requirements is of primary importance. This may involve meal planning, that is, selecting foods that the patient likes, as well as foods that are nutritional. The patient's tray should be checked after each meal for foods or liquids not taken. If the appetite is poor or the patient is unable to eat, the physician must be informed so that dietary supplements, nasogastric feeding (Fig. 15-5), or hyperalimentation may be ordered if necessary.

The patient who is unable to suck through a straw

may be fed with a spoon or with a rubber-tipped syringe. Dentures should be replaced as soon as it is safe to do so, because the patient will feel more comfortable and be able to eat better. The patient's teeth should be brushed or cleaned with an applicator after he eats.

The patient must not be given too much at one time, because overloading the stomach may cause vomiting. The danger in vomiting is aspiration. Some patients cannot tolerate more than 200 ml. at a time and will need to be fed more frequently than those who can take more.

Whatever is the patient's capacity, he should ingest an adequate diet in liquid form. Protein, carbohydrate, fat, and caloric needs can be met through tube feedings. If the patient's skin seems dry, his mouth is cracked, and he shows other signs of dehydration, the physician should be consulted about an increase in fluid intake. Water or fruit juice may be given between his scheduled feedings.

Mouth Care. Good care of the mouth is essential, especially in patients who are not alert or who are unable to give their own oral care. The edentulous (without teeth) patient will need dentures cleaned at least twice a day. At times when dentures are not worn, they should be placed in a *safe* place and mouth rinses offered frequently, at least after every meal. The comatose patient's mouth is often wide open, because he breathes through it. His mouth becomes dry, saliva sticks to his teeth, and his lips crack without frequent mouth care. The patient's teeth will need special care; inflammation of the gums (gingivitis) and other gum problems occur rapidly if the teeth are not thoroughly cleaned. A soft toothbrush is best, especially if the gums are sore and bleeding. The lips are to be kept moistened, especially if dry or cracked. Swabs soaked in glycerine to which a few drops of lemon juice are added can be used to moisten and soften the lips.

Positioning. If the patient's condition keeps him from changing position in bed, a position change every 2 hours is necessary. This procedure offers several preventative measures. It (1) prevents contractures, (2) prevents pneumonia, (3) prevents damage to nerve plexuses, and (4) prevents decubitus ulcers.

Contractures (Fig. 15-6) are avoided by passive exercising of immobile limbs that are not exercised because of paralysis or because of a decreased level of consciousness. A footboard is used to prevent footdrop and shortening of the calf muscles. Support to the wrists by means of splints or alignment with pillows may prevent wristdrop. Adequate support of the head is attained with the use of a small pillow; if this is not available, a regulation size pillow is placed under the head and shoulders. As the patient is turned, his breathing pattern alters. He may be stimulated to take a deeper breath and fill resting alveoli with air. The circulatory pattern also alters. More blood can enter the skin areas that were partially deprived of circulation when they were pinched between the bone and the bed. As the patient is turned, the arm and the leg that have been lying motionless under him for the previous 2 hours may be exercised. It is necessary to pay particular attention to the position of the feet every time the patient's position is changed. The physical therapist is a valuable resource person for information regarding methods that may be used to prevent contractures.

Hypostatic pneumonia, which is due to a pooling of secretions in the lungs, may be prevented by turning the patient routinely, that is every 2 hours. The

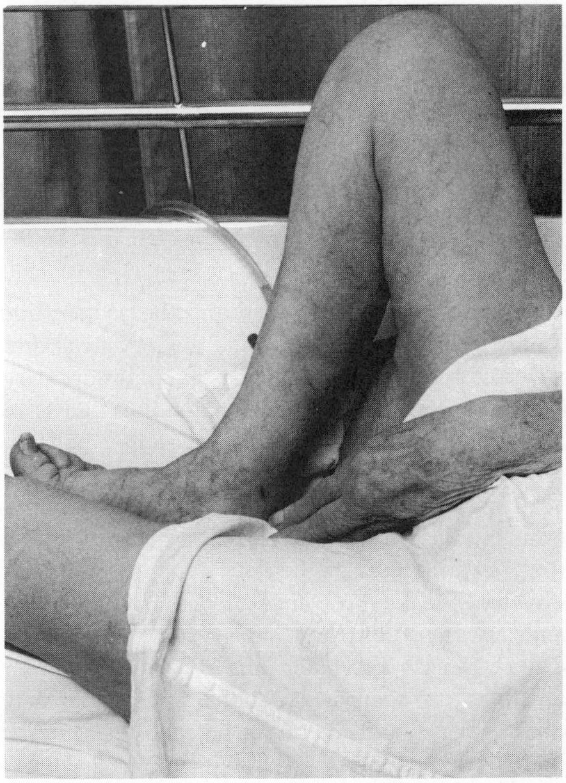

figure 15-6. Contracture of the right leg in a patient cared for at home after a CVA. The patient was brought to the hospital after development of extensive decubitus ulcers. (Photograph—D. Atkinson)

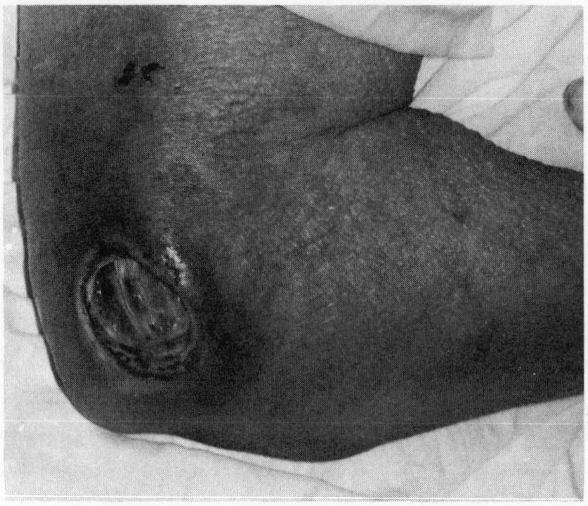

figure 15-7. Decubitus of the elbow in a patient with a CVA cared for at home. This patient was admitted to the hospital for treatment of multiple decubitus ulcers. (Photograph—D. Atkinson)

unconscious patient should be kept off his back; this is especially important when the coughing and swallowing reflexes are absent.

Injury to nerve plexuses, especially the brachial plexus (a group of nerves in the lower part of the neck and axilla) can be prevented by a slight rotation of the lower shoulder and a positioning of the lower arm away from, rather than under, the body.

Prevention of decubitus ulcers (Fig. 15-7) requires an intensive nursing approach and the cooperation of all nursing personnel. Each time the patient is turned, bony prominences are gently massaged. If necessary an alternating pressure mattress or flotation pad is used. Pillows are used for support of the upper part of the body when there is a tendency for the patient to roll back from the assigned position. The head is supported by a small pillow; regulation size pillows may induce contractures of the neck and shoulder muscles as well as make breathing difficult by pushing the head forward.

Skin Care. The older patient usually has dry skin and the use of soap has a tendency to further dry the skin. Soaps should be used sparingly except when washing the perineal area. If excessive dryness and flaking is a problem, emollients (skin softeners) such as Alpha Keri can be added to the bath water. Excessive use of talcum powder on the perineal area, groin, and body creases should be avoided, since powder has a tendency to cake and further irritate the skin. Powder should always be applied sparingly and alcohol and other drying agents avoided. Brief rubbing of reddened areas is a good assignment for a family member who is visiting the patient and is eager to do something to help. Explaining the importance of preventing skin breakdown will help the visitor feel that he is making a real contribution to the care of the patient.

Changes in vital signs and levels of consciousness should be watched. It should be determined if the pupils are equal in size, and if they accommodate to light. Skin color and muscle tone must be noted. Increasing spasticity may indicate increasing cerebral involvement. Changes in pulse, respiration, or blood pressure may precede or accompany a new pathologic process. Rigidity of the neck sometimes indicates involvement of the meninges. Daily descriptions of the patient's response to his environment should be in the nurse's notes.

Eye Care. The eyes should be checked daily for corneal drying, especially in the elderly or unresponsive patient. Normally, the cornea has a "wet" or shiny appearance. When blinking is absent or there is a reduction in tear formation, the cornea appears dull. This abnormality should be reported to the physician who may order ophthalmic ointments, eye drops, or the use of an eye patch. If an eye patch is ordered it is necessary to change it daily, looking at the eye for such signs of irritation as redness and excessive dryness.

Bowel and Bladder. The comatose patient as well as patients with other neurological disorders may lose control of the bowel, the bladder, or both. An indwelling catheter may be necessary when bladder control is lost. Constipation may also be a problem and may go unnoticed unless there is an accurate record of bowel movements recorded on the patient's chart. If there has been no bowel movement for several days, if the stool appears hard, or there are episodes of persistent diarrhea without an apparent cause, the physician should be informed. The perineal and anal areas must be kept scrupulously clean. A record of intake and output may be necessary.

Dependency. *The unconscious patient is totally dependent.* He is powerless to move and to prevent asphyxiation. He has lost both position sense and the ability to catch himself if he starts to fall out of bed. He may be cold, but he cannot cover himself or protect himself from a draft. He needs protection. The side rails of his bed should be put up every time the patient is alone. If a nurse is changing his position alone he should be turned toward, not away from her.

Because the patient does not respond, it cannot be assumed that he does not hear, think, and feel. He may be aware of others even though he cannot indicate that he is. His environment should be peaceful and quiet. Nothing should be said in his presence that you do not wish him to hear. He should be told what is happening even though there is no indication that he understands. Some patients with neurological disorders first begin to make contact with the outside world in response to talk directed to them when they appear to be entirely unresponsive.

Helping the Family. The care of the unconscious patient is a difficult experience for the physician, the nurse, and the patient's family. A person once well is now unable to speak, to feed himself, or to think. When there is no chance for cure, the hopelessness of the situation can be very difficult for the family.

It is the responsibility of the physician to explain to the family the extent of damage to the patient and to encourage a less expensive means of care than that offered by the general hospital. It is the responsibility of the nurse to give the best care possible. The nurse may be able to help the family accept the fact that no amount of medical or nursing therapy may restore the patient to his original mental and physical state. The family requires support and time to go through the process of grief so that they can accept the situation.

Meningitis

The meninges are three layers of membranes that lie between the bones of the skull and the brain tissue. The *dura mater,* the outermost layer, lines the skull; the *arachnoid,* the middle layer, is separated from the pia mater by the subarachnoid space, which is filled with cerebrospinal fluid; the *pia mater,* covering the brain, is a highly vascular membrane. Meningitis means inflammation of the meninges.

Etiology. The causative organism can be any bacteria, but meningococcus, streptococcus, staphylococcus, and pneumococcus are the most common causative organisms of meningitis. The infectious organisms reach the meninges by way of the bloodstream or by direct extension from infected areas such as the middle ear or the paranasal sinuses.

Signs and Symptoms. The signs and symptoms of meningitis are: elevated temperature, pain and stiffness of the neck (nuchal rigidity), nausea, vomiting, aversion to light (photophobia), headache, restlessness, irritability, and in some instances convulsions. Severe irritation of the meninges may cause opisthotonus—an extreme hyperextension of the head and arching of the back. The patient with *meningococcal* meningitis may have multiple petechiae on the body. In some people, symptoms of meningitis develop slowly, whereas in others the symptoms develop rapidly.

Treatment and Nursing Management

When the patient has been admitted to the hospital, a lumbar puncture is done to establish the diagnosis and to identify the organism. A blood culture also may be taken.

Intravenous fluid therapy and antibiotics are started immediately. Antibiotics are given intramuscularly and perhaps directly into the subarachnoid space of the spinal cord (intrathecal injection). Drug therapy for meningitis may be continued after the acute phase of the illness is over to prevent the recurrence of infection of the meninges. Corticosteroid therapy may be used for the dangerously ill patient. After the meningitis episode is over, the physician may search for the primary focus of infection and take steps to eradicate it, if possible.

During the early stage of meningitis the patient is very sick. Side rails, careful monitoring of vital signs, cooling measures if his temperature goes too high, attention to hydration and nutrition, and observation of his color, his alertness and his muscle tone are required.

Most adults with bacterial meningitis will recover without sequelae, due to the use of antibiotics. When complications occur, they are usually serious. The infection may be overwhelming, and the patient may die. Neurological complications, such as damage to cranial nerves, and especially visual and auditory deterioration, may take place.

Encephalitis

Encephalitis is an infectious disease of the central nervous system characterized by pathological changes in both the white matter and the gray matter of the cord and the brain.

Etiology. Encephalitis can be caused by bacteria, fungi, or viruses. Poisoning by drugs, chemicals like lead or arsenic, or carbon monoxide clinically may closely resemble encephalitis but are referred to by the term *encephalopathy.*

The disease can occur after any viral infection elsewhere in the body, such as measles, smallpox, or rabies, or after vaccination. In endemic or epidemic forms it is caused by a filtrable virus. Some of these viruses have been identified, such as the St. Louis virus, the Western equine virus, and the Eastern equine virus. Some viruses are transmitted by ticks; others, by mosquitoes.

PATHOLOGY. There is severe, diffuse inflammation of the brain, with intense lymphocytic infiltration, especially around the blood vessels of the brain. In patients who die, and in some who do not, there is extensive nerve cell destruction.

SYMPTOMS. The onset of viral encephalitis is usually sudden. The patients are admitted to the hospital with fever, severe headache, stiff neck, vomiting, and drowsiness. Lethargy is a prominent symptom and coma or delirium may be present. The patient may have tremors or convulsions; rarely, spastic or flaccid paralysis; usually irritability, incoordination, and muscular weakness; sometimes, incontinence, spasm of the muscles of the jaw, or eye symptoms, such as sensitivity to light, involuntary eye movements, double vision, or blurred vision.

TREATMENT AND NURSING MANAGEMENT

As there is no known specific antiviral measure in existence yet, treatment for encephalitis is symptomatic. Application of sponges or hypothermia treatment may be ordered to reduce fever. The patient's room should be dimly lighted, quiet, and free from excitement. Intravenous therapy is usually necessary. Accurate intake and output records are important. Because the patient may be comatose, a nasogastric tube may be inserted to provide nourishment. Suctioning to prevent choking or aspiration of secretions, and mouth care are important. An indwelling urethral catheter may be inserted to keep track of the patient's output and to keep the bed dry. The patient is kept clean and turned frequently. As is true with any delirious or comatose patient, side rails should be kept in place. The patient's eye symptoms, tremors, and mental state, as well as any changes in his condition must be reported. Patients with extreme respiratory difficulty may require mechanical assistance with respiration.

Table 15-4.
The types and causes of parkinsonism

TYPE	CAUSE(S)
Paralysis agitans	Idiopathic (unknown)
Secondary or symptomatic parkinsonism	Drugs (example, phenothiazines), head injuries, poisons, encephalitis

Herpes zoster or "shingles"

Herpes zoster is an acute viral infection caused by the same virus which causes chickenpox. Those who have never had chickenpox and are in contact with someone who has the disease appear to be susceptible, as are those who have lost some of the naturally acquired immunity to chickenpox. Nursing personnel who have not had chickenpox should not be assigned to care for a patient with herpes zoster.

The disease usually begins with pain and intense itching of the skin, followed in several days by the formation of vesicles (blisterlike elevations). The pain, itching and vesicular eruptions follow the path of sensory nerves; usually eruptions are unilateral. The pain, in some instances severe, may persist for several weeks. Scarring can also occur.

TREATMENT AND NURSING MANAGEMENT

Treatment is symptomatic; there is no effective, specific drug for this or most viral infections. Analgesics, corticosteroids—orally or as ointments or lotions, and other liquid preparations that have a drying effect on the lesions may be ordered.

Nursing management is aimed at keeping the patient as comfortable as possible. Clothing should be loose, and wool or rough materials should not be worn close to the affected areas. Topical medications are usually ordered to be applied liberally. If tincture of benzoin, collodion or calamine lotion is prescribed, a dressing should not be applied. These solutions encourage adherence of the dressing to the skin, making removal of the dressing difficult and painful. Also included in a program of care is bed rest, a planned program of physical therapy, and the prevention of muscle contractures and loss of muscle tone. A cradle or footboard is used to keep bedding off feet and legs.

Parkinson's disease (paralysis agitans)

Parkinsonism (Parkinson's disease, paralysis agitans) was first described by Dr. James Parkinson in 1817. The term *parkinsonism* is now more commonly used, since it encompasses the various causes of this disorder (see Table 15-4).

PATHOLOGY. Parkinson's disease primarily affects the basal ganglia and their connections. The main pathway of the basal ganglia is the extrapyramidal tract, comprising the system of motor nerves responsible for automatic movements like blinking, walking, eating, posture, muscle tone, and the movements of facial expression. Idiopathic parkinsonism is thought to be due to a deficiency of dopamine, a neurohormone, in the basal ganglia of the brain.

ETIOLOGY. The cause of the classic syndrome of Parkinson's disease is unknown, and as yet even the nature of the pathological changes it causes in the nervous system is not entirely clear.

SYMPTOMS. The most common form of parkinsonism is idiopathic and usually begins after age 50. Early signs include stiffness, tremors of the hands which are described as "pill-rolling" (a rhythmic motion of the thumb against the fingers), and difficulty in performing movements. Usually tremors decrease when movement is voluntary, for example, when picking up an object. Some patients may experience the reverse effect, that is an increase in tremors during voluntary movements. This is called an intention tremor.

As the disease progresses, tremors of the head, a masklike expression, stooped posture, monotonous speech, shuffling gait, and weight loss are seen. The shuffling gait, with difficulty in turning or redirecting forward motion, is a typical manifestation of the disease. Arm swinging while walking is almost nonexistent. The symptoms of secondary parkinsonism are similar to those of the idiopathic type; rhythmic and involuntary movements of the tongue, the jaw, the neck and the extremities, along with facial grimaces may also be seen.

The symptoms progress so slowly that there may be a lapse of years between the time of the patient's first symptom and the time of diagnosis. The symptoms may start on only one side of the body, and later become bilateral. The spread to the other side may occur quickly, or it may be delayed for as long as 15 years.

Rigidity is more widespread through the muscles of the body than is tremor. There is a slight but continuous flexion of all limbs. Reflexes and the power of contraction are not affected, but speed of movement is.

In late stages of the disease, when jaw, tongue and larynx are affected, the speech becomes slurred, and food is chewed inadequately and swallowed with difficulty. Rigidity that is not controlled by drug therapy, physical therapy, or surgery, can lead to contractures. There is increased salivation sometimes accompanied by drooling. In a small percentage of patients, the eyes roll upward or downward and stay there against the patient's will (*oculogyric crises*) perhaps for several hours or even a few days. Pain may occur. The spasm of the ocular muscles may be regular—e.g., occurring once a week—or there may be 10 years between attacks. This peculiar, frustrating symptom is not found in any other disease known to mankind.

PROGNOSIS. Parkinson's disease progresses slowly. A patient may have the disease 20 years or more. Because of their disability, patients are susceptible to respiratory disease.

TREATMENT AND NURSING MANAGEMENT

Treatment is aimed at prolonging independence and preventing dependence. Drugs such as levodopa and anticholinergic agents such as benztropine (Cogentin) and cycrimine (Pagitane) often reduce the intensity of symptoms. Physical therapy, occupational therapy, patient and family education, and counseling are rehabilitation measures concurrent with drug therapy. Surgery has been employed in selected cases; however, levodopa has reduced the need for surgical attempts to alleviate symptoms.

Nursing management is aimed at encouraging independence. Many with this disease are admitted to the hospital for other problems or because of the debilitating effects of the disease such as severe contractures, fractures from falling, pneumonia, or extensive decubitus ulcers. Physically, the patient may have become difficult to care for at home and is admitted to the hospital because skilled nursing care is needed. Transfer to a nursing home or skilled nursing facility may even be necessary. Rehabilitation in the advanced stages of the disease is difficult and, usually, only minor progress is achieved. Decreased debilitation and prevention of secondary problems such as pneumonia and decubitus ulcers is often the main focus of treatment in advanced cases. Those in less advanced stages of the disease are usually more amenable to rehabilitation.

Many patients are diagnosed and started on medical management in a physician's office or a clinic. The initiation of rehabilitation and patient and family education rests with the physician who may delegate some teaching responsibility to other professional staff in these facilities. The role of the nurse in rehabilitation of the patient with parkinsonism is described in

Table 15-5.
The nurse's role in rehabilitation of the patient with parkinsonism

MINIMAL PHYSICAL DISABILITY

Physical activity and ambulation should be encouraged.

Exercise of the extremities is important. The type of exercise may be suggested by the physical therapist and must be demonstrated to the patient.

Self-care activities should be encouraged but must be done gradually. The patient should sit for activities such as shaving, grooming, bathing, and so on.

MODERATE PHYSICAL DISABILITY

The patient should be assisted with ambulation several times a day.

Exercise of the extremities is necessary but passive exercises should be done if the patient is unable to move or exercise his legs.

Participation in daily self-care is to be encouraged, with assistance when needed.

ADVANCED DISABILITY

The patient should be allowed to do as much as possible even though participation in any activity is minimal.

Total dependence is to be avoided as long as possible.

If eating is difficult, a soft diet and ample time to eat will be necessary.

If feeding becomes necessary, the patient should be fed slowly.

A suction machine should be placed in the room since difficulty in chewing and swallowing poses the threat of aspiration.

Table 15-5. The patient is encouraged to lead as normal a life as possible, with emphasis on the importance of exercise and self-care. Drugs administered for parkinsonism are capable of causing a wide variety of side effects requiring careful observation of the patient, especially when therapy is first instituted. Since some patients have a poor appetite, a well-balanced diet is necessary to maintain nutrition. Adequate fluid intake is important, especially in those in an advanced stage of the disease who may neglect taking fluids because tremors make holding a glass difficult. Constipation may be a problem, making stool softeners necessary to produce soft, formed stools. Ample time must be allowed when the patient is participating in his own care. These patients move slowly and cannot be hurried. To do so only creates a stressful situation.

PHYSICAL THERAPY. Although it cannot halt progression of the disease, physical therapy can result in the patient's maintaining greater ability for self-care. Physical therapy is not indicated for tremor, but is of great value in rigidity. Here, as always, early and consistent treatment will be more beneficial.

THE LONG-TERM VIEW. The patient should be helped by his family, friends, or the professional staff only when he is unable to perform a movement by himself. It is important that stress, anxiety and fatigue, all of which make the symptoms worse, be kept to a minimum, and the family can help. When the patient is not present, the nurse might discuss with them his needs for serenity and peace of mind.

Parkinson's disease is discouraging for patient, family, and nurse. It is a long-term affliction without remission in its symptomatology. The drooling disgusts the patient, the blank face and the slowed movements make social interchange difficult, and the rigidity is anxiety-provoking and frustrating. There are many areas in which treatment facilities are scarce or nonexistent.

Yet, the nurse can point out to a discouraged patient that present-day drug therapy does control many of the symptoms and research on new drugs is proceeding.

Epilepsy

Epilepsy was described by Hippocrates as long ago as 400 B.C., but modern study and treatment of the disorder began only about a century ago. Attitudes toward epilepsy have delayed both study and treatment. Until recent times epileptics were considered to be possessed by good or evil spirits; fear of the disease was the rule, not study of it.

Epilepsy may be defined as an *abnormal* electrical disturbance in one or more specific areas of the brain. Epilepsy can be divided into two general groups: (1) *idiopathic* or primary epilepsy and (2) *symptomatic* or secondary epilepsy. The term "idiopathic" means of unknown cause. The majority of convulsive disorders (another term for the epilepsies) falls into this class. Symptomatic epilepsy is a convulsive disorder in which the cause *IS* known or is at least suspected, such as a convulsive disorder resulting from a brain tumor or uremia. Presumably, once the cause of symptomatic epilepsy is removed, the disorder will be corrected. There are different types of convulsive disorders or epileptic seizures, each characterized by a specific pattern of events: *grand mal, petit mal, psychomotor,* and *focal/jacksonian.*

TYPICAL GRAND MAL SEIZURES are characterized by a sequence of events beginning with a prodromal phase, which may or may not be present in all patients. The prodromal phase consists of vague emotional changes such as depression, anxiety, or nervousness. This may last for minutes or hours and then be followed by an *aura,* which usually precedes the seizure by a few seconds. The aura may be sensory, that is an odor or sound, or it may be a sensation such as weakness or numbness. In those who experience an aura, the aura is most always the same. The aura is related to the anatomical origin of the seizure.

The aura is followed by the epileptic cry, caused by spasm of the respiratory muscles and muscles of the throat and glottis. This cry immediately precedes the loss of consciousness and the ensuing tonic and clonic phases of the convulsion. The tonic phase is a rigid contraction of the muscles; the clonic phase, an alternate contraction and relaxation of muscles result-

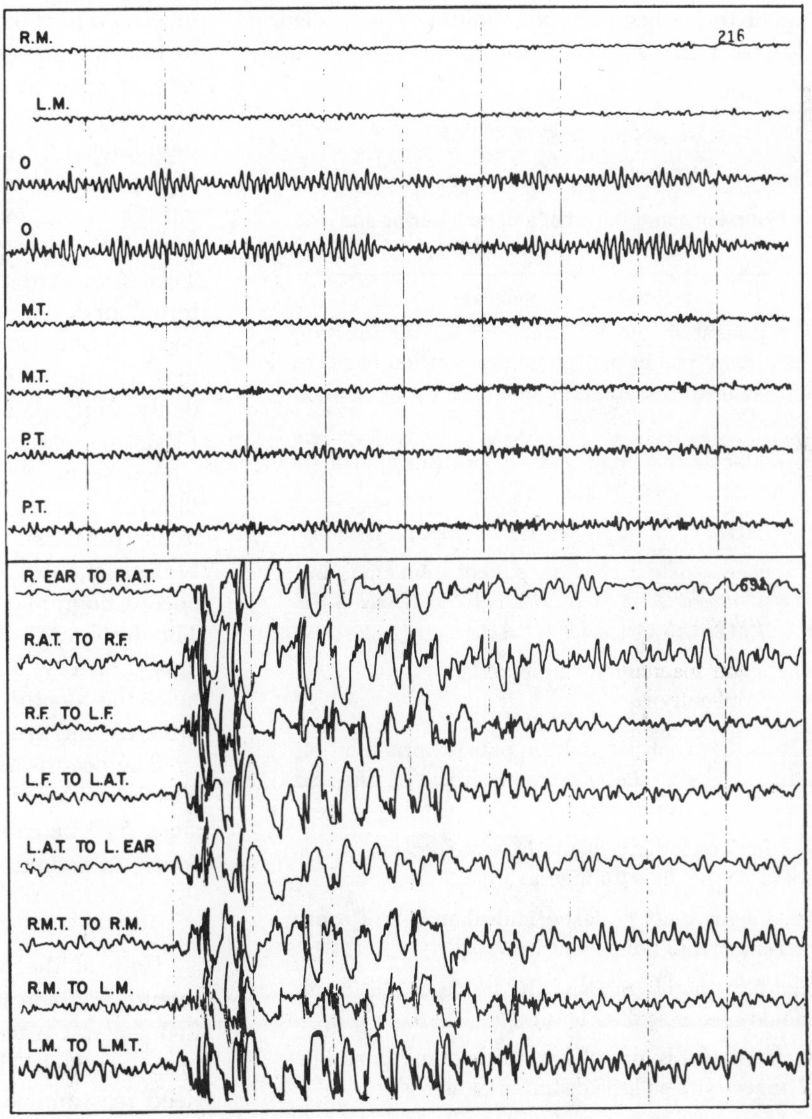

figure 15-8. Contrast of a normal electroencephalogram with that of an epileptic patient during a grand mal seizure. Note the sharp, spiky waves recorded during the seizure. (Dr. Julius Korein, New York, N.Y.)

ing in jerking movements and thrashing of the arms and legs. The skin becomes cyanotic and breathing is spasmodic. Saliva mixes with air resulting in "frothing" at the mouth. The jaws are tightly clenched and the tongue and inner cheek may be bitten. Urinary and/or fecal incontinence usually occurs. The clonic phase may last up to a minute or more and then gradually subside, to be followed by the postictal state. This phase of the seizure may vary; headache, fatigue, deep sleep, confusion, nausea, and muscle soreness may be experienced. Many fall into a deep sleep for several hours.

Petit mal seizures are characterized by a brief loss of consciousness, during which time physical activity ceases. The individual stares blankly, his eyelids may flutter, lips move and there may be a slight movement to his head and extremities. These seizures usually last 1 to 15 seconds and the individual rarely falls to the ground. Petit mal is more common in children.

Table 15-6.
Nursing management of a patient during and after a gland mal seizure

During the Seizure:

The patient should be turned on his side to keep the airway patent and prevent aspiration of saliva and vomitus. Remove oral secretions by suctioning, if possible.

Any objects that may obstruct breathing must be removed: pillows, bedding, clothing.

Restrictive clothing should be loosened, if possible.

It is necessary to protect the patient from injury but *it is dangerous to FORCIBLY RESTRAIN THE EXTEMITIES OR THE HEAD.*

The nurse must *stay with the patient.*

After the Seizure:

The bed is kept flat and the patient turned on his side until he awakes. The room should be dim and noise kept to a minimum.

Restrictive clothing should now be loosened if this could not be done during the attack.

Vital signs must be taken immediately and every half-hour until the patient is awake.

The lips, the tongue, and the inside of the mouth should be checked for injury.

If the patient is incontinent, the bedding should be changed with as little disturbance as possible.

Psychomotor attacks are characterized by periods of automatic activity: asocial behavior—for example, removing one's clothes; inappropriate or purposeless behavior—for example, puffing the cheeks or smacking the lips. The pattern of behavior remains the same and is repeated each time the seizure occurs. Auditory, visual, or olfactory hallucinations may also be a part of this seizure.

Focal or jacksonian seizures (also called marching seizures) are characterized by convulsive twitching or jerking movements that begin in one area of the body and spread or "march" to other areas. For example, a seizure may begin in the left foot and spread up to the leg and to the left side of the body. A seizure could also begin in the face and spread downward to the opposite side of the body, since nerves decussate or cross at the level of the medulla. Consciousness may or may not be lost. This type of seizure may be followed by a grand mal seizure.

Status epilepticus is a rapid progression of convulsive grand mal seizures which the patient undergoes without regaining consciousness between them. This is an extremely dangerous condition; unless it is terminated, the patient will die. Status epilepticus may occur spontaneously and for no known reason but may also occur if anticonvulsant medications are suddenly stopped. Intravenous barbiturates or diazepam (Valium) may be administered to terminate the attack.

Diagnosis. Epilepsy may be the easiest or the most difficult disorder to diagnose, depending on the symptoms. Recurring grand mal seizures present a very typical picture. Irregular tracings on the electroencephalogram confirm the diagnosis (Fig. 15-8, p. 187). The history of the onset of the patient's illness, his family history, and a careful neurological examination help the doctor to differentiate between idiopathic epilepsy and symptomatic epilepsy.

The occurrence of a single convulsion is never conclusive evidence that a person has epilepsy. Convulsions may be caused by a variety of disorders, such as severe infections with high fever.

Nursing management

Care of the patient during and after a grand mal seizure is given in Table 15-6. The patient with petit mal seizures usually requires no special care during or after an attack. Those having psychomotor attacks may need reassurance after the seizure due to mental confusion. This also applies to those who have had a focal or jacksonian seizure but have not lost consciousness.

The patient must not be forcibly restrained during a grand mal seizure as this can result in fractures of the arms, legs, or shoulders. If the nurse is present *before* the tonic phase (the rigid or stiffening part of the convulsion) an oral airway can be inserted. A padded tongue blade can also be used and is placed between the upper and lower molars. The tremendous pressure created by the clamping of the jaws can splinter a tongue blade if it is not inserted correctly. Keeping the patient on his side with his head turned downward will prevent the tongue from obstructing the pharynx.

It is most important that there is accurate documentation of *all observed* activity before, during and after the convulsion. While this can be done in narrative form, seizure records can also be developed and used by nursing personnel.

Discharge Teaching. Discharge teaching and public education are two very important nursing responsibilities. The newly diagnosed epileptic will need a thorough explanation of his disease; this is best done initially by the physician and should include the type of epilepsy the patient has, the medications necessary, and the precautions, if any, to be taken. Points that can be included in the teaching plan are:

- The importance of medication, which in most instances must be taken throughout one's life
- The seriousness of omitting or stopping medication
- The side effects of the medication(s), which should be reviewed after the physician's original explanation
- The necessity of routine visits to the physician's office or clinic
- The hazards of operating a motor vehicle or performing potentially dangerous tasks until seizures are under control with medication
- The importance of wearing Medic-Alert tags or other medical identification

Social, emotional, and economic implications of epilepsy

Many epileptics suffer more acutely from the stigma attached to epilepsy than from the symptoms themselves. Every life situation is tinged with the dread of an attack and the fear of what others will think. The family often is ashamed that the patient has epilepsy. Because of the familial predisposition to epilepsy, family members often feel that the disorder of a relative is a reflection on them and make every effort to conceal it.

The questions of marriage and childbearing may arise. The individual may be helped in making these decisions by personal counseling based on consideration of his condition.

Finding and keeping a job present tremendous problems for the person with epilepsy. There is a false impression that epileptics are of subnormal intelligence. Although some persons with epilepsy experience alteration in their mental functioning, many are nevertheless coping satisfactorily with work, home, and community responsibilities. The proportion of epileptics who have severe impairment of intellectual functioning, due to brain damage, and who are therefore unable to function adequately in work and other community situations is very small. Some people with epilepsy have unusual intellectual gifts, but may lack the opportunity for advanced education and work commensurate with their talents.

Persons with epilepsy who have frequent, severe seizures can be employed only in controlled situations, such as sheltered workshops. It has been estimated that this group comprises only 15 percent of persons with epilepsy.

Emotional strain is often a factor in precipitating seizures, making a satisfying home and family life and suitable work important assets to persons with epilepsy.

Multiple sclerosis

Multiple sclerosis (sometimes abbreviated MS) is a chronic, progressive disease of the nervous system. It is also called a demyelinating disease because myelin, a fatty substance, or phospholipid) surrounding some nerves in the central and peripheral nervous systems undergo degeneration and loss of myelin. Myelin is thought to act as an insulator, enabling nerve impulses to pass along a nerve fiber. Loss of myelin and subsequent degeneration and atrophy of nerve axons interrupts transmission of impulses along these fibers.

At first the lesions formed by destruction of myelin are temporary; later they are permanent. Symptoms often subside during early phases of the illness, and the patient may seem to be perfectly healthy for several months or even years. But with each reappearance the symptoms tend to be more severe and to last longer. These periods of growing better and then growing worse again are called remissions (getting better) and exacerbations (getting worse). They form a characteristic pattern.

INCIDENCE. Multiple sclerosis is a disease of youth and early middle life. The highest incidence occurs between the ages of 20 and 40. Men and women are affected about equally. The disease is more common in northern temperate zones than it is in warm climates; it is more common in the northern parts of the United States and in Europe than the southern regions.

CAUSE. The cause of multiple sclerosis is unknown. Some theories implicate allergy, infection, and emotional stress.

SYMPTOMS. Usually, symptoms appear gradually, and early symptoms vary greatly from patient to patient. There may be a slight weakness or dragging of an extremity, which soon passes, or a transitory blurring of vision or double vision. Often these seemingly minor symptoms are dismissed as a result of fatigue or strain. Later, when the doctor questions the patient, he may recall these episodes. Just as the symptoms themselves vary, their intensity and duration differ. Some patients have severe, long-lasting symptoms early in the course of the disease, whereas others may experience only occasional and mild symptoms for several years after onset.

Common symptoms of multiple sclerosis are:

- Blurred vision
- Diplopia (double vision)
- Nystagmus (involuntary movement of the eyeball)
- Blindness
- Weakness, clumsiness, numbness and tingling of an arm or leg; ataxia (motor incoordination)
- Paralysis, usually of lower extremities (paraplegia)
- Disturbance of bowel function and of bladder function—incontinence or retention
- Intention tremor (the hand trembles when the patient uses it)
- Emotional lability
- Slurred, hesitant speech

TREATMENT

There is no cure for multiple sclerosis; nor is there any single treatment that reliably relieves symptoms. The problem of treatment is complicated by the uneven and unpredictable course of the disease.

Research is being carried on in many parts of the country to try to determine the cause and to develop specific therapy for multiple sclerosis. Organizations like the National Multiple Sclerosis Society are active in programs of education and research.

The patient with multiple sclerosis should be helped to maintain the best possible general health, so that he may withstand his illness better. Infections, such as colds or influenza, and emotional upsets may precipitate exacerbations of the disease.

Here are some important measures that the patient can observe to maintain his general health:

- Get plenty of rest. Do not continue an activity to the point of fatigue. Stop and rest; then resume the activity.
- Avoid infections. (For instance, try to stay away from people who have colds.)
- Eat a nourishing diet, with enough meat, milk, eggs, and fresh fruits and vegetables. Eat regularly.
- As far as possible, avoid situations that you know are upsetting.
- Keep on doing things that are enjoyable, but find ways to make them less strenuous, so that they do not produce fatigue.

MANAGEMENT OF THE DISEASE; PROGNOSIS

People can live a long time with multiple sclerosis. Living for 20 years after the diagnosis has been established is not unusual. Usually the patient with multiple sclerosis gradually develops more severe symptoms and shorter remissions. Weakness of a limb may progress gradually to paraplegia. Incontinence of urine may develop, and slight visual disturbances may progress to total blindness. The activity of the patient gradually is modified as these changes occur—for example, from walking to wheelchair to bed.

Although many patients experience gradual worsening of their symptoms, this is not invariably the case. Some patients have the disease in mild form, and do not experience increasing severity of their symptoms. Some people who have had the disease for 15 years are able to continue their usual activities. The prognosis is decidedly variable.

Nothing is to be gained by insisting on bed rest before the symptoms of the patient require it. If a patient has influenza, bed rest is an important aid to recovery. But if he has multiple sclerosis, confining him to bed before it is absolutely necessary not only fails to halt the disease, but also leads to depression, boredom, and such physical complications as decubitus ulcers. The patient should be helped to maintain normal activity as long as he can.

EMOTIONAL RESPONSES. Mood swings (emotional lability) are common among patients with multiple sclerosis. The patient may feel ecstatic one minute, and shortly later declare that life is not worth living. Two possible explanations have been given for this state. The patient may experience fluctuations of mood because of damage done to his nervous system or because of his deep anxiety about his illness and prognosis. Both may contribute to alternating euphoria and depression.

COMPLICATIONS. Some patients show symptoms of impaired intellectual functioning late in the course of the illness. For instance, loss of memory, difficulty in concentrating, and impaired judgment may occur. As the disease progresses, the patient is subject to many complications. With the knowledge that paralysis and incontinence often occur, it is possible to foresee the complications to which the patient is especially vulnerable:

- Pneumonia. It is not unusual for pneumonia to be the immediate cause of death. The patient is very susceptible to infection because of his limited activity, shallow breathing, and general debility. People with respiratory infections must be kept away from the patient. He must be encouraged to breathe deeply and to cough up mucus. He should be helped to change his position frequently.
- Decubitus ulcers. Incontinence and immobility, along with general body wasting (cachexia), make him an easy prey to decubitus ulcers. An indwelling catheter (to prevent soiling), changes of position, and massage help to keep the skin in good condition.
- Deformities. These often occur because of weakness and paralysis. Joints should be put through full range of motion daily. Position and body alignment require careful attention.

Headache

Headache is one of the commonest ailments of mankind. Headache is a symptom and not a disease in itself. It may be due to emotional tension, concussion, sinusitis, or brain tumor—to name only a few possible causes.

Rational therapy of headache starts with understanding and, if possible, removing the cause. Treatment may involve such measures as prescription of glasses, drainage of an infected sinus, or psychotherapy. People who have occasional headaches resulting from fatigue or emotional stress often find that rest and analgesics, such as aspirin, help to relieve the symptom.

MIGRAINE

Migraine is a particular type of headache believed to be due to initial constriction and subsequent dilation of cerebral arteries. The underlying cause of the condition is not fully understood, but it has been noted that emotional stress plays an important part in precipitating attacks. There is also a marked familial tendency toward the disease.

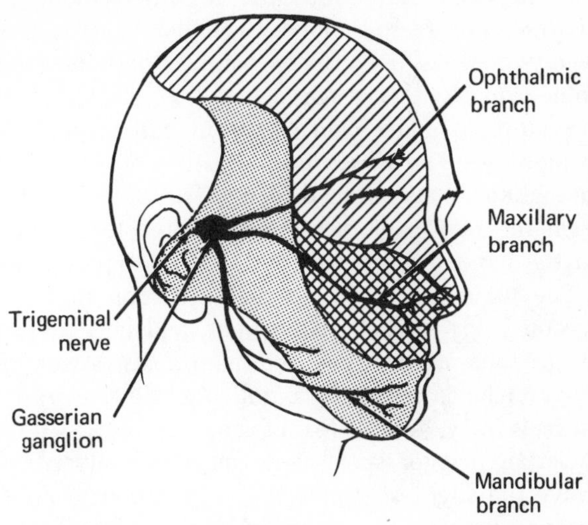

figure 15-9. Areas innervated by the three branches of the trigeminal nerve. These are the areas that become painful in tic douloureux.

The attack usually begins with feelings of malaise, irritability, and fatigue. Pallor and puffiness of the face may occur. Just before the headache begins, some patients experience visual disturbances, such as irregular patterns (scintillating scotomata) before their eyes. The headache usually starts on one side, but it may involve the entire head before the attack is over. Patients describe the pain as "throbbing" or "bursting." The headache is severe, and it often is accompanied by nausea and vomiting. The patient may be incapacitated for one day or even several days. Often light increases the anguish. Many patients must lie in bed in a darkened room until the attack subsides.

Treatment of migraine should include a thorough medical and neurological examination, as well as investigation of the patient's social and personal background. Following evaluation, the physician may prescribe drugs such as ergotamine and caffeine (Cafergot) or methysergide (Sansert). Antiemetics may be necessary if nausea and vomiting become acute during an attack. There are some patients who respond best to tranquilizers.

Trigeminal neuralgia (tic douloureux)

The fifth (trigeminal) cranial nerve has three major branches: mandibular, maxillary, and ophthalmic (Fig. 15-9). It is a major sensory and motor nerve, important to mastication, facial movement, and sensation. For reasons not fully understood, it occasionally becomes exquisitely painful, particularly in people over 50 years of age.

SYMPTOMS. The pain comes in paroxysms, each lasting about 2 to 15 seconds, and they are so painful that patients have been driven to suicide. During a spasm the face may twitch, tears come to the eyes, and the hand may rise to the face, without touching it. The patient has learned that a certain facial expression helps to shorten the bout, and he maintains the grimace as long as the pain lasts. After the paroxysm he is left with a dull afterglow, a tongue that feels furry, and the fear of the next attack.

Certain trigger spots cause an attack when they receive the slightest stimulus: the vibration of music, a passing breeze, or a change of temperature. Patients are understandably reluctant to wash that side of the face, and men remain unshaven. The forehead over the eyebrow is a common trigger spot when the ophthalmic branch of the nerve is affected. If the trigger zone is in the angle of the mouth, the patient gulps a mouthful of food, has a paroxysm, and pauses while he gathers courage for the next swallow.

Treatment

Mild analgesics rarely relieve pain. Narcotic analgesics may be necessary, although continued use can result in addiction. Phenytoin (Dilantin) and carbamazepine (Tegretol) have proved of value in some cases. For some patients surgery is the only satisfactory solution. There are three usual approaches:

- Alcohol is injected into the gasserian ganglion in the dura mater or into the branches of the nerve. This injection paralyzes the nerve, causing loss of sensation, movement and pain. The effect wears off in about 6 months, and then the nerve can be injected again, or it can be cut. With each injection the effect lasts a shorter time because of the scarring from the previous treatments.
- The dura is stripped off the ganglion. There is no loss of sensation in the face, but there may be a crawling sensation or other paresthesias.
- Partial section of the root of the ganglion is the standard operation. The effect is the same as that from the injection of alcohol into the ganglion, but it is permanent. A creeping, crawling, burning, or tingling sensation may be present, but it tends to decrease in time. When the ophthalmic branch is cut, the corneal reflex is lost. Because the patient no longer blinks normally, there is danger that he will develop a corneal ulcer.

Nursing management

PREOPERATIVE. Temperature extremes stimulate the trigger zone; therefore, food and fluids should be tepid. The patient should be given food that is easy to swallow. After he eats, he may not be able to rinse his mouth. He may be able to use an applicator, but the nurse should not attempt to give him mouth care if this will stimulate pain. The patient should talk as little as possible, since facial movement can start the pain. Ventilation of the room is important. Breezes and drafts must be avoided. A sign should be placed on the patient's bed that it is not to be jarred. His face should not be touched in any way. Hair brushing on the affected side may have to wait until after surgery. The patient may be exhausted from fighting the pain and need assistance with bathing, dressing, and other personal hygiene.

Preoperatively, the hair is shaved to a point about 4 inches above the ear. Surgery is performed under local or general anesthesia, with the patient in a sitting position.

POSTOPERATIVE. The elderly patient may have vasomotor changes from the sitting position in which the operation was performed. Vital signs are taken as ordered until they are stable. The head of the bed is elevated 12 inches or more to avoid a change from the operative position. Because the dura mater was entered, the dressing should be checked for the yellow stain of cerebrospinal fluid leakage. The patient may have a headache from the loss of cerebrospinal fluid during surgery. It is vital to look for any change in the responsiveness of the patient that may indicate hemorrhage or a clot in the brain. Often patients undergoing this surgery are elderly, and may have a preexisting cardiovascular problem.

If the ophthalmic branch was severed, the eye on the operative side will be bandaged for one or two days. When the dressing is removed, eye irrigations with sterile saline may be ordered.

Eating becomes a new problem. The patient may bite his tongue and drool without realizing it, food gets caught in his mouth, and his jaw deviates toward the operative side. Until he becomes used to the altered sensation, he may have difficulty swallowing. Since the patient may be elderly, and aspiration of fluid or food may lead to a fatal pneumonia, postoperatively he should be supervised when he first begins to swallow. He must be encouraged to take small sips, and to concentrate on what he is doing.

After he has eaten, the inside of the mouth should be checked for particles of food that may remain and set up a site of infection. The best way to teach the patient to rinse his mouth and to brush his teeth after eating is to have him do this after each meal in the hospital. He should make regular visits to his dentist, because he will not feel the warning pain of a cavity. A pocket mirror placed at the dinner table so that the patient can observe his operative side will help him to eat in a neater way, and it may make him feel less shy about eating with others.

Most patients develop a painless herpetic rash over the distribution of the nerve. Usually, it subsides in about a week. The physician may order local application of tincture of benzoin or camphorated oil.

The side effects of numbness and loss of muscle power are annoying, and they require adjustment. This can be aided by the nurse's understanding of the daily living problems posed by the symptoms.

General nutritional considerations

- Meeting the daily nutritional requirements of the patient with a long-term or disabling neurological disorder is an important aspect of nursing care.
- The patient's tray should be checked after *each* meal. If he is eating poorly the nurse should try to find out why. The problem should be reported to the physician. A consultation with the dietician may also be warranted.
- Patients unable to take sufficient food orally may require nasogastric feedings or hyperalimentation.
- The patient with trigeminal neuralgia, multiple sclerosis, or any neurological disorder which prevents proper chewing of food will usually require a soft or soft-bland diet.

General pharmacological considerations

- Patients allergic to *iodine* cannot receive radiopaque dyes containing iodine. Many of the dyes used in x-ray contrast studies contain iodine. A thorough allergy history must be taken before the patient has an x-ray contrast study using a product containing iodine.
- Patients receiving anticholinergic-like drugs in the treatment of parkinsonism may complain of a dry mouth and throat, which are expected side effects of these drugs. These drugs are contraindicated in those with glaucoma or benign prostatic hypertrophy.
- Levodopa is frequently used in the treatment of Parkinson's disease. This drug has many side effects some of which include mental changes, weakness, gastrointestinal disturbances, or dry mouth.
- Patients taking levodopa must be cautioned against the use of vitamin preparations. Only those vitamins prescribed by the physician are to be taken as the use of pyridoxine—vitamin B_6—which is found in most all vitamin preparations will reverse the effects of levodopa. This will result in a return of the symptoms of parkinsonism.
- The physician selects the anticonvulsant drug(s) that will best suit the patient. The drugs used in the treatment of epilepsy have many side effects; some, such as blood dyscrasias, are serious.
- Anticonvulsant drugs are given alone or in combination with other anticonvulsant drugs. The patient must be made aware of the many side effects of each preparation he is taking as well as what to do if side effects occur.
- Patients with epilepsy must be instructed in the importance of *continual* medication so that they do not stop taking the drug or omit a dose.
- Migraine headaches may be treated with ergotamine and caffeine (Cafergot) which is taken *as soon as* the headache starts. Methysergide (Sansert) may be used to prevent attacks of migraine. The effectiveness of both preparations varies with the individual.

Bibliography

Bates, B.: *A Guide to Physical Examination.* Philadelphia, Lippincott, 1974.

Blackwell, C. A.: PEG and angiography: A patient's sensations. Am. J. Nurs. 75:264, February, 1975.

Blount, M. and Kinney, A. B., guest eds.: Neurological and neurosurgical nursing. Nurs. Clin. North Am. 9:591, December, 1974.

Carini, E. and Owens, G.: *Neurological and Neurosurgical Nursing,* ed. 6. St. Louis, Mosby, 1974.

CONN, H. F., ed.: Current Therapy. Philadelphia, Saunders, 1975.

COOPER, C.: Anticonvulsant drugs and the epileptic's dilemma. Nurs. '76, 6:44, January, 1976.

DIPALMA, J. R.: Radiopharmaceuticals: Nuclear-age drugs for diagnosis and treatment. RN 75:59, March, 1975.

GARCIA, W. A.: When your patient suffers a seizure. RN 75:45, February, 1975.

GUTHRIE, H. A.: *Introductory Nutrition*, ed. 3. St. Louis, Mosby, 1975.

HARKNESS, L.: Bringing epilepsy out of the closet. Am. J. Nurs. 74:875, May, 1974.

HOSLINS, L. M.: Vascular and tension headaches. Am. J. Nurs. 74:846, May, 1974.

KINTZEL, K., ed.: *Advanced Concepts of Clinical Nursing*. ed. 2. Philadelphia, Lippincott, 1977.

LLINAS, R. R.: The cortex of the cerebellum. Sci. Am. 75:56, January, 1975.

MAZZOLA, R. and JACOBS, G. B.: Brain tumors: Diagnosis and treatment. RN 75:42, March, 1975.

POSNER, J. B.: Diagnosis and treatment of metastasis to the brain. Nurs. Dig. 3:58, November-December, 1975.

RODMAN, M. J. and SMITH, D. W.: *Clinical Pharmacology in Nursing*. Philadelphia, Lippincott, 1974.

SHEARER, D., COLLINS, B. and CREEL, D.: Preparing a patient for EEG. Am. J. Nurs. 75:63, January, 1975.

SCHERER, J. C.: *Introductory Clinical Pharmacology*. Philadelphia, Lippincott, 1975.

TAYLOR, R. B.: *A Primer of Clinical Symptoms*. Hagerstown, Harper and Row, 1973.

THOMAS, B. J.: Modern treatment for an old complaint—Headache. RN 38:20, October, 1975.

CHAPTER 16

The patient with cerebrovascular disease

On completion of this chapter the student will:

- Explain the pathophysiology of cerebrovascular disease.
- Contrast arteriosclerosis with atherosclerosis and identify the pathophysiology of each.
- Describe the symptoms of cerebrovascular disease and the early symptoms of a cerebrovascular accident.
- Discuss the nursing management of the patient with a ruptured cerebral aneurysm.
- Discuss nursing management during the acute phase of a cerebrovascular accident.
- Identify the various methods of rehabilitation of the patient with a cerebrovascular accident.

Cerebrovascular disease

Cerebrovascular disease, or disease of the blood vessels of the brain, is one of the major medical problems affecting adults in the United States. The frequency of cerebrovascular disease increases with age, thus as the life span increases it is expected that the incidence of cerebrovascular disease will increase.

PATHOPHYSIOLOGY. The pathophysiological basis for cerebrovascular disease involves the lessened ability of the arteries to carry blood to the brain cells. Cerebral nerve cells are extremely sensitive to a lack of oxygen; in a few minutes complete ischemia leads to destruction of cells that have been deprived of oxygen. These changes are irreversible; cerebral nerve cells that have been destroyed do not regenerate.

ATHEROSCLEROSIS AND ARTERIOSCLEROSIS. The pathological processes which impair the ability of the blood vessels to nourish the brain are primarily atherosclerosis and arteriosclerosis. In *atherosclerosis* fatty plaques (*atheromas*) are gradually deposited in the intima of the artery, causing the lumen to become narrowed and in some instances occluded. This process roughens the normally smooth lining of the artery, making it more prone to the development of clots that adhere to the atherosclerotic plaques. Such clots may form gradually and increase in size until they occlude a vessel (thrombosis), or they may travel in the bloodstream and become lodged in a narrowed portion of the blood vessel, cutting off the flow of blood (embolism) (Fig. 16-1).

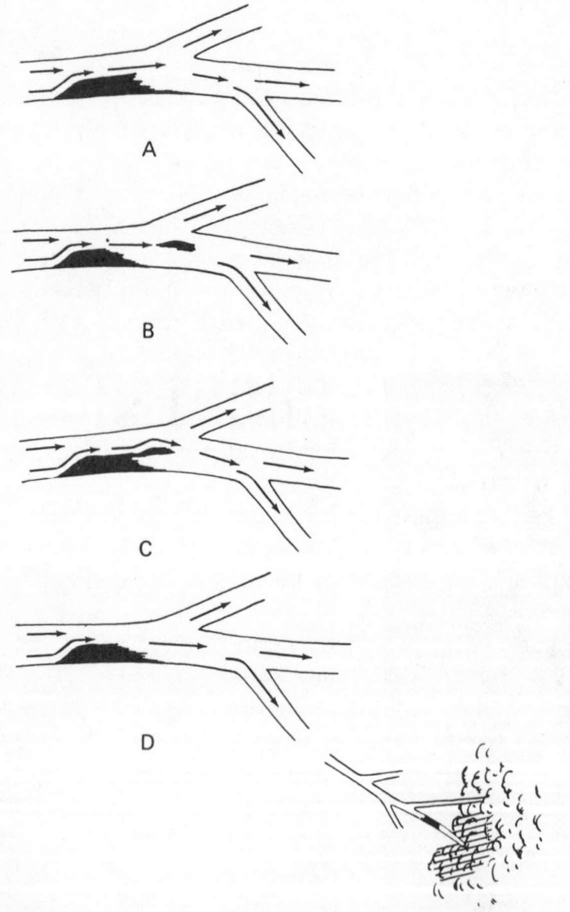

figure 16-1. (A) A thrombus forms in a vessel. (B) The force of the flowing blood over the clot helps to break off a piece from it. (C) The embolus is loose in the bloodstream and can travel to any tissue fed by connecting blood vessels. (D) The embolus is pushed into a small terminal vessel, completely occluding it and causing anoxia of the tissue served by the occluded vessel.

In *arteriosclerosis* there is loss of elasticity of the artery and thickening of the intima of the artery. The combined effects of arteriosclerosis and atherosclerosis lead to a reduction of the artery's ability to transport blood. When the blood supply is completely cut off to an area of the brain, the normal tissues are destroyed and replaced by scar tissue. This region of the brain is referred to as an *area of infarction*. The episode itself in which an area of the brain undergoes infarction is called a *cerebrovascular accident*. Such an episode usually occurs suddenly, with prompt development of symptoms of brain damage. The lay term for the condition is *stroke*.

SYMPTOMS. The severity of the patient's symptoms depends on the extent of brain damage and its location. Damage to the brain in the area concerned with vision will result in visual impairment; damage in the area involved with speech will result in speech impairment. The following symptoms are typical of organic brain disease:

- Impaired memory, especially of recent events.
- Impaired attention and concentration.
- Impaired abstract thinking.
- Circumstantiality. (For example, the patient introduces topics into his conversation that seem unrelated to the main point.)
- Lability of affect. (For example, the patient suddenly cries without apparent reason.)
- Perseveration. (For example, the patient may be asked to close his eyes. He does so. Then he is asked to raise his arms. Instead he again closes his eyes.)

SPECIAL PROBLEMS OF PATIENTS WITH CEREBROVASCULAR DISEASE

Cerebrovascular disease is typically a condition of later life; consequently, its incidence is rising sharply because of the increased number of older persons in the population. Many advances have been made in the care and treatment of these patients. The importance given to rehabilitation after a cerebrovascular accident and the possibility of surgical treatment have made it possible for some of these patients to live fuller lives now than in previous years. A tendency exists, however, to ignore the needs of patients who, because of the extent of their disease or the unavailability of effective treatment, continue to have marked impairment of physical and mental functioning.

The number of such patients is growing rapidly. Many of them are in nursing homes; many continue to live in their own homes. Whether they live alone, share a home with others, or live in homes for the aged, the problems involved in their care are difficult. An increasing share of nurses' time is spent caring for these patients. This is especially true of nurses employed in nursing homes and public health agencies. Efforts to care for these patients are often hampered because of the general apathy of many groups, both lay and professional, an apathy which may stem from feelings ot hopelessness. Nevertheless, there are ways in which nurses can help patients and their families to deal with the problem of organic brain disease.

Nurses who work successfully with these patients are able and willing to appraise the patient's condition for what it is. If it is unlikely that 98-year-old Mrs. Winters will be gainfully employed, or that she ever will be able to care for herself again, what *is* possible? Instead of a bed bath, would it be possible to lift her into the tub? A tub bath would afford her the opportunity for stimulation of circulation, which might minimize the likelihood of decubitus ulcers, as well as provide her with relaxation and a feeling of personal freshness. Instead of dozing all day in her chair and spending restless nights, could she, by having someone to talk with and an interesting view to watch, be helped to remain awake part of the day and to sleep better at night? Why not take her to the porch on pleasant days? Is there a half-forgotten skill, such as knitting, which she could use if she were provided with the materials and simple directions?

Recognition of the Complexity of Behavior. Patients who have cerebrovascular disease are usually very much aware of the changes occurring in their abilities, unless their disease has progressed to the point that awareness has been lost or blunted. For example, the patient's family may be talking and laughing together about an incident that occurred yesterday. The patient is painfully aware that he should know what the joke is about, but he doesn't. Observing that he is not laughing, his wife may say reproachfully, "Why, that happened only yesterday, Arthur. Don't you remember?" Nurses, too, can point up to the patient his lack of memory or his confusion by comments like "But it was only this morning that I asked you not to drink anything until the test was over. Now the test is ruined." Such small humiliations are commonplace in the lives of those with cerebrovascular disease. The patient's symptoms by their very nature are likely to prove to be irritating to others. The impatience shown by others can increase the patient's feeling of being unwanted and a burden.

In caring for such a patient the nurse should make every effort not to demand of him abilities that he lacks. As she works with the family, she can help them to do likewise. For example, the patient's wife may tactfully mention to her husband, as the group begins to laugh and she detects a puzzled look on his face, the event that is the cause of the laughter. Such measures help the patient to feel more at ease in his relationships with others.

It is important to remember, however, that motivation for behavior is complex, and that it grows not only from conscious thought processes but also from unconscious ones. If the patient's wife has been angry with her husband for many years, she may find ways to humiliate him, even though she is consciously aware of the kind or thoughtful thing to say in a given situation. Nurses also respond to patients in ways that are not wholly congruent with an intellectual grasp of their patients' needs. Recognition of the complexity of these factors does not lessen the need for their thoughtful consideration, but it does imply that one should not expect all problems to be solved by an intellectual approach.

Changes and Orientation. The realization of these patients that they suffer some confusion and memory loss tends to intensify their feelings of insecurity and fearfulness. Since changes in environment or being alone in the dark may accentuate their fears and increase their confusion, it is important to keep the patient's environment as unchanged as possible. For example, transfer from one room to another or contact with an entirely strange staff should be avoided when possible. Keeping a light on in the patient's room at night helps him to avoid the increased confusion that can result if he is left in a darkened room. Careful and, if necessary, repeated orientation to the location of the bathroom or his own room may help a patient who has been newly admitted to a nursing home.

Dependence and Independence. Because of their

infirmities, aged persons with cerebrovascular disease tend to be dependent, emotionally and physically, on those who care for them. This tendency must be recognized and dealt with; otherwise, it readily engenders situations in which the patient clamors for more of the nurse's attention, while she insists that he is too demanding. For example, when a patient is newly admitted to a nursing home, it is important to recognize that his efforts to gain the attention of the nurse are necessary to help him feel more secure and to assure him that those responsible for him care about him. By accepting and dealing with the patient's efforts to gain attention, the nurse can help him gradually to feel safer, then slowly help him to increase independence.

Families

The families of patients with cerebrovascular disease are particularly in need of the nurse's help. To a greater extent than many other disabilities, brain damage severely taxes interpersonal relationships. Sometimes these difficulties are avoided rather than faced. Many families fail to visit a member with cerebrovascular disease if he is in a nursing home; or if he lives at home, they find ways to exclude him from most of their activities. Too frequently, such reactions by the family are censured by physicians and nurses; instead, the family needs help in dealing with the problem.

An important point for the nurse to remember in dealing with the family is that usually they are doing the best that they can in the situation. Reproaching them not only fails to help but may result in their showing even more rejection of the sick relative. Allowing them opportunities to discuss, if they wish, some of the problems they are experiencing and showing them ways that can help to provide more satisfactory care for the patient often enable the family to be more understanding and to accept the illness better. The nurse and the physician can help the family to acquire information that is valuable in making decisions concerning long-term care. However, the making of such decisions—for example, whether to care for the patient at home or in a nursing home—should follow an appraisal by the family of their own resources and the needs of the patient.

Evaluation of Orientation. A difficult problem for families and nurses is the fluctuation in the patient's mental status. Some patients with cerebrovascular disease are well oriented at some periods and grossly confused at others. Those who care for the patient must become accustomed to evaluating the patient's state of orientation and adapting their approach accordingly. If the patient typically is well oriented in the morning, this time can be used to talk over plans with him or to provide instruction or encouragement with a hobby. In evaluating the patient's orientation, it is important to distinguish between the ability to make stereotyped responses like "Hello, how are you?" and the ability to think abstractly. Many patients with brain damage are able to continue to respond in stereotyped phrases, but have impaired ability to think through current problems. Because a patient can smile brightly and say, "Good morning," it is sometimes assumed that he is more intellectually capable than he is. In such instances nurses and family members often expect him to do things that actually are beyond his ability.

Another problem involves the patient's ability to perceive emotionally the significance of events. He may, for example, say without emotion, "My son was killed last week." Those who do not understand that he is ill may reproach him for being heartless, whereas actually the disease process has blunted his perception of the significance of events.

Cerebrovascular accidents (CVA's) or "strokes"

The most common cerebrovascular disease is a cerebrovascular accident (CVA) or "stroke." The most common causes of a cerebrovascular accident are cerebral embolus and cerebral thrombus. Atherosclerosis and arteriosclerosis may contribute to the formation of a cerebral thrombus. Cerebral hemorrhage is another cause of cerebrovascular accident (Fig. 16-2). Common causes of cerebral hemorrhage (also called intracranial hemorrhage) are rupture of cerebral aneurysms, usually in the circle of Willis; rupture of a cerebral vessel; hemorrhagic disorders such as leukemia; aplastic anemia; and tumors of the brain. The role of hypertension in cerebrovascular accidents is not entirely clear but it is thought to involve the narrowing of cerebral vessels which is frequently seen in hypertension. Narrowing of cerebral vessels reduces the amount of blood traveling through them, which may ultimately result in cerebral ischemia and infarction.

Signs and symptoms

The signs and symptoms of a cerebrovascular accident are highly variable and will depend on the area of the brain involved. In most instances, onset is sudden; the level of consciousness may range from lethargy and mental confusion to deep coma; the blood pressure may be severely elevated but in some instances symptoms of shock may be present. The patient may also experience a severe headache along with nausea and vomiting. Breathing may be difficult and there may be paralysis, speech disturbance, and memory impairment. Occasionally symptoms may be milder—headache, fatigue, weakness, numbness and tingling of an extremity, and mental confusion.

Immediately after a *severe* cerebral hemorrhage the patient is unconscious, his face often is brick red, and his breathing is stertorous and difficult. On the paralyzed side the cheek blows out with each respiration. The pulse usually is slow but full and bounding. Initially, blood pressure is likely to be elevated. The patient may proceed into deeper and deeper coma until he dies. He may remain comatose for days or even weeks, and then recover. However, the longer the coma, the poorer the prognosis. Pneumonia is the most common cause of death during prolonged coma.

When the accident is due to cerebral embolism, there are neurological symptoms, usually without loss of consciousness, although the state of consciousness may be altered.

Sometimes cerebrovascular accidents occur without warning. In other instances the patient suffers from such symptoms as dizzy spells, headache, unusual fatigue, or disturbances of speech or vision. Usually, the significance of such premonitory symptoms is recognized only retrospectively, when the physician questions the patient or his family about his health just before the CVA.

If the patient survives a major cerebrovascular accident, symptoms will depend on the extent and the severity, as well as the location, of the resulting brain damage. Some areas of the brain may have suffered from hypoxia and then recover as the supply of oxygen and other essential elements carried by the blood improves; other areas have died from anoxia. During the early stage it is not possible to tell whether the symptoms will be permanent or temporary. Improvement in neurological symptoms can occur for at least six months after the accident—a point of encouragement for the patient, and a reason for the nurse's doing everything possible to prevent deformities and to help the patient to maintain and to improve his contact with others and his orientation to his surroundings.

Hemiplegia. The most common neurological sequela is hemiplegia. A hemorrhage or clot in the right side of the brain causes the patient to have a left hemiplegia, because there is a crossover of nerves in the pyramidal tract as they lead from the brain down the spinal cord. A right-handed person is left-brain dominant, and a left-handed person may be right-brain dominant.

The speech center of a right-handed person is also located in the left side of the brain, and the speech center of a left-handed person is on the right side of the brain. It is not uncommon for the hemorrhage or clot responsible for the patient's hemiplegia to cause aphasia by cutting off the blood supply to the patient's cerebral speech center. A right-handed person developing a right hemiplegia might have aphasia, since the speech center is in the left hemisphere.

Other symptoms of a cerebrovascular accident

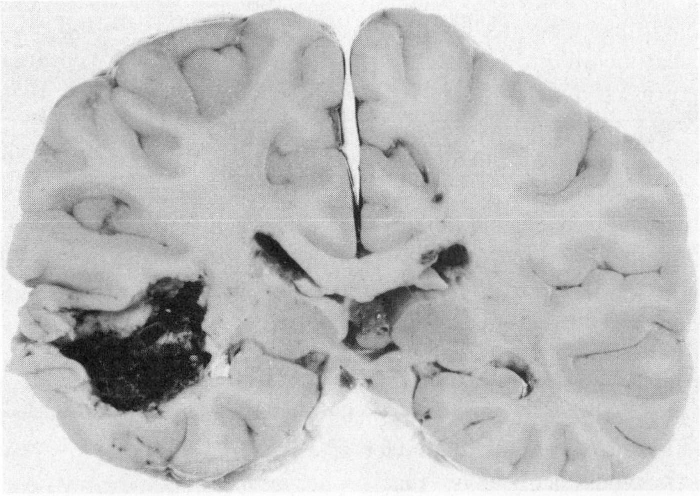

figure 16-2. Postmortem specimen of a cerebral hemorrhage of the right temporal lobe. (Courtesy P. S. Milley, M.D. Photograph—D. Atkinson)

Table 16-1.
Some types of aphasia

Receptive	
	Auditory aphasia (symptom: difficulty in understanding the spoken word)
	Alexia (symptom: difficulty in reading)
Expressive	
	Motor (symptom: difficulty in speaking)
	Agraphia (symptom: difficulty in writing)

include confusion, emotional lability, and hemianopsia, which refers to a condition in which the patient can see only half of the normal visual field. He cannot see, with either eye, what is going on to the right or to the left as he looks straight ahead. This is due to damage to the visual area of the cerebral cortex or its connections to the brain stem (optic radiations). This symptom like other symptoms resulting from cerebrovascular accident may subside completely, partially, or not at all.

APHASIA. The loss of the usual ability to use or to understand spoken and written language is called *aphasia* (Table 16-1). Although aphasia may exist without intellectual impairment, in aphasia resulting from a cerebrovascular accident there is usually evidence of some intellectual impairment in all but the mildest forms.

Until aphasia is seen, it is a very difficult syndrome to believe. In one type of aphasia a patient may know what a pencil is, if he is shown one. If it is handed to him, he will write with it; but he cannot think of the word "pencil." He says, "Rag—sweater—miniature—wife." He cannot think of the correct name. The patient may be able to conceive the symbol, but he cannot express the word "pencil." This type of aphasia is *expressive aphasia.*

Any type of vascular disorder or tumor can cause aphasia if it involves the speech center in the brain. The patient may, to his horror, find that he has lost not only his speech, but, if he also has an auditory aphasia, that the words people speak to him are as garbled as an unfamiliar foreign language. On the other hand, the patient frequently does not realize that what he is saying is not what he thinks he says. He then is mystified, and sometimes he becomes angry, at the seemingly strange behavior of others, who say, "What?" when he believes that he has asked a perfectly logical and intelligible question.

TRANSIENT ISCHEMIC ATTACKS (TIA's). Transient ischemic attacks or TIA's are brief, fleeting attacks of neurological impairment due to disease (usually atherosclerosis) of cerebral blood vessels. Impaired circulation, due to a narrowing of the blood vessels by atherosclerotic plaques, momentarily deprives part of the brain of an adequate supply of oxygen. The symptoms will vary according to the area(s) affected: numbness, tingling, weakness, speech difficulty, or blurred vision may be experienced.

Treatment varies and is directed toward the cause, if known. If atherosclerosis of the carotid artery is the cause, removal of the plaque (carotid endarterectomy) is indicated. If cerebral vessels are involved or if the patient is not a candidate for surgery, anticoagulant therapy may be instituted.

Transient ischemic attacks are indications of cerebrovascular disease and are a warning that a cerebrovascular accident could occur at any time.

DIAGNOSIS

In an attempt to identify the cause of the cerebrovascular accident and thus to select those patients whom surgery may help, a lumbar puncture may be performed. A stroke caused by hemorrhage will show blood in the cerebrospinal fluid, whereas a stroke from a thrombosis will not.

Cerebral angiography may be done. An electroencephalogram or a pneumoencephalogram may also be performed.

MEDICAL TREATMENT

Anticoagulant therapy of cerebral thrombosis and emboli may be used in selected patients in the hope that it will discourage further formation of thrombi at the place of their origin and, therefore, prevent pieces of clot from breaking off and becoming emboli. Anticoagulants are always contraindicated in hemorrhage.

In many cases, treatment is symptomatic, as once death of brain tissue has occurred, nothing can be done medically or surgically to repair the damage. What can be done involves an intensive medical program aimed primarily at rehabilitation and prevention of future cerebrovascular accidents, if possible. Some forms of intracranial hemorrhage, e.g., ruptured cerebral aneurysm, can be treated surgically.

Cerebral insufficiency due to extracranial vessel occlusion

The four major arteries supplying the brain are the two vertebral and the two internal carotid arteries. In about 30 percent of the patients with cerebral ischemia, an atheroma of one of these vessels obstructs the flow of blood to the brain. The sections of blood vessel proximal and distal to the atheroma are often relatively normal.

Sometimes atheromas occur in more than one vessel, or the vessels in the neck may be normal, and the infarction results from atherosclerosis involving only the small vessels in the brain itself.

Treatment and Nursing Management. Following diagnosis—based on the history, the neurological examination, and studies of the vessels by angiography—the surgeon removes the offending atheroma, perhaps with a patch graft of the vessel, or he may bypass the obstruction with a shunt. The patient comes to the recovery room with a dressing on his neck.

Postoperative nursing care includes observations for a change in neurological symptoms from the patient's preoperative status. Important symptoms for which to watch include headache, increased confusion, return or loss of ability to move an extremity, facial asymmetry and aphasia. These symptoms may indicate the formation of a thrombus in the surgical area. The physician must be contacted immediately if any of these symptoms occur.

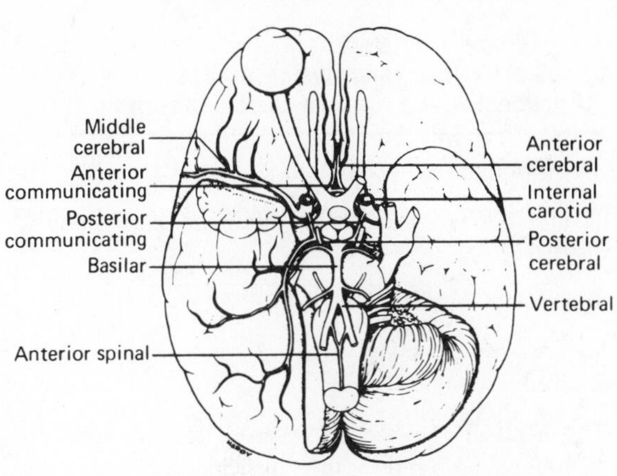

figure 16-3. The circle of Willis as seen at the base of a brain which has been removed from the skull.

Aneurysms of the blood vessels of the brain

Aneurysms are formed by the outpouching of blood vessel walls, which may occur in cranial vessels. Most cerebral aneurysms occur in the circle of Willis (Fig. 16-3) and are called berry aneurysms. These are thought to be congenital and may rupture at any time, often without warning. The symptoms of a ruptured aneurysm include severe headache, dizziness, nausea, and vomiting. These symptoms may be followed by a loss of consciousness. Bleeding from a berry aneurysm will result in blood in the subarachnoid space with grossly bloody spinal fluid.

Treatment. The presence and location of an aneurysm are identified by cerebral angiography. As the danger of further hemorrhage from the weakened aneurysmal sac is great, particularly in the first weeks after the initial hemorrhage, surgical repair may be attempted. The operation is not without hazard, because manipulation of the small cerebral vessels may result in increased vasospasm or thrombosis and cerebral infarction. Usually, the risks of surgery are less than the dangers of recurrent hemorrhage.

Surgery involves a wrapping or clipping of the aneurysm in an attempt to control further episodes of bleeding. Some aneurysms are inoperable because of their anatomical location and must therefore be treated medically. Medical treatment is usually employed until the bleeding has stopped. Medical treatment and nursing management are given in Table 16-2, p. 202.

Postoperative Nursing Care. The patient is observed for increased intracranial pressure, which may mean intracerebral hemorrhage, and for neurological symptoms on the side of his body opposite the site of the surgery. The nurse talks to the patient, observing for language difficulties that may indicate the beginning of aphasia, and frequently tests the movement and the strength of the muscles on the opposite side of the body. Facial and pupillary symmetry is also noted. *Any change* in the patient, no matter how slight, must be reported to the physician as soon as possible.

Arterial Clamp. As an alternative to direct repair of the aneurysmal sac when collateral circulation is believed to be adequate, a Crutchfield or a Selverstone clamp may be applied to a carotid artery. The purpose is to obstruct the blood flow to the vessel on which there is an aneurysm, thus reduce the pressure in the sac and so prevent rupture. Sometimes the clamp is tightened all at once, or the doctor may prefer to gradually tighten the clamp over a period of several days in the hope that collateral circulation will have a chance to develop. In either case, when the clamp finally occludes the artery, the patient should be observed frequently, perhaps as often as every 15

Table 16-2.
Medical treatment and nursing management of the patient with a ruptured cerebral aneurysm

Absolute bed rest is maintained.

The room is kept dim, with a minimum of noise and disturbance.

Visitors are limited.

Vital signs are taken every 2 to 4 hours or as ordered.

The head of the bed is elevated; the amount of elevation is ordered by the physician.

The patient is observed for signs of increased intracranial pressure: rise in blood pressure, slowing of pulse, full and bounding pulse, change in the level of consciousness, headache, vomiting with or without nausea, change in the pupil size and reaction to light, decrease in the respiratory rate.

Coughing, straining at stool are to be avoided.

Intake and output records are kept. Urinary incontinence or retention may require an indwelling catheter.

Drug therapy: analgesics for headache, stool softeners, antihypertensive drugs if blood pressure is elevated.

Elastic stockings may be used to prevent thrombophlebitis, a complication of prolonged bed rest.

Passive exercises and back rubs are *not given* unless specifically ordered by the physician.

minutes, for aphasia or hemiparesis, which may result if the circulation to the brain is inadequate. If this occurs, the clamp must be opened promptly to prevent permanent brain damage. The doctor may instruct the nurse in this procedure, as she is usually the first to discover signs of ischemia, and speed is important. If some time has passed before signs of cerebral ischemia are discovered, removal of the clamp may be done more safely on the exposed vessel in the operating room, because a clot may have formed proximal to the clamp and be embolized to the brain when the clamp is unscrewed. The patient is not really out of danger until after the clamp has been tightened for 48 or more hours.

General points in the nursing management of patients with cerebrovascular accidents

Objectives in the treatment and nursing care of the patient with a cerebrovascular accident include maintenance of body functions and prevention of complications, such as pneumonia, decubitus ulcers, and contractures. These considerations are applicable to any unconscious patient.

Management of the patient with a cerebrovascular accident begins with the formulation of short- and long-term goals. The immediate goals of nursing management (Table 16-3) are aimed at meeting the pa-

Table 16-3.
Nursing management of the patient with a cerebrovascular accident: acute phase

The patient's position is changed every 2 hours.

If unconscious, the patient is turned from side to side and kept off his back.

The head of the bed is slightly elevated.

The patient's mouth is suctioned as necessary to clear secretions.

An oropharyngeal airway is used if the patient is unconscious, if his breathing is difficult, or if the tongue is obstructing the back of the throat.

Vital signs: temperature every 1 to 4 hours; blood pressure, pulse, respirations every 1 to 2 hours.

Hypothermia measures are initiated if the patient's temperature is elevated: hypothermia blanket, tepid sponges, aspirin (suppository) may be used.

Oxygen is administered if the patient is cyanotic.

Measures are taken to prevent contractures and deformities: use of footboard, hand rolls, trochanter rolls, pillow between the knees, alternating pressure mattress, flotation pad, lamb's wool padding.

Intake and output measurements are kept.

Indwelling urethral catheter is used if the patient is incontinent.

Intravenous fluids and/or tube feedings are used until fluid and food can be taken orally.

tient's basic needs and preventing complications. Long-term goals focus on the return of the individual to society with maximum functional ability. Realistically, the latter goal is not always possible, especially in those who have had extensive cerebral damage.

Family visits

The family make the decision on how long to stay with the patient in light of his condition and their own reactions to the experience. Some family members wish to be present as much as possible. One consideration is that, if the condition of the patient changes markedly, or if he dies, they will be with him at the critical time. Family members should be helped to be as comfortable as possible. Comfortable chairs should be provided, and the locations of the coffee shop, the telephone, and the visitors' bathroom pointed out. Above all, convey to them that they should not hesitate to call the nurse whenever they believe her presence is needed. Some family members do not undertake a prolonged vigil at the bedside, perhaps because of responsibilities for children or their need to get away from the stressful environment to regain their composure. If they decide not to stay, assure them that you will call if there is a significant change in the patient's condition. In either case try to be perceptive of the family's reaction to the experience, and avoid implying that there is one correct way for them to behave in relation to length and frequency of visits.

The return of consciousness

As the patient recovers from coma, the head of the bed may be elevated further. If the hand was affected, a roll of gauze or a rubber ball placed in the hand may help to prevent the clawlike contracture deformity that so frequently follows a cerebrovascular accident (Fig. 16-4). If the patient has any movement at all, encourage him to squeeze the ball periodically for exercise. As the patient sits up more, special attention is paid to the skin of the buttocks, in an attempt to prevent skin breakdown. Change of position and frequent massage continue to be necessary. The patient's feet should press against a footboard. Beware of footdrop and outward rotation. The physician may ask that a light splint be used on an extremity, if contractures seem to be forming.

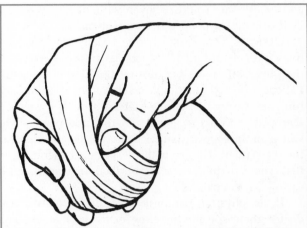

figure 16-4. A ball placed in the spastic hand may help prevent contractures and keep the hand more in a position of function. It may be necessary to bandage the ball lightly in place. If this is done, inspect the hand frequently to make sure that the fingers have not curled up between the gauze and the ball, causing the gauze to cut into the skin or to impede the circulation.

With continued improvement

As the patient who has had a cerebrovascular accident improves, he may be able to eat and drink, although some of what he takes will run out of the paralyzed side of his mouth. He may not be able to swallow well. Embarrassment, when he feels that he is drooling like a baby, can be minimized by turning him on his unaffected side during meals and putting only small amounts of food in the side of his mouth that has the best control. This method of feeding will also help to minimize the possibility of aspirating the food.

As the patient recovers, he should be taught not to strain while moving his bowels. Straining may result in a repeat hemorrhage. The physician should be told of the difficulty; a laxative or an enema may be ordered.

Anticipation of Needs. As the patient recovers, he becomes aware of new limitations, and the discovery is frightening. Perhaps one reason that most people fear paralysis is that they have no assurance their needs will be met. A patient's throat is parched, and he cannot ask for a drink. He lies on his arm until it is painfully cramped, and is powerless to move or to complain. A patient wishes to tell his wife not to cry, but cannot speak.

Do the little extra things that will make your patient more comfortable. Put a piece of ice in his drink, adjust the pillows, elevate or lower the bed to his exact satisfaction, and rub an aching shoulder as you change his position. If his mouth is dry, and he is allowed extra fluids, bring him a glass of water or juice. Anticipate what is needed before the patient has to try to ask you. If he vomits, his mouth will have a sour taste, and mouth care sould be given without his asking for it. If appetite is poor, give frequent snacks.

EXERCISE AND AMBULATION. Many doctors have their patients ambulate as soon as possible. Whether the physician orders bed rest or ambulation, keep the patient in enough motion to maintain muscle tone and function, but not so active that he tires. If a physical therapist is available, he is the resource person who will plan, in cooperation with the physician, exercises for the patient. Confer with the physical therapist, so that you can follow the prescribed treatment while caring for the patient.

If no physical therapist is available, consult the doctor about specific exercises for the patient. Perhaps he will be permitted to go through range-of-motion exercises several times a day—actively on the unaffected side and passively on the affected side (Fig. 16-5). Teach the patient to massage and to stretch the fingers of the affected hand with his unaffected hand several times daily. Work toward having the patient passively exercise his affected arm with his good arm; thus both arms are exercised at once. Early use of exercise not only serves to prevent contractures and wasting of unused muscles but also implies to the patient that he is not going to be a hopeless cripple.

If you are the one who is responsible for the early ambulation of the patient, have someone else—preferably a strong person—assist you the first time that you help the patient out of bed. This arrangement will make both you and the patient feel more secure. Remember that the patient who has lived for a while with his hemiplegia has found ways of moving that are effective for him, but the newly paralyzed patient does not know what he can and cannot do.

Let the patient sit at the edge of his bed for a minute, to become accustomed to the upright position. If dizziness is prolonged, help him to lie down again, and consult the doctor. Tell the patient just what the

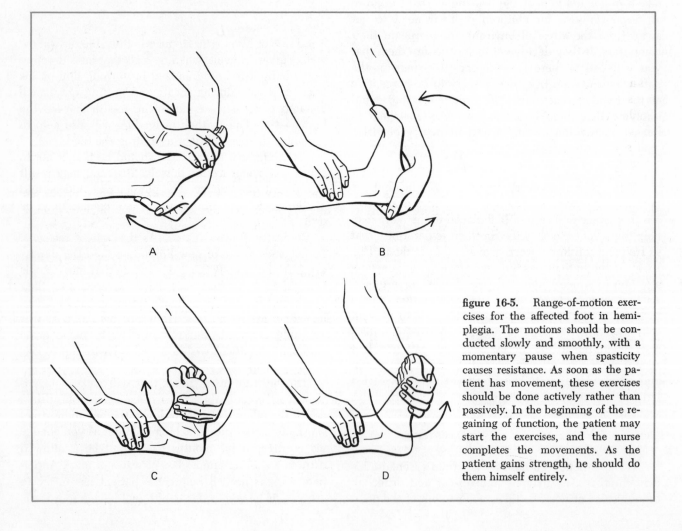

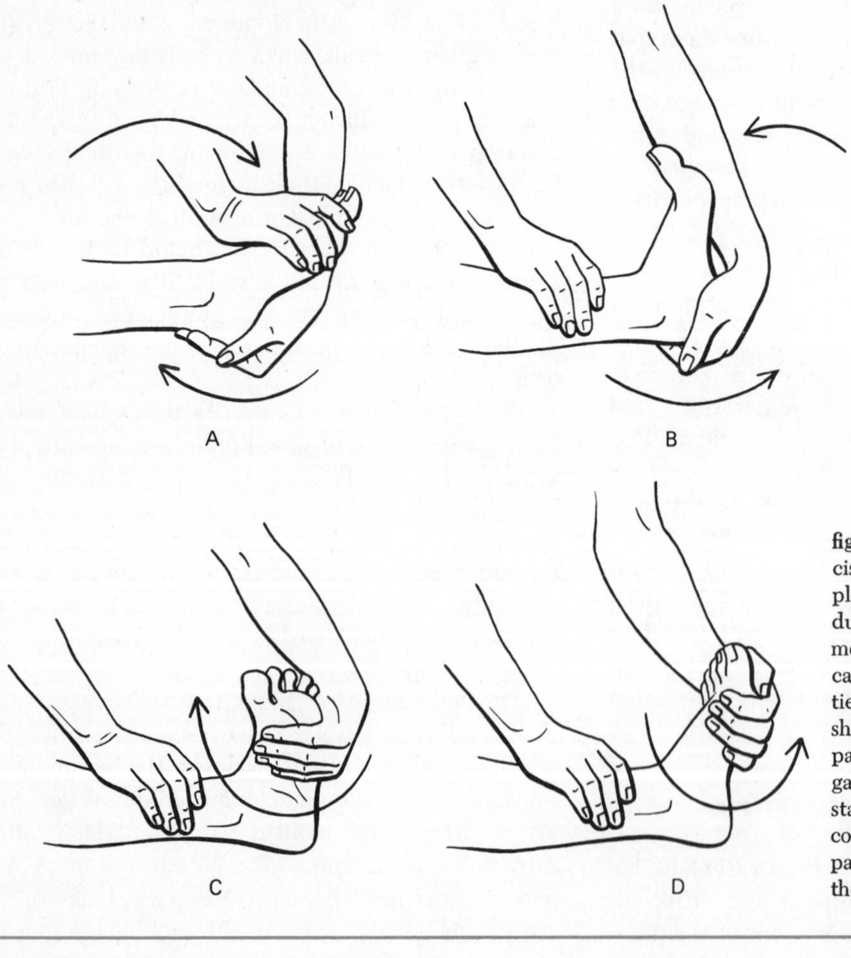

figure 16-5. Range-of-motion exercises for the affected foot in hemiplegia. The motions should be conducted slowly and smoothly, with a momentary pause when spasticity causes resistance. As soon as the patient has movement, these exercises should be done actively rather than passively. In the beginning of the regaining of function, the patient may start the exercises, and the nurse completes the movements. As the patient gains strength, he should do them himself entirely.

sequence of movement will be, so that you will both be moving in the same direction. If the patient is not faint or dizzy, put his robe on while he is sitting up. Put the sleeve on his affected arm first (it would be much more difficult for him to maneuver his affected arm into the second sleeve). Later, in the same manner, the patient learns to get dressed. Stand at the patient's unaffected side and support him from that side. Support the side that helps the patient to steady himself. While you hold him firmly, let the patient step onto the footstool and then to the floor with his unaffected foot. The one or two steps to a chair are probably enough for the first day. When helping the patient return to bed, tell him to step up on the footstool with his unaffected foot. The other is still too weak to lift his entire body. Many hospitals have beds that are adjustable in height. If this type of bed is being used, place the bed in the lowest position and help the patient to place both feet on the floor. This type of bed makes the use of a footstool unnecessary; the procedure is easier for the patient and the nurse, and it is safer.

Slowly, the patient may graduate under the guidance of the physical therapist to parallel bars, a walker (Fig. 16-6), a crutch, and a cane. Make the goal of each day's activity one that is attainable, even if it is only one more step. Walking is a primitive activity, something that the patient doubtless has taken for granted for years. To lose it is disheartening. To the patient every small success in regaining mobility is a point of great encouragement for the future; every failure may be a sign that the future is hopeless.

Care of an Affected Arm. If the patient's arm on the affected side is completely paralyzed, consult the physical therapist concerning positioning of the arm when the patient is up. Usually, a sling is recommended to keep a completely paralyzed arm from dangling while the patient is out of bed. If a sling is used, teach the patient to remove his arm from it at intervals and to provide passive range-of-motion exercises for the paralyzed arm with his unaffected arm (Fig. 16-7, p. 206). It is usually recommended that the arm be left out of the sling if there is any function in the arm, no matter how feeble. Any hint of movement should be persistently nurtured.

Rehabilitation

An early start at rehabilitation is one of the best ways to prevent depression. The patient should never be given the impression that there is no use in training muscles up to their full capacity. It is also important

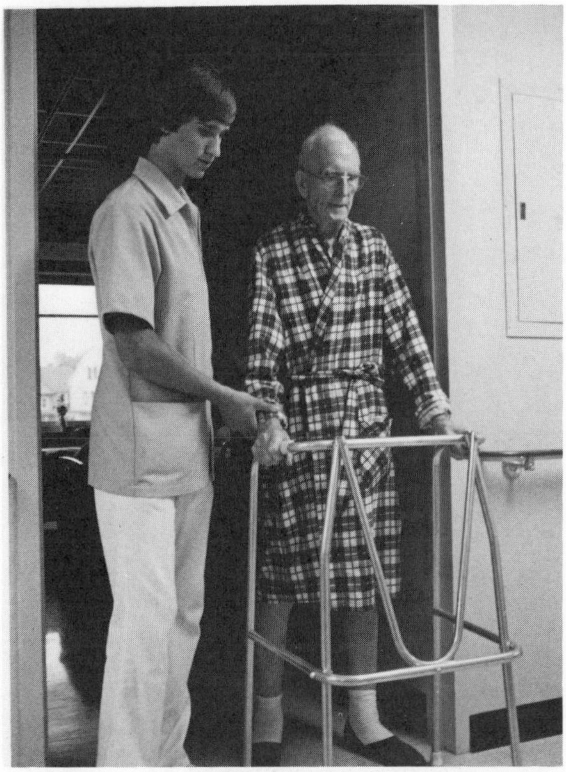

figure 16-6. The patient with a cerebrovascular accident may need to ambulate with the use of a walker. When the patient first uses the walker a member of the nursing team should stay with him. (Photograph—D. Atkinson)

for the patient to take a realistic account of what he can do, and what he cannot, so that he can plan his life; however, no one knows at the beginning how much function can be recaptured. Some patients recover completely. Every step forward is nurtured, encouraged, and enlarged (Fig. 16-8, p. 206). After about six to eight months the patient's limitations, if any, will be more clear.

Family attitudes are of the utmost importance. If family members become upset in his presence, his newly labile emotions (based on the recent brain damage) will make him easily subject to depression. Then it will be more difficult to help him to recover from his depression and to work toward further function. A stable emotional environment is essential for the patient who is recovering from a cerebrovascular accident. Bouts of sudden, uncontrolled weeping should not be infectious to those around him.

The family can help the patient with a retraining program if they are instructed in the necessary steps

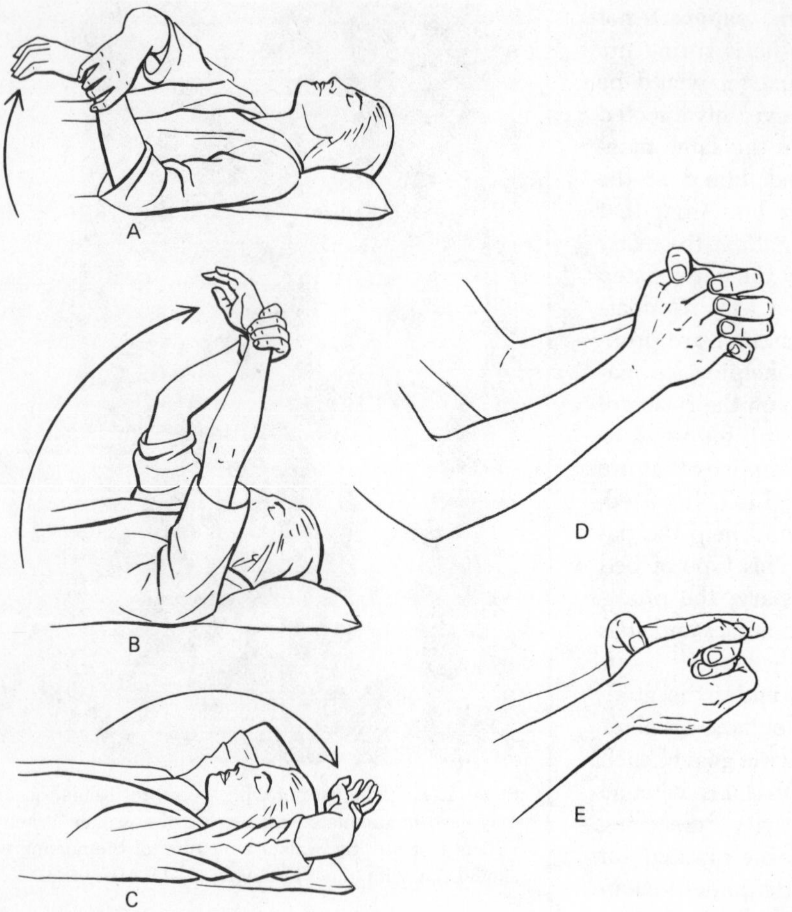

figure 16-7. Exercises of the affected hand and the affected arm that the hemiplegic patient should learn to do himself. (A), (B) and (C) The affected arm is grasped at the wrist by the unaffected hand and is raised over the head. (D) and (E) The unaffected hand is slipped into the spastic hand, and slowly in turn each finger is extended.

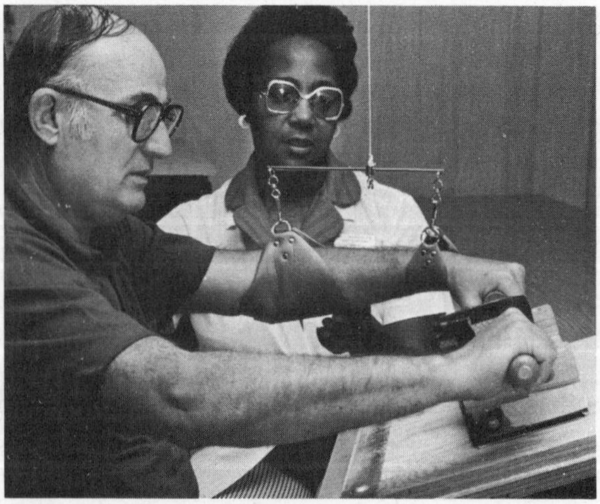

figure 16-8. Physical therapy and occupational therapy are used in the rehabilitation of the patient with a cerebrovascular accident. (Photograph—D. Atkinson)

by the physician and the nurse, and if *their* emotional needs for support and help are recognized and dealt with by the professional staff, relatives, friends, and clergy. Family members may understand what will catch the patient's attention. One patient may like stamp collecting; another, gathering recipes.

If the family is large and live near each other, and if they typically come to one another's aid in crises, the care of the patient can be shared in terms of both its emotional impact and its daily time-consuming activities, such as helping the aphasic patient read aloud. But in many instances such family assistance is not available, especially when the patients are elderly. When the patient does not have family members available and willing to help him, supplementary arrangements, such as the services of a visiting homemaker or a church worker, must be sought.

Long-Term Treatment. If the patient is overweight, he is advised to reduce. If he smokes, he is advised to stop, or if this is impossible, to decrease his smoking. Moderate exercise that does not lead to fatigue is recommended and excessive use of alcohol discouraged.

For some patients only a part-time job is advisable, due either to problems of general fatigue or to residual disability. Other patients continue to work full-time, but curtail social and family activities to gain necessary additional rest.

Some patients find it impossible to accept the physician's recommendations. Older persons with cerebrovascular disease frequently have lost some of the adaptability that would make it possible to follow suggestions for changes in their way of living. Sometimes they reject a treatment regimen simply because it is not acceptable, although they recognize it may be ideal for most patients. Unfortunately, sometimes the patient's inability to follow a regimen suggested by his physician is viewed as sheer stubbornness rather than as the result of years of gradually developing a way of life that the patient cannot suddenly relinquish —possibly, too, because of problems in adaptability due to brain damage. Most patients manage best when they have opportunity to consider the suggestions made to them without feeling undue pressure from others to change themselves or their way of living (Fig. 16-9). Patients who have habitually overeaten, for example, ordinarily do not suddenly eat sparingly. The patient who has made work the center of his existence and the means of helping to fill needs not met in other areas of his life will not be likely to agree to give up work until conditions force him to do so. Although nurses and physicians of necessity place health needs first in advising patients, the patient himself may decide that he would rather live in his accustomed way, however unwise it may seem in relation to his health, in order to fulfill other needs which for him may take precedence—such as the need to be self-supporting. In such instances the physician and the nurse help the patient to carry out those aspects of treatment which he can accept.

Speech Rehabilitation. Like retraining for arm movement and walking, speech rehabilitation is most effective when it is begun early. Ideally, the patient's speech problem is evaluated carefully and promptly by a speech therapist, and a program developed in which the nurse can collaborate with the speech therapist. Although the nurse is not in a position to carry out the detailed evaluation of the type of aphasia from which the patient suffers or to set up a program of therapy, there are ways that she can help the patient in the interim before speech therapy is started or in the absence of a speech therapist. In either instance the nurse should consult with the physician. For instance, the physician who has assessed the patient's neurological status can help the nurse to understand the type of aphasia from which the patient suffers, whether the patient's intellectual functioning has been affected, and to what extent.

Ways in which the nurse can help the patient with aphasia are as follows:

- Because the patient has problems of association (between word and subject, between word and concept), talk to him and expect response from him. Do not tire him; on the other hand, do not work in silence, guessing

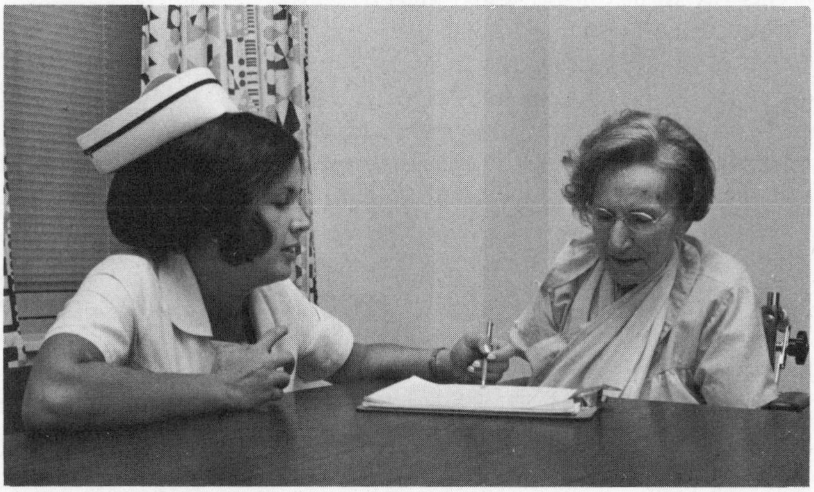

figure 16-9. The nurse can teach the older patient who has had a cerebrovascular accident without placing undue pressure on the patient, giving her time to consider suggestions regarding necessary changes in her way of living. (Photograph—D. Atkinson)

at what he wants and accepting only nonverbal communications, such as hand signals. "Do you want a blanket, Mr. Jones? Here is a blanket. *You* say: 'Blanket.'" Continuously, strengthen associations.

- Even if hurried, the nurse must seem calm and unhurried. The patient is frightened by his loss of speech, and feels inadequate in not being able to talk. Any impatience or haste on your part will inhibit him even further. Wait quietly and pleasantly while he struggles with a word. Praise him, if it comes out, but do not show impatience if he is unsuccesssful.
- Never be tempted to treat him like a child, even though the tasks he must relearn are those that children learn. He is not a child, and he does not think like one.
- Capitalize on what speech he has. If he can say his dog's name, but not his own, build sentences that he can copy, using the dog's name and ask him questions that he can answer with the dog's name. Be sure to point out his successes to him.
- Do not shout. He's not deaf.
- Set attainable goals. One sound may be worked on for weeks before it is mastered.
- Involve the family as much as possible in the early stages of rehabilitation. They may catch an attitude of hope from you, and you can show them how to help with retraining.
- Minimize distraction while you are helping the patient with his speech. Since he has difficulty concentrating due to his illness, working with him in an area where others are talking loudly or where a radio is playing adds unnecessarily to his difficulty and quickly leads to fatigue and frustration.
- Be aware of your own reactions to the speech difficulty. Work with these patients can be taxing and frustrating for the nurse. If you work with the patient to a degree that exceeds your ability to tolerate the effort and stress, you will show impatience and frustration, which in turn can lead the patient to become discouraged or resentful. In general, both patient and nurse function best when speech practice periods are brief and interspersed with other activities.
- Because social isolation is such a common response to this disability, help both the patient and his family to feel that, his physical condition permitting, there is no reason for him to live without friends, parties, and outings. Group speech therapy often is the first contact that a patient has with others, but it should not be the only contact.

Care of the patient with a stroke is a tremendous nursing challenge. The nurse's knowledge, dedication, and willingness to persevere can be crucial in determining whether the patient can resume his accustomed responsibilities.

General nutritional considerations

- When able to take oral food and fluids, the patient with a cerebrovascular accident should be given a soft diet.
- Adequate time should be allowed for the patient to be fed or to feed himself. If self-feeding is difficult, but a part of rehabilitation, small portions of food and between-meal feedings may be more conducive to eating.
- If the patient is unable to feed himself, he must be offered fluids between as well as with meals. If dietary intake is poor, nutritious fluids as well as water should be provided.

General pharmacological considerations

- Anticoagulant therapy with heparin, which is given parenterally, or with an oral anticoagulant may be indicated for some patients with a cerebrovascular accident.
- If the patient is receiving heparin:
  Early in therapy the dose is ordered according to the patient's response;
  Clotting time determinations (Lee-White, partial thromboplastin time, or PTT) measure the patient's response to therapy;
  If the drug is administered by the subcutaneous route the site of injection *should not be massaged before or after* the drug is given;
  The most notable side effect of heparin is hemorrhage;
  Protamine sulfate should be readily available in case it becomes necessary to reduce the effects of heparin.

- If the patient is receiving oral anticoagulants:
  - The dose is adjusted according to the patient's response;
  - The patient's response is determined by prothrombin levels; for example, the prothrombin time determination;
  - Optimum therapeutic results are obtained when prothrombin levels are 1½ to 3 times the normal control value;
  - Bleeding can occur at any time, even when the prothrombin level appears to be within safe limits. The patient is observed for evidence of bleeding: easy bruising, nosebleeds, excessive bleeding from small cuts, blood in the urine or stool, etc.;
  - The antidote for oral anticoagulants is vitamin K, which should be readily available in parenteral form.
- Stool softeners, such as Surfak and Colace, may be ordered to prevent constipation and straining. Straining increases intracranial pressure which must be avoided in some neurological disorders.
- The senile or brain-damaged patient may be difficult to manage; he may be noisy, confused, or uncooperative, and tranquilizers or sedatives may be ordered. If at all possible, one should try to determine the reason for the patient's confusion before resorting to these drugs.

Bibliography

American Heart Association: In a nutshell—a guide for stroke rehabilitation in the community hospital. EM 597.

Carbary, L. J.: Aiding the patient with aphasia. Nurs. Care 9:22, January, 1976.

Dayhoff, N.: Soft or hard devices to position heads? Am. J. Nurs. 75:1142, July, 1975.

Drury, J. H.: Handbook of range of motion exercises. Nurs. '72, 2:19, April, 1972.

Fowler, R. S. and Fordyce, W.: Adapting care for the brain-damaged patient. Am. J. Nurs. 72:1832, October, 1972.

Gilmore, S. E.: Your aphasic patient . . . communicating. J. Prac. Nurs. 25:18, October, 1975.

Grey, H. A.: The aphasic patient—How you can help him. RN 70:46, July, 1970.

Jacobansky, A. M.: Stroke. Am. J. Nurs. 72:1260, July, 1972.

Maddox, M.: Subarachnoid hemorrhage. Am. J. Nurs. 74:2199, December, 1974.

McNeil, F.: Stroke! Nursing insights from a stroke-nurse victim. RN 38:75, September, 1975.

Oradei, D. M. and Waite, N. S.: Group psychotherapy with stroke patients during the immediate recovery phase. Nurs. Dig. 75:26, May–June, 1975.

Pfaudler, M.: After stroke: Motor rehabilitation for hemiplegic patients. Am. J. Nurs. 73:1892, November, 1973.

Ransohoff, J.: Treatment of supratentorial aneurysms. Current Concepts of Cardiovascular Disease, Vol. VIII, No. 5, September–October, 1973.

Skelly, M.: Aphasic patients talk back. Am. J. Nurs. 75:1140, June, 1975.

Stevens, C. B.: *Special Needs of Long-Term Patients.* Philadelphia, Lippincott, 1974.

Stoicheff, M. L.: Communicating with the aphasic patient. Nurs. Dig. 75:18, March–April, 1975.

CHAPTER—17

The patient with spinal cord impairment

On completion of this chapter the student will:

- Name the various types of lesions and injuries to the spinal column.
- Identify the causes of cord and spinal nerve root compression.
- Describe the care of a patient with a laminectomy.
- Describe the care of a paraplegic patient and a quadraplegic patient.
- Prepare a nursing care plan for a paraplegic patient and a quadraplegic patient including the long-range aspects of nursing management and rehabilitation.
- Discuss the problems encountered by the paraplegic patient and the quadraplegic patient.

Areas of function of the spinal cord

The two main functions of the spinal cord are (1) to provide centers for reflex action and (2) to provide a pathway for impulses to and from the brain. The *sensory fibers* enter the *posterior* portion of the cord; the nerve fibers that transmit *motor*

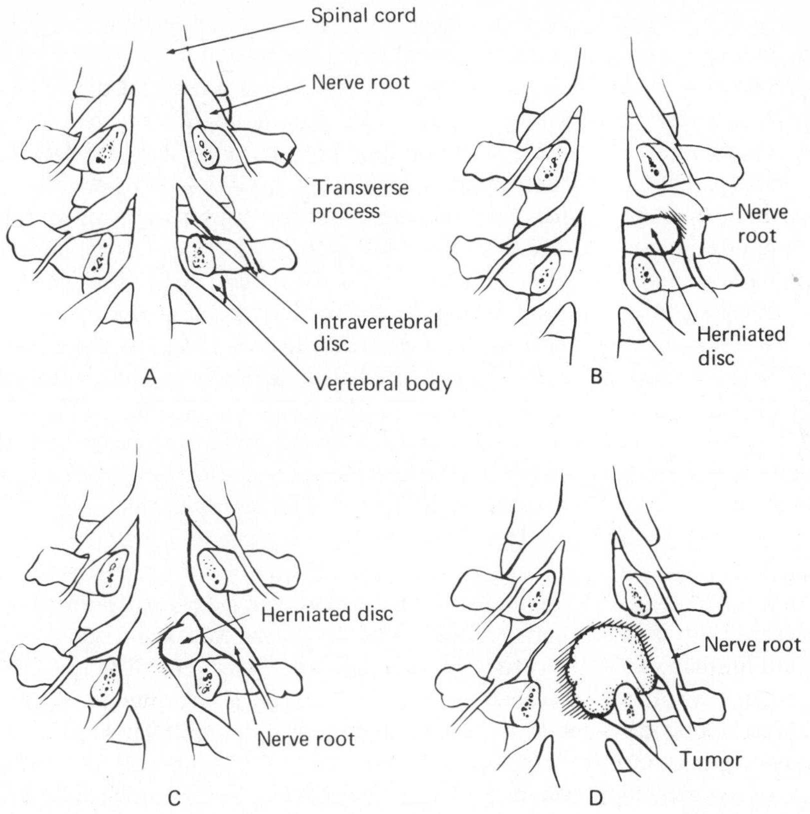

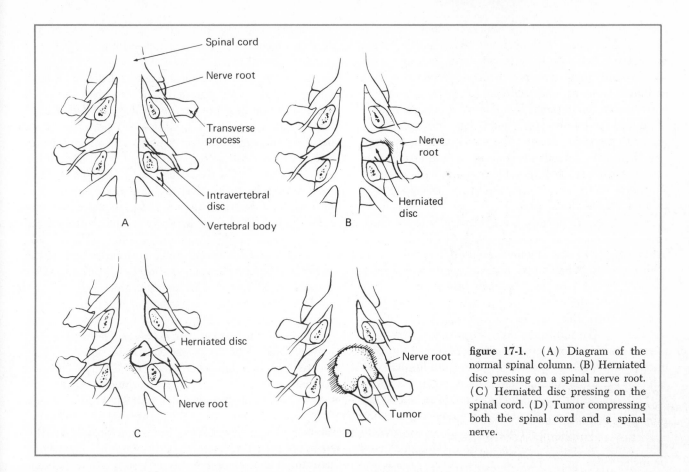

figure 17-1. (A) Diagram of the normal spinal column. (B) Herniated disc pressing on a spinal nerve root. (C) Herniated disc pressing on the spinal cord. (D) Tumor compressing both the spinal cord and a spinal nerve.

impulses run outward to the peripheral nerves from the *anterior* portion of the cord.

A lesion on the posterior horn cells of the cord can result in hypoesthesia (diminished sensation) and anesthesia (no sensation). A lesion on the anterior horn cells can result in muscle weakness, paralysis, and spasticity. Disturbance of motor and/or sensory function occurs below the level of the injury (i.e., its location in the spinal column).

Hence, the degree of injury and it location determine the extent of the disability. If the injury is high in the cervical region, respiratory failure and death follow paralysis of the diaphragm. Midcervical injuries result in breathing only by diaphragmatic movement, since the muscles of the upper thorax are paralyzed. Thoracic vertebrae are seldom injured, because they are protected by the rib cage. The 5th and 6th cervical vertebrae and the 1st and 5th lumbar vertebrae are especially vulnerable to injury; therefore, injury to the cord at these levels is frequent.

The severity of the injury to the cord also determines how much function will be lost. When the cord is completely severed, function is lost permanently below the level of the injury. If the damage to the cord is partial, some function may be maintained or at times regained.

Causes of cord and spinal nerve root compression

Lesions of the spinal cord are of two basic types: (1) those involving the spinal cord or *intramedullary* lesions and (2) those of tissues that surround the spinal cord or *extramedullary* lesions. Whatever the lesion, it is the pressure on the cord that causes the symptoms (Fig. 17-1). Symptoms may begin on one side and become bilateral as the disease progresses.

The pressure may be caused by:

TRAUMA. Violence to the back may fracture and/or collapse one or more vertebrae. A bone fragment pressing into the cord can interfere with the transmission of nerve impulses. Even if there is no fracture, momentary compression of the cord can lead to edema, which will further compress the cord. In this instance, symptoms may disappear gradually as edema subsides. Trauma may lead to bleeding within the cord; because the blood has no place in which to drain, its mass forms a hematoma that occupies space and squeezes the nerve roots. An injury to the cord, such as a gunshot wound, may sever nerve fibers. When this kind of injury happens, and the complete severance of the cord results, the patient is completely and permanently paralyzed and loses sensation below the site of the injury to the cord. Because the tracts of the nerves are cut, there is no effective regeneration, and attempts to suture the pieces together have not been successful. Vertebral fracture may be caused by osteoporosis or tuberculosis of the spine.

HERNIATED INTERVERTEBRAL DISC. Discs of cartilage act as cushions between the bones of the spine. Their spongy center (nucleus pulposus) is encased in a fibrous coat. When stress, age, or disease weakens an area in the coat or in a ligament attachment to the vertebra, and the nucleus pulposus becomes thickened and hardened, the disc herniates, causing pressure on the nerves. The most common site of the protrusion is one of the three lower lumbar discs. Because the cord ends at the level of the first or the second lumbar vertebra (L 1, 2), herniated lumbar discs compress spinal nerve roots rather than the cord itself. Pain along the distribution of the sciatic nerve is a common symptom. Anything (straining, coughing, lifting a heavy object) that causes increased pressure within the spinal cord intensifies the pain. Pain is more severe when the nerves are stretched, such as when the patient, while lying flat on his back, tries to lift his leg up without bending his knee. Also, there may be weakness and changes in sensation. The symptoms tend to be recurrent rather than steady, at least in the beginning of the disease.

TUMORS. Tumors of the spinal cord and surrounding areas may be primary, that is, originating in this area, or metastatic, that is, spreading from another site. Signs and symptoms depend on the level involved—cervical, thoracic, or sacral. Symptoms may include weakness, paralysis, numbness, or tingling, all of which appear below the level of the tumor.

CERVICAL SPONDYLOSIS. In this disease the hypertrophic osteoarthritic ridging of cervical vertebrae can cause cord compression.

Treatment and nursing care

CONSERVATIVE THERAPY

BED REST. The patient with a herniated intervertebral disc is often treated first with conservative measures. For several weeks he may be placed on bed rest with a firm mattress and bed board. The patient may also be placed in traction and may be allowed out of traction several times a day.

A patient with rupture of a cervical disc may have a sandbag at either side of his head to help keep his head in the midline position. Pain is relieved by drugs, the application of heat, traction, and bed rest. Since part of the pain is due to muscle spasm, muscle relaxant drugs may be prescribed. Heat applied to the affected area may also be a comfort to the patient, but care should be taken that the skin does not become burned, since there may be numbness and other sensory changes in that area. Early in the course of the illness, the physical therapist may come to the bedside to save the patient the strain of getting on and off the stretcher. Heat, massage, and stretching exercises under water may be included in his program.

TRACTION by Buck's extension or pelvic traction for a lumbar herniated disc, and a cervical halter or tongs implanted into the skull for a cervical herniated disc, may be used to decrease muscle spasm, which may be severe. Traction also increases the distance between adjacent vertebrae. It may be continuous or intermittent, with 5 to 30 pounds of weight. The traction keeps the patient in bed in good alignment, and some patients find that it relieves their pain. Sometimes this treatment is so effective that the patient is symptom-free for a period of months or years. Some patients return to the hospital for several weeks in traction once or twice a year, when symptoms recur.

The patient's situation suggests his nursing needs: for example, in Buck's extension, special attention to the skin of his legs; relief of pain and boredom; range-of-motion exercises in unaffected limbs.

Lying relatively still in bed with 6 or 10 pounds of weight pulling on each leg can be uncomfortable and boring, especially if the patient is no longer in pain. The physician usually regulates the time intervals in which the patient on intermittent traction is allowed out of traction. Occasionally he is permitted bathroom privileges. Some patients remove the weights during the periods when traction is prescribed. In other instances, the physician allows the patient to remove the traction at his own discretion. In either case, the patient must be assisted with reapplying the traction.

When reapplying traction, the weights should be supported and lowered gently so that the patient does not receive a jolt. A pillow may be placed under the legs in such a way that the heels do not rub against the sheets. In pelvic traction, thick abdominal pads are placed over the iliac crest. While the nurse gives skin care she observes for symptoms of increasing compression on the cord (when the herniation is above L 1–2) or the root. Is the affected leg weaker? Does the patient say that he has less sensation in that leg, or has more pain?

When out of traction and moving in bed the patient should roll from side to side without twisting the spine. However, if his symptoms are not severe it is difficult for him to remember to move in this way. Sudden movement that strains or twists the spine should be avoided. When the patient first gets out of bed, bending over to put his slippers on or to pick up something, twisting his body, such as turning to step over the edge of a bathtub, and quick motions should be avoided. He may need to wear a lumbosacral brace or support.

Surgery

If conservative therapy fails to relieve symptoms of a ruptured intervertebral disc, surgery is considered. For spinal cord tumors, surgery is the treatment of choice. The operative procedure is a *laminectomy* which may or may not be followed by a spinal fusion. In a laminectomy the posterior arch of a vertebra is removed to expose the spinal cord. Then the surgeon can remove whatever lesion is causing blockage: a herniated disc, a tumor, a clot, or a broken bone fragment.

If a spinal fusion is performed, a piece of bone is taken from another area, such as the iliac crest, and grafted onto the vertebrae. The fusion stabilizes the spine weakened by degenerative joint changes, such as osteoarthritis, and further weakened by the laminectomy. Fusion results in a firm union; mobility is lost, and the patient has to become accustomed to a permanent area of stiffness. When a portion of the lumbar spine is fused, the patient usually becomes unaware of stiffness after a short time because motion increases in the joints above the fusion. There is usually more limitation of motion when the area of fusion is in the cervical spine. Spinal fusion also may be done for such orthopedic conditions as fractures and dislocations of the spine and Pott's disease (tuberculosis of the spine).

Preoperative Care. Before surgery the care of the patient is similar to that of a patient being treated conservatively. When the patient has spinal compression, whatever the cause, specific observations of function and sensation should be made. The nurse will note, and chart, what activity and which position increases pain, and any gain or loss in motion or sensation since the last observation.

The patient is instructed in and encouraged to practice such exercises as deep breathing and "log rolling" before the operation so that he has experience with the pattern to follow afterward.

Laminectomy—Postoperative Care. Postoperative management of the patient with a laminectomy is given in Table 17-1. While deep-breathing exercises are an important part of care, the patient should cough only when he needs to, since coughing increases pressure within the spinal canal. Watch for signs of compression due to edema or hemorrhage at the operative site. Compression of the cord will cause changes of motility or sensation from that point downward. Inspect the dressing for leakage of spinal fluid as well as for bleeding.

Incisional pain can usually be relieved by narcotics. Surgery for a herniated disc will abolish the pain that was due to stretching the nerve, but a few patients will continue to have backache, especially after standing for long periods. When there has been irritation of the nerve by pressure exerted by the herniated disc or by surgery, the pain may last for some time postoperatively.

One of the most important principles of care after

Table 17-1.
Postoperative nursing management of the patient with a laminectomy

Blood pressure, pulse, respirations are noted every 15 minutes until stable, then every 4 hours. Temperature is taken every 4 hours.
The patient does deep-breathing exercises hourly while awake.
The bed is kept flat.
The patient is log-rolled.
Support the back with pillows when the patient is on his side. Use pillows against the shoulders and buttocks. *Do not* press pillows against the surgical dressing.
Check the dressing for evidence of bleeding each time the patient is repositioned.
Analgesics are administered as ordered.
Intake and output measurements are kept.
Urinary retention may require catheterization or an indwelling urethral catheter.

a lumbar laminectomy is to have the patient rest his back as much as possible. Twisting, turning and jerking the back are not conducive to healing. The first postoperative order concerning the position of the patient may specify that he not be turned for the first 8 hours, that his position be supported with sandbags, and that he is to be kept flat for 12 hours. It is usually the surgeon's wish that the patient not help himself turn in bed for the first two days postoperatively, and he is turned "log fashion." Before he is turned, the bed is flattened, and he makes himself stiff as a log, with his arms at his side. Then the nurse rolls him over all at once, without bending his spine. A turning sheet is helpful, especially early in the postoperative period. Get help if the patient is heavy. Usually patients feel safer when they are allowed to participate in the turning process. At first a patient may be limited to listening to the nurse explain just how the turning will be carried out, to be as comfortable and safe as possible. Later, he will be taught to turn himself, log fashion. It is essential to avoid any abruptness in the turnings, either in manner or the movement of the patient. Most patients greatly fear that they will be moved in such a way that the results of the operation will be compromised, or that they will suffer much pain. Therefore, one proceeds slowly, with the patient's full knowledge, and his participation insofar as possible, in order to lessen anxiety by helping him have more control. Support the patient's position in good alignment with pillows. Look at his spine in the new position. If it is not straight, use small propping pillows until it is. The surgeon usually allows the patient to have a pillow under his head. The patient may be placed in a bivalve cast, made preoperatively.

The patient should not lift his hips and for this reason a fracture bedpan should be used. If a regular bedpan is used, the patient should roll into the bedpan, and his back should be supported with pillows. Try to anticipate what the patient will need, and put it close enough to him so that he will be able to reach it without stretching.

The beginning of ambulation varies with the surgery and the physician's preference; some patients ambulate as early as the day after surgery. A back brace may be worn during ambulation and should be applied while the patient is still lying in bed. A thin cotton shirt should be worn under the brace, no part of which should contact the skin, and there should be no wrinkles to leave marks on the skin. If the doctor does not want a shirt to be worn under the brace, there should be smooth padding where the brace touches the skin.

To help the patient into a brace, have him lie on his side. Center the stays on his back, and have him roll onto the garment. While he is still lying down, after the support has been snugly fastened in place, assist the patient across the bed, so that when he sits up, his feet will be over the edge. Help him to sit up, without straining or twisting his back. In such a support, the patient has to keep a straight back. Also, encourage him to use his muscles to maintain good posture. The stronger the back muscles become, the more support they can give to the operative site, and the less the patient will need the external support of the brace.

Exercises in some form will be prescribed. Such calisthenics as lifting the arms and legs off the floor simultaneously from a prone position are boring. Because swimming is equally effective in strengthening the muscles and is enjoyable to many people, it may be recommended by the doctor.

After a lumbar laminectomy, patients are more comfortable and better supported when they sit in a straight chair rather than an easy chair.

Patients should be taught not to bend over from the waist; instead, they should lower the body by bending the knees while they keep the spine straight.

Laminectomy With Spinal Fusion—Postoperative Care. A patient who has had a spinal fusion is usually kept on postoperative bed rest longer than the patient who has had a simple laminectomy. Even greater care must be taken that the fusion patient does not twist his back while the fused bones unite.

Occasionally, this patient is placed in a spica cast, from his knees to his chest. The cast may be applied several days after surgery. This interval is provided to permit visualization of the operative site to detect bleeding or drainage. During the time between surgery and the application of the cast the patient may be encouraged to move his arms, but extreme care is taken that his spine is kept straight at all times.

A patient who has had a spinal fusion may have two wounds: the wound in the spinal column and the wound in the donor site (although sometimes the bone for the graft is taken from a bone bank). If bone was taken from the patient's leg, he wears an elastic bandage on that leg as long as there is swelling, possibly for several weeks. Be sure that the patient knows how to apply the bandage himself before he leaves the hospital.

Cervical Spine. A patient with injury or surgery of the cervical spine may not be turned at all without special equipment, such as Crutchfield tongs, a brace or halter, or a Foster or Stryker frame. Two sandbags may be placed along his head or neck to keep the cervical spine straight. If turning is allowed, two people will be needed to turn him, one at the head and one at the hip. When the patient lies on his side, put a small pillow under his neck to keep the cervical spine straight. Watch for respiratory distress. Edema of the cervical cord or the spinal nerves may temporarily paralyze the respiratory muscles. If this should occur, a tracheostomy may be performed, followed by the use of a respirator.

After injury or surgery of a cervical disc, traction may be applied with a head halter. Sometimes, the patient can remove the head halter when he sleeps, and sometimes he is ordered to use it continuously. When he improves after surgery, he may wear a rigid collar to decrease neck motion.

Thoracic Spine. When surgery has been performed on the thoracic spine, a figure-of-8 dressing may be applied postoperatively. Because the dressing may constrict the axillary vessels, the radial pulses are checked every hour. The patient is cautioned not to stretch his arms until healing is well advanced.

Resumption of Activities. When spinal fusion has been performed, the resumption of activities is gradual for six months to a year, after which the patient can usually resume full activity. After a laminectomy without spinal fusion the patient is gradually allowed to do light work, but usually he should do no lifting for a year, and may never be able to lift heavy objects. The light objects he does lift should be held close to his body to avoid back strain.

Paraplegia

The word *paraplegia* usually calls to mind a picture of a war-wounded veteran in a wheelchair. This picture is only partly true, for civilians become paraplegics, too. Paraplegia is paralysis of both lower extremities; *quadriplegia* is paralysis of all four extremities. The term paraplegia is sometimes used to include both paraplegia and quadriplegia (Fig. 17-2).

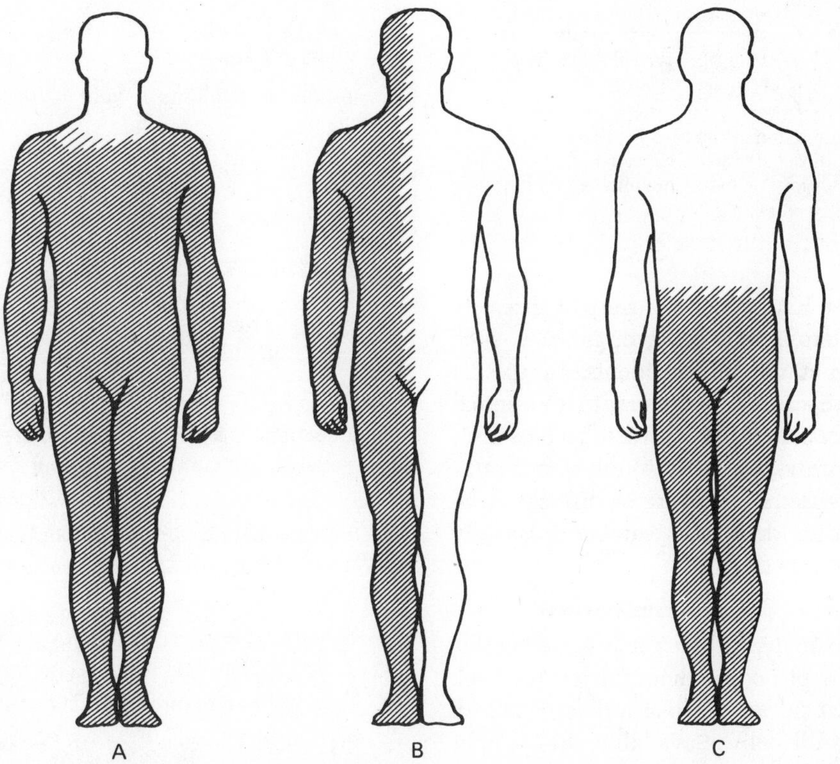

figure 17-2. These diagrams illustrate three common types of disability: (A) quadriplegia, (B) hemiplegia, and (C) paraplegia. The shaded areas indicate the parts of the body that are affected. The location and the extent of the paralysis depend on the location and the severity of the injury. The diagrams are oversimplified. A patient may have some remaining function in an affected part.

Table 17-2.
Level of injury to spinal cord and neurological findings

Injury to	Findings
Cervical Spine	
C-1, C-2, C-3	Usually fatal
C-4	Quadriplegia, respiratory difficulty
C-5 to C-8	Variable function of neck, shoulder, and arm muscles. No function in lower extremities
Thoracic Spine	
T-1 to T-11	Paraplegia—occasionally leg braces can be used when injury is to lower thoracic spine
Thoracic-Lumbar Spine	
T-12 to L-3	Paraplegic; wheelchair with leg braces

Note: Complete transection of the cord results in symptoms additional to those of partial transection, which may produce only sensory or motor loss or hemiplegia.

The cause may be any one of a variety of diseases, such as multiple sclerosis and polio, or injuries, such as those sustained in automobile accidents. Paraplegia and quadriplegia are caused by injury to the spinal cord. When the injury comes from disease, such as multiple sclerosis, the paralysis is likely to develop gradually. The paralysis caused by fracture or dislocation of vertebrae due to an accident or a war injury usually occurs suddenly.

Early treatment

First Aid. If an injury to the spine is suspected, the patient should be placed, without flexing his back or neck, on a firm, flat surface, such as a door or board. Do not move him until help is available, and a firm, flat support on which he can be carried has been obtained. Never permit bystanders to pick up the injured person hastily, thus flexing his spine, as careless moving may cause further damage to the cord. Proper first aid may mean the difference between his being able to walk and having to spend the rest of his life in a wheelchair. Treatment for shock may also be required as a first-aid measure.

After the patient has been admitted to the hospital, the doctor will determine the extent of the injury by physical and x-ray examinations (Table 17-2). If the vertebrae are so injured that they are squeezing or crushing the cord, measures may be taken to relieve the pressure of the bones on the cord.

Nursing management

The general points of nursing management are given in Table 17-3.

Positioning. During the period immediately after

Table 17-3.
Basic management of the patient with a spinal cord injury

Proper alignment of the spine *must* be maintained at all times.

Special attention is given to pressure points: heels, buttocks, shoulders, elbows.

The patient does deep-breathing exercises hourly while awake.

A suction machine is kept in the room in case of aspiration.

Passive exercises (if ordered) are instituted to prevent deformities, muscle contractures, ankylosis of joints.

If turning is allowed, log roll the patient: fold the patient's arms across his chest, place a pillow between the legs, support the head and neck, remove the pillow under the head, and turn.

The bottom sheet is kept free of wrinkles.

Injections are given above the area of paralysis (if possible) as circulation is poor below the area of injury.

Intake and output measurements are kept.

Adequate nutrition and fluid intake are maintained.

Elastic stockings for the legs may be ordered to improve circulation and enhance the return of venous blood to the major veins. The stockings are removed and reapplied once or twice a day.

Neurological evaluation of the patient's status is made every 1 to 4 hours, depending on the patient's condition; evaluation includes: vital signs, movement and presence or absence of sensation in the extremities, size and equality of pupils, level of consciousness.

spinal cord injury the patient is seriously ill and requires a great deal of care and observation. When nerve impulses to the skin are interrupted, the skin's normal response to injury is diminished. The paralyzed patient cannot engage in the almost constant movement that is normal, even during sleep, and that protects the skin from pressure sores. Decubitus ulcers form easily in these patients, become infected easily, and heal very slowly. Unless his position is changed frequently, decubitus ulcers will result. Eventually, the patient is taught to inspect his own skin. The Stryker or Foster frame and the CircOlectric bed make it easier to turn helpless patients (Figs. 17-3 and 17-4).

Complications. Deformities readily develop unless special precautions are taken. Footdrop is a frequent complication because of paralysis of the lower extremities. A footboard must be used from the very beginning to prevent footdrop.

Because the patient is unable to move about, his breathing is shallow, and he fails to cough up respiratory secretions. Therefore, he is predisposed to the development of respiratory complications, such as pneumonia. Changing the patient's position frequently and encouraging him to breathe deeply and to cough up respiratory secretions are important in preventing respiratory complications. IPPB treatments may be indicated for some patients.

Observations. The areas affected by paralysis must be observed carefully. Does the patient have sensation in those parts? Can he feel that water during his bath is warm or cold? Can he feel the pressure of the nurse's hand? Can he move the part? At first the paralysis is flaccid (limp); later it becomes spastic. Severe uncontrollable reflex spasms of the muscles are frequent; the muscle movement is spasm and not the return of voluntary function. Physical activity may help decrease spasm. Passive exercises and changes of position, when they are used regularly, also reduce spasms.

Many patients have pain in the affected area, even though sensation in the usual sense has been lost. The pain is associated with scar formation or irritation around a nerve root. In most patients the pain decreases gradually with recovery from the initial injury.

At first the patient will not perspire below the point of injury. Later, he may perspire profusely and require frequent bathing.

Site of Injections. When possible, intramuscular injections should be given above the level of the paralysis. Because capillary circulation is sluggish below

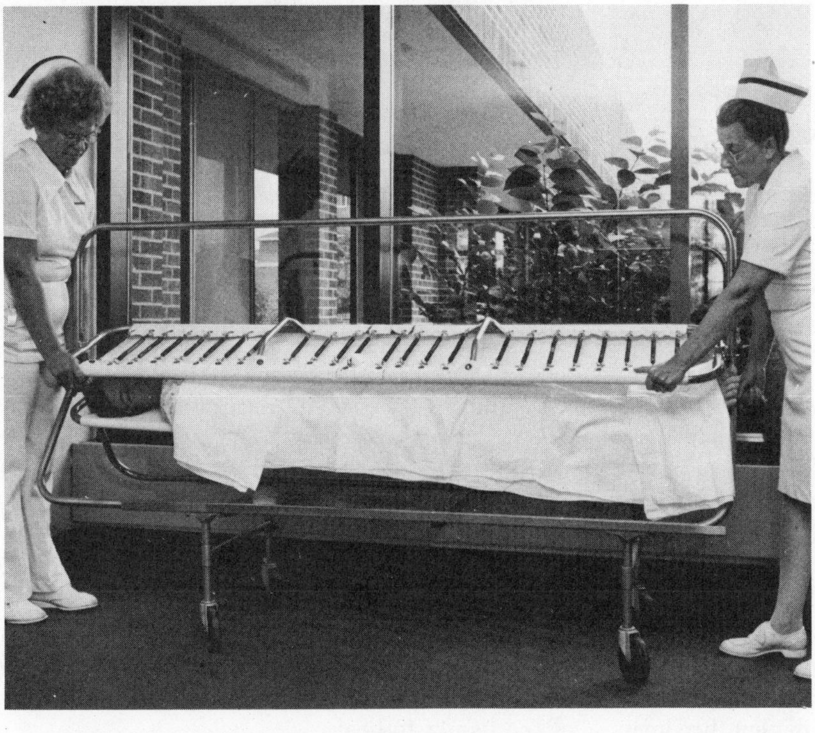

figure 17-3. The Stryker frame may be used for the paralyzed patient. The patient can be turned from prone to supine. In this photograph, the nurses are getting ready to turn the patient to a prone position by placing the frame on top, securing it, and then rotating it. With the patient in a face down position the frame that had supported his back is removed. (Photograph—D. Atkinson)

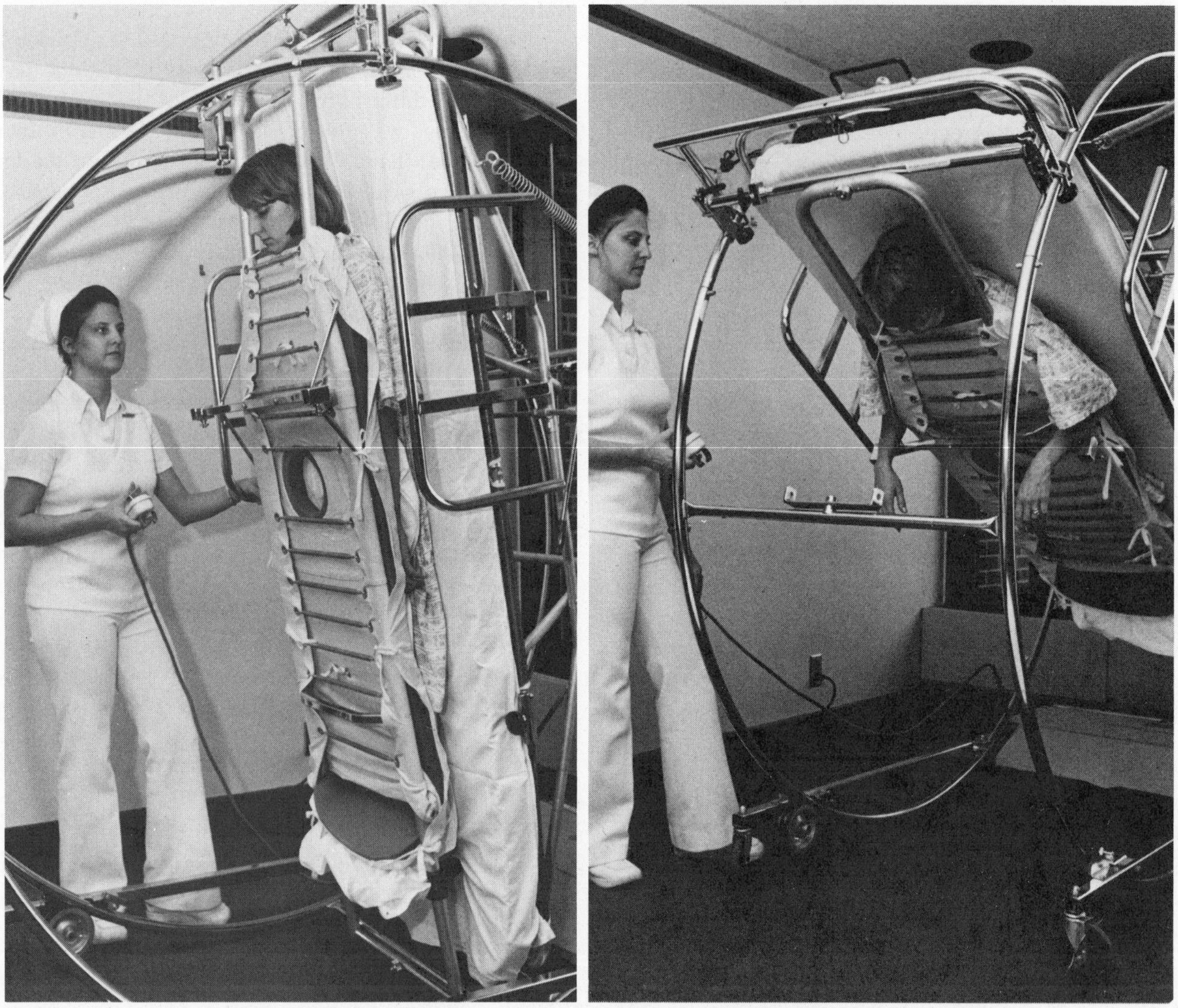

figure 17-4. The CircOlectric bed permits vertical rather than lateral movement seen in the Stryker frame in Fig. 17-3. The nurse has prepared the patient for a prone position. After the bed is in place, a table can be put underneath so that the patient can use her personal belongings, read, etc. (Photograph—D. Atkinson)

the injury, the medicine will be less well absorbed, and injury to the tissues due to the injection is more likely to occur.

ELIMINATION. Cord compression can interfere with the patient's control over bladder and bowel. There may be incontinence or retention of feces, and fecal impactions are frequent. At first there is usually retention of urine; later the patient voids involuntarily. Even when the patient is incontinent there is often some retention of urine. A retention catheter is used in the bladder. If the bedding of the patient becomes wet, the likelihood of decubitus ulcers increases. Enemas may be given daily or every other day to evacuate the bowel and to lessen the problems of fecal impaction or incontinence.

FLUIDS AND FOOD. The fluid intake and the nutrition of the patient must be maintained. High-fluid intake helps to lessen the possibility of urinary-tract infections and calculi. High-protein foods are important in controlling decubitus ulcers, because they help to keep the tissues healthy, and they increase the ability of the tissues to heal.

Psychological problems

As the patient begins to recover from the overwhelming physical injury, he gradually becomes aware of what has happened to him. He finds that he is unable to move parts of his body. Because he can no longer feel these parts, he must look to see if they are still there. Psychological trauma is intense. The body image must be changed. Now, instead of viewing himself as a whole, healthy person, the patient must recognize that part of his body is permanently useless. At first, most patients react with depression and withdrawal. They lie and stare into space, and they show no interest in people and events around them. During this period it is better to emphasize quiet presence, empathy, and attention to physical needs, than it is to adopt a cheer-him-up campaign. It will take time for the patient to recover from the psychological as well as the physical hurt of so devastating an experience.

The patient recognizes his complete dependence on others, and he is fearful because he can no longer help himself. He wants someone near him day and night. Particularly if he is a quadriplegic, his helplessness is extreme. He must be bathed, toileted and dressed—just like an infant. His mind is active, though, even if his body is not.

The nurse may be able to help him by being a good listener. When the patient is ready to talk about how angry or discouraged he is, he does not need advice; he does not need cheering up. He needs someone who can help to lift the burden by accepting how he feels. A patient who tells a nurse that he wishes only for death may not tell her that again if her response is, "Oh, you have lots to live for. You can read, and you have two lovely children," or if she says, "Don't talk like that. Where there's life, there's hope." The patient will still feel as hopeless as he did. He just will not discuss that subject with that nurse again.

The nurse who can reply, "You feel pretty discouraged," or "You don't see much purpose in life now," by implication is telling the patient that she understands how deeply he is discouraged, and that there is nothing wrong about feeling as he does. If his feelings are accepted by the nurse, the patient may be able to express himself further, and afterward he may be able to give the nurse some clue as to how she can help him.

Incontinence poses a tremendous problem. Very early in life human beings are taught to maintain high standards of personal cleanliness. Much is made of the shamefulness of not controlling excretory functions. An adult who becomes unable to control these functions often feels shamed and disgraced—even though intellectually he understands the reason for the lack of control. Incontinence poses a social problem, too. Patients are very sensitive to the reaction of others. Many paraplegics are constantly fearful that an embarrassing accident will occur while they are with others, or that other people will detect odors from catheters and urinals. Hence, bowel and bladder rehabilitation is highly important, not only for physical reasons, such as preventing decubitus ulcers, but also for its effect on morale; it helps the patient to overcome the threat of embarrassment, and so helps him to feel more like his adult, independent self.

The paraplegic male may be impotent; such patients suffer a severe blow to their manhood. They may feel that they are being regarded with scorn and derision. Some women patients are able to have children. Questions about sexual functioning must be answered individually by each patient's doctor, since the degree of normal function will be determined by the particular nature and extent of the illness. Both the patient and the wife or husband should have an opportunity to discuss this subject with the doctor.

In addition to disturbances of sexual and reproductive function, opportunities for meeting people are usually curtailed and opportunities for marriage decreased. The patient does not conform to the ideals of musculine or feminine attractiveness made fashionable by society. For instance, women must wear braces, use crutches, and wear low-heeled oxfords to walk. A tall, well-built man who develops paraplegia no longer appears tall when he sits in his wheelchair.

The paraplegic is subject to a great deal of frustration. He cannot move about freely, and in many situations he must rely on others to help him. A quadriplegic may be unable to light his own cigarette, but he may have an even greater desire to smoke than he did before his injury, when his attention was absorbed by many activities.

Because of his disability he is less able than most other people to get away from situations that are irritating or frightening or to "work off steam" by physical activity. With his mobility decreased and his frustration increased, it is not surprising that the paraplegic often flies into a rage over apparent trifles. Sometimes the frustration of not finding someone to light his cigarette is just too much after all the other discouraging situations.

Rehabilitation

The aim of rehabilitation is to help paraplegics and quadriplegics to use their remaining capacities to the fullest and to avoid complications resulting from the disability. For example, decubitus ulcers seriously interfere with the program of rehabilitation. The patient who develops a large ulcer on the sacrum must return to bed and lie on his abdomen to relieve pressure on the part.

An important part of the role of the nurse in rehabilitation involves helping the patient to avoid complications, so that he can profit from the rehabilitation program. The nurse can help by:

- Giving good skin care; being alert for beginning signs of pressure sores; placing a foam-rubber cushion in the wheelchair to help to relieve pressure.
- Teaching the patient about skin care, change of position, massage, and the importance of inspecting paralyzed areas daily. Because the patient cannot feel the discomfort caused by a beginning decubitus ulcer, he must be especially observant. Patients should use a mirror to inspect parts that they cannot see.
- Maintaining good body alignment; putting joints through a full range of motion (see Chapter 16): flexion, extension, abduction, adduction, internal rotation, external rotation, pronation, supination.
- Encouraging high-fluid intake; using careful aseptic technique when irrigating catheters.
- Showing sensitivity to the emotional needs of the patient; encouraging but not forcing him toward self-care; allowing him to express his feelings concerning the disability.

Positioning. The will of the patient, plus the help of skilled therapists, can mean the difference between invalidism and independence. Paraplegics can learn to put on their own braces and to move from bed to wheelchair. Because of the tremendous effort required to walk (the patient must raise the entire weight of his body, plus the weight of the braces, with his arms), most paraplegics use the wheelchair most of the time and walk only short distances. However, it is important for the patient to assume upright posture at intervals during the day, whether or not he is able to walk. Quadriplegic patients who cannot stand or walk may be placed in an upright position with the aid of a tilt table or by using a CircOlectric bed. This position helps the patient to breathe more deeply, relieves pressure on the sacral region, relieves spasms, and helps to prevent urinary calculi and osteoporosis. The patient often feels dizzy and faint the first few times that he assumes an upright position. He must be watched carefully and protected, so that he does not fall. The pooling of blood in the abdominal area is a factor in causing postural hypotension. The application of an abdominal binder and elastic stockings to the legs before the patient gets up helps to prevent dizziness and faintness. When a tilt table is used, patients are strapped to it, and it is tilted gradually until the patient is standing erect.

Parallel bars help to support the patient whose upper extremities are unaffected. Therefore, he can support his own weight by grasping the bars. With the help of parallel bars, paraplegic patients can learn to balance themselves and to practice skills that will later be useful in crutch walking.

Bowel Rehabilitation. The rehabilitation of the bowels and the bladder is of crucial importance in helping the patient to move toward independence. Many patients can achieve self-controlled emptying of the bowels and the bladder, provided that they and those who care for them exert the persistent effort required to achieve this goal. Control of the bowels usually is easier to achieve than control of the bladder. The following steps are useful in helping patients to achieve self-controlled emptying of the bowel:

- Encourage the patient to drink plenty of liquid and to eat foods that produce bulk, such as fresh fruits and vegetables. Teach him not to eat foods that normally cause him to have loose stools.
- Help the patient to plan to go to the toilet at a certain time each day. Select a time that will later fit into his own schedule for self-care.
- Allow the patient privacy and sufficient time to have a bowel movement.
- As soon as he is able, encourage the patient to go to the bathroom rather than to use the bedpan. The physical activity involved in getting out of bed often helps the patient to move his bowels. Using the bathroom has psychological value, too, with its indication of self-help rather than helplessness.

Enemas and suppositories may be needed at first. For example, the patient may be given a small enema each day at the same time. He later may find that inserting a suppository just before the time for defecation will result in a normal bowel movement. Later his bowel function may become regulated so well that he has normal bowel movements without the aid of enemas or suppositories.

Giving an enema to a paraplegic patient requires skill. Be very careful in checking the temperature of the solution, and gentle in inserting the rectal tube.

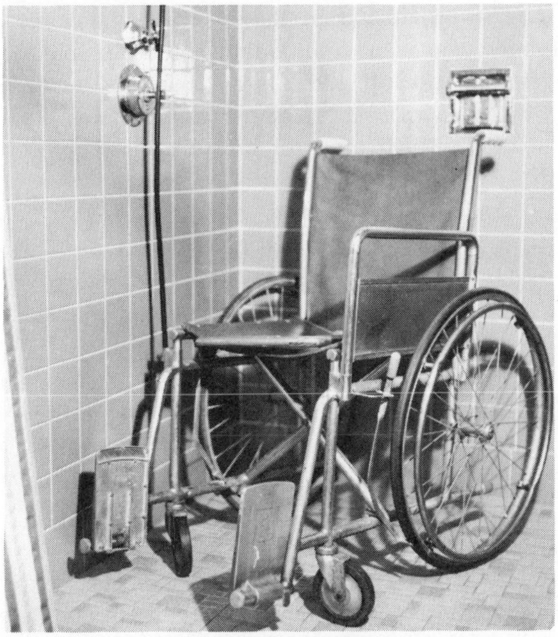

figure 17-5. Bathing. An extra wheelchair is stationed permanently in the shower stall. The stall is wide, allowing plenty of room for the wheelchair. One can sit in the wheelchair and bathe without assistance. Water for the shower comes through the hose seen at the left. If the water suddenly becomes too hot or too cold, the rubber hose can be directed away from the body. Some paraplegics use a chair or a stool rather than a wheelchair in the shower. Sitting under the shower is much easier than getting in and out of a bathtub.

The inability of the patient to feel means that he is more, not less, vulnerable to trauma. Because the patient cannot retain the solution during the administration of the enema, use some device to prevent the solution from running out as fast as it runs in. One device consists of a hard rubber ball with a hole in it. The rectal tube is passed through the ball, and, as the enema is given, the ball is held close to the patient's body. Provide ahead of time for leakage of the solution during the enema. Regardless of the technique, some leakage is likely to occur. For example, the bed can be protected by a large rubber sheet.

Bladder Rehabilitation. The control of the bladder is more difficult to establish, but many patients can achieve it. (See Chapter 35 for a discussion of rehabilitation of patients who are incontinent of urine.)

Prognosis depends upon many factors. The level of the cord injury, the occurrence of complications, the patient's motivation and perseverance, and the quality of care he receives are important influences upon prognosis. Many paraplegics are able to go home, to care for themselves, and in some instances to resume work.

Nursing Guidelines. Helping paraplegic and quadriplegic patients to resume living that is as normal as is possible presents a tremendous challenge and equally great rewards. It is not an easy kind of nursing. Here are some suggestions on how to help the patient:

- Let the patient do as much as he can for himself. Arrange the environment so that self-care is encouraged (feeding devices, keeping belongings handy, and so on). It will take him longer to do it himself than it will for you to do it for him. Try to arrange the schedule to allow him extra time for such activities as feeding himself.
- Avoid pushing the patient. Great sensitivity is required to know when he is ready to attempt something new. These tasks look easy to us. Activities of daily living (ADL), such as eating, bathing, and dressing, seem elementary (Fig. 17-5). Do not be surprised and try not to show disappointment on days when he seems to regress.
- Encourage the patient to be up and about, to get dressed, to go to the dining room, the bathroom, the recreation rooms. Try to help him to achieve as nearly normal living as is possible. Remember that these activities are very fatiguing, especially at first, when the patient is not used to them, and plan for rest periods as well as activity.
- Partial self-care may not be as dramatic, but it is just as important a goal as the more complete rehabilitation of a less disabled person. Think what a difference it makes to the patient and his family if he can feed himself or pick up a telephone to call for help. Learning these skills may mean the difference between having to have a family member stay with him constantly and being able to be left alone.
- All the emphasis on activity and on being with others often makes patients long for a few moments to themselves. Do not insist that the patient be busy and with other people every minute. Everyone needs a balance of solitude and companionship.

The environment—hospital and home

The patient's environment is important. Whether he is at home or in the hospital, his recovery is slow, and he is less free to move from one place to another. Some paraplegics must spend a long time in the hospital. The significance of the environment is much greater for these patients than for those who return home after a few days.

Because physically disabled patients need special facilities, they often are grouped together in hospitals. Relationships among these patients affect rehabilitation. Attitudes are contagious, and the role of the nurse involves working not only with individuals, but also with groups of patients. Each individual is facing severe emotional strain. Patients find various ways of expressing their feelings about the disability.

Patients and staff get to know one another very well over the many months, and even years, in which they are together. This can be a rewarding, valuable experience—really knowing the patient and his family and home situation and having the opportunity to work with him and to see his progress over a longer period of time.

However, there are some pitfalls in caring for long-term disabled patients. Identifying some of them will help you to avoid them.

- Do not play favorites. These patients are very sensitive to any show of favoritism, and they are quick to resent it. Treat all alike in the sense that they have equal call on your knowledge and skill. Treat each differently in the sense that each patient has his own unique needs.
- Remember that you are the patient's nurse, not a family member or a pal. The relationship of nurse and patient sometimes tends to become confused when the nurse has cared for the patient over a long period of time.
- Note how the patients get along with one another. Place them near those whose company they seem to enjoy.
- Avoid regimentation. For some the hospital is now the only home that they have.

In one way the home environment is less restricted than that of the hospital; in other ways it may be more so. At home the patient can have visitors at any hour, and he can arrange his own schedule for sleeping and waking, and so on. On the other hand, if his home does not have facilities that help him to get about, he may spend all his time in one room.

Home is the usual environment—and usually the best one—provided that the patient has a home and a family who want him. Going home is a major step in rehabilitation. It presents the challenge of helping the disabled patient to adjust to his home and his community. What kinds of problems may the patient face?

- How will my family feel about me?
- Will I be a burden to them?
- Will my friends forget me?
- Will I be able to manage without the doctors and nurses around?
- What if I'm alone in the house and something happens—like a fire? In the hospital there's always someone around to help.

The patient and his family will need help in planning for his homecoming. The home situation will need to be evaluated; often a public health nurse or a social worker makes this evaluation. She notes the physical environment—the stairs, the bathroom, etc.—as well as the attitude of the family toward the return of the patient.

After the patient returns home, continued care and supervision will be needed. The patient may be seen regularly by his private doctor or at a clinic. The public health nurse may continue the teaching begun in the hospital, showing the family how to adapt care to the home situation, as well as carrying out treatments, such as injections or dressings. In some communities physical therapists are available who come to the patient's home and continue the program started in the hospital.

General nutritional considerations

- High fluid intake is necessary for the immobilized patient with a spinal cord injury.
- In order to increase the fluid intake, fluids other than water may be offered. If there is no special dietary restriction, the patient may also have carbonated beverages, ice cream, broths, flavored gelatin.
- If the patient appears to have a problem with excessive gas when drinking carbonated beverages, the beverage can be allowed to stand open for several hours and then served cold. This will eliminate some of the carbonation.
- A high-protein diet is essential to the prevention of skin breakdown.

■ It may be necessary to offer foods in small amounts, with between-meal feedings, to meet daily nutritional requirements.

■ The hospital dietitian may be needed to help the patient select foods high in protein. The dietitian can also plan meals that are appetizing and include the patient's own food preferences.

■ Foods that provide bulk, including fruits, vegetables, and bran and other cereals, are usually included in the diet of the patient on a bowel rehabilitation program.

General pharmacological considerations

■ Muscle-relaxing drugs such as carisoprodol (Soma) or the tranquilizer diazepam (Valium), which has muscle-relaxing properties, may be prescribed for patients with a herniated intervertebral disc, back strains, and spasms of the muscles of the back.

■ Bowel rehabilitation of the paraplegic or quadriplegic patient may include the use of suppositories or enemas. Suppositories used include glycerin suppositories, which soften the stool in the lower rectum, and bisacodyl (Dulcolax), which stimulates peristalsis in the terminal section of the large colon. Enemas may include plain water, glycerin and Fleet Brand enema.

■ With the patient on his side, a suppository is gently inserted past the rectal sphincter. If the patient reflexly expels the suppository soon after insertion, it may be necessary to tape the patient's buttocks together in an effort to keep the suppository in place. The tape is then removed at the time the suppository is expected to work.

■ Enemas are given slowly as paraplegic and quadriplegic patients are unable to *voluntarily* retain the enema solution. If a small amount (approximately 1 to 2 ounces) of the fluid is given, followed by a waiting period (which varies from patient to patient), the patient may be able to retain a sufficient amount of the enema solution.

Bibliography

ANDERSON, L. et al.: *Nutrition in Nursing.* Philadelphia, Lippincott, 1972.

CARINI, E. and OWENS, G.: Neurological and Neurosurgical Nursing, ed. 6. St. Louis, Mosby, 1973.

COSGRIFF, J. H. and ANDERSON, D. L.: *The Practice of Emergency Nursing.* Philadelphia, Lippincott, 1975.

HENDERSON, G. M.: Teaching-learning for rehabilitation of the spinal cord-disabled individual. Nurs. Clin. North Am. 6:655, December, 1971.

HINKHOUSE, A.: Craniocerebral trauma. Am. J. Nurs. 73:1719, October, 1973.

HOLVEY, D. N. and TALBOTT, J. H., eds.: *Merck Manual of Diagnosis and Therapy,* ed. 12. Merck, Sharp and Dohme Research Laboratories, 1972.

JIMM, L. R.: Nursing assessment of patients for increased intracranial pressure. Nurs. Dig. 75:4, July/August, 1975.

KINTZEL, K., ed.: *Advanced Concepts of Clinical Nursing,* ed. 2. Philadelphia, Lippincott, 1977.

McCAY, D. R.: How to care for your laminectomy patient. J. Prac. Nurs. 25:27, September, 1975.

SCHERER, J. C.: *Introductory Clinical Pharmacology.* Philadelphia, Lippincott, 1975.

TUCKER, S. M. et al: *Patient Care Standards.* St. Louis, Mosby, 1975.

VORHEES, J.: The lingering danger of head injuries. RN 75:43, April, 1975.

CHAPTER—18

The patient with visual and hearing impairment

On completion of this chapter the student will:

- Describe simple rules for daily care of the eyes.
- Differentiate between the medical and allied personnel concerned with the care of the eyes, the performance of eye examinations and refractions, and the dispensing of optical prescriptions.
- Identify the instruments used in testing the eyes for glaucoma.
- Describe basic first aid given to those with eye injuries.
- Discuss some of the problems encountered by the blind, the partially sighted, and those with hearing impairments.
- Describe the types of refractive errors and how these errors may be treated with optical prescriptions.
- List common eye diseases and disorders and describe the signs, symptoms, and nursing management of patients with these disorders.
- Describe the nursing management of patients undergoing eye surgery.
- Define the two basic types of hearing loss.
- List common disorders of the external, middle, and inner ear and describe the signs, symptoms, and nursing management of each.

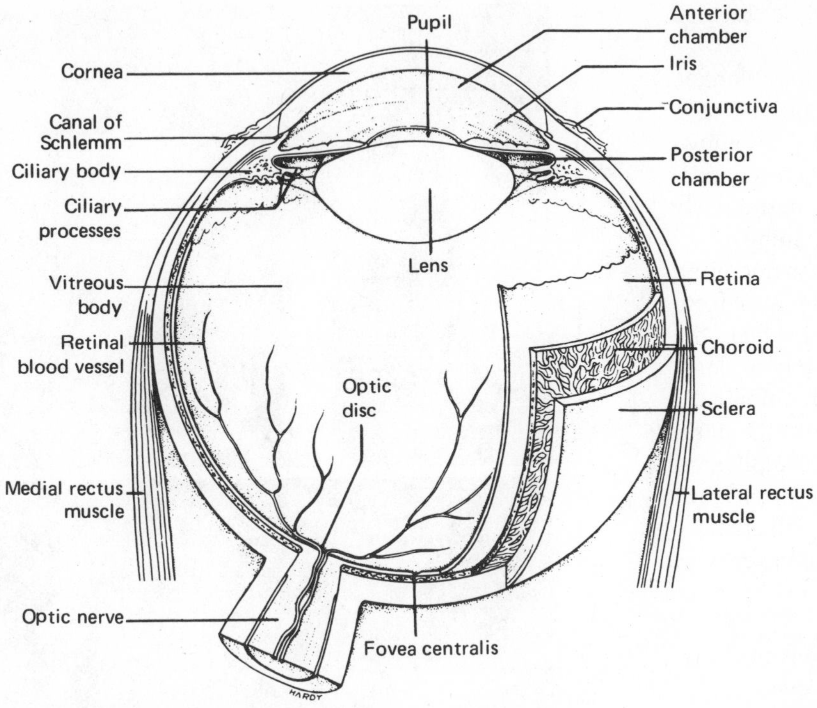

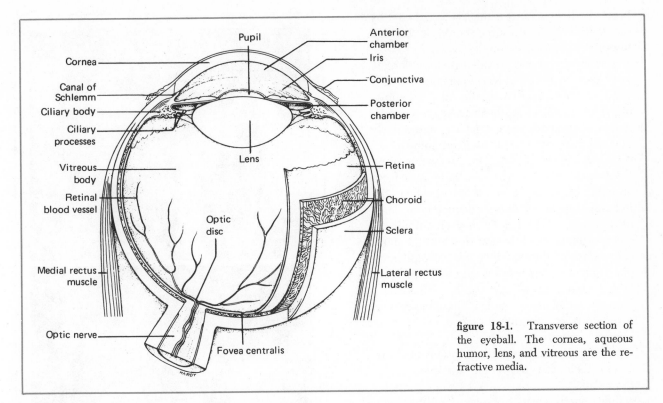

figure 18-1. Transverse section of the eyeball. The cornea, aqueous humor, lens, and vitreous are the refractive media.

Many people are confused by the terms *optician, optometrist, ophthalmologist,* and *oculist.* An *optician,* like a pharmacist, fills prescriptions given by a doctor. In this instance the prescription is for glasses. The optician has the prescribed lenses made and sees that the glasses are properly fitted. An *optometrist* is one who has had special training in testing vision for refractive errors and in prescribing and fitting glasses to correct such errors. Because he is not an M.D., he is not permitted to prescribe medications for the eye or to diagnose or treat eye diseases. The terms *ophthalmologist* and *oculist* are synonymous and refer to a medical doctor who has had special training in the diagnosis and treatment of eye diseases, including refraction and the prescription of glasses.

Important structures of the eye are shown in Fig. 18-1.

Instruments. The physician uses an instrument called an *ophthalmoscope* to examine the interior of the eye. After the lights in the room have been turned off, the doctor holds the ophthalmoscope close to his eye and to the patient's eye, and looks through the instrument.

The ophthalmoscope must not be sterilized by boiling or autoclaving, because it contains many small lenses. Since the ophthalmoscope does not come into direct contact with the patient's eye, sterilization after each use is not necessary.

A tonometer is used to test the pressure within the eyeball. Increased intraocular pressure is a sign of glaucoma. Two methods of tonometry are commonly employed (Fig. 18-2). With the Schiotz tonometer, the patient is usually seated in a treatment chair, and the chair is tilted to a reclining position. A local anesthetic is dropped into the eye to anesthetize the cornea. The tonometer, a small metal instrument, is then placed gently on the cornea. The moving pointer indicates the intraocular pressure. Because the footplate of the tonometer touches the eye, it must be sterilized before use with each patient. In the past few years another method known as applanation tonometry has become increasingly used by ophthalmologists because of its greater accuracy.

Tonography is a recently devised method of recording intraocular tension over a period of 4 minutes, during which time a specially sensitive Schiotz-type tonometer is allowed to rest on the eyeball. The tonometer in this instance is attached to an electric recording device. This test is of value for diagnosis of early glaucoma and for confirming that known glaucoma is being satisfactorily controlled by treatment.

Eye Care. Simple rules for the daily care of the eyes include the following:

- Have a good light when reading, writing, sewing or other close work is being done.

Place the light so that a shadow is not cast by the hands. The light source should be shielded to prevent direct glare on the eyes.

- Rest the eyes periodically when prolonged fine work is being done. Looking out of a window at intervals rests the eyes by allowing them to focus on distant objects (relaxation of accommodation). Looking continuously at small print or tiny stitches is fatiguing.
- General health is important in maintaining the health of the eyes. For example, a form of night blindness, a condition in which the individual is unable to see adequately in darkness, is related to a deficiency of vitamin A. (The adjustment of the eye to see in the dark, called *dark adaptation,* involves a complicated photochemical process in the retina.) Epithelial tissues of the eye also are affected by vitamin A deficiency, and, if the deficiency is severe, the cornea may be so damaged that blindness results.
- Avoid the use of nonprescription eyedrops unless their use has been approved by a physician.
- Keep hands away from eyes. Rubbing the eyelids causes irritation and may introduce infection.
- Avoid direct exposure of the eyes to sunlamps. They can burn the lids and the cornea, as can excessive exposure to sunlight at the beach or on snow-covered ground. Ultraviolet rays can cause painful burns that are not apparent for several hours after overexposure.

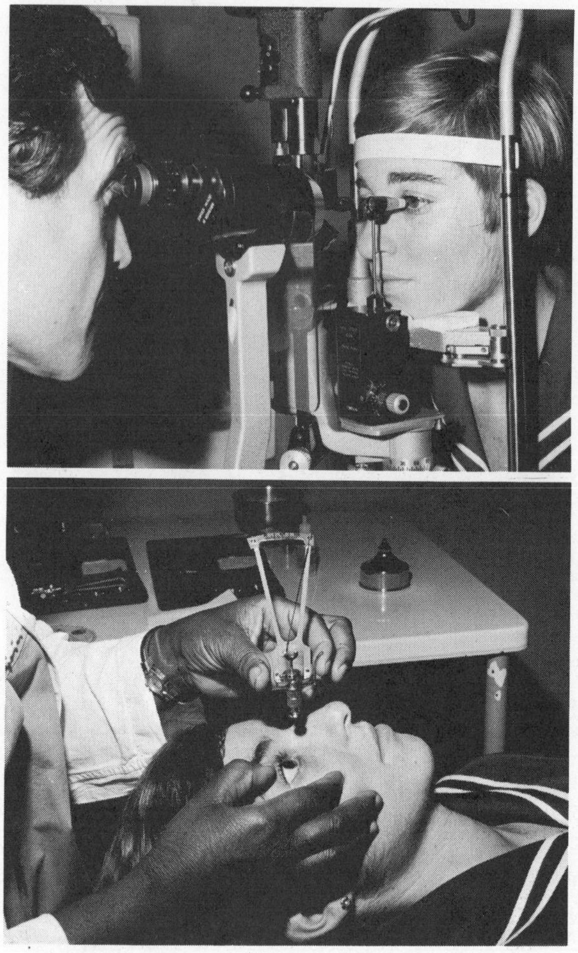

figure 18-2. (*Top*) Intraocular pressure measured with the Goldmann applanation tonometer. (*Bottom*) Intraocular pressure measured with the Schiotz tonometer. (Raymond Harrison, M.D.)

First aid

Foreign Body in the Eye. Almost everyone has suffered the exquisite discomfort of a foreign body in the eye. A cinder barely large enough to see feels like a boulder when it gets in the eye. A foreign body can be removed by the nurse if:

- It is not on the cornea.
- It has not penetrated the eyeball (for instance, a sharp splinter of metal or wood that has pierced the eyeball).
- It is removed readily by a sterile applicator.

The first requisite is a good light. Remind the patient not to rub the eye. This is an urge that is hard to resist when a foreign body is present, but it may lead to further injury and irritation or to imbedding the particle, making it difficult to remove. Wash your hands thoroughly. Then, with the patient seated, examine the eye, including the inside of the upper and lower lids. To evert the upper lid, lay a toothpick swab just back from the edge of the upper lid, grasp the lashes gently but firmly with your other hand, pull the upper lid slightly outward from the eye and turn it upward, exposing the underside of the lid.

When you locate the tiny particle, touch it gently with a sterile swab moistened in clear water or sterile saline. (The latter is preferable, if it is available.) If the particle is not readily removed in this manner, avoid further attempts to remove it. Picking at it with the swab can push it into the tissues and may injure the eye. Explain to the patient that the services of an ophthalmologist are needed, and help the patient to make arrangements for further care, either in the doctor's office or at an eye clinic. Assure the patient that this referral does not necessarily mean that there is anything seriously wrong, but only that the doctor's skill is needed to remove the particle safely. A similar explanation can be made if the foreign body is on the cornea. Attempts to remove it could lead to scarring of the cornea and to diminished vision. The doctor's skill and delicate instruments can remove the particle with the least possible injury to the cornea.

Irrigating the eye with sterile saline is also sometimes effective in removing a foreign body. An irrigating tip attached to a flask of sterile saline may be used for this purpose, in a manner similar to that used when acids or other irritants are splashed unexpectedly into the eye.

After the particle has been removed, the patient usually continues to feel some irritation. An oval eye pad applied over the closed lids with tape affords relief. Instruct the patient not to rub the eye, and, if it is not completely comfortable within a short time (an hour or so), to visit an ophthalmologist.

CHEMICALS. Splashing an irritating chemical, such as bleach, into the eye is another common emergency. The eye should be flushed copiously with water to remove the chemical as promptly as possible. If sterile saline is available, use it, but do not delay the irrigation to obtain it. Use plain tap water instead. If the accident occurs in the home or at work, take the patient to the nearest sink or water fountain, and have him hold his eyelids open while the water cleanses the eye. The importance of speed cannot be overemphasized, because the longer the chemical is in contact with the eye, the more damage it does. The same procedure is followed if an eyedrop is instilled into the wrong eye, or if the wrong kind of medication is used. After the eye has been irrigated, the patient is instructed to close his eye, and an eye pad is applied over the lid and held in place with tape. The patient is taken immediately to an ophthalmologist or to a hospital emergency room for further treatment. Assure the patient that everything possible is being done to avoid any further injury to his eyes.

Usually, further irrigation with sterile saline is carried out at the doctor's office or the clinic. A flask of sterile saline is hung on an infusion pole about 6 inches above the eye, and, by means of rubber tubing and an irrigating tip, copious amounts of the solution are used to flush away the harmful chemical. The patient may be draped with a plastic apron to prevent wetting the clothing. The return flow is caught in a large emesis basin. The patient lies on a cot or is seated in a chair that can be placed quickly in a reclining position. The flow of solution is directed from the inner canthus to the outer canthus, so that it does not flow into the opposite eye. If both eyes must be irrigated, it is preferable to have two nurses, or a nurse and an assistant, work simultaneously. If this is not possible, the person performing the irrigation switches the flow from one eye to the other frequently, so that both eyes are irrigated as quickly and thoroughly as possible. The upper lid is everted and any solid particles, such as lime, are carefully washed out.

The visually handicapped

Visual disorders are extremely common. So many people wear corrective glasses that the need for them is not usually considered a disability. However, the vision of some individuals cannot be improved by glasses or any other type of treatment. Their defective vision may have been caused by injury or by a disease, such as glaucoma. Regardless of its cause, poor vision affects the individual's emotional, social and vocational life. The incidence of visual handicaps rises markedly with increasing age.

Visual acuity is expressed as a fraction and is based on a standard of "normal vision." For example, to the person with 20/200 vision, letters readable to the normally sighted at 200 feet are readable at distances no greater than 20 feet. If you have 20/70 vision, you must be within 20 feet of letters large enough for one with normal vision (20/20) to read at 70 feet, in order to read them.

The term *blindness* is used for many legal purposes when central visual acuity is 20/200 or less in the better eye, even when corrective glasses are worn. Those with severe restrictions in the field of vision also are referred to as "blind." For instance, the patient may be able to see only an area the size of a book page at a distance of 20 feet. Those who have visual acuity between 20/70 and 20/200 in the better eye, with the use of glasses, are often referred to as "partially sighted."

The partially sighted

Contrary to the beliefs of many patients and families, the use of the eyes by the partially sighted does not necessarily harm or strain them. Some refuse to read with a special magnifying glass for fear of further reducing their vision. The patient should be guided by his ophthalmologist's advice concerning how much to use his eyes. Practice in using a special lens, either as a hand lens or fitted into eyeglass frames, can help the patient to make the most effective use of his remaining vision. The chief objectives in the rehabilitation of partially sighted individuals include:

- Preservation of the remaining sight by treatment, if possible, of the underlying disorder.
- Making the fullest possible use of the remaining vision by special lenses, large type, or holding the object closer to the eyes.

The patient's visual ability and the type of aids that might help him are evaluated carefully. Vocational preparation is undertaken in the light of the patient's ability to see. For example, a severe visual handicap would make the job of a bus driver a hazard for everyone concerned, whereas certain types of factory work could be performed efficiently and safely. The partially sighted individual should be assisted and encouraged to work at a suitable occupation and to help to take care of his home and family. Ingenuity and willingness to try new ways of doing things can help the individual to maintain his independence.

The blind

Misconceptions

For centuries blindness has been shrouded in mystery. Many myths have developed, such as that blind people develop extraordinary powers of hearing and touch to compensate for the loss of vision. Tests of these senses among blind and sighted people have not shown the blind to have unusual perception in the other senses. It is now believed that blind people learn to make more effective use of their other senses in their effort to interpret their environment. For example, the blind person learns to be especially aware of tones of voice. This helps him to recognize changes in other people's moods, although he cannot see facial expressions. Most of us could learn to make greater use of auditory and tactile stimuli, but our ability to see makes this effort seem to be less necessary.

Orientation and aids to self-care

How can we as nurses help a blind person to take his place in the community? Often, the nurse works with newly blind persons. These patients, just like others who have lost a part of themselves, usually show sadness and depression, a natural reaction to loss. At this time the patient needs a feeling of support and encouragement—someone to listen when he feels like expressing his feelings, someone to guide his first faltering steps, so that his clumsiness will be less embarrassing and less dangerous.

Gradually, the patient is helped to orient himself to his room in the hospital or at home. Where is the chair? The dresser? He is helped to form a mental image of his surroundings and gradually to move about his room without assistance.

At mealtime he is told where the food is on his plate. Likening the location of the food to the numbers on the face of a clock is helpful. In Figure 18-3 the meat is at 9 o'clock, the potato at 3 o'clock and the vegetable at 6 o'clock. Placing the patient's food on his plate in the same position day after day will help him to become adept at finding it. Other articles should be kept in the same position at each meal—for example, the napkin always on the left, near the fork, and the milk always on the right, near the knife. The patient is given as much help as is necessary to avoid repeated spilling and discouragement. At first he will need help in buttering bread, cutting meat and pouring beverages. Gradually, he masters even these tasks. Many blind people can eat with little or no assistance, once they have been oriented to the location of the food and the tableware.

Remember to tell the patient when something has been moved or is different from usual. Explain that the easy chair has been placed on the other side of the room, or that he is having spaghetti instead of meat, potato and vegetable. Leave the doors open wide or completely closed. The patient is likely to bump into a partly opened door.

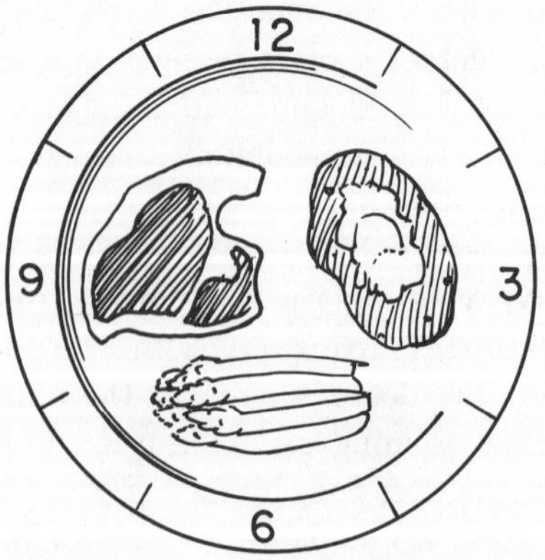

figure 18-3. Telling the patient that his meat is at 9 o'clock, potato at 3 o'clock, and vegetable at 6 o'clock helps him to locate them on his plate.

Let the patient *gradually* assume responsibility for his own grooming. Bathing, combing hair, shaving, and brushing the teeth are all activities that he can learn to do himself. Keep his toilet articles in the same place. Never move them without telling him. If his electric razor is always in the top drawer and his towel on the rack nearest the sink, see that no one moves them. The patient at first will require tactful assistance. If he has missed part of his whiskers, tell him so gently and help him to learn to feel his skin to make sure that his shave is complete.

Reading is an invaluable pastime for persons with all sorts of disabilities. Blind people can read, too, but methods for doing so must be adapted to their particular needs. Braille is a system of raised dots that the patient can feel with his fingertips (Fig. 18-4). The dots are arranged in different ways to signify letters of the alphabet and punctuation marks. The use of Braille requires learning and a great deal of patience. Information about securing Braille books may be obtained from the Library of Congress, Washington, D.C. Agencies for the blind, such as the American Foundation for the Blind, and state agencies for the blind can provide information about teachers of Braille, many of whom go directly into the patient's home. Braille watches are also available (Fig. 18-4). The blind person feels the hands and the raised characters on the face of the watch with his fingertips.

Talking books are long-playing records that allow the patient to listen to recordings of books and even some magazines. Talking books are available for purchase or loan. Information concerning talking books is available from the Library of Congress, Washington, D.C., from state agencies for the blind, and from the public library.

Special typewriters are available that type Braille, making it possible for blind people to write to one another. Blind people use a regular typewriter when they write to their sighted friends. They use the same touch system as sighted people. Also, handwriting is possible. Some blind people lay a ruler underneath the line of writing to keep it straight.

The newly blind person typically reacts with depression to the loss of his vision. Gradually, with assistance and support, he may move through this grief reaction to the point where he is ready to learn to become as independent as possible. Some patients react initially with denial of their disability; these

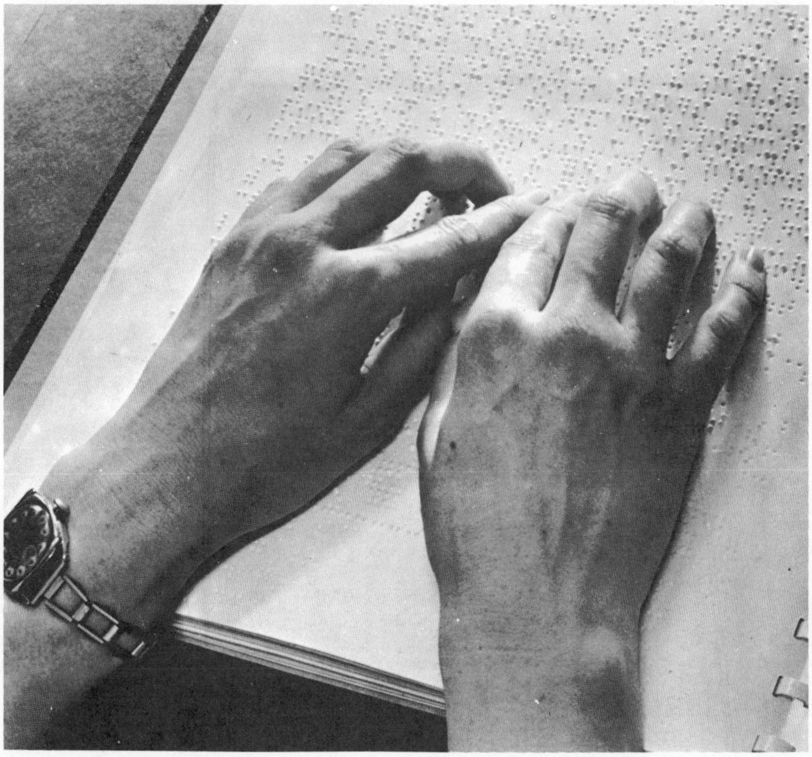

figure 18-4. A page of Braille. Note the raised dots and the placement of the fingers on the page. Note also the special watch with dots in place of numerals. It has no crystal, and the user can tell the time by feeling the relationship of the hands and the dots. (American Foundation for the Blind, Inc., New York, N.Y.)

patients are especially disadvantaged, as they must first be helped to recognize the fact of their disability.

AIDING BLIND TRAVELERS. Nurses can help and teach others to aid blind travelers by:

- Resisting the impulse to rush up and try to help. If the blind person seems to be managing well, he will appreciate being allowed to continue to do so, rather than being whisked across the street, often opposite to where he wishes to go, by an impulsive "helper."
- Courteously asking the blind person how we can help him, if he seems lost or uncertain. If he requires directions, remember that he cannot see landmarks like "the big church on the corner." He can count the streets that he crosses and then turn left or right.
- Avoiding any fuss that would embarrass him and call attention to his disability. Unobtrusive, thoughtful help—offering him a seat in a crowded bus or preventing him from being pushed—is appreciated. When you guide a blind person, let him take your arm. Walk slightly in front of him, so that the movement of your body when you stop or step up or down will give him advance warning of what to expect. Seizing the blind person's arm and pulling him along is a common mistake. It is destructive of his dignity and is likely to throw him off balance. Encourage the blind person to walk erect and to turn his head toward the person speaking to him.
- Seeing-eye dogs have given mobility and independence to the blind. These animals are allowed in most areas where pets are not ordinarily permitted, such as buses and department stores.

COURTESIES AND ATTITUDES

Certain courtesies smooth the way for the blind person and his sighted companions. When you address the blind person, especially when he is with a group, call him by name to save him the embarrassment of not knowing you are speaking to him. He cannot see that you are looking in his direction. Speak to him before touching him, so that he will realize you are there, and what you are going to do. For instance, the sighted hospitalized patient can observe the syringe in your hand, and he knows even before you tell him that he is about to receive an injection. The blind patient has no such way of preparing himself, and he is especially dependent on others for an explanation of what is about to happen, and what is expected of him. Tell the patient when you are entering or leaving the room, so that he is spared the uncomfortable realization that he has been talking to someone who has already left. Teach the patient to turn on the light at a certain time each evening when he is alone. This will prevent others from the startling experience of unexpectedly finding him sitting in a dark room, when they were not aware that he was there.

Some people are afraid of the blind, and avoid contact with them. Perhaps they feel a certain eeriness in the lack of normal eye contact. Some blind people have learned that a handshake helps to overcome this when they meet people for the first time. Shake the blind person's hand when he extends it, but remember that he cannot see your hand if you initiate the handshake. In the latter instance, you will have to reach for his hand.

The only thing that blind people have in common is the inability to see. They differ from one another in other ways, just as sighted people do. The patient must be helped to maintain his individuality, and he must not, because of his handicap, be expected to conform to some nebulous personality considered appropriate for "the blind." Blind people rely on us, not for pity, but for help in resuming independent lives despite the handicap. The one ingredient that has often been lacking, despite many charitable enterprises for the benefit of the blind, is true acceptance by the sighted community.

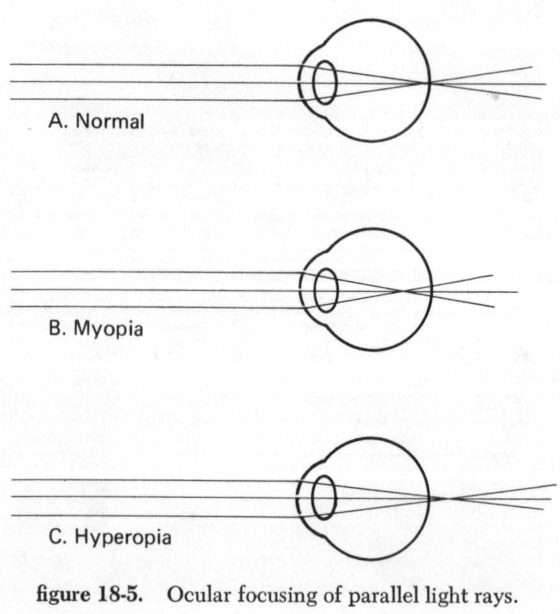

figure 18-5. Ocular focusing of parallel light rays.

Refractive errors

The cornea, the aqueous humor, the lens, and the vitreous body constitute the *refractive media* of the eye. Ocular refraction is the process by which rays of light are "bent" so that they will focus on the retina. Normally, all the refractive media are transparent.

Refractive errors are the commonest type of eye disorder, resulting when the refractive media do not converge light rays to a focus on the retina (Fig. 18-5). Many refractive errors have a tendency to be inherited.

Myopia (nearsightedness) usually results from elongation of the eyeball. Because of the excessive length of the eyeball, light rays focus at a point in the vitreous humor before reaching the retina.

Hyperopia (farsightedness) results when the eyeball is shorter than normal, causing the light rays to focus at a theoretic point behind the retina.

Astigmatism results from unequal curvatures in the shape of the cornea or, sometimes, of the lens. Vision is distorted. For example, a straight object may appear to be slanted. Often a person has both astigmatism and myopia or hyperopia. Astigmatism is corrected by cylindrical lenses.

Myopia, hyperopia, and astigmatism can cause diminished and blurred vision. The individual with myopia must bring things close to his eyes to see them, whereas the person with hyperopia usually can see objects better at a distance. The conditions are corrected by lenses that bend light rays in a way that compensates for the patient's refractive error.

The shape of the lens is changed by the action of the ciliary muscle, thus providing the eye with a focusing mechanism. This process is known as *accommodation.* The lens is elastic and pliable in youth and early adult life. In middle life and old age it becomes more rigid.

Presbyopia is caused by the gradual loss of the elasticity of the lens which leads to a decreased ability to accommodate to near vision. Small objects and print must be held farther and farther away to be seen clearly, because the eye has lost the ability to adjust the shape of the lens to permit clear vision of close objects. The person trying to read may comment jokingly, "My arms aren't long enough any more." The loss of accommodation begins in youth and progresses gradually. By the time the person is in his 40's, the loss is sufficiently marked to interfere with reading, sewing, and other close work.

Bifocals often are prescribed. They are really two pairs of glasses in one. The lower part of the glass is for near vision; the upper part, for distance vision. The glasses permit the wearer to see both near and distant objects clearly. A further refinement is the use of trifocals (3 kinds of lens in 1 glass), which some patients find even more effective for viewing objects at various distances. Some persons who have never needed glasses previously use "reading glasses" that enable them to see close objects. Bifocals with a plain upper portion are sometimes used by those who need no distance correction, so that glasses do not have to be removed and replaced constantly. Halfmoon or "half-eye" lenses attain the same purpose.

Nurses are frequently asked such questions as "Are contact lenses safe?" and "Are certain eyedrops any good?" Often, too, nurses are the first to be consulted after accidents at work or at home, such as when a neighbor splashes bleach into her eyes. In such situations nurses need to know what first aid to give, how to instruct others to give it, if necessary, and when to refer the patient to the doctor.

Contact lenses are tiny, almost invisible plastic lenses that fit directly on the cornea, separated only by the tear film from the eye itself. They are worn by people who object to the appearance of conventional glasses in frames and by those with special needs that can be met more adequately by contact lenses. Some patients who have had cataracts removed benefit from the use of contact lenses.

The most common dangers involved in the use of contact lenses are injury to and infection of the cornea. Patients who express interest in contact lenses should be referred to the ophthalmologist. If it is decided that the patient is a suitable candidate for contact lenses, he is carefully fitted with them and is instructed by the doctor in their use. A special type of contact lens known as a scleral lens fits the entire front of the eyeball. These lenses are sometimes prescribed for treatment of certain diseases of the cornea or conjunctiva. Athletes sometimes wear scleral lenses.

Eyedrops. People who ask about the use of eyedrops to soothe the eyes can be told that such preparations approved for sale without prescription are generally (but by no means always) harmless in themselves, but that harm can come from using any such preparation as a substitute for medical attention when the eyes are persistently irritated or uncomfortable. Allergy, the need for glasses, and even beginning glaucoma may cause discomfort. Those who experience itching, burning, or other discomforts of their eyes should consult an ophthalmologist.

Cataract

A cataract is a condition in which the lens of the eye becomes opaque (no longer transparent), thus reducing the amount of light reaching the retina. The lens is a small, transparent structure that lies behind the iris. It is enclosed in an elastic membrane called the *capsule*. The lens is one of the refractive media through which light passes. Normally, the lens is not visible; we see only the dark spot which is the opening (pupil) through which light passes. When the lens becomes opaque, it becomes visible as a white or a gray spot behind the pupil.

Vision diminishes as the lens becomes opaque. The process usually advances slowly, and eventually it leads to loss of sight. If both eyes are severely affected, the patient becomes blind. Cataract is, in fact, the most common cause of blindness.

Cataracts may be congenital, they may be caused by injury to the lens, or they may be secondary to other diseases of the eye. When cataracts occur in response to injury, usually they develop quickly. Most cataracts, however, are caused by degenerative changes associated with the aging process, and they tend to develop slowly. Although some people develop cataracts in earlier life, the incidence of the condition rises steadily with advancing years. Cataracts are especially common among persons in the 7th, 8th, and 9th decades of life. A high incidence of cataracts occurs among patients with certain diseases, such as diabetes. A family history of cataracts is often pronounced.

The treatment of cataract involves surgical removal of the lens when vision is sufficiently impaired; changing eyeglasses does not give any improvement. No way has yet been found to restore the lens to its normal transparency. Removal of the lens is necessary because its opacity prevents light rays from reaching the retina. The lens may be removed by the intracapsular method (removal of the lens within its capsule) or by the extracapsular method (removal of the lens, leaving the posterior portion of its capsule in position). The choice of method is made by the surgeon after considering the patient's age and the degree of opacity of the cataract. The operation is often done under local anesthesia, but general anesthesia is sometimes used and has certain advantages especially in the case of a very apprehensive patient. A recent development has been the use of a probe cooled to very low temperatures. The cataract is partially frozen and extracted in contact with the cold probe. This technique is known as cryosurgery.

Table 18-1.
Nursing management of the patient having cataract surgery

The patient is kept in bed as ordered by the physician.
The bed is usually kept flat or in low Fowler's position.
The patient does deep-breathing exercises every 2 hours. Do not encourage coughing.
Straining is to be avoided.
If nausea and vomiting occur, an antiemetic is indicated.
Check the dressing. Report *any* drainage or signs of bleeding immediately.
Reinforce the eye dressing and/or the tape anchoring the dressing when necessary.

Another method of removal is phaco emulsification, which uses ultrasound to break the lens into minute particles which are then removed by aspiration. With this method, the patient usually returns to full activity in a short time.

After the lens has been removed, the patient must wear a strong lens (eyeglass) to take its place. The correcting lens causes the patient to see objects about one third larger than a normal eye sees them. If the lens has been removed from both eyes, the patient can continue to use both eyes simultaneously. However, if only one eye has had the lens removed, the patient must use only one eye at a time. Contact lenses usually solve this problem. Some patients can be fitted with a contact lens for the aphakic eye (the eye from which the lens has been removed). The use of the contact lens lessens the difference in the size of the image perceived by each eye and makes binocular vision possible.

Postoperative nursing management of the patient having surgical removal of a cataract is given in Table 18-1.

The patient is usually kept on bed rest, with the bed flat or in a low Fowler's position. The head may be positioned with sandbags. The length of time the patient is kept in bed will vary and can be from 4 hours to 1, 2, or more days.

Two major complications of cataract extraction are loss of vitreous humor and hemorrhage. Loss of vitreous humor can occur during or after surgery; it is serious, because vitreous does not regenerate, and its loss may cause serious damage to the eye. Hemorrhage can injure the delicate structures of the eye. Special care is taken during the postoperative period to prevent straining, such as straining at stool, and sudden movement or jarring of the head, which might lead to hemorrhage or opening of the incision.

Glaucoma

The *anterior chamber* of the eye lies between the cornea anteriorly and the iris posteriorly. The anterior chamber is filled with *aqueous humor,* a transparent fluid that nourishes the lens and the cornea. At the outer margin of the anterior chamber, between the iris and the cornea, lies the angle of the anterior chamber. It is at this angle that the aqueous humor drains through sievelike structures into the canal of Schlemm and, from there, into the general circulation. A balance is achieved between the amount of aqueous humor formed by the ciliary body and the amount drained out of the eye. This balance helps to maintain normal intraocular pressure.

Glaucoma is a condition that results from increased intraocular pressure due to a disturbance of the normal balance between the production and the drainage of the aqueous humor that fills the anterior chamber.

Glaucoma may be classed as primary or secondary:

Primary glaucoma

- Open-angle glaucoma, also called chronic simple glaucoma;
- Closed-angle glaucoma, also called narrow-angle or acute congestive glaucoma. There are acute and chronic forms of this type of glaucoma.

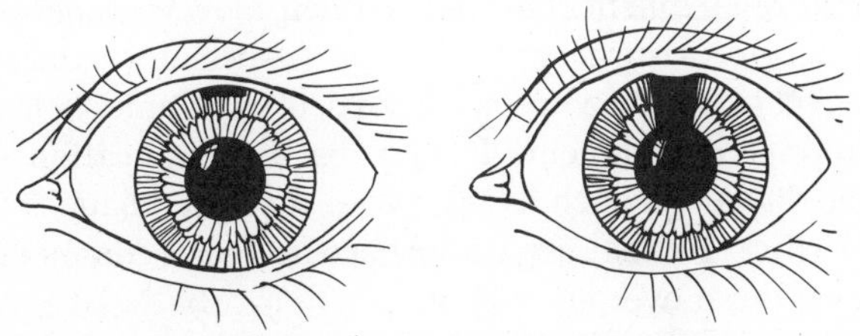

figure 18-6. (A) Appearance of the eye after peripheral iridectomy. (B) After keyhole (sector) iridectomy.

Secondary glaucoma

- Glaucoma due to tumors, injury, hemorrhage, inflammation, etc.

Although glaucoma can occur at any age, it is most common over 40. Anatomic abnormalities and degenerative changes play a part in causing glaucoma. Its appearance sometimes seems to be related to emotional stress. Glaucoma is much more common among people who have a family history of glaucoma.

Prompt diagnosis and treatment are of the utmost importance in preventing loss of vision. Everyone should be examined regularly for early indications of glaucoma.

Acute glaucoma

Symptoms include severe pain in and around the eyes, blurred vision, and the appearance of halos (colored circles), particularly around lights. The attack also may be accompanied by nausea and vomiting and a steamy appearance of the cornea. Acute attacks can occur suddenly, with little or no warning.

Drug Therapy. Miotics (drugs that constrict the pupil) are given at once to pull the iris away from the drainage channels, so that drainage of aqueous can resume, thus reducing the intraocular pressure and relieving the symptoms. Acetazolamide (Diamox), a carbonic anhydrase inhibitor, may be given to slow the production of aqueous fluid, thus helping to decrease the intraocular pressure. Drugs are likely to be used just before and during surgery, in order to lessen intraocular pressure thus rendering the operation safe. Analgesics are given to relieve pain, and the patient is kept at complete rest.

Surgery. Early surgical intervention usually is indicated to relieve acute glaucoma and to prevent further attacks. *Iridectomy* is performed to relieve the symptoms of acute closed-angle glaucoma: a section of iris is removed, thus preventing it from bulging forward, crowding the chamber angle and obstructing the drainage of aqueous fluid. Thus, a permanent entrance to the drainage canal is achieved. Two types of iridectomy are the *peripheral,* in which a small section of iris is removed at the periphery, and the *sector* or *keyhole,* in which a larger segment of iris is removed (Fig. 18-6).

Chronic glaucoma

Symptoms. Chronic glaucoma occurs more frequently than acute glaucoma. Often, symptoms are absent, or they are not so dramatic and therefore are more readily disregarded. The patient may have occasional periods when he sees rings around lights, has blurred vision, and experiences some discomfort or aching of the eyes. These mild symptoms are sometimes precipitated by prolonged watching of TV or moving pictures, or by emotional upsets. Sometimes, a reduction in the field of vision is the first indication of chronic glaucoma. The patient may fail to see things on either side and appear to be awkward or clumsy by bumping into doors or furniture. The impairment of peripheral vision is a hazard if the person drives a car, because he is unable to see pedestrians or vehicles that are off to the side. Sometimes the patient's family are the first to notice this visual defect, perhaps after narrowly escaping a highway accident.

DRUG THERAPY. Patients who exhibit such symptoms should seek medical attention promptly. As in acute glaucoma, miotics, such as eserine or pilocarpine, are used. Newer long-acting miotics include echothiophate iodide (Phospholine iodide), which requires instillation only once or twice in 24 hours. Epinephrine is also used as eyedrops. Carbonic anhydrase inhibitors, such as acetazolamide (Diamox), are often prescribed. Some of these patients require iridectomy if chronic angle-closure is present. When medical treatment is no longer effective, surgery is considered.

SURGERY. Drainage operations frequently performed for chronic glaucoma include sclerectomy, trephination, iridencleisis and thermal sclerostomy.

GENERAL MEASURES

All patients with glaucoma (even those who have had surgery) require continued care and examinations as recommended by the ophthalmologist. Certain general measures also can help to control the condition. The patient should be instructed to:

- Avoid *all* drugs containing atropine. This includes prescription as well as nonprescription drugs. Some preparations advertised as beneficial for symptoms of a cold or an allergy contain atropine.
- Maintain regular bowel habits. (Straining at stool can raise intraocular pressure.)
- Avoid emotional upsets, and especially avoid crying, which increases intraocular pressure.
- Avoid heavy lifting. (This, too, can raise intraocular pressure.)
- Limit activities that make the eyes feel strained or fatigued.
- Keep an extra supply of prescribed drugs on hand for vacations, over holidays, or in case some is spilled.
- Carry a card stating that he has glaucoma, so that necessary therapy can be continued even if he is sick or hurt.

Extreme care must be taken in administering eyedrops to any patient and especially to patients with glaucoma. Usually, a miotic is ordered to constrict the pupil. If through error a mydriatic, such as atropine, is given, the resulting dilation of the pupil can further obstruct drainage of aqueous humor, precipitating an acute attack that could result in permanent blindness. *No amount of caution is too great to prevent such a tragedy.* Notice carefully which eye is to receive the medication, read the doctor's order and the label on the bottle carefully, and identify the patient before instilling the drop in his eye.

Detached retina

The *retina*, the innermost coat of the eye, lies inside the choroid. The retina is composed of a pigmented outer layer and an inner sensory layer. The two layers are held very closely together; however, there is a potential space between them. The sensory layer of the retina receives visual stimuli that are then transmitted to the brain by the optic nerve. The pigmented layer is in close contact with the choroid, through which both layers of the retina receive their blood supply.

In detached retina the sensory layer becomes separated from the pigmented layer of the retina. The separation of the two layers of the retina deprives the sensory layer of its blood supply. Vision is lost in the affected area, because the sensory layer is no longer able to receive visual stimuli. Fluid (vitreous humor) flows between the separated layers of the retina, holding the layers apart and causing further separation.

Retinal separation is usually associated with a hole or a tear in the retina, which results from stretching or from degenerative changes in the retina. Often, retinal detachment follows a sudden blow, a penetrating injury, or surgery on the eye (especially cataract removal). Loss of vitreous is particularly liable to lead to retinal detachment. It may be a complication of other disorders, such as advanced diabetic changes in the retina. Retinal separation occurs more commonly among those over 40.

SYMPTOMS. The patient often notices definite "gaps" in his vision or areas in which he cannot see. Sometimes, he has the feeling that a curtain is being drawn over his field of vision, and he commonly sees flashes of light. The sensation of spots or moving particles before the eyes is common. Complete loss of vision may occur in the affected eye. The patient has no pain, but he is usually extremely apprehensive.

Although the prognosis is guarded, it is now more favorable because of the advances in surgical treatment.

DIAGNOSIS AND TREATMENT. Prompt diagnosis and treatment are essential. After examining the patient's retina with the ophthalmoscope and establishing the diagnosis, the doctor usually recommends prompt admission to the hospital. The physician's orders on admission usually include rest and the use of mydriatics to dilate the pupil, thus facilitating further examination.

Surgical intervention may include several methods utilized to reattach the separated retina: cryosurgery, electrodiathermy, photocoagulation (use of a laser beam) and the scleral buckling procedure.

After surgery the patient is kept on complete bed rest for 1 day or longer. In some instances the physician may order sandbags placed on both sides of the head for immobilization. The patient should not be turned or moved unless movement is ordered. If both eyes are covered, the patient should always have a call light within reach. Before going home, the patient is instructed to avoid jarring or bumping his head, and not to do any heavy lifting. Usually, he is advised to wear dark glasses for several weeks, thereby preventing the discomfort from bright light that occurs after treatment with mydriatics.

Other common eye disorders are listed in Table 18-2.

Table 18-2.
Common eye disorders

CONDITION	DEFINITION	TREATMENT
Uveitis	Inflammation of the uveal tract (iris, ciliary body, choroid)	Mydriatics, antibiotics, hot compresses
Conjunctivitis (pinkeye)	An inflammation of the membrane that lines the eyelids and covers the front of the eyeball, except the cornea	Depending on cause: antibiotics or avoidance of allergen, antihistamines
Keratitis	Inflammation of the cornea	Antibiotics, chemotherapeutic agents, cycloplegics
Hordeolum (sty)	An infection at the edge of the eyelid which originates in a lash follicle	Hot compresses; occasionally, surgery and antibiotics may be necessary
Chalazion	Infection and firm swelling of the gland in the eyelid that helps to maintain the normal tear-film on the eyeball	Surgical excision
Ectropion	Turning out of the eyelid	Usually surgical
Entropion	Turning in of the eyelid	Usually surgical
Ptosis	Drooping of the upper eyelid	Usually surgical

Sympathetic ophthalmia

Injury of one eye sometimes results in the development of severe inflammation of the fellow eye. This rare condition is called *sympathetic ophthalmia.* Typically several weeks after serious injury to one eye, the other eye develops severe uveitis that eventually may lead to loss of sight.

The cause of sympathetic ophthalmia is unknown. It is most likely to occur after penetrating injuries of the eyeball. Therefore, it is sometimes necessary to remove a severely injured eye (enucleation) without delay, in order to avoid risk to the unaffected eye with the possibility of the loss of sight in both eyes. Recently, however, corticosteroids have proved to be so effective that enucleation often is avoided.

Often, enucleation is resisted by the patient and his family. Frequently, they feel that while the patient still has the eye, there is hope that it will heal. Removal of the eye means irreparable loss of the use of that eye, as well as the trauma accompanying the loss of a part of oneself. Such decisions in many cases are made more difficult by the fact that they follow an accident that already has caused pain and fear and has threatened loss of sight. Because the mechanism of sympathetic ophthalmia is mysterious, it is difficult for a patient to believe that such a thing could happen to the unaffected eye.

The nurse can help the patient and his family by letting them express their fears and disbeliefs and ask questions. It is essential that the nurse know just what the doctor has told the patient and his family. She then can repeat this explanation, or, if the patient seems not to understand, the nurse can talk the matter over with the doctor.

Enucleation

Removal of the eye also may be necessary when the eye has been destroyed by injury or disease, or if a malignant tumor develops. Fortunately, malignant tumors of the eye are not common. However, removal of the eye is necessary when a tumor is discovered, to prevent the spread of malignant cells to other parts of the body. Sometimes, the eye is removed to relieve pain, when it has been severely damaged by injury or disease, and is blind.

The terms *enucleation* and *evisceration* have different meanings. *Evisceration* means removal of the contents of the eyeball, leaving the sclera in place. *Enucleation* means removal of the entire eyeball.

When enucleation is performed, a ball made of metal or plastic usually is buried in the capsule of connective tissue from which the eyeball has been removed. The eye muscles attach to this capsule and give movement to the ball that it now contains. After the tissues have healed, a glass or plastic prosthesis, shaped like a shell, is placed over the buried ball. The shell is painted to match the patient's remaining eye, and it is the part that is sometimes referred to as a "glass eye."

Depression is common after the operation. No amount of explanation or reassurance erases the fact that the patient has lost his eye, and that the loss is irretrievable. Most patients are gradually able to accept the result of enucleation, and they become interested in acquiring a prosthesis.

After enucleation, a pressure dressing is applied. The patient is observed carefully for any symptoms of bleeding or infection. The dressing is changed by the surgeon. Usually, the patient is allowed out of bed the day after the operation.

When healing is complete (approximately 2 to 4 weeks), the patient is fitted with the shell. The patient learns to insert and remove the prosthesis himself. Usually, he removes it before going to bed at night, and he inserts it the next morning. When the patient is learning to insert and to remove the prosthesis, he should hold his head over a soft surface, such as a bed or a well-padded table, so that the shell will not be broken if it is dropped. The shell is cleansed gently after removal, and it is kept in a safe place where it will not be scratched or broken.

Nursing management of the patient with an eye disorder

Any eye disease, injury, or operation can be upsetting and even frightening because of its possible effect on vision. The patient can be helped by careful explanation of his condition and the treatment or surgery to be instituted.

Some patients experience photophobia. Turning the bed so that it does not face the window and adjusting the blinds to keep out direct sunlight are important comfort measures. Often, the patient is instructed to wear dark glasses to protect his eyes from excessive light and glare.

Preoperative care

Many patients with eye disorders come to the hospital for surgery. At the time of admission the patient may have diminished or absent vision; sometimes, he enters the hospital in the hope that his vision will be improved by an operation. In other instances the patient has useful vision on admission, but, because of the kind of operation to be performed, both eyes may be covered during the immediate postoperative period. Since the eyes move together, it is often necessary to cover both eyes to provide rest for the eye that has had surgery.

Admission Procedure. The admission procedure should be modified to help both types of patient. If the patient cannot see, make a special effort to help him to become oriented to his surroundings. Introduce him to the other patients in the room. If he is able, allow him to walk about his room with assistance, noting the location of the furniture, the bathroom, and particularly the call light, so that he knows how to call for help when he needs it. A walk in the hall, during which the location of other rooms, nurses' station, and lounge are pointed out, also helps him to form a mental picture of his new surroundings.

If, on the other hand, the patient can see and later will have both eyes covered, help him to use his sight to the greatest advantage in orienting himself to his room, his neighbors, and the area as a whole. The next day, when his eyes are covered, he will be able to recall the layout of his new surroundings, and he will feel less lost and confused. If both eyes are to be covered, even though only one will actually have surgery, it is important to explain this to the patient, so that

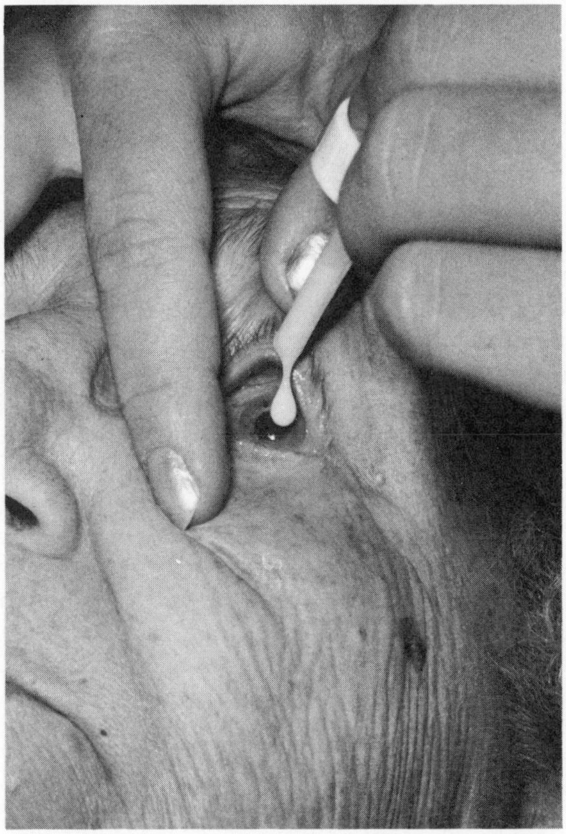

figure 18-7. When eyedrops are instilled, the patient looks up. The lower lid is gently everted as the drop is placed just inside it. (Photograph—D. Atkinson)

later he does not fear that some injury or complication has befallen his unaffected eye.

SEDATION. Usually, the preoperative preparation includes sedation to ensure rest the night before surgery and relaxation before the patient goes to the operating room. Elderly patients should be observed carefully after sedatives have been administered. Sometimes, the patient becomes disoriented and restless after the administration of sedatives, particularly the barbiturates.

EYEDROP TECHNIQUE. Often, eyedrops, such as antibiotics or mydriatics, are ordered at specified intervals. When you instill an eyedrop, have the patient lying down or seated, with his head tilted backward. Rest against the patient's forehead the hand in which you are holding the dropper (Fig. 18-7). (Your little finger and the side of your hand rest against the patient's forehead, while your thumb and forefinger grasp the dropper or the plastic squeeze bottle containing the medication.) This position helps to steady your hand and provides control of the dropper. The dropper never should be poked toward the patient's eye without resting the hand on the patient's forehead; if the patient moves suddenly, the dropper could be thrust into his eye. The patient is asked to look up, the lower lid is gently everted, and the drop is placed just inside the lower lid. The patient is asked to close his eye gently, allowing the medication to bathe his eye. The drop should not be allowed to fall on the cornea, which is very sensitive. Plastic squeeze bottles are often used in place of droppers. The medication is instilled into the eye directly from the bottle. The procedure for holding the bottle and inserting the drop is the same as that described in relation to the dropper.

OTHER CONSIDERATIONS. Sometimes, an enema is ordered the evening before surgery, particularly if it is desirable for the patient to avoid the exertion of moving his bowels the first day or two after surgery.

If the patient's head must be kept very still postoperatively, it is important to plan ahead, so that as much care as possible can be given before surgery and preparations can be made that will permit the patient to lie quietly with the least possible discomfort. For example, the male patient should shave before his operation. The female patient should have her hair carefully combed and held back from her face. Braiding the hair helps to keep long hair neat. A contour sheet fits better than an ordinary sheet, and stays smooth longer without frequent need for pulling and tightening it.

Any respiratory condition, such as allergy or infection, that might cause sneezing or coughing is treated before the patient has surgery to minimize the possibility of sneezing and coughing after surgery. Sneezing or coughing can cause hemorrage during the early postoperative period.

Eye surgery on adults is often performed under local anesthesia. Preoperative sedation helps to lessen the patient's apprehension during the procedure, and he is able to respond and to cooperate with the surgeon. For example, he can follow directions, such as "Look up." The use of local anesthesia formerly had the advantage of lessening the likelihood of postoperative nausea and vomiting. Vomiting produces strain and may cause hemorrhage or separation of the incision. With modern anesthetic techniques and the use of new drugs, however, there should be no nausea or vomiting after general anesthesia. This is especially advantageous in cataract surgery.

Postoperative care

Postoperative care is directed toward the prevention of hemorrhage or the disruption of the surgical wound. Pressure or trauma to the eye or the head, such as that resulting from jarring or suddenly turning the head, is avoided. The patient is encouraged to move his arms and his legs, but he is discouraged from raising his head or turning it suddenly.

In Bed. After surgery the patient is moved carefully and gently from the operating table to a cart or to his own bed. Placing him directly in his own bed means that he is moved only once, and that he does not have to be moved to a stretcher and then to his bed.

The patient is wheeled back to his room. If both eyes are covered, it is important to show him the location of his call light and to assure him that he is back in his own room. Whether or not both eyes are covered, side rails should be kept in place. Older people, especially, are likely to become confused and to attempt to get out of bed.

Keeping both eyes covered provides rest for the operated eye. Some older people, however, become restless and disoriented when they are unable to see. It is very important to stay with the patient as much as possible. A few words spoken frequently and the touch of your hand help the patient to realize that he is not alone, and they help to keep him in contact with his environment. Many patients need frequent gentle reminders not to touch the dressing or to lift the head. Often the assurance of someone's presence can help the patient to relax enough to fall asleep. Sometimes, a family member can help by sitting quietly at the patient's bedside and assuring him that someone is there.

When a patient with both eyes covered becomes extremely excited and disoriented, attempting to climb out of bed over the side rails, the unoperated eye is uncovered as an emergency measure. Usually, the ability to see helps the patient become oriented, and it calms him enough to be able again to cooperate. Restraining the patient or giving him additional sedation often makes him more disoriented in such circumstances. It is important to check with the surgeon beforehand concerning the measures to be taken if the patient becomes disoriented.

If the patient vomits, his head should be turned gently to the side to prevent aspiration of vomitus, but the head should not be raised. Measures that help the patient to avoid vomiting, sneezing, and coughing should be used. For example, he is not given anything by mouth if he feels nauseated, since this may lead to vomiting. If he experiences nausea, this symptom should promptly be reported to the surgeon. He may prescribe the injection of a drug, such as chlorpromazine (Thorazine), to relieve the nausea and to lessen the possibility of vomiting. Often a p.r.n. order for an antiemetic drug is given.

The patient who must maintain a fixed head position has to be fed. Often the diet is restricted to fluids on the day of surgery to avoid nausea, vomiting, and the facial movements required by chewing. Usually, a soft diet is permitted on the day after surgery. The patient is fed until the surgeon indicates that the fixed head position is no longer necessary, and until the unaffected eye is uncovered.

Specific postoperative orders differ widely, depending on the type of operation and the preferences of the surgeon. Before giving nursing care to any patient who has had eye surgery, you should be able to answer each of the following questions. Most of the information can be obtained directly from the doctor's order sheet. Conferences with the doctor and the head nurse will also help you to learn the answers.

- May the patient have a pillow?
- May the head of the patient's bed be elevated? If so, how much?
- May the patient turn? If so, to which side may he turn?
- May he brush his teeth, or should mouth care be limited to rinsing his mouth with mouthwash?
- How soon may he be shaved?

Everything must be done for the patient in a slow, gentle way. Explanation is important, particularly if both the patient's eyes are covered. Saying your name helps the patient to learn who you are by the sound of your voice. Avoid jarring the bed, because sudden movements can startle the patient and may even injure his eye.

Diversion helps the long hours to pass more quickly. It also helps to keep the patient in contact with his environment. A radio becomes a real companion to a patient who cannot see.

If the patient is unable to turn for several days, certain adaptations in his care will be necessary. The sheets are kept as clean and smooth as possible without changing them. If necessary, a small disposable pad may be placed under the patient's buttocks and changed as necessary merely by sliding it in and out when the patient raises his hips. Assistance with the

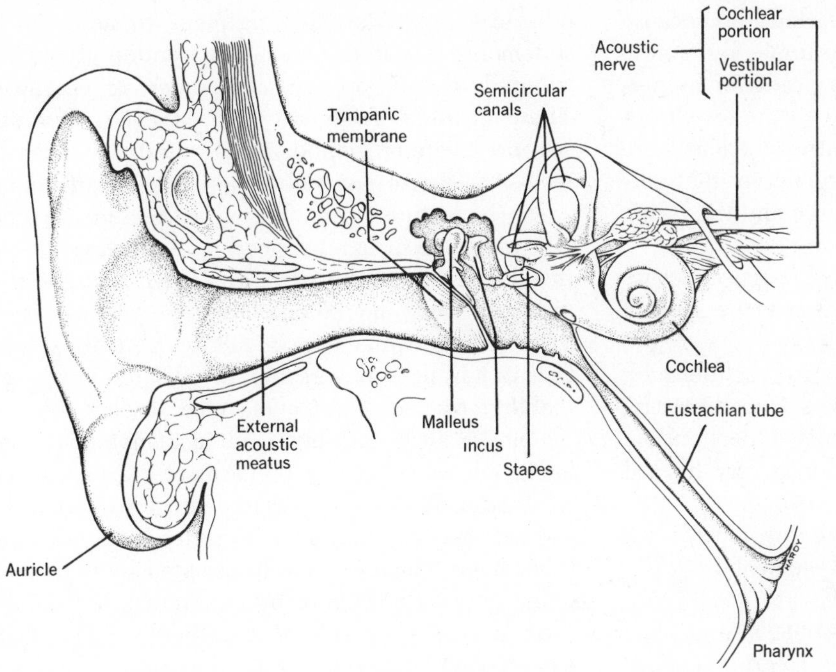

figure 18-8. Diagram of the ear, showing the external, middle, and internal subdivisions.

use of the bedpan and the urinal is important, so that the patient does not raise his head. The sacrum may be massaged gently by slipping the hand under the patient's back when he raises his hips slightly off the mattress. If prolonged bed rest is prescribed, an alternating pressure mattress, or a flotation pad, may be necessary.

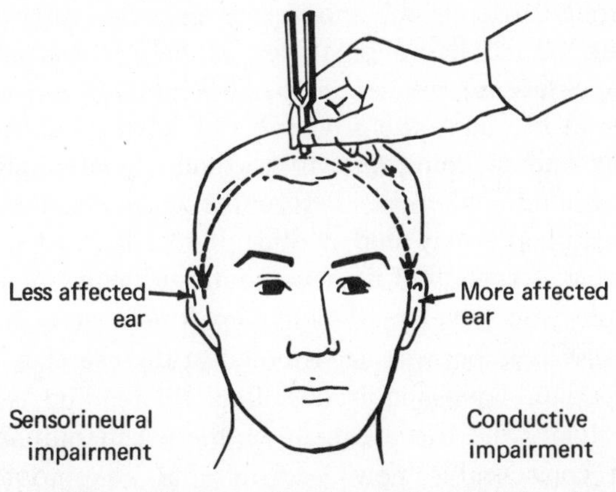

figure 18-9. When a vibrating tuning fork is placed against the forehead of the patient with conductive hearing loss, the tone sounds louder in the more affected ear; whereas to the patient with sensorineural hearing loss, the tone sounds louder in the less affected ear.

Out of Bed. The length of time that the patient must remain in bed varies. Often he is allowed out of bed a day or two after surgery, and the unoperated eye is uncovered. Sometimes, he must remain quietly in bed for a week or even longer. Usually, his appetite returns to normal when he is allowed up and can feed himself. He also finds it easier to move his bowels when he can assume a more normal position on a commode chair or a toilet. Sometimes, the doctor orders an enema, gentle laxative, or stool softener to help to reestablish regular elimination. Straining at stool must be avoided, because it may lead to hemorrhage or strain the wound in the operated eye.

Hearing impairment

Hearing loss may be divided into two types: conductive and sensorineural (Figs. 18-8 and 18-9). *Conductive hearing loss* or *conduction deafness* is caused by any disease or injury that interferes with the conduction of sound waves to the inner ear. For example, an accumulation of cerumen in the auditory canal or the failure of the ossicles to vibrate may cause conductive hearing loss. *Sensorineural hearing loss* or *sensorineural deafness* (sometimes called "nerve deafness") results from the malfunction of the inner ear, the auditory nerve, or the auditory center in the brain. The prognosis is better in conductive hearing loss because often its cause can be treated—for example, by removing excess cerumen from the auditory canal or by performing surgery to restore the ability of the ossicles to vibrate. Persons with conductive deafness benefit more from the use of hearing aids, since the organs that perceive sound, such as the auditory nerve and the brain, are able to function.

A recent cause of sensorineural deafness is exposure to loud music. This type of deafness may be seen in the musicians as well as in the listeners.

Sensorineural deafness is usually irreversible and, thus far, is beyond surgical correction. Unfortunately, these patients frequently have difficulty understanding speech and therefore can be helped to a very limited degree by a hearing aid.

Some patients have *mixed hearing loss,* a combination of conductive and sensorineural elements.

The Patient with Hearing Loss

Communication and Attitudes. Hearing loss can seriously impair a person's ability to protect himself and to communicate with others; thus it can keep him out of touch with his environment. Perhaps most of us do not realize how often sounds warn us of danger. For example, the failure to hear the sounds of a fire or an approaching car could lead to serious injury. Listening to what others say is a vital element in all human relationships. Everyday life is accompanied by a background of sounds that we hear without being aware of them. The sound of others moving about the house or of traffic in the distance helps us to feel part of a dynamic world and to feel more alive ourselves. The loss of this aspect of hearing has profound effects on the patient, who may describe having a feeling that "the world is dead." The loss of this auditory background is believed to contribute significantly to the depression that so commonly occurs after a patient loses his hearing. Besides serving to keep us in tune with the world, the auditory background noises serve as cues to changes that are occurring in the environment, thus helping us to become ready to meet and cope with these changes. Because he lacks these cues, the deaf person often feels vaguely insecure. While he is very keenly aware of his inability to hear conversation, he may be unaware of the reason for his feeling of insecurity. Explanation of this relationship can help the patient to cope with this reaction.

Whereas blindness usually is obvious to others, deafness usually is not. The person with impaired hearing looks very much like everyone else, and so his quizzical expression, his frequent requests to have statements repeated, and his inattention often are attributed to stubbornness, ill temper, or eccentricity. These attitudes frequently persist even after others become aware of the individual's disability. Such comments as "He can hear when he wants to" are common.

Such attitudes are unusual in relation to people who are blind or handicapped in other ways. Just why this difference exists is not clear. The less visible nature of hearing loss may be one factor. People may become irritated when one who seems to have no disability fails to join in a conversation or talks too loudly. (The inability to hear their own voices causes some deaf people to speak too loudly or in monotonous tones.)

People with hearing impairment are very sensitive to these attitudes. Many flatly refuse to wear a hearing aid, because they feel it carries a stigma. On the other hand, glasses are well accepted by most people. Some persons with hearing loss refuse to admit that they have the disability and thereby they deprive themselves of the help that they require. For example, in addition to helping the patient hear, the hearing aid can serve useful purposes by calling attention to the disability, thus encouraging others to speak more slowly and more distinctly and indicating that problems in communication are due to hearing deficit rather than to intellectual impairment.

Factors Influencing Rehabilitation. The age at which hearing loss occurs, as well as the severity of the impairment, affects rehabilitation. If a person has been born deaf, his education and his opportunities for marriage, friendship, and career may be jeopardized unless he has had a great deal of help in learning to compensate for the handicap. Those who become deaf later in life have the advantage of having heard normally and of being able to become educated, start a home, and find a job before the onset of deafness. Older people may find it difficult to adjust to loss of hearing, especially if it occurs quite suddenly. Whereas people who develop hearing impairment early in life usually have become accustomed to the use of a hearing aid or have acquired skill in lip reading during childhood, the development of these capabilities entails considerable new learning and adaptation for older persons.

There are many ways of helping people with hearing loss. Many patients are taught speech reading. They learn to watch facial movements so closely and skillfully that they can understand what is said. Often the patient does not catch every word; however, he understands enough to enable him to follow the conversation. The term *speech reading* is preferred by many to *lip reading,* because the skill actually encompasses not only reading lips but also noting facial expressions and gestures. The person who uses speech reading can be helped if others face him when they speak, so that he can see their lip movements and facial expressions.

Another way of helping people who use speech reading is to mention briefly and tactfully the topic of the conversation that he is following. For example, if a lively discussion about baseball is taking place, turning to him and saying distinctly, "We are discussing baseball" will help him to follow the conversation. If the patient does not understand you, restate the thought in different words. Some words are more difficult to "read" than others, and changing the wording often helps the speech reader to understand what is meant. Avoid dropping your voice at the end of a sentence. Pronounce new or unfamiliar words with special care. Do not try to talk to the patient when you have something in your mouth, and avoid placing your hand over your mouth while speaking.

Shouting is seldom a help. Often it only confuses and embarrasses the patient. Speak somewhat more loudly, but emphasize slowness and distinctness of speech. Above all, try not to show excitement or impatience when the patient fails to understand. Treat the disability as you would any other—accept it, and do everything that you can to help the patient to compensate for it. If he speaks too loudly, tell him so tactfully, so that he can learn to modulate his voice.

Hearing aids

Modern hearing aids are battery-operated sound amplifiers with a transistor circuit. Adjustable volume and tone controls are provided, so that the wearer can adapt the aid to changing conditions.

Although hearing aids have helped many people, they do not restore normal hearing. In general, they do not provide as good a correction for the hearing loss as glasses provide for faulty vision. And unlike glasses, hearing aids require considerable time and effort to learn to use. The failure to understand these facts has led many persons to become discouraged and to abandon the use of the aid.

Because sound is considerably modified as it passes through the aid, it will approximate—but not duplicate—the sound that the patient remembers hearing before he became deaf. The range of tones is greatly reduced. However, the sounds are sufficiently similar to be interpreted correctly by most patients. The aid has the disadvantage of amplifying background noise as well as the sounds that the patient wants to hear. Amplified background noises are distracting, particularly to patients who have not become accustomed to the aid.

Despite these disadvantages, the modern hearing aid opens new vistas to many patients with hearing loss. Constant improvements are being made in these instruments, so that they are not only less conspicuous but more efficient. Their very efficiency poses a problem in adjustment. Patients sometimes find that the sudden increase in their ability to hear is quite startling. They must become accustomed to the sounds of everyday experiences all over again. (However, this is an adjustment that most people are delighted to make!)

Here are some ways that nurses can help patients to obtain the best possible results from a hearing aid:

- Direct the patient to an otologist or an otologic clinic for help in determining whether an aid is likely to benefit him, and if so, what type of aid would be most useful.
- Avoid building up unrealistic hopes about the help that a hearing aid can give. Stress the need for patience and training in the use of the aid.
- Encourage the patient to follow the directions given him by his doctor or by the manufacturer of his instrument.
- If a patient with hearing difficulty is admitted to the hospital, find out whether or not he uses an aid. If he does, ask his family to bring it to him. In the stress of illness the aid may be forgotten, and its absence can make the patient's adjustment to the hospital all the more difficult.
- Give your patient time to adjust his hearing aid, if he needs to, before speaking with him.
- Remember that the aid is very valuable to the patient, besides being expensive. Protect it from loss or injury when the patient is unable to do so—for example, when his illness is severe, or when he is in the operating room.

Disorders of the external auditory canal

The external auditory canal extends from its own orifice in the auricle to the tympanic membrane. The canal is approximately an inch long and contains the ceruminous glands.

The external auditory canal is subject to a variety of annoying disorders (Table 18-3). Usually, these are discomforts rather than threats to life or hearing. However, if they are not carefully and adequately treated, these disorders may involve the middle ear and become serious problems. Unskilled attempts at removing cerumen or foreign bodies may perforate the eardrum and push the material into the middle ear.

The nurse never should irrigate a patient's ear without specific orders from the doctor. Sometimes, nurses working in otologic clinics are specially instructed by a physician, and may be delegated to perform the irrigation after he has examined the ear (Fig. 18-10). Emphasis is placed on this, because patients often ask nurses to perform ear irrigations without medical direction.

INSECTS IN THE AUDITORY CANAL. Insects occasionally enter the canal. Although they usually fly out again, sometimes they remain inside. Their fluttering and buzzing are agonizing. Holding a flashlight to the ear often draws the insect out by attracting it to the light. A few drops of alcohol or mineral oil may be effective in killing the insect; turning the head to the side may help the dead insect to float out of the meatus. If these measures are not successful, the patient should be taken immediately to a doctor or a hospital emergency room. Never try to remove the insect with forceps or tweezers.

Conditions of the middle ear

The middle ear is a small, air-filled cavity in the temporal bone. Stretched across the middle ear cavity from the tympanic membrane to the oval window lies a chain of small bones called *ossicles*—the malleus, the incus and the stapes—joined together by small ligaments and attached to the tympanic membrane by the handle of the malleus (see Fig. 18-8). The footplate of the stapes fits into the oval window, held in position by a ligament that allows free motion for the transmission of sound. The medial wall of the middle ear has two openings that communicate with the inner ear, the oval window (fenestra ovalis) and the round window (fenestra rotunda). Sound waves pass into the external ear and its canal and strike the tympanic membrane, causing it to vibrate. The vibrations are transmitted by way of the mechanical linkage of malleus, incus, and stapes to the oval window. The motion of the footplate of the stapes in the oval window agitates the perilymph and the endolymph, thus stimulating the sensitive sound receptors of the organ of Corti, in the inner ear.

Table 18-3. Common disorders of the external auditory canal

External Auditory Canal Disorder	Treatment
Impacted cerumen	Warm water irrigations following ear examination by physician
Furuncles (boils)	Antibiotics, local application of heat, analgesics
External otitis	Ear drops containing antibiotics

Otosclerosis

Otosclerosis is a common cause of hearing impairment among adults. It results from bony ankylosis of the stapes, which interferes with the vibration of the stapes and the transmission of sound to the inner ear. Fixation of the stapes occurs gradually over a period of many years. The hearing loss usually becomes apparent to the patient during the second and the third decades of life and is more common among women. Heredity is an important causative factor; the majority of patients have a family history of the disease. The underlying cause of otosclerosis is unknown.

The progressive loss of hearing is the most characteristic symptom. The patient notices this symptom when it begins to interfere with his ability to follow conversation. The patient has particular difficulty in hearing others when they speak in soft, low tones, although he can hear adequately when the sound is loud enough. *Tinnitus* (a ringing or buzzing in the ears) may appear as the loss of hearing progresses. Tinnitus, which can occur in any type of hearing loss, is especially noticeable at night, when the surroundings

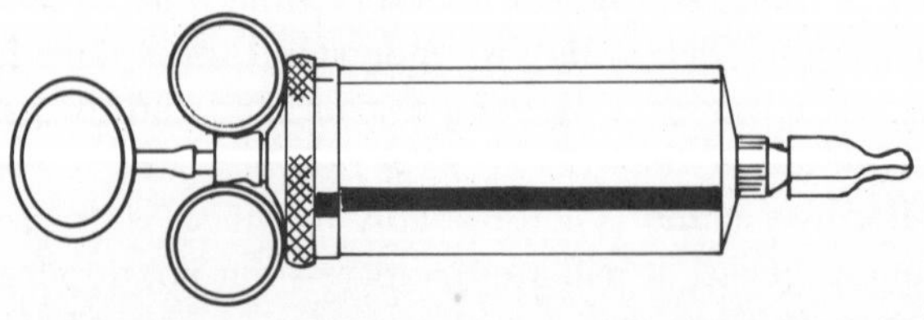

figure 18-10. Pomeroy syringe, usually used by the physician when he is removing cerumen by irrigation.

are quiet, and it can be very distressing to the patient.

The diagnosis is made by an otologist after noting the family history, examining the ears, and testing the hearing. Although the hearing loss in otosclerosis is of the conductive type, often with progression of the disease, involvement of the cochlea supervenes and the hearing loss becomes a mixed type.

Although at present there is no cure for otosclerosis, the hearing loss can be corrected by surgery and the use of a hearing aid. The potential success of surgery, as well as the ability to wear an aid, depends greatly on the severity of the sensorineural involvement; the prognosis is best when the hearing loss is purely conductive.

Stapes Surgery. In a procedure known as stapedectomy, surgeons remove the entire stapes and replace it with a prosthetic device composed of such substances as fat, Teflon, or a vein.

The surgery is carried out using very fine instruments and an operating microscope designed specifically for surgery on the ear.

Occasionally the ear may ooze immediately after surgery. The nurse should notify the doctor but should not attempt to stop the bleeding by additional pressure on the canal packing as this pressure may dislocate the prosthesis.

Whether the patient will be allowed to turn and which side (operated or unoperated) he can or cannot lie on will be stated by the surgeon in the postoperative orders. It is very important that this order is followed.

Dizziness or nausea may be noted, and antiemetics are usually ordered. If fever, headache, severe pain, excessive drainage, or extreme dizziness is noted, the physician should be notified immediately. When ambulation begins, the patient may have some vertigo for a short time and should therefore have assistance when he begins walking. Handrails in corridors and bathrooms are important in preventing falls and in giving the patient a greater feeling of security. The total period of hospitalization is usually brief; the patient may sometimes be discharged on the fourth postoperative day. He is cautioned not to blow his nose suddenly or violently, as this action may dislodge the prosthesis or loosen the eardrum before healing has taken place, or may result in infectious matter being blown up into the eustachian tube to the middle ear. He is cautioned to keep water out of the ear as this, too, may lead to infection. The physician usually orders an ear plug (a small piece of cotton) to be placed in the ear after the packing is removed. The cotton is gently placed in the outer ear canal and never pushed into the ear. Use of this ear plug may be ordered for a week or more after the packing is removed. It is usually changed once or twice daily. After healing has occurred the patient may shower, swim, and engage in practically all activities. Many surgeons restrict their patients from deep-water diving and caution against flying with a head cold, because severe pressure changes may dislodge the prosthesis.

A patient may be discouraged if hearing does not return immediately after surgery, thus creating concern regarding the success of surgery. He should be encouraged to talk this over with his physician; the nurse can also explain that the packing in the ear and the swelling of tissues after surgery decrease the sound reaching the middle ear.

Infections

The middle ear connects with the nasopharynx by way of the eustachian tube, which serves to equalize the air pressure on either side of the tympanic membrane. Upper respiratory infections spread readily from the nose and throat to the ear through this tube. Children are especially vulnerable because of the more nearly horizontal position of the eustachian tube during childhood. However, adults can and do develop ear infections, and in addition they suffer from the same consequences of ear infections as children. Before the development of antibiotics, ear infections often caused considerable damage to the ear. Use of antibiotics has created another problem: microorganisms are becoming resistant to them, and we are again faced with some infections for which the available antibiotics are of limited benefit.

Serous Otitis Media. This condition, in which fluid forms in the middle ear, can result from obstruction of the eustachian tube. The obstruction itself may be caused by infection, allergy, tumors, or sudden changes in altitude, such as sudden descents in an airplane in which case the condition is sometimes referred to as aero-otitis media. Measures that help prevent aero-otitis media include avoidance of flying while suffering from a head cold. Chewing gum, yawning, or repeated swallowing during descent open the eustachian tubes.

The Valsalva maneuver—a pinching of the nostrils while at the same time trying to blow air through the nose—is usually successful in equalizing the pressure on both sides of the eardrum.

The symptoms of serous otitis media include a feeling of fullness, diminished hearing, pain, and hearing one's own voice echoing in the involved ear. If allowed to remain, the fluid thickens and scars form, with resulting permanent hearing loss.

Treatment is surgical, by means of a simple *myringotomy*—an incision of the eardrum. This aids in release of the fluid trapped in the middle ear. A tiny plastic tube may be inserted into the eardrum to provide an opening should fluid again form.

Acute Purulent Otitis Media. This acute infection of the middle ear usually results from the spread of microorganisms to the middle ear through the eustachian tube during upper respiratory infections. Pus collects in the middle ear, causing increased pressure which, in turn, causes bulging of the eardrum.

The symptoms include fever, ear noises, malaise, severe earache, and diminished hearing. Using an otoscope, the doctor notes that the eardrum is red and bulging. Sometimes, it has perforated, and pus is present in the auditory canal. Prompt treatment usually can avoid rupture of the eardrum. Rupture often causes a jagged tear that heals slowly, sometimes incompletely, and with considerable scarring. Such scarring can interfere with the vibration of the drum, causing diminished hearing.

To prevent spontaneous rupture, the doctor may perform a myringotomy, letting the pus escape. This eases the pressure and relieves the throbbing pain. The incision heals readily with very little scarring. At first the discharge from the ear is bloody, and then it is purulent. The doctor may order eardrops to facilitate drainage. He may ask the nurse to wipe the external portions of the canal with a dry sterile applicator. Cotton plugs should not be stuffed into the ear, because it is important for the pus to drain. The external ear must be cleaned frequently. Applying petrolatum to the skin helps to prevent excoriation. A small piece of cotton may be placed loosely at the meatus to help to absorb the drainage. It should be changed frequently. The drainage may continue for several days.

Culture and sensitivity tests are performed on specimens of the purulent material to determine which antibiotics will be effective against the organisms. Antibiotics are given to control the infection. Fluids are encouraged. Rest and the avoidance of chilling are important until all symptoms of the infection have subsided.

The complications of acute purulent otitis media include mastoiditis (the middle ear connects with the mastoid process by complex passages through which infection can travel), scarring and/or permanent perforation of the eardrum, and hearing loss. The infection also may spread to the meninges, causing meningitis, or it may become chronic (chronic otitis media). Other complications include labyrinthitis, indicated by nystagmus, vertigo, nausea and vomiting; lateral sinus thrombosis (spread of the infection to the large veins at the base of the brain), causing clot formation and septicemia. Infection may injure the facial nerve and cause facial paralysis. Brain abscess may result from the extension of the infection to the brain.

These complications almost always occur when otitis media goes untreated. With prompt and correct treatment, complications are rare.

Patients with perforated eardrums are prone to repeated infections throughout life. Often a chronic infection develops that is difficult to cure, and that spreads throughout the ear and the mastoid process. Patients who have perforated eardrums should avoid getting water in the ear, since this readily causes infection. Special precautions must be taken when they are bathing. Custom-molded ear plugs plus a bathing cap are sometimes recommended to keep water out of the ears during swimming or bathing. Some physicians advise their patients who have perforated eardrums not to swim at all, because of the risk of severe infection if water should enter the middle ear. Patients with questions concerning this matter should be referred to the physician.

Plastic surgery (myringoplasty) is usually successful in repairing the perforated drum. In one technique the edges of the perforation are cauterized, and a patch of bloodsoaked Gelfoam is used as a scaffolding over which new tissues grow until they have completely filled in the defect.

Subsequent repeated and chronic infections, with all their risk of spreading the infection to the brain and the loss of hearing, may be avoided if the drum can be repaired.

Chronic Otitis Media. This preventable condition usually results from neglect, incomplete treatment of acute otitis media, or repeated attacks of acute otitis media with organisms that are resistant to antibiotic therapy. The patient usually has a chronic discharge from the ear, a reduction of hearing, and sometimes a slight fever. Treatment with antibiotics may be effective in controlling the infection. However, when it has persisted for a long time, destruction occurs in the middle ear and the mastoid process. Such patients have marked loss of hearing, and often they are in danger of spread of the infection to the brain. Surgery is usually recommended to eradicate the disease and to prevent further complications. Often, a radical mastoidectomy is necessary to remove the diseased tissue.

Mastoiditis. The spread of the infection to the mastoid process can occur in either acute or chronic otitis media. The symptoms of *acute mastoiditis* include pain and tenderness over the mastoid process, chills, fever, malaise, and headache. The treatment includes prompt administration of antibiotics and sometimes, if there is not a favorable response to medical treatment, simple mastoidectomy. Through a postaural (behind the ear) incision, the surgeon removes the infected mastoid cells. Hearing impairment usually does not occur.

Chronic mastoiditis carries a less favorable prognosis. Chronic infection in the mastoid process leads to destruction of the tissue, causing hearing loss. The infection usually involves the middle ear also, since chronic otitis media frequently causes chronic mastoiditis. Often, radical mastoidectomy is necessary to remove the diseased tissue. Usually, the hearing is reduced markedly because of the necessity for removing important structures. The diseased mastoid cells are removed, as well as the incus, the malleus and the eardrum. The middle ear and the mastoid become one cavity. The stapes is left in position to protect the entrance to the inner ear. Just how radical the operation must be depends on the extent of the infection. The more extensive the surgery, the greater the hearing loss. Surgical procedures have been developed recently that preserve important structures. These delicate operations are performed under magnification, and they require a great deal of time, patience, and surgical skill.

Principles in the management of any patient after ear surgery

Regardless of the specific nature of the operation, certain principles are applicable to the care of any patient after aural surgery. These may be summarized as follows:

- Make sure that the external ear and the surrounding skin are meticulously clean. Excess cerumen will be removed from the canal by the doctor.
- Injury to the facial nerve may occur during ear surgery. Note whether the patient can wrinkle his forehead, close his eyes, pucker his lips and bare his teeth. Report any inability to perform these movements. If these signs appear immediately after surgery, there probably has been damage to the facial nerve. If the paralysis appears after 12 to 24 hours postoperatively, it is probably due to edema; the doctor may recommend loosening the ear dressing and administering anti-inflammatory drugs.
- Strict adherence to aseptic techniques is essential. Because the ear is so close to the brain, any infection may endanger the patient's life. Antibiotics may be ordered to help prevent infection. Instruct the patient to keep his hands away from the dressing, which is changed only by the surgeon. Observe the dressing for drainage.
- Vertigo is common, due to the temporary effects on the body-balancing function of the semicircular canals. Special measures should be employed to protect the patient from falling. Side rails and handrails should be used, and the patient should be helped out of bed. Vertigo is very distressing. Explain that this symptom is not unusual after ear surgery, and that it will subside gradually.
- Instruct the patient not to blow his nose. During the postoperative period, nasal secretions should be wiped off the end of the nose without blowing it. Blowing the nose can permit infectious material to enter the operative area through the eustachian tube or may dislodge prostheses or grafts in the ear.

Disorders of the inner ear

The inner ear, or labyrinth, is a very complicated structure that lies deep in the temporal bone. It consists of a series of cavities and canals. The bony canals and spaces constitute the bony labyrinth. These canals are lined with periosteum and enclose the much smaller membranous labyrinth. The space between the two is filled with *perilymph.* The membranous labyrinth is filled with *endolymph.* The movement of this fluid stimulates the nerve endings of both branches (vestibular and cochlear) of the auditory nerve. There are two sections to the inner ear: an anterior portion, the cochlea; and a posterior portion, the semicircular canals.

Disorders of the inner ear are difficult to treat. Inner-ear deafness is of the sensorineural type, which usually cannot be helped by surgery and only occasionally by hearing aids. The auditory center in the brain, the inner ear, and the auditory nerve may be injured by drugs (such as streptomycin), tumors, systemic diseases (such as measles), prolonged exposure to loud noise, and the aging process. Management involves the prevention of further injury, if possible, and training in speech reading.

MENIERE'S DISEASE. The cause of Ménière's disease is unknown, and the pathological changes responsible for the symptoms are not entirely clear.

This condition is characterized by severe vertigo, tinnitus, and progressive hearing loss. It usually involves only one ear. An attack may last from a few minutes to weeks. The attacks occur with alarming suddenness. Often, the patient becomes afraid to leave his home lest he have an attack in public. For some patients, continued employment becomes impossible.

Symptomatic treatment includes the use of a low-sodium diet to lessen edema. Sedatives may help to relieve apprehension. Such drugs as dimenhydrinate (Dramamine) may lessen the symptoms. Bed rest is usually necessary during an acute attack. Some patients recover spontaneously from the disorder, or it may be so incapacitating that the labyrinth is destroyed surgically to relieve the symptoms. Ultrasonic waves have been used to destroy the labyrinth. Another type of operation has been developed that establishes permanent drainage of excessive endolymph from the inner ear into the subarachnoid space around the brain.

The nursing care of the patient with Ménière's disease is challenging. Every effort must be made not to aggravate the symptoms or to precipitate attacks by sudden movement. The patient should not turn over quickly, and the bed should be protected from excessive movement. All movements must be explained carefully beforehand and then carried out slowly. Protection from falls is essential when the vertigo is severe. It is important to use side rails when the patient is in bed and to give him assistance when he is out of bed. Foods and fluids are accepted better if they are offered frequently and in small amounts, and if the patient's preferences are considered.

General nutritional considerations

- Placing the food on the plate and putting napkin and utensils in the same position every day will help the blind person become adept at feeding himself.
- Tell the patient who is blind where the food is located on his plate, likening the location to the numbers on the face of a clock.
- For the newly blind patient, foods which are easy to eat and unlikely to spill will help him gain confidence in his ability to be self-sufficient.

General pharmacological considerations

- Use of nonprescription eyedrops may be disguising a more serious eye condition. Approval of a physician for the use of these products (for "tired" eyes, itching of the eye, redness of the eye) should be obtained.
- Miotic drugs in ophthalmic form are used to treat glaucoma. These drugs constrict the pupil and pull the iris away from the drainage channels. When these drugs are used the pupils appear constricted or pinpoint.
- Acetazolamide (Diamox) may be ordered for the patient with glaucoma in an effort to reduce intraocular pressure.
- Patients with glaucoma must avoid atropine and medications containing atropine. Popular nonprescription cold and allergy remedies contain atropine or atropine-related drugs. This warning should be included in the discharge teaching of all patients with glaucoma.
- External auditory canal disorders may be treated with antibiotics in the form of ointment or eardrops.
- The microorganisms responsible for middle ear infections may be resistant to some antibiotics. The patient should be encouraged to contact the physician if the infection does not appear to improve.
- Treatment of Ménière's disease may include drugs used for motion sickness such as dimenhydrinate (Dramamine). Various other drugs, such as antihistamines, diuretics, and sedatives, may also be used.

Bibliography

BALLINGER, W. F. et al: *Alexander's Care of the Patient in Surgery*, ed. 5. St. Louis, Mosby, 1973.

BRUNNER, L. and SUDDARTH, D. et al: *Lippincott Manual of Nursing Practice*. Philadelphia, Lippincott, 1974.

FERNSEBNER, W.: Early diagnosis of acute angle-closure glaucoma. Am. J. Nurs. 75:1154, July, 1975.

FULTON, M. et al: Helping diabetics adapt to failing vision. Am. J. Nurs. 74:54, January, 1974.

GUTIERREZ, A.: Nursing care during cataract removal by phaco emulsification. AORN J. 18:929, November, 1973.

HIRTH, K.: Beyond the curtain of silence. Am. J. Nurs. 74:1060, June, 1974.

Jordan, H.: The use of the argon laser photocoagulator in retinal surgery, AORN J. 18:914, November, 1973.

Patient assessment: Examination of the eye; programmed instruction. Am. J. Nurs. 74:2039, November, 1974.

Saunders, W. H. et al: *Nursing Care in Eye, Ear, Nose and Throat Disorders,* ed. 3. St. Louis, Mosby, 1974.

Shiery, S.: Insight into the delicate art of eye care (pictorial), Nurs. '75 5:50, June, 1975.

Tucker, S. M. et al: *Patient Care Standards.* St. Louis, Mosby, 1975.

Zucnick, M.: Care of an artificial eye. Am. J. Nurs. 75:835, May, 1975.

UNIT FIVE

Threats to adequate respiration

- The patient with disease of the nose or the throat
- The patient with acute respiratory disorder
- The patient with chronic respiratory disorder

CHAPTER—19

The patient with a disease of the nose or the throat

On completion of this chapter the student will:

- Discuss disorders of the nose and sinuses and the medical and surgical management of each.
- Describe early symptoms of cancer of the larynx.
- Discuss the emotional impact of radical surgery which is often necessary for cancer of the larynx.
- Prepare nursing care plans for a patient with a tracheostomy and a patient with a laryngectomy.
- Describe the ways to teach the laryngectomy patient how to clean and care for his laryngectomy tube.

Disorders of the sinuses and the nose

The lateral walls of the nasal cavity are formed by three bony protuberances on either side—the superior, the middle, and the inferior turbinate bones. Between the turbinates are grooves that contain the openings through which the sinuses drain. There

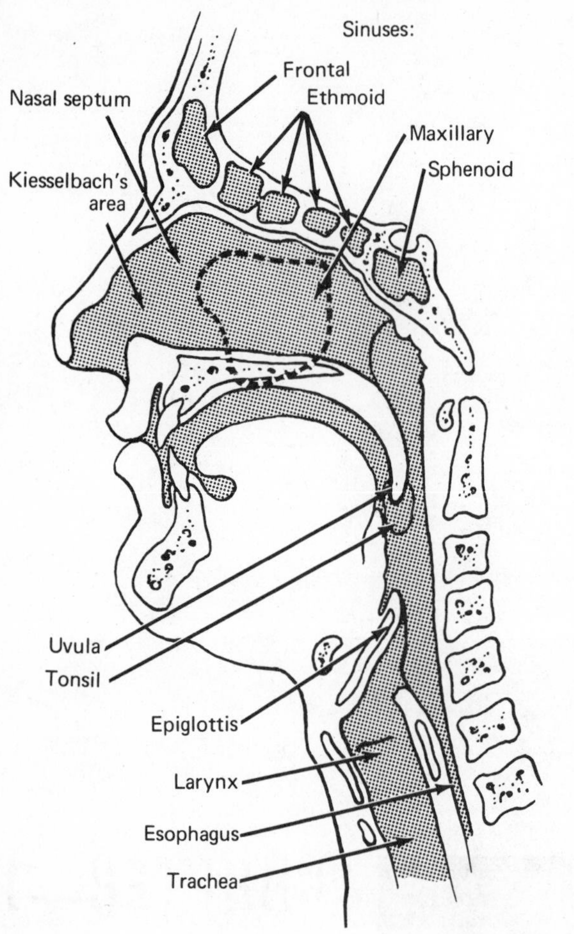

figure 19-1. Some important structures of the nose and the throat.

are three pairs of openings (meatus)—superior, middle, and inferior—each beneath its respective turbinate. The entire nasal cavity is lined with a highly vascular mucous membrane, the surface of which is composed of ciliated columnar epithelial cells. Interspersed with the columnar cells are numerous goblet cells that secrete mucus which is carried back to the nasopharynx by the movement of the cilia.

The paranasal sinuses are extensions of the nasal cavity into the surrounding facial bones. The lining of these sinuses is continuous with the mucous membrane lining of the nasal cavity. These sinuses are located in the frontal, the ethmoid, the sphenoid, and the maxillary bones. Their functions are to lighten the weight of the skull, and to give resonance to the voice.

The two frontal sinuses lie within the frontal bone, extending above the orbital cavities. The ethmoid bone contains a honeycomb of small spaces known as the ethmoid sinuses, or cells, located between the eyes. The sphenoid sinuses lie behind the nasal cavity. The maxillary sinuses (antra of Highmore) are located on either side of the nose in the maxillary bones. They are the largest of the sinuses, and most accessible to treatment (Fig. 19-1).

The olfactory area lies at the roof of the nose; directly above is the cribriform plate which forms a portion of the roof of the nose, and the floor of the anterior cranial fossa. Therefore, trauma or surgery in this area carries risk of injury or infection to the brain.

Sinusitis

Sinusitis is an inflammation of the sinuses. A maxillary sinus (antrum) most often is affected. Sinusitis is caused principally by the spread of an infection from the nasal passages to the sinuses and by the blockage of normal sinus drainage (Fig. 19-2). Lessened resistance to infection is an important predisposing factor. Emotional strain, fatigue and poor nutrition increase one's susceptibility to sinusitis. Sinusitis that accompanies or follows the common cold illustrates the role played by infection and obstruction. Because the mucous membrane lining of the nasal passages and the sinuses is continuous, infection spreads readily from the nose to the sinuses.

Anything that interferes with the drainage of the sinuses predisposes to sinusitis, because the trapped secretions readily become infected. Allergy frequently causes edema of the turbinates and, therefore, frequently leads to sinusitis. Nasal polyps and deviated septum are other common causes of faulty sinus drainage.

Sinusitis can lead to serious complications, such as spread of the infection to the middle ear, the brain, and also, to bronchiectasis and asthma. Nurses should encourage the prompt treatment of conditions that predispose to sinusitis, such as allergy and polyps, and should emphasize the importance of early medical attention when sinusitis occurs.

Treatment. Acute sinusitis frequently responds to conservative treatment designed to help the patient to overcome the infection. Bed rest, ample fluid intake, steam inhalations, local heat application, and salicylates for the relief of pain often are effective. Antibiotic therapy may be necessary in some instances.

Vasoconstrictors such as phenylephrine (Neo-Synephrine) nosedrops may be used; however, misuse of nosedrops and other medications can make the

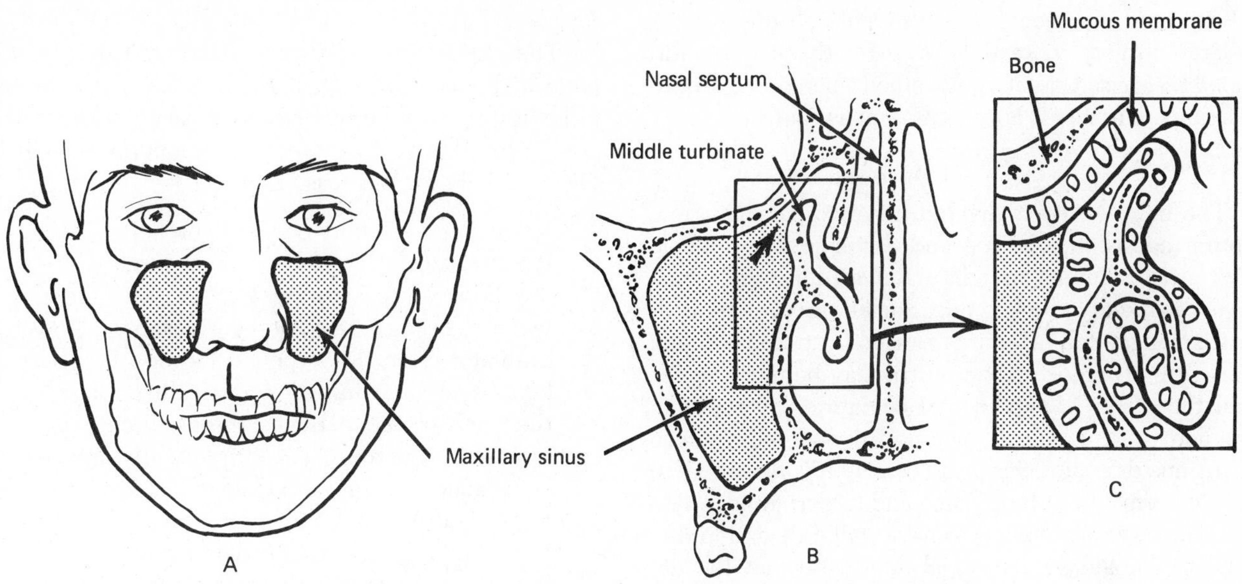

figure 19-2. Edema can cause obstruction of sinus drainage. (A) Location of maxillary sinuses. (B) The maxillary sinuses normally drain through the openings that lie under the middle turbinates. Note that the opening for the drainage is nearest the upper portion of the sinus. (C) Edema, such as that which commonly accompanies upper respiratory infections, can obstruct the opening and prevent normal sinus drainage.

condition worse. Many preparations for sinusitis can be purchased without a prescription, and some individuals may have a tendency to overmedicate. When nosedrops are applied too frequently or over too long a period, they provide shorter and shorter periods of relief, and are followed by "rebound" congestion of the turbinates, making the problem of obstruction worse. The nurse who observes prolonged indiscriminate use of these preparations can perform a real service by advising the person to consult his physician. Vasoconstrictors may be absorbed systemically and should be used with caution. Patients with hypertension should seek their physician's advice before using these preparations.

Many "cold tablets" contain antihistamines which thicken nasal secretions; while this action may temporarily decrease the discomfort of profuse nasal secretions, it can lead to failure of the sinus to drain adequately, due to the thickened secretions. Secretions thus trapped readily form a focus for continuing infection.

If the lack of drainage has resulted in the accumulation of pus, the maxillary sinus often is irrigated to remove the purulent material and to promote drainage. Usually, a special catheter can be inserted through the normal opening under the middle turbinate.

Surgery may be indicated in treatment of chronic sinusitis. An opening may be made in the inferior meatus to provide sinus drainage. This relatively simple operation is called an *antrotomy,* or antrum window operation. A more radical procedure occasionally is done through the mouth, above the upper teeth. This is called the Caldwell-Luc operation. The diseased mucous membrane lining of the sinus is removed, and a new opening is made into the inferior meatus of the nose, so that adequate drainage can occur.

Nurses can avoid, and help others to avoid, the attitude that sinusitis is something to "put up with," and that nothing can be done about it. Modern treatment can prevent much needless misery, as well as help to avoid chronic sinusitis and serious complications such as bronchiectasis.

Polyps

Polyps are grapelike swellings that are believed to result from chronic irritation, such as that caused by infection or allergy. When polyps grow in the nose, they obstruct nasal breathing and sinus drainage. They are removed under local anesthesia. Unfortunately, polyps tend to recur, and the patient often must undergo surgery more than once for the same condition. The excised tissue is examined microscopically to determine whether it is benign or malignant.

Deviated septum

The nasal cavity is divided into two passages by a septum consisting of bone and cartilage. Few people have an absolutely straight nasal septum, and some have a markedly crooked one. Sometimes the crookedness is congenital; often it is caused by trauma. When the septum is crooked, one nostril may be much larger than the other. Marked septal deviation can result in complete obstruction of one nostril and interference with sinus drainage. Surgical correction is necessary to restore normal breathing space and to permit adequate sinus drainage. Patients who have septal deviation due to injury should seek medical advice, so that the deformity can be corrected, and chronic sinusitis avoided.

The operation performed for deviated septum is called a *submucous resection* (SMR). After a local anesthetic has been administered, the surgeon makes an incision through the mucous membrane and removes the portions of the septum that are causing obstruction. When surgery is completed, both sides of the nasal cavity are packed with gauze, which usually is left in place for 24 to 48 hours. A moustache dressing (a folded piece of gauze applied under the nostrils and held in place with adhesive tape) is applied to absorb any bloody drainage.

General postoperative nursing management

Regardless of the particular operation performed on the nose, the principles of postoperative nursing management are similar.

Adequate preoperative instruction may help to allay some of the patient's fears, thus providing for a smoother postoperative course. For instance, the prospect of surgery on any part of the face may cause considerable anxiety over the possibility of a changed appearance. The physician usually advises the patient that his appearance will return to normal after the postoperative edema and discoloration subside.

Another fear common among patients who have surgery under local anesthesia is that they will experience pain during surgery. The nurse can reassure such patients that they will receive enough local anesthesia to prevent pain but that they may feel some pressure. If the patient has many questions about his surgery, he should be encouraged to discuss these matters with his physician.

The patient should also be instructed that he will have to breathe through his mouth for a day or two following surgery because there will be packing in his nose. The patient's postoperative temperature will be taken rectally for this reason.

- The nurse should be alert for hemorrhage, the major complication of nasal surgery. It is not unusual to saturate two or three moustache dressings; there is considerable bloody drainage after this type of surgery. A flashlight is used to inspect for trickling blood in the back of the patient's throat. Blood pressure and pulse are checked frequently and the moustache dressings are changed as necessary.
- The patient and his environment are kept neat. There is no need for blood-stained shirts, soggy moustache dressings, or soiled tissues to be in plain sight.
- The patient is instructed to spit out drainage so that the amount and character can be noted. Some swallowing of blood is usual after nasal surgery, and the patient may even pass a tarry stool postoperatively.
- The patient is protected from falling by bed side rails until the effects of sedation have worn off. He is assisted the first few times that he gets out of bed.
- The head of the bed is elevated to a 45-degree angle to decrease edema and to promote more comfortable breathing.
- The patient is encouraged to help himself as much as possible, for example, by applying cold compresses to his nose.
- Mouth care and oral fluids are important nursing measures. Old blood can give a foul odor and taste to the mouth, and dryness of the mouth is inevitable during mouth breathing.
- The patient should not be forced to try more than liquids and soft foods until after the packing has been removed. This period lasts only a day or two, and afterward the patient quickly resumes a normal diet.
- Occasionally, nasal packing slips back into the throat causing gagging and discomfort. The surgeon should be advised of the situation. In emergency treatment for packing that has slipped back into the throat and obstructs breathing, the nurse has the patient open his

mouth, then grasps the packing with forceps and pulls it out through the open mouth.

- An enema may be ordered preoperatively to empty the lower bowel, so that swallowed blood will pass through the gastrointestinal tract more quickly after surgery. Cathartics may be ordered postoperatively for the same purpose.
- Sedatives and/or analgesics may be necessary during the postoperative period to control pain, apprehension and restlessness. However, nasal surgery is usually relatively painless; mentioning this to the patient preoperatively can help allay fear of pain.
- As hemorrhage can occur, the patient is told not to blow his nose until given permission to do so by his physician.

Epistaxis (nosebleed)

Most nosebleeds occur in Kiesselbach's area, a plexus of capillaries located on the anterior part of the nasal septum. Epistaxis may result from picking the nose or from local trauma, such as any kind of blow. Also, it may result from diseases, such as rheumatic fever, hypertension, or blood dyscrasias. Epistaxis resulting from hypertension is likely to be especially severe and difficult to control.

Nosebleed is a common occurrence and is usually not very serious, but it is often very frightening for both the person experiencing it and those who witness it. Every nurse should be familiar with simple first aid for epistaxis. Merely applying pressure by holding the soft parts of the nose firmly between thumb and forefinger for several minutes is often effective in controlling bleeding. The patient should sit with his head tilted slightly forward to prevent the blood from running down his throat; he is instructed to breathe through his mouth, and firm pressure is applied. The sitting position usually is preferable, because it lessens the possibility of fainting, as well as the fatigue and the discomfort caused by standing. Also, the flow of blood to the head is lessened by keeping the head elevated while the patient is sitting. The patient can be shown how to apply pressure, and often he can control the bleeding himself if it occurs while he is alone. If the bleeding is severe, a basin must be provided to catch the blood. The patient should be instructed not to swallow blood that may run into his mouth and throat, but to spit it out. If the bleeding is slight, tissues or a handkerchief may be sufficient to prevent soiling the clothing. Applying cold compresses to the bridge of the nose sometimes is helpful.

If the bleeding is profuse, or if it does not stop within a few minutes, the physician should be called. He may place cotton pledgets saturated with epinephrine 1:1,000 in the nostril, and also apply pressure. If the bleeding cannot be controlled, the nasal cavity may have to be packed with gauze to apply continuous pressure for approximately 24 hours. Sometimes, it is necessary to cauterize the bleeding areas.

Laryngitis

The larynx, or *voice box* is made of a more or less rigid framework of cartilages held together by ligaments. Except for the vocal cords, the interior of the larynx is lined by ciliated mucous membrane that is continuous with the mucous membrane of the pharynx and the trachea. The cartilaginous framework of the larynx consists of the *thyroid,* the *arytenoid,* and the *cricoid* cartilages.

On each lateral wall of the laryngeal cavity are two horizontally placed folds of mucous membrane—the ventricular folds, or false cords and the vocal folds, or true vocal cords. The latter are the lower of the two. The larynx and the air passages of which it forms a part constitute an air column that produces sounds of varying pitch. However, the larynx cannot produce words. The sounds made by the vibrating vocal cords are molded into speech by the pharynx, the palate, the tongue, the teeth, and the lips.

Laryngitis is an inflammation and swelling of the mucous membrane lining of the larynx. Laryngitis often accompanies upper respiratory infections, and it is due to the spread of the infection to the larynx. Laryngitis also can be caused by excessive or improper use of the voice or by smoking. The symptoms include hoarseness or, sometimes, the inability to speak above a whisper. A cough and a feeling of throat irritation commonly accompany laryngitis.

Sometimes the diagnosis is made by the patient on the basis of the symptoms alone. If the condition persists, the individual should seek the advice of a physician. Most physicians believe that hoarseness which persists more than two weeks warrants a laryngoscopic examination, by which the larynx can be examined visually. Indirect laryngoscopy is the visualization of the larynx by means of a laryngeal mirror held in the pharynx while a light is directed onto the mirror. In direct laryngoscopy, a laryngoscope (a hollow instrument with a light at its distal end) is passed to the larynx after the patient's throat has been anesthetized. Nursing management before and after direct laryngoscopy is similar to that of a patient having a bronchoscopy. The prompt investigation of the cause of persistent hoarseness is essential, because this symptom may be due to cancer of the larynx.

The treatment of laryngitis involves voice rest and the treatment or the removal of the cause. The meaning of the term "voice rest" should be explained to the patient. It means writing what he wishes to communicate rather than speaking. It must be emphasized that whispering is as bad as talking. Voice rest facilitates the healing of the inflamed mucous membranes, and, when the condition is due to an upper respiratory infection or to brief overuse of the voice, it is usually the only specific treatment required.

Cancer of the Larynx

Cancer of the larynx is most common among people over 45. Men are affected more frequently than women. Although the cause is unknown, it is believed that chronic laryngitis, irritants such as alcohol, cigarette smoke and industrial pollutants, habitual overuse of the voice, and heredity may predispose to the condition.

Symptoms. Persistent hoarseness usually is the earliest symptom. Often this is slight at first and is readily ignored. Also, the patient may have a sensation of a swelling or a lump in his throat, followed by dysphagia (Fig. 19-3) and pain when he is talking. If the malignant tissue is not removed promptly, the patient develops symptoms of advancing carcinoma, such as weakness, weight loss, and anemia. The importance of consulting a physician for any persistent hoarseness or difficulty in swallowing cannot be overemphasized. Patients who seek treatment early have a good chance of cure, because cancer of the larynx usually does not metastasize as early as cancer in other parts of the body.

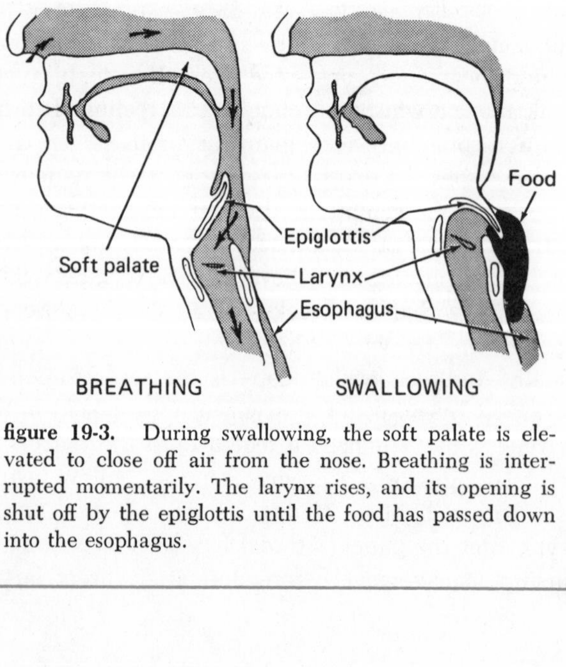

figure 19-3. During swallowing, the soft palate is elevated to close off air from the nose. Breathing is interrupted momentarily. The larynx rises, and its opening is shut off by the epiglottis until the food has passed down into the esophagus.

Diagnosis. The diagnosis is established by laryngoscopy, biopsy and x-ray films.

Treatment. The surgical removal of the tumor, and often the entire larynx, is necessary. Radiotherapy also may be employed. If the tumor is discovered promptly, the surgeon sometimes can remove it without removing the entire larynx; this less radical procedure is called *laryngofissure*. Because laryngofissure does not involve a removal of the total larynx, but only a portion of it, the patient does not lose his voice. However, his voice is husky. In more advanced cases total laryngectomy is necessary. If the disease has spread to the cervical lymph nodes, radical neck dissection (removal of the lymph nodes and the adjacent tissues) also is performed. Patients who have total laryngectomy have a permanent tracheal stoma or opening because after surgery the trachea does not connect with the nasopharynx. The larynx is severed from the trachea and removed completely. The only respiratory organs in use thereafter are the trachea, the bronchi, and the lungs. Air enters and leaves through the tracheostomy; the patient will no longer feel air entering his nose. The anterior wall of the esophagus connects with the posterior wall of the larynx, and consequently it must be reconstructed. Tube feeding facilitates healing by avoiding muscular activity and irritation of the esophagus.

Nursing management of a laryngectomy patient

Preoperative Preparation. The physician explains the need and the expected extent of the surgery to the patient preoperatively. If total laryngectomy is necessary, the patient often is shocked and dismayed at the prospect of losing his voice. (Even the temporary loss of the ability to communicate verbally with others causes a great deal of anxiety.) A detailed explanation of the measures that will be used to help the patient to communicate with others is important before surgery is performed. For example, the patient should know that he can write messages immediately after surgery, and that he will have a call light that will be answered promptly. As soon as he recovers from the surgery sufficiently, he may be taught *esophageal speech,* a method of speaking by regurgitating swallowed air. Some patients are unable to learn esophageal speech and an artificial (electronic) device may be used to produce speech. There are several different portable models available.

How much the patient is told during the preoperative period depends on the surgeon. The patient must be told that the loss of voice will be *permanent.* Although most surgeons give a careful, detailed explanation of the procedure prior to surgery, some patients may tell the nurse that they did not know they would lose their voice. Many times the patient was depressed or had refused to accept the diagnosis of cancer and the need for radical surgery when the physician was explaining the procedure.

A visit from someone who has undergone laryngectomy and has mastered esophageal speech often does more to convince the patient that such speech is possible than all the explanations given by his physician and the nurse.

The patient should understand that he will be fed through a nasogastric tube postoperatively. It will remain in place until sufficient healing has occurred. The patient can usually look forward to eating normally after the tube has been removed.

The patient is told that he will have a permanent tracheostomy, or opening in his neck, and that he will be taught how to care for this opening before he is discharged from the hospital.

Postoperative Nursing Management. The patient who has had a laryngectomy may or may not have had a radical neck dissection. Radical neck dissection is performed when the tumor has extended beyond the larynx and includes the removal of lymph nodes, muscles, and other structures adjacent to the larynx. General nursing management for the patient who has had a laryngectomy is given in Table 19-1.

On his return from the operating room, the patient is positioned on his side until he wakens. A heavy pressure dressing may be placed over the surgical area, although some surgeons prefer to use a minimal amount of dressing. Drainage catheters may be placed under the skin to remove excess fluid accumulation. These catheters are connected to a suction device as soon as the patient returns from surgery. The surgeon will specify the type of suction to be used.

Pain is relieved with analgesics; however, narcotic analgesics are avoided because they depress respirations. While all postsurgery patients experience varying degrees of pain, those with radical neck dissections usually have less pain than patients with other types of major surgery because the sensory nerve endings are severed during surgery. These patients may respond to non-narcotic analgesics such as propoxyphene (Darvon) or pentazocaine (Talwin) especially after the first few postoperative days. A small pillow or a folded towel placed under the patient's head and shoulders relieves tension of the suture line; full pillows are to be avoided.

Once the patient appears interested in communicating with the nursing staff, he should be provided with a Magic Slate or a pad and pen. The nurse should make every attempt to require as brief an answer as possible.

One of the biggest fears the patient has is that of suffocation. *At all times* the stoma must be kept patent and free of obstruction. The patient is suctioned when-

Table 19-1.
Postoperative nursing management of the patient who has had a laryngectomy

Maintain patent airway: Suction every hour and as needed; clean inner cannula of the laryngectomy tube every 2 hours and p.r.n.; keep objects (dressings, bed linen, and so on) away from the stoma.

Elevate head of bed.

Prevent extremes in movement of the head. Support the patient's head when moving or changing position.

Increase humidification of inspired air by means of a tracheostomy mist collar, ultrasonic mist unit, or any other device that will serve this purpose.

Keep a spare laryngectomy set at the bedside.

Turn the patient and assist him to cough and deep breathe every 2 hours. Check vital signs every 2 to 4 hours.

Clean the area around the stoma every 4 hours and p.r.n., using hydrogen peroxide. Rinse with normal saline and be sure area is dry.

If drainage catheters are placed under the skin, connect them to suction such as Gomco or Hemovac. Empty and measure contents every 8 hours.

Check intake and output.

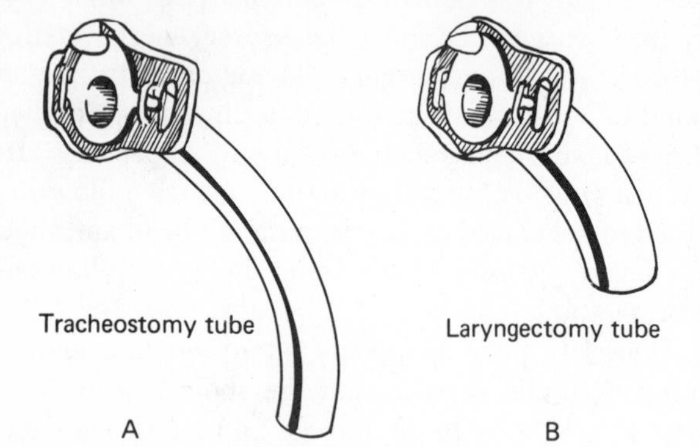

figure 19-4. Both tubes come in different sizes.

ever mucus obstructs the laryngectomy tube (Fig. 19-4), and suctioning must be attended to *promptly* lest the patient panic. All potential obstructions to the patient's air supply will understandably produce severe anxiety in the laryngectomy patient. In time, the patient can be taught to suction himself with the aid of a mirror.

As noted previously, after laryngectomy, the patient is fed through a nasogastric tube, usually for about a week (Fig. 19-5). However, some surgeons now discontinue the nasogastric feedings and begin oral feedings as early as the second postoperative day. When the patient can swallow, he is allowed sips of water. When he is able to swallow fluids without difficulty, the nasogastric tube is removed. The patient is permitted soft foods and fluids. Gradually, he is permitted to resume a normal diet.

Nasogastric tube feedings. Patients unable to swallow but able to digest foods placed in the stomach may be fed liquids through a nasogastric tube passed through the nose to the stomach. A patient fed this way can maintain good water and electrolyte balance and be well nourished. The amount and the type of tube feeding is ordered by the physician. The food passed through the tube is a liquid form of an ade-

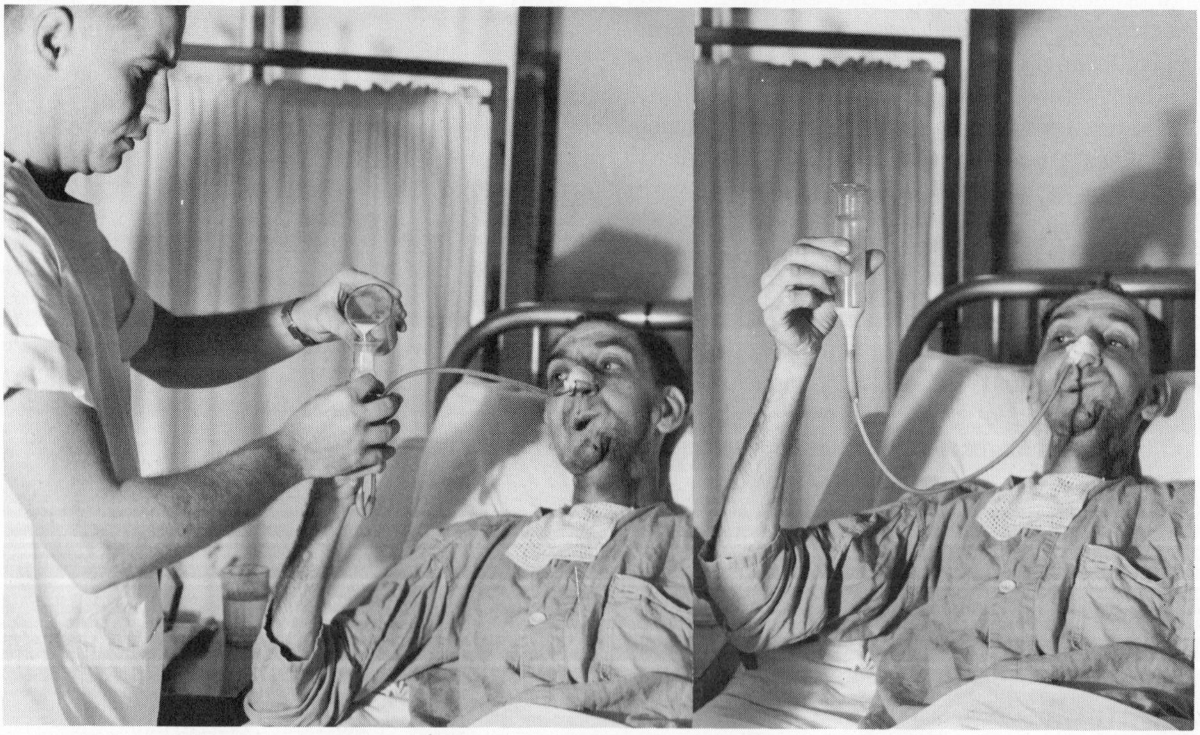

figure 19-5. (*Left*) The nurse is shown pouring the tube feeding into an Asepto syringe, which is being used as a funnel. The tube is kinked while the syringe is being filled. Note the damp mesh square that the patient is wearing over his tracheostomy tube. Facial deformity has resulted from the extensive surgery that was necessary to treat his condition. (*Right*) The feeding is permitted to flow through the tube by gravity. Before the syringe is empty, more of the feeding will be added. The patient is encouraged to help with the procedure.

quate diet. The patient does not taste the mixture. Feedings may be ordered at 1, 2, or 4 hourly intervals.

Caution must be used to avoid aspiration, especially when tube feedings are given to a comatose patient, or one who is disoriented or restless. Before feeding, the tube is checked to make sure that the end is well situated in the stomach. Some tubes are marked with black lines. When the black line is at the nose, the end of the tube is in the stomach. Even if the tube has no such line, the nurse can tell if it has pulled out by seeing whether or not the adhesive tape that holds it in place has been disturbed.

Tube feedings are warmed to body temperature and are allowed to flow in by gravity through an Asepto syringe, a funnel, or a 50 ml. syringe. After the feeding is finished, it is followed by a syringe full of clean water to rinse the tube and to prevent food particles from lodging in the tube and turning sour. The patient is given mouth care and observed for irritation of the nostril through which the tube passes.

Oral medications may be crushed thoroughly, mixed with water, and administered through the nasogastric tube. Water is always administered through the tube after the medication has been instilled, otherwise, the patient will not receive the entire dose, because part of the medicine will remain in the tube.

The patient is taught to administer his own tube feedings as soon as he is able. He is instructed never to let the funnel become empty during the feeding (since this would allow air to enter his stomach) and to clamp the tube carefully after administering the feeding. Many patients fold the tube over on itself, and secure it with an elastic band. A heavy metal clamp is not desirable, because its weight is uncomfortable and tends to pull the tube out.

Later Postoperative Period. The patient may be allowed up and about as much as he wishes after the fourth or fifth postoperative day. He bathes himself, administers his own feedings, suctions, and is shown how to clean his inner cannula. From this point on, the nurse spends less time in direct physical care and more in teaching the patient to care for himself. Besides the techniques of suctioning and cleaning the inner tube, the patient must learn what foods he may eat when he returns home. (At first, soft foods and liquids are easier to swallow; gradually he resumes normal diet.) He also may learn acceptable ways of camouflaging his tube if he wishes. A scarf helps to keep dust and dirt out of the trachea, as well as to make the tracheostomy less obvious. A scarf made of smooth material, such as silk or rayon, may be worn loosely; fabrics that have fuzz must be avoided, since small fibers can be drawn into the tube.

The patient with a permanent tracheostomy must prevent water from entering the tracheal opening, since it would flow down his trachea to his lungs. He never can go swimming, and he must be careful to prevent entrance of water into the tracheostomy during his bath.

Instruction and emotional support help the patient to mobilize his defenses and to begin to learn how to cope with the effects of the operation. Many cities have Lost Cord Clubs—groups of people who have had a laryngectomy and who help one another cope with the disability. Many of the club members visit others who are hospitalized for laryngectomy, and they distribute literature that offers practical help and encouragement to others with the condition. Patients can find out about the club nearest them by contacting the American Cancer Society, 219 East 42nd Street, New York City 10017, or by contacting their local chapter of the Society, as listed in the telephone book.

Nursing management of patients with a tracheostomy

These patients require almost continuous nursing care immediately after surgery. Not only are they unable to speak, but they must breathe through a new opening in their tracheas. A tube is placed in the tracheal opening.

Tracheostomy without laryngectomy may be necessitated by any condition, such as allergy or infection, that causes edema and results in obstruction of the patient's airway. In such situations the tracheostomy is performed as an emergency measure to create a new opening through which the patient can breathe. The operation may be performed at the bedside, or even outside the hospital, when the patient's condition suddenly requires it. However, in most instances it is possible and preferable to prepare carefully for this operation and to perform it in a methodical way before the patient's respiratory distress is so acute that his life is in jeopardy. Nurses can help by promptly reporting respiratory difficulty to the physician, so that the needed care can be given immediately. Patients who have had a tracheostomy without a laryngectomy can speak by taking a breath, briefly covering the tube with a finger, uttering a word or two, and then removing the finger to resume breathing.

Tracheostomy tubes come in several sizes and may be made of metal (sterling silver or stainless steel), disposable plastic, or rubber. If the tube is metal, it

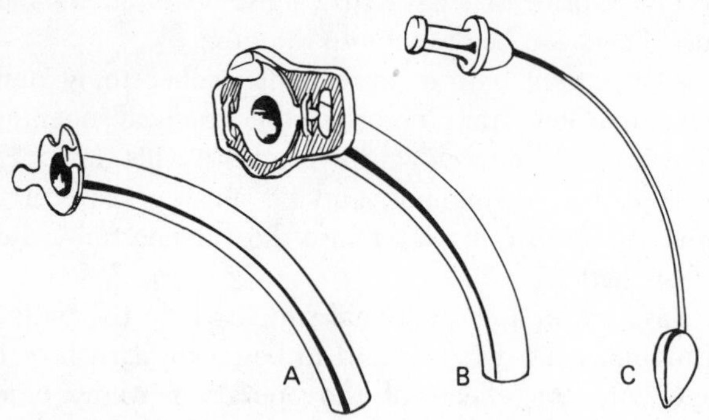

figure 19-6. A tracheostomy or laryngectomy tube has three parts: (A) inner tube, (B) outer tube, and (C) obturator.

usually consists of three parts—an outer tube, an inner tube, and an obturator (Fig. 19-6). Before the outer tube is inserted into the tracheal opening, the obturator is placed in the tube. The lower end of the obturator protrudes from the end of the tube to be inserted. The protruding end of the obturator is smooth, facilitating insertion. Since the obturator obstructs the lumen of the tube, it is removed immediately, once the tube is in place. The parts of the tubes are not interchangeable; they fit only one particular tube. If one part is lost, the entire set is useless. Therefore, each part, including the obturator, is carefully accounted tor is placed in the tube. The lower end of the obturator usually is taped to the patient's wrist when he returns from the operating room, so that it is returned to the unit with the patient.

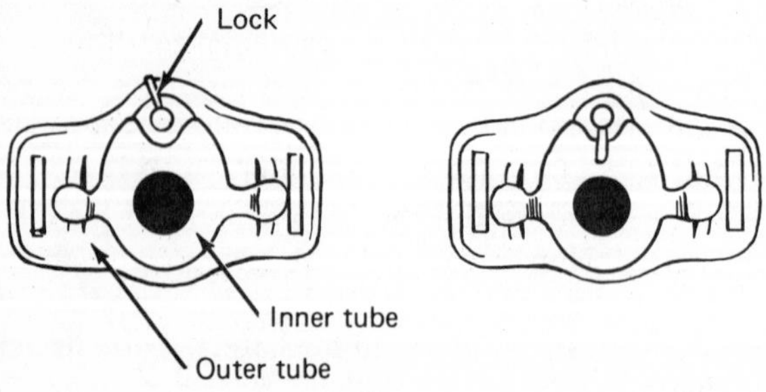

figure 19-7. The inner tube fits snugly into the outer tube. Turning the lock up with the finger makes it possible to remove the inner tube for cleaning. Turning the lock down keeps the inner tube securely in place. The inner tube always is locked in place after it is reinserted.

The cuffed tracheostomy tube is another type of tube that may be used, especially when mechanical ventilation (use of a respirator) is necessary. The cuff is inflated with air to provide a snug fit in the stoma. The physician will specify the amount of air to be injected into the cuff, as the amount of air determines the seating of the cuff in the trachea.

The inner tube slides inside the outer tube. It is removed by the nurse as often as necessary, cleaned, and replaced. The nurse must always be sure that the inner tube is locked securely in position after she reinserts it (Fig. 19-7). Various methods are used for cleaning the inner tube. Because dried mucus sticks inside, merely rinsing the tube with water is not sufficient. The lumen must be wiped as well. Some nurses use a piece of bandage threaded through the tube to clean the inside; others prefer a small brush. Soap and cold water, or hydrogen peroxide plus friction applied with a brush, aids in the removal of secretions. The tube always should be held up and inspected to be sure that it is clean and dry before it is reinserted.

In the immediate postoperative period, the *inner* tube may have to be removed as often as every half hour. Before the inner tube is reinserted, the outer tube is thoroughly suctioned. The inner tube should be cleaned promptly and reinserted. Otherwise, the outer tube will collect secretions. The outer tube is left in position. The entire tube usually is changed by the physician daily or several times a week.

An extra tracheostomy set always is kept at the patient's bedside, since immediate change may be necessary if the patient's tube becomes blocked with mucus that cannot be removed by suction or removal of the inner cannula. Each time the physician changes the patient's metal tube, the one that has been removed is scrubbed thoroughly with soap and water and sterilized by boiling. It is then ready for reuse. Often, the tube is placed in a jar and labeled with the patient's name. The tubes come in various sizes, and it is important that the patient always have the correct size at his bedside.

The outer tube is held snugly in place by tapes inserted in openings on either side of it and tied at the back of the patient's neck. These tapes always should be tied securely in a knot. A bow may be added if desired. If the knot is not tied securely, the patient can cough the tube out. This is a very serious occurrence if the edges of the trachea have not been sutured to the skin, as is the case in a temporary tracheotomy. If the outer tube accidentally comes out, the nurse immediately inserts a tracheal dilator (Fig. 19-8) to hold the edges of the opening apart until the physician arrives to insert another tube. A tracheal dilator is kept at the bedside at all times. The tube should never be forced back in. If force is used, the patient's trachea may be compressed (by pushing the tube alongside the trachea, thus compressing the trachea, rather than inserting the tube into the stoma). Such action could cause asphyxiation. It is essential that the nurse try to remain calm if the patient's tube should come out and she cannot easily re-insert it, and remember to hold open the stoma with a tracheal dilator until the physician arrives.

Many patients wear a "bib" of folded gauze or mesh over the tube as a camouflage. If the material is kept damp, it helps to humidify the inspired air. The bib never should be made of the kind of gauze that has a layer of cotton inside, since bits of cotton easily are sucked into the tube. It is important not to let any material hide the condition of the tube. Unless the nurse is alert to this possibility, a badly crusted tube much in need of being cleaned and changed may be overlooked.

A gauze dressing is placed under the tube to absorb the secretions. Gauze squares usually are used for this purpose. A slit is cut halfway through the square, so that the gauze can fit around the tube. This piece of gauze should be changed as often as necessary (Fig. 19-9).

The patient's respiratory passages react to the creation of the new respiratory opening with irritation, excessive secretion of mucus, and formation of crusts of dried mucus. The inspired air passes directly into the trachea, the bronchi and the lungs without becoming warmed and moistened by passing through the nose. The copious respiratory secretions that characteristically occur immediately after the new opening has been made are a threat to the patient's life. They may clog the only remaining breathing passage—the tracheostomy—and quickly cause death by asphyxia. The patient is usually very much aware of this possibility, and often he is terrified of being left alone even for a moment. Constant vigilance and care are necessary during the immediate postoperative period to keep the tube patent and to reassure the patient. He is taught to care for the tube himself as soon as possible; the ability to care for himself is the patient's most effective defense against the fear of a blocked airway.

A suction machine is placed in readiness before the patient returns from surgery, and it is kept at his bedside at all times. Mucus is gently suctioned from the tube by a No. 14 or No. 16 (F.) vented or Y sterile catheter, inserted gently into the lumen of the tube. Suction is not applied while the catheter is on the way down the trachea, because this causes unnecessary irritation of the lining of the trachea. Instead, suction is commenced once the catheter has been passed, and suctioning is continued while the catheter is withdrawn slowly. As the catheter is withdrawn it is rotated, so that the openings in the catheter can remove mucus more effectively. This procedure may be necessary as often as every 5 to 10 mintues in the immediate postoperative period.

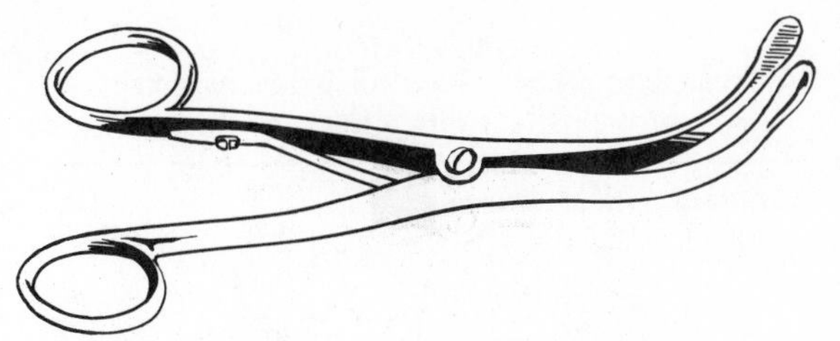

figure 19-8. Tracheal dilator.

Cleanliness of all equipment used in caring for the tracheostomy is essential. The hands are washed before suctioning the patient, and equipment kept at the bedside exchanged frequently (at least every 24 hours) for fresh supplies. Poor technique may lead to postoperative pneumonia by spread of infection to the lungs. If it is necessary to suction through the nose or

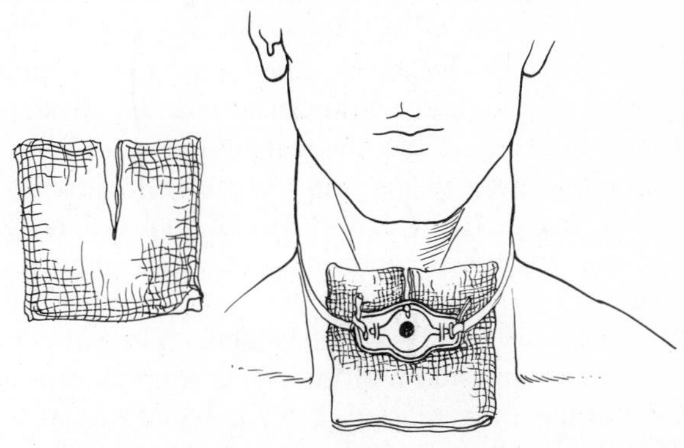

figure 19-9. Gauze squares, slit halfway down, are placed around the tube to catch secretions. These dressings are changed by the nurse as often as necessary. Note the tapes that hold the outer tube in place. The tapes are tied in a knot at the back of the patient's neck.

Table 19-2.
Immediate postoperative nursing management of the patient with a tracheostomy

Maintain patient airway.
Suction p.r.n. with a Y or vented catheter.
Clean inner cannula as needed—usually every 2 to 4 hours.
Administer heated mist to inspired air.
Place bed in semi-Fowler's position.
Clean skin around stoma every 4 hours and p.r.n. and replace dressing (see Fig. 19-9).
Provide a means of communication: pen and pad, Magic Slate.
Check vital signs every 4 hours or oftener, depending on the patient's condition.
Check intake and output.

the mouth, another catheter (not the one used for the tracheostomy) should be used. Disposable catheters lessen the danger of transmitting infection via catheters.

If the airway becomes completely obstructed, the patient will become markedly cyanotic, restless, and frightened, and will die within a few minutes if the obstruction is not relieved. First aid is of the greatest urgency, with the primary focus placed on establishing adequate ventilation by removal of the obstruction. The physician is notified immediately by one member of the nursing team while someone remains with the patient and attempts to relieve the obstruction. The removal of the tracheostomy tube followed by suctioning may be lifesaving. Consultation with the physician ahead of time concerning the first aid measures acceptable for the nurse to perform for each individual patient is essential. The nurse then will know which patients may have their tubes removed as an emergency measure.

Immediate Postoperative Period. The patient is positioned on his side until he reacts from anesthesia. When he has fully reacted, and his blood pressure is stable, the head of the bed is elevated to a 45-degree angle. This position decreases edema and makes breathing easier. At first the patient is very apprehensive and restless. However, the constant presence of the nurse usually helps him to feel more secure. Frequent suctioning and cleaning of the inner tube and providing a means of communication also are reassuring. In the immediate postoperative period, writing messages is the only means of communication left to the patient. A Magic Slate is useful for this purpose, because the words can be erased promptly by raising the plastic cover, and the tablet is ready for reuse. The patient should not be left unattended during this early postoperative period, because he is unable to care for his own tube, and he could quickly experience respiratory obstruction from copious secretion of mucus. Leaving him alone may lead to panic, if not suffocation, and may frighten him so much that rehabilitation will be difficult.

Opiates usually are ordered sparingly, because of their tendency to depress respiration. Fortunately, this type of surgery does not ordinarily cause a great deal of postoperative pain. When narcotics are given, the nurse should note carefully their effect on respiration and report any respiratory depression. The patient is observed for cyanosis and dyspnea, as well as for other postoperative complications, such as shock and hemorrhage.

General nutritional considerations

- Nasogastric tube feedings may be employed after a laryngectomy.
- The first feedings are usually dilute or approximately ½ calorie per ml. These feedings are given slowly and at body temperature. Some physicians may prefer the feeding be at room temperature rather than body temperature. The physician indicates the amount to be given in the first feeding.
- The amount given for each feeding is increased if the patient tolerates the amount given in the previous feeding. If the patient complains of gastric distress or has diarrhea, he may not be tolerating the tube feedings.
- Tube feedings may need additional supplements of certain vitamins and minerals. These may be added at the time of the feeding or added by the dietary department when the feeding is prepared.

General pharmacological considerations

- Many of the nonprescription over-the-counter (OTC) drugs available for seasonal allergies contain one or more antihistamines which can thicken nasal secretions and lead to inadequate sinus drainage and consequent infection of the sinuses.

- Indiscriminate use of nosedrops which most always contain an adrenergic agent which shrinks the nasal membranes can lead to "rebound" congestion, which may be worse than the original problem.
- Profuse nasal bleeding may be controlled by the direct application of epinephrine, usually as a 1:1,000 solution, to the nasal membrane.
- Patients with a radical neck dissection usually have less pain postoperatively than other patients with major surgery and may be given non-narcotic analgesics, such as pentazocine (Talwin). If narcotics are necessary, the respiratory rate is counted before giving the drug. The drug is withheld if the respiratory rate is below 10 or 12 per minute.

Bibliography

Behrens, J., et al, eds.: Laryngectomy: Paving the way to successful adjustment (pictorial). Nurs. '74, 4:60, June, 1974.

Brunner, L. S. and Suddarth, D. S.: *Textbook of Medical Surgical Nursing,* ed. 3. Philadelphia, Lippincott, 1975.

De Weese, D. D. and Saunders, W. H.: *Textbook of Otolaryngology,* ed. 4. St. Louis, Mosby, 1973.

Ferrer, M. I.: How to recognize sick sinus syndrome. Consultant 14:149, October, 1974.

Komorn, R. M.: Laryngectomy and surgical vocal rehabilitation (pictorial). AORN J. 17:73, June, 1973.

Lauder, E.: Towards total rehabilitation. Nurs. Dig. 3:50, March-April, 1975.

Lawless, C. A.: Helping patients with endotracheal and tracheostomy tubes communicate. Am. J. Nurs. 75:2151, December, 1975.

Loré, J. M.: *An Atlas of Head and Neck Surgery,* ed. 2, Vol. 1-2. Philadelphia, Saunders, 1973.

O'Dell, A. J.: The administration of airway humidification. Nurs. '74, 4:66, April, 1974.

Saunders, W. H., et al: Nursing Care in Eye, Ear, Nose and Throat Disorders, ed. 3. St. Louis, Mosby, 1974.

Shafer, K. N., et al: *Medical-Surgical Nursing,* ed. 6. St. Louis, Mosby, 1975.

CHAPTER—20

The patient with acute respiratory disorder

On completion of this chapter the student will:

- **List the various tests used in the diagnosis of respiratory disorders.**
- **Discuss the importance of arterial blood studies in the evaluation of acute and chronic respiratory disorders.**
- **Discuss the etiology, symptoms, treatment, and nursing management of the patient with pneumonia and pleurisy.**
- **Discuss the etiology, symptoms, and treatment of influenza with regard to the hospitalized and nonhospitalized patient.**
- **Recognize the seriousness of chest injuries and describe the treatment given to patients with various types of chest injuries.**

Respiratory disorders are the most frequent type of acute illness. Who has not experienced the "common cold"? Much of the time in the basically healthy person, milder respiratory infections result in unpleasant symptoms and the inconvenience of loss of time from work, school, or social activities. However, a similar infection which develops as a complication of another disease, or in the elderly person, or in a person with chronic respiratory impairment may make the difference between life and death. If such a patient recovers, convalescence is prolonged and costly.

One of the most vital needs is a continuous supply of oxygen (Figs. 20-1 and 20-2). Severe disease in the network of the respiratory passages can interfere with the oxygen supply. Because many respiratory conditions can be prevented to a certain extent, the nurse needs to know what causes them to develop, how they are spread, how their severity can be reduced, and how to care for the patient who becomes acutely ill.

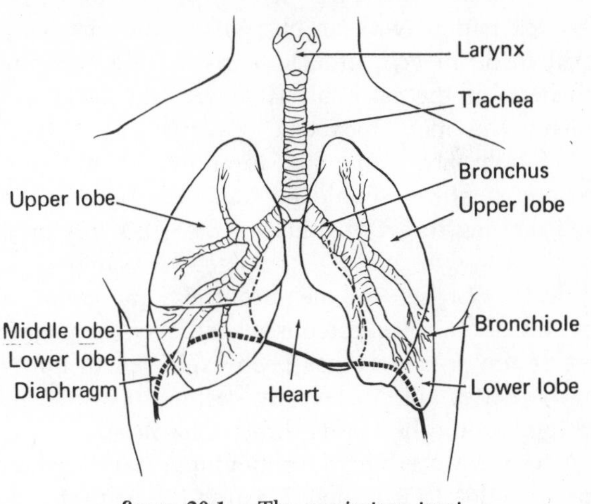

figure 20-1. The respiratory tract.

Diagnostic tests

X-RAY. X-ray of the chest is secondary only to the physician's stethoscope in the diagnosis of acute respiratory disorders. Often, when the physical examination of the patient fails to reveal a respiratory disorder, small lesions may be noted on the chest x-ray.

Under normal circumstances, the x-ray examination is performed in the radiology department. When the patient is too ill to be transported to the radiology department, a chest film may be obtained at the bedside with the use of portable x-ray equipment. Modern portable x-ray equipment has reduced unnecessary patient radiation exposure to a minimum. The nurse helps to position the patient according to the directions of the x-ray technician.

Use of an EMI or other type of scanner for computerized axial tomography produces axial views of any part of the body. By viewing the lungs in a different perspective, tumors and other lung disorders are often diagnosed during the early stages of the disease. These body scanners also pinpoint the location of a lesion with far more accuracy than conventional x-ray procedures.

FLUOROSCOPY. This examination enables the physician to view the thoracic cavity with all its contents in motion. Usually, the patient stands in front of the machine, and may need help in moving to the machine from the wheelchair. Currently, many hospitals are equipped with special image intensifiers on their x-ray equipment which are capable of displaying a continuous motion study of the chest on a television screen.

BRONCHOSCOPY. The physician may elect to use a bronchoscope for direct visual examination of the trachea, the two major bronchi, and multiple smaller bronchi in both the diagnosis and therapy of acute respiratory disorders. The bronchoscope is a hollow instrument which can be passed into the trachea under local anesthesia. Through the lumen of the bronchoscope the physician may pass suction tubes in order to obtain secretions for culture and Papanicolaou cell studies. If required, special biopsy forceps can be introduced and specimens obtained for direct pathologic evaluation. In life-threatening circumstances, such as

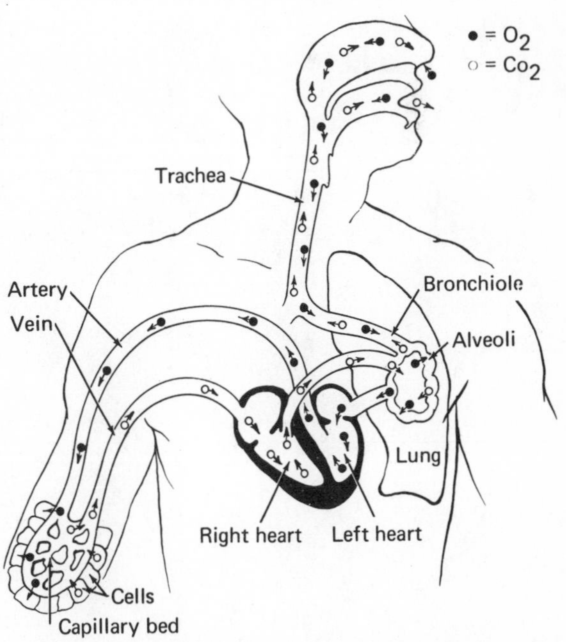

figure 20-2. Inspired oxygen, drawn in through the nose, can be traced into the alveoli, the left heart and the capillary bed; and carbon dioxide can be traced from the capillary bed to the right heart, the lung and out of the body.

when a foreign body has been aspirated or when a very sick patient with an obstructing mucous plug is too ill to be moved, bronchoscopy can be performed anywhere in the hospital. However, the location of choice is the operating room.

Before bronchoscopy the patient should have mouth care and dentures should be removed. He is usually given nothing to eat or drink for 8 to 12 hours before bronchoscopy to avoid the danger of vomiting and aspiration. Lights in the bronchoscopy room are dimmed, and a towel often is placed over the patient's eyes. If the procedure has been explained to him, he may be better able to help by keeping his neck muscles relaxed and breathing through his nose.

After the procedure, the patient may have increased secretions due to irritation. Because the gag reflex has been temporarily abolished, he is given nothing by mouth for several hours. Supplied with a sputum cup and tissues, the patient should be encouraged to expectorate and to clear the secretions as often as necessary. Following bronchoscopy, his throat may feel irritated for several days and he is advised to talk as little as possible. Some bloody mucus usually is expectorated after the test.

Complications of bronchoscopy include laryngeal edema—which may be so severe that the patient requires a tracheostomy—and bleeding, if a biopsy has been taken. Red streaks of blood may be expected after biopsy, but frank bleeding requires the immediate attention of the physician.

Bronchography. After the pharynx and larynx have been anesthetized, the physician introduces a catheter into the trachea by either the nasal or oral route, and it is positioned above the bifurcation. A radiopaque oil is then injected into the trachea via the tube, and the patient is tilted in various positions so that the dye flows throughout the bronchial tree. X-ray films (bronchograms) are then taken that reveal the radiopaque outlines of the bronchi and bronchioles. The airways of both the right and the left lung can be studied at one session. However, the physician usually prefers to perform a complete evaluation in two sessions because, with different views of the chest, opacified airways may overlie each other and confuse the diagnosis. If tracheobronchial secretions are profuse, postural drainage may be necessary before the examination to clear mucus and to enable better visualization of smaller bronchi. The patient should be informed of the discomfort that he may experience during the procedure and should be advised not to cough during instillation of the contrast material since this may drive the dye into the alveoli. Sedation may be ordered. Following bronchography, postural drainage may again be required to remove excess oil. The

Table 20-1.
Blood gas analyses

Blood Gas Study	Measures	Normal Range
PaO_2 (also written as PO_2)	Partial pressure of oxygen in the arterial blood	80 to 100 mm. Hg
$PaCO_2$ (also written as PCO_2)	Partial pressure of carbon dioxide in the arterial blood	38 to 42 mm. Hg
pH	Hydrogen ion concentration	7.35 to 7.45
HCO_3^-	Bicarbonate ion concentration	22 to 26 mEq. per L.
SaO_2	Percentage of oxygen hemoglobin is carrying related to total amount it could carry	95 percent arterial blood 70 to 75 percent mixed venous blood

newer contrast media, however, are absorbed by the body and the lungs are usually clear within 12 to 24 hours. Frequently, bronchography follows bronchoscopy, and the care of the patient is similar.

RESPIRATORY FUNCTION TESTS. These studies may be divided into two components. The first is the analysis of the physical phenomena involved with the movement of the air in and out of the chest. The second is a measure of the effectiveness of the mechanical processes. The first group includes the vital capacity, maximum breathing capacity, timed vital capacity, and the forced midexpiratory flow rate. These measurements are obtained during various respiratory maneuvers. The *vital capacity* is a measure of the amount of the air a patient can expire following a maximal inspiration. The normal range is 3,500 to over 5,000 ml., but is significantly dependent upon age and sex. The pattern of the vital capacity as recorded by the respirometer can then be related to time, permitting measurement of the *timed vital capacity* and the various flow rates. Edema, pain, fibrosis, and space-filling lesions, such as cancer, can lower vital capacity. The *maximum breathing capacity* (MBC) is the most air that a patient can voluntarily move in and out of the lungs within a period of one minute. This study is a measure of the airway resistance within the lungs and is reduced in patients with asthma and chronic obstructive pulmonary disease. The MBC, however, is a very strenuous test and many patients with acute respiratory disease perform poorly due to fatigue.

The primary tests for the assessment of the effectiveness of *ventilation* (the movement of air in and out of the lungs) are measures of the partial pressures of oxygen and carbon dioxide in the arterial blood.

Blood gas studies may be performed on patients with respiratory disorders as well as on any patient that is acutely ill. These studies are the measurement of oxygen, carbon dioxide, and hydrogen in either venous or arterial blood. Most, though not all, blood gas studies are performed on arterial blood. Two of these studies—the PaO_2 and the $PaCO_2$—measure the partial *pressure* or *tension* of oxygen and carbon dioxide in the blood. (See Table 20-1 for a list of blood gas analyses.)

Patients with respiratory disorders have varying degrees of electrolyte imbalance. When the $PaCO_2$ is *elevated,* the patient has *respiratory acidosis.* This disorder is seen in patients with chronic obstructive pulmonary disease, inadequate ventilation with a mechanical ventilator, or in any patient with a decreased respiratory *rate.* When the $PaCO_2$ is *low,* the patient has *respiratory alkalosis.* This disorder is seen in those with nervousness, anxiety, or in any condition causing hyperventilation or a rapid respiratory rate.

Oxygen is present in the blood as a gas dissolved in plasma and combined with the hemoglobin of red blood cells. The greatest amount of oxygen in the blood is contained in the hemoglobin. If the PaO_2 is decreased, body tissues will not receive sufficient oxygen. Oxygenation of body tissues depends on (1) the amount of oxygen in arterial blood and (2) the ability of the heart to pump oxygenated blood to all parts of the body. Thus, patients with respiratory disorders can neither get oxygen into the blood nor relieve the blood of carbon dioxide—a waste product of cellular metabolism. Also, patients with cardiac disorders cannot adequately pump oxygenated blood to all areas of the body because of the inefficiency of the pump (the heart).

The pH measures the acidity or alkalinity of the blood. A pH of 7.0 is neutral, that is neither acid or alkaline. A pH *above* 7.0—for example, 7.42—is alkaline; one *below* 7.0 is acidic. The body is normally alkaline with a normal pH of 7.35 to 7.45.

Bicarbonate (HCO_3^-) is influenced by metabolic changes in the body. Elevation of the serum bicarbonate indicates *metabolic alkalosis*; decrease of serum bicarbonate indicates *metabolic acidosis.*

The SaO_2 indicates the ability of hemoglobin to carry oxygen. If a disease of the lungs prevents a proper exchange of the gases oxygen and carbon dioxide, the SaO_2 will be decreased.

SPUTUM EXAMINATION. Samples of bronchial secretions frequently are collected and sent to the laboratory. The microscopic examination of appropriately stained smears may reveal casts, cancer cells, or pathogenic organisms. If an attempt is to be made to grow the organisms in a culture, the collecting receptacle must be sterile, and both the nurse and the patient should be careful not to contaminate the inside of the collection bottle. Because negative smears do not necessarily indicate the absence of disease, repeated examinations may be ordered on successive days. Sometimes 24-hour specimens are collected. Sputum specimens should be raised from deep in the bronchi, such as the sputum first expectorated in the morning. The patient's mouth should be cleaned first, so that no saliva or old food particles are expectorated into the collecting receptacle. Color, consistency, odor, and quantity of sputum should be noted and charted. The appearance of blood should be reported to the physician. A waterproof, waxed sputum cup, or a wide-mouthed bottle should be used and is kept at the patient's bedside. The patient is instructed to keep the outside of the container free of contamination by the secretions. The cup or bottle should be covered to keep air-borne organisms and odor inside and to prevent the contents from being easily viewed. The specimen is refrigerated, if there is a delay in sending it to the laboratory.

For aesthetic reasons, the sputum container is covered with paper.

Analysis of Gastric Contents. Because pathogenic organisms causing lung disease frequently are swallowed, the fasting contents of the stomach may be examined. This diagnostic procedure may be used when tuberculosis is suspected.

Pneumonia

An acute illness caused by inflammation or infection of the lungs, pneumonia is characterized by a productive cough, chest pain, and fever.

Pathology

Coarse hairs at the entrance of the nose filter larger foreign particles from the inspired air. The mucous membrane that lines the respiratory passages is lined with a layer of ciliated epithelium, and its tiny, hair-like projections trap debris and microorganisms that enter with air. A sticky mucous secretion gathers these foreign bodies together. Then the motion of the cilia carries the foreign particles into the pharynx, where they are either swallowed or eliminated through the nose or the mouth. Irritation of the respiratory passages due to noxious gases or large foreign particles stimulates additional secretions, sneezing, and coughing—all of which help to expel foreign particles and accumulated mucus. The defenses of the respiratory tract against infection are so efficient that not until the body is weakened, or the noxious stimuli are overwhelming, do the lungs become infected.

When bacteria enter the alveoli they act as irritants and cause the production of fluid which fills the alveolar sacs. The fluid is an excellent culture medium and, as organisms grow in the fluid-filled alveolar sac, the body responds, as it does to all infections, by pouring more fluid into the area. The previously filled alveolus spills some fluid into the adjoining sac, and pneumonia spreads. The infected fluid moves into the bronchioles, and as the patient breathes and coughs, more alveoli become filled.

The final stage of the process, consolidation, is a filling of the alveoli with thick exudate, so that an

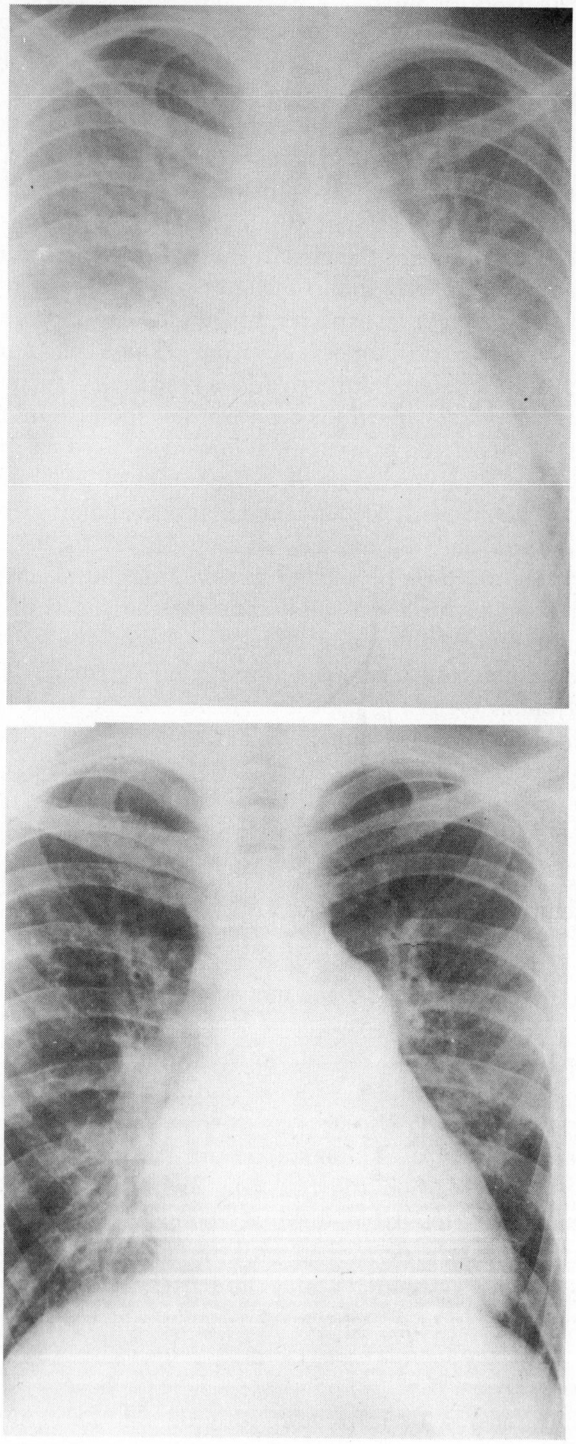

figure 20-3. (*Top*) Right lobar pneumonia. Note the consolidation of the right lower lobe. The left lung field is essentially normal. (*Bottom*) Complete resolution of the pneumonia after two weeks of antibiotic therapy. (Department of Radiology, Methodist Hospital of Brooklyn)

exchange of gases is impossible in these areas of the lung. When the pleura becomes infected, the patient has a severe, stabbing chest pain as the inflamed tissues rub over each other with each inspiration.

As the disease spreads, the mucous membranes of the nose, the pharynx, the trachea, and the bronchi become inflamed, as are the alveoli of the lungs. Secretions containing mucus, serum, fibrin, and cast-off cells exude from the membranes. As inflammation proceeds, blood oozes from the membrane and colors the sputum to the characteristic rusty color. Irritation of the mucous membrane with the collection of secretions causes coughing. At first, the cough may be dry and unproductive, but later the secretions are mucopurulent, and then they are rusty. Coughing and expectoration help to prevent clogging of the bronchi with mucous plugs.

When the inflammation is confined to one or more lobes of the lung, it is called *lobar pneumonia* (Fig. 20-3). Patchy and diffuse infection scattered throughout both lungs is called *bronchopneumonia.* Pneumonia caused by the pneumococci usually leads to lobar rather than bronchopneumonia.

Etiology

Pneumonia can be caused by many different types of organisms, such as viruses, rickettsiae, streptococci, staphylococci, fungi, and Friedländer's bacilli. However, the most common causative organism is the pneumococcus (*Diplococcus pneumoniae*). This bacterium is common in the air. It often can be cultured from the throats of healthy persons. It causes illness when the resistance of the individual is lowered, or when the person is exposed to an extraordinarily large concentration of the organisms or to particularly virulent organisms. *Staphylococcus aureus* is responsible for 1 to 5 percent of bacterial pneumonias.

Pneumonia can be caused by a group of organisms called *Mycoplasma pneumoniae.* For many years bacteria could not be cultured from secretions of patients with this type of illness. The disease was then called primary atypical pneumonia or "virus" pneumonia. It is now known to be caused by the mycoplasma, one of the smallest organisms that can be grown in cell-free media. The disease is also known as Eaton's agent pneumonia.

Hypoventilation of lung tissue over a prolonged period of time—as happens when a patient lies quietly in bed, breathing with only a part of his lungs over a prolonged period—can result in the accumulation of bronchial secretions and cause hypostatic pneumonia. Pure oxygen, if inhaled for a period of several days, can result in atelectasis or collapse of the lung. The collapsed segment then becomes susceptible to bacterial invasion and can be the site of a pneumonic infiltrate. Smoke particles and other air pollutants, such as nitrogen dioxide, can cause irritation of the linings of the air passages and create the setting for bacterial invasion. If the epiglottis does not close completely on swallowing, and fluid or other food particles are aspirated into the bronchial tree, an acute chemical pneumonitis can result followed by bacterial infection and classical pneumonia. People who are unconscious because of anesthesia, coma, sedation, or alcoholic intoxication are prone to pneumonia because the epiglottal reflex is slowed and because hypoventilation with retention of fluid occurs.

Nursing implications

When suctioning is indicated, it should be done promptly, before the mucus is aspirated. Nasogastric feedings to a comatose patient are dangerous if the tip of the tube should slip up above the epiglottis, or if the patient regurgitates. Fluids never should be poured into the mouth of an unconscious person. The thin, slippery secretions of a head cold (unlike bacteria breathed in with dusty air) are less likely to be rejected from the body by the cilia, and, therefore, may reach the alveoli, establishing an initial infection. Likewise, oily substances are not easily passed upward by ciliary action and may fill alveoli with fluid in which bacteria can grow. This is the reason that saline nosedrops are preferable to those in an oil base.

Symptoms

The onset of bacterial pneumonia is sudden. Without warning symptoms, the patient experiences severe, sharp pain in his chest, rapid prostration, and often a shaking chill that gives way to a fever going as high as 106°F.

Irritation of the tissues of the respiratory tract produces a cough that is painful, since it causes movement of the chest wall and a consequent rubbing together of the two pleural layers. As noted previously, the sputum often is rusty in color. Breathing also causes pain, and the patient tries to breathe as shallowly as possible.

In bacterial pneumonia the alveoli become filled with exudate. Bronchitis, tracheitis, and spots of necrosis in the lung may follow. In pneumonia caused by mycoplasma, there is thickening of the alveolar septa and partial filling of the alveoli with exudate. As the inflammatory process continues, there is more interference with the exchange of gases between the bloodstream and the lungs. With an increase in the carbon dioxide content of the blood, the respiratory center in the brain is stimulated, and breathing becomes more rapid and shallow. The patient is more comfortable and better able to breathe while he is sitting up.

If the disease process is not halted, the patient becomes sicker and perhaps delirious. If the circulatory system is unable to maintain the burden of decreased gaseous exchange, the patient may die from heart failure or asphyxia.

The fever of mycoplasmal or viral pneumonia resolves by lysis; that is, it slowly returns to normal. Viral pneumonia also differs from bacterial pneumonia in that the blood cultures are sterile, the sputum may be more copious, the chills are less frequent, and the pulse and the respirations are characteristically slow.

The course of viral pneumonia usually is less severe than that of bacterial pneumonia, although the patient is far from comfortable. In viral pneumonia the mortality rate is low, but it rises when bacterial pneumonia occurs as a secondary infection. Often, the patient with viral pneumonia is weak and ill for a longer time than the patient with successfully treated bacterial pneumonia.

Diagnosis

The diagnosis of pneumonia is made usually through the clinical signs and symptoms. Sputum and blood cultures are done immediately to identify the causative organism. Since the organism may not be present in early cultures, several cultures usually are ordered. Sputum for culture should be collected before antibiotics are given, since the choice of the antibiotic will depend on the positive identification of the organism. If antibiotic therapy is started before the specimen is taken, it may mask the organism. If a physician has ordered that an antibiotic be given after the collection of a sputum specimen, and difficulty is encountered in obtaining the specimen, the physician should be consulted concerning whether or not the antibiotic should be started. Cultures of the sputum require at least 24 to 48 hours to grow.

A chest roentgenogram will be ordered. The pattern and extent of pulmonary infiltration may be extremely valuable to the physician in the diagnosis and treatment of the pneumonia. A consolidated lobe of the lung may be characteristic of a pneumococcal pneumonia while the presence of multiple pulmonary abscesses is the hallmark of staphylococcal pneumonia.

The laboratory is also helpful in establishing the etiology of the pneumonia. Gram stain of a sputum smear will separate gram-positive from gram-negative organisms and frequenty the specific organism can be tentatively identified on the microscope slide pending culture. The white blood cell count is useful because it is most often normal or below normal in mycoplasmal infection while the elevation may be dramatic in staphylococcal pneumonia.

Treatment

The specific antibiotics chosen for treatment depend on the sensitivity of the causative organism to their action. Sometimes, an organism will be encountered that does not respond to any available antibiotics. If the infecting organism has not been identified, broad-spectrum antibiotics, that is, antibiotics that are effective against a large number of organisms, may be ordered.

Supportive Therapy. Other treatment of the patient is primarily supportive, including bed rest to enable the body to use all its powers for fighting the disease. Fluids in large quantities are ordered to replace those lost through increased respiration and perspiration. If the patient cannot tolerate them by mouth, intravenous fluids are given.

For cough and chest pain, codeine, 30 mg. or 60 mg., may be ordered. Codeine depresses respirations less than does morphine. Toxic effects include nausea, vomiting, constipation, and excitement.

If the inflammatory process is far advanced, the patient may have considerable respiratory difficulty and be cyanotic. The humidification of the inspired air is usually very helpful in liquefying secretions and is best administered by a cool-mist vaporizer. A nasal catheter or cannula is usually ordered for supplementary oxygenation. In the presence of severe infection with thick, abundant secretions, the physician may perform endotracheal intubation or tracheostomy. These techniques make suctioning easier, and also permit more effective ventilation by a positive pressure breathing apparatus.

Intravenous fluids are ordered when the patient is vomiting or unable to eat. Antibiotic medication may be ordered by the intravenous route, into the IV bottle, sparing the patient repeated injections. The nurse observes that the intravenous flow rate is at the speed ordered to deliver the required amount (dose) of the drug over the prescribed period of time.

Nursing management of pneumonia patients

The patient admitted to the hospital with pneumonia usually is very sick and very uncomfortable. He is likely to be frightened, have great difficulty in breathing, and experience sharp pain on inspiration. The head of the bed is elevated and the pillow placed lengthwise, so that it supports the entire back and helps expand the chest. A pillow across the upper portion of the patient's back will tend to bend him forward and lessen the expansion of his chest.

Temperature, Pulse, Respiration. These are taken on admission and every 4 hours. An increase of temperature to over 103° F. or below 98.6° F. should be reported to the physician immediately, since these signs are warnings of a drastic change in the patient's condition. A sharp increase or a sharp decrease in pulse rate warns of circulatory complications and also is reported. The character as well as the rate of respirations is observed closely. Increasingly labored respirations indicate very rapid progress of the disease and are often a sign that more drastic treatment measures are required. It is characteristic for the patient to grunt with each expiration. Temperature is taken rectally, since coughing and oral breathing render oral readings grossly inaccurate. Hypothermia measures, that is, the use of aspirin, tepid sponge baths, or a hypothermia blanket may be ordered for fever over 102° F. or 103° F. The patient should not be exposed to a draft or chill during a sponge bath.

Medications and Treatment are planned so that the patient is disturbed as little as possible. Antibiotics are given on time to maintain consistent blood levels. Nursing care is planned so that when the nurse gives the patient medication she also gives him mouth care and fluids, changes his position, and takes his vital signs, thus allowing for uninterrupted rest periods. Although the daily bath should be omitted during the acute phase to avoid tiring the patient, a back rub and fresh linens are essential. Also, to avoid chilling, the patient's pajamas and linen are changed every time they become wet with perspiration.

Food and Fluids. Fluids should be offered in small quantities and at frequent intervals. Since the ingestion of food may stimulate coughing, fluid should not be offered after a coughing spell. Ice chips may be used to moisten the mouth if fluids are not tolerated orally. Frequent mouth care is essential to prevent stomatitis. The lesions of herpes simplex often appear around the mouth. The physician may order only fluids or a light diet for the acutely ill patient. A regular diet is resumed when the appetite returns, and the patient's condition improves.

Elimination. If the patient's urinary output is not consistent with intake, the discrepancy should be reported to the physician. Since abdominal distention and paralytic ileus are complications of pneumonia, bowel movements should be observed and recorded, and the abdomen should be watched for distention. Distention pushes the diaphragm up, so that it presses on the base of the lungs at a time when they are especially in need of space for expansion.

Expectoration. When the patient is disturbed for medications or for treatment, he is encouraged to cough up mucus. Whenever he coughs, whether voluntarily or by reflex, the nurse places her hands on his chest where it hurts, using firm pressure to splint the chest. This will decrease the pain a little and help the patient to be more willing to cough. Some patients are shy about expectorating in the view of another person, but the infected sputum should not be swallowed. Care is taken to make sure that the patient does not cough directly into the nurse's face; there are live organisms in the sputum. A sputum cup with a cover is provided if the sputum is to be saved for inspection or measurement. If not, disposable tissues and a paper bag in which to dispose of them may be used instead. This equipment is kept within easy reach, so that the patient does not have to exert himself to reach it. The sputum cup or paper bag is changed at least twice a day, handled with great care, and sealed so that the infection is not spread.

Restlessness. The patient is observed closely for signs of restlessness. The nurse listens to his respirations, looks at his color, notes whether he is restless. If he is, the nurse asks him to tell her why. She may be able to relieve his pain, to help him to cough out some sputum, or to change his position. Restlessness may be a prelude to delirium. The physician is informed at once if delirium should occur. The patient is protected with padded side rails and with restraints when they are ordered.

Isolation. In some hospitals, patients with pneumonia (particularly staphylococcal pneumonia) are isolated during the acute phase.

Some physicians believe that the spread of pneumonia is prevented by this measure; other physicians believe that handwashing and ordinary cleanliness are sufficient to prevent the spread of infection. In either case, medical asepsis is enhanced if the nurse wears an isolation gown over the uniform when giving direct care. The patient needs to be protected from secondary infection. The nurse should wash her hands before caring for him, as well as before leaving the unit. Visitors with head colds should be excluded from the room.

If isolation is not used, care should be taken that

the patient's roommates are not in a high-risk group, such as the aged, postsurgical patients, or those with chronic obstructive pulmonary disease.

CONVALESCENCE. With the administration of antibiotics, symptoms usually subside rapidly during the first 48 to 72 hours, and the patient feels much improved. However, he will be weak and tired. He is kept in bed for several days after his temperature has returned to normal. He then is helped gradually to resume normal routine and self-care. A follow-up roentgenogram usually is ordered to make sure that the disease process is clearing.

COMPLICATIONS OF PNEUMONIA

Complications of pneumonia are seen more rarely today than in the past, since antibiotics usually reverse the disease process early. Congestive heart failure is a serious complication. On occasion a patient's temperature may fall within two days, but his pulse may remain fast. Even though the fever is gone, the lung pathology and the other symptoms remain. The patient is still acutely ill.

Empyema, the collection of pus in the pleural space, and pleurisy (see below) may occur. Symptoms include continued fever and other signs of infection. The pain in the chest is usually at the site of infection. Empyema is treated with the antibiotics that are specific for the invading organisms. This is determined through thoracentesis and bacteriological examination of the fluid obtained.

The invasion of the bloodstream by organisms, which occurs during periods of septicemia while the patient is having a chill, makes the entire body accessible to the organisms. A secondary focus of infection may be established, resulting in endocarditis, meningitis, or purulent arthritis.

Atelectasis, or the collapse of the lung, is caused by the plugging of a bronchus with mucus. Encouraging the patient to cough and changing his position frequently will help to prevent this complication.

Otitis media, bronchitis, or sinusitis may complicate recovery, especially from atypical pneumonia, by the spread of the organisms to these organs.

PREVENTION OF PNEUMONIA

Because colds can lower resistance and lead to more serious infections, such as pneumonia, patients in hospitals should be isolated promptly at the first signs of a cold. It is especially important that colds be treated promptly and carefully in people with increased susceptibility—for example, alcoholics and older persons. Health personnel with colds, including nurses, should remain at home.

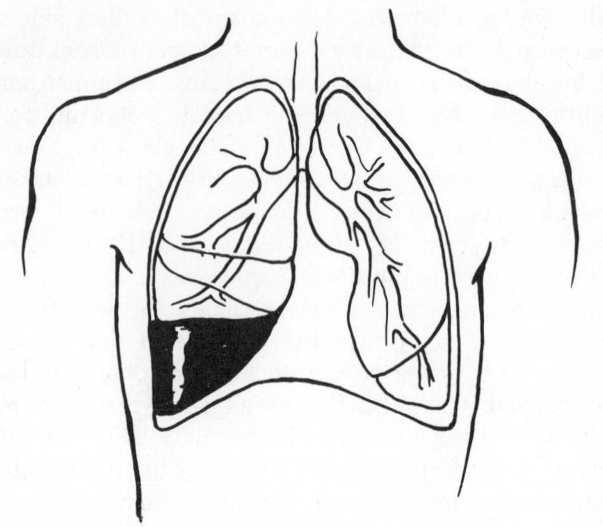

figure 20-4. Fluid in the pleural space can compress the lung.

Nurses have a particular responsibility to prevent hypostatic pneumonia. Every patient on bed rest is a candidate for this disease, especially the heavily sedated, comatose, and elderly patients. All patients should be encouraged to move and exercise. If they are unable to do so, their positions are changed at regular intervals. Patients should take several deep breaths at least every hour during the day.

Pleurisy

PATHOLOGY

Pleurisy is an inflammation of the *pleura,* the membrane that covers the lungs in two layers. Pleurisy occurs as a complication of pulmonary disease. Two forms are seen: acute fibrinous or dry pleurisy, in which only small amounts of exudate are formed during the inflammatory process; and *pleurisy with effusion,* in which large amounts of fluid are secreted and collect in the space between the pleural layers (Fig. 20-4). There may be so much fluid that the lung is collapsed partially on that side, and there is pressure on the heart and the other organs of the mediastinum. Dry pleurisy is seen most commonly in pneumonia, in which the inflammatory process spreads from the lung to the parietal pleura. Pleurisy with effusion may result from tuberculosis, carcinoma of the lungs, cardiac and renal disease, systemic infections, pneumonia, and pulmonary embolism. The pleura becomes thick, swollen, and rigid. The visceral pleura has no pain fibers, but the parietal pleura does. Very sharp pain occurs when the two surfaces of the pleura rub over each other during respiration. As fluid is formed, this pain gradually subsides; but the patient has a dry cough, fatigues easily, and may get out of breath.

Treatment and nursing management of pleurisy patients

The care of the patient with pleurisy is similar to that of the patient with pneumonia. Bed rest is required. The room should be warm and well ventilated. The patient needs encouragement to cough. The nurse can help by firm pressure at the painful spot. Positioning the patient on the side of the effusion helps to splint the painful area and also encourages the expansion of the other side of the rib cage. A heating pad or hot-water bag over the painful area may be ordered for comfort.

If there is a great deal of fluid with respiratory embarrassment, the fluid may be removed by thoracentesis. The nurse prepares the equipment, including that needed for the collection of specimens. She watches the patient closely during the thoracentesis for signs of weakness, excessive diaphoresis, increased respirations or dyspnea, pain, chill, nausea, coughing, or shock. Any symptoms are reported to the physician, who then proceeds more slowly or discontinues the treatment. It may be necessary for the nurse to support the weakened patient in position. He should be comfortable so that he can remain immobile during the procedure. Leaning forward over a pillow-padded bed table is generally a helpful position.

Influenza

Influenza ("Flu") is an acute respiratory disease of short duration caused by one of several related and yet distinct viruses.

Influenza occurs chiefly in epidemics, although sporadic cases appear between epidemics.

Epidemics can be predicted, and vaccines are available, but significant protection against influenza epidemics is not yet a reality.

Most patients recover. Fatalities usually are due to bacterial complications, especially among pregnant women, the aged or debilitated and those with chronic conditions, such as cardiac disease. During an epidemic, the death rate from pneumonia and cardiovascular disease rises.

Symptoms

The incubation period is 2 to 3 days, and the onset is sudden, with considerable individual variation in symptoms. The patient looks acutely ill and complains of chilliness, severe headache, muscular aching, and fever. There may be anorexia, weakness, and apathy, as well as respiratory symptoms, sneezing, sore throat, dry cough, nasal discharge, and herpetic lesions of the lips and the mouth. Severe disease causes prostration and may lead to vasomotor collapse. Fever, 100° to 103° F., persists about 3 days, but other symptoms usually continue for 7 to 10 days. Cough may persist longer.

The return to normal activities should be gradual, because of the amount of prostration typical of influenza. Overexertion and chilling should be avoided. The patient should not return to work until all symptoms have subsided, including the cough.

Complications include tracheobronchitis, caused by damage to the ciliated epithelium of trachea and bronchi; bacterial pneumonia; and cardiovascular disease. Staphylococcal pneumonia is the most serious complication.

Treatment and nursing management of influenza patients

Bed rest in a warm, well-ventilated room is recommended until the temperature is normal and for 1 or 2 days afterward. Temperature, pulse, and respirations are taken every 4 hours. Copious amounts of fluid, given frequently, may include fruit juices and broths; a regular diet is given as soon as the patient's appetite returns. Acetylsalicylic acid (aspirin), 0.3 to 1.0 gm., may be given every 4 to 6 hours for headache and muscular aching. Steam or cool vapor inhalation eases a dry cough. The physician may order codeine 30 to 60 mg. every 6 hours, as needed, to control coughing.

The viruses that cause influenza are transmitted through the respiratory tract. Hospitalization is not recommended in uncomplicated cases, because of the possibility of exposing the patient to a secondary bacterial infection. The patient is observed for signs of increasing fever, elevated pulse rate, chest pain, difficulty in breathing, change in the amount and the quality of the sputum—particularly, whether it is purulent or rusty—and for the sudden occurrence of chest pain. A prompt report of any of these symptoms is made to the physician.

Common cold

A large number of filterable viruses cause colds. Immunity is of very short duration, and incubation is short. Extraneous factors, such as fatigue, chilling, emotional upset, exposure to irritating gases or allergens—all of which affect the nasal mucosa—are believed to lower the natural resistance, facilitating invasion by the virus.

SYMPTOMS. Although there is considerable individual variation in the symptoms, they may include sneezing, chilliness, headache, watery eyes, and a dry scratchy throat, followed by copious nasal discharge, sore throat, hoarseness, and cough. There may be a slight fever. The cold lasts from 4 to 14 days, with symptoms gradually subsiding.

TREATMENT. Bed rest is perhaps the most important aspect of the treatment, since it restricts contact with others and limits the spread of the cold. It is particularly important for the individual who may be susceptible to complications—infants, aged and debilitated individuals, and those whose temperature is elevated. Ordinarily, the otherwise healthy adult does not remain confined to bed, although he should get extra rest and avoid contact with others. Fluids in large amounts are helpful. Petroleum jelly around the nose and the mouth will relieve chapping.

Individuals who have a tendency to develop a secondary bacterial infection may benefit from prophylactic antibiotic therapy. This group includes patients with asthma, chronic obstructive pulmonary disease, and other chronic lung ailments. Aspirin, 0.3 to 0.6 gm., may be given every 4 to 6 hours for the relief of general discomfort. Although nosedrops or inhalers obtained commercially may help to relieve some of the nasal congestion, indiscriminate use of them is harmful as many of them contain drugs that affect the body systemically, or they cause local irritation of the mucous membrane of the nose.

Injuries of the chest

FRACTURED RIBS are a common form of injury to the chest. They may be caused by a hard fall or by a blow on the chest. Automobile accidents are a frequent cause. Although rib fractures are very painful, they usually are not serious unless injury to other structures results. For example, the sharp end of the broken bone may tear the lung or blood vessels. If the injury involves fractured ribs without other complications, the patient often is permitted to return home after treatment. The usual treatment includes supporting the chest with an elastic bandage or adhesive strapping to minimize the pain, and the administration of analgesics. Sometimes a regional nerve block is necessary to relieve the pain. If the patient is treated on an outpatient basis, it is important for him to understand that:

1. He should breathe as deeply as possible; his natural inclination will be to take very shallow breaths to minimize pain.
2. He should take the analgesic as ordered, in order to minimize the pain, to promote rest, and to permit more normal breathing.
3. He will probably breathe more comfortably in a sitting position than when he is lying flat.
4. If he experiences sudden, sharp chest pain or difficulty in breathing, he should call his physician at once.

BLAST INJURIES, such as those that result from compression of the chest by an explosion, cause serious injury to the lungs by rupturing the alveoli. Death often results from hemorrhage and asphyxiation. The treatment includes the provision of complete rest and the administration of oxygen.

PENETRATING WOUNDS of the chest are also very serious. An open wound may permit air to enter the thoracic cavity, causing *pneumothorax*. If the wound is large, it may cause a sucking noise as air enters and leaves the chest cavity. Applying an airtight dressing is an important first-aid measure to prevent the entrance of more air into the chest cavity. Air also may enter the pleural space from an injury to the lung tissue. For example, the sharp end of a broken rib may tear the lung tissue, permitting air to enter the pleural space. Many chest injuries involve both pneumothorax and *hemothorax* (blood in the pleural space).

When medical aid has been obtained, the air and the blood are aspirated from the pleural space by thoracentesis. Sometimes a chest catheter is inserted and attached to closed drainage. Later it may be necessary to perform a thoracotomy to repair or to remove injured tissues. Foreign bodies that have entered the chest should be removed only by the physician. Their presence in the wound may prevent the entrance of air, and their removal without medical aid may cause pneumothorax.

All chest injuries are serious or potentially serious, and any patient with a chest injury must be observed for dyspnea, cyanosis, chest pain, weak and rapid pulse, and hypotension—all signs and symptoms of respiratory distress. The patient with a chest injury is examined by a physician as soon as possible after the injury.

General nutritional considerations

- The patient undergoing a bronchoscopy is usually placed on NPO for 8 to 12 hours prior to the test to avoid the danger of vomiting and aspiration. The patient should be informed that he must not eat or drink and given an explanation of the reasons for this precaution.
- Fluids should never be given by mouth to an unconscious person.
- The patient with increased respirations (e.g., with pneumonia, influenza, or a cold) should be encouraged to drink extra fluids to replace those lost through increased respiration and perspiration.
- IV fluids may be necessary for the patient who is too ill to eat or drink.
- Frequent feedings of juice, broth, and eggnog may help supplement the patient's increased nutritional needs.

General pharmacological considerations

- Antibiotics may be ordered for the patient with a respiratory infection; however, a culture and sensitivity are usually done to identify the organisms causing the infection. Once the organisms are identified and the sensitivity to various antibiotics determined, the antibiotic proven to be effective will be prescribed.
- Antitussive agents (drugs used to relieve coughing) and mucolytic agents (drugs used to reduce thickness and tenacity of sputum) may be ordered for patients with respiratory disorders.
- The indiscriminate use of nonprescription cough medicines may do more harm than good. Coughing is nature's way of clearing the respiratory passages of mucus; depressing the cough reflex may cause a pooling of secretions and further problems.

Bibliography

Alexander, M. M., et al: Physical examination: chest and lungs (pictorial), part 12. Nurs. '75, 5:44, January, 1975.

Baum, G. L., ed. *Textbook of Pulmonary Diseases*, ed. 2. Boston, Little, Brown, 1973.

Boyce, B. A.: Respiratory care terminology, part 1. Clinical Newsletter 1:1, January, 1976.

Delaney, M. T.: Examining the chest, part 1: The lungs. Nurs. '75, 5:12, August, 1975.

Gordon, R., et al: Image reconstruction from projections. Sci. Am. 233:56, October, 1975.

Hudak, C. M., et al: *Clinical Care Nursing*. Philadelphia, Lippincott, 1973.

McCormick, K. A. and Birnbaum, M. L.: Acute ventilatory failure following thoracic trauma. Nurs. Clin. North Am. 9:181, March, 1974.

New, P. F. J.: Computed tomography: a major diagnostic advance. Hosp. Prac. 10:55, February, 1975.

Pnemonia with a new look (pictorial). Emer. Med. 6:64, December, 1974.

Scherer, J. C.: *Introductory Clinical Pharmacology*. Philadelphia, Lippincott, 1975.

Tilkian, S. M. and Conover, M. H.: *Clinical Implications of Laboratory Tests*. St. Louis, Mosby, 1975.

Tinker, J. H.: Understanding chest x-rays. Am. J. Nurs. 76:65, January, 1976.

Traver, G.: Assessment of the thorax and lungs. Am. J. Nurs. 73:466, March, 1973.

CHAPTER—21

The patient with chronic respiratory disorder

On completion of this chapter the student will:

- Describe the symptoms and medical and nursing management of the patient with allergic rhinitis, chronic and acute bronchitis, and bronchial asthma.
- Identify and discuss the criteria for chronic obstructive pulmonary disease (COPD).
- Formulate a nursing care plan for a patient with chronic obstructive respiratory disease.
- Describe the symptoms and medical, surgical, and nursing management of patients with bronchiectasis, empyema, lung abscess, and lung cancer.
- Draw and label the parts of the underwater seal drainage and describe the nursing management of the patient with an underwater seal drainage.
- Formulate a nursing management plan for patients with: (1) a pneumonectomy, (2) a lobectomy, and (3) a thoracotomy.
- Discuss the relationship of cancer of the lung and acute and chronic lung diseases to smoking, air pollution, and other possible causes of these disorders.
- Discuss the case finding, treatment, and basic long-term management of the patient with tuberculosis.

Any change in the size, shape, or function of the body is apt to cause anxiety. When the usually automatic function of breathing enters awareness and becomes a struggle, a vicious cycle often ensues. The dyspneic patient is anxious because he cannot breathe normally, and the more anxious he becomes the more difficult it is for him to breathe. When the nurse uses measures which facilitate the patient's breathing (such as mechanical devices and drugs), the patient becomes more relaxed and anxiety is reduced.

The incidence of serious chronic respiratory disease is increasing. Although the reasons for this increase have not been definitely determined, two important contributing factors appear to be smoking and air pollution.

The nurse demonstrates concern about chronic respiratory disease by participating in programs and other educational efforts to eradicate or minimize smoking as well as environmental air pollution.

Allergic rhinitis

DEFINITION. Allergic rhinitis is a term used to describe the reaction of the nasal mucous membrane to various allergens commonly found in the environment. The allergic response is characterized by swelling of the nasal mucous membrane, sneezing, and increased nasal secretions. Other terms such as hay fever or rose fever have been used to describe the allergic response secondary to specific allergenic substances. Allergic rhinitis may occur seasonally and be specifically related to pollens, or it may develop on a perennial (nonseasonal) basis where the reaction is due to other environmental antigens such as dust or feathers.

ETIOLOGY AND PATHOLOGY. The condition is caused by allergy to a specific antigen (see Chapter 3 on allergy). When the symptoms are seasonal, allergic rhinitis usually is caused by pollens from weeds, trees, or grasses. Perennial allergic rhinitis may be due to dust, feathers, and animal danders. The allergen-antibody reaction occurring in the nose causes immediate release of histamine that affects the local tissues of the nose by causing edema, itching, and a watery discharge. The eyes and the pharynx may also be affected.

INCIDENCE. Allergic rhinitis is common in persons who have an allergic background. Often there is a family history of allergy, although the specific allergen may vary among different members of the same family. Allergic rhinitis can occur at any age; although it tends to recur in the same individual for an indefinite period, its course over a lifetime is variable. One person may have the onset of symptoms at puberty; another may develop symptoms for the first time in middle life. It is possible for the symptoms to subside without apparent cause or to subside and be replaced by other allergic manifestations such as asthma.

SYMPTOMS. The patient usually experiences itching of the nose, eyes, throat, and roof of the mouth. This is accompanied by sneezing, a profuse watery discharge, and tearing of the eyes. Marked swelling of the nasal mucosa may cause complete obstruction of the nasal airway, making breathing difficult. During a full-blown episode of allergic rhinitis, a feeling of malaise accompanies the episode. Symptoms due to pollen are more severe on clear, windy days and during early morning and evening hours.

DIAGNOSIS. Allergic rhinitis is diagnosed through a careful history of events related to the attacks. Symptoms may appear only a few weeks at the same season each year, leading the doctor to suspect pollen, or they may have their onset when a new pet or a new object is introduced into the environment. Skin testing is helpful in determining which substance is causing symptoms and, frequently, the patient may be allergic to several different substances. Physical examination and microscopic examination of nasal secretions are also helpful in diagnosis. The nasal mucous membrane usually appears edematous and pale. An abundance of eosinophils is found typically in nasal secretions.

TREATMENT. The most effective treatment is avoidance of the allergen. However, it is often very difficult to completely avoid all contact with the various allergens in the environment. For the majority of patients, treatment centers around desensitization, antihistamines, and diminishing contact with the allergen.

Contact with pollen can be diminished by remaining indoors, away from open windows on windy days, and by using an air conditioner, although some individuals may find an air conditioned atmosphere increases the severity of symptoms. Should the allergic rhinitis be of the perennial type and due to animal danders or feathers, using a foam rubber pillow and finding a new home for the pet may result in complete remission of symptoms. For those persons whose interest in the outdoors or love of a pet outweighs the desire for total relief, desensitization will often diminish the symptoms. Antihistamines frequently give temporary relief. Corticosteroid preparations may be used in *severe* cases of allergic rhinitis.

COURSE AND PROGNOSIS. Allergic rhinitis is most severe when exposure to the allergen is at its height. Fatigue and emotional strain tend to aggravate the symptoms. Because the edema may block drainage of the sinuses, sinusitis sometimes complicates allergic rhinitis. Obstruction of the eustachian tube results in middle ear infection, a common finding in allergic rhinitis. Should infection of the nasal mucosa intervene during an acute episode, nasal polyps may develop. These polyps further tend to obstruct the nasal air passages, resulting in difficult breathing. Some patients may go on to develop asthma as a consequence of their disease. Although allergic rhinitis is not a threat to life, it is a major cause of discomfort. Effective treatment, usually desensitization, cannot eradicate the condition, but can add greatly to the patient's comfort and decrease the likelihood of sequelae.

Bronchial asthma

DEFINITION. Asthma is derived from the Greek word for panting and is used clinically to mean shortness of breath. Bronchial asthma is typified by paroxysms of shortness of breath, wheezing, cough, and the production of thick, tenacious sputum. The onset and the duration of the acute episode vary markedly among individuals. The duration may be brief, lasting less than one day, or extend into prolonged periods of several weeks.

SYMPTOMS AND PATHOPHYSIOLOGY. The triad characteristic of the acute asthmatic state consists of spasm of the smooth muscle of the bronchi and the larger bronchioles, swelling of the mucosal lining, and thick bronchiole secretions. The degree of airflow obstruction is directly related to the severity of the above mechanisms. Once the air has entered the alveoli, air trapping takes place since the bronchioles and bronchi narrow during the expiratory effort. The attempt to move air across a narrowed orifice results, as in the playing of any reed instrument, in the production of musical tones. This is the classical wheezing that the physician hears on auscultation of the chest and which may be audible without the stethoscope. The patient is usually aware of the wheezing and reports it as one of his symptoms. Every breath becomes an effort and during the acute episode the work of breathing is greatly increased. The patient may suffer from a sensation of suffocation. Frequently, a classical sitting position is assumed with the body leaning slightly forward and the arms at shoulder height. This position facilitates expansion of the chest as well as more effective excursions of the diaphragm. Because life depends on the power to breathe, fear accompanies the symptoms. Unfortunately, fear and anxiety tend to intensify the symptoms rather than relieve them.

The effort to move trapped air within the alveoli is accompanied by a marked prolongation of the expiratory phase of respiration. Coughing commences with the onset of the attack, but is ineffective in the early stage and only as the attack begins to subside is the patient able to expectorate large quantities of thick, stringy mucus. Usually, the skin is pale; however, if the attack is very severe, mild cyanosis of the lips and nailbeds may be noted. Perspiration is usually profuse during an acute attack. Following spontaneous or drug-induced remission of the episode, examination of the lungs commonly reveals normal findings and it is frequently impossible to diagnose bronchial asthma by physical signs without observation during the acute attack. Occasionally, however, the acute state can intensify and be resistant to all therapy, progressing into "status asthmaticus."

ETIOLOGY. Prominent among the causes of asthma are antigen-antibody reactions as seen in allergy, infection, and emotional stress. These factors vary in importance in different patients, but with careful observation all three components may be found active at the same time. Bronchial asthma has been divided into two separate groups. The first is extrinsic asthma, which occurs chiefly in response to allergens such as pollen, dust, spores, or animal danders. Intrinsic asthma is the second type and has been associated with upper respiratory infection or emotional upsets.

INCIDENCE AND COURSE. Asthma may occur at any period in life. Approximately 50 percent of all asthma occurs prior to the age of 10. A significant relationship between bronchiolitis in the first year of life and the development of bronchial asthma in early childhood has been noted. Extrinsic asthma is the most common form noted in childhood and young adulthood. Intrinsic asthma due to recurrent infection frequently related to chronic sinusitis or chronic bronchitis is most frequently seen after the age of 40. Asthma may be limited to occasional attacks and the patient is usually symptom-free in the interim.

TREATMENT OF BRONCHIAL ASTHMA

Symptomatic treatment is given at the time of the attack. The long-term care of the patient involves measures to control the cause of the illness. Thus, treatment of allergy, infection, and emotional disorders may all play a part in the therapy.

Oxygen Therapy. Oxygen is usually not necessary during an acute attack. This is because most patients with bronchial asthma are actively hyperventilating. Rarely, particularly after a long bout of asthma, some patients may develop cyanosis. Oxygen may then be given by nasal catheter, mask, or, preferably, intermittent positive pressure breathing. Thus, the nurse does not automatically reach for oxygen for the patient in the acute asthmatic state unless cyanosis is present. Oxygen administration should be prescribed for each patient, as drugs are prescribed. The physician should specify how the oxygen is to be administered, that is, by mask, nasal catheter, or some other means and the liter flow to be used.

The nurse should explain to the patient the reason for the mask or the catheter. By providing an explanation, as well as remaining with the patient initially until he gets adjusted to the oxygen and equipment, the nurse will help to allay the patient's anxiety and reduce the fear of suffocation. Intermittent positive pressure breathing employing equipment such as the Bird or Bennett Respirator may greatly aid the patient by taking over the work of breathing and promoting better alveolar ventilation.

Bronchodilators. The bronchodilator preparations are usually divided into two groups: the adrenergic drugs and aminophylline. Adrenergic medications are most commonly used in the treatment of acute bronchial asthma; they include such drugs as epinephrine (Adrenalin) and isoproterenol (Isuprel). These agents tend to reduce bronchospasm by causing relaxation of the smooth muscle lining the bronchi and the larger bronchioles.

Epinephrine and isoproterenol are extremely effective bronchodilators when given by nebulizer. Delivering the bronchodilator by nebulizer directly into the lung has the advantage of providing maximal effect on the bronchial musculature. Although side effects do occur, they are limited as compared with subcutaneous injection. Since the effectiveness of the nebulized bronchodilator is dependent on the dose and proper delivery of the drug into the lung, specific instructions must be given to the patient. The drug should not be diluted by the addition of water or any other agent. It has been shown that the effectiveness of the nebulized bronchodilator is dependent solely on its concentration. Therefore, if the 0.5 ml. of drug is diluted with 2 ml. of saline, the overall effectiveness of the therapy will be one-fifth of that expected.

The usual dose of the aerosol using a hand nebulizer is one or two sprays delivered to the tracheobronchial tree every 4 hours. The tip of the nebulizer, whether hand-bulb or aerosol type, is placed in the open mouth. The nurse instructs the patient not to close his lips around the nebulizer. Then, while breathing in, the patient squeezes the bulb or presses on the aerosol can. In this manner, the nebulized material is carried with the airstream into the trachea, bronchi, and bronchioles. Without proper instruction, many patients will close their mouths around the mouthpiece and while breathing through the nose, deliver the drug. This results in deposition of the bronchodilator in the oral cavity and absorption by the mucosa of the mouth. The principal effect will then be on the cardiovascular system with very little relief of respiratory symptoms. Because the pressurized aerosol form is so readily available, overmedication can become a problem. Obviously, these agents must be used with great caution in individuals who have cardiac disease.

The nurse explains to the patient and family the purpose of the drug, when and how it should be used, and why it should not be overused. They should be aware that harmful, systemic side effects of the drugs can occur and when these should be reported to the physician. The physician should also be informed when the usual dose of the aerosol seems to be ineffective. The public health nurse can give the patient overall health supervision and specific instruction in the use of drugs at home. Especially if the patient is elderly or handicapped, the family needs instruction and support to assist him.

Aminophylline is effective in reducing bronchospasm. It is most useful when administered intravenously in a dose of 0.25–0.5 gm. The doctor injects the drug slowly over a period of approximately 10 minutes in order to avoid a sudden drop in blood pressure, with dizziness, faintness, palpitation, and headache. For prolonged in-hospital use, the dose of aminophylline may be given over an 8-hour period in 500 ml. to 1,000 ml. of intravenous fluid. The use of aminophylline as a rectal suppository is valuable and effective. Most patients develop anorectal irritation, however, if the dose exceeds 0.5 gm. every 12 hours. The nurse observes whether and to what extent symptoms are relieved and whether there is anorectal irritation.

Humidification of the inspired air is extremely important in the therapy of the bronchospastic state. It has been shown that dehydration of the respiratory mucous membrane may by itself lead to attacks of bronchial asthma. The use of steam or cool vapor humidifiers has proved effective. The value of humidification becomes evident as the attack subsides and the patient brings up thick, tenacious sputum. Liquefication of the secretions promotes more effective clearing of the airways and a rapid return to normal.

A large daily intake of fluids also helps the patient to bring up secretions and serves to replace fluid lost by profuse perspiration during the acute attack. The initiative for increasing fluid intake rests with the nurse who must continually offer the patient fluids. The exhausted dyspneic patient often cannot reach for and take them himself.

Sedatives and Tranquilizers. These drugs are frequently used to control anxiety during the acute attack. However, care must be taken to avoid depression of respiration and the cough reflex. The anxiety that accompanies the acute attack is related to the patient's inability to breathe. To sedate the patient simply to relieve anxiety prior to relieving the respiratory distress may intensify the symptoms and, if the respiratory center is sufficiently depressed, death may occur. Narcotics, because of their respiratory depressant effects, are not used unless preparations have been made for mechanical support of respiration.

Nursing measures that help to lessen the patient's apprehension include:

- Staying with him, if possible.
- Listening to his concerns.
- Indicating by words and actions that his condition does not unduly alarm those caring for him.
- Providing him with a way to signal for help, answering calls promptly, and observing him when he does not call.
- Doing nothing to indicate within the patient's hearing that his attack is unusually severe or is not responding to treatment.
- Checking with the doctor if there is doubt concerning administration of sedatives to provide mental and physical rest. The patient is thus spared any anxiety resulting from indecision on the nurse's part.

Corticosteroids are not generally used in the treatment of the patient with uncomplicated bronchial asthma. Medical opinion holds that bronchodilators, when used promptly, can be as effective as corticosteroids but without serious side effects. Should the disease progress, the doctor may order these drugs by the oral route.

If the acute asthmatic state is complicated by an infection, the doctor orders antibiotics. Because most infections of this type are gram-positive, penicillin or one of the penicillin derivatives is the drug of choice. Many allergists believe that all bronchial asthma is complicated by infection and now prescribe antibiotic therapy even in the absence of clinical signs and symptoms of infection.

Environment. The asthmatic patient's environment should be as free as possible of factors which contribute to respiratory infection. Nurses or visitors with upper respiratory infection should avoid contact with the patient. The patient should be protected from exposure to allergens that may have set off attacks or that may continue to perpetuate them. Thorough cleanliness of all inhalation therapy equipment is urgent.

Long-term care

Efforts must be made to determine the cause of the attacks. If the patient's history and his diagnostic tests indicate that allergy is an important causative factor, treatment by avoidance of the allergen, by desensitization, or by antihistamines may be used.

Common inhalants that may cause asthma are dust, feathers, pollens, and animal danders. It is important to keep the patient's environment as free as possible from substances to which he is allergic. Air conditioners are very helpful in eliminating pollen as well as in controlling temperature and humidity. Feathers and down frequently cause symptoms, thus pillows made of synthetic fibers or foam rubber are preferable. Flowers also may aggravate the symptoms. When family or friends express a desire to send gifts to the patient, the nurse may suggest tactfully that the gift be something other than flowers.

The control of infection plays a major role in the care of patients with asthma. Frequently, the patients are susceptible to respiratory infections, and these infections tend, as the patients say, "to go to the chest." Patients should avoid factors that predispose to respiratory infections, such as exposure, fatigue, and contact with persons who have colds. Respiratory infections, when they do occur, should be treated promptly. Antibiotics are often necessary.

Emotional stress is likely to be a causative factor in asthmatic attacks. Adjustments in home or job situations may be helpful in relieving stress. Psychotherapy may help the patient to understand and to handle his emotional reactions better; it may be suggested by the doctor, if the patient's attacks seem closely related to emotional factors.

The maintenance of good general health is important in reducing the frequency of attacks and in helping the patient to achieve the maximum benefit from his treatment. Rest, optimum diet, and a balance of work and recreation are important.

Nursing management of the asthmatic patient

Seeing a patient in extreme respiratory distress may be a frightening experience for the nurse. The patient is very anxious and looks to those who care for him for support and reassurance. Since it is the nurse who spends the greatest amount of time with the hospitalized patient, a large measure of this support and reassurance becomes a nursing responsibility.

Although the extreme dyspnea, wheezing, and struggle for breath make it appear that the patient will not survive, most patients who have acute asthmatic attacks do recover. Most attacks are temporary and short; thus the nurse, on the basis of this understanding, can help the patient to feel that his attack will subside. Occasionally, however, asthmatic attacks are very prolonged or recur in rapid succession. This condition is called *status asthmaticus*. Most patients do not die during an asthmatic attack; nevertheless it is true that death sometimes occurs. The patient often fears that each breath will be his last. He may describe a feeling of suffocation or of drowning. It should be remembered that the spasm of the patient's bronchi is causing marked interference with a vital function. The nurse should avoid giving glib and superficial reassurance and must recognize that, although emotional factors may precipitate attacks in some patients, the patient who is having an attack is very ill. Such attitudes as, "It's all in his mind—he could snap out of it if he wanted to," betray a gross misunderstanding, and seriously interfere with the nurse's ability to care for patients with asthma.

Initial Care. The patient's greatest concern is his breathing; nursing care must involve nothing that would increase the difficulty in breathing. Measures should be taken, before the doctor arrives, to make the patient more comfortable. Routine admission procedures may need to be modified temporarily. For instance, it would be most unwise to place an oral thermometer in the patient's mouth for an admission TPR, since the patient needs to breathe through his mouth. Recognizing that a sitting position makes breathing easier during an asthmatic attack, the nurse should not insist that the patient lie in bed, and assist him to assume the position that is most comfortable for him.

Because of the patient's anxiety during the attack, the nurse should stay with him, if possible, and convey through manner and actions that someone is there to help him. There are many small ways in which the nurse can demonstrate this: replacing a moist nightgown with a dry one, showing the patient the call bell, and assuring him that, when he rings, someone will come.

Since most patients with asthma already feel closed in, it is important to avoid intensifying this sensation by drawing curtains around the bed or closing the doors and the windows. It is wise not to ask the patient to answer any unnecessary questions, because respiratory difficulty is made worse by an attempt to talk. The nurse should observe and chart rate and character of respirations, pulse, color, cough, sputum, emotional state, and diaphoresis.

Continuing Care. What nursing management will be needed after the physician leaves? Since the patient has been frightened, and is now in a strange environment, it would be wise to keep a dim light on in his room at night and to encourage him to signal the nurse whenever it is necessary. Rest and adequate fluid intake are important. As he becomes assured that his breathing has improved, he will probably be comfortable with the head of the bed elevated. If plenty of fluids are provided within easy reach, and the patient is encouraged to drink them, the increased fluid intake will help secretions become less tenacious and will replace the fluids lost through perspiration. Tissues and a sputum cup should be provided, and the patient should be encouraged to expectorate the mucus.

It is not unusual for the patient with asthma to signal the nurse repeatedly for apparently insignificant requests. Frequent use of the call bell is particularly likely at night or when the patient has had a recent attack and usually indicates that he is anxious and wants someone to stay with him. It is true that the nurse has many patients to care for and cannot spend as much time with the patient as might be desirable. Regardless of how much time the nurse has, it can be spent more effectively by devoting attention to what the patient really seems to need. Spending 10 or 15 minutes with the patient, allowing him to express some of his fears and to ask questions concerning his condition may require no more time than answering the call light a dozen times to adjust the window, and is more effective in helping the patient rest.

Observations for Toxic Effects of Drugs. This is an important nursing function. It is especially necessary when the patient is receiving repeated doses of epinephrine, which may cause palpitation, nervousness, trembling, pallor, and insomnia.

Bronchitis

Acute bronchitis is a disease characterized by inflammation of the mucous membranes lining the major bronchi and their branches. Frequently, the inflammatory process also involves the trachea, and is then referred to as tracheobronchitis. The most common cause of acute bronchitis is viral infection. Frequently starting as an upper respiratory infection (URI), the inflammatory process extends into the tracheobronchial tree, with direct involvement of the mucous linings. This involvement takes the form of inflammatory change with the production of increased amounts of mucus by the secretory cells of the mucosa. Usually the disease is self-limiting, lasting approximately 3 to 4 days, with symptoms that initially include a dry, nonproductive cough that later becomes productive of a mucopurulent sputum, fever, and malaise. It is treated simply by bed rest, salicylates, and a light, nourishing diet with plenty of liquids. Humidifiers are used, because dry air aggravates the cough. Occasionally, secondary bacterial invasion takes place and the previously mild infection may now become a serious bacterial infection with the production of a thick purulent sputum and a cough that may persist for several weeks. While antibiotics are not generally ordered for the treatment of acute bronchitis of viral etiology, the doctor usually interprets the establishment of the secondary invader in the tracheobronchial tree as an indication for culturing the sputum and starting antibiotic therapy. A period of 2 to 3 days will be required prior to the sputum culture report. During this time period, the doctor may order a broad-spectrum antibiotic. He may change the antibiotic medication later depending on the sputum culture report. Acute bronchitis may be complicated by laryngitis with hoarseness and, occasionally, loss of voice, and sinusitis. These secondary areas of infection will usually subside as the bronchitis subsides.

Although acute bronchitis is most often related to an infectious process, chemical irritation due to noxious fumes (sulfur dioxide, nitrogen dioxide, smoke, and other air pollutants) can also cause acute bronchitis. The disease may be further complicated by the development of bronchial asthma. Nursing management of the patient with acute bronchitis is similar to that in any acute respiratory infection with emphasis on rest and prevention of secondary infection, as well as prevention of the spread of infection to others.

Chronic bronchitis

Chronic bronchitis is characterized by the hypersecretion of mucus by the bronchial glands as well as a chronic or recurrent respiratory infection. It is a serious health problem with symptoms that develop gradually and go untreated for many years until the disease is well established. A chronic cough, often attributed to smoking, may persist and gradually grow worse. The cough is frequently disregarded and early treatment delayed.

Etiology and Incidence. Multiple factors in the causation of chronic bronchitis have been recorded. The development of the disease may be insidious or may follow a long history of bronchial asthma or an acute respiratory infection, such as influenza or pneumonia. Air pollution is a major cause of chronic bronchitis, as evidenced by the extremely high incidence of disease in areas of heavy pollution. The role of cigarette smoking cannot be overemphasized. Smoking characteristically causes hypertrophy of the mucous glands and hypersecretion. The mucosal surface of the tracheobronchial tree is lined by small hairs called cilia. These cilia play a significant role in clearing the air passages of the lung of mucus and secretions. Their function is specifically to propel excess secretions to the trachea, where a cough or other method of clearing the throat will rid the body of this material. Many air pollutants, such as sulfur dioxide and smoke, have been shown to significantly alter cilial activity with retention of secretions the end result. These secretions form plugs within the smaller bronchi and are excellent culture media. Infection readily ensues. A chronic infection of the airway can then result in further increases in mucus secretion and, ultimately, in areas of focal necrosis and fibrosis.

Individuals who are exposed to large amounts of irritating dusts and chemicals are very likely to develop chronic respiratory diseases such as bronchitis. For instance, coal miners are especially prone to develop chronic bronchitis. Although the disease may occur at any age, it is most frequently seen in middle age and is usually the result of many years of untreated, low-grade bronchitis.

Symptoms. A cough is usually the earliest symptom, and is accompanied by the expectoration of thick, white mucus that is usually attributed to cigarette smoking. The cough is ordinarily most marked on arising and prior to going to bed. Acute respiratory infections are frequent during the winter months. All colds tend to "settle in the chest" and may persist for several weeks or more. As the disease progresses, the sputum may become purulent, copious, and occasionally streaked with blood after a severe paroxysm of coughing. Although the patient may have a sensation of heaviness in the chest, dyspnea is usually not a symptom of uncomplicated chronic bronchitis. In fact, pulmonary function tests are frequently normal. The general health is usually maintained and the physical examination may be remarkably normal.

Diagnosis. The patient's history is very important. The physician can usually make the diagnosis by evaluating the duration of the patient's symptoms, the circumstances under which they started, the patient's employment, his previous respiratory diseases, and his smoking history. Physical examination, x-ray examination of the chest, fluoroscopy, and pulmonary function tests may be normal. Examination of the sputum, particularly the volume expectorated per day, may be helpful in assessing the severity of the disease. Sputum culture may be of therapeutic interest. All the above studies must be obtained in order to exclude bronchogenic carcinoma, bronchiectasis, tuberculosis, and other diseases where cough is a predominant feature.

Treatment. Management of patients with chronic bronchitis requires long-term planning and attention to detail. Patients may be disappointed to learn that there is no miracle drug that can wipe out chronic bronchitis. If chronic infection is present, all treatment is usually palliative in nature. However, careful treatment can do much to minimize symptoms and prevent complications.

In general, the essence of treatment is directed toward the prevention of recurrent irritation of the bronchial mucosa either by infection or chemical agents. The smoking of tobacco in any form should be immediately discontinued, since it is virtually impossible to prevent exacerbation and progression of the disease during active smoking. The patient must be helped to realize that even one cigarette may cause marked irritation of the mucosa and can by itself lead to bronchospasm.

With only slight readjustment in the diet, most individuals do not gain additional weight following cessation of smoking. The anxiety that accompanies the discontinuation of tobacco usually diminshes when other appropriate outlets for tension relief are substituted, such as small but repetitive motor actions. If the patient's work involves exposure to dust and chemical irritants, a change of occupation may be necessary. It is impossible to escape from the air pollution of urban areas. However, in the patient's home, air conditioning with filtration of incoming air often can result in marked reduction of sputum production and cough. The maintenance of optimal general health and the prevention of other respiratory infections are very important in maintaining the patient's resistance. A diet that contains adequate protein, vitamins, and other nutrients is important, as well as sufficient rest and the avoidance of emotional strain. There is usually no need for any change of climate and, although some individuals may derive relief from living in a warm, dry climate, it is better that the patient live in an area where the relative humidity is maintained at a moderate level so as to assist in the liquefication of secretions and prevent mucous plugs. In fact, maintenance in the home of a high relative humidity, between 40 and 50 percent, is considered a prerequisite for good treatment, especially in the winter months.

The specific therapy is directed toward the prevention of recurrent infection and the suppression of chronic infection. In the late stages of chronic bronchitis the infection is usually persistent and antibiotic therapy may become a lifelong therapeutic measure.

Course and Prognosis. Although the disease commences with the hypertrophy in the mucous glands in the bronchi, it frequently progresses to chronic inflammatory changes with fibrosis and structural damage. Without adequate treatment, chronic bronchitis may progress into a more severe form of chronic obstructive pulmonary disease with progressive destruction of the alveolar linings of the lung and the capillary bed. With adequate control, many patients can be maintained for the rest of their lives without further progression of the illness. The aim of the treatment is to arrest the disease and to prevent further destruction of tissue.

Chronic obstructive pulmonary disease (COPD)

Emphysema

Definition. The term "pulmonary emphysema" has been used for many years to define the *clinical* triad characterized by marked shortness of breath with persistent breathlessness even at rest, a chronic cough productive of large quantities of mucoid sputum that may be purulent, and intermittent episodes of expiratory wheezing. This triad of symptoms is nonspecific and can be seen in patients suffering with bronchial asthma as well as chronic bronchitis. By contrast, the term "emphysema" refers to a specific morphological change in the lung that is characterized by overdistention of the alveolar sacs, rupture of the alveolar walls, and the destruction of the alveolar capillary bed. Currently, any patient presenting the above symptoms is diagnosed as having chronic obstructive pulmonary disease (COPD). This title was selected in order to provide a more suitable term for the clinical labeling of this group of patients. Chronic obstructive pulmonary disease can be subdivided into two groups: (1) chronic bronchitis, and (2) generalized obstructive lung disease. The latter is further subdivided into reversible obstructive lung disease, such as asthma, and irreversible or persistent obstructive pulmonary disease of the type pathologically described as pulmonary emphysema. Since the symptoms in asthma, chronic bronchitis, and other obstructive disease may all be present concurrently, the term COPD can encompass the symptoms of all three disease states. Further subdivision is unnecessary for the treatment of the disease, and a definitive diagnosis must often await thorough morphological examination.

ETIOLOGY. The exact cause of chronic obstructive pulmonary disease is unknown. The frequent association of chronic bronchitis with the development of severe COPD suggests more than a casual relationship. Possible causative factors previously cited in the section on chronic bronchitis are of obvious importance. These include smoking, respiratory infection, air pollution, and allergy. Although a direct relationship between cigarette smoking and chronic obstructive pulmonary disease has not been established, many individuals with this disease are heavy smokers. The constant irritation of the tracheobronchial tree and the suppression of normal cilial function in the respiratory airways predisposes the respiratory tract to chronic infection. Repeated pulmonary infection can result in alteration of lung structure and destruction of pulmonary tissue. Inner pollutants such as nitrogen dioxide and sulfur dioxide result in chronic irritation of the tracheobronchial linings and may cause permanent changes. The industrial exposure to coal dust, asbestos, cotton fibers, and molds and fungi has resulted in COPD. Hereditary factors have also been incriminated in the causation of COPD. The disease is more prevalent and of greater morbidity and mortality in men than in women. Aging may play a role in the causation of this group of diseases. A normal manifestation of the aging process is overaeration of the lung and enlargement of the alveolar sacs. Destruction of alveolar walls and change in the pulmonary capillary bed has not been noted, however, as part of the aging process.

PATHOLOGY. The lungs in chronic obstructive pulmonary disease are large and do not collapse when the thorax is opened. Large air sacs or bullae may be seen over the surface of the lung. The cut surface of the lung reveals large air spaces everywhere, giving a moth-eaten appearance. On microscopic examination, the walls of the alveoli are broken down, resulting in one large sac rather than multiple small air spaces. The capillary bed previously located within the alveolar walls is destroyed and much of the tissue replaced by fibrous scarring.

SYMPTOMS. Exertional dyspnea is usually the first symptom of COPD. As the disease progresses, the breathlessness may continue even at rest. A chronic cough is invariably present and is productive of mucopurulent sputum. Inspiration is difficult because of the rigid chest cage and the patient must use the accessory muscles of respiration to maintain normal ventilation. Expiration is prolonged, difficult, and often accompanied by wheezing. In advanced emphysema, respiratory function is markedly impaired. The appearance of the patient is quite characteristic. He looks drawn, anxious, pale, and speaks in short, jerky sentences. He sits up, often leaning slightly forward, and appears markedly dyspneic. Often the veins in his neck distend during expiration.

In advanced COPD, the patient may have loss of memory, drowsiness, confusion, and loss of judgment. These changes are due to the marked reduction in oxygen reaching the brain, and the increased amount of carbon dioxide in the blood. If untreated, the level of carbon dioxide in the blood may reach toxic levels, resulting in lethargy, stupor, and finally coma. This is called carbon dioxide narcosis.

DIAGNOSIS. A thorough history will usually reveal many of the symptoms of chronic obstructive pulmonary disease. The disease can be diagnosed on the basis of the history alone. Physical examination may reveal classical signs that can be confirmed on x-ray films and through fluoroscopy. Tests of pulmonary function may indicate characteristic changes.

Blood gas studies are useful in assessing the state of blood gas exchange across the lung.

PREVENTION, TREATMENT, AND CONTROL. The prevention of COPD is directly related to the control of cigarette smoking as well as more effective public health measures against air pollution. Prompt and effective treatment of conditions that predispose to pulmonary obstructive disease is essential. Educating the public to the necessity for medical evaluation of minor respiratory symptoms, such as "morning cough"

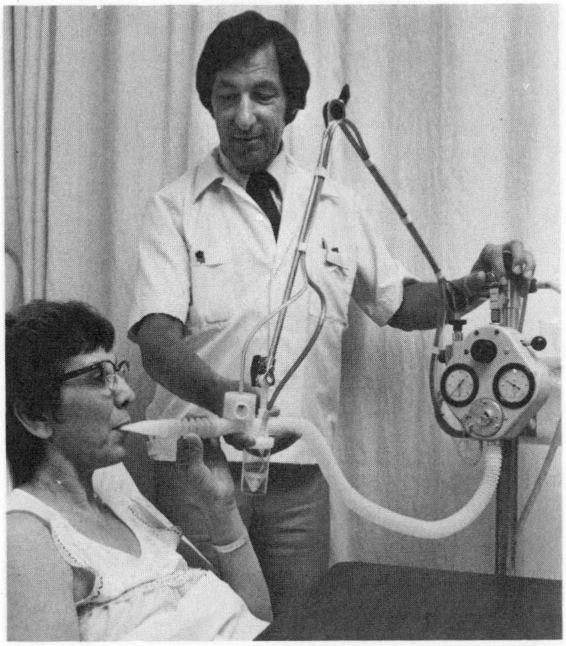

figure 21-1. Intermittent positive pressure breathing (IPPB) is frequently used to improve aeration of the lungs in the patient with COPD or the postsurgical patient. (Photograph—D. Atkinson)

or "smoker's cough," is important in breaking the chain of events leading to emphysema.

Symptomatic treatment is similar to that in chronic bronchitis. Efforts to increase pulmonary ventilation by reducing bronchospasm include the use of such medications as epinephrine and aminophylline. Unfortunately, as patients reach advanced states of the disease, the bronchospastic component may be negligible and not responsive to bronchodilator therapy. The use of expectorants, humidity control, and postural drainage is necessary to remove the excess respiratory secretions. The control of infection is important. This may be achieved by measures to increase the individual's resistance, by avoiding contact with those suffering respiratory infection, and by the use of antibiotics. It must always be remembered that the lung in COPD is chronically infected.

During acute exacerbations of the illness, therapy with antibiotics alone or with additional drugs may be ordered. Oxygen may be necessary in severe obstructive disease if the arterial oxyhemoglobin saturation is significantly reduced. However, the use of oxygen in high concentrations can be dangerous if the level of carbon dioxide in the patient's blood has increased. The respiratory center of the brain is usually sensitive to the level of carbon dioxide in the blood; if the level increases slightly, the respiratory rate and the depth increase to eliminate the excess carbon dioxide. If, however, the carbon dioxide level is chronically elevated, the respiratory center becomes insensitive to carbon dioxide changes. Under these circumstances the level of oxygen in the blood becomes a regulatory factor—the hypoxic drive to respiration. As long as the level of oxygen saturation of the blood is low, the patient will tend to breathe effectively in order to maintain oxygenation. Should the patient suddenly be given 100 percent or any other high concentration of oxygen by mask or other means, the hypoxic drive to respiration is lost and the respiratory rate will drop. This leads to the further retention of carbon dioxide, apnea, and death. The safest method for the administration of oxygen to the patient with COPD is by nasal catheter or cannula, with the oxygen flow rate set at no more than 2 or 3 liters per minute. If the patient's color improves but he becomes increasingly somnolent, he may be approaching respiratory arrest.

Intermittent positive pressure with compressed air or oxygen is frequently used to provide a more adequate aeration of the lungs (Fig. 21-1). The many types of equipment available fall into two groups, pressure-cycled and volume-cycled. Pressure-cycled equipment is regulated by a gauge which registers the pressure developed by the on-rushing air in the trachea and the major airways. When the inflow pressure equals the pressure set at the machine, the machine shuts off and expiration starts. The volume of air delivered to the patient is dependent on the generated pressure and may vary from minute to minute in the very ill patient. The volume-cycled respirators do not rely on pressure as a sensing device and are not pressure regulated. The physician simply decides the volume of air to be delivered during each respiratory cycle. This technique insures the continued delivery of a known quantity of air under all circumstances. While the pressure-cycled apparatus may be used with either mask or mouthpiece, volume-cycled equipment can only be effectively applied via a tracheostomy or an endotracheal tube. It is important for the nurse to become familiar with the equipment before undertaking the care of the patient. Information concerning the particular type of equipment in use may be obtained from the physician, the inhalation therapy department, the head nurse, the hospital procedure manual, or from information supplied by the manufacturer.

As the disease progresses, the patient is usually forced to curtail activities and may have to retire early with less pay. The husband who is a patient may have to relinquish his role as breadwinner to his wife. If the patient is not helped by competent medical and nursing management, there may be a progressive loss of sleep, appetite, weight and physical strength. The patient often has many somatic complaints, and may show signs of depression and anxiety based on fear of suffocation.

Nursing management of emphysematous patients

Nursing care of patients with severe pulmonary emphysema demands judgment and skill. These patients have severe limitations on their physical activity. Even moving from bed to chair can cause extreme dyspnea. In contrast with asthmatic patients, whose attacks usually are interspersed with periods of relative well-being, patients with far-advanced pulmonary emphysema receive little respite from their respiratory distress. For many of these patients the severe curtailment of their daily activities and their enforced dependence on others are made more difficult by the realization that their condition is not likely to undergo marked improvement. Helping such patients to live with their disability without misleading them demands sensitivity and tact. It is essential that the nurse understand what the physician has told the patient concerning his condition and prognosis, so that the patient is spared the added anxiety of receiving conflicting information.

An approach that emphasizes day-to-day progress, however slight, often helps these patients to continue treatment. For example, noting that the patient walked to the bathroom this week, whereas last week he found it impossible to do so, can be a point of encouragement. Patients who are highly motivated are better able to profit from whatever treatment is available and, despite their severely damaged lungs, are able to make the best possible use of their remaining pulmonary function.

The illness is often a discouraging one. Emphysema is believed to be closely linked to smoking, and many of these patients express sadness and bitterness at not having been able to stop smoking before illness became incapacitating. Helping such patients to stop smoking even at this point and to follow the physician's recommendations concerning other aspects of treatment can result in greater symptomatic relief than was originally thought possible.

Therapeutic breathing exercises (Fig. 21-2) emphasize the effective use of the diaphragm, thus relieving the compensatory burdens on the muscles of the

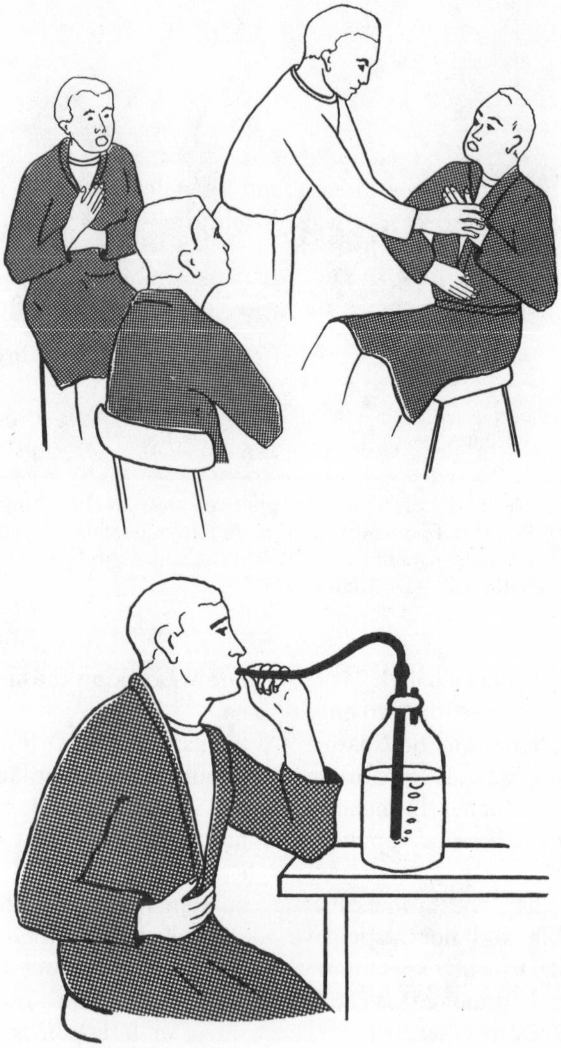

figure 21-2. Breathing exercises help to improve the patient's respiratory function. (*Top*) The physical therapist teaches patients abdominal breathing. Placing one hand on his chest and the other on his abdomen helps the patient to recognize when he is doing the exercise correctly. During abdominal breathing the movement of the abdomen is felt with each breath, whereas the chest remains quiet. (*Bottom*) A blow bottle like this one can be prepared easily for use at home or in the hospital. The long glass tube extends below the water and is connected to rubber tubing, through which the patient blows. By taking deep breaths and exhaling, the patient causes the water to bubble vigorously.

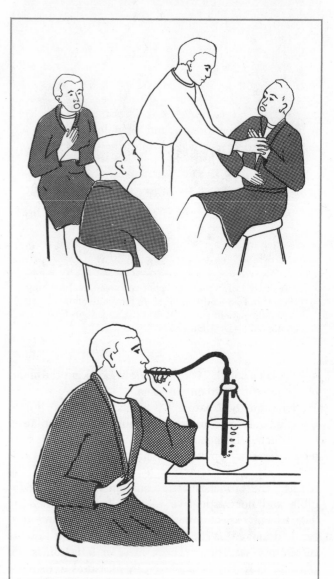

upper thorax. The patient is taught to let his abdomen rise as he takes a deep breath and to contract the abdominal muscles as he exhales. He can feel whether he is doing the exercise correctly by placing one hand on his chest and the other on his abdomen. During abdominal breathing his chest should remain quiet, and his abdomen should rise and fall with each breath. Other exercises include practice in blowing out candles at various distances and blowing some small object, such as a pencil or a piece of chalk, along a table top. Patients are encouraged to exhale more completely by taking a deep breath and then letting the body bend forward at the waist while they exhale as fully as possible.

POSTURAL DRAINAGE (Fig. 21-3) helps to remove secretions by gravity. The exact position of the patient during the treatment will depend on the location of the lesions to be drained and will be ordered by the physician. Usually recommended is 5 to 15 minutes three times a day in each prescribed position while inhaling slowly and blowing the breath out through the mouth.

For some patients postural drainage may require the head-down jackknife position but a number of other positions in bed are designed to drain a specific bronchopulmonary segment. For example, the upper lobes are drained in the sitting position. Leaning 30° forward drains the posterior upper lobe segments. Leaning 30° backward drains the anterior segments. If the bed it gatched in the center or two pillows are placed under the patient's hips so that his head is about 30–45° from the general body axis and the patient is positioned on his abdomen, the posterior lower lobe segments can be drained. Lying on the back in this position drains the patient's anterior lower lobe segments, and lying on either side drains the lower lateral segments.

Patients are assisted as necessary to assume each position and are encouraged to cough between positions. A sputum cup, tissues, and a call bell are made available. Pulmonary physiotherapy measures by a prepared nurse or therapist include gentle shaking or vibrating during expiration over the segment being drained and gentle but firm clapping or percussion

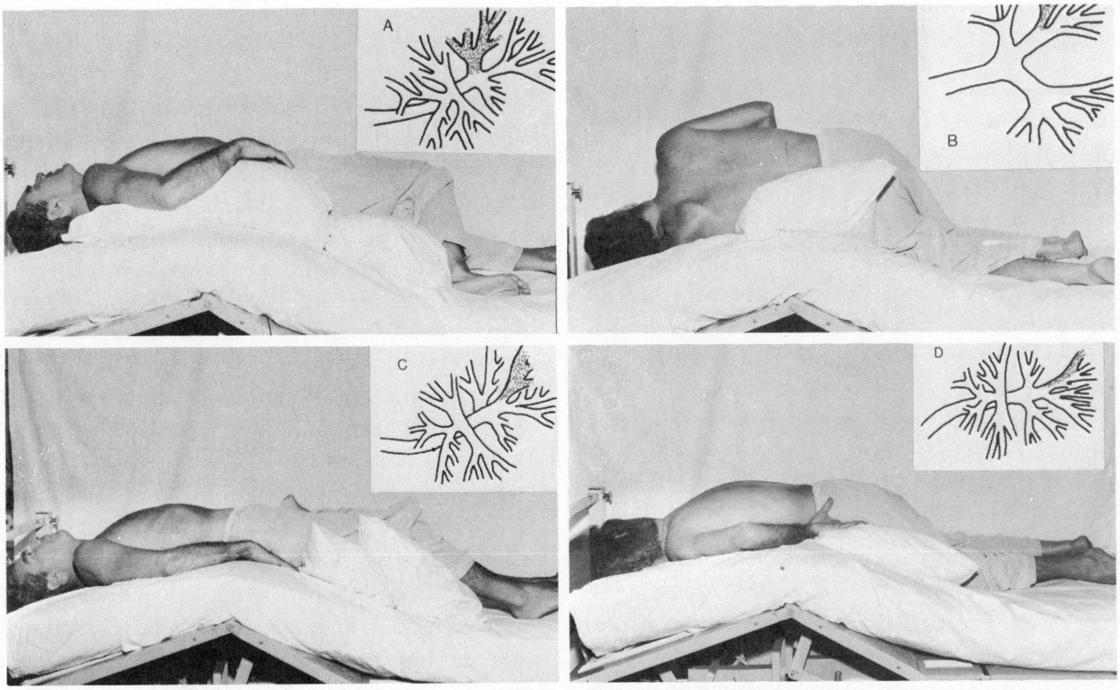

figure 21-3. (A) Postural drainage of the right middle lobe of the lung. (B) Postural drainage of the lateral basal segment of the right lower lobe. The patient is placed on the unaffected side. (C) Postural drainage of the anterior basal segment of the right lung and the anterior and medial basal segments of the left lung. (D) Drainage of the posterior segments of the right or left lower lobe bronchi. (Ayers, S. M. and Giannelli, S.: *Care of the Critically Ill*, New York, Appleton-Century-Crofts)

with cupped hands on the chest wall over the segment. These measures help to loosen secretions which are then moved by gravity to the trachea where they can be coughed up or suctioned.

Patients vary in their ability to tolerate postural drainage. For aged and debilitated patients, the procedure may need to be modified, so that the head is not placed too low, and the length of time that the position is maintained is shortened. Special care and observation of elderly or weak patients is important during and after postural drainage. The patient should be observed very frequently, and assisted to resume normal position when the treatment is over. Afterward, he should rest. Dizziness and falling are likely to occur if the patient gets up or if these precautions are not taken. Younger, more vigorous patients may be able to carry out the procedure with little or no assistance after they have done it a few times with the nurse's help.

Mouth care is important after the treatment, because sputum leaves an unpleasant taste and odor in the mouth. Note the amount and type of sputum that the patient expectorates during and immediately after the treatment.

Postural drainage should not be attempted after meals, because nausea and vomiting may result.

Bronchiectasis

Bronchiectasis is a chronic infectious disease in which structural changes in the bronchial walls result in saccular dilatations of the bronchi. Purulent material collects in these dilated areas. The expulsive power of the affected areas is diminished, and the purulent material tends to remain in the dilated bronchi.

Etiology. Infection is the principal cause. Bronchopneumonia and chronic sinusitis are possible precursors of bronchiectasis. Congenital weakness of the bronchi may be a contributing factor. The disease often begins in early adulthood and progresses slowly.

Symptoms. Patients with bronchiectasis cough and expectorate foul, greenish-yellow sputum. Coughing is most severe when the patient changes position, as on arising in the morning or lying down at night. The amount of sputum produced in one paroxysm varies with the stage of the disease and may be 200 ml. or more. The expectoration of the foul sputum leaves an unpleasant odor in the mouth and on the breath, making careful oral hygiene especially necessary. Fatigue, loss of weight, and anorexia are common. Hemoptysis may occur.

Diagnosis. Diagnosis of bronchiectasis is made by patient history and physical examination plus x-ray examination, including a routine x-ray film of the chest and a bronchogram.

Treatment. The treatment of bronchiectasis includes drainage of the purulent material from the bronchi. Antibiotics are used to contol infection, and may be prescribed for long periods. Postural drainage is performed to remove secretions from the lungs. Humidification is often necessary to aid in the raising of the thick, tenacious sputum.

Surgery may be required for severe cases providing involvement of the disease is limited to one or two areas of the lungs. It is usually not performed if the affected area is extensive. By removing the diseased area(s), healthy lung tissue is protected against future involvement.

When bronchiectasis is confined to a relatively small portion of the lung, a cure may be achieved by this surgical removal of the diseased portion. Medical treatment is palliative, since the damaged bronchi do not return to normal, but for patients with extensive disease of both lungs, this is the only treatment that is possible.

Empyema

Empyema is a general term used to denote pus in a body cavity. However, it refers most frequently to pus within the thoracic cavity (thoracic empyema). Empyema results from infection, which causes the formation of pus. Infection may follow trauma or preexisting diseases, such as pneumonia, tuberculosis, or lung abscess. Before the introduction of antibiotics, empyema was a frequent complication of pneumonia. Symptoms of empyema include fever, pain in the chest, dyspnea, and malaise. Diagnosis is made by x-ray examination and by aspiration of purulent fluid during thoracentesis.

Initial treatment often consists of antibiotics, given both parenterally and into the pleural space, and aspiration of pus by thoracentesis. Sometimes closed drainage of the empyema cavity is used. Open drainage may be used when pus is very thick, and when the walls of the empyema cavity are strong enough to keep the lung from collapsing during the time that the chest is opened. One or more soft rubber tubes may be placed in the opening to promote drainage. The wound is then covered by a large absorbent dressing that is changed as necessary. The drainage of the pus results in a drop in temperature and general symptomatic improvement.

If empyema is inadequately treated, it may become chronic. A thick coating may form over the lung, preventing its expansion. Decortication (removal of the coating) allows the lung to re-expand.

Lung abscess

An abscess, a localized area of suppuration, may occur in the lung as a result of the aspiration of a foreign body or of respiratory secretions after surgery. Lung abscesses also may follow pneumonia or a mechanical obstruction of the bronchi, such as that due to cancer. Lung abscess can be prevented in the unconscious patient by the avoidance of aspiration of secretions and the avoidance and prompt treatment of obstructions and infections in the respiratory tract.

Symptoms of lung abscess include chills, fever, weight loss, and cough productive of purulent or bloody sputum. Clubbing of the fingers often occurs in chronic cases.

The treatment of lung abscess involves drainage of the abscess, control of infection, and measures to increase the body's resistance. Sometimes, postural drainage and the use of antibiotics prove sufficient; in other instances, surgical drainage of the abscess may be necessary. The portion of the lung containing the abscess may be removed surgically.

Pneumoconiosis

Pneumoconiosis is an inclusive term describing any disease of the lung caused by the inhalation of dust, although it usually refers to diseases caused by the inhalation of silica (silicosis) or asbestos (asbestosis). Pneumoconiosis is common among persons working in industries in which exposure to these substances is prolonged, such as mining, stonecutting, and manufacture of products using asbestos.

Only the tiny particles of dust reach the lung; the larger ones are trapped in the respiratory passages. Therefore, the tiny particles are the most hazardous; they cause irritation and gradual fibrosis of lung tissue. The lung tissue loses its elasticity: reduced vital capacity, with dyspnea and cough, results. Tuberculosis has a very high incidence among persons who have silicosis. The diagnosis of pneumoconiosis is based on the history of exposure (usually over a prolonged period), roentgenography, and pulmonary function studies.

Treatment. Treatment of pneumoconiosis is usually conservative because the disease is widespread rather than localized. Surgery is rarely of value. The primary focus is on prevention, with frequent examination of those working in areas where dust is present in high concentration. Also, industry is encouraged to remove dust from the working area, when possible. Workers found to have early signs of the disease should change occupations.

Cancer of the lung

Incidence. Carcinoma of the lung has shown marked increase in incidence during the last several decades. More accurate diagnosis may be partly responsible; the growing number of older persons in the population, the popularity of cigarette smoking, and the increasing air pollution in industrial centers may be other factors contributing to higher incidence. Carcinoma of the lung is approximately 6 times more common in men than in women. Most patients are over 40 when the disease is discovered. It has been noted that the incidence of carcinoma of the lung is especially high among those who suffer from chronic bronchitis, and that many of these chronic bronchitis sufferers have been heavy smokers for many years.

Pathology and Symptoms. Bronchogenic carcinoma, a malignant tumor arising from the bronchial epithelium, is the most common type of lung cancer. The tumor usually produces no symptoms at first; however, as it enlarges, the patient may experience cough productive of mucopurulent or blood-streaked sputum. The cough may be slight at first and be disregarded or attributed to smoking. As the disease advances, the patient experiences fatigue, weight loss and anorexia. Dyspnea and chest pain occur late in the disease. Hemoptysis is not uncommon.

Diagnosis. An early diagnosis of cancer of the lung is difficult, since symptoms often do not appear until the condition is well-established. Routine x-ray examinations of the chest particularly in persons over 40, are recommended as part of the physical examination to detect carcinoma of the lung in the early, asymptomatic stage. Other diagnostic measures include bronchoscopy, biopsy, examination of sputum, and surgical exploration.

Treatment. Surgical removal of the malignant tissue offers the only type of cure and usually is successful only in the early stages of the disease. Depending on the size and the location of the tumor, lobectomy or pneumonectomy may be performed. Radiation therapy may be helpful in slowing the spread of the disease and in providing symptomatic relief. Chemotherapy is used to slow the course of the disease and to alleviate symptoms.

Course and Prognosis. The prognosis is poor unless the condition is treated early. Since cancer of the lung presents few warning symptoms during the period when cure is possible, the mortality rate is high. Metastasis occurs to the mediastinal and cervical lymph nodes, the esophagus, and the opposite lung. The patient with advanced carcinoma of the lung with metastases is very ill. Marked wasting of tissues, pain, dyspnea, and cough are present.

Postoperative management of chest surgery patients

Postoperative nursing measures

In addition to the general principles of postoperative care that apply to any patient who has had surgery, the opening of the thoracic cavity requires certain special postoperative nursing measures. Preoperative care of this group of patients is similar to that of other preoperative patients. However, because of the specialized procedures that the patient experiences postoperatively, and because his participation is essential to the success of his postoperative regimen, giving careful instruction to the patient concerning what to expect is especially important. The array of special equipment required for postoperative care can be very frightening if the patient does not understand its purpose; he must be aware that its use after chest surgery is usual and does not indicate a complication.

One particularly significant problem of chest surgery is its interference with normal pressure relationships within the thoracic cavity. When the chest is opened, the air from the atmosphere rushes in, due to the negative pressure which normally exists in the thoracic cavity. The entrance of air under atmospheric pressure collapses the lung, causing serious impairment of respiratory function. By administering anesthesia and necessary oxygen through an endotracheal tube, collapse of the lung is prevented.

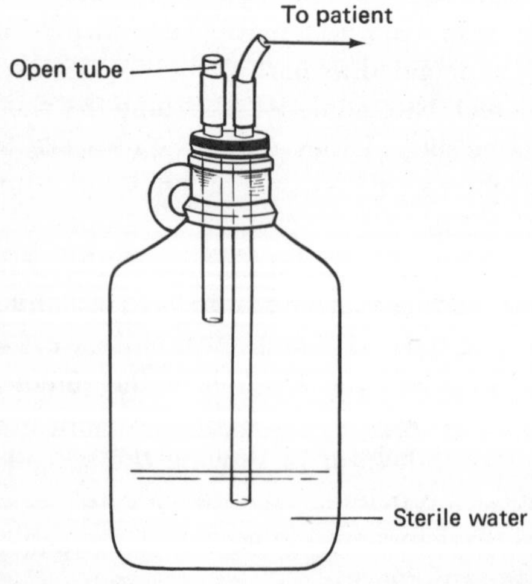

figure 21-4. A one-bottle underwater seal drainage. The tube leading to the patient is *always* under water. As the patient inhales and exhales the level of the water rises and falls in this tube.

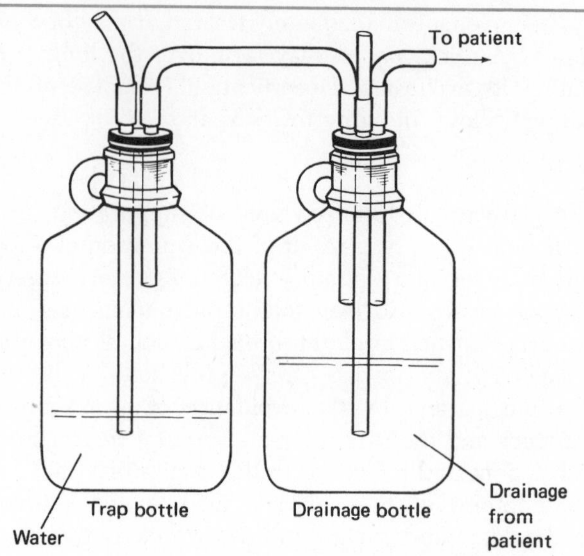

figure 21-5. The two-bottle underwater seal.

After chest surgery it is usually necessary to continuously drain secretions and blood from the thoracic cavity. Accumulation of blood and other fluids within the chest would prevent the necessary re-expansion of the lung. Drainage ordinarily must be carried out by the closed (underwater) method (Figs. 21-4, 21-5, and 21-6). In an open drainage system air would enter the thoracic cavity, for it would be sucked in every time

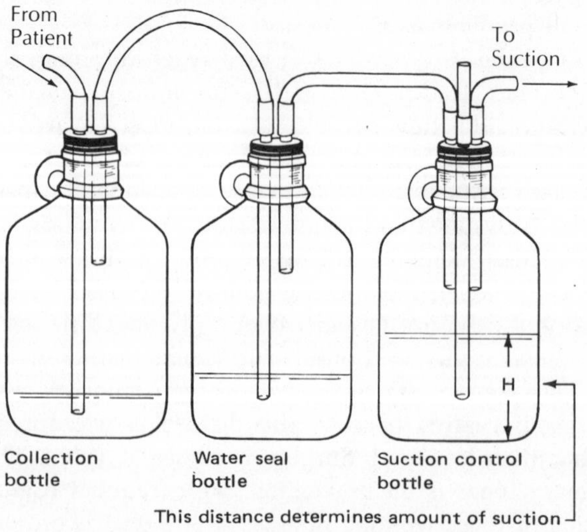

figure 21-6. Three-bottle suction apparatus.

Table 21-1.
Postoperative management of the patient with chest surgery: thoracotomy, lobectomy, pneumonectomy

The nurse:

Maintains patent airway.

Administers oxygen as ordered.

Suctions as ordered and p.r.n.

Turns the patient and has him cough and deep breathe as ordered (usually q1h).

Does *not* turn the pneumonectomy patient on his *unoperated* side unless the physician specifically states this position can be used.

Splints (supports) the chest when the patient coughs.

Administers IPPB treatments as ordered.

Records blood pressure, pulse, respirations as ordered or at own discretion, depending on the patient's condition and any changes noted.

Checks for respiratory depression 20 to 30 minutes after the administration of narcotic analgesics. *Any* respiratory depression should be reported immediately.

Records intake and output.

Checks chest tubes and drainage bottles every one-half to one hour; looks for drainage, bubbling, and a rise and fall of water in the tube going to the patient. The amount of chest tube drainage is added to the intake and output record.

Checks surgical dressing.

Checks for swelling and crepitation around the site of insertion of the chest tube(s); outlines any areas of swelling with a pen.

the rib cage expanded. The air entering from the atmosphere would collapse the lung further. Open drainage of the thoracic cavity, which permits air to flow back into the chest, is used only when adhesions have formed that prevent the collapse of the lung.

Closed drainage of the thoracic cavity is accomplished by means of a catheter placed in the pleural space during surgery. Postoperatively it is allowed to drain under water into a bottle. By keeping the end of the drainage tube always under water, air is prevented from being drawn up through the catheter into the pleural space. A sterile drainage bottle, into which a measured amount of sterile water has been poured, is used for this purpose. The drainage bottle is connected by tubing with a control (trap) bottle, used to regulate the amount of suction being applied. The trap bottle is connected by rubber tubing with a suction device. The doctor regulates the amount of suction being applied by adjusting the position of a tube in the control (trap) bottle. The length that this tube is submerged under water in the trap bottle determines the amount of suction applied. The trap bottle is used because usually the amount of suction applied by the ordinary suction device is too great to be applied to the chest catheter. Therefore, the trap bottle lessens to the desired extent the degree of suction applied. The water in the trap bottle (in contrast with that in the chest drainage bottle) need not be sterile.

Any break in the system, from either loosened or broken bottles, would present the hazard of air entering the tubing and being drawn up into the pleural space. All connections of stoppers and tubing are taped carefully to minimize the possibility, for instance, of having the end of a catheter slip off a glass connecting tip. Placing the drainage bottle in a holder is another precaution. The holder helps to protect the bottle from being knocked over and broken. More elaborate devices are also available to hold the bottles. A clamp must always be in readiness so that, if any break in the system occurs, the chest tube can be clamped immediately as close to the chest wall as possible. The clamp is placed where it can be easily seen.

Preventing fluids from flowing up through the catheter and entering the pleural space is also essential. While connected for drainage, the chest drainage bottle is *never* raised from floor level. Raising the bottle could result in a flow of fluid to the pleural space.

Often two chest catheters are used—one anteriorly and one posteriorly. In this instance two bottles are used into which the chest drainage flows, and each is labeled *anterior* or *posterior*. Two clamps are kept in readiness in case of any break in the drainage systems—one for each chest catheter. The amount and character of the drainage in each bottle is noted and recorded separately.

The principles illustrated here are essentially the same even though different kinds of chest drainage apparatus may be used. Commercial products are also available, with all parts of the drainage apparatus assembled and presterilized.

The drainage tube must be patent to allow for the

necessary escape of fluids from the pleural space. Clogging of the catheter, which may occur if a blood clot lodges in it, or if it becomes kinked, will cause the drainage to stop. This will prevent the lung from re-expanding normally, and it may cause the position of the heart and the great vessels to shift (mediastinal shift). In the first hours immediately after surgery the nurse must be constantly alert to the functioning of the drainage system so that, if a malfunction occurs, precious minutes will not be lost in correcting it.

The fluid in the long glass tube in the drainage bottle will fluctuate with each respiration; bubbling will occur in the drainage bottle if the system is working properly. Failure of the fluid to fluctuate in the long glass tube may mean that the catheter is clogged, or that the lung has completely re-expanded. During the early postoperative period the former possibility is more likely. In some hospitals, milking the drainage tube from the patient toward the drainage bottle to remove an obstruction is considered a nursing responsibility. If drainage is not resumed by milking the tube, the physician should be notified at once. An x-ray film (made by a portable machine) may be ordered to determine whether the failure of the fluid to fluctuate is due to re-expansion of the lung.

It is important to check the color and the amount of chest drainage frequently and to note the condition of the dressings over the operative area. Although some bloody drainage is expected through the catheter postoperatively, it should not appear bright red or be copious. In some hospitals, measuring and emptying the drainage bottles is a nursing function; in others, the physician assumes this responsibility. If the nurse is to empty the drainage bottle, she should first clamp the chest catheter close to the patient's chest. The stopper is then removed from the bottle and the contents measured.

It is important to subtract from the total amount of drainage the amount of sterile water originally placed in the bottle. A sterile bottle to which sterile solution has been added to cover the end of the drainage tube is placed in position, the stopper is inserted and the clamp removed from the chest catheter. Drainage must be re-instituted promptly, so that the catheter does not become clogged or the necessary drainage delayed.

On occasion air escapes from the chest into the subcutaneous tissues and an area of swelling may be noted above or below the dressing. Upon palpation, a crackling sensation (crepitation) is felt with the fingertips. While a small amount of air in the subcutaneous tissues is sometimes seen, any increase should be reported to the physician. The area is marked with a pen for future comparisons.

Patients find it difficult to cough and deep breathe because of the pain experienced in performing these tasks. Incisional support may relieve some of the discomfort, but many patients still find these tasks painful. Large doses of narcotics, and sometimes even normal doses, are avoided as respiratory depression can occur. When an analgesic is administered, the respiratory rate is checked 20 to 30 minutes after the administration of the drug.

Effect on the patient

What does the patient see when he regains consciousness? Usually he sees a transfusion running, several drainage bottles beside his bed, suction equipment, and oxygen. He has a tube running into his nose (for oxygen), tubes running out of his chest, and a tube carrying fluids into a vein in his arm. Many other types of equipment also may be in use, such as monitoring devices which continuously record his ECG on a screen, hypothermia equipment, and a monitoring device which indicates his rectal temperature.

Patients who have had chest surgery need nurses who are familiar with the equipment, who have operated it enough to be at ease with it, and who can center their attention on the patient. The nurse's manner of sureness and confidence as she performs necessary tasks can convey a feeling of confidence to the patient which no words, in the absence of technical skill, can convey.

Nursing management of patients with chronic respiratory disorders

The nursing management of patients with chronic respiratory disorders requires patience, attention to detail, and the ability to maintain interest and hope when progress is slow.

The patient's *general health* is important in his struggle with chronic respiratory illness. It is important to teach him and his family the principles of optimum nutrition and to help them to plan rest, recreation, and suitable work for the patient. Often patients feel there is little use in these measures, and an important aspect of nursing care involves communicating the belief that treatment is worthwhile. Most of the gains will come about slowly, as a result of prolonged and painstaking effort in the maintenance of general health, regular visits to the doctor or the clinic, and faithfully following instructions concerning medications, breathing exercises, rest, activity, and avoidance of infection. Helping the patient to establish a regular routine, whether he is cared for in the hospital or at home, is important in helping him to maintain therapy over long periods. It is not unusual for patients to follow the treatment carefully for the first few days or weeks and then gradually to abandon it when dramatic improvement does not ensue.

Smoking is contraindicated in chronic respiratory disease.

Observation of the patient for changes in symptoms is necessary. It is important to note the amount of coughing, the amount and the character of sputum, the degree of dyspnea and/or wheezing, as well as the patient's color, weight and appetite. Instructing him in oral hygiene and helping him to carry this out before meals may improve his appetite, particularly if he is raising considerable sputum.

The patient's *attitude* is very important in his improvement. Sometimes, emotional factors have played an important part in causing the disease. Whether or not this is the case, prolonged breathing difficulty often causes feelings of helplessness and despair. Patients who have formerly been active and self-sufficient may feel severely crippled by their inability to walk up a flight of stairs without gasping for breath. Although the disability is less immediately obvious than the amputation of a limb it may be no less distressing to the patient.

In collaboration with the physician and others who care for the patient, the nurse may help him *to adjust his activities* within the framework of his tolerance. Although it is undesirable for the patient to undertake strenuous exertion, neither is it wise for him to abandon all his interests and his activities. The latter course leads to invalidism. Adjustments in the patient's schedule can help him to continue his accustomed activities.

The nurse must carefully observe the patient for *complications and progression of his illness.* Increased dyspnea, cough, and sputum are important, as are symptoms of respiratory infection, such as chills and fever. Right heart failure (cor pulmonale) may occur because of increased resistance in the pulmonary vascular bed, which in turn increases the work of the right ventricle. Symptoms of heart failure include edema and cyanosis, as well as dyspnea, orthopnea, and cough.

Pulmonary tuberculosis

Incidence and Predisposing Factors. The death rate from tuberculosis has declined markedly in recent years. This marked reduction in mortality has led some people to the false assumption that tuberculosis is no longer an important health problem. Although progress has been made in fighting tuberculosis, the disease is by no means conquered.

Resistance to the disease varies considerably with age. Infants and very young children have poor resistance to the infection, and with the onset of puberty there is a marked rise in the incidence of tuberculosis.

The fact that tuberculosis is more common among persons of low social and economic status reflects the effects of poorer living standards. Overcrowding and poor hygienic conditions make the spread of the disease more likely.

Tuberculosis morbidity and mortality vary widely in different sections of the country. The highest incidence tends to occur in the most densely populated areas.

The incidence of tuberculosis is especially high among alcoholics because of health and social problems associated with alcoholism—for example, malnutrition.

Etiology. The presence of *Mycobacterium tuberculosis,* the tubercle bacillus, is a necessary cause of the disease, but usually it is not the only cause. In contrast with the number of people who have at some time been infected with the tubercle bacillus, only a very small proportion ever become ill from tuberculosis.

Many factors predispose to the development of tuberculosis. When the body's resistance is lowered, through such factors as inadequate rest and poor nutrition, or when the organisms are sufficiently virulent and numerous, the clinical disease may develop.

Tubercle bacilli are aerobic, gram-positive and acid-fast. They are rod-shaped and can be identified by microscopic examination of sputum and other body substances. Although the bacilli can live in the dark for months in particles of dried sputum, exposure to direct sunlight kills them in a few hours. The organism is difficult to kill with ordinary disinfectants. Tubercle bacilli are killed by pasteurization (30 minutes at 62° C.), a process widely used in preventing the spread of tuberculosis by milk and milk products.

Tuberculous infection is transmitted most commonly by direct contact with a person who has the active disease, through the inhalation of the droplets from coughing, sneezing, and spitting. By far the most important means of spread is inhalation of organisms. The disease is primarily airborne, a point of relevance for protective techniques.

Signs and Symptoms. The onset of tuberculosis is insidious, and early symptoms vary somewhat from person to person. For a long time the patient may have no symptoms; symptoms often do not appear until the disease is well advanced. This fact further emphasizes the need for routine examinations for the detection of tuberculosis.

Early symptoms of tuberculosis are often vague, and they may be readily dismissed. Fatigue, anorexia, weight loss, and slight, non-productive cough are all symptoms that can be attributed to overwork, excessive smoking, or poor eating habits; however, they are also early symptoms of tuberculosis. Elevation of temperature, particularly in the late afternoon and evening, and night sweats are frequent as the disease progresses. The cough often becomes productive of mucopurulent and blood-streaked sputum. Hemoptysis, the coughing up of blood, may occur. Marked weakness and wasting are characteristics of later stages of the illness; dyspnea may be a late symptom. Chest pain may result from the spread of infection to the pleura.

Diagnosis

Diagnostic tests for tuberculosis consist chiefly of tuberculin skin tests, chest x-ray examinations, and examinations of sputum and other body substances.

Tuberculin Tests. A positive tuberculin test is evidence that a tuberculous infection has existed at some time, somewhere in the body. In relation to tuberculosis the word *infection* is used to indicate that the organisms have entered the body and the body has reacted to them. This may or may not lead to active disease. Since most such infections with the tubercle bacillus do not result in disease, a positive test is not necessarily an indication of the development of active clinical disease.

The chief value of tuberculin tests lies in case finding. By means of tuberculin tests it is possible to discover persons who have been infected by the tubercle bacillus and to perform further tests on them to determine whether clinical disease is present.

The Mantoux Test. Tuberculin may be administered in several ways. The most exact, since an accurately measured dose can be given, is the Mantoux test. Two types of tuberculin are in use: Old tuberculin (OT), which contains some impurities; and purified protein derivative (PPD), made by a newer process that produces a purified, stable substance. Purified protein derivative is used most frequently today.

Other Tuberculin Tests. Other methods of performing tuberculin tests are the *patch test* (Vollmer) and the *scratch test* (Von Pirquet), neither of which is now in common use. Formerly, they were used rather commonly in mass tuberculin testing, particularly of school children.

Tuberculin tests using *multiple-puncture technique* have largely replaced the patch and the scratch tests. Various companies manufacture equipment for multiple puncture tests. Some of those commonly used in this country include the tine, the Sterneedle, and the Monovacc tests. The advantage of these tests is that the equipment comes individually sterilized, packaged, and ready for use. No syringes or needles are necessary. The tine test is administered by pressing a small disk firmly against the palmar surface of the patient's forearm. Tiny prongs that have been impregnated with tuberculin pierce the skin. The test causes scarcely any discomfort. Multiple-puncture tests are read after 48 to 72 hours with the area of induration measured in millimeters.

Sputum Examination. Microscopic examinations of sputum to detect acid-fast bacilli are often carried out when tuberculosis is suspected. The patient is instructed to cough deeply, so that the specimen will not consist merely of saliva. Most patients find that they are most likely to expectorate sputum when they first get up in the morning; therefore, this is the best time for them to obtain a specimen. A wide-mouthed specimen bottle is used for this purpose. It is important to see that the outside of the bottle is free from contamination and to avoid contamination of the specimen with other organisms. Specimens of sputum are often obtained for culture of the organism (growing it on a suitable laboratory medium). This test takes 4 to 8 weeks to complete.

Since it is possible that tubercle bacilli, although present, may not be recovered in a single specimen, serial tests of sputum are often ordered. It is important to explain to the patient the necessity for repeated tests so that he will not become irritated or apprehensive by the request for more than one test.

Gastric lavage or gastric aspiration may be used to determine the presence of the organisms, particularly among patients who have difficulty raising a sputum specimen for examination. It is believed that the mechanism whereby tubercle bacilli reach the stomach from the lungs is that sputum is raised and is not expectorated but swallowed.

Treatment

Chemotherapy is the most important aspect of treatment for tuberculosis. Occasionally, advanced disease or the failure to respond to medical treatment may indicate the need for surgery. Rest and a nutritious diet are also important in the therapeutic regimen.

Bed rest is no longer considered necessary for most patients. It is usually prescribed only for seriously ill patients and for those who have had recent hemoptysis. Rest, in the sense of relief from worry and strain, continues to be important. If the patient is tense and anxious, worried about his prognosis or his family, he will be unable to rest.

If the patient is not accustomed to accepting responsibility for his own health, it is difficult, but extremely important, to help him learn how to follow his treatment, and to assist him in adapting his mode of life to his treatment. Drug therapy is of no use unless the patient can be helped to realize the necessity for taking prescribed medications over a long period.

Chemotherapy. Drugs have made recovery more rapid, and have provided a chance for the arrest of the disease for those with advanced lesions, but they do not provide a guaranteed cure. Their usefulness lies in the ability to decrease the growth and multiplication of the tubercle bacillus, thus giving the patient's body a chance to overcome the disease. Two factors make drugs less than ideal: toxicity and the tendency of the tubercle bacillus to develop resistance to the drugs. Combined therapy with two or more drugs decreases the problem of drug resistance, increases to some extent the tuberculostatic action of the drugs, and lessens the toxicity of the drugs for the patient.

All tuberculostatic drugs should be given for long periods without interruption, since healing is slow and resistance to drugs may be increased by interrupted treatment. Lapses in the administration of these drugs can be serious, and the patient should understand the importance of taking his drugs regularly.

Usually, the greater period of drug therapy (in some instances, the entire period) is carried out while the patient is at home. The patient must be aware of the necessity for returning regularly to the physician's office or clinic for follow-up care. In addition to other aspects of treatment and assessment carried out at these periodic visits, tests of the sensitivity of the patient's organisms to the drugs he is taking must be performed, and the toxicity of the drugs for the patient must be evaluated.

Surgical Treatment. Surgical treatment may be required for patients with advanced disease or for those who do not respond to medical treatment. Resistance of organisms to chemotherapeutic agents is an important factor in lack of response to medical treatment.

Radical surgery, such as pneumonectomy, is less frequent than formerly; there is increasing use of operations that remove only a portion of the lung. When the disease is located primarily in one section of the lung, that portion may be removed by *segmental resection* (removal of a segment of a lobe) or by *wedge resection* (removal of a wedge of diseased tissue). If the diseased area is larger, *lobectomy* (removal of a lobe) may be done. In some cases the entire lung is so diseased that a pneumonectomy is necessary.

Nursing management in general hospitals

Relatively short-term care of patients with tuberculosis in general hospitals is becoming more common. This practice could be increased if greater attention were given to the use of safe and effective procedures for preventing the spread of tuberculosis. Too often patients with tuberculosis are unnecessarily transferred to a chest hospital many miles from home, when they do not require extended hospitalization or highly specialized procedures. Nurses can, by their own attitude of rational concern about measures to prevent the spread of infection, and by careful adherence to protective measures, foster care of patients with tuberculosis in general hospitals.

Nurses have a key role in aiding the tuberculosis patient in the general hospital to have a positive experience. He can be helped to learn more about his illness, to understand the ways he can participate in protecting others from infecton, and to establish a treatment regimen which he can later carry out at home.

Fostering the patient's participation, by instructing him in such measures as "covering his cough," and disposing of sputum can increase his feelings of self-esteem and responsibility toward himself and toward others.

Rehabilitation

One of the earliest measures in rehabilitation is helping the patient and his family to accept the reality of the diagnosis so that they will recognize the need for instruction and treatment. It may take the patient some time to accept the fact that he has tuberculosis; the nurse's supportive attitude may help him in his adjustment.

The nurse can find many ways of helping the patient to bridge the gap betwen dependence on care during illness and independent living. The gradual resumption of independence as the illness improves is important.

The period of disability from tuberculosis is considerably shorter now than it was a few years ago. It is therefore especially important to help the patient and his family participate in the plan of treatment as soon as possible. The objective is to minimize the interruption in the patient's life due to tuberculosis, so common until recently. Although drug therapy must be continued for an extended period, most patients are able to resume their usual activities within a relatively short time.

Casefinding and control

Since tuberculosis in the early stages is frequently asymptomatic, screening devices such as tuberculin tests and x-ray films are used to discover the disease in apparently healthy people. It is recommended that all children and adults have tuberculin tests as part of the yearly physical examination, and that chest x-ray films be taken of those who show a positive reaction.

Early diagnosis is essential to bring the patient's illness under control, for his welfare as well as that of his associates and the community as a whole.

BCG and isoniazid as prophylaxis

For people who are exposed to the disease frequently or who may be particularly vulnerable to it, BCG (bacille Calmette Guérin) vaccine is sometimes recommended. This vaccine is made from living, attenuated tubercle bacilli and is given to those who react negatively to tuberculin. Although it offers some protection, BCG cannot be relied on for the complete prophylaxis of the disease.

Isoniazid is being used as prophylaxis against development of active tuberculosis among those in whom the tuberculin reaction recently has changed from negative to positive. For example, in one program of prophylaxis, all persons whose tuberculin reaction has changed from negative to positive within the past 6 months are advised to have treatment with isoniazid for one year. The education of the public and improved living and working conditions have helped to reduce the incidence of tuberculosis.

General nutritional considerations

- Adequate fluid intake is of great importance in reducing tenacious secretions.
- If at all possible, meals should be timed so that the patient is rested.
- Adequate nutrition is a key point in maintaining good general health which will reduce the patient's susceptibility to recurrent infections.

General pharmacological considerations

- Some of the most common OTC (*o*ver *t*he *c*ounter or nonprescription) medications purchased are preparations advertised for colds and allergies. While these drugs may benefit some, they are not indicated for everyone and in some instances may be harmful. These preparations may contain atropine or other cholinergic blocking agents which are contraindicated in patients with glaucoma and prostatic hypertrophy. Patients should be cautioned to avoid these drugs and consult their physician if they require medication.
- Bronchodilators may be used in the treatment of asthma. They include adrenergic drugs and aminophylline. Epinephrine and isoproterenol (Isuprel) are two adrenergic agents.
- Epinephrine is usually given subcutaneously or by nebulization; isoproterenol, by nebulization or sublingually. Both drugs dilate the bronchi and therefore relieve bronchospasm. Aminophylline is administered intravenously for acute attacks and may be given rectally or orally once the acute attack has subsided. Corticosteroid preparations may also be used in the treatment of asthma, either orally or parenterally.
- Side effects of adrenergic drugs include: tachycardia, hypertension, anxiety, restlessness, and palpitations. When aminophylline is given intravenously, it *must* be given *slowly*. Rapid injection can result in hypotension, cardiovascular collapse, and arrhythmias.
- Antibiotics may be necessary to control chronic infection in those with chronic obstructive pulmonary disease (COPD).
- Patients with respiratory disease should be advised to check with their physician before using OTC antitussive preparations (drugs used to prevent coughing). These drugs suppress the cough reflex and are contraindicated in diseases such as bronchiectasis and emphysema.
- When a narcotic is administered to patients

who have had thoracic surgery, the respiratory rate is counted *before* and 20 to 30 minutes *after* the drug is given. If the respiratory rate falls below 10 at either time, the physician must be notified.

- Drugs used in the treatment of tuberculosis include: aminosalicylic acid (PAS), isoniazid (INH), cycloserine (Seromycin), streptomycin, ethambutol (Myambutol), capreomycin (Capastat), rifampin (Rimactane) and viomycin (Viocin).
- Antitubercular drugs are usually given over long periods of time. The importance of drug therapy, that is, adhering to the dose schedule and not omitting the drug, must be emphasized during patient teaching. The *only* way drug therapy is of value is when medications are taken exactly as prescribed.

Bibliography

Bates, B.: *A Guide to Physical Examination.* Philadelphia, Lippincott, 1974.

Barstow, R. E.: Coping with emphysema. Nurs. Clin. North Am. 9:137, March, 1974.

Breathing reconditioning exercises for your COPD patient. Patient Care 8:140, February 15, 1974.

Brunner, L. and Suddarth, D. S.: *Lippincott Manual of Nursing Practice.* Philadelphia, Lippincott, 1974.

Collart, M. E. and Brenneman, J. K.: Prevention of postoperative atelectasis. Am. J. Nurs. 71:1982, October, 1971.

Conn, H. F., ed.: *Current Therapy.* Philadelphia, Saunders, 1975.

Egan, D.: *Fundamentals of Respiratory Therapy,* ed. 2. St. Louis, Mosby, 1973.

Foley, M. F.: Pulmonary testing. Am. J. Nurs. 71:1134, June, 1971.

Fuhs, M. F. and Stein, A. M.: Better ways to cope with C O P D. Nurs. '76, 6:29, February, 1976.

Kudla, M.: The care of the patient with respiratory insufficiency. Nurs. Clin. North Am. 8:183, March, 1973.

Moody, L.: Asthma—physiology and patient care. Am. J. Nurs. 73:1212, July, 1973.

Patient Care in Tuberculosis, Publ. No. 45-1414. National League for Nursing, New York, 1973.

Nett, L. M. and Petty, T. L.: Why emphysema patients are the way they are. Am. J. Nurs. 70:1251, June, 1970.

Petty, T. L.: *Intensive and Rehabilitative Respiratory Care,* ed. 2. Philadelphia, Lea and Febiger, 1974.

Rodman, M. J. and Smith, D. W.: *Clinical Pharmacology in Nursing.* Phliadelphia, Lippincott, 1974.

Weg, J. C.: Tuberculosis and the generation gap. Am. J. Nurs. 71:495, March, 1971.

UNIT SIX

Insults to cardiovascular integrity

- The patient with a blood or lymph disorder
- The patient with heart disease: anatomy; diagnostic tests
- The patient with heart disease
- The patient with inflammatory or valvular disease of the heart
- The patient with cardiovascular disease: coronary artery disease; functional heart disease; hypertension
- The patient with peripheral vascular disease: thrombosis and embolism

CHAPTER 22

The patient with a blood or lymph disorder

On completion of this chapter the student will:

- Discuss the common tests utilized for diagnosing blood disorders.
- List the more common causes and symptoms of iron-deficiency anemia.
- Describe the various types of anemia and the treatment and nursing management of each.
- Discuss the various types of leukemia and the treatment and prognosis of each.
- Discuss the emotional impact of leukemia on the patient and his family.
- Develop a nursing care plan for a patient with leukemia.
- Discuss the etiology, symptomatology, and nursing management of the blood disorders purpura, hemophilia, polycythemia vera, agranulocytosis, and multiple myeloma.
- Discuss the etiology, symptomatology, and nursing management of the lymph disorders lymphosarcoma, Hodgkin's disease, and infectious mononucleosis.

Part 1: Blood disorders

The term *blood dyscrasias* often is used to describe a large group of disorders affecting the blood. (*Dyscrasia* is derived from Greek words meaning *bad* and *mixture.*) Although all blood dyscrasias affect the blood in some way, the disorders themselves are manifestations of many different pathologic processes. For instance, leukemia is believed to be due to malignant changes; anemia may be due to a variety of causes, such as blood loss, inadequate formation of red blood cells, or increased destruction of red blood cells. Regardless of the pathology, disorders of the blood lead to many similar symptoms and nursing problems, and they necessitate many similar kinds of diagnostic tests. For example, many of these patients exhibit a tendency to bleed that may be due to reduction in the number of platelets (leukemia) or a disturbance of the coagulation of blood (hemophilia). Whether bleeding is due to leukemia or hemophilia, nursing problems involving management and observation of the patient with a tendency to bleed are similar.

Common diagnostic tests

Samples of blood are often examined for the number of cells and the amount of hemoglobin (Fig. 22-1). The number of white blood cells, platelets, and red blood cells per cubic millimeter is compared with the normal values. Frequently, the relative number of the different types of white cells is of diagnostic importance, and a differential count of white blood cells is ordered. The size and the shape of the cells, as well as their number, may be significant. Red blood cells of normal size are called *normocytic,* abnormally small ones are called *microcytic,* and abnormally large ones are called *macrocytic.* The amount of hemoglobin contained in the erythrocytes may be contrasted with the normal, using the terms *hypochromic* (less hemoglobin than normal) and *hyperchromic* (more hemoglobin than normal).

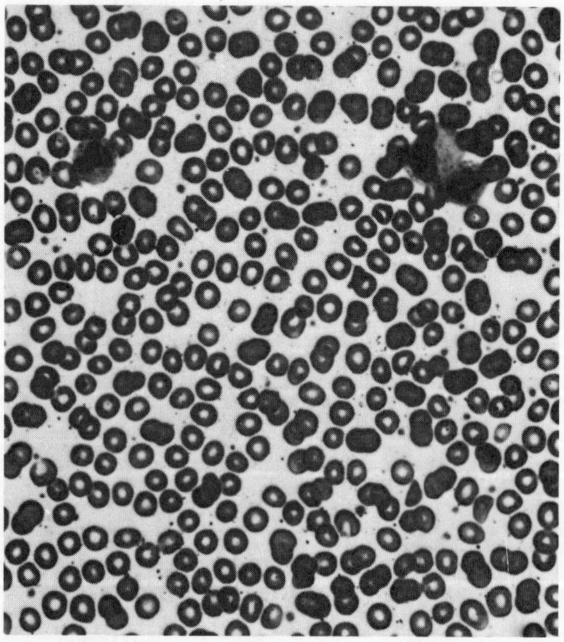

figure 22-1. Normal blood cells (magnified × 450). (Photograph—D. Atkinson)

Since many patients with blood dyscrasias tend to bleed, the site of the puncture should be inspected frequently to make sure that there is no oozing. The patient usually is instructed to apply firm pressure to the site for a few minutes after the blood has been withdrawn.

Sternal Puncture. Specimens of bone marrow are very useful in studying the formation of blood cells; these specimens can be obtained from the sternum or the iliac crest. The patient lies on his back or on his side. The skin over the area is cleansed and a local anesthetic injected. A needle is inserted into the marrow of the bone. A dry, sterile 5 to 10 ml. syringe is attached, and specimens are withdrawn. The patient may feel discomfort when the specimen is taken, as well as apprehension and a feeling of pressure when the needle is inserted. (A special needle is used that is short and strong; there is generally a guard on the needle that will prevent it from being inserted too far.)

The nurse has two important functions during this procedure: assisting the physician and making the patient as comfortable as possible. The necessary equipment is outlined in the nurse's hospital procedure manual. After preparing the equipment and assisting with the explanation of the procedure, the nurse positions and drapes the patient, and assists the physician by handing him equipment, adjusting the lighting, and labeling the specimens. As with any test or treatment that is uncomfortable or upsetting, a few words or a smile of encouragement help the patient.

Capillary Fragility Test. This test is done to determine how easily the capillaries rupture. In some blood dyscrasias, capillary fragility is increased, leading to tiny hemorrhagic spots (*petechiae*) under the skin. The physician wraps a blood-pressure cuff around the patient's arm, inflates it to a point between the patient's diastolic and systolic blood pressure, and leaves the cuff inflated for 15 minutes. After he removes the cuff, the physician examines the skin distal to the area where pressure was applied. Normally, only one to two petechiae per square inch are noted. If the patient's capillaries are abnormally fragile, many petechiae will be found. Usually, the physician explains that the development of some tiny red spots on the skin is to be expected when the cuff is removed.

Changes in the blood often accompany other disorders. Anemia may be the first warning of cancer, or it may be the first clue to the discovery of a peptic ulcer that has been causing the persistent loss of small amounts of blood. Finding an abnormal blood count is only the beginning. To treat the patient effectively, the physician must first discover the cause of the condition.

Patients can be helped by explaining the need for medical care, encouraging them to have whatever diagnostic tests are necessary, and showing them the folly of succumbing to the lures of advertising and trying remedies that can waste their money or provide false assurance while a serious disease continues undiscovered.

Anemia

The term *anemia* means that the patient has a decrease in the number of red blood cells and a lower than normal hemoglobin level. The number of red blood cells normally present varies with age, sex, and altitude. Infants have more red blood cells per cubic millimeter than adults. Women have fewer erythrocytes per cubic millimeter than men; normally women average about 4,500,000 red blood cells per cubic millimeter of blood; men average 5,000,000 per cubic millimeter. The difference between men and women in the number of red blood cells is most noticeable during the reproductive years. People who live at very high altitudes have an increased number of red blood cells.

Erythrocytes perform the important function of carrying oxygen from the lungs to the tissues, and carbon dioxide from the tissues to the lungs. The red color of the blood is caused by hemoglobin, which is contained in the erythrocytes. Hemoglobin combines with oxygen to form oxyhemoglobin. The average amount of hemoglobin is 14.5 to 15.0 Gm. per 100 ml. of blood. Men have slightly more hemoglobin than women. As the blood passes through the lungs, oxygen is taken up and carbon dioxide is released. Oxygenated blood is bright red and is carried by arteries and capillaries to all tissues of the body. After the oxygen has been released from the hemoglobin for use by the tissues, the hemoglobin is called "reduced hemoglobin." The blood at this time looks dark red and is returned by the veins to the heart and to the lungs, where the carbon dioxide is released and the blood reoxygenated.

Anemia can be caused by loss of blood and by destruction or faulty production of red blood cells and hemoglobin. Blood loss can occur suddenly and copiously, as in severe hemorrhage from a severed artery, or it may result from slow but persistent bleeding from hemorrhoids or a peptic ulcer. Conditions that can lead to chronic blood loss, such as hemorrhoids or uterine tumors, should be treated promptly to avoid the development of anemia. Bleeding also results in the loss of iron from the body, since iron is contained in the hemoglobin. Normally, the body saves and reuses the iron for the production of new hemoglobin after the worn-out red blood cells have been broken down. By increasing its production of erythrocytes, the body can compensate for some degree of loss or destruction of erythroctes; anemia becomes manifest only when the body is unable to increase its production of erythrocytes sufficiently to compensate for these losses.

Hemolysis (the destruction of red blood cells) leads to a reduction of their number. It is believed that, normally, each red blood cell survives for about four months. Old red blood cells are destroyed in the spleen, the bone marrow, and the liver. The body is constantly making new red blood cells and destroying old ones, so that the number is kept fairly uniform. In hemolytic conditions, the red blood cells do not survive as long as they normally do. They may survive only two weeks. The increased destruction of red blood cells leads to anemia. Hemolysis may be caused by infection, abnormal red blood cells, transfusion of incompatible blood, or exposure to harmful chemicals.

Inadequate production of red blood cells can be due to an injury to the bone marrow (for example, by toxic effects of drugs) or to the lack of necessary materials (such as iron, folic acid, vitamin B_{12}) for the formation of red blood cells and hemoglobin. Anemia also may be caused by other diseases, such as cancer.

Regardless of the cause, symptoms of anemia are similar and are due largely to the inability of the blood to transport sufficient oxygen to the tissues. Fatigue, anorexia, faintness, and pallor are typical signs of anemia.

Iron-deficiency anemia

Iron is necessary for the production of hemoglobin. Iron-deficiency anemia occurs frequently among persons whose need for iron is increased. Less than 10 percent of the iron obtained from food is absorbed. During periods of rapid growth, at the onset of the menses, and during pregnancy, there is increased need for iron, which often results in anemia unless additional iron is obtained. It is sometimes difficult to provide for these increased needs by dietary measures alone, although correction of a faulty diet, if it exists, is an important aspect of treatment. Iron-deficiency anemia is characterized by red blood cells that are microcytic and hypochromic.

Treatment involves the administration of extra iron. Iron causes the stools to appear black, and patients are always informed of this fact, so that they will not fear that the color indicates gastrointestinal bleeding. Iron is given occasionally in liquid form. It should be taken through a straw; otherwise it will stain the teeth. Foods high in iron are important in the diet. The patient may have to force himself to eat at first, because the anemia causes anorexia.

Pernicious anemia

An intrinsic factor normally present in the stomach secretions is necessary for the absorption of vitamin B_{12} found in food. Vitamin B_{12} is necessary for the normal maturation of red blood cells. Patients with pernicious anemia lack this intrinsic factor, which normally is contained in the gastric juice.

The body requires such small amounts of vitamin B_{12} that most people have an adequate supply in their food. Animal proteins, such as meat, milk, eggs, and cheese, contain vitamin B_{12}, and even a small daily intake of these foods ensures an adequate supply of the vitamin.

This point is stressed, because some patients mistakenly believe that pernicious anemia can be cured by diet, and that medication will no longer be necessary. Patients with pernicious anemia do need an adequate diet to maintain general health, and instruction in what constitutes such a diet is indicated if the patient's nutrition is poor. Yet dietary treatment alone is not sufficient. Everyone must help the patient to understand this. Probably, the crux of the problem lies in helping the patient to understand that different types of anemia require different kinds of treatment. The patient with pernicious anemia may have a neighbor with iron-deficiency anemia, whose condition responded quickly to the administration of iron and an improved diet, and who, therefore, could stop taking the medication.

In contrast, patients with pernicious anemia must have regular injections of vitamin B_{12} to control the disease, because their lack of the intrinsic factor in gastric secretions prevents the adequate absorption of vitamin B_{12} from food.

Diagnosis of pernicious anemia is established by the patient's history and symptoms and by studies of his blood and bone marrow.

Treatment. Vitamin B_{12} (cyanocobalamin) is given intramuscularly in a dosage that is adequate to control the disease. No toxic effects have been noted from the use of vitamin B_{12}.

Other Considerations. In addition to the usual symptoms of anemia, patients with pernicious anemia occasionally develop a sore tongue and mouth, digestive disturbances, and diarrhea. The anemia may be so severe that the patient experiences dyspnea on the slightest exertion. Jaundice often occurs. Personality changes are not unusual, especially when the disease is severe. Often the patient is irritable, confused, and depressed. Such changes are most likely to be noted by the patient's family, who often observe that "He just isn't himself lately." Fortunately, personality changes usually disappear promptly with treatment.

If the condition is not treated promptly, the patient develops degenerative changes in the nervous system, sometimes referred to as *combined system disease.* Numbness and tingling of the extremities and ataxia are common. Vibratory and position sense may be lost. Symptoms of neurological damage may improve somewhat, but permanent damage sometimes occurs before treatment is begun. The earlier the diagnosis and the more prompt the treatment, the greater is the likelihood of escaping permanent neurological damage. Physical therapy may be of benefit.

Nursing Management. During the severe phase of the illness, nursing management involves keeping the patient warm and at rest. Despite anorexia, the patient is encouraged to take easily digested, nutritious foods and fluids. Soft foods that are not highly seasoned are preferable, especially if the patient's mouth is sore.

Neurological symptoms should be watched for and reported if they occur. The prevention of falls is particularly important if the patient is ataxic. Questions concerning the possibility of recovery from neurological symptoms are referred to the patient's physician. Some of these symptoms may subside or improve, but the patient may need help in accepting some permanent residual disability. Because the patient may be ill and weak, he may not have normal resistance to other illnesses and infections. He should be protected from contact with those who have any type of infection.

Some patients are more likely to take the injections with the frequency recommended by the physician if a member of the family is taught to administer the medication. If such instruction cannot be arranged, the patient must return to the physician's office or clinic or have the injections given by a community health nurse. If the patient has been hospitalized, plans for continued treatment should be made before he leaves the hospital. It is of paramount importance that he and his family understand the necessity for continued therapy.

Anemia due to blood loss

Blood contains cells and liquid (plasma) in approximately equal volume. It has been estimated that the total blood volume is approximately one-thirteenth of the body weight. An adult weighing 154 pounds has about 6 quarts of blood. Normally, the quantity of blood circulating in the body is kept relatively constant at all times.

Blood loss, either acute or chronic, causes anemia. Sudden severe bleeding leads to *hypovolemia* (diminished volume of circulating blood) and shock. The most effective treatment involves the replacement of lost blood by transfusions. If blood loss is chronic, as may be the case in uterine tumors or hemorrhoids, the main treatment is that of the underlying condition causing the bleeding. Depending on the amount of the blood lost, the treatment may include transfusion and/or administration of iron to help the body to compensate for the blood loss. Continued care and observation are necessary for any patient who has experienced blood loss. Sometimes, the patient does not understand the reason for continued care, and, once the emergency is over, he continues to experience fatigue and weakness due to anemia that might have been readily corrected had he realized the importance of returning to the physician's office or to the clinic.

Anemia due to destruction of red blood cells

A reduction in red blood cells and hemoglobin may be caused by hemolysis. The life span of the red blood cells is shortened; the cells die more rapidly than they normally should. An example of hemolytic anemia due to an abnormality of the red blood cells is *sickle cell anemia* (Fig. 22-2). This hereditary disease occurs chiefly in blacks. In addition to the classic symptoms of anemia, the patient with this condition may develop chronic leg ulcers and attacks of fever and pain in the abdomen or the extremities. There is no cure for sickle cell anemia. Transfusions are given as palliative treatment, but life expectancy usually is decreased.

Acquired hemolytic anemia (autoimmune hemolytic disease) is due to the development within the patient's body of substances harmful to his erythrocytes. These patients are treated by corticosteroids. In some patients the steroid can be withdrawn after several weeks; in others, not for several months. Sometimes splenectomy is performed. Transfusions may be necessary.

One group of hereditary hemolytic anemias is referred to generally as *thalassemia.* Thalassemia major, or Cooley's anemia, has a high incidence in the Po valley (Italy) and on islands of the Mediterranean. Treatment of the various forms of thalassemia is symptomatic. Frequent transfusions may be required.

Hemolysis often accompanies severe infections, such as malaria and subacute bacterial endocarditis. Rapid hemolysis is accompanied by chills, fever, prostration, headache, and gastrointestinal disturbances. Jaundice follows, due to the rapid destruction of erythrocytes and the escape of hemoglobin into the plasma. Hemolysis can be caused also by transfusions of incompatible

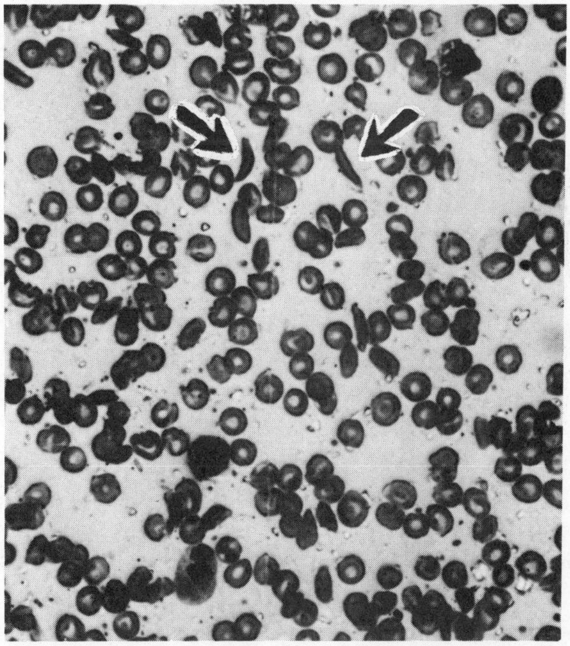

figure 22-2. An example of abnormal blood cells. This sample demonstrates sickle cell anemia (magnified × 450). (Photograph—D. Atkinson)

blood and by administration of certain drugs, such as quinine.

Treatment of hemolytic anemia is that of the underlying condition—for instance, stopping the transfusion or the drug and giving supportive treatment, such as oxygen, or treating whatever infection may be present. Transfusions may be necessary to replace red blood cells and hemoglobin.

Aplastic anemia (bone marrow failure; aregenerative anemia)

Erythrocytes, granular leukocytes (granulocytes) and platelets are formed in the bone marrow. *Aplastic anemia* is the term used to describe a condition in which the activity of the bone marrow is depressed, and red blood cells, white blood cells and platelets are not adequately produced. The formation of one or all of the three elements may be impaired, with varying degrees of severity. Aplastic anemia is a serious toxic manifestation of certain drugs, such as streptomycin, chloramphenicol (Chloromycetin), and nitrogen mustard. This condition also occurs without known cause. Major clinical signs of aplastic anemia are anemia, leukopenia (decreased leukocytes) and thrombocytopenia (decreased platelets) which result in fatigue, weakness, exertional dyspnea, lowered resistance to infection, and a tendency toward bleeding. Patients with aplastic anemia are very ill, and the death rate is high. In treating the condition, every effort must be made to prevent infection. Reverse isolation may be necessary. If the white blood cell count falls extremely low, special isolation procedures such as the use of a laminar airflow room may be used.

The causative agent, if it is known, is removed. Repeated transfusions are given to supply erythrocytes and hemoglobin. Usually, antibiotics are given to help to prevent infection. The objectives of treatment are to supply the missing elements of the blood and to prevent or to treat the infection or the bleeding, in the hope that the patient will recover his ability to produce the blood cells. If the bone marrow has been so damaged that this recovery is impossible, death will result.

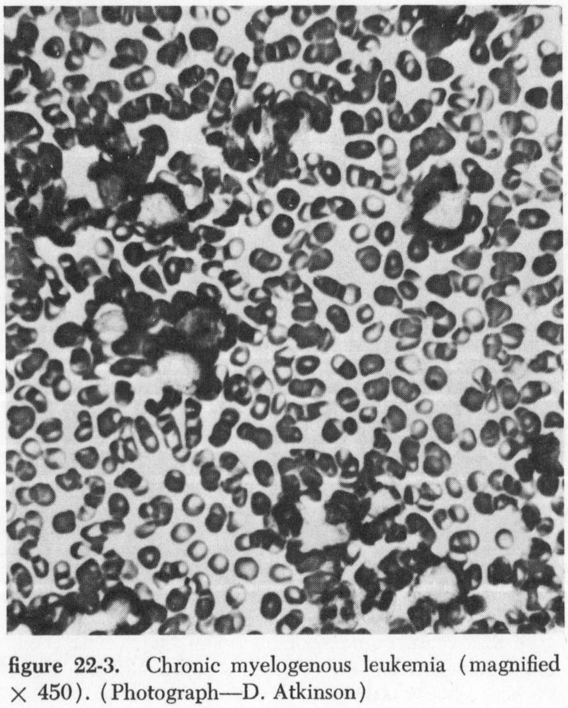

figure 22-3. Chronic myelogenous leukemia (magnified × 450). (Photograph—D. Atkinson)

Leukemia

There are three types of leukocytes (white blood cells): *lymphocytes, monocytes,* and *granulocytes.* Normally, there are between 5,000 and 7,000 leukocytes per cubic millimeter of blood. Fighting infection is one important function of the leukocytes, and they increase in number during most infections. This increase is called *leukocytosis.*

Lymphocytes are produced in the lymphatic tissue; granulocytes are produced chiefly in the bone marrow. It is believed that the different types of leukocytes survive varying lengths of time. Much remains unknown concerning the life span of various kinds of leukocytes. At the end of their life span the leukocytes die and are replaced by the new white blood cells that are constantly being formed.

Blood platelets (*thrombocytes*) are concerned with the clotting of the blood. Normally, there are approximately 300,000 platelets per cubic millimeter of blood. It takes blood about 5 minutes to clot in a test tube. This laboratory test is often referred to as "coagulation time" or "clotting time."

Leukemia usually is a fatal disease characterized by a marked increase in the number of leukocytes (Fig. 22-3). This rampant increase in white blood cells is not useful to the body. The patient is less, rather than more, able to cope with infections. Although he has more leukocytes, they are immature and, therefore, are not effective in fighting infections. The rapid proliferation of leukocytes and of the tissues that produce them results in the diminution of the number of erythrocytes and platelets. The patient eventually suffers from severe anemia, and the reduction in platelets leads to bleeding. The cause of leukemia remains unknown.

Acute leukemia

Symptoms. In acute leukemia, symptoms begin abruptly. The onset often coincides with an acute upper respiratory infection. Ordinarily, attention is directed at first to the symptoms of sore throat, fever, or rhinitis, whereas the seriousness of the underlying illness is unsuspected. Sometimes, the patient is admitted to the hospital for the treatment of the respiratory infection, and the discovery of an unusually large number of leukocytes in the routine-admission blood count is the first clue to the existence of the disease. Sometimes unusual pallor, weakness, fatigue, or bleeding warn that the illness involves more than a cold or tonsillitis, and examination of specimens of blood and bone marrow confirms the diagnosis. The leukocyte count can reach 30,000 or even 50,000 per cubic millimeter.

Anemia is usually severe and causes pallor, weakness, and fatigue. The number of platelets is reduced, causing a tendency to bleed. Bleeding may be internal or external. Common sites from which bleeding occurs include nose, mouth, gastrointestinal tract, and vagina. The tendency to bleed also may be reflected by the persistent oozing of blood after such a minor injury as the administration of an injection. Usually, fever is present, particularly as the disease advances. Occasionally, the patient will develop a spontaneous temporary remission of symptoms, perhaps lasting several months. More often, the symptoms grow progressively and steadily worse.

Treatment. Although there is no cure, treatment gives respite from the symptoms. The patient is given repeated blood transfusions to increase his red blood cells and his hemoglobin. Antineoplastic drugs—alone or in combination—are used to produce a state of remission. These drugs interfere with the multiplication of cells, particularly of cells undergoing rapid proliferation, such as the leukocytes of patients with leukemia. They are highly toxic and can impair the formation of all blood cells, including erythrocytes and platelets. Other toxic effects include anorexia, nausea, vomiting, and diarrhea. The patient's blood picture is watched very carefully while these drugs are being administered. Antibiotics are given to treat the secondary infections that are the common complications of the illness.

The patient eventually becomes resistant to all forms of treatment, and becomes severely ill with weakness, fever, bleeding, and, often, secondary infections such as pneumonia. Often death occurs within a few weeks after the patient develops resistance to drug therapy.

Chronic leukemia

Onset and Symptoms. The two most common types of chronic leukemia are lymphocytic and granulocytic. Both conditions have an insidious onset. In chronic lymphocytic leukemia, the total leukocyte count is increased, with the largest proportion of the increase in the lymphocytes. Often the disease commences with the painless enlargement of one or several lymph nodes in neck, axilla, or groin. The patient develops anemia, characterized by fatigue, palpitation, pallor, and dyspnea. A decrease in platelets is reflected in a tendency to bleed. Often the spleen is enlarged (*splenomegaly*).

Marked splenomegaly is often the earliest symptom of chronic granulocytic leukemia. The patient may notice a swelling in his left upper quadrant and a sense of heaviness in his abdomen. The largest proportion of the increased leukocytes consists of granulocytes. The patient develops anemia and thrombocytopenia.

In both types of chronic leukemia the patient may, with treatment, live five years or longer. However, eventually he no longer responds to treatment; he becomes very weak, has a tendency to bleed, and develops fever. Secondary infections, such as influenza or pneumonia, are common.

Treatment. The treatment of chronic leukemia is basically the same as for acute leukemia, that is, the administration of one or more drugs to produce a state of remission.

Nursing management of patients with leukemia

Management of patients with leukemia makes particular demands on the nurse's insight and adaptability. Newer drugs can cause dramatic changes in the course of the disease. A patient admitted to the hospital with acute leukemia may appear moribund—pale, weak, bleeding, and feverish. Two weeks later, as a result of treatment, he may be up and about and ready to go home. Often he continues to feel well for months or even years after the original diagnosis.

Long-range planning is important. When the patient feels well, he is encouraged to continue his usual activities—at school, at work, or at home. The disease has been temporarily checked; in other words, the patient is in a state of remission but the disease has not been overcome. Sometimes, the patient is aware of his diagnosis and prognosis; in other situations, the family knows, but the patient does not.

The remission of symptoms in leukemia is often quite dramatic and poses somewhat different problems from those of the patient with cancer. For instance, a 20-year-old who feels well is usually active, busy, and very much involved in planning for his career and establishing his own home and family. If he has acute leukemia, such plans and activities will be short-lived. Most people who work with these patients believe that they should be helped and encouraged to live as full, normal lives as possible. Activity in itself is not harmful, and staying at rest will neither slow the course of the disease nor alter the eventual outcome. The patient should take every precaution to avoid infections, such as colds, and he should seek medical care promptly if he develops the symptoms of any illness. Sufficient rest and an adequate diet are important in preventing secondary infections.

To advise the patient to live as fully and as normally as possible gives no recognition of the agonizing decisions that face patients who know they have leukemia. If the patient is engaged, he may wonder whether going ahead with the marriage would be fair to his fiancée.

The patient and others intimately affected by his illness must make these decisions after learning as much as they can about the disease and its prognosis. For every patient, as long as he lives, there is the hope and the possibility that a cure will be found before death occurs.

Life expectancy is longer for patients with chronic leukemia. Because they tend to be older when the disease appears, concern is more likely to be with helping them to maintain their usual occupations and home life than with making decisions concerning career and marriage. Nevertheless, with both types of patients, there is the tremendously important need to help them to maintain their will to live and determination to keep on trying despite an uncertain future.

The patient must understand the importance of returning regularly to the physician's office or clinic. Frequent examinations of the blood and sometimes of the bone marrow are essential, both in the light of the patient's disease and of the treatment that he is receiving. Emphasis should be placed on the importance of these examinations in helping him to stay well rather than on the possible complications from drug therapy.

Usually, the patient is admitted to the hospital several times over a period of a few years. Each time that he leaves, he is improved, although often he is not as strong as he was in the early phase of his disease. However, the time comes when his illness strikes for the last time—this time to win. Usually, the patient and his family are well aware when this time has come.

During the Final Illness. Sometimes the patient is cared for at home, so that he can remain with his family and in familiar surroundings. Private-duty or community-health nurses help to provide care in the home.

The nurse's role involves helping the family to endure the emotional and physical strain of the patient's illness. Frequently, the family appreciates the opportunity to do things that help the patient or add to his comfort. Feeding him or bringing in a dish of his favorite food gives the family opportunities to express their love and their concern. The sensitive nurse can encourage such participation without giving the family any less support and help and without pushing them to become involved in the aspects of care that are too upsetting or too emotionally taxing for them.

The death of a young person is usually harder to accept than that of an older person. Young people with acute leukemia are often surrounded by family members who are deeply grieved and shocked. The staff, too, feel the helplessness of watching a young person die. Usually, the physician and often the nurses have worked with the patient for several years and know him well. The care during the patient's last illness demands of them a high degree of compassion and an awareness and a control of their own feelings.

Everything possible is done to help the patient and his family. Does a member of the family want to stay all night? Move a lounge chair into the room and give him a pillow and a blanket. The quiet, reassuring presence of a loved one may mean more to the patient than anything else and should be permitted whenever possible. Ordinarily, the patient is permitted diet as desired. However, if his mouth is sore and bleeding, it is best to exclude rough or highly seasoned foods.

The patient's clergyman often provides comfort and help, both for the patient and his family. The nurse shows him, by being courteous and helpful, that his important contribution is recognized.

Physical Care. The physical care of the patient is demanding. *Bleeding* may occur suddenly and severely. Develop the habit of watchfulness. Always look at the contents of the bedpan, the urinal, and the emesis basin before emptying them. They may contain a large, tarry stool, indicating gastrointestinal bleeding, or bloody urine, or blood-streaked saliva from the mouth and the gums. Epistaxis (bleeding from the nose) is common. Report bleeding promptly. Whenever it is possible (as in the case of epistaxis), try to stop the bleeding by applying pressure and elevating the part. Pulse and blood pressure are important indicators of internal bleeding. Watch for a rapid, weak pulse and a sudden drop in the blood pressure. Observe the patient's color, and watch for purpuric spots.

Keep the patient's nostrils clean with moistened applicators in order to limit the patient's need to manipulate them. Instruct the patient to blow the nose gently if this is necessary so as not to rupture a fragile vessel.

Extreme caution should be taken if cuticle scissors, a blade razor, or other sharp instruments are used.

Note the patient's *temperature* frequently. Because an accurate reading is so important, the temperature should be taken rectally, unless this method is contraindicated by some rectal disease. If fever is high, the physician may order tepid sponge baths or salicylates to help reduce the temperature and to make the patient more comfortable.

The patient's *skin* will bruise easily, and the administration of injections may cause the oozing of blood and ecchymoses. Never give two injections when one will suffice. (Check with the physician to determine which drugs prescribed for the patient may be combined in one syringe.) Never use any larger gauge needle than is necessary to inject the medication. Apply firm pressure over the site of the injection after the withdrawal of the needle to control bleeding. Handle the patient with extreme gentleness when you are bathing or turning him. Frequent turning and skin care are important in preventing decubitus ulcers.

Disorientation may develop quite suddenly. Be alert for this, and keep side rails on the bed whenever the patient appears confused and might try to get out of bed. Falls are serious, because they may precipitate internal or external bleeding.

Protect the patient from *infection* as carefully as if he were a newborn infant. Wash your hands before caring for him. Often it is desirable to wear a clean gown over your uniform to protect the patient from organisms that may be carried on your clothing. Staff members and visitors who have any kind of infection, such as colds or boils, should not enter the patient's room.

Frequent, gentle *mouth care* is important. If the gums bleed easily, avoid using a toothbrush. Cotton swabs are less likely to cause bleeding and can be used for cleansing. Allowing the patient to rinse his mouth frequently and cleansing the mouth with moistened cotton applicators help to avoid the distressing and the lips. Frequent oral hygiene also helps to prevent infection of the raw, oozing mucous membranes odors and taste caused by old blood around the mouth of the mouth. Make sure that your technique is scrupulously clean when giving mouth care—clean hands, clean applicators, and fresh solution. Mouthwash, saline or glycerine may be used.

Report symptoms of infection promptly. Be alert for a sudden rise in temperature and for chills, cough and purulent exudate from the sores around the mouth.

Watch for *toxic effects of drugs*. Often the patient is given powerful and potentially dangerous drugs. The physician must steer a narrow course between helping and hurting the patient. The nurse can help by watching for the toxic effects of the drugs and reporting them promptly.

Transfusions are often necessary. When assisting with a transfusion, be sure to check the label on the blood carefully, to prevent the administration of incompatible blood. Observe the patient frequently during the transfusion. See that the blood runs at the rate recommended by the physician. If the patient shows any symptoms that might indicate an allergic reaction to the blood, or that possibly he is receiving the wrong blood, follow hospital procedure regarding the status of the blood transfusion. Some hospitals and physicians prefer that the blood transfusion be stopped and normal saline given to keep the vein in use until a physician decides the nature of the problem. Watch especially for chills, cyanosis, rise in temperature, dyspnea, orthopnea, pain in the lumbar region, restlessness, or urticaria.

Sometimes it is noted that family members, once they learn that death is inevitable, gradually withdraw their emotional involvement from the ill person, probably as a way of attempting to cope with a situation that makes overwhelming demands on them. It is especially important for physicians and nurses to recognize the burdens that families face in such situations. By helping the family to cope with the experience, physicians and nurses may make it more possible for the family to contribute to the patient's comfort during his last days, as well as to provide the family with support that can aid them, not only during the final days of illness, but afterward, as well, in dealing with their grief. Some ways in which such help can be given include:

- Providing an atmosphere in which the family members can discuss, if they wish, some of their feeling and concern, and providing this opportunity not only in the patient's presence, but away from the bedside, as well.
- Making it possible for the family to participate in some aspects of the patient's care, but avoiding exposing them to situations (such as massive bleeding or care of incontinence) which can add greatly to their anguish.
- At all times demonstrating concern and compassion as well as skillful care of the patient.

Purpura

The term *purpura* refers to small hemorrhages in the skin, the mucous membranes, or the subcutaneous tissues. The hemorrhagic area may be tiny, as when petechiae occur, or it may be larger and result in ecchymoses of various sizes. Purpura results either from lack of platelets or from abnormality of the blood vessels. For example, certain diseases (leukemia), or the administration of x-ray therapy or certain drugs can depress the formation of platelets. Lack of ascorbic acid can damage the blood vessels, thus leading to bleeding. Treatment of all of these conditions involves discovering and treating the cause of the purpuric lesions. Often the purpuric spots are only one symptom of a tendency to bleed. The patient may suffer severe or even fatal hemorrhages in other parts of his body.

Idiopathic thrombocytopenic purpura is characterized by a reduction in platelets, the development of purpuric lesions (petechiae and ecchymoses), and bleeding from other parts of the body, such as the nose, the oral mucous membrane, and the gastrointestinal tract.

Patients with idiopathic thrombocytopenic purpura often recover spontaneously. Adrenocorticotropic hormone (ACTH) and cortisone are used frequently to provide symptomatic relief until the patient recovers from the disease. Transfusion of platelets as well as blood may be necessary to supply additional platelets in a hemorrhagic emergency, but generally are of limited usefulness. (Platelets cannot survive in stored blood.) If the patient does not recover spontaneously, splenectomy may be performed. This operation is useful, because the spleen (for reasons not fully understood) may be destroying too many platelets. The removal of the spleen often results in a rise in the platelet count and relief of the symptoms. The patient is observed carefully postoperatively for any symptoms of hemorrhage.

Nursing Management. Nursing management of the patient with purpura is essentially the same as that for any patient who has a tendency to bleed. It is imperative that these patients be protected from even the slightest injury because extensive bleeding can occur even with the slightest trauma.

Hemophilia

Hemophilia is a hereditary disease characterized by prolonged coagulation time, which results in persistent and sometimes severe bleeding. It results from deficiency of the antihemophilic factor normally present in blood plasma. The disease is transmitted from mother to son as a recessive sex-linked characteristic. Although women rarely develop the disease, they can inherit the trait, which, when it is passed on to a male infant, results in the development of the disease.

Hemophilia occurs with varying degrees of severity. Mild forms sometimes go unrecognized for years, until unusual bleeding is noted after an injury. Usually, however, bleeding is noted in infancy and childhood. There is persistent oozing of blood after slight injuries, such as a pin prick or a tiny cut. Often, bleeding occurs into joints, eventually damaging the joint and leading to deformity and limitation of motion. Relatively minor surgical procedures, such as tooth extraction, carry considerable risk and must be performed in a hospital. Transfusions usually are necessary even when minor surgery is performed.

Life expectancy is considerably shortened by the disease; many patients do not reach adulthood. On the other hand, those with mild hemophilia may lead full and productive lives despite the illness. Treatment includes avoidance of injury, transfusions of fresh blood or frozen plasma, and the application of thrombin to the bleeding area. Other measures to help to control the bleeding include direct pressure over the site of the bleeding and sometimes the use of cold compresses. Cold precipitated concentrate of antihemophilic factor is also used in the treatment of hemophilia. This preparation enables hemophiliacs to control accidental bleeding by obtaining an intravenous injection of the concentrated factor.

Polycythemia vera (primary polycythemia)

Polycythemia vera is a disease characterized by the excessive production of red blood cells and hemoglobin. The number of white blood cells also is increased. Its etiology is unknown. The patient may have 10 million red blood cells per cubic millimeter rather than the normal 5 million. The increased number of cells in the blood makes it more viscous than normal and leads to increased blood volume and to a tendency to develop thrombi. When clots cut off the blood supply to the tissues, areas of infarction result. The thrombosis of cerebral vessels is common.

Often the color of the face, and especially of the lips, is a reddish-purple. Fatigue, weakness, headache, and dizziness are common. The patient may bleed excessively after minor injuries, perhaps because of the engorgement of his capillaries and his veins. Splenomegaly commonly occurs. The condition usually has an insidious onset and a prolonged course.

The treatment involves measures to reduce the volume of the circulating blood, to lessen its viscosity, and to curb the excessive production of the red blood cells. Frequent medical examinations are important to determine the course of the disease and the patient's response to therapy.

A phlebotomy may be performed at intervals. Usually 500 ml. of blood is removed from the vein at a time. This is one instance in which bleeding the patient still has a legitimate place in modern medical treatment.

Radiophosphorus and radiation therapy are sometimes administered to decrease the production of the blood cells in the bone marrow. Antineoplastic drugs may be administered to curb the excessive activity of the bone marrow.

The patient is encouraged to continue his usual activities as long as he is able. He is observed carefully for symptoms of thrombosis. The patient is advised to limit his dietary intake of iron, since this limitation may lessen to some degree the production of the red blood cells.

Agranulocytosis

Agranulocytosis is a condition characterized by a decreased production of the white blood cells. Agranulocytosis may result from the toxic effects of drugs, such as sulfonamides, tranquilizers, aminopyrine, and barbiturates.

The symptoms of agranulocytosis include fatigue, fever, chills, headache, and the appearance of ulcers on the mucous membranes of the mouth, the throat, the nose, the rectum, or the vagina.

The prognosis is related to the cause of the condition. When the cause can be determined and promptly removed, and when the treatment can be commenced immediately, the patient usually recovers.

The treatment includes removing the causative factor—for example, stopping the drug that is producing the toxic effect. Severe infection usually occurs promptly, and the patient, if he is untreated, is powerless to fight the pathogens. Antibiotics are given to control infection. Careful medical aseptic technique is important in preventing the spread of pathogenic organisms to the patient. Meticulous handwashing and the wearing of clean gowns and masks while caring for the patient are necessary. The removal of the drug often may result in the resumption of the normal production of the white blood cells.

Multiple myeloma

Multiple myeloma is a malignant disease of plasma cells in which the cells infiltrate the bone marrow and result in single or multiple tumors.

Onset and Symptoms. The disease develops slowly. Usually the first symptom is a vague pain in the pelvis, spine, or ribs. As the disease progresses the pain may become more severe and localized. As the bone marrow is replaced by tumors, pathological fractures may occur. In addition, the patient may also show a decreased resistance to infection and anemia due to bone marrow destruction. Diagnosis is made by skeletal x-ray studies which reveal "punched-out" bone lesions. Urine samples will show the presence of M-type globulin (Bence-Jones protein).

Treatment and Nursing Management. Treatment is symptomatic as there is no cure for this disease. Pain is controlled with analgesics, with the stronger analgesics reserved for the terminal stages of the disease. Ambulation is an important part of therapy because the loss of calcium from the bone (osteoporosis) increases the amount of calcium in the blood (hypercalcemia) and urine (hypercalciuria). As osteoporosis can be made worse by immobilization, ambulation may prevent one of the complications of hypercalcemia and hypercalciuria—renal damage. The increased intake of fluids is also important as this measure may also prevent renal damage due to hypercalcemia and the precipitation of protein in the renal tubules. *Ambulation and adequate hydration are extremely important and must be stressed* during the hospital stay as well as when the patient is preparing for discharge.

Anemia is treated with blood transfusions and infections managed with antibiotics. Chemotherapy with antineoplastic agents may reduce the size and growth of the tumors. Back braces may be necessary when there is spinal involvement and body casts (which are usually bivalved) are used when there is extensive involvement and pathological fractures.

Part 2: Related disorders

Lymphosarcoma

Lymphosarcoma is characterized by overgrowth of lymphocytes in the lymph nodes, spleen, and lymphoid tissues in other parts of the body. As is true in other forms of neoplastic disease, the overgrowth of tissue (in this instance of lymphocytes) is unruly and, unless it can be completely eradicated, ultimately fatal. Lymphosarcoma is more common in older people than in the young.

SYMPTOMS depend on the site of lymph node involvement. Lymph node enlargement typically occurs in cervical, axillary, and inguinal regions. For example, if cervical lymph nodes are enlarged, dyspnea and dysphagia can result from pressure on nearby structures. In the final stages of illness the patient develops fever, cachexia, bleeding, and vulnerability to infection.

TREATMENT includes primarily irradiation, corticosteroid, and chemotherapy with such agents as nitrogen mustard. Surgical removal of involved lymph nodes may be performed. The objectives of therapy are to control the growth and the spread of the disease and to provide symptomatic relief during the course of the illness, which may last from several months to several years. It is questionable whether patients are ever cured of this disease; it is considered likely that even patients who experience unusually long remissions will eventually succumb.

Hodgkin's disease

Hodgkin's disease is characterized by the painless enlargement of the lymph nodes. Usually, the cervical nodes are involved first; inguinal and axillary nodes usually are affected later.

The cause of Hodgkin's disease is unknown. The disease is more common among men than women. It occurs most frequently during young adulthood. Like acute leukemia, Hodgkin's disease is a particularly tragic condition, because it so often claims the lives of young people.

Although some patients survive ten years or longer, most succumb in four or five years. It has been stated that patients whose disease is localized to one section of the body may occasionally be cured with present treatment methods, such as irradiation.

The diagnosis of Hodgkin's disease is established by a biopsy of an affected lymph node. The pathologist notes the changes that are typical of Hodgkin's disease, including the presence of a particular type of abnormal cell (Reed-Sternberg cell).

SYMPTOMS. The early symptoms of Hodgkin's disease include the painless enlargement of one or several lymph nodes. As the nodes enlarge, they often press on adjacent structures. Enlarged retroperitoneal nodes can cause a sense of fullness in the stomach and epigastric pain. Marked weight loss, anorexia, fatigue, and weakness occur. Chills and fever are common. Sometimes the patient develops marked anemia and thrombocytopenia, which results in a tendency to bleed. The resistance to infection is poor, and staphylococcal infections of the skin and respiratory infections often complicate the illness. Pruritus is a common symptom. Patients who receive treatment usually have remissions that may last months or even years. However, symptoms recur, and eventually they cause death from respiratory obstruction, cachexia, or secondary infections.

TREATMENT. The treatment of Hodgkin's disease includes x-ray therapy, corticosteroids, and antineoplastic drugs. Antibiotics are given to fight secondary infections. Transfusions may be necessary to control anemia.

The nodes may be subjected to intensive x-ray therapy to reduce their size. Although irradiation of a node may be followed by a remission, the disease usually returns and continues its progressive course.

The nursing care of patients with Hodgkin's disease is similar to that of patients with leukemia.

Infectious mononucleosis

Infectious mononucleosis is a condition that affects lymphoid tissues primarily. Lymph node enlargement is typical, accompanied by malaise, fever, sore throat, and headache. The cause of the disease is unknown, although viral etiology is suspected. Infectious mononucleosis occurs most commonly among college students. The incubation period is about six weeks.

Diagnosis is based on the symptoms, the presence of lymphocytosis, and a positive heterophil agglutination test. The latter two diagnostic tests are performed on samples of the patient's blood.

There is no specific treatment for this disease, which is usually self-limited. Rest, optimal diet, and prevention of secondary infection are important. Secondary infections, if they occur, may be treated with antibiotics. The average course of the disease is four weeks, after which most patients experience a period of weakness and fatigue of variable duration. Nursing management involves provision of rest and quiet recreation, measures to avoid secondary infection, and guidance in gradual resumption of activities after recovery. Young people who have missed school work need help in planning their return to a full schedule gradually, instead of trying to resume school and make up what they have missed while still feeling below par.

General nutritional considerations

■ Patients with iron-deficiency anemia may be treated with iron administered either orally or parenterally, *or* iron and a diet high in iron and protein. Liver is one food high in iron and may be given two or more times per week.

■ Pernicious anemia *cannot* be successfully treated by diet alone. This type of anemia is treated by the administration of vitamin B_{12} and a well-balanced diet.

■ Patients who develop an aplastic anemia usually develop oral lesions and should be given a soft bland diet.

General pharmacological considerations

■ Patients receiving iron orally for iron-deficiency anemia must be told that their stools will have a black color while taking this drug.

■ Iron administered orally may irritate the stomach and cause mild to severe gastric distress. Patients should be advised to take this product with or immediately after meals. The enteric-coated form of iron appears to cause less gastric distress.

■ Vitamin B_{12} (cyanocobalamin) is used to vitamin is given frequently and in large doses. Once the patient's symptoms have stabilized, smaller doses are given at two to four week intervals.

■ Some drugs can cause aplastic anemia. Any time the nurse notes drug literature warning of the possibility of a blood dyscrasia or bone marrow depression during the use of the drug, treat prenicious anemia. Early in treatment the she observes the patient closely for any signs of a blood disorder. Patients receiving drugs capable of causing bone marrow depression should have weekly blood studies (usually a CBC).

■ Most drugs used to treat leukemia, multiple myeloma, and Hodgkin's disease are extremely toxic and can depress bone marrow. Reliable references (Hospital Formulary, PDR, and so on) should be consulted for the many side effects of these drugs.

■ If a drug affects the hematopoietic (blood-forming) system there may be (1) a decrease in red blood cells (anemia), (2) a decrease in white blood cells (leukopenia), and (3) a decrease in platelets (thrombocytopenia).

■ Drug-induced anemia may require blood transfusions. Leukopenia, if severe, means the patient cannot fight infection and antibiotics may be necessary. In some instances, the leukopenia is so severe that antibiotics are unable to control an infection. Thrombocytopenia results in easy bruising and bleeding tendencies. Transfusions of platelets may be necessary.

Bibliography

Dougherty, W. M.: *Introduction to Hematology.* St. Louis, Mosby, 1971.

Eisenhauer, L.: Drug-induced blood dyscrasias. Nurs. Clin. North Am. 7:799, December, 1972.

England, J. M.: Pernicious anaemia. Nurs. Mirror 139:52, August 30, 1974.

French, R. M.: *Guide to Diagnostic Procedures,* ed. 4. New York, McGraw-Hill, 1975.

Goth, A.: *Medical Pharmacology,* ed. 5. St. Louis, Mosby, 1970.

Kübler-Ross, E.: *Death: The Final Stage of Growth.* Englewood Cliffs, N.J., Prentice-Hall, 1975.

Lund, D.: *Eric.* Philadelphia, Lippincott, 1974.

Memorial Sloan-Kettering Cancer Center, Behnke, H. D., ed.: *Guidelines to Comprehensive Nursing Care in Cancer.* New York, Springer, 1973.

Platt, W. R.: *Color Atlas and Textbook of Hematology.* Philadelphia, Lippincott, 1969.

Rodman, M. J. and Smith, D. W.: *Clinical Pharmacology in Nursing.* Philadelphia, Lippincott, 1974.

Schumann, D. and Patterson, P.: *Multiple myeloma.* Am. J. Nurs. 75:78, January, 1975.

———: The adult with acute leukemia. Nurs. Clin. North Am. 7:743, December, 1972.

Shafer, K. N., et al: *Medical-Surgical Nursing,* ed. 6. St. Louis, Mosby, 1975.

Tilkian, S. M. and Conover, M. H.: *Clinical Implications of Laboratory Tests.* St. Louis, Mosby, 1975.

CHAPTER—23

The patient with heart disease: anatomy; diagnostic tests

On completion of this chapter the student will:

- **Discuss the emotional impact of heart disease on the patient and his family.**
- **Describe the basic anatomy of the cardiopulmonary system.**
- **List overt symptoms of cardiac patients that may indicate a change in cardiac status.**
- **Discuss patient preparation for diagnostic tests related to the cardiovascular system.**

People often have intense reactions to the diagnosis of heart disease. Some may be frightened out of all proportion to the seriousness of the condition and become helpless invalids, when all that the doctor has suggested is a slowing down of the hectic pace of their lives. Others may verbally acknowledge the doctor's recommendations and yet drive themselves all the harder, getting less sleep than ever and smoking twice as much. Such patients seem to be saying by their actions—and often they express the thought in words when they are given an opportunity—"What's the use? Nothing can be done for it anyway. When your heart goes, that's it, and I may as well get as much fun as I can out of life in the time that I have left."

All too often the patient is discouraged from talking about his condition—particularly his feelings concerning it. Nor are such discussions easy for those who minister to the patient. Being able to listen without catching some of his anxiety demands the utmost in skill, tact, and self-understanding. Nurses may tell patients, "Now don't you worry about your heart! Just let us do the worrying." Such comments will not relieve anxiety and may even intensify it by preventing its expression. Instead of denying the patient's natural concern, we should allow him to discuss his worries and to learn more about his condition and treatment.

What are some of the things that patients and those who care for them fear most about heart disease? Sudden death or even a "sudden turn for the worse" is one. Such sudden changes are by no means limited to heart disease; nevertheless, almost everyone has heard and read about a person who was apparently in excellent health and then died suddenly of a "heart attack." (The term "heart attack" has no precise medical meaning, but it is often used to refer to myocardial infarction). The very unpredictability of some types of heart disease forms a basis for fear and uncertainty. Fear of sudden and dire symptoms may make the patient afraid to go on a trip or to continue working—even though the doctor has assured him that his condition does not warrant curtailment of such activities.

Despite the sudden onset of some types of heart disease, by far the largest proportion of patients find that their disease has become a lifetime companion. Many of these people continue to lead active, useful lives, though chronically ill, while others become incapacitated.

The care of chronically ill cardiac patients is difficult and, in a different way, demanding, too. Teaching the patient to care for himself and guiding him in planning his activities and following his treatment require patience and understanding. The nurse must be willing to work with a situation that may improve slowly and almost imperceptibly, or possibly not at all. Despite rapid progress in the treatment of heart disease, there are still some patients who cannot be helped by present medical knowledge. Some of them are older people whose failing hearts no longer respond to treatment. Others are young people whose hearts have been functioning under great handicap, such as the severe damage that results from rheumatic fever. These patients need support and care as their independence and well-being gradually diminish. All too often the attitude of doctors and nurses working with patients who do not respond to treatment is pessimistic if not fatalistic. At such times our patients need us the most. Caring for the patient does not stop even when there seems little likelihood of cure.

Epidemiology

In this country cardiovascular disease is the leading cause of death. The number of people succumbing to heart disease mounts steadily as age increases. Heart disease is an especially serious problem among the aged, and because of the increased life span more and more people are living long enough to develop it. Improved diagnostic methods have indicated that deaths once attributed to "old age" now may be classified as deaths from heart disease. When age has greatly weakened the body and the time of death draws near, some one organ of the body must give way first, precipitating death. Often this organ is the heart.

Structure (anatomy) of the cardiopulmonary system

The heart is a four-chambered muscular pump about the size of a fist. It can be viewed as a master pump to which is attached a system of tubes for outflow and inflow, namely, the aorta and pulmonary arteries, and the vena cava and pulmonary veins (Fig. 23-1).

The heart is anchored in the mediastinum, under and a little to the left of the midline of the sternum. (The part of the heart directly under the sternum is the right ventricle, which is significant to the dynamics of external cardiac compression.) The heart's lower border lies on the diaphragm and forms a blunt point extending to the left, which is called the apex of the heart.

Three distinct layers of tissue make up the heart wall. The bulk of the heart consists of specially constructed muscle tissue known as the *myocardium.* Covering the myocardium on the outside and adherent to it is the *pericardium.* Lining the interior wall of the heart is a delicate layer of endothelial tissue known as the *endocardium.* This is the layer that the blood directly contacts.

The term cardiac cycle means a complete heartbeat, consisting of contraction (systole) and relaxation (diastole) of both atria plus contraction and relaxation of both ventricles. The two atria contract simultaneously; then, as they relax, the two ventricles contract and relax, instead of the entire heart contracting as a unit; this gives a kind of "milking" action to the movements of the heart.

Though having different kinds of work to do, and working under different pressures, both sides of the heart work in unison. The left atrium receives newly oxygenated blood from the lungs via four pulmonary veins. This oxygenated blood flows during diastole into the left ventricle through the mitral valve, and during atrial systole, there is a squeezing down of additional blood into the ventricle before the valve closes.

Attached to the mitral valve are cord-like structures known as chordae tendinae which in turn attach to two major muscular projections from the left ventricle known as papillary muscles. During contraction of the left ventricle these muscles also contract, thereby providing tension on the mitral valve and preventing prolapse or invagination of the mitral valve back into the left atrium. If this were to happen, as it sometimes does when the papillary muscles are involved in a myocardial infarction, blood would flow not only forward into the aorta but also backward into the left atrium through an incompetent mitral valve (mitral regurgitation).

During ventricular systole, the blood is pumped through the aortic valve into the aorta from which it then flows under pressure into many smaller arteries, thence to arterioles. Arterioles branch into capillaries which permeate the tissues of each individual organ and are in intimate contact with the cells of those tissues. Oxygen and metabolic foods are delivered to the cells through this complex circulatory network. The thin walls of the capillaries, their tremendous surface area, and their tiny size, all allow for rapid exchange of gases and metabolic substances between the blood and cells. After this exchange takes place, deoxygenated venous blood is transported back to the heart under low pressure by the veins.

Veins from all organs of the body drain into the superior or inferior vena cava, and, along with blood from the coronary veins, empty into the right atrium of the heart. Then this venous blood is pumped into the right ventricle through the tricuspid valve. From this chamber it is pumped through the pulmonary artery into the pulmonary or lesser circulation. This smaller circulatory unit is responsbile for the exchange of oxygen and carbon dioxide. Blood leaving the right ventricle flows through the pulmonary artery to the pulmonary capillaries. Here, carbon dioxide, which has built up in the venous blood because of its release from the tissue as a metabolic end product, is transferred from the blood into the lung spaces (alveoli) and is exhaled. The venous blood takes on oxygen by coming in contact with inspired air. After this exchange of oxygen and carbon dioxide has taken place, the oxygenated blood is transported through four pulmonary veins to the left side of the heart.

Though the structure of the pump itself and the complex lengthy system of arteries and veins are impressive, the entire cardiopulmonary system is designed to serve as a transport system to provide oxygen and other nutrients and to remove metabolic end products from the *individual cells.*

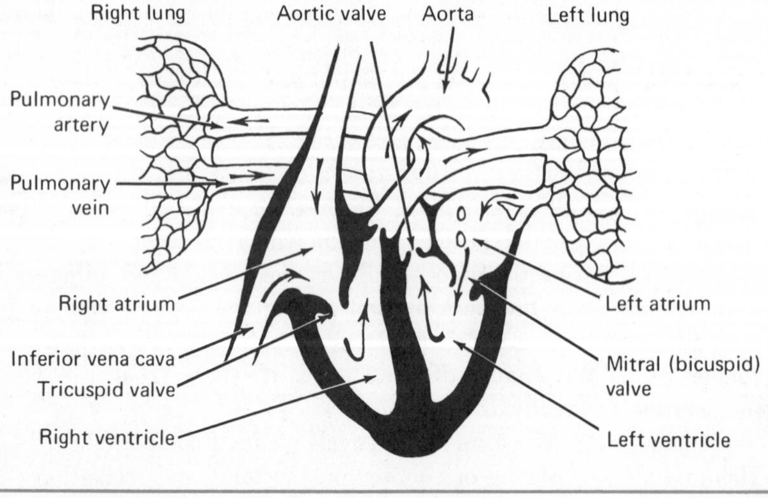

figure 23-1. Diagram illustrating the flow of the blood through the heart and the lungs. The path can be observed by starting at the vena cava and following the arrows through the right atrium, the right ventricle, the pulmonary artery, the lungs, the pulmonary vein, the left atrium, the left ventricle, and into the aorta.

Observations of signs and symptoms

Insufficient blood supply to the heart is an important factor in some kinds of heart disease. It is often indicated by chest pain, pallor, apprehension, and sweating. The location, intensity, and duration of the pain should be noted; the patient is placed at rest, and the symptoms are reported immediately.

Various symptoms appear in congestive heart failure, the condition in which the heart is unable to keep pace with the demands made on it. If the right side of the heart is in failure, edema of the extremities will be noted. The edema is usually first seen in the feet and ankles, but, as the heart becomes increasingly weak, it may be noted in the legs and sacral area. If the left side of the heart is in failure, fluid accumulates in the lungs, causing congestion. Insufficient oxygenation of the blood may be reflected in a variety of respiratory symptoms, such as cyanosis, cough, dyspnea, and orthopnea (difficulty in breathing in a flat position). The patient is observed for cyanosis around the lips and the nailbeds. If the patient becomes dyspneic, he is placed at rest with his head elevated.

Observation of temperature, pulse, blood pressure, and respiration is particularly important in caring for the cardiac patient. Symptoms often change suddenly. Significant symptoms, such as changes in heart rate and rhythm, may manifest themselves only at brief intervals, and it is important that *any* change be reported and recorded.

Temperature. Fever is characteristic in some types of heart disease, particularly in acute myocardial infarction, rheumatic fever, and subacute bacterial endocarditis. Patients with these conditions should have their temperatures taken rectally, since this method provides the most accurate reading. Though a rectal temperature is more accurate, oral temperatures might be ordered to avoid vagal stimulation from the insertion of the rectal thermometer. Vagal stimulation can produce slowing of the heart (bradycardia) and other cardiac arrhythmias such as heart block, especially in the patient with acute myocardial infarction. If obtaining the more accurate rectal temperature is still necessary, care should be taken that the thermometer is well lubricated and inserted gently. An eye on the electrocardiographic monitor or a finger on the patient's pulse will give evidence of excess vagal stimulation, which should be reported.

Pulse. When the nurse takes the pulse, she notes not only its rate but also its rhythm and its quality. Is the rhythm regular? If not, does the irregularity have a pattern? For example, an unusually long interval after every fourth beat, or alternating weak and strong beats, may be noted. Is the pulse strong, or does it seem weak and hard to detect? Can it be easily obliterated by the pressure of the fingers? Is the pulse bounding? Does it seem to be striking forcefully against the fingers?

The pulse rate is not always the same as the heart rate. Some of the beats may be too feeble to produce a pulsation in the radial artery. Counting the radial pulse of such a patient is equivalent to counting only the strong beats. Listening to his heart with a stethoscope may indicate that his heart is beating 90 times a minute, rather than the 60 beats per minute that were counted when the radial pulse was taken. The difference between the apical (heart) rate and the radial rate is known as the *pulse deficit.* It can be detected by taking an apical-radial pulse. One nurse counts the beats as she listens over the apex of the patient's heart with a stethoscope. (The apex of the heart is the lowermost point of the left ventricle.) Usually, it is easiest to hear the heartbeat over the apex (fifth intercostal space in the left midclavicular line). The stethoscope is placed near the left nipple or, in mature women, under the left breast. Simultaneously, another nurse counts the radial pulse. Both nurses count for at least a full minute. Both figures are charted. If a pulse deficit exists, the number of beats at the radial artery is fewer than that of the apex. The apical rate is most significant in a patient with pulse deficit. For example, when the nurse counts the pulse prior to administering digitalis, she should not report that the pulse is below 60 until the *apical* rate has been taken.

Today, many hospitalized cardiac patients receive continuous electrocardiographic monitoring. The monitor will indicate the patient's heart rate and rhythm but not the quality of the beat; the quality can be ascertained by feeling the pulse. Correlating pulse quality with the cardiac monitor provides useful information. The cardiac rhythm on the monitor, for example, can look normal but the cardiac output, reflected in a weak, thready pulse, can be low. Also, the monitor pattern might be irregular but the pulse and other data show that the patient can maintain sufficient cardiac output. By correlating cardiac monitor data with the feel of the patient's pulse while the patient is on the monitor, the nurse is better able to detect arrhythmias by feeling the pulse when the patient is off the monitor.

Blood pressure readings are important, because diseases of the heart are often closely associated with changes in blood pressure. For instance, a drop in

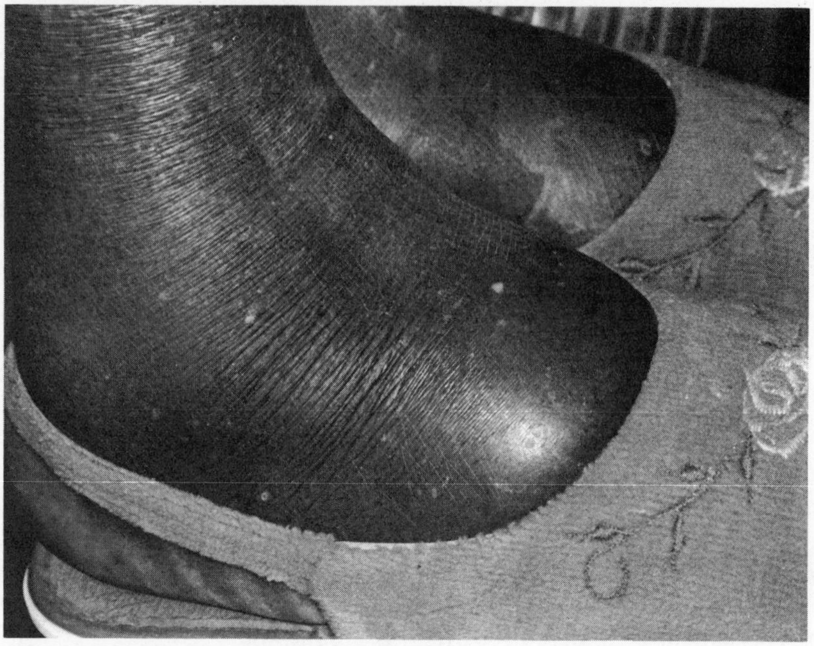

figure 23-2. The patient with cardiac disease may have edema of the feet and ankles. (Photograph—D. Atkinson)

blood pressure frequently follows acute myocardial infarction. The patient should be sitting or lying in a comfortable position, and the systolic and diastolic readings should be noted and recorded carefully. Blood pressure is taken in both arms on admission and once a day. Any discrepancy should be reported. In charting, it is good practice to identify the arm(s) used to determine the blood pressure.

RESPIRATIONS. Careful observation of the rate and character of respiration is important. Some nursing studies have shown that inaccuracy in reporting respiration is so widespread that the results of the procedure are of little value. Too often, also, the nurse focuses only on rate, although other observations are equally significant. While counting the rate for a full minute, the *quality* of respiration should be observed. Is the patient's breathing easy or labored (dyspneic)? Are his respirations deep or shallow, wet or dry, wheezing or quiet? Does he use his neck muscles or abdominal muscles to help him breathe? Is the rate faster than normal (tachypnic)? Is he restless or confused? (This can indicate oxygen lack.) Does he have late signs of hypoxia, such as cyanosis or orthopnea? Does he have Cheyne-Stokes-type breathing?

EDEMA. Note edema, particularly in dependent parts of the body such as the feet and ankles (Fig. 23-2), and over the sacrum. Edema often accompanies congestive heart failure. The blood is not pumped efficiently, and venous blood that is being returned to the heart by the large veins cannot be received promptly and pumped by the right side of the heart. As a result the venous blood being returned to the heart dams up in the veins. The inefficient return of the blood to the heart causes congestion in the veins and the collection of extra fluid in the tissues.

Fluctuations in weight are important indications of edema. A gain in weight often means that edema is increasing, and not that the patient is growing "fatter," in the usual sense of the term. Loss in weight often reflects the desirable and needed loss of excess fluid that has collected in the tissues. If a daily weight is ordered, the patient should be weighed at the same time each day and with the same amount of clothing. The recording of weight should be as accurate as possible. A pound more or less may indicate that edema is increasing or decreasing.

Diagnostic tests

ELECTROCARDIOGRAM (*ECG*)

The electrocardiogram is a graphic record of electric currents generated by the heart muscle (Fig. 23-3). The record is made by a special instrument, called an *electrocardiograph*, which measures and records these currents. The 12-lead ECG is especially useful in determining the nature of myocardial damage and in interpreting arrhythmias. Connections are made between the machine and the patient by means of electrodes placed at various points in the patient's body. A special conducting jelly is rubbed on the points of contact. The electrodes are placed on the outside of the skin, usually on the wrists, ankles, and chest, in a number of combinations. The leads that go to the extremities are strapped in place. The chest lead is held in position by the technician using a suction cup.

No special preparation for the test is needed other than explaining it to the patient, but since the test does involve the heart the explanation should be individualized to prevent undue anxiety. The nurse should explain that the test is completely painless, and that it merely records the electrical currents of the heart. Otherwise, patients who are having it done for the first time may feel uneasy when they see wires being attached to them, and may wonder whether they are about to receive some kind of electric shock.

THE ROLE OF THE NURSE.

- The nurse helps the patient to understand what to expect. (For example, the patient should know that the ECG is often repeated in order to aid the physician in following the course of the illness.)
- In addition to the usual information, such as the patient's name and room number, the request slip should state whether or not the patient is receiving digitalis, quinidine, or any cardiac drug, as these drugs produce changes in the electrocardiogram that resemble those seen in disease. Since some drugs other than cardiac drugs may affect the heart, it is good practice to record *all* drugs being taken by the patient, on the request slip.
- The nurse introduces the technician to the patient and makes sure that the patient is comfortable and ready for the test.
- The nurse stays with the patient, if he is very ill, during the test. This is especially important if the patient is anxious, dyspneic, or in pain.
- A copy of the electrocardiogram will be placed on the patient's chart along with a sum-

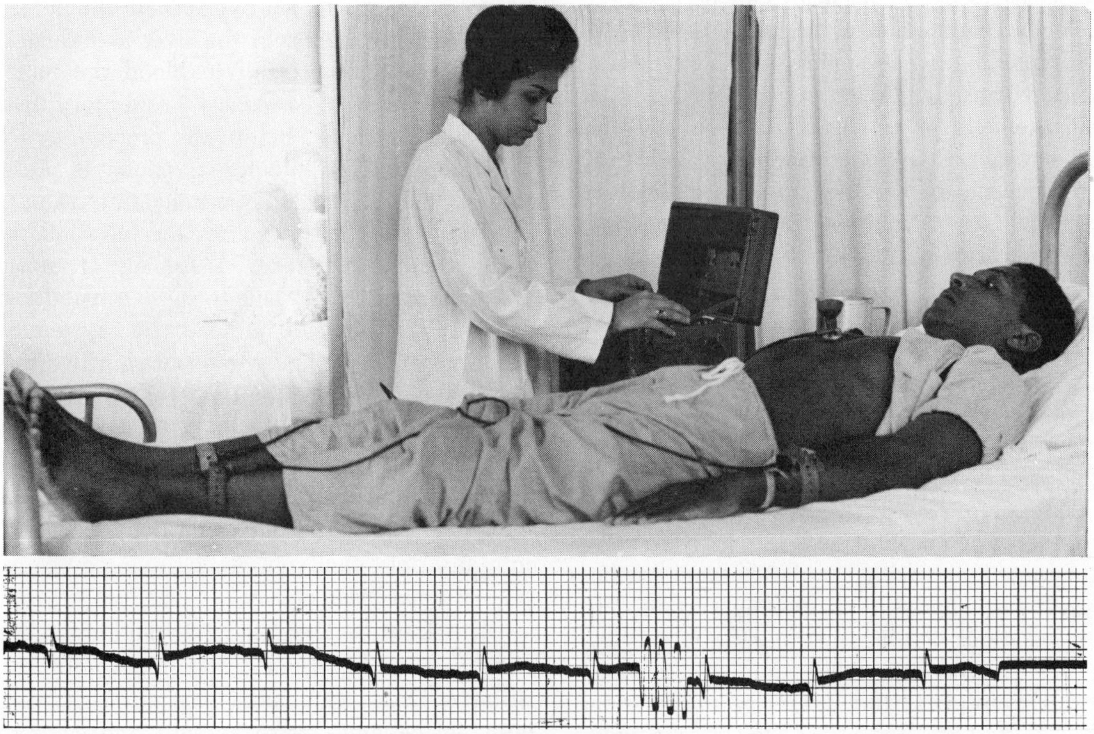

figure 23-3. (*Top*) Technician taking an ECG. Leads have been placed on arms, legs and chest. (*Bottom*) A sample of the graphic record obtained by electrocardiography.

mary of the physician's findings. For example, the statement may indicate recent damage to the myocardium that has resulted from coronary occlusion, or it may describe a disturbance in heart rhythm. All nurses should develop the habit of reading the written summary. The findings may significantly affect the nursing care plan.

Vectorcardiogram

Spatial vectorcardiography is a type of electrocardiography in which the heart's forces are represented by arrows and loops, rather than by waves and complexes.

Heart damage can sometimes be inferred from the oscillographic loop when it is inapparent or questionable in the conventional electrocardiogram.

The vectorcardiogram is obtained by a specially trained technician and interpreted by a cardiologist. Preparation of the patient is similar to that for the electrocardiogram.

X-ray tests and fluoroscopy

Fluoroscopy is frequently helpful in the examination of the heart, because the heart can be observed in action. X-ray examination of the chest has the advantage of providing a permanent record. For example, it is often useful in determining the extent of cardiac enlargement. When heart function is inefficient, the heart enlarges—a mechanism that helps the heart to compensate or to keep up with circulatory load. No special care other than an explanation is required before or after the taking of x-ray films or before or after fluoroscopy.

Angiocardiogram

An intravenous angiocardiogram is a test in which a radiopaque dye is injected into a vein, and its course from the right heart to the lungs, back to the left heart and out the aorta is recorded by a rapid series of x-ray pictures. The pictures reveal not only the size and the shape of these structures but also the sequence and the time of their filling with blood. The angiocardiogram is used particularly in diagnosing certain congenital abnormalities of the heart and the great vessels. This test is used only when simpler diagnostic measures fail to provide the necessary information. Breakfast is omitted the morning of the test, and sedative and antihistaminic drugs are administered ½ to 1 hour before the patient is taken to the x-ray department.

Arteriograms

Aortogram. Dye is injected into the aorta, and x-ray films are taken to outline the abdominal aorta and the major arteries in the legs; dye also may be injected into other vessels to help to visualize them in the x-ray pictures.

Peripheral Arteriogram; Coronary Arteriogram. Dye is injected into the femoral or the popliteal artery, and x-ray films are taken to diagnose occlusive arterial disease. In deciding whether or not a patient is a candidate for surgery for the relief of myocardial ischemia, a catheter is passed through an artery, such as the right femoral artery, to the heart, dye is injected through the catheter into various coronary arteries, and serial films are taken. The physicians look for localized blockage of a coronary vessel which may be amenable to surgery. After the test there is a greater chance for bleeding than after a venipuncture. A pressure dressing is applied. Patient activity is restricted for 12 hours. The nurse observes for bleeding, arrhythmias, and peripheral circulation.

Allergic reactions and other complications

During and after such tests as the three immediately above, in which a dye is used, the nurse watches for allergic reactions to the dye, including urticaria, flushing of the skin, fall in blood pressure, nausea, vomiting and, less commonly, respiratory distress and anaphylactic shock. Before the procedure, a skin test may be performed to determine possible allergy to the dye, so that severe allergic reactions can be avoided.

For 5 to 10 minutes after the injection of the dye the patient experiences a feeling of intense heat throughout his body. Due to sudden blood vessel dilation he may develop a headache. Systemic allergic reactions are most likely to occur shortly after the dye has been administered, while the patient is in the x-ray department. However, when the patient returns to his room, the nurse should observe him for any symptoms of delayed systemic reaction. Watch for adequate urinary output when dye has been injected into an artery or a vein, as the dye may cause a temporary renal insufficiency.

The treatment of allergic reactions includes epinephrine, antihistamines, and oxygen for respiratory distress. Drugs to combat allergic reactions, such as epinephrine and antihistamines, and equipment for giving oxygen should be available.

Other emergency resuscitation equipment such as a defibrillator, an "Ambu" or other breathing bag, and a tracheostomy set, likewise is kept available for immediate use. The patients undergoing the tests are likely to have cardiac impairment. A continuous ECG is usually taken during the tests to monitor the patient's condition. Frequent check is kept of the patient's pulse. Cardiac arrhythmia—ventricular fibrillation is the most common—and cardiac arrest have been known to occur.

Thrombosis and irritation of the artery into which the dye was injected also may occur, and the dye may cause irritation if it leaks beneath the skin. Check the pulse distal to the site of injection in the search for a clot or spasm of the vessel. The absence of a pulse on that side requires the immediate attention of the physician. The artery used for the injection should be observed for pain and swelling. Tenderness over the artery is usual and disappears in 1 or 2 days.

The tests are tiring. An angiocardiogram, for example, may take 2½ hours. On returning from the x-ray department the patient should be given the opportunity to rest in a quiet atmosphere.

Operative permits are required for most of these procedures.

Cardiac catheterization

Cardiac catheterization involves passing a long flexible catheter into the heart and the great vessels. As the catheter enters the various chambers, the pressures are measured, and samples of the blood are obtained and analyzed for the content of oxygen and carbon dioxide. For example, the oxygen content of the blood in the right atrium is higher than normal when there is an atrial septal defect—a hole in the septum that separates the atria. The test is usually performed to aid in the diagnosis of congenital defects.

A team, usually comprising several physicians, a nurse, and technicians, performs the test. During the test the nurse functions as an assistant to the physicians, and she reassures the patient, making him as comfortable as possible. The patient lies supine on a table in a special room equipped with x-ray and fluoroscopy machines. The procedure usually takes from 1 to 3 hours; the table is covered with a foam rubber pad, and the patient is positioned carefully, so that he will be as comfortable as possible.

Usually, the room is darkened at intervals during the test to facilitate the use of the fluoroscope. However, a device called a *fluoroscopic image amplifier,* or image intensifier, sometimes makes it possible to perform this test in a lighted room.

Ordinarily, the adult patient is not anesthetized (the walls of blood vessels have no fibers that transmit pain), but is given a sedative before the test. Breakfast is withheld on the morning of the test. The patient may have some slight discomfort at first from the cutdown and the insertion of the catheter. As the catheter enters the chambers of the heart, he may experience some irregularity of heart rhythm that resembles a feeling of fluttering or "butterflies in the chest." If this should occur, the patient is reassured that the sensation will pass, and that there is no cause for alarm. The patient may cough when the catheter is passed up the pulmonary artery. If so, he is told that the sensation will pass quickly. However, despite sedation the patient often is alert and apprehensive, and he is very much aware of the slightest sensation that is out of the ordinary.

When the procedure is over, the catheter is withdrawn gently, and the patient returns to his room with a small sterile dressing over the site of the cutdown.

Cardiac catheterization is not without danger, although most patients experience no complications, except possibly a transient arrhythmia during the actual procedure. The patient's pulse is checked frequently after the catheterization has been performed. Rapidity or irregularity of the pulse should immediately be reported to the physician. The site of the cutdown should be watched afterward for any tenderness or inflammation. Pulmonary edema and air embolism are rare complications. Sometimes the patient's temperature is elevated for a few hours after the test. The patient is usually kept on bed rest for the rest of the day.

Bibliography

Andreoli, K. G. et al: *Comprehensive Cardiac Care: A Text for Nurses and Other Health Professionals,* ed. 3. St. Louis, Mosby, 1975.

Armington, Sister C. and Creighton, H.: *Nursing of People with Cardiovascular Problems.* Boston, Little, Brown, 1971.

Brunner, L. S. and Suddarth, D. S.: *Textbook of Medical-Surgical Nursing,* ed. 3. Philadelphia, Lippincott, 1975.

Coats, K.: Noninvasive cardiac diagnostic procedures. Am. J. Nurs. 75:1980, November, 1975.

Delaney, M. T.: Examining the chest. The heart, Part 2 (pictorial). Nurs. '75, 5:41, September, 1975.

Gillete, E.: Heartbeat—the rhythm of life (pictorial). Nurs. Care 8:24, June, 1975.

Kelly, Sister P.: Diagnostic tests: What should we tell the patient? Nurs. '74, 4:15, December, 1974.

Kinztel, K. C., ed.: *Advanced Concepts in Clinical Nursing,* ed. 2. Philadelphia, Lippincott, 1977.

Lawson, B.: Clinical assessment of cardiac patients in acute care facilities. Nurs. Clin. North Am. 7:431, September, 1972.

Sparks, C.: Peripheral pulses. Am. J. Nurs. 75:1132, July, 1975.

CHAPTER—24

The patient with heart disease

On completion of this chapter the student will:

- **State the causes and mechanisms of congestive heart failure.**
- **Describe the symptoms of congestive heart failure.**
- **List the tests employed in the diagnosis of congestive heart failure.**
- **Prepare a nursing care plan for the patient with congestive heart failure and acute pulmonary edema.**

Congestive heart failure

Heart failure develops when the heart is unable to meet the demands of the body. In effect, the heart has become an inefficient pump. The term *congestive* is often used in describing heart failure, because the inefficient circulation leads to the congestion of many organs with blood and tissue fluid.

Heart failure can occur with varying degrees of severity. When symptoms are slight, the patient may be able to be up and about without having any marked symptoms. In contrast, the patient in severe heart failure is critically ill. A patient can go through varying degrees of heart failure, and with treatment he can often recover from it. When the patient shows symptoms of heart failure, his condition is described as *decompensated*—that is, his heart is not able to compensate or to make up for the demands placed on it. When the treatment succeeds in enabling the heart to keep up with the circulatory load, the symptoms disappear, and the condition is described as *compensated*. Often, however, the abnormality of the heart that led to heart failure remains, and unless the patient has continued treatment, he may again develop the symptoms of congestive heart failure.

Causes of congestive heart failure

Congestive heart failure may result from many different forms of heart disease. It usually develops gradually, as the result of strain placed on the heart by congenital defects, diseases of the heart and blood vessels, or other diseases that overburden the heart. For example:

- Rheumatic fever can damage the heart valves, and the strain of pumping a sufficient amount of blood through the damaged valves may cause heart failure.
- A branch of a coronary artery may become occluded and cut off the blood supply to a portion of the heart muscle (myocardial infarction). The efficiency of the heart as a pump is impaired and congestive heart failure may develop.
- The pericardium may become inflamed, and later scarred and constricted. Constriction can interfere with heart action by pressing on the heart and so lead to heart failure.
- Hyperthyroidism, if it exists for many years, can cause a normal heart to fail because of the excessive demands placed on it by the very rapid heart action that occurs in hyperthyroidism.

The treatment of congestive heart failure involves locating the cause and, if possible, correcting it. Sometimes, cure of the underlying condition is impossible, and treatment consists entirely of measures designed to help the heart to continue to function as efficiently as possible despite the underlying disease. Thus, an abnormality of a valve damaged by rheumatic fever may be corrected surgically. If surgery is not possible, medical treatment designed to help the heart to function despite the valvular lesion would constitute the treatment. The treatment of hyperthyroidism can cure congestive heart failure due to the overactive thyroid.

Particularly in older age groups congestive heart failure is frequently brought about by a combination of factors. The blood vessels may gradually lose their elasticity (a condition called *arteriosclerosis*), and the lumen of the arteries may slowly grow smaller due to the fatty deposits in the walls of the arteries (*atherosclerosis*). Elevation of the blood pressure is common among older persons. In time, these vascular changes can lead to congestive heart failure by interfering with the blood supply to the heart muscle and by causing the heart to pump blood through vessels that have become narrowed and inelastic. The heart itself is not exempt from the process of aging. Gradually, with advancing age, cardiac reserve is lessened, and the heart becomes less able to withstand the effects of injury or disease. Congestive heart failure, then, is not a separate disease; rather it is a pathological state resulting from a variety of conditions that impair heart function. Although the immediate treatment of congestive heart failure is the same regardless of the cause, the treatment of the underlying condition can involve a variety of measures, both medical and surgical, designed to relieve or to cure it.

The process of congestive heart failure

Disturbances of one part of the heart, if they are severe enough or last long enough, eventually affect the entire circulation. The process of congestive heart failure from mitral stenosis is one example of the process of congestive heart failure:

- Narrowing of the mitral valve impedes the flow of the blood from the left atrium to the left ventricle.
- The left atrium, because it cannot empty normally, becomes enlarged, and the pressure within this chamber of the heart increases.
- This increased pressure, in turn, causes the lungs to become congested with fluid, because the distended left atrium cannot effectively receive the oxygenated blood coming to it from the lungs.
- Lung congestion results in the inefficient oxygenation of the blood. The patient develops dyspnea, cough, orthopnea, and sometimes hemoptysis. These are symptoms of left-sided heart failure.

- Because of the congestion in the lungs, it becomes harder for the right ventricle to pump blood to the lungs. The right ventricle must pump more forcefully to overcome the resistance of the lungs to the blood coming from this ventricle.
- The right ventricle eventually becomes unable to keep up with its work. It cannot pump the blood effectively, and the right side of the heart becomes congested with blood.
- Venous blood returning to the right side of the heart cannot be pumped to the lungs quickly and efficiently enough because of the failure of the right side of the heart. Congestion develops in the large veins leading to the heart and eventually in other organs and tissues of the body as the result of inefficient venous return.
- Dependent edema, such as that of the feet and the ankles on standing, appears. The abdomen may become distended with fluid (ascites). The liver, too, becomes edematous and enlarged. Presacral edema may be present in the patient on bed rest. The veins in the neck become distended. These are symptoms of right-sided heart failure.

This is only one example of the process of congestive heart failure. In each type of heart disease the process is somewhat different, depending on the location of the heart damage and its severity. Yet the process is similar in that, although one part of the heart and the circulation is primarily affected at first, the process, if it continues, eventually affects the entire circulation. The sequence in which symptoms appear reflects the sequence of physiological disturbance. Symptoms of either right-sided or left-sided heart failure may appear first; eventually, symptoms of failure in both sides will usually be present.

Patients with congestive heart failure retain excessive amounts of sodium, which contributes to the problem of edema by holding water in the tissues.

Symptoms of congestive heart failure

Often the patient notices that he is unusually tired after work that previously had not caused fatigue. Some patients find that dyspnea on exertion is their first symptom. For instance, a person who lives on the second floor may find that he becomes short of breath and has to rest on the landing before he attempts the second flight of steps. He may notice that he has difficulty breathing while he is lying flat, and he begins to use two or even three pillows. Cough, occasionally productive of blood-streaked sputum, may occur.

The patient may notice that his feet and ankles are swollen, particularly at the end of the day, when he has been standing and walking (Fig. 24-1). This swelling usually disappears during the night when his feet and his legs are elevated, but the fluid can shift to the lungs or sacral region.

Actually, the edema does not really disappear. It is just distributed differently due to the patient's posture and is therefore less noticeable. When he stands, his ankles will gradually swell again. By the time that

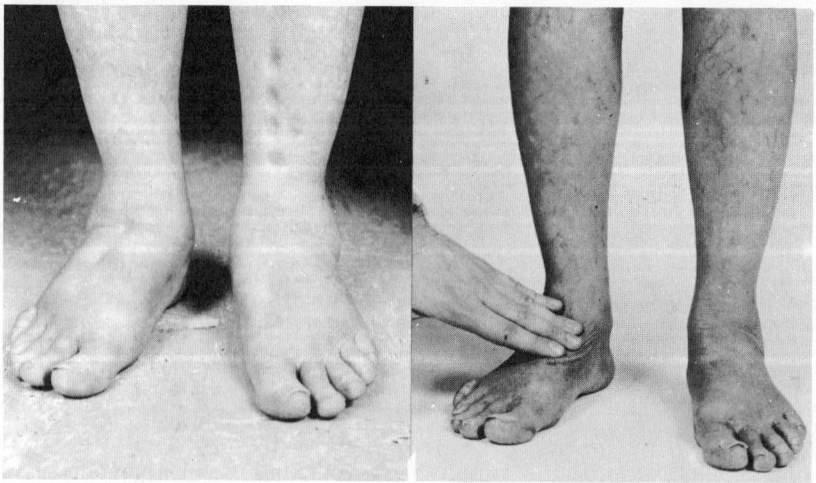

figure 24-1. (*Left*) Pitting edema of feet and lower legs. (*Right*) The same patient after treatment relieved the edema. (CIBA Pharmaceutical Company)

the edema becomes noticeable, the patient usually has retained 10 or more extra pounds of fluid in his tissues. These extra pounds, which actually are due to the retained fluid, show up on the scale when the patient is weighed. His apparent gain in weight is not in the usual sense of increased fat or muscle tissue. Although the patient's weight gradually increases, he usually is losing rather than gaining fat and muscle tissue. When this process has continued for a time, the patient often looks strangely out of proportion. The lower parts of his body (the ankles, legs, and eventually thighs and abdomen) become swollen and heavy, whereas the face and the upper parts of the body look thin and wasted. When edema is relieved by treatment, his family and friends often are amazed at how thin and frail he looks.

Edema of the feet and legs rarely causes pain, but it makes the legs feel heavy, clumsy, and tired. It is usually described as "pitting edema," because, when pressure is exerted, the part that has been pressed will become indented. The indentation gradually disappears after the pressure has been released. Edema of other areas, though it is less visible, often causes symptoms of the dysfunction of the organs involved. For example, distention of the liver and other abdominal viscera may cause flatulence, anorexia, and nausea. The collection of fluid within the lungs and the pleural space leads to dyspnea and sometimes to persistent cough.

Some patients with congestive heart failure experience Cheyne-Stokes respirations. This symptom is believed to be due to poor circulation to the brain, causing the respiratory center in the brain to become less sensitive to the amount of carbon dioxide in the blood. Irritability, restlessness, and decreased attention span may occur when the condition is very severe. These symptoms are due to impaired cerebral circulation, and they may progress to stupor and coma before death.

Diagnosis

Because congestive heart failure can be produced by various diseases of the heart, any test or combination of tests used for cardiac patients may be ordered in an effort to discover the underlying cause of congestive heart failure. For example, in addition to the history and the physical examination, the patient may have electrocardiograms, x-ray examination and fluoroscopy of his chest, or cardiac catheterization.

Two tests—measuring the venous pressure and the circulation time—are done especially to determine the congestion and the slowing of the circulation so typical of congestive heart failure.

Measuring Venous Pressure. The technique of measuring arterial pressure, which is usually referred to as "taking the blood pressure," is a familiar one. Measuring venous pressure is done less often, and it may be less familiar. The doctor performs this test, and the nurse may assist. First, the patient's arm is positioned at the same level as his heart by supporting the arm with a pillow or a rolled blanket. The doctor performs a venipuncture, and to the needle and the syringe he attaches a water manometer that has had sterile normal saline placed in it. A three-way stopcock connects the syringe, the needle, and the manometer. When the manometer is in place, the stopcock is adjusted to allow the saline from the manometer to flow into the patient's vein. The pressure in the vein will permit only a certain amount of the saline to run in. When the saline stops entering the vein, the level of the saline left in the manometer is read. The normal venous pressure ranges from 7 to 14 cm. of water. It is increased in congestive heart failure.

Measuring Central Venous Pressure. The most accurate measurement of venous pressure is obtained when a catheter is inserted into a peripheral vein and threaded into the right atrium. This is called central venous pressure or CVP. The catheter is connected via a three-way stopcock to a water manometer and an intravenous infusion bottle, and serial readings are taken. Central venous pressure is recorded as the height of the fluid column in the manometer when it is filled with fluid from the infusion bottle. When the venous pressure is not being read, the three-way stopcock is adjusted so that the intravenous fluid runs through to keep the catheter patent. Since venous pressure decreases slightly on inspiration and increases slightly on expiration, oscillations of the fluid level in the manometer occur with the patient's breathing. Normal central venous pressure is 5 to 12 cm. of water. Central venous pressure is increased in congestive heart failure.

Normally the external jugular veins in the neck are collapsed above the level of the suprasternal notch when a person sits or stands. Distention of these veins indicates that the pressure within them is elevated.

Measuring Circulation Time. The circulation time is determined by the intravenous injection of a substance that can be tasted by the patient when it reaches his tongue. Sodium dehydrocholate (Decholin), which causes a bitter taste, or sucrose, which causes a sweet taste, may be used. The substance is injected into a vein in the arm, and the time interval between the injection and the patient's tasting the substance is called the *arm-to-tongue time*. Normally, this is less than 15 seconds. The test is timed by a stopwatch, after careful instruction of the patient to signal as soon as he tastes the substance. In congestive heart failure the circulation time is prolonged.

Treatment

The treatment of congestive heart failure involves measures to help the heart to function as effectively as possible and to relieve the symptoms produced by the inefficient circulation:

> The patient is helped to rest. His heart may be able to meet the demands of the body at rest, but be unable to cope with the demands placed on it by physical or emotional stress. Sedatives are sometimes necessary to help the patient to rest.
>
> The abnormal retention of sodium is combated by limiting the patient's intake of sodium, whether in food or drugs.
>
> Digitalis is given to slow the heart rate and to strengthen its beat. These two actions help the weakened overburdened heart to pump blood more efficiently.
>
> Diuretics are given to rid the body of the excess fluid and the sodium that have been stored in the tissues. Paracentesis is sometimes necessary to relieve ascites.
>
> Oxygen is ordered to improve ventilation when oxygenation is impaired by congestion and sluggish circulation through the lungs.

Nursing management

Nursing management involves a variety of abilities (Table 24-1). When the patient is admitted with acute congestive heart failure, nursing care involves speed, assurance, and technical skill in quickly providing oxygen and medications. The nurse has the responsibility for observing the critically ill patient and for notifying the doctor of changes in his condition. When a patient is suddenly admitted to the hospital in a critical condition, the need for reassurance is especially great. Because the situation demands speed and action, the nurse quickly assists the doctor with emergency treatment.

Detailed explanations are deferred until the patient improves. At first he is too sick to take in complicated explanations, and care must be given quickly. For example, instead of giving a detailed explanation of why oxygen is necessary, the nurse assures the patient that it will help his breathing, deftly applies it, and stays with the patient. A quiet, "All right, now just breathe in and out," until the patient becomes accustomed to the oxygen mask or other device, conserves the patient's energy and helps him to realize that it really does help him to breathe and will not smother him. Seeing prompt, competent, compassionate care given to a loved one gives the family assurance that they are leaving the patient in the hands of people who know enough and care enough to help him, and that whatever happens, they will do their best for him.

The nurse has to be alert for possible complications and their prevention. Because of the danger of thrombophlebitis in patients who are confined to bed, the knee gatch is not raised. A footboard is used to prevent footdrop and to keep the patient from sliding down in bed when the head of the bed is raised. Feet and legs should be maintained in good alignment. Good skin care, along with a foam-rubber pad, an alternating pressure mattress, flotation pad, or sheepskin, helps to prevent decubitus ulcers.

Intake and output are carefully recorded. If the patient has an order for daily weights, this procedure

Table 24-1.
Nursing management of the patient in congestive heart failure

Blood pressure, pulse, and respirations are taken as ordered or q1-2h.
Temperature is taken q4h.
Intake and output are measured.
Intravenous fluids are regulated to avoid rapid infusion.
Weight is measured daily.
The patient's position is changed q2h.
The head of the bed is elevated to a position of comfort (do not raise foot gatch).
Oxygen is administered as ordered.
Any changes are reported immediately.
If oral fluids are allowed, they are given at room temperature.

Table 24-2.
Signs of electrolyte depletion

Signs of Hypokalemia	Signs of Hyponatremia
Muscle cramps	Oliguria, anuria
Muscle weakness	Decreased skin turgor
Cardiac arrhythmias	Dry mucous membranes
Postural hypotension	Hypotension
Apathy, malaise	Tachycardia
Anorexia	Apprehension
Vomiting	
Abdominal distension, paralytic ileus	
Thirst	
Shallow respirations	

Scherer, J. C.: *Introductory Clinical Pharmacology.* Philadelphia, Lippincott, 1975, p. 106.

is performed at the same time daily (before breakfast). Similar clothing or bed clothing should be incorporated each time the patient is weighed.

Rest is very important. The nurse does not fall into the trap of assuming that her patients receive poor care if they do not have a complete bath every day. Rather, she selects aspects of care that are most important at the time. Provision for rest at intervals during care is important.

Careful note is taken of the degree of the ankle edema, the dyspnea or cyanosis, and the quality and rate of both apical and radial pulse. The pulse is checked before digitalis is administered. If signs of digitalis toxicity are present, such as an apical pulse below 60 or above 90 per minute, irregular rhythm, or premature ventricular contractions, the physician should be notified before the drug is given.

It is important to know the predicted time of effect of the diuretic given the patient. Diuretics administered intravenously may initiate diuresis in 5 to 10 minutes, with the peak volume in 30 to 60 minutes. The oral drugs may produce a peak urinary volume in about 2 hours. Sudden diuresis can result in bed wetting or in acute urinary retention. The bedpan or urinal should be offered, and the bladder checked for distention. Urinary frequency and urgency are very tiring, especially on the first day of hospitalization. Female patients should be assisted to get on and off the bedpan; male patients should be checked closely, so that they have an empty urinal when they need it. Patients should be watched for signs of electrolyte depletion (Table 24-2).

Each time the patient's activities are increased, or when supportive therapy is withdrawn, he is observed for any difficulties or problems. New activities are undertaken gradually. The patient's first activity may involve merely taking a few steps to the chair. In addition to checking the pulse, the nurse can choose this time to make the patient's bed, so that someone is nearby if he becomes fatigued and needs to go back to bed.

Oral fluids are given at room temperature as extremely cold fluids and foods can trigger a cardiac arrhythmia. Although this is more likely to occur in patients with a myocardial infarction, some physicians prefer to limit the intake of cold fluids and foods in all cardiac patients during the acute phase of the disease.

Teaching

As soon as the patient recovers from his acute symptoms, the nurse begins to use opportunities for teaching. For instance, when the patient first asks for salt, the nurse explains that many foods in their natural state contain some salt. Later, when the patient feels better, the necessity of limiting the salt intake is explained. Also included in this explanation is a list of foods that are high in sodium. The patient is also cautioned to avoid *all* drugs not prescribed or approved by his physician. This warning is based on the fact that many drugs, including nonprescription drugs, contain sodium.

The patient's limitations should also be explained. For example, he may need to reduce some of his physical activities on a permanent or temporary basis. He will need to know precisely what he can or cannot do. While this explanation is initially given by the physician, it is the nurse who reinforces it.

The patient is also told to weigh himself every morning, always wearing similar clothing. The physician may wish the patient to keep a record of his daily weight and bring this record each office visit. Daily weights are a general indication of the efficacy of medical treatment. If the weight rises, it is possible that the patient is retaining excess fluid.

Diet

Low Sodium Diets. The dietitian can talk with the patient or family member several times about the sodium content of various foods, the kind and the amount of food that can be consumed each day without exceeding the amount of sodium permitted, and the variety of other seasonings that can be used. The nurse can help the patient to understand that foods which contain relatively large amounts of sodium must be eliminated from the diet. Depending on the amount of sodium specified in the doctor's prescription, it may be necessary to use foods containing moderate amounts of sodium in very small amounts. The patient must understand that it is the sodium rather than the salt per se that has to be limited. This distinction will help him understand why he must not take any drugs—prescription or nonprescription—without first consulting his physician. The patient whose sodium intake is restricted cannot, for example, take a teaspoonful or two of sodium bicarbonate to relieve indigestion.

The amount of sodium allowed varies. Patients on very low sodium intake should be watched, especially in hot weather, for symptoms of sodium deficit (hyponatremia). When the patient perspires a great deal, he may need more sodium than his diet provides. If symptoms of hyponatremia appear, the doctor may increase the allowance of sodium.

Many prepared foods have salt added in the process of canning or freezing. The patient should cultivate the habit of reading labels on all prepared foods. Other forms of sodium, such as sodium benzoate, baking powder, and sodium propionate, are contained in many prepared foods.

When the patient asks for a snack between meals, it is easy to forget that the amount of sodium must be considered. Discuss this addition to the daily diet with the dietitian and consider the amount of sodium in the snack as part of the patient's daily allotment. Give only foods known to be virtually free of sodium, such as fresh fruit. The patient should consult his doctor before using any salt substitute, such as those substitutes containing potassium chloride. Excess potassium (hyperkalemia) can cause cardiac arrhythmias. The nurse can recommend the use of other seasonings, such as lemon juice or onion juice.

The nurse can find out the patient's favorite foods in order to help keep as many as possible in his diet. The nurse works with the doctor to clarify the order. ("Just how many grams of sodium may he have, doctor?") She keeps the doctor and the dietitian informed about how the patient is eating and reacting to the diet.

Dietary Potassium. Some patients are instructed to increase their dietary intake of potassium. Foods high in potassium include fresh fruit juices, except apple and cranberry, most whole fruits such as bananas, but only if they are fresh or dried, nuts, high protein foods such as meat or fish, nonstarchy vegetables such as spinach, milk solids, and whole grain cereals. Foods low in potassium include fats, carbohydrates including starchy vegetables, apples and cranberries, and products made from them, and canned fruits.

Drugs

Digitalis preparations are very powerful drugs, and an incorrect dose is a very dangerous one. Read the label very carefully and know the average dose of the particular preparation that is being given. Relatively large doses of these preparations may be given at the beginning of therapy in order to quickly achieve a therapeutic effect. This is called *digitalization.* A daily, smaller dose is then given that is sufficient to maintain therapeutic amounts of digitalis in the body. This is called the *maintenance dose.* Many patients take digitalis preparations for years. It has helped many cardiac patients to control their disease and to live comfortably. Patients especially need to know that they should not discontinue their medication when they feel well, or take more than the prescribed dose when they don't feel well.

Toxic effects can occur from digitalis preparations. They tend to appear gradually. The patient is generally instructed to consult the physician if he experiences sudden loss of appetite for 24 hours, unexplained nausea or vomiting, unusual palpitation or change in pulse, or sudden disturbance in color vision. If early symptoms are noted and reported to the doctor, more serious toxic effects can usually be avoided.

In severe potassium deficiency with digitalis intoxication (hypokalemia) potassium may be given intravenously. The usual rate of administration is 40 mEq. every 8 hours. The maximum rate is 40 mEq. every 2 hours.

Discharge teaching

Discharge teaching is discussed with the physician early in the hospital stay so that the patient and family have the opportunity to ask questions.

Examples of teaching points for a patient with congestive heart failure might be:

- Digitalis preparations are to be taken as ordered by the physician. Any loss of appetite, any nausea, or any vomiting or irregular heart action should be reported to the doctor.

- If approved by the physician, a large glass of orange juice is to be taken every morning to guard against the development of hypokalemia, a complication of diuretic therapy.
- Any recurrence of symptoms is to be reported to the doctor—for example, edema of the ankles, dyspnea, unusual fatigue.

Acute pulmonary edema

Pulmonary edema represents an acute emergency and is often associated with heart disease. The weakening of the left ventricle, which may be caused by such conditions as acute myocardial infarction, arteriosclerotic heart disease, or rapid cardiac arrhythmias, makes it incapable of maintaining sufficient output of blood with each contraction. However, the right ventricle continues to pump blood toward the lungs. The pulmonary capillaries and the alveoli become engorged, because blood continues to flow to the lungs and is not adequately and promptly pumped into the systemic circulation by the left ventricle. Sometimes, the lungs become rapidly filled with fluid. This condition can occur in patients who have congestive heart failure; it may be triggered by some unusual exertion or by slipping down in bed during sleep. (Lying flat may cause edema to settle in the lungs, which are then lower than the rest of the body.) Acute respiratory distress develops. This is termed paroxysmal nocturnal dyspnea.

Acute pulmonary edema can also result from injury to the lung tissue, such as blast injuries, causing many small hemorrhages within the lung, and from conditions in which the drainage of the pulmonary secretions is impaired. For example, chronic pulmonary diseases, such as emphysema, may lead to the obstruction of the respiratory passages when the patient is unable to cough up secretions. Pulmonary edema also may be caused by the inhalation of irritants, such as ammonia.

Patients with acute pulmonary edema experience anxiety, restlessness, sudden dyspnea, wheezing, orthopnea, cough (often productive of pinkish, frothy sputum), cyanosis, and severe apprehension. Respirations sound moist or "gurgling."

The relief of these symptoms is urgent. The patient literally can drown in his own secretions during an attack of acute pulmonary edema. Every effort is made to relieve the congestion in the lungs as quickly as possible.

The doctor's orders may include measures to provide physical and emotional relaxation, to relieve hypoxia, to retard venous return to the heart, and to improve cardiovascular function.

- Provide physical and emotional relaxation.

  Morphine or meperidine (Demerol) is often ordered intravenously to lessen apprehension. Morphine, particularly, seems to help to relieve the attack by depressing higher cerebral centers, thus relieving anxiety and slowing the respiratory rate. In addition, morphine promotes muscular relaxation to reduce the work of breathing. The patient should be permitted to stay in the position most comfortable for him, usually sitting up. Avoid anything that would increase his feeling of breathlessness and choking. Do not pull curtains around his bed or close the window if the patient indicates he wants it open. If it is possible, have someone else talk to the doctor, so that you do not have to leave the patient. If you must leave, tell the patient you will be right back, and be right back.
- Relieve hypoxia and improve ventilation.

  To raise the rate of oxygen diffusion across the fluid barrier of edema in the alveoli, 100 percent oxygen through a positive pressure, nonrebreathing type of mask may be ordered initially. This helps to prevent further engorgement of the lungs with fluid. Later, a nasal catheter, or nasal cannula, may be substituted. Apply the mask quickly, but do not forget a brief word of explanation and reassurance to the patient, who is already afraid of suffocation, and who may be made more so by the sudden application of the mask. Be sure there is a firm seal between the mask and the patient's face, but guard against pressure damage to the patient's skin. Frequent drying of the skin will minimize this risk. Oxygen must always be humidified to prevent the drying of secretions and further impairment to ventilation.

  Aminophylline may be administered intravenously to dilate the bronchi and to make breathing easier, and to lessen pulmonary-capillary transudate.
- Retard venous return to the heart.

  Measures may be taken to decrease the volume of circulating blood, thus helping to relieve the congestion of blood and fluid in the lungs. These measures consist of wet or dry phlebotomy, the use of an intermittent positive pressure ventilator, and the use of morphine. Wet phlebotomy of approximately 500 ml. of blood may be performed, or rotating tourniquets may be used to trap blood in the extremities, so that it is not returned to the already overburdened and congested heart and lungs, a so-called "dry" phlebotomy.

When rotating tourniquets are used, they may be applied clockwise or counterclockwise, provided that they are always rotated in the same direction throughout the treatment. The tourniquet is applied tightly enough to interfere with venous return and not tightly enough to cut off arterial circulation. If a rubber tourniquet is used, check the pulse in the extremity after applying the tourniquet. If the pulse has been obliterated, the tourniquet has been applied too tightly, and it should be loosened. If blood-pressure cuffs are used, inflate each cuff to a point between the patient's systolic and disastolic blood pressure.

The exact procedure to be used varies, and it will be specified by the doctor. Tourniquets may be rotated every 15 minutes, although in some instances the doctor may order more frequent rotation. If 15-minute intervals are used, each extremity will have had the tourniquet on it for 45 minutes and will have been free of the tourniquet 15 minutes (Table 24-3 and Fig. 24-2).

The patient's extremities will become swol-

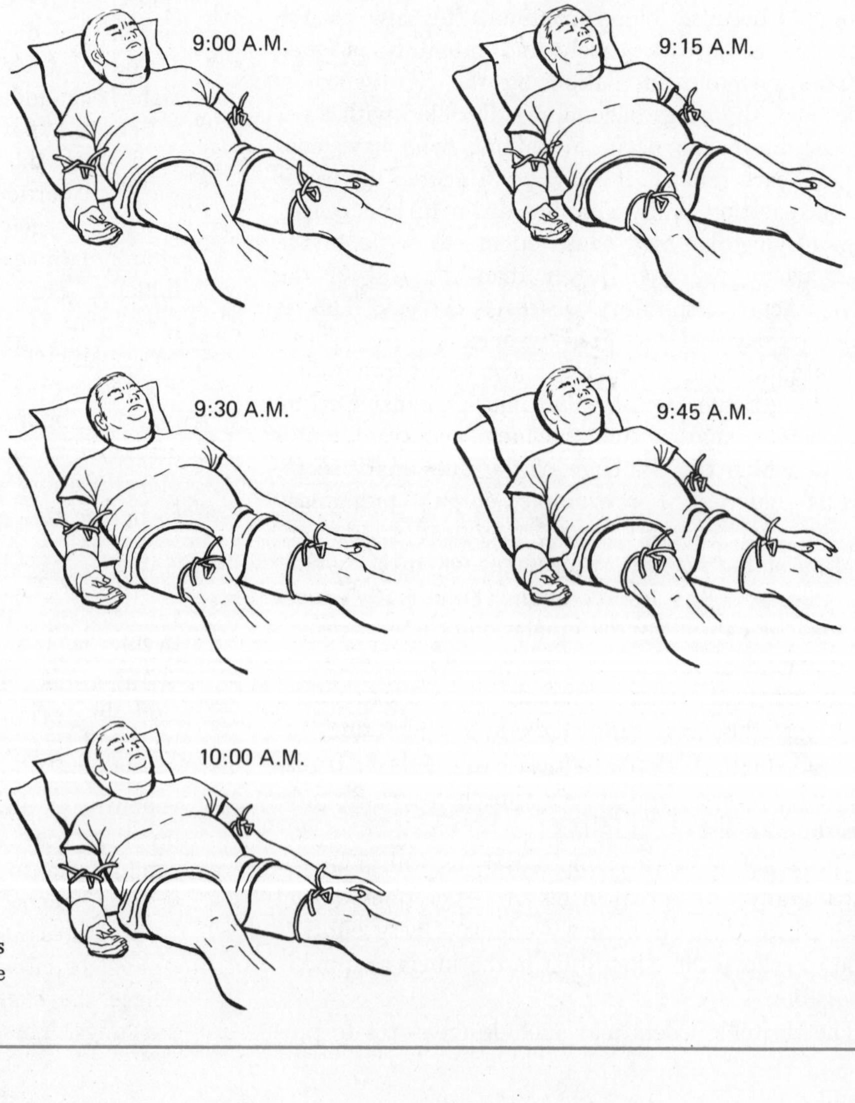

figure 24-2. Rotation of tourniquets at 15-minute intervals. (See Table 24-3.)

Table 24-3.
Plan for rotating tourniquets

Time A.M.	Right Leg	Left Leg	Left Arm	Right Arm
9:00	off	on	on	on
9:15	on	off	on	on
9:30	on	on	off	on
9:45	on	on	on	off
10:00	off	on	on	on

len, mottled, and uncomfortable due to engorgement with venous blood. Explain to the patient that the swelling will disappear when the tourniquets are removed. Check the pulse in the extremity frequently, to be sure that the circulation to the part is adequate.

When the tourniquets are to be removed, follow the same rotation already established and remove one tourniquet every 15 minutes, so that by the end of 45 minutes all tourniquets will have been removed. *Never remove all tourniquets at once.* To remove them all at the same time would cause a sudden increase in the amount of circulating blood, with a return of more blood to the heart and the lungs than they can handle, causing another attack of pulmonary edema. If the extremities do not return promptly to their normal appearance when the tourniquets have been removed, notify the doctor.

Several models of electrically operated automatic rotating tourniquet machines are currently available. The use of such a machine saves nursing time since there is no need to change the velcro-fastened blood pressure cuff-type tourniquets once they are applied. Inflation and deflation time is automatically cycled. The machine is more efficient since it eliminates the variability in technique and cuff pressure which results when more than one person manually applies rubber tourniquets. Human failure resulting from "forgetting" to rotate the tourniquets or not being able to get back to the patient on time is eliminated.

Blood pressure can be taken easily using the pressure gauge on some machines or, on others, by disconnecting an arm cuff from the machine and attaching a sphygmomanometer to it. The same observations relative to arterial circulation and discontinuance of therapy are necessary.

Some physicians advocate mechanical positive pressure breathing (IPBB) during inspiration to reduce venous return to the heart in the treatment of acute pulmonary edema. Normally, the intrathoracic pressure of spontaneous respiration is negative. When this negative pressure is replaced by positive pressure, venous return to the heart is reduced. The doctor determines flow-rate, pressure, and inspiratory/expiratory ratio in order to arrive at an intrathoracic net positive pressure which will impede venous flow. (If the patient is hypotensive, further reduction of venous return to the heart is contraindicated.) IPPB has the additional benefit of assisting ventilation in all lung segments and is an effective means of administering oxygen.

- Improve cardiovascular function.

When the attack of pulmonary edema is due to congestive heart failure, other measures for the treatment of this condition may be begun promptly, if the patient has not already been receiving them. For example, digitalization with a rapid-acting preparation and the injection of a rapid-acting, potent diuretic may be ordered.

General nutritional considerations

- Patients with congestive heart failure are usually placed on sodium-restricted diets. The degree of restriction may depend on the severity of the disease, the patient's response to other forms of therapy, and the presence of edema.
- Patients on diuretic therapy may be required to eat or drink food or fluids high in *potassium.* Examples of such foods are: apricots, bananas, lima beans, liver, and celery. Orange juice is also high in potassium.
- Patients who must restrict the amount of sodium in their diets, or who are on any other type of cardiac diet such as one which limits dietary intake of foods high in fat, should be seen by the dietitian before discharge from the hospital. The patient needs a detailed explanation of: (1) foods allowed, (2) foods to

be avoided, (3) how to read food labels, (4) the various ways sodium and fats can be listed on a food label, and (5) seasonings that may be used in place of salt.

General pharmacological considerations

- Digitalis preparations, which include digitalis, digoxin, digitoxin, and other related glycosides of digitalis, are indicated in the treatment of congestive heart failure. These drugs have the ability to increase the force of contraction of cardiac muscle.
- Digitalis preparations are potent drugs capable of causing various side effects. There is a narrow margin between a full therapeutic effect and drug toxicity. Thus, the patient must be observed for signs of digitalis toxicity not only during the initial period of therapy but throughout the entire hospitalization.
- The signs of digitalis toxicity are: anorexia, nausea, vomiting, epigastric discomfort, diarrhea, abdominal cramps, blurred vision, halos around dark objects, disturbance in green/yellow vision, headache, and change in pulse *rate* and *rhythm*. A patient with digitalis toxicity may have one or more of these signs.
- If signs of digitalis toxicity are noted, they are reported at once and the drug withheld until the patient is seen by his physician.
- Patients receiving digitalis preparations should have an apical-radial rate taken for 1 full minute before the drug is given. (If the patient is on a cardiac monitor this is not necessary.) This method of determination is used during the first few days of therapy or until the patient is digitalized. Once the patient is on maintenance therapy, a radial rate will usually suffice. The drug is not given if the pulse rate is below 60 unless the physician has indicated otherwise. The drug is also withheld if there is a change in cardiac rhythm or there are signs of digitalis toxicity.
- Diuretic therapy is often necessary in patients with congestive heart failure. Patients receiving these drugs should be observed for signs of hyponatremia, hypokalemia, and dehydration.
- For patients taking diuretics, discharge teaching should include the signs and symptoms of electrolyte and water loss and the importance of adhering to the medication schedule prescribed by the physician. Teaching may also include the eating of foods high in potassium.
- Patients receiving emergency drug therapy for acute pulmonary edema must be observed for results of drug therapy and side effects of the drugs administered. Many of the drugs given for this disorder are given by the intravenous route and occasionally in large doses; thus the importance of patient observation. Drugs that may be administered are: morphine, aminophylline, digoxin (or other digitalis preparations) and adrenergic drugs for hypotension.

Bibliography

ANDERSON, L. et al: *Nutrition in Nursing*. Philadelphia, Lippincott, 1972.

ANDREOLI, K. G. et al: *Comprehensive Cardiac Care: A Text for Nurses and Other Health Professionals,* ed. 3. St. Louis, Mosby, 1975.

ARMINGTON, SISTER C. and CREIGHTON, H.: *Nursing of People with Cardiovascular Problems*. Boston, Little, Brown, 1971.

BAXLEY, W. E.: Acute pulmonary edema. Emer. Med. 5:132, July, 1973.

CLARK, N. F.: Pump failure. Nurs. Clin. North Am. 7:529, September, 1972.

CONN, H. F., ed.: *Current Therapy*. Philadelphia, Saunders, 1975.

COSGRIFF, J. H. and ANDERSON, D. L.: *The Practice of Emergency Nursing*. Philadelphia, Lippincott, 1975.

HABAK, P. A. et al: Rotating tourniquets: How effective in left heart failure? (pictorial), Part 1. RN 38: ICU/CCU 1-2+, January, 1975.

HOLVEY, D. N. and TALBOTT, J. H.: *Merck Manual of Diagnosis and Therapy,* ed. 12. Merck, Sharp and Dohme Research Laboratories, 1972.

RAMSEY, M. A., ed.: The failing heart. Nurs. '72, 2:18, October, 1972.

RASMUSSEN, S. et al: The pharmacology and clinical use of digitalis. Cardiovasc. Nurs. 11:23, January/February, 1975.

REDDING, J. S. et al: Management of pulmonary edema (pictorial), AORN J. 21:659, March, 1975.

RODMAN, M. J. and SMITH, D. W.: *Clinical Pharmacology in Nursing*. Philadelphia, Lippincott, 1974.

SANDERSON, R.: *The Cardiac Patient: A Comprehensive Approach*. Philadelphia, Saunders, 1972.

SHAFER, K. N. et al: *Medical-Surgical Nursing,* ed. 6. St. Louis, Mosby, 1975.

SPENCER, R.: Problems of drug therapy in congestive heart failure. RN 35:46, August, 1972.

CHAPTER—25

The patient with inflammatory or valvular disease of the heart

On completion of this chapter the student will:

- **Discuss the etiology, diagnosis, medical treatment, sequellae and nursing management of the patient with rheumatic fever.**
- **Describe prophylactic measures that prevent rheumatic fever in patients with streptococcal infections and the prevention of recurrence of the disease in those with a history of rheumatic fever.**
- **List the serious complications of any valvular disease.**
- **Discuss the etiology, pathology, treatment, and nursing management of patients with bacterial endocarditis.**
- **Contrast the symptoms of acute and chronic pericarditis and describe the treatment of each.**

Patients with cardiac diseases such as rheumatic fever or rheumatic valvular disease, bacterial endocarditis, or pericarditis share certain commonalities. These disorders are inflammatory and often follow infection elsewhere in the body, leaving the patient too weak to cope with additional physical and psychosocial threats. The treatment process is not dramatic but rather slow and tedious. The diseases are frequent among young adults who must forego their usual job, civic, and family and social responsibilities for a long period, sometimes with loss of income. All such diseases carry an uncertain future.

The extent of the damage often is not fully manifest during youth, but may lead to symptoms later in life when the individual experiences additional stressors, such as another illness, childbearing, or the aging process.

Rheumatic fever and rheumatic heart (valvular) disease

Rheumatic fever is usually found most among those between the ages of 5 and 15. It sometimes occurs in late adolescence or young adulthood, particularly in persons with a history of the disease in childhood; it is rare after the age of 25 except when crowded living conditions favor streptococcal infections.

Rheumatic fever often leads to permanent damage to the heart and valves with subsequent chronic valvular heart disease. *Rheumatic heart disease* refers to the cardiac manifestations of rheumatic fever, either in the acute phase or the later stage of chronic damage. In caring for adults we are concerned primarily with rheumatic heart disease. At one time rheumatic heart disease was the commonest form of organic heart disease in persons under 50 in the United States. Between 1944 and 1965, however, the death rate from acute rheumatic fever in the United States showed a decline of 90 percent, primarily due to vigorous treatment with penicillin.

Cause

The precise cause of rheumatic fever is unknown, but it is believed to be related to streptococcal infection. Rheumatic fever is a systemic response found in 3 percent of persons infected with group A hemolytic streptococci. Why three people in every 100 are affected and 97 escape is an unsolved mystery. A previous attack increases the risk of recurrent attacks following streptococcal infection. It often follows such conditions as pharyngitis, tonsillitis and scarlet fever. Some investigators have noted a strong familial tendency, but this is sometimes attributed to the spread of streptococcal infection within a family.

Rheumatic fever is most prevalent during cool, damp weather, and its incidence is greater in the northern sections of the United States than in the South. Such differences may be related to the higher incidence of streptococcal infections during cold, damp weather. Poor living conditions, such as crowding and poor diet, seem to increase the incidence of rheumatic fever by lessening individual resistance to infection and increasing the likelihood of the spread of the streptococcal infection.

Diagnosis

No single diagnostic test proves that a patient has rheumatic fever. The doctor makes the diagnosis after he has carefully evaluated the patient's personal and family history, his symptoms, and certain physical and laboratory findings that are useful in the diagnosis of rheumatic fever. In the last group are the following:

- Subcutaneous nodules. These appear as small round or oval lumps under the skin. Not all patients with rheumatic fever have these nodules. When they occur, they are considered characteristic of the disease.
- Increased sedimentation rate. The rate at which the red blood cells settle to the bottom of a tube is increased in rheumatic fever. The particular usefulness of this test lies in the tendency of the increased sedimentation rate to persist even after other evidences of active disease have subsided. The sedimentation rate is more useful in determining whether the disease is still active than it is in indicating whether the disease is rheumatic fever.
- Leukocytosis and anemia. These are characteristic during an acute rheumatic infection.
- C-reactive protein. This protein substance, which is not normally present in the blood, appears in a variety of infections, including rheumatic fever.
- An increase in antistreptolysin-O titer indicates a recent hemolytic streptococcus infection.
- Other laboratory tests that may be ordered are antihyaluronidase titer, antifibrinolysin titer, and SGOT.
- Abnormal electrocardiogram. During the course of rheumatic fever the ECG frequently shows rhythm disturbances and other cardiac changes and is an aid in assessing the presence and the severity of cardiac damage.
- Abnormal heart sounds. An example is heart murmurs. Murmurs can indicate a change in valve configuration or myocardial dilatation.

Often it is hard for the patient to understand that there is no single definite test for rheumatic fever, and that varied and repeated tests are necessary to establish the diagnosis. The nurse can help the patient and his family by encouraging the continuation of the tests recommended by the doctor. Also, the nurse participates in the explanation of various diagnostic procedures, and sometimes she assists with the collection and the labeling of specimens.

Active rheumatic fever

Symptoms

Rheumatic fever affects the connective tissue in many different areas of the body. Therefore, symptoms often are widely distributed, involving the joints, the heart, and the nervous system. In one patient most of the symptoms may be related to the nervous system, whereas in another patient the inflammation of the joints may be severe. Sometimes, the disease is so mild that it escapes detection, or it is so atypical in its symptoms that many and repeated tests, plus very careful observation of the patient, are necessary to confirm the diagnosis.

The disease may appear 1 to 4 weeks after a streptococcal infection. It may be gradual in onset, with slowly increasing fatigue, anorexia, weight loss, lassitude, and slight fever, or it may begin suddenly with acute swelling and inflammation of one or many joints, moderate fever, malaise, and pallor. Joint symptoms often are described as *migratory polyarthritis*, meaning that the condition moves from one joint to another, eventually involving many joints in the body.

Epistaxis (nosebleed), abdominal pain, a rash resembling giant hives but which does not itch, and subcutaneous nodules may be part of the patient's symptomatology.

Cerebral lesions can be associated with neurological symptoms such as chorea. Chorea occurs in childhood, especially in girls, and it is characterized by uncontrollable, uncoordinated, purposeless movements. These symptoms usually disappear entirely after a period of rest and supportive care. Children who have chorea should be observed carefully for symptoms related to cardiac function.

Pulmonary and pleural lesions can also occur.

The amount of the cardiac involvement is of great concern in rheumatic fever, because the heart can develop permanent deformity as a result of the disease. The involvement of the heart varies from patient to patient. Typically, patients with rheumatic fever have tachycardia out of proportion to the degree of fever. Some experience palpitation associated with rapid heart action. Pain over the heart sometimes occurs. Myocarditis (inflammation of the heart muscle) and pericarditis (inflammation of the sac enclosing the heart) account for most of the cardiac symptoms that occur during the acute phase of the disease. If the involvement of the heart is severe enough, its function will be impaired, and the patient with active rheumatic fever may show symptoms of congestive heart failure or cardiac arrhythmias.

The endocardial involvement consists of inflammation of the endocardium and valve leaflets. Characteristic vegetations (verrucae) appear in the valves. There is edema and inflammation of the valve ring which heals with scar formation. This can seriously deform the delicate valve structures and result later in chronic valvular disease manifested by cardiac enlargement, congestive heart failure, and rhythm disturbances.

As a result of clots or a piece of valve breaking off and entering the general circulation, cerebral emboli or peripheral arterial occlusions can develop.

Treatment

Rest is very important during the active stage of rheumatic fever. The patient is kept in bed. Some physicians allow bathroom privileges if the disease seems mild. If cardiac involvement occurs, it does so within the first 2 weeks of the illness in 80 percent of patients who develop this complication. However, the effects of activity beyond strict bed rest during acute rheumatic fever have not been definitely determined. Most physicians prefer that bed rest be maintained until all signs and symptoms of active disease have subsided. The patient's emotional state is considered, too. If he becomes restless and discontented after many weeks of strict bed rest, the doctor may permit him to be taken to the bathroom once daily in a wheelchair. The chance to get out of bed, carried out in such a way that it entails as little exertion as possible, may boost the patient's morale and help him to comply with the order for extended rest.

Rest is both facilitated and made more difficult by other aspects of treatment. Salicylates and corticosteroids promptly and effectively relieve the symptoms, but they do not cure the underlying disease. The patient feels better, and although the lessening of the joint pain and the fever helps him to rest more comfortably, it also makes him wonder why he needs to rest at all. It is hard for him to understand that feeling well is not necessarily indicative of being well.

Medication. The first principle in the treatment

of active rheumatic fever is the eradication of the Group A beta hemolytic streptococcus. Penicillin is the drug of choice. Erythromycin may be used if the patient is sensitive to penicillin. Throat cultures may be ordered at various times after the onset of treatment to confirm eradication of the organism.

Salicylates are very effective and have been used for many years for the symptomatic relief of rheumatic fever. Usually, fairly large doses are necessary to control the symptoms.

Corticosteroids promptly and effectively relieve the symptoms of rheumatic fever; like salicylates, they do not cure the disease. Their effectiveness in decreasing damage to the heart is being studied. It has been suggested that the prompt administration of these drugs, by decreasing the inflammation, may lessen damage to the heart.

DIET is important in helping the patient to overcome the disease. Because patients with rheumatic fever tend to have poor appetites, frequent small meals may be tolerated better than three large ones. A liberal fluid intake is important. Sodium may be restricted to prevent edema due to corticosteroids, or if the patient develops congestive heart failure.

Nursing management

Skillful nursing management can make the difference between a fretful, restless patient, one who defies the physician's recommendation of rest, and a patient who is able to tolerate the restricted activity.

Here are a few brief reminders of ways in which the nurse can help:

- Smooth, sure, unhurried movement by the nurse prevents additional pain in the patient's swollen, painful joints. The possibility of sudden jerky motions may be lessened through the use of temporary supporting splints or pillow support of the extremities, especially when the patient is turned.
- Unnecessary restrictions should be avoided and those that are necessary should not be carried out in a punitive manner. Most patients with rheumatic fever are young people. They are accustomed to activity, and they need gradually increasing independence.
- The physician should decide what kind of activity and what kind of diversion the patient may have. Reading and television help to pass the time, as do hobbies such as painting.
- The patient must be made to understand the reason for the restriction of activity. If he is a student, he should be encouraged to keep up with his studies, providing the physician permits this.
- All measures for keeping bed patients comfortable should be applied: the extra long back rub; placing his feet in the basin when they are washed; a bottom sheet tucked in to stay smooth all day; attention to details of personal grooming. The patient's gown and his bedding must be dry. If he perspires freely, several changes a day may be needed. Careful massage over bony prominences, and a frequent change of position are helpful.
- The nurse should be prepared for the patient's ups and downs. Any young person who has to curtail so many pleasures and so many of the normal experiences of growing up is bound to become discouraged and angry at times.
- The patient may need help to develop self-discipline and concern for others. A prolonged illness can interfere with the development of these abilities and attitudes, and as a consequence, the patient's relationships with others may suffer.

The nursing care of patients with chronic rheumatic heart disease involves observation for the symptoms of congestive heart failure (dyspnea, cough, orthopnea, edema, fatigue) and for symptoms that might indicate the recurrence of rheumatic infection or any streptococcal infection (fever, sore throat, swollen painful joints, malaise).

Rheumatic heart (valvular) disease

A series of thin but strong valves ensures that the blood, in passing through the heart, does not seep back and reverse its direction of flow. A valve separates the atrium from the ventricle on each side of the heart, preventing blood from passing back into the atrium each time the ventricle contracts. Valves also prevent blood that is pumped into the aorta and the pulmonary artery from flowing back toward the heart. The name of the artery is used to describe its valve; these valves are the *pulmonary* valve and the *aortic* valve.

ENDOCARDITIS (inflammation of the lining of the heart, including the lining of the heart valves) is the type of rheumatic involvement of the heart that leads to permanent scarring and deformity. As an end result of endocarditis, heart valves, particularly the mitral and the aortic valves, become scarred, and function inefficiently. Damage to the valves can be found even after attacks of such mildness that the patient does not recall having had the disease. Often such lesions are detected by the doctor many years later during a routine physical examination. If the deformities of the valves are slight, these patients may continue to be asymptomatic, requiring no treatment and no limitation of their physical activity. If the deformity of the valves is considerable, the patient's heart function may in time become sufficiently impaired that the heart can no longer keep up with the circulatory load, and the patient will develop symptoms of congestive heart failure. These symptoms may appear first when the patient encounters some unusual strain, such as pregnancy, an infection, or unusual physical exertion. Atrial fibrillation is another disorder that may occur in patients with rheumatic heart disease.

Mitral Stenosis. The mitral valve lies between the left atrium and the left ventricle (see Fig. 23-1, p. 312). It has two leaflets. In the healthy heart these open with each pulsation of the atrium to allow the blood to flow from the left atrium into the left ventricle, and then they close as the ventricle fills.

The most common cause of stenosis (narrowing) of the valve is the inflammation and scarring of the leaflets as a result of rheumatic fever. The leaflets stick together and are prevented from opening all the way, as they should. They tend to become progressively thicker. The opening narrows, so that the blood in the atrium does not have time to flow into the ventricle. The atrium cannot then empty to receive a new full load of blood from the pulmonary artery and veins. To compensate, the atrium contracts harder and enlarges. Pressure is exerted backward through the blood vessels of the lungs. Pressure builds up in the pulmonary artery (pulmonary hypertension), which carries blood from the right ventricle to the lungs. Eventually, pressure also increases in the right ventricle. Because it usually takes less force to pump blood through the lungs than through the rest of the body, the walls of the right ventricle are thinner than the walls of the left ventricle. In long-standing mitral stenosis the walls of the right ventricle get thicker. When, through hypertrophy, the muscular walls no longer meet the demands of the increased work caused by the narrowed mitral valve, pressure is passed to the right atrium, and to the entire venous system of the body. The liver and the lungs become congested; edema of the legs appears. Because the ventricles are not receiving a normal amount of blood to pump through the body, the organs are not getting sufficient nourishment. The patient tires easily and becomes dyspneic. He suffers the progressive disability of cardiac failure.

Another symptom of this condition is lowered systolic blood pressure. The patient often appears emaciated. Although he may gain weight due to edema, he has poor appetite, and is chronically tired and listless.

Mitral stenosis is the most common aftermath of rheumatic fever. Two-thirds of all patients with mitral stenosis are females.

Treatment. The symptomatic relief of congestive heart failure is often an important part of the treatment of patients with mitral stenosis. Surgical treatment is possible. However, not all patients with mitral stenosis are suitable candidates for surgery. Usually excluded are those whose condition is so slight that it does not cause symptoms, or so severe or of such long duration that profound changes in the heart and the lungs have occurred. The earlier the operation, the

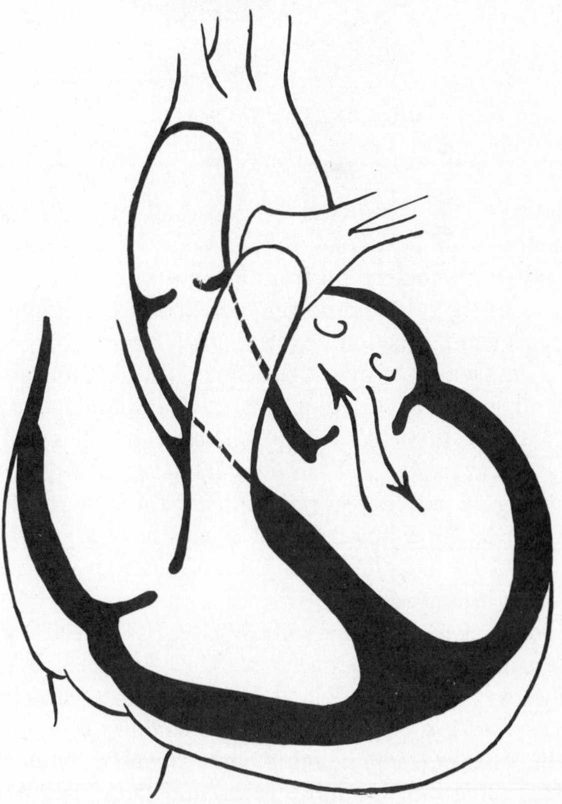

figure 25-1. Mitral insufficiency. The inadequate valve allows blood to return to the left atrium.

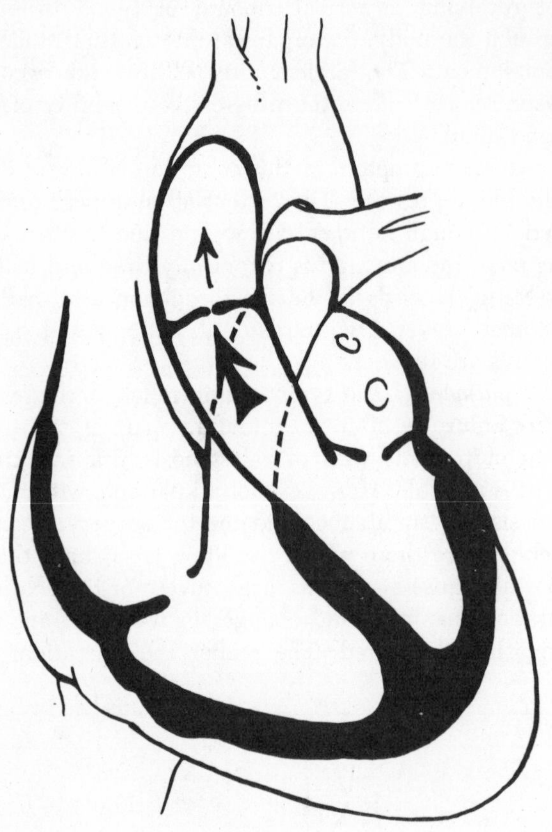

figure 25-2. Aortic stenosis.

greater is the likelihood of cessation of symptoms. Patients who have had one episode of cerebral or peripheral embolization from a piece of clot or valve but are in good condition nonetheless are candidates for surgical correction.

The usual operative treatment of mitral stenosis is commissurotomy, valvuloplasty, or valve replacement.

Mitral Insufficiency. Insufficiency of a valve means that it does not close completely, consequently allowing blood to regurgitate back through it (Fig. 25-1, p. 333). A hole remains when the valve is supposed to be completely closed. Any heart valve may become insufficient.

Insufficiency of the mitral valve is caused most commonly by rheumatic fever. The left ventricle becomes overfilled with blood because each contraction of the ventricle fails to empty the chamber through the aorta. Instead, some blood is pushed back through the mitral valve into the left atrium, and then leaks back into the ventricle. The walls of the ventricle become distended, and the patient may suffer from left ventricular failure.

Among the operations performed to correct mitral insufficiency are suturing loose valves and the implanting of a prosthetic valve to restore unidirectional blood flow.

Aortic Stenosis. The 3-leaf aortic valve is between the aorta and the left ventricle. The cusps may be thickened, stiffened, and eventually calcified after rheumatic fever, although the aortic valve is affected less commonly than the mitral valve (Fig. 25-2). In older patients aortic stenosis may be caused by arteriosclerosis.

When there is stenosis of the aortic valve, the work of the left ventricle is increased. More force is needed to push blood through the narrowed opening. The supply of blood passing through the narrowed valve may be insufficient to nourish the brain and the muscles of the heart. In this instance the patient will present symptoms of dizziness, fainting, and anginal pain from insufficient blood in the coronary arteries. Instead of being full, the radial pulse is weak. It seems to crawl against the finger rather than to hit it. Characteristically, angina and syncope occur before heart failure. Surgery should be considered before the patient reaches the late stages of the disease and suffers dyspnea, a congested liver, and dependent edema, as the left ventricle enlarges, and heart failure occurs.

Aortic Insufficiency. Aortic insufficiency can be caused by rheumatic heart disease, by subacute bacterial endocarditis (especially when it is superimposed on a valve already damaged by rheumatic fever), and by syphilis. When the aortic valve is incompetent and does not close tightly, blood flows through it during systole, dropping back into the ventricle instead of moving forward through the aorta. This backflow results in a decrease in the amount of circulating blood and an increase in the amount of blood in the ventricle. The patient may have a "pistol-shot" pulse, which consists of a pronounced pulsation and then an extraordinarily long interval before the next sharp beat. The left ventricle hypertrophies and goes into failure. The patient is aware of palpitation, a throbbing sensation in the head, and dyspnea related to the failure of the left ventricle.

Aortic insufficiency is the most serious of valvular diseases. It can cause sudden death, even before left ventricular failure, due to ventricular fibrillation.

Prevention of rheumatic fever

Mass throat culture programs and appropriate antibiotic therapy result in a decreased incidence of acute rheumatic fever. The nurse acts as a case finder and also gives leadership to community efforts to prevent the spread of streptococcal infections in throat culture programs underwritten by voluntary or state funds. Financial support is also given by various health agencies for rheumatic fever prophylaxis.

Every possible measure is taken to prevent further streptococcal infections in patients who have had rheumatic fever, because every such infection carries with it the high possibility of recurrence. Each new attack brings the threat of heart damage. Some doctors recommend that the siblings of patients with rheumatic fever also have prophylactic treatment. The prevention of this disease is extremely important, because there is at present no cure. It causes serious heart disease among many young people, often interfering with their plans for a career, marriage, and family life; and sometimes it results in severe illness and death during what should be their most productive years.

Most doctors agree that prophylactic medication should be taken for at least 5 years following the most recent attack of rheumatic fever and be reinstituted prophylactically if the patient undergoes dental surgery or other stressful experiences where the risk of streptococcal infection is increased. Some preventive measures are:

- Avoidance of contact with persons who have upper respiratory infections. Although this cannot always be accomplished, the person who has had rheumatic fever should take reasonable precautions.
- Reporting to the physician any symptoms, such as sore throat and fever, that might indicate a streptococcal infection.
- Regular visits to the doctor's office or clinic for careful cardiac follow-up after the attack is over.

Prognosis and rehabilitation

Many people recover from attacks of rheumatic fever with little or no permanent heart damage. When death occurs, it is usually due to severe cardiac damage resulting in congestive heart failure. The later in life the first attack occurs, the better is the prognosis, since the likelihood of repeated attacks diminishes with age, and recurrence after the age of 25 is very unlikely. It has been estimated that approximately 25 to 50 percent of patients who have had rheumatic fever develop some degree of permanent heart damage.

Although lack of awareness of the symptoms of rheumatic fever may result in insufficient medical care, greater recognition of the problem has led to earlier diagnosis and more thorough treatment for many children whose illness might once have been dismissed as "growing pains." Because of improved diagnosis and treatment, the outlook for people with rheumatic fever is more favorable than it was a generation or two ago. Recurrences of rheumatic fever have decreased markedly due to the prophylactic use of antibiotics among those who have had an attack.

Continuing nursing management involves:

- Education of the patient concerning his abilities and his limitations, in the light of the degree of heart damage, and helping the patient to learn to live within his limitations.
- Teaching the patient what symptoms to watch for and to report, if they should occur (for example, fever, sore throat, ankle edema, fatigue).

The plan of rehabilitation depends on the degree of heart damage and the patient's reaction to his experience with the illness. Those patients who do not develop heart disease after rheumatic fever are encouraged to live active lives. Their only reminder of the disease is the need for preventing further attacks. Because rheumatic fever so frequently results in heart disease, it is hard for some of these patients to believe that their hearts can tolerate normal activity.

Invalidism can become a way of life, especially in illnesses like rheumatic fever and rheumatic heart disease that impose prolonged restrictions on the patient's living. Some patients through fear are unable to break away from this pattern even when their physical condition no longer makes it necessary.

Bacterial endocarditis

Previously, bacterial endocarditis (inflammation of the membrane that covers the heart valves and lines the cavities of the heart) was usually fatal. The recovery of a large proportion of patients through the use of antibiotics is one of the most dramatic achievements of modern medicine.

Bacterial endocarditis may be acute or subacute. The acute condition has a more abrupt onset and a more rapid course, whereas the subacute form has a gradual onset, and the duration of the illness is usually longer. In subacute bacterial endocarditis the infecting organisms also tend to be less virulent. Modern therapy, with emphasis on prompt diagnosis and control of the infection, has so altered the course of the disease that the terms "acute" and "subacute" are now less frequently used to describe this disease.

Incidence

People whose heart valves have been damaged are most vulnerable to bacterial endocarditis. The majority of patients who develop it have had rheumatic fever. The relationship between rheumatic heart disease and bacterial endocarditis is so marked that bacterial endocarditis is often considered a complication of rheumatic heart disease. The condition also occurs in those who have congenital defects of the heart. Although it may occur at any age, bacterial endocarditis is most common during young adulthood and early middle life.

Etiology and pathology

Transient bacteremia occurs fairly commonly in the lives of most people—for example, after tooth extraction. In most instances the organisms are quickly overcome by the body's own defenses. However, patients with damaged heart valves are especially prone to develop bacterial endocarditis after such relatively safe experiences as the pulling of a tooth, cystoscopy, childbirth, or an upper respiratory infection. Organisms that invade the bloodstream after such occurrences tend to settle on damaged heart valves, where they multiply and produce vegetations (verrucae)—clumps of material composed of bacteria, necrotic tissue and fibrin, which accumulate on the affected heart valves. These vegetations are *friable* (easily broken). Pieces of the vegetation tend to break off and travel in the bloodstream. They are then called *emboli*, and they may damage other organs by occluding blood vessels, thus interfering with the organ's blood supply.

A variety of bacteria can cause bacterial endocarditis. *Streptococcus viridans* and *Staphlococcus aureus* are two of the organisms most frequently responsible for this disease.

Today the pattern of bacterial endocarditis is changing. An increased incidence is evident in populations such as those undergoing heart surgery with cardiopulmonary bypass and heroin and morphine addicts who use the intravenous route of injection.

Maintenance of strict surgical asepsis is an essential task of the team involved in insertion of cardiac pacemakers, cardiac catheterization, or cardiac surgery, if the complication of bacterial endocarditis is to be avoided.

Signs and symptoms

Often the disease has an insidious onset, with slight fever, malaise, and fatigue. The patient may ignore the early manifestations of the illness, attributing them to colds or overwork. Early diagnosis and treatment are important. Patients—particularly those with rheumatic or congenital valvular defects—should report promptly to their doctors any fever, malaise, or other symptoms of infection; they may have bacterial endocarditis or a recurrence of rheumatic fever.

As the condition advances, the patient often develops a muddy, sallow complexion, sometimes described as the color of *café au lait*. His fever becomes more marked and more frequent, and often it is accompanied by chills and sweats. Pronounced weakness, anorexia, and weight loss are common. Petechiae, tiny reddish-purple hemorrhagic spots on the skin and mucous membranes, are characteristic. Anemia and slight leukocytosis are common. Heart murmur is present in the vast majority of patients.

Embolism, resulting in the occlusion of a blood vessel by a clump of vegetation that has broken away from the heart valve, may cause sudden disturbances in many organs of the body, such as the brain, kidney, or the lungs.

Clubbing of the fingers and the toes may appear later in the course of the illness. The symptoms of congestive heart failure may appear, either during the active infection or afterward, as a result of the damage to the valves during the illness. Often this development is best described as further damage to the heart valves, because many of the patients already have some valvular damage.

Diagnosis

The physician carefully evaluates the patient's history, particularly regarding rheumatic heart disease or congenital defects and any recent operation, injury, or illness. He orders blood cultures in an attempt to discover the organism circulating in the blood. Often several blood cultures are required before the organism is found. Occasionally, no bacteria are found despite repeated blood cultures, although the patient has a history and symptoms that are typical of the disease. In these instances the diagnosis is made as carefully as possible on the basis of other evidence, but the treatment with antibiotics cannot be as precisely planned when the sensitivity of the organism to various drugs is not known.

Treatment and nursing management

Large doses of the antibiotic to which the organism is sensitive are given. For example, a patient may receive 4 to 20 million units of penicillin daily in divided doses intramuscularly or via a continuous intravenous infusion. Treatment is continued for 3 to 4 weeks.

The drugs must be given on time, exactly as ordered, so that a sufficient amount of the drug will be maintained continuously in the patient's blood. The patient must be observed carefully for any toxic reactions to the drugs, and they should be reported if they occur. Rotating injection sites is essential when so many injections are given, so that one area does not become traumatized from repeated injections. Even the most stoical patients grow weary of repeated injections. The nurse's skill, patience, and encouragement can help patients continue the lifesaving treatment.

If the patient is receiving his antibiotics intravenously, he will have an intravenous line inserted for the duration of treatment to avoid frequent venipunctures. The antibiotic may be given either in divided doses (with a "keep-open" infusion running between doses) or by continuous drip. The venipuncture site should be observed for signs of inflammation; that is, redness and swelling above or below the needle site. The intravenous solution should be checked hourly (or more often, if necessary) for the flow rate or number of drops per minute. The prescribed amount of solution must be infused each hour in order to maintain a therapeutic blood level of the drug administered.

Supportive care is important in helping the patient to overcome the infection. Usually, bed rest is ordered at first. When the patient begins to improve, he is permitted gradually to go to the bathroom and later to be up and about. While the patient is on bed rest, he should be spared exertion and kept as comfortable as possible. Prompt changes of bedding that becomes damp from perspiration are required. The patient should be encouraged to eat, and particularly, to drink fluids; fluids are especially important because of the fever and sweating.

It is important to observe the patient carefully. Note fluctuations in temperature. The temperature is usually taken rectally every 4 hours. Changes in the rate and the quality of the pulse and the appearance of any new symptoms, such as petechiae, should be noted. Signs and symptoms of an embolus are especially significant.

As symptoms subside, the patient will be allowed increased activity. Activities are stopped short of fatigue.

When the antibiotic treatment is discontinued, the patient should be observed for any recurrence of the symptoms. Sometimes, although the infection seems to be conquered, it flares up again after the drugs have been discontinued. Then the treatment has to be resumed and continued until the infection has been eradicated. Nowhere is the need for skilled nursing management more evident than in the care of patients with bacterial endocarditis, who are seriously ill and subject to a variety of complications that may appear without warning.

Prognosis

It has been estimated that about 90 percent of patients with bacterial endocarditis can recover from the infection. Much depends on the sensitivity of the organism to available drugs. The amount of pre-existing heart damage as well as that which results from the attack, also affects the prognosis. Some patients have the infection controlled by drugs, but not before heart damage or embolization has occurred. These patients may be incapacitated by or succumb to congestive heart failure or damage inflicted on the vital organs by emboli.

Prevention

Any patient with damaged heart valves should have antibiotics just before and for a short time after any event that might cause bacteremia, such as a tooth extraction or childbirth. The patient must understand that this precaution is a lifelong necessity. Unfortunately, bacterial endocarditis does not provide immunity to further attacks. Patients who develop the condition are usually those whose previous valvular damage predisposes them to it. They will continue to be vulnerable to this disease as long as they live.

Pericarditis

Covering the myocardium on the outside is a loose fitting inelastic sac known as the *pericardium*. The outermost layer is the fibrous pericardium. The innermost layer, or that adhering to the myocardium, is the visceral layer or epicardium. The pericardial space contains a few drops of pericardial fluid which lessens the friction between the myocardium and the pericardium. Since the pericardium does not stretch, overdilatation of the heart during diastole cannot take place.

Inflammation of the pericardium (pericarditis) can result from infection, trauma, or neoplasms. Blood, excess fluid, or pus can accumulate in the pericardial space and produce partial or complete cardiac tamponade with fall in cardiac output or death. Sections of

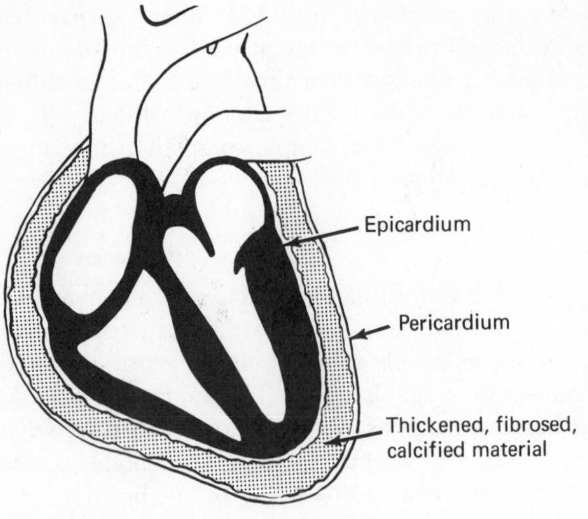

figure 25-3. Pericarditis. Normally, the epicardium and the pericardium slide over each other easily. They are lubricated by a small amount of fluid, which in pericarditis is replaced by thicker material that can cause the surfaces to adhere.

the epicardium and pericardium can adhere and cause chronic constrictive pericarditis (Fig. 25-3).

Acute pericarditis

Pericarditis can be caused by an infection from any organism. For example, tubercle bacilli and streptococci can cause a purulent pericardial exudate. Infection from a virus, pneumonia, or a lung abscess can spread to the pericardium. Myxedema and uremia can produce a nonbacterial, serofibrinous pericarditis. In acute pericarditis there may be sharp pain, aggravated by moving and breathing, due to the rubbing together of the two inflamed surfaces. A pericardial friction rub can usually be heard with a stethoscope and is the most striking sign.

The pain of acute pericarditis is very similar to the pain of acute myocardial infarction—sudden, severe, beginning over the sternum, and radiating to the neck and left arm. However, the pain of the patient with pericarditis is usually increased by rotating the chest or deep breathing and is relieved by sitting up and leaning forward. In contrast, the pain of acute myocardial infarction is not usually influenced by position, movement, or breathing. Acute pericarditis is a disease of the younger age group (15 to 35 years) and is generally preceded by an upper respiratory infection or hay fever.

X-ray films may show dilatation of the heart with pericardial effusion. Serum enzyme changes are confusing in that they are similar to those of acute myocardial infarction.

If there is sufficient fluid in the pericardial space to compress the heart, there may be signs of congestive heart failure and a pulse that is weaker on deep inspiration (*paradoxical pulse*).

Coronary precautions are usually taken until myocardial infarction is ruled out. Treatment depends on the underlying cause. Rest, analgesics, antipyretics, and other supportive treatment are given.

Chronic constrictive pericarditis

Patients may have no symptoms and no disability, even when there is some adherence of the two linings. However, as scar tissue forms in chronic constrictive pericarditis, there is compression of the heart (as there is when fluid is present in the pericardial sac) that prevents the ventricle from filling fully. The cardiac output of blood is decreased, even though the heart rate increases to compensate. The patient tires easily and eventually shows such signs of cardiac failure as hepatomegaly, dyspnea, edema, and distention of the superficial veins, especially of the neck.

Treatment. When there is fluid in the pericardial sac, the surgeon may aspirate it (pericardial paracentesis), or if there is pus in the sac, he may incise the pericardium and insert a drain. A chronic accumulation of fluid may be treated by making a pericardial opening (window), thus allowing the fluid to drain into the pleural space. Constrictive pericarditis is treated surgically by removing the binding pericardium (pericardectomy or decortication) to allow more adequate filling and contraction of the heart chambers.

The surgical nursing management of the patient having pericardectomy is similar to that of other patients undergoing cardiac surgery.

Postpericardiotomy (postcardiotomy) syndrome

A febrile illness with symptoms and signs characteristic of acute pericarditis may develop 1 to 3 weeks after the pericardium has been surgically opened. It is thought to be due to reaction to the presence of fibrin and blood in the pericardial sac. In most patients the episode resolves spontaneously in 1 to 3 weeks. Analgesics and antipyretics may be ordered as well as corticosteroid therapy.

General nutritional considerations

- Patients with rheumatic fever may have anorexia due to the illness or prolonged periods of inactivity. Frequent small feedings may improve the dietary intake.
- A diet low in sodium may be prescribed for patients with rheumatic fever to prevent edema due to corticosteroid therapy or if the patient develops signs of congestive heart failure. A low-sodium diet may prove unpalatable to the young patient and in such cases a consultation with the dietician is needed to provide foods or seasonings that improve the taste of food.

General pharmacological considerations

- Penicillin is the drug of choice in the treatment of rheumatic fever. This drug may be given prophylactically after the disease process has subsided to prevent infection.
- The nurse must be aware of the most common side effects of penicillin: rash, itching, and urticaria. If these or any other symptoms are apparent, the drug must be withheld until the physician has been consulted.
- Salicylates are effective in relieving the fever and joint discomfort of rheumatic fever. Fairly large doses may be necessary and the patient may note symptoms of salicylism (see page 332).

Bibliography

BATES, B.: *A Guide to Physical Examination.* Philadelphia, Lippincott, 1974.

BEESON, P. B. and McDERMOTT, W.: *Textbook of Medicine,* ed. 14. Philadelphia, Saunders, 1975.

BRETT, B.: The prevention of rheumatic fever. Canad. J. Public Health 63:486, November-December, 1972.

BRUNNER, L. S. and SUDDARTH, D. S.: *Textbook of Medical-Surgical Nursing,* ed. 3. Philadelphia, Lippincott, 1975.

BUCHHOLZ, P. K. et al: Understanding the ECG. RN 35:38, February, 1972.

DOYLE, E. F.: Rheumatic fever—a continuing problem. Nurs. Dig. 3:23, January-February, 1975.

FITZGERALD, W. R.: Changing pattern of infective endocarditis. Health 11:31, Winter 74-75.

FRENCH, R. M.: *Guide to Diagnostic Procedures,* ed. 4. New York, McGraw-Hill, 1975.

GOTH, A.: *Medical Pharmacology: Principles and Concepts,* ed. 7. St. Louis, Mosby, 1974.

GUYTON, A.: *Textbook of Medical Physiology,* ed. 4, Philadelphia, Saunders, 1971.

JOHNSON, A.: A continuing threat: Rheumatic fever. Nurs. '74, 4:51, March 1974.

LIKOFF, W.: Differential diagnosis of some common cardiovascular diseases. Hosp. Med. 9:8, June, 1973.

OAKLEY, C. M.: Infective endocarditis. Nurs. Times 70:1150, July 25, 1974.

SCHULTZ, W. L. and MUHA, K.: Penicillins in review. Nurs. Care 8:17, November, 1975.

SILVERMAN, M. E.: Physical signs in infective endocarditis (pictorial). Hosp. Med. 9:94, January, 1973.

TILKIAN, S. M. and CONOVER, M. H.: *Clinical Implications of Laboratory Tests.* St. Louis, Mosby, 1975.

CHAPTER—26

The patient with cardiovascular disease: coronary artery disease; functional heart disease; hypertension

On completion of this chapter the student will:

- **Discuss the pathophysiology of coronary artery disease.**
- **Describe the signs, symptoms, and treatment of angina pectoris.**
- **Discuss the drug therapy instituted for angina pectoris and how drugs relieve symptoms of the disease.**
- **Define hypertension and discuss the terminology used to describe it.**
- **Discuss the physiological control of arterial pressure.**
- **Define the criteria used to diagnose hypertension.**
- **Describe the general treatment of hypertension.**
- **Discuss the rehabilitation of the patient with heart disease.**

Coronary artery disease

Coronary circulation

The myocardium has its own blood supply through a system of coronary arteries (Fig. 26-1). Blood flows through these vessels and through branches over the outer surface of the heart, then

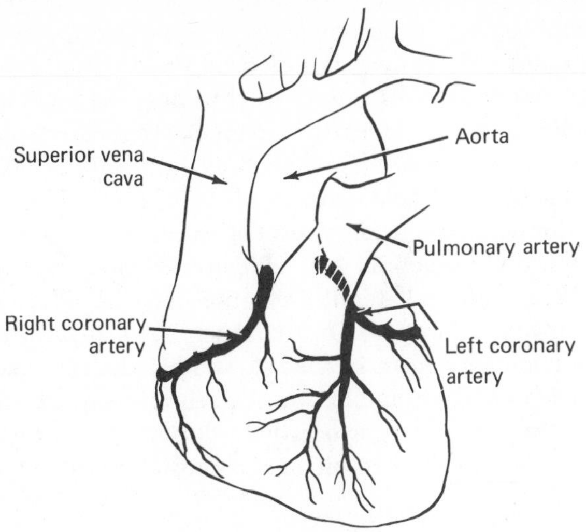

figure 26-1. Anterior view of the heart, showing the right and left coronary arteries that supply the myocardium with blood.

into smaller arteries and capillaries in the cardiac muscle and finally back to the systemic circulation through the coronary veins which empty into the coronary sinus in the right atrium.

Usually there are two main coronary arteries, a right and left, and these originate from the aorta immediately above the aortic valve. Thus the coronary arteries get the first supply of the rich, oxygenated blood leaving the left ventricle. The myocardium is nourished with very little overlap of vessels from one region to another. If a coronary artery is acutely blocked, few other vessels can take over the blood supply to the area served by the blocked artery and the viability of the myocardial tissue is threatened. During the course of slowly advancing atherosclerotic disease of the coronary arteries, or with time, after an acute coronary occlusion, preexisting anastomotic channels open up and grow into the involved area. In the person with coronary heart disease the rate of development and the extent of this new collateral circulation is of critical importance in the survival and viability of myocardial tissue.

Hypoxia, or diminished oxygen supply to cells, is one of the best stimulants to myocardial blood supply. Thus the person with slowly progressive coronary atherosclerosis may have developed some collateral vessels over the course of time which may hold him in good stead in the event of a sudden occlusion of a major vessel. However, the young man who never had the need or opportunity to develop collaterals has a greater chance of dying instantly following a coronary occlusion due to the sequelae of overwhelming oxygen lack to a critical portion of the myocardium.

Like other arteries in the body, the coronary arteries may develop degenerative changes or disease. The pathologic change most responsible for coronary artery disease is atherosclerosis—the gradual deposition of substances, such as lipids and calcium, within the walls of the arteries, making them narrower. Cholesterol is one of the lipid substances believed to be implicated. The lipid deposits are often called *plaques*. Coronary artery disease is more common among people over 50, but it may occur in younger people. A familial tendency toward early development of the condition has been noted. During early middle life men are affected much more frequently than women.

At rest, normal myocardial blood flow may be maintained despite considerable coronary artery narrowing; however, the ability to increase this flow sufficiently during exercise in order to meet the increased metabolic needs of the heart may be markedly impaired. Beyond the narrowed segment, the vessels supplied by the artery dilate. Because of this vasodilation and the development of a good collateral circulation, people with significant coronary atherosclerosis may be fairly asymptomatic and their disease may go unrecognized during their lifetime, particularly if they lead a sedentary existence. During exercise or emotional stress with increased cardiac workload, however, the normal coronary arterial vasodilation which usually allows myocardial blood flow to increase proportionately can no longer occur, since the local capillary bed is already in a maximally dilated state. Under these circumstances the myocardial demand for oxygen and metabolic nutrients exceeds the ability of the coronary circulation to supply them, and clinical manifestations of coronary heart disease such as chest pain of cardiac origin (angina pectoris) may then ensue.

Epidemiology

Approximately 600,000 people die each year from heart disease, the leading cause of death in America. Many of these deaths are premature in the sense that the victims are young or middle-aged adults with basically sound myocardiums. For each fatality, there are two nonfatal but disabling events. The disease is most serious because its ravages affect the prime productive years of life. The patient, his family, and society as a whole suffer from the loss of productivity.

Coronary artery disease is thought to be due to

multiple causative factors rather than to a single cause. Considerable study is being directed toward the discovery of measures to diagnose coronary artery disease before an acute myocardial infarction occurs and to develop ways of decreasing, or at least arresting, the process of atherosclerosis before damage occurs to the muscle of the heart.

Factors which when present are thought to increase the risk of coronary artery disease are:

- Age.
- Sex. (The incidence of coronary artery disease in women rises after the menopause and becomes similar to that among men.)
- Family history of coronary disease.
- Hypertension.
- Rise in serum cholesterol and triglyceride levels.
- Obesity.
- Cigarette smoking.
- Lack of physical activity.
- Personality-behavior patterns.
- Emotionally stressful situations.
- Other diseases, such as gout and diabetes mellitus.

A number of pamphlets explaining risk factors for the lay public, as well as for the professional, are available from the local affiliates of the American Heart Association.

Pathophysiology

The symptoms of coronary artery disease result from an insufficient supply of blood to the myocardium. Like other muscles, the myocardium requires more blood when it works hardest—as is the case during physical exertion or emotional stress. Blood supply through narrowed arteries may be sufficient for a body that is at rest, but not adequate for some of the more strenuous activities of daily living.

If the normal vessels or collateral circulation is not adequate for the needs of the heart during exertion, symptoms of *myocardial ischemia* develop.

Coronary occlusion, or the closing of an already narrowed coronary artery, can occur from a variety of mechanisms. Usually a clot lodges in the vessel. This is called a *coronary thrombosis.* Occlusion can also result from a gradually increasing build-up of atherosclerotic plaques. A sudden loss of blood supply to a portion of the myocardium from an occluded coronary artery often leads to necrosis (death) of that portion of the muscle of the heart. The area of necrotic tissue is called a *myocardial infarction.* This condition is usually accompanied by persistent, severe pain and clinical evidence of dead heart tissue. *Coronary insufficiency* is a term used to describe a clinical condition in which cardiac pain is frequently more severe than typical angina pectoris, but death of heart muscle does not take place.

Coronary occlusion does not necessarily result in myocardial infraction. A small coronary vessel may be occluded, but collateral circulation may be adequate to prevent infarction. On the other hand, myocardial infarction may occur in conditions other than coronary occlusion; for example, drastic curtailment of the blood supply to the myocardium during shock or general anesthesia can result in myocardial infarction.

Angina pectoris

The chief symptom of myocardial ischemia is pain. When ischemia and the resulting pain are fleeting, as is often the case during periods of stress when the blood supply is briefly inadequate for the heart's increased needs, the condition is called *angina pectoris.*

Characteristics. Attacks of angina pectoris are characterized by sudden chest pain or pressure, which may be most severe over the heart under the sternum (substernal). Sometimes, the pain radiates to the shoulders and arms, especially on the left side, or to the jaw, neck, or teeth. Some patients may deny that they have "pain," but will describe other sensations such as tightening in the chest, a squeezing, choking feeling in the upper chest or throat, indigestion, or burning in the epigastric region.

The patient may experience dyspnea, pallor, sweating, and faintness. Although the intensity of the pain and the apprehension that it arouses may make minutes seem like hours, the attack usually lasts less than five minutes. Sometimes, the patient seems to "freeze" —the pain makes him suddenly stop whatever he is doing, and he waits, tense and motionless, for it to subside. The attacks characteristically occur during periods of physical or emotional stress. Sometimes, a particular activity almost invariably brings on an attack. For one patient this might be the morning walk to his train; for another, an argument with his wife.

In some patients the severe pain comes without any apparent relation to meals, activity, rest, excitement, or anything that is under patient's control. These patients are prone to a particularly helpless feeling, because there seems to be little that they can do to lessen the frequency of the attacks.

The pain usually subsides as soon as the patient rests, thus lessening the need of the heart for blood. Most patients quickly discover this, and they need no further urging to stop their activity. Occasionally, a patient may feel that if he just ignores it and refuses to "give in to it," the pain will disappear. The pain is a warning that the myocardium is not receiving enough blood.

Heeding the warning may help the patient to avoid serious illness or even sudden death. The possibility of the sudden death of patients who have angina pectoris is very real. The underlying problem of atherosclerosis and diminished circulation makes the heart especially vulnerable to serious arrhythmias and myocardial infarction which may cause sudden death.

The patient need not lie down to rest. In fact, lying down often increases his sensations of breathlessness. Merely stopping the activity and standing or, if it is possible, sitting quietly for a few minutes usually suffices. Some patients with angina learn to cease their activity quite inconspicuously—for example, by pausing in a walk and appearing to look in a store window or by merely sitting down quietly and waiting for the attack to subside. If you are with a patient who often has had attacks in the past, take your cues from him. Help him to find a place to rest, locate any medication that the doctor has prescribed, and stay quietly and calmly with him, assuring him by your presence and manner that the attack soon will be over. If the pain does not subside within 10 to 15 minutes, keep the patient at rest and call his doctor.

Treatment

Drugs. Nitroglycerin is often used to relieve attacks that do not disappear quickly with rest. This drug is also used to prevent anginal attacks and is given sublingually. The tablets are designed to dissolve quickly under the patient's tongue. Nitroglycerin relieves the pain within 2 or 3 minutes. The duration of effect is also brief, usually about half an hour. Sometimes nitroglycerin may cause a throbbing headache, flushing, and nausea; usually these side effects can be minimized by decreasing the dose. A patient who is not accustomed to taking nitroglycerin should remain seated for a few minutes after taking the medication since some people experience a feeling of faintness. If they take the drug while they are seated, fainting and injury due to falls can be prevented.

When a patient is about to undertake an activity that usually causes anginal pain, taking a nitroglycerin tablet a few minutes beforehand often will prevent the attack. Nitroglycerin is a safe drug; many patients take it for years without ill effect. Other drugs that may be used in the treatment of anginal attacks are dipyridamole (Persantine), erythrityl tetranitrate (Cardilate), and isosorbide (Isordil).

Surgery. Surgical attempts to correct the pathology caused by the diseases of the blood vessels that serve the muscle of the heart have been directed mainly toward improving vascularization, because the basic problem of coronary artery disease is insufficient blood supply to the muscle of the heart. Two techniques are used: the saphenous vein coronary artery bypass and the internal mammary artery bypass graft. In both procedures a blood vessel is used to bypass the diseased portion of a coronary artery.

Daily Activities. Often the doctor advises the patient to stop smoking, because of the association of smoking with the increased risk of coronary artery disease.

Patients with angina are advised to eat small meals rather than large ones, as large meals increase cardiac output and so may precipitate attacks of angina. Regular exercise, such as walking out of doors, is often beneficial in promoting collateral coronary circulation, thus lessening the frequency and the severity of attacks. Overweight patients usually benefit from weight reduction.

Many patients continue to live active, productive lives despite attacks of angina pectoris. Vasodilators and careful regulation of activity may decrease the frequency and severity of the attacks. For instance, the patient who has attacks of angina every morning while he is walking to the railroad station may find that leaving the house earlier, walking more slowly, and taking a nitroglycerin tablet will prevent the attack.

Some patients find that their symptoms remain the same for years. In others the atherosclerosis advances rapidly, and anginal attacks become more frequent and severe despite treatment. These patients are crippled by such severe interference with blood supply to the heart that everyday activities must be curtailed.

The patient with angina faces the problem of finding his level of tolerance for activity and then learning to live within that level. Data obtained from the patient's performance on various tests in a cardiac work evaluation clinic are most helpful to the physician.

The patient also has to learn to live with the ever-present possibility of an attack. For some patients the fear aroused by the attack is worse than the pain. Some feel each time that an attack comes, "Well, this is it." Some react by being more angry at the necessary curtailment of their activity than afraid. All who care for the patient must strive to relieve and, if possible, to prevent the symptoms. They will need to help the patient to strike a reasonable compromise with his condition: to avoid the one extreme of giving up all activity and allowing his entire life to revolve around the possibility of an attack and the other extreme of refusing to acknowledge that his heart places some definite restrictions on the amount of exertion that he can undertake safely. Because the prognosis is so variable—the patient may live for years, or he may die suddenly because of the poor circulation to his heart—he is encouraged to live each day as it comes, to take reasonable precautions, and to continue with his activities, provided that they do not precipitate attacks of angina.

Functional heart disease

Anxiety can produce a variety of physical discomforts. Symptoms associated with heart disease also can be produced by anxiety, and they are referred to as functional heart disease.

Careful examination is essential to rule out organic heart disease and to assure the patient that his heart is normal. Regular, complete physical examinations are especially important. Because the patient is known to have had a functional disturbance, early symptoms of organic disease may be ignored or attributed to the functional disorder.

The treatment of functional heart disease involves:

- Carefully evaluating the factors, both in the patient's personality and in the environment, that seem to be related to the attacks.
- Providing symptomatic relief while the underlying causes of the condition are investigated. In functional heart disease, relief might be obtained by a vacation or by the use of sedatives or tranquilizers.
- Gradually helping the patient to understand that his symptoms may be due to anxiety and that treatment involves helping him to recognize and to deal with his emotional problems, and sometimes modifying his environment.

New and taxing situations often provoke symptoms, such as dyspnea, fatigue, and chest pain. Treatment involves a gradual and lifelong process of reeducation, in which the patient is helped by his doctor and, ideally, by his family, his employer, and his friends. Referral to a psychiatrist may be necessary.

The patient with hypertension

The term *hypertension* may be used in a general sense to describe any condition of elevated tension or tonus and, as such, is a sign. However, it commonly refers to a disease entity characterized by sustained elevation of arterial pressure. The systolic, diastolic, and mean arterial pressure may be elevated.

The lack of certainty about the future is a condition of life—particularly so for patients with hypertension, in which the development of complications is to some extent unpredictable. Hypertension hastens the onset of atherosclerotic coronary and cerebrovascular disease. The patient may be fortunate and live comfortably for many years, or he may be less fortunate and suffer a cerebrovascular accident or cardiac failure. In either case he and his family may need nursing help in living each day as fully and as hopefully as possible, avoiding, on the one hand, the extremes of ignoring the illness and failing to follow treatment and, on the other hand, dwelling on its possible consequences to the point that there is no joy in living.

Arterial blood pressure

Systolic blood pressure is determined by the rate and volume of ventricular ejection and the ability of the aorta to distend. Normally the walls of the aorta are elastic and yield to the volume of blood which bursts into it on ventricular contraction. In older persons with a rigid, atherosclerotic aorta, however, systolic blood pressure may be quite elevated due to loss of this elasticity. Systolic hypertension is a response to change in central hemodynamics.

Diastolic blood pressure is the pressure recorded during the period of ventricular relaxation. It depends on the peripheral resistance and the diastolic filling interval. If arterioles are constricted, blood will have to be at an increased pressure to flow through the constriction. On the other hand, if the arterioles are wide open, then there will be brisk blood flow and diastolic pressure will fall rapidly. Diastolic hypertension is a response to change in peripheral hemodynamics.

The mean arterial pressure is the average pressure tending to push blood through the system's circulation. It is usually slightly less than the average of the systolic and diastolic pressures, however, since arterial pressure is nearer to diastolic level during the greater portion of the pulse cycle. Mean arterial pressure is important from the point of view of tissue blood flow since it takes into account systemic resistance, blood flow, and blood pressure. A high mean arterial pressure can be produced by a high systolic pressure and a normal diastolic pressure, or a normal systolic pressure and an elevated diastolic pressure, or when both pressures are elevated.

PULSE PRESSURE is the difference between the systolic and diastolic pressures. The magnitude of the pulse pressure largely determines the forcefulness and volume of the radial pulse felt at the wrist. Factors which *increase* the systolic pressure, such as a rigid, atherosclerotic aorta, or factors which decrease the diastolic pressure, such as a slow heart rate, will increase the pulse pressure. A strong bounding pulse reflects a wide pulse pressure.

Factors which *decrease* the systolic pressure and increase the diastolic pressure will decrease the pulse pressure. A rapid, weak, and thready pulse reflects a decreased or narrowed pulse pressure. This is the case in shock.

PHYSIOLOGICAL CONTROL OF ARTERIAL PRESSURE

Arterial pressure is regulated by the autonomic nervous system, the kidneys, and the endocrine glands. Normal blood pressure for adults ranges from about 100/60 to 140/90. Although a progressive increase in blood pressure with age has been frequently noted in the United States, this is not invariably true. The reasons for the changes in blood pressure in advancing age are not fully understood.

Blood pressure normally fluctuates with changes in posture, exercise, and emotion. It is lowest when an individual is sleeping, slightly higher when he is awake but lying down, higher still when he is sitting up, and elevated even further when he is standing. Exercise and emotional stress cause elevation of blood pressure. These normal fluctuations show the importance of measuring blood pressure under similar conditions. For example, the patient's blood pressure should not be taken before he has been out of bed one morning, and the next morning while he is sitting in a chair immediately after he has taken a shower. The nursing care plan should designate the circumstances for taking the patient's blood pressure so that conditions are most nearly duplicated.

HYPERTENSIVE DISEASE

A person having a sustained systolic pressure of 150 mm. Hg or above and a sustained diastolic pressure of 90 mm. Hg or above is usually considered hypertensive. Hypertension is a serious condition because it increases the workload of the heart and causes damage to the arteries by excessive pressure brought about by increased resistance of the arterioles to the flow of blood. Congestive heart failure, myocardial infarction, stroke, and renal failure are serious sequelae of hypertension.

When cardiac abnormality (such as electrocardiographic or x-ray evidence of enlargement of the left ventricle) is present with the elevated blood pressure, the term *hypertensive heart disease* is used. When extracardiac vascular damage is present without heart involvement, the term *hypertensive vascular disease* is used. When both heart and extracardiac pathology are present with hypertension, the appropriate term is *hypertensive cardiovascular disease.*

Hypertension is divided into two main categories: primary (or essential) hypertension and secondary hypertension.. The cause of *primary hypertension* is unknown. About 90 percent of hypertensive patients have the primary or essential type.

Secondary hypertension is a term used to describe a variety of conditions in which elevation of blood pressure is secondary to some known cause. Pheochromocytoma (a tumor of the adrenal gland) is an example of a condition causing secondary hypertension. The condition is corrected by the removal of the tumor. The phentolamine (Regitine) test, histamine test, and determination of catecholamines in the urine or blood are diagnostic aids.

Secondary hypertension is also associated with such conditions as toxemia of pregnancy, increased intracranial pressure, congenital blood vessel and heart malformations, and diseases of the kidney such as glomerulonephritis, pyelonephritis, and polycystic disease. Only 10 percent of persons with hypertension are estimated to have the secondary type.

Secondary hypertension may be treated with drugs, diet, and sodium restriction, but when possible the cause of the hypertension is removed. For example, a patient who has a pheochromocytoma may be treated with drugs until such time as the tumor can be removed.

PRIMARY (ESSENTIAL) HYPERTENSION

Primary hypertension is characterized by sustained elevation of the diastolic pressure. A diastolic pressure of 90 mm. Hg or greater is generally accepted as a cut-off point for diagnosis.

The term *malignant hypertension* is used to describe the condition when it has an abrupt onset and is followed rapidly by severe symptoms and complications. The prognosis is poor. Most untreated patients live only a few months to 1 or 2 years. Death is frequently caused by damage to heart, brain, or kidneys, resulting from the very high blood pressure which may rise rapidly to the range of 250/150.

SYMPTOMS. The onset is very gradual; usually, hypertension is first discovered during a routine physical examination. Because of the insidious onset, it is hard to say when the disease begins. Persons in their 30's and 40's may be discovered to have a sustained elevation in blood pressure without any symptoms. Often the condition is present for 10 or 15 years before the patient experiences any discomfort or complications.

One patient may experience no discomfort, whereas another with a similar blood pressure reading may complain of headache, dizziness, fatigue, insomnia, and nervousness. Headache is often described as throbbing or pounding. The person may have nosebleeds (epistaxis), blurring of vision, or spots before the eyes. Angina pectoris or shortness of breath may be the first clue to hypertensive heart disease.

Hypertensive disease, unfortunately, may not be diagnosed until the patient becomes ill from its complications. The heart may enlarge, and eventually the patient may develop congestive heart failure. Many of the complications arise from hemorrhage or occlusion of blood vessels supplying important organs. The atherosclerotic process is increased by hypertension. Hemorrhage from the tiny arteries in the retina may cause marked visual disturbance or blindness. Cerebrovascular accident may result from hemorrhage or occlusion of a blood vessel in the brain. Myocardial infarction may result from occlusion of a branch of a coronary artery. Impaired circulation to the kidney is believed to be related to the frequency of degenerative kidney disease among hypertensive patients.

THEORIES ABOUT ETIOLOGY. Among the many theories concerning the cause of primary hypertension are:

- *Heredity.* Many investigators have noted a strong familial tendency toward the development of primary hypertension.
- *Fluid-Electrolyte Metabolism.* A disturbed relationship among salt intake, body fluid-electrolyte metabolism, and renal-adrenal function has been observed in many studies, but the results are inconclusive.
- *Emotional Stress.* Patients with hypertension are sometimes described as having particular difficulty expressing and dealing with their aggressive impulses. Although they are outwardly calm and composed, inwardly they may be in a turmoil.
- *Obesity.* It has been noted that overweight persons have a higher incidence of hypertension than those of normal weight.

INCIDENCE. Hypertension is presently estimated to affect approximately 10 percent of the adult population. There is a markedly higher proportionate incidence among blacks than whites. The incidence of hypertension is also higher in those subjected to emotional stress.

PREVENTION. Despite the lack of knowledge concerning the etiology of primary (essential) hypertension, the information available from current epidemiologic studies affords a useful basis for its prevention. Factors that increase the risk of hypertensive disease are:

- Race.
- Obesity.
- Positive family history.
- Blood pressure lability in young adulthood.
- Family and/or personal history of diabetes mellitus.

Measures to decrease the risk in susceptible populations may help to forestall the development of symptoms or curtail advancement of the disease.

People with a family history of hypertension or those who have shown transient elevations of blood pressure (often considered to be indicative of a tendency to the disease) may be helped by:

- Having a periodic health examination at least annually.
- Correcting obesity and maintaining efforts to remain lean and trim through a nutritious diet and physical exercise.
- Moderating salt intake—about 5 Gm. per day instead of 15 to 20 Gm.
- Learning to deal more effectively with problems at work, at home, or elsewhere. Some people may need professional assistance. If, for some reason, the patient doesn't learn to cope with situations causing stress, it may become necessary for him to avoid certain stress-producing situations.
- Improving general health habits, if the patient has been taking them lightly. Plenty of sleep, rest and relaxation may prove to be a tremendous help in controlling the condition.

Treatment and nursing management

Many forms of treatment are available that often help to lower the blood pressure and to prevent, or at least to delay, discomfort and complications.

The objective of medical care is sustained nutritional-hygienic-pharmacological management in order to prevent major complications. For example, weight reduction and moderate salt restriction suffice to lower blood pressure in a significant number of patients, although the reason is not clear.

Drugs. Drugs do not counteract the cause of the pressure elevation. Rather, they relax constricted arterioles so that the high arterial peripheral resistance is reduced. The doctor prescribes the drug which will keep the pressure at a near normal level. Combinations of drugs may be used. The more potent drugs have more serious side effects and are reserved for patients with severe, sustained hypertension.

Nursing Implications. When hypotensive drugs are administered, observe the patient carefully for side effects, and promptly report them if they occur. Since some drugs may cause postural hypotension, the patient may feel weak, faint, or dizzy when he changes position. To lessen this discomfort he should be instructed to rise from a sitting or lying position slowly. When he arises in the morning, he first should sit on the edge of the bed a few moments and then stand. Teach him to sit or, preferably, to lie down promptly if he feels faint. Getting off his feet will help the feeling to subside, as well as prevent injury from fainting and falling.

Some patients, especially those who are receiving very potent hypotensive drugs, are taught by the nurse or physician to record their own blood pressure, usually sitting and standing, while they are at home. A family member may be taught to take the patient's blood pressure. Then therapy can be planned and adjusted according to multiple blood pressure recordings made in the patient's usual surroundings. Make sure that the patient is in the desired position when you are taking the blood pressure. For instance, some doctors will ask you to check it each morning before the patient arises; others will ask you to take it with the patient standing.

Often the patient seeks repeated reassurance and explanation from the nurse. Find out what the doctor has told the patient about his particular condition, so that you can be as helpful to the patient as possible. Avoid the pitfalls of giving your patient information for which he is not prepared or for withholding information that he has long considered necessary for self-care.

For example, a patient who has been admitted for diagnosis and who asks you his blood pressure, should not be told, "It's 160/120." Such information, in the absence of a definite diagnosis and an explanation from his doctor, could be very upsetting to him. On the other hand, a patient who has had the condition for years and who has been taking and recording his own blood pressure at home may be justifiably irritated if you refuse to tell him his blood pressure reading. There is no substitute for knowing what the doctor has told the patient about his condition.

When the patient learns that he has hypertension, he needs a great deal of explanation and reassurance concerning its possible consequences. Almost everyone has heard of people who have had strokes or heart attacks that were attributed to high blood pressure. Often the patient's first thought is that such a catastrophe is about to befall him. The doctor usually helps the patient to understand the course of the disease, and he explains how the patient can help himself.

Working with hypertensive patients gives the nurse an opportunity to participate in long-term care that may help the patient to live longer and more comfortably. This care places a premium on the nurse's ability to teach, to listen, and to guide the patient in following his treatment. The treatment in a sense becomes a way of life for the patient. It continues for years, with gradual adaptations, according to the patient's condition.

Nursing Management of the Patient with Secondary Hypertension. Nursing management is essentially the same as for the patient with essential hypertension but may also include preparing the patient for surgery (if surgery is indicated as part of the treatment) or for extensive medical treatment such as renal dialysis.

Rehabilitation of patients with heart disease

The rehabilitation of the cardiac patient presents some particular problems and challenges. Heart disease is not an obvious disability. In some ways this aspect helps the patient to resume his previous relationships and activities; on the other hand, it may make it harder for others to recognize his limitations.

Specific, knowledgeable advice helps the patient guide himself back to health in an orderly fashion. To return to his job and recreation successfully, he and the physician, nurse, family, employer, and others need to know what the goals are each step of the way. If the patient understands the goals, and they are his goals, and if he receives guidance in achieving them, he is likely to have a high level of motivation. When family and health team members are more certain about the plan of rehabilitation, they are less apt to advise the patient to restrict his activities unnecessarily. This lessens the tension and worry which sometimes can be far worse than the sickness and it also can help promote more positive relationships among the patient, family, and health team.

All who care for the patient—doctors and nurses, as well as family members—must guard against the insidious temptation to protect themselves by overprotecting the patient. They may have a tendency to assume total responsibility for anything that may happen to the patient, forgetting that there are many unpredictable events over which human beings have no control. For the cardiac patient, rehabilitation means evaluating how much and what kind of activity the patient's heart will allow him to do and helping him to live as fully and contentedly as possible within these limitations.

Helping the cardiac patient extend his physical independence benefits him emotionally and socially as well. The earlier physical rehabilitation is initiated, the less likely is the patient to develop satisfaction in the secondary gains of illness such as overdependence or disability income benefits.

Physical rehabilitation of the cardiac is concerned with:

- Achieving maximal physical capacity through a program of physical training and conditioning. This is especially applicable to those patients with coronary artery disease.
- Balancing the energy costs of the activities the patient will engage in with his energy capacity.
- Decreasing the energy cost of various activities so that he can negotiate the physical environment in which he functions; for example, reorganizing the cardiac homemaker's kitchen so that energy expenditure can be minimized.

Some overall points in rehabilitation

For many cardiacs, especially those men with atherosclerotic coronary artery disease, the concept of cardiac rehabilitation—returning to as near normal as possible—may well mean doing more physically after a "heart attack" than before. Lack of regular physical exercise could have been one of the major factors leading to the illness. Exercise is of extreme importance in reconditioning the heart muscle. Its efficiency improves just as any other muscle which is made to work harder. Exercise is prescribed on a regular basis with gradually increasing loads. The danger is to move ahead too rapidly with the possibility of overload. Thus, specific graded programs are essential for safety.

Though patients with compensated congestive failure and those following cardiac surgery require rehabilitation, the vast majority of patients today requiring conditioning programs are those with coronary artery insufficiency or myocardial infarction. In addition to a prescribed physical conditioning program, the patient is strongly urged to cease smoking since smoking results in increased catecholamine secretion (epinephrine and norepinephrine) which causes the myocardium to use more oxygen. Many studies have indicated that smoking is associated with increased pulse rate and some deviation of blood pressure.

Avoiding or correcting obesity is important, since overweight can increase strain on an already damaged heart. Diets that limit calories often are prescribed with restrictions in sodium and cholesterol frequently necessary. The nurse can work with the dietitian in teaching the patient the rationale of the diet, as well as helping him to plan appetizing menus that conform to the diet prescription.

Rehabilitation also involves learning how to minimize emotional tension; in some cases, it may be necessary for the patient to avoid certain stress situations. Emotional tension leads to catecholamine secretion, which is oxygen wasting and can result in serious cardiac arrhythmias.

The same principles are used in the rehabilitation of the cardiac homemaker. After an assessment of functional capacity is made, and the energy costs of various household activities are learned from the charts, a matching of "cost" and "capacity" can be carried out. The patient and doctor decide what activities are most essential in the light of the patient's welfare and that of her family. The nurse can assist by evaluating methods used in an activity and helping the patient to adopt methods that will produce a satisfactory result with a minimum of strain and fatigue.

Although housework is important, it is not the only consideration in the rehabilitation of the cardiac homemaker. The strains of pregnancy, childbirth and child rearing may present special problems for the woman with heart disease. Social activities and jobs outside the home have to be considered, too.

On the other hand, doing various household tasks can actually help in rehabilitation. Housework can be viewed as a form of exercise and doing routine things may serve as a tension reliever. Most housework is not too heavy in terms of caloric expenditure and the problem is lessened if labor-saving devices such as a clothes washer and dryer are available.

The need for a broader viewpoint in relation to the employment of cardiacs has been highlighted by the more widespread use of careful physical examinations, x-ray examinations and even electrocardiograms before employment. Many persons who have slight cardiac abnormalities and few, if any, symptoms are being discovered. This is a good trend, since treatment can be initiated in the early stages of heart disease, with the possibility of preventing serious illness. However, this trend could work a hardship for some people, if employment is denied or discontinued without considering the worker's capabilities.

The person with heart disease who lives and works within the limits of his capacity is usually healthier and happier than the person who gives up his accustomed pursuits. Idleness is no guarantee of long life, and in fact may hasten death.

Nursing implications

Nurses in many fields of practice can assist in the cardiac's rehabilitation program throughout all its phases by doing the following:

- Watching for danger signals accompanying increased activity such as anginal pain, palpitation, dyspnea, dizziness, undue fatigue, arrhythmias, inordinate rise in pulse rate or prolongation of its return to its resting level at the end of a period of activity. Discussing these with the doctor before the patient repeats the activity is necessary.
- Listening to the patient as he talks about his illness—what led up to it, what the acute illness means to him, and what he thinks about the future. Helping the patient to establish realistic goals and to assess his strengths and assets as well as his losses and liabilities can assist him in a realistic way to make the most of what he has.
- Using a positive though realistic approach to the patient. For example, when asking the hospitalized patient to move his legs and feet, emphasize the need to maintain the muscles in good condition since these will have to carry him when he starts to walk again, rather than placing emphasis on the prevention of venous thrombosis and emboli.
- Working with the vocational counselor, psychologist, physicians, nurses and other team members in various settings so that the best program for the individual cardiac patient can be achieved.
- Being aware of the facilities available in the community for vocational evaluation, retraining, and placement, such as the State Rehabilitation Commission.
- Recognizing that the patient is the driving force for his own rehabilitation. The team makes his potential evident and provides encouragement and continued support.

General nutritional considerations

- The patient with hypertension may be told to limit his sodium intake. This limitation may range from avoiding obviously salty foods and not using salt at the table to a sodium-restricted diet.
- The patient should be shown how to check food labels for sodium which may be listed as "salt" or a form of "sodium" such as mono*sodium* glutamate.
- The amount of sodium allowed in a sodium-restricted diet may be stated as a 500-, 1000-, or 2000-mg. sodium diet. An example of sodium in a common food: there are approximately 240 mg. of sodium in a pint of whole milk.
- The patient on a severe sodium-restricted diet (the 500- or 1000-mg. diet) should see a dietitian for an explanation of dietary allowances.

General pharmacological considerations

- Patients with angina usually receive a vasodilator, usually one of the nitrites. Included in the nitrite group are nitroglycerin, erythrityl tetranitrate (Cardilate) and isosorbide dinitrate (Isordil).
- Nitrites are capable of producing a variety of side effects. The most common are headache, flushing, dizziness, lightheadedness, weakness, and gastrointestinal distress. These effects are more commonly seen with sublingual nitroglycerin. In some instances symp-

toms disappear with continued use of the drug.

- For some patients the side effects of nitroglycerin may prove annoying and produce varying levels of anxiety, which in turn could cause angina, thereby negating the therapeutic effect of the drug.
- Various drugs may be used to treat hypertension: diuretics, ganglionic blocking agents, adrenergic blocking agents, veratrum alkaloids, sedatives, and tranquilizers.
- Patients receiving antihypertensive drugs for the first time should have their blood pressure taken every 1 to 4 hours, especially if hypertension is severe and a potent antihypertensive agent is administered. Those with mild to moderate hypertension may only require blood pressure determinations daily or b.i.d.
- Patients receiving antihypertensive drugs may experience postural hypotension early in therapy and therefore should be cautioned about this side effect. The patient can minimize symptoms of postural hypotension by rising slowly from a lying or sitting position.

Bibliography

Aagaard, G. N.: Treatment of hypertension. Am. J. Nurs. 73:621, April, 1973.

Allendorf, E. J. and Keegan, M. H.: Teaching patients about nitroglycerin. Am. J. Nurs. 75:1168, July, 1975.

Andreoli, K. G. et al: *Comprehensive Cardiac Care: A Text for Nurses and Other Health Professionals*, ed. 3. St. Louis, Mosby, 1975.

Barry, E. M. et al: Hospital program for cardiac rehabilitation. Am. J. Nurs. 72:2147, December, 1972.

Bean, P.: The nurse: Her role in cardiopulmonary rehabilitation. Heart Lung 3:587, July-August, 1974.

Beeson, P. B. and McDermott, W., eds.: *Textbook of Medicine*, ed. 14. Philadelphia, Saunders, 1975.

Carbary, L. J.: Hypertension: No. 1 cardiovascular disease. Nurs. Care 8:10, September, 1975.

Clark, N. F.: *Normal Conduction System and the Electrocardiogram: A Programmed Instruction Unit*. Philadelphia, Davis, 1975.

Cooper, T.: Hypertension: The silent killer, Part 1. J. Prac. Nurs. 23:23, November, 1973.

Deberry, P. et al: Teaching cardiac patients to manage medications. Am. J. Nurs. 75:2191, December, 1975.

Finnerty, F.: Aggressive drug therapy in accelerated hypertension. Am. J. Nurs. 74:2176, December, 1974.

Germaine, C.: Exercise makes the heart grow stronger. Am. J. Nurs. 72:2169, December, 1972.

Hellerstein, H. K.: Rehabilitation of the postinfarction patient. Hosp. Pract. 7:35, July, 1972.

Kintzel, K. C., ed.: *Advanced Concepts in Clinical Nursing*, ed. 2. Philadelphia, Lippincott, 1977.

Martin, H. L.: Rehabilitation following a first coronary occlusion. Med. Insight 6:8, April, 1974.

Rodman, M. J.: Drugs used in cardiovascular disease: Treating hypertension, Part 2. RN 36:41, April, 1973.

Scherer, J. C.: *Introductory Clinical Pharmacology*. Philadelphia, Lippincott, 1975.

Sharp, L. and Rabin, B.: *Nursing in the Coronary Care Unit*. Philadelphia, Lippincott, 1970.

Taif, B.: Diet planning in coronary care. J. Prac. Nurs. 26:22, April, 1976.

CHAPTER—27

The patient with peripheral vascular disease: thrombosis and embolism

On completion of this chapter the student will:

- Define, in broad terms, peripheral vascular disease.
- Name the types of peripheral vascular disease commonly seen in the hospital and outpatient setting.
- Describe the symptoms and the medical or surgical treatment of a specific peripheral vascular disease.
- Formulate a nursing care plan for a patient with a specific peripheral vascular disease.
- Discuss the discharge teaching for patients with peripheral vascular disease.
- Define and differentiate between thrombosis and embolism.
- Describe and recognize symptoms of thrombotic and embolic episodes.
- Describe the medical and/or surgical treatment of a thrombus and embolus.
- List and define the types of aneurysms.
- Discuss the methods of surgical treatment of aneurysms and postoperative nursing management following a revascularization procedure.

The term *peripheral vascular disease* refers to diseases of the blood vessels that supply the extremities. Whether the disease involves the veins, arteries or lymphatics, or all of these, patients with peripheral vascular disease experience a number of similar problems. Pain is common, but the kind of pain may vary. For example, the patient with an ulceration often experiences constant and severe pain, which interferes with his ability to sleep and to carry on his usual life activities. While the pain of varicosities may not be as acutely intense, the heaviness and burning interfere with the patient's ability to concentrate, and restrict his activities. Constant pain undermines morale and affects the patient's response to his surroundings, his associates, and his medical treatment.

The long-term nature of peripheral vascular disease is discouraging. Treatment is tedious, and often painful, and healing is slow. A small ulceration that may be looked upon by the hospital staff as relatively "minor" compared with more dramatic patient conditions is a tragedy to the patient if he loses his ability to walk. It may require months of treatment for healing to take place. Worry about finances, loss of job, and suspension of family and civic responsibilties compounds the patient's burden.

Peripheral vascular disease is especially common among older people. Many of the disorders are chronic and tend to be progressive with advancing age. Often, only palliative treatment is possible. Management consists of a multitude of detailed measures to control the disease, to halt its progress, and to prevent complications.

The nurse must have a great deal of patience and willingness to carry out the detailed management that can mean the difference between invalidism or continued ability to carry out daily activities. Often, the patient requires treatment for the rest of his life. He is faced with the management of a condition that usually necessitates changes in his mode of living for years, not merely for weeks or months.

Many of these patients have multiple diagnoses. Peripheral vascular disease is often only one manifestation of a widespread vascular disorder affecting many different organs. For instance, the patient may have suffered myocardial infarction due to atherosclerosis of coronary vessels, and he may have failing vision due to vascular changes in the tiny blood vessels of the retina. Diabetics are especially prone to arteriosclerosis and atherosclerosis. Plans for nursing management must encompass not only the peripheral vascular disease, but also any other disorders from which the patient is suffering.

Patients with peripheral vascular disease often are obliged to change the type of work they do. Among the types usually contraindicated are those involving considerable outdoor exposure to cold, prolonged standing, or repeated trauma to the feet. Indoor, sedentary occupations are the most suitable. However, a change of job is frequently difficult or impossible for the older person. Often, illness carries the threat of prolonged disability, loss of earning power, and, as a consequence, lessened personal independence. Retirement from active work may be necessary earlier than had been anticipated.

Helping the patient to stop smoking is an important aspect of nursing care, as smoking aggravates the symptoms of peripheral vascular disease.

Although the patient may require hospitalization for acute exacerbations of his illness or for complications arising from the condition, the bulk of care usually is carried out at home. Therefore, the teaching of self-care and the arranging for continued medical and nursing supervision through the physician, the clinic, and the community health nurse are of special significance.

Understanding the factors that may hamper or facilitate peripheral circulation is essential in caring for patients with peripheral vascular disease. It is important to know whether the arteries, veins, lymphatics, or all three are involved in the disease process, and what pathological changes are responsible for the symptoms. For instance, the idea that elevating the legs always improves circulation is erroneous. Elevating the legs promotes venous and lymphatic return; it does not improve—it actually reduces—the blood supplied by the arteries.

Errors in positioning the patient can be avoided by:

- Basic understanding of the dynamics of circulation to the extremities.
- Understanding of the patient's particular disease.
- Frequent conferences with the patient's physician, so that specific procedures concerning important details, such as positioning the patient, can be fully discussed.

If in doubt about positioning the patient, it is best to have him keep his legs flat on the bed rather than elevated or dependent (lower than the heart) until the opportunity arises to discuss the matter with the physician.

Ischemia

Ischemia is the term used to describe a lack of blood supply to meet the needs of the tissues. Excessive vasoconstriction can lead to diminished flow of blood resulting in ischemia. Gradual occlusion of the lumen of the artery by fatty deposits (atherosclerosis) can slowly and inexorably reduce the amount of blood that the arteries can deliver. Such occlusion may be speeded by formation of a blood clot at the atherosclerotic site (thrombosis). Regardless of the particular pathology responsible for the decreased blood flow, certain changes in the ischemic part will occur if the diminished blood supply is severe and persistent.

- Coldness. Ordinarily, the body feels warm to touch, because of the presence of warm blood. When the blood supply is markedly decreased, the part is cold to touch and also feels uncomfortably cold to the patient.
- Pallor. The normal pink hue of the skin is due to the blood in superficial vessels. Diminished arterial blood supply causes pallor.
- Rubor (redness). Redness—usually a reddish-blue color—results when the superficial blood vessels have been injured by anoxia or coldness and remain dilated. The extremity is both blue-red and cold, rather than pink and warm, as it normally should be.
- Cyanosis (blueness). Cyanosis indicates that the blood in the part contains less than the normal amounts of oxygen. Cyanosis usually results from a blood supply that is diminished and yet not diminished sufficiently to cause blanching.
- Pain. Pain is characteristic when the blood supply is not adequate for the requirements of the tissues. Pain that occurs only after a certain amount of exercise is called *intermittent claudication.* The patient may walk a block and then have to stop because of severe aching in his calf muscles. His arteries are not able to deliver the amount of blood required by his legs during this exercise. The pain disappears when the patient rests, but it promptly returns when he repeats the same amount of exercise. Pain occurs even at rest (rest pain) when sudden occlusion of an artery by an embolus occurs, because there is not sufficient blood supply to sustain the tissues even when no exercise is undertaken.
- Trophic changes. These are abnormal changes in the skin and the nails due to impaired circulation. The skin becomes smooth, shiny, taut, dry, and hairless. It has very little resistance to infection.

Measures to increase the blood supply

In what general ways can the blood supply to an extremity be increased? How may these measures be utilized in the management of patients with diminished blood supply to an extremity?

- Position. The flow of arterial blood to the limb is improved when the part is dependent or at least flat, rather than raised. Raising the extremity will further diminish the amount of blood reaching the part.
- Warmth. The kind of warmth that merely insulates the extremity from a cold environment may be safely used. Warm gloves and socks are examples. Extra heat provided by hot-water bags, hot foot soaks, or heating pads never should be used. Often, the patient has diminished sensation in the part, making him less able to note when excessive heat is applied and, therefore, placing him in even greater danger of being burned.
- Interrupting sympathetic stimuli. Interruption of sympathetic stimuli to the extremity prevents vasoconstriction. Sympathetic stimuli may be removed temporarily by sympatholytic drugs.

  Permanent interruption of sympathetic stimulation is achieved by cutting the nerve (sympathectomy), with resultant decrease in vasoconstriction.
- Vasodilators. To be effective, vasodilators must have more than a fleeting action. Alcohol and papaverine are examples of drugs used to cause vasodilation. The usefulness of vasodilators is limited by the fact that organic changes, such as arteriosclerosis, often make the vessels incapable of dilating. Thus, diseases characterized by spasm of vessels or vasoconstriction respond best to vasodilators.
- Prevention of clot formation. If clots are impeding circulation, anticoagulants may be given to prevent further clot formation.
- Avoidance of vasoconstriction. Nicotine leads to vasoconstriction; therefore, smoking or the

use of tobacco in any form is contraindicated in any patient with diminished arterial circulation. Exposure to cold causes vasoconstriction and should be avoided whenever possible. The constriction of vessels by pressure must also be avoided. For instance, sitting with the knees crossed causes pressure on popliteal vessels and lessens further the blood supply to the legs.

- Exercise. If exercise does not cause greater demand for blood than the body can supply to the extremity, it is beneficial. Mild exercise with frequent rest periods is usually recommended. Pain is a warning that the patient has exercised more than his blood supply will allow; he should stop and rest.
- Replacement or bypass of diseased arteries using synthetic vessels or veins (grafts). When successful, surgery of this type produces the most rapid and dramatic improvement possible.

Arteriosclerosis and atherosclerosis

Arteriosclerosis and atherosclerosis commonly accompany the aging process. *Arteriosclerosis* refers to the hardening and the loss of elasticity of the arteries. *Atherosclerosis* refers to the deposition of fatty plaques (composed chiefly of cholesterol) inside the artery and is the most common cause of peripheral arterial disease. These plaques gradually reduce the size of the lumen, resulting in partial or complete obstruction of the artery and in impairment of the blood supply to the part of the body served by the artery.

Arteriosclerosis and atherosclerosis affect many different parts of the body. Heart, brain, and kidneys, as well as extremities, may be involved.

Frequently, one extremity is affected more severely than the other, although the circulation to both legs and both feet usually is impaired. It is believed that the loss of elasticity and the deposition of fatty substances occur gradually over many years. The process usually is not advanced enough to cause symptoms until late middle life or old age.

The rate at which the changes occur varies in different persons. Patients with diabetes mellitus suffer these changes quite early in life. Other factors that may influence the age of onset and the severity of the condition are heredity and diet. Some authorities assert that a diet high in fat, particularly in cholesterol, may contribute to the occurrence of atherosclerosis. Patients with a family history of vascular disease may be especially prone to develop the condition.

Symptoms. The symptoms are those of ischemia of the feet and the legs. These symptoms have already been discussed and can be briefly summarized as follows:

- Color changes (pallor, rubor, cyanosis).
- Coldness.
- Absent or diminished pulse.
- Trophic changes in skin and nails.
- Susceptibility to infection, lessened ability to fight infection, tendency to develop ulcers and gangrene.
- Pain—intermittent claudication and pain at rest. Cramping pain may occur at night, particularly in the calf muscles.
- Numbness and tingling.

Treatment. Treatment may be summarized as follows:

- Keeping the parts warm, such as by wearing warm clothing, but avoiding excessive warmth and taking special precautions to avoid burns.
- Cleanliness; prompt medical care of even minor cuts or infections.
- Avoiding such factors as exposure to cold and smoking, that cause vasoconstriction.
- Moderate exercise, provided that it does not exceed the patient's tolerance.
- Avoidance of prolonged standing or sitting in a position that places pressure on the legs, particularly pressure in the popliteal space.
- Resting with the legs somewhat lower than the rest of the body. Elevating the head of the bed accomplishes this and facilitates the flow of blood to the legs.
- Buerger-Allen exercises. These exercises involve elevating the feet and the legs until the feet blanch, lowering them until they appear red, and then resting with the legs and the feet in a horizontal position. The patient performs the exercises while he is lying on a bed or sofa, first raising the legs, then dangling them over the side of the bed; and finally resting with his legs flat on the bed. The length of time that the patient is to spend in each position and the number of times the exercise is to be repeated are specified by the physician. The patient is instructed to watch the

color of his legs and feet and to lower them as soon as they turn white. Blanching indicates an inadequate blood supply. Maintaining this position could harm the tissues. Walking and active foot exercises may be prescribed by the physician instead of Buerger-Allen exercises.

- Measures to lessen vasoconstriction. Because vasoconstriction often is not a prominent factor in causing the symptoms, the use of these measures frequently gives disappointing results. However, adrenergic blocking drugs like tolazoline (Priscoline) and azapetine phosphate (Ilidar), vasodilators such as cyclandelate (Cyclospasmol) and alcohol may be used. A sympathectomy may be tried.
- Treatment of ulcers and infections by cleansing, use of antibiotics, and all the measures previously mentioned to improve circulation.
- Surgical procedures. Procedures such as endarterectomy (removal of an atherosclerotic plaque from the lumen), bypass operations, and the replacement of diseased vessels with prostheses made from synthetic materials are sometimes effective in increasing the blood supply to the part.
- Possibly resorting to amputation if gangrene occurs.

There is no cure for arteriosclerosis. Such measures as meticulous attention to personal cleanliness and avoidance of injury and exposure often can preserve the extremity, as well as lessen the patient's discomfort.

Treatment for leg ulcers

Ulcers often complicate peripheral vascular disease, and they require a great deal of care. Because ulcers tend to heal very slowly, the patient and those who care for him may become discouraged. Meticulous technique is especially important when carrying out prescribed care, such as the application of ointments and dressings. No care is too great in preventing further infection.

Patients with peripheral vascular disease are especially vulnerable to infection. They develop infection readily, and their ability to control it and to heal wounds is so lessened by poor circulation that gangrene and amputation are not unusual. The nurse uses the most careful technique possible, and teaches the patient to do so. Washing the hands thoroughly before starting to care for the lesion, applying prescribed medication with a sterile tongue blade to sterile gauze, and then laying the gauze and medication against the ulcer are examples of simple techniques that can lessen the problem of infection. The patient is taught not to touch the side of the gauze that he places next to the ulcer.

When the patient has a leg ulcer, he often must stay off his feet for weeks or even months. Part or all of this time may be spent in the hospital. Diversion is very important as hours and weeks pass slowly, and the patient often worries about finances, his family and his job. The nurse should take the time to listen, when he expresses some of his worries and fears—perhaps of amputation or of losing his job.

Helping to lessen the patient's pain

Pain may cause restless days and agonizing nights. The pain tends to be chronic, but it occurs with special severity at certain times of the day. Narcotics usually are avoided, if possible, because of the long-term nature of the condition and the consequent danger of addiction. Salicylates may give relief, particularly when they are used in combination with measures to improve circulation, such as changes in position, exercise, warmth, and vasodilators.

It is important to remember that the reluctance to use narcotics stems from the danger of addiction; it does not mean that the pain is trivial. As much concern and effort to relieve pain are required for these patients as for any others on the ward. All too often the patient senses a slackening of interest, and he may have the impression that his pain is not as dramatic, or given as careful consideration, as that of a postoperative patient. Its chronicity makes the pain harder rather than easier to bear. The pain itself is added to the fatigue from many sleepless nights and the uncertainty about when the symptoms will abate. Prolonged pain can set nerves on edge and make the patient seem irritable or demanding.

What can the nurse do to help to lessen the patient's pain?

- Use any measures that are approved by the physician to improve circulation. For example, placing the legs in a dependent position often helps. Let the patient put his legs over the side of the bed, and be careful that this position does not also cause pressure from the edge of the bed against the popliteal space, since this pressure could further impair circulation. Give him a stool or a chair on which to support his feet, so that the pressure behind his knees is relieved.

▪ Make sure that his feet do not become chilled. If he gets up at night to put his legs over the edge of the bed or to sit in a chair, be sure that he wears his warm socks and has a blanket over his legs and his feet.

▪ Give p.r.n. analgesics promptly when they are needed. A dose given about one-half hour before a dressing change or soak may make the pain of the treatment easier to bear.

▪ Flexibility in carrying out the care is important. If the patient was awake most of the night and has just gone to sleep, do not waken him for his bath just because it is 8 A.M. If he is restless at night, try to place him where he will be least likely to disturb others, so that the emphasis can be on helping him rest.

▪ Place a foam rubber or lamb's wool pad under the heels to help to prevent necrosis—a frequent complication in patients with peripheral vascular disease.

▪ Nurses carry major responsibility for the patient's safety as well as his comfort. Patients with peripheral vascular disease are especially prone to burns. A thermoregulated cradle to warm the patient's foot is far safer than an ordinary cradle, in which a light bulb has been placed. The temperature in thermoregulated cradles can be set according to the physician's instructions (95° F. is usual), and it can be maintained constant as long as it is

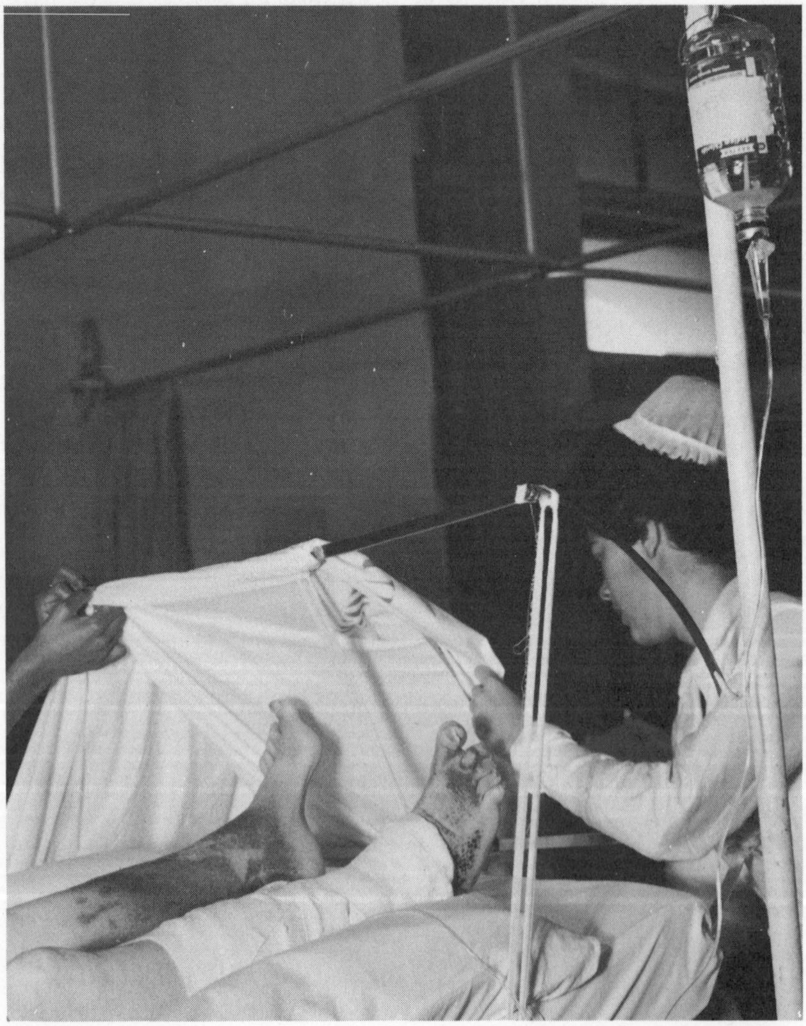

figure 27-1. A bed cradle keeps the weight of the covers off the patient's feet. Note the discoloration of the skin and the thickening of the nails that occur typically in patients with peripheral vascular disease. The pillows under the patient's legs have been protected with plastic covers. The dressing is being kept wet with enzymes used to dissolve clots and fibrinous exudates. The enzymes pass through the tubing to the dressing.

desired. The Aquamatic pad is another example of a device that can be used to apply heat safely.

- A bed cradle or a footboard may be used to keep the weight of the bedding off the feet (Fig. 27-1).
- Test the temperature of the bath water with a bath thermometer before having the patient place his feet in the bath basin or the bathtub (95° F. is a safe temperature). Instruct him to do the same when he goes home. Placing the feet in bath water that is too hot may result in a severe burn or even the loss of a leg.
- Use external heat only as specified by the physician. Patients with peripheral vascular disease should never have a hot-water bag applied—especially not to their feet—without the physician's specific order.

The patient will see concern for his welfare reflected in promptness, in measures concerning warmth and position and in manner, all of which convey a feeling of caring.

Foot care

If the patient is feeble, has poor vision or an unsteady hand, someone must assume the responsibility for inspecting his feet regularly, bathing them, and trimming the nails. A member of the family may give this care, or, if the patient lives alone, the community health nurse can visit him weekly to provide this important care, as well as continued instruction and encouragement in the care that he can still perform himself.

The services of a chiropodist are valuable in managing such problems as cutting thickened, brittle nails. The patient should explain that he has peripheral vascular disease and give the name of his physician. These measures enable the chiropodist to carry out treatment with consideration of the patient's impaired circulation, as well as to confer with the patient's physician concerning particular needs and problems.

Teaching the patient and his family

The nurse has an important role in teaching the patient and his family. The following instructions are applicable to most patients with peripheral vascular disease:

- Keep your feet clean. Wash them once a day, and inspect them regularly for cuts or bruises. Wear clean socks or stockings daily.
- Avoid having your feet constantly moist, because constant moistness predisposes to infections, like athlete's foot.
- Trim nails regularly, at least once a week. Nail clippers and emery boards are safer to use than pointed scissors. *Never* use a razor blade for this purpose. Cut the nails straight across.
- Don't treat cuts, corns, or calluses yourself. Ask your physician's advice. If you accidentally cut your foot, cleanse the wound with 70 percent alcohol, apply a dry sterile dressing, and see your physician. Never apply any medication, such as corn plasters, to your feet without first consulting your physician.
- If your feet are dry, apply lotion or cream after bathing. Applying alcohol and prolonged soaking increase dryness and should be avoided.
- Wear comfortable shoes that fit. Heels that are too high cause pressure on the toes. Sneakers make the feet perspire and are not advisable. A comfortable shoe with good support and a leather sole is preferable. Shoes made of soft leather with rounded rather than pointed toes help to prevent pressure and friction.
- Socks and stockings should be large enough to avoid any tightness or pressure. Avoid bulky darns that could cause pressure and irritation of your foot.
- Never wear circular garters and avoid garments that cause constriction around the thigh.
- Never go barefoot, even at home. There is too much chance of cutting or bruising your feet. "Thong" sandals do not give adequate protection to the feet.
- Avoid positions that cause pressure on the legs. Do not curl your legs under you when you are sitting, or cross your knees. The edge of the chair should not come right behind your knees.
- Follow your physician's directions concerning exercise. If walking causes pain, learn to judge distances, so that you stop and rest before pain occurs. Walking slowly will enable you to walk farther without experiencing pain.
- Avoid prolonged standing. Unless your physician has advised otherwise, alternate rest with mild exercise, such as walking.

- Keep your feet warm, and avoid excessive heat. An extra blanket at the foot of your bed, warm socks, and fleece-lined boots are examples of safe ways to keep your feet and your legs warm. Test bath water before you get into the tub. Never use an electric heating pad, hot-water bag, hot foot soak, or electric blanket without the advice of your physician.

These general instructions are modified and supplemented in the light of each patient's particular program of treatment. Most patients are advised to stop smoking; many are on special diets, such as reducing diets, low-cholesterol diets (in atherosclerosis), or diabetic diets. Instruction concerning diet is an important part of the teaching program for such patients. The patient is encouraged to follow his physician's instructions concerning medications.

If a sympathectomy has been performed, the patient should understand that the affected extremity will no longer perspire. Dryness of the skin can be prevented by applying cream or lotion frequently. If Buerger-Allen exercises have been prescribed, it is necessary that the patient understand how often to do them, how long the legs are to remain in each position, and how to support the legs when they are elevated. He can rest them against the wall beside the bed or against the back of a sofa.

Raynaud's disease

Raynaud's disease is characterized by periodic constriction of the arteries that supply the extremities. The digital arteries of the hands and the feet commonly are affected. Nose, ears, and chin are involved less commonly.

The underlying cause of Raynaud's disease is not entirely clear. The condition is much more common among women than men, and it usually occurs in young adults. Familial predisposition may play a part in causing the disease.

Symptoms. The attacks occur intermittently and with varying frequency, but especially with exposure to cold. The hands become cold, blanched, wet with perspiration, and they feel numb and prickly. Awkwardness and fumbling are noted, especially when fine movements are attempted. After the initial pallor, the hands, and especially the fingers, become deeply cyanotic. The cyanosis often is accompanied by aching pain. Usually, the patient learns that the attack can be relieved by placing the hands in warm water or by going indoors, where it is warm. The warmth relieves the vasospasm, and blood rushes to the part. The skin in the deprived areas becomes flushed and warm, and the patient has a sensation of throbbing.

In the early stages of the disease, the hands usually appear perfectly normal between attacks. The disease does not necessarily progress to cause severe disability. In many instances the symptoms are mild, and they may even improve spontaneously. However, when the disease is severe and of long duration, cyanosis of the fingers may persist between the attacks, and trophic changes gradually may occur. Ulcers and superficial gangrene may appear at the fingertips and are exquisitely painful. The fingers are especially vulnerable to infection. Healing of even minor lesions is often slow and uncertain.

Treatment. The treatment of Raynaud's disease involves avoiding the factors that precipitate attacks. The patient is instructed to avoid chilling. It is important to encourage the patient to dress warmly without sacrificing style and attractiveness. Smoking is contraindicated since it causes vasoconstriction.

The patient also should be helped to recognize situations that cause emotional upset. Often, counseling is effective in helping the patient to change the environment and/or ways of reacting to it, in order to minimize stress.

Adrenergic blocking drugs, such as tolazoline (Priscoline) and phenoxybenzamine (Dibenzyline) often are prescribed to relieve spasm of the arteries, thus providing greater blood supply to the tissues. Vasodilating drugs are also useful in preventing or relieving the attacks.

Sympathectomy is sometimes performed when the disease is severe and progressive, and when medical treatment fails to relieve the condition. The areas from which sympathetic stimuli have been removed will no longer perspire. The patient is instructed to apply cream frequently to prevent excessive dryness of the skin.

Thromboangiitis obliterans (Buerger's disease)

The name of this disease describes the pathology—inflammation of blood vessels associated with formation of clots and with fibrosis of arteries. This condition leads to the obstruction of the blood vessels. The disease affects primarily the arteries and the veins of the lower extremities. The upper extremities occasionally are involved.

The cause of thromboangiitis obliterans is not definitely established. It is far more common among men than women, and it usually has its onset during young adulthood.

Symptoms. The patient notes that one foot or both feet are always cold. Intermittent claudication is a common symptom. Usually, the symptoms fluctuate in severity with attacks of acute distress often being followed by remissions, during which the disease is quiescent.

Cyanosis and redness of the feet and legs may be noted. Frequently, the color is a mottled purplish-red. Ulcers that heal slowly or progress to the development of gangrene may occur, particularly at the toes and the heel. (Fig. 27-2). Trophic changes in the skin and nails are characteristic when circulation has been impaired for a considerable period. Phlebitis is common. Pain at rest occurs when circulation has been seriously impaired, and particularly when ulcers have formed. Although the disease usually is most pronounced in one leg and foot, both legs usually are affected to some degree.

Treatment. The use of tobacco in any form is contraindicated, and it should never be resumed, even if the symptoms of the disease abate. The resumption of smoking leads to an exacerbation of the disease. The patient is instructed to avoid chilling. Warm socks, boots, and gloves are essential in cold weather. Prolonged standing should be avoided. Sometimes, these requirements mean that the patient must change his job. The prevention of injury and of infection of the extremities is very important.

Exercise is helpful in stimulating circulation, provided it is not excessive and does not cause pain. Buerger-Allen exercises, walking, and active foot exercises may be prescribed by the physician.

Adrenergic blocking agents such as tolazoline (Priscoline) and phenoxybenzamine (Dibenzyline) may be ordered. Analgesics often are required to lessen pain. Since the disease is chronic, the physician attempts to control the pain without narcotics because of the danger of addiction.

The vasodilating effect of heat may be utilized, if the heat is properly applied. Heat is not set above body temperature, and no appliance should be used in which the amount of heat cannot be reliably regulated. Some physicians allow their patients to use electric blankets, provided the blankets are in good condition, and the temperature can be regulated safely. Thermoregulated heat cradles may also be used, if they are kept at, or slightly below, body temperature.

The patient's legs are kept horizontal or dependent, except during Buerger-Allen exercises or while the patient is on the oscillating bed, if these measures have been prescribed. Elevating the legs increases ischemia, and, therefore, causes or increases pain.

A sympathectomy may be performed to relieve vasospasm. If lesions occur on the extremity and become infected, antibiotics are ordered to help to control the infection. Enzymes, such as streptokinase-streptodornase, are ordered sometimes to debride the lesion. If the circulation becomes so impaired that gangrene results, amputation may be necessary.

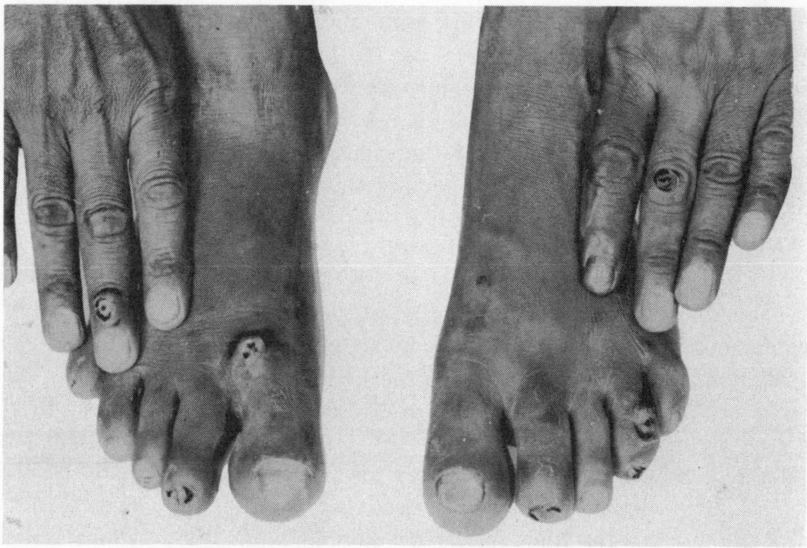

figure 27-2. Thromboangiitis obliterans, with gangrenous ulcers. (Vakil, R. J., and Golwalla, A.: *Clinical Diagnosis,* Bombay, Asia Publishing House)

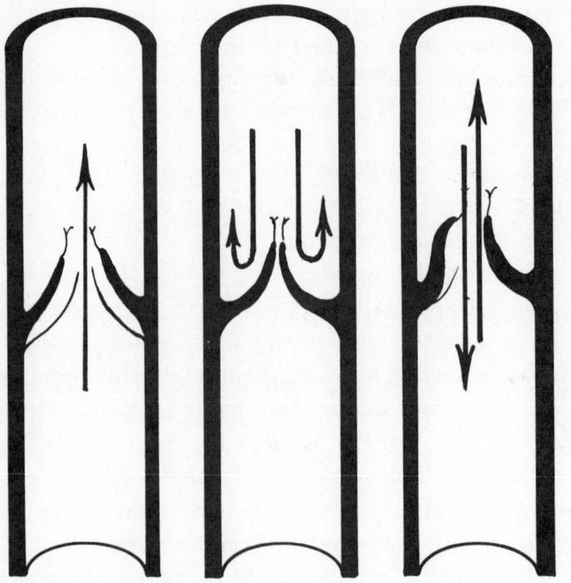

figure 27-3. Competent valves in the veins permit the blood to flow toward the heart and prevent the flow of the blood in the opposite direction. Incompetent valves, by failing to close tightly, permit the blood to flow in both directions.

Varicose veins

Veins serving the extremities have valves that keep the blood flowing in one direction only. The closure of successive sets of valves along the veins keeps the blood moving up toward the heart and prevents it from seeping down toward the feet.

Varicose veins are dilated, tortuous veins. Blood collects in these veins and cannot be returned efficiently to the heart. The valves of the veins are incompetent (Fig. 27-3). They close incompletely or not at all, and blood is permitted to seep backward, rather than being propelled always onward toward the heart. This seepage causes further congestion of the part with venous blood and further distention of the veins. The saphenous veins of the legs commonly are affected. Varicose veins occur in other parts of the body, such as the rectum (hemorrhoids) and the esophagus (esophageal varices).

Some people have a familial tendency toward varicose veins. The valves of the veins become incompetent early in life, resulting in the development of varicosities. Men as well as women suffer from varicose veins—a point sometimes overlooked because men's trousers conceal their legs. Often, the condition first manifests itelf when other factors impair venous return. For example, pelvic tumors or pregnancy may exert pressure on the veins, causing interference with venous return. Prolonged standing aggravates the condition, because the venous return is impaired further by the force of gravity. The action of the leg muscles during exercise, such as vigorous walking, aids venous return. Anything that causes constriction or pressure on the legs makes varicosities worse. Obesity contributes to inefficient venous return by placing excess weight on the legs. Thrombophlebitis sometimes leads to the development of varicose veins, because the valves of the veins may be damaged during the inflammatory process. Often several of these factors combine to produce varicose veins.

Symptoms. When blood is not returned efficiently from the legs, it tends to collect in the saphenous veins. Because these veins are superficial and less well supported by surrounding tissues, they are especially prone to distention. The deeper veins of the legs are better supported by muscles. The veins become swollen and tortuous. They can be seen under the skin as dark blue or purplish swellings. The patient's legs feel heavy and tired and often become edematous, particularly after prolonged standing. There may be cramping pains. Inefficient venous return causes congestion of the tissues of the leg and the foot. This congestion leads to diminished arterial blood supply and results in impaired nutrition of the tissues with consequent reduction in their ability to resist infection and to allow wounds to heal. Minor injuries readily become infected and ulcerated. The healing of such lesions is slow and uncertain.

Treatment. The treatment of varicose veins usually is surgical. One frequently used procedure is *ligation and stripping*. The affected veins are ligated, severed from their connections, and removed. The entire great saphenous vein, which extends from the groin to the ankle, usually must be removed. In the course of stripping, numerous small incisions are made on the leg. These incisions are covered with sterile dressings, and elastic bandages are applied firmly from the foot to the groin. The operation may be performed under local or general anesthesia.

The patient returns from the operating room with the elastic bandages in place. The foot of the bed may be elevated in the immediate postoperative period to aid venous return. The operative sites are observed for bleeding. If any is noted, manual pressure is applied over the bleeding area, the leg elevated, and the physician notified.

Early ambulation is an important aspect of postoperative treatment as it stimulates circulation and helps to prevent venous thrombosis. If the patient asks how the blood will be returned from the leg "now that my veins have been removed," he is told that the blood will be returned by the deep veins of his leg, which are still working efficiently.

The patient is helped to understand that walking is a part of postoperative treatment and *early* ambulation is very important. The nurse should be sure to stay with him the first few times that he gets up. His legs will feel clumsy and painful. This, plus the effect of preoperative medications and anesthesia, makes it especially important to protect the patient from falls.

As a rule, the patient remains in the hospital only 2 or 3 days. After the immediate postoperative period, nursing management involves helping the patient to plan his activities so that he takes frequent short walks, alternating with periods of rest in bed and in the chair. If elastic bandages are used, they must be checked regularly and reapplied as it is necessary, because they tend to become loose when the patient walks about. At first these bandages are changed and reapplied by the surgeon; later they are changed by the nurse.

Before discharge from the hospital, the patient is instructed in the correct procedure for applying the bandages, because he ordinarily is advised by the physician to continue their use at home. After returning home, the patient is instructed by the physician concerning how long to wear elastic bandages, and when to begin to wear elastic hosiery.

The postoperative period provides an excellent opportunity for the patient to learn how to minimize the possibility of the recurrence of varicosities or (if only one leg was affected) their development in the other leg. The patient has already found that he has a tendency to varicose veins and, therefore, must make every effort to control and, if it is possible, to prevent them in the future. Unfortunately, many patients cherish the belief that the operation will make further precautions unnecessary. The importance of follow-up care at the physician's office or clinic should be emphasized, and the patient should be encouraged to follow the physician's directions concerning future care.

General instructions given by most physicians include:

- Whenever possible, the patient should elevate the legs when sitting.
- He should avoid prolonged standing. For example, it is better to walk about at the bus stop than to stand still.
- Circular garters or tight girdles should not be worn.

If the patient is obese, the physician usually recommends a reducing diet.

VARICOSE ULCERS. Varicose ulcers usually appear on the lower leg over a vein. It is believed that the ulcer is usually caused by inflammation of the vein and the surrounding tissues. This inflammatory process impairs the blood supply to the overlying skin and leads to the development of an ulcer.

Varicose ulcers are painful and disabling, since elevation of the leg usually must be maintained in order to facilitate venous repair and promote healing. The treatment involves primarily the treatment of the varicose veins that have led to the formation of ulcers. Every effort should be made to persuade patients to have treatment before ulcers develop. The ulcers are slow to heal and have a tendency to recur. Sometimes a gelatin paste boot (Unna's paste boot) is applied, and the patient is permitted to walk about. The principle is similar to that of an elastic bandage or stocking. The boot, which consists of a circular gauze bandage saturated with a special paste, is applied while the patient's foot is elevated. It dries and "sets" after about 20 minutes, and it provides firm support, compressing the superficial varicose veins and facilitating the return of the venous blood through the deeper veins of the leg.

Thrombophlebitis and phlebothrombosis

Thrombophlebitis means inflammation of a vein accompanied by clot formation. *Phlebothrombosis* refers to the presence of clots in a vein that has little or no inflammation.

AVOIDING VENOUS STASIS. Venous stasis predisposes to the development of both of the above conditions. The factors contributing to venous stasis are inactivity after surgery or any illness, heart failure, and pressure on the veins in the pelvis or legs.

Unless leg exercises are contraindicated by the patient's condition, all patients who are unable to walk should have leg exercises while they are in bed. Active exercises are preferable, for example, bending the knee, rotating the foot at the ankle, and wiggling the toes. However, if the patient is unable to carry out these active exercises, passive exercise may be given by the nurse. Pressure should not be applied to the legs. For example, pillows and blanket rolls should not be placed behind the knees, and the knees should not be elevated for prolonged periods. Prolonged sitting is inadvisable, because the chair may cause pressure behind the knees. Convalescent patients should alternate sitting with walking about the room or lying on the bed. The vague instruction, "Move your legs often," or "Don't sit in the chair too long" is not effective in motivating patients who are in particular danger of developing thrombophlebitis—for example, fresh postoperative or aged patients. Specific instructions, such as, "Bend your knee this way [demonstrate] five times," is far more likely to result in the patient's actually performing the exercise. It is important to observe and to encourage the patient in this exercise throughout his period of inactivity. Brief instruction given only once is easily overlooked or forgotten, especially when a patient is tired or in pain. The activity plan should be recorded on the nursing care plan so that all who care for the patient will carry it through.

Elderly patients and those with heart disease, infections, or dehydration are susceptible to thrombophlebitis. And it does not occur only in hospitals. Prolonged sitting on airplane flights, on bus rides, or in front of a TV has led to thrombophlebitis. The importance of changing position frequently and of exercising the legs at intervals cannot be overemphasized.

Wrapping the legs with elastic bandages or wearing elastic stockings or support hose may help to prevent thrombophlebitis in susceptible persons by giving added support to the veins and facilitating venous return from the legs. Sometimes, anticoagulants are given to patients who are especially susceptible to thrombophlebitis in an effort to prevent the development of thrombi. Elevating the foot of the bed aids venous return, and this measure is sometimes used to prevent thrombophlebitis.

SYMPTOMS. The symptoms of thrombophlebitis include pain, heat, redness, and swelling in the affected region. Usually, the legs are involved. If there is marked interference with deep venous return, the leg becomes markedly swollen and may have a mottled bluish color. Often, the patient has systemic symptoms of fever, malaise, fatigue, and anorexia.

Phlebothrombosis produces few, if any, symptoms, since inflammation is slight or absent. Sometimes, the leg suddenly becomes swollen and cyanotic, calling attention to the condition. The patient may experience pain in the calf on dorsiflexion of the foot (Homan's sign).

TREATMENT. The treatment of thrombophlebitis usually includes complete rest of the leg and promotion of venous return by elevating the foot of the bed. Keeping the leg at rest and avoiding massage help to prevent clots from being dislodged and traveling in the bloodstream. The affected part *never* is rubbed since rubbing might dislodge a clot and result in embolism.

Some difference of opinion exists among physicians concerning the advisability of elevating the leg, and keeping it at complete rest. Specific orders concerning the position of the part and the amount of activity permitted should be obtained.

Warm (95° F.) wet packs may be ordered to lessen pain and decrease inflammation. Frequently, anticoagulants are ordered to prevent further clot formation. Sometimes, the clot is removed surgically, or the vein is ligated in order to prevent the clot from moving to another area of the body such as the lungs or brain.

When symptoms have subsided, the patient gradually is permitted more activity. The leg is elevated for only part of the day, and the patient is allowed to walk about. Usually, elastic bandages or elastic stockings are advised at first to give support and to promote venous return. The condition frequently subsides completely, and the patient may resume his accustomed activities. The illness and the convalescent period often last several weeks or even several months. The patient requires encouragement to continue treatment as long as it is necessary. Diversion helps the time to pass more quickly and lessens the restlessness and the impatience that so often accompany restricted physical activity.

Lymphedema

Lymph is similar in composition to tissue fluid and plasma. A system of vessels called *lymphatics* carries tissue fluid from the body tissues to the veins. Obstruction of lymph vessels causes accumulation of tissue fluid in the affected part. Edema (often massive) occurs, resulting in deformity and poor nutrition of the tissues. This condition is called *lymphedema.*

Lymphedema usually occurs in the legs and the genitalia. It also occurs frequently in the arms, particularly in patients who have had radical mastectomy.

Lymph vessels can be damaged in a variety of ways. For example, filarial worms may invade lymph channels, causing a condition known as *elephantiasis.*

Burns and excessive radiation can damage the lymphatics and cause lymphedema. Some children are born with inadequate lymph channels, although the edema may not manifest itself until puberty. Carcinoma often spreads by way of the lymph channels. Often, the lymphatics are damaged, either by the malignancy or by the extensive surgery required to cure it. The infection of lymph channels by such organisms as the streptococcus also can lead to lymphedema. Lymphedema can also follow repeated bouts of phlebitis and supervening streptococcal (erysipeloid) infection. With each attack more permanent scar tissue accumulates and edema fluid becomes trapped in small "fibrous" lakes.

The symptoms of lymphedema include enlargement due to edema of the affected part and tight, shiny skin. Sometimes, the skin becomes thickened, rough, and discolored. Because nutrition of the tissues is impaired, ulcers and infection are common.

The treatment of lymphedema consists of removing the cause, if possible. Rest, prevention of reinfection and drug therapy may be used. The obstruction of lymphatics caused by such injuries as burns can be corrected sometimes by surgery.

Mild cases of lymphedema may respond to symptomatic treatment. The affected part is elevated at intervals to promote lymphatic drainage. An elastic bandage or an elastic stocking is worn when the part is dependent. Massage starting at the toes or the fingers and moving up toward the body may be helpful.

Thrombosis and embolism

When an embolus reaches a blood vessel that is too small to permit its passage, the vessel is occluded, and blood is prevented from flowing through the rest of the vessel. The tissues lying beyond the obstruction are deprived of their blood supply. Thrombosis of a blood vessel means that a clot has formed within the vessel. Often, the clot enlarges, causing partial or complete obstruction of the vessel. Clots form relatively easily in arteries whose lining has become roughened and narrowed from atherosclerosis.

Symptoms. The symptoms of an embolism affecting the extremities are due to ischemia of the tissues that depend on the obstructed vessel for their blood supply.

If the curtailment of blood supply is drastic, the extremity suddenly becomes white, cold, and excruciatingly painful. Normal arterial pulse is absent below the area of the obstruction. The patient may feel numbness, tingling, or cramps. Surrounding vessels go into spasm. These symptoms are followed by a loss of sensation in the affected area of the extremity and a loss of the ability to move the part. Unless the obstruction is promptly relieved, necrosis of tissue occurs and necessitates amputation. Symptoms of shock frequently occur if a large vessel has been obstructed. When a small vessel is occluded, symptoms of ischemia, such as pallor and coldness, occur, but they are less severe.

Initial Treatment. To save the part, treatment must be *immediate.* Patients who already are hospitalized have a better chance for cure, since treatment is available immediately. The symptoms usually occur suddenly.

The extremity is placed in a dependent position to facilitate some possible blood flow to the part. The part is kept at complete rest. The patient is kept warm, since chilling may lead to further vasospasm, thus further decreasing the blood supply to the extremity. The extremity is wrapped to prevent radiation of heat. Direct heat is never applied to ischemic tissues, because it may burn the skin and accelerate the development of gangrene. The nurse calls the physician immediately, and describes the symptoms accurately and concisely. She assures the patient that the physician is coming, and that she will stay with him in the meantime.

The physician may order an immediate injection of heparin to help to prevent the development of further clots or the extension of those already present. An attempt may be made to improve the circulation by dilating the blood vessels. Vasodilating drugs may be used for this purpose. A block of the sympathetic nerves, usually by injecting procaine into the sympathetic ganglia, may relieve vasospasm. A narcotic may be ordered to relieve the pain and to lessen the patient's apprehension.

Surgery. If, as a result of this treatment, the extremity does not regain normal color and warmth, surgery is performed. Surgery may be done under local anesthesia, except when a clot has become stuck at the bifurcation of the aorta into the iliac arteries. In an embolectomy the vessel is cut above the clot, the clot is suctioned out, and the vessel sutured together. In an endarterectomy, the intima also is resected. When necessary, a temporary bypass shunt is created to maintain circulation while the diseased segment is repaired. Sometimes the problem is solved surgically by a permanent bypass graft.

Nursing Management. Both preoperatively and postoperatively, the patient with an acutely occluded vessel needs to be constantly attended. The pain is severe, and the patient is apprehensive. Postoperative observations include:

- Checking blood pressure every hour or as ordered.
- Observing the extremity for color, temperature every half hour or as ordered.
- Checking the pulse(s) in the involved extremity every half hour or as ordered.
- Checking the surgical dressing for drainage.

The location of each peripheral pulse can be marked with a pen, thereby making it easy to locate the pulse(s). Any change in the quality of a peripheral pulse or the sudden absence of a pulse should be reported immediately. The vessel that was operated on may become plugged again due to clot formation from surgical trauma. When normal circulation has been reestablished, the part becomes warm and normal in color and sensation.

The nurse observes for bleeding on the bandage, a drop in blood pressure, and a rapid pulse, as the patient may have been given anticoagulants and, therefore, must be observed for signs of bleeding.

Exercise of the affected part is not given postoperatively unless specified by the surgeon. Chilling of and pressure on the affected extremity are avoided. The knees should not be elevated and pillows should not be placed under the knees unless the surgeon specifically orders them, as pressure on the legs may impair circulation and lead to thrombosis.

Pulmonary embolism

An embolus is any foreign substance, such as a particle of fat or a clot, that travels in the bloodstream. A clot that has formed in a vein becomes dislodged and travels toward the heart and lungs. Often, the clot occludes one of the pulmonary vessels, causing infarction. If the blood vessel is large and the area of infarction is extensive, the patient may go into acute cor pulmonale (right heart failure). Complete cardiovascular collapse (cardiac arrest) may follow and the patient may die despite resuscitative attempts.

In addition to thrombophlebitis and phlebothrombosis, predisposing conditions to pulmonary embolism are recent surgery, confinement to bed rest, fracture or trauma of the lower extremities, the postpartum state, and debilitating diseases.

If the occluded blood vessel is small, the patient may experience chest pain, dyspnea, wheezing, tachypnea and tachycardia, cough, hemoptysis, and cyanosis.

An ECG and chest x-ray examination may be ordered. Their results are suggestive, but not specifically diagnostic. They are used in conjunction with the results of a lung scan and angiogram. A pulmonary radioisotope scan would show an area of hypoperfusion, but the physician needs to distinguish this from other causes such as tumor or pneumonitis.

The patient is treated with heparin and other measures such as complete rest, oxygen, and analgesia. Heparin prevents the extension of the thrombus in the pulmonary artery and prevents the development of additional thrombi in the veins from which the embolus arose. Heparin is preferably given intravenously, initially in higher doses than usually recommended for anticoagulation since there is evidence that high initial dosage decreases mortality.

For massive embolus, embolectomy may be performed using cardiopulmonary bypass to support the circulation, while the embolus is being removed.

Since the embolus to the lungs passes through the inferior vena cava, it can be interrupted by various means if pulmonary embolus is recurrent. Because of the problem of severe venous stasis and edema in the lower extremities following ligation of the inferior vena cava, methods which attempt to stop large emboli without blocking blood flow have been devised. These include plication of the inferior vena cava (stitching folds between the walls), creation of a suture filter, or application of a smooth or serrated plastic clip around the vessel.

Pulmonary embolism is a greater danger in phlebothrombosis than in thrombophlebitis, because the absence of inflammation makes clots less likely to adhere to the vein and more likely to be dislodged and to travel in the bloodstream.

Surgical conditions of the blood vessels

It is a good rule to assume that the patient with a vascular disease has other circulatory problems. Anything that affects one blood vessel may have repercussions throughout the entire cardiovascular system, and patients should be cared for with this in mind. For example, observations of the blood pressure and of the rate and the quality of the pulse may give important clues to pathology elsewhere in the system.

Aneurysms

The middle layer, or *media,* of the wall of an artery is elastic, allowing for pulsation with every heartbeat. When the elasticity is weakened by disease or trauma, an outpouching (*aneurysm*) of the wall is created (Fig. 27-4). The aneurysm grows progressively larger under pressure of the blood. Some aneurysms become very large, and they exert relentless pressure on surrounding structures. Untreated, some aneurysms lay down layer on layer of clots, but the overwhelming majority become larger and larger until they rupture.

When the walls of the aneurysm contain deposits of calcium, the exact location of the outpouching can be seen on a roentgenogram. Aortography may be done to positively identify the size and exact location of the aneurysm.

Aneurysms may cause pain. Other symptoms may be related to pressure on nearby structures. For example, a thoracic aortic aneurysm can cause bronchial obstruction, dysphagia, or dyspnea. An abdominal aortic aneurysm can produce nausea and vomiting from pressure exerted on the intestines, or it may cause back pain from pressure on the vertebrae. Sometimes it can be felt as a pulsating mass. Sometimes an aneurysm of a superficial vessel can be seen as a pulsating bulge. Sometimes aneurysms go undetected, producing no symptoms until the patient has a massive hemorrhage.

Aneurysms are treated surgically whenever it is possible; there is no other cure. Rupture of an aneurysm is a surgical emergency. In some instances the rupture produces almost instant death. Heparin is used during these procedures to control the formation of thrombi. The diseased vessel is clamped off above and below the aneurysm while surgical repair is in progress. If the aortic arch is involved, the situation may call for, or the surgeon may elect, to divert the bloodstream from the work site temporarily by the use of a heart-lung machine. Bypass also may be used when the surgery would interrupt the circulation to important organs, especially the kidneys.

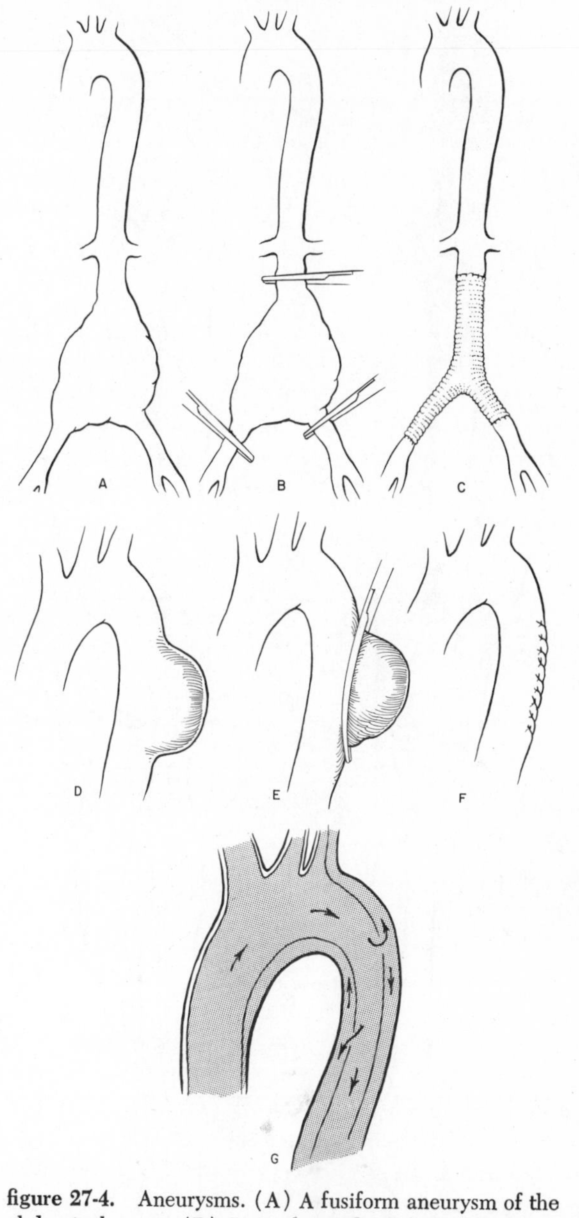

figure 27-4. Aneurysms. (A) A fusiform aneurysm of the abdominal aorta. (B) It is clamped off before removal. (C) Replacement with a graft. (D) Sacciform aneurysm. (E) Clamping before suturing. (F) The sutured vessel. (G) Dissecting aneurysm. In this instance blood is seeping between the layers of the vessel wall through two holes.

Atherosclerosis

When calcified plaques of atherosclerosis ulcerate and cause thrombosis, a vessel can become completely filled, so that no blood flows through the vessel. The discovery of the location of the site of the occlusion is aided by an arteriogram or an aortogram. The surgical treatment includes an endarterectomy, a bypass graft, a shunt, or a replacement graft.

Nursing management following revascularization procedures

A bypass or replacement graft, a shunt, and an endarterectomy are revascularization procedures performed on diseased blood vessels. The preoperative and postoperative management of a patient undergoing vascular reconstructive surgery is similar to that of a patient who has had heart surgery. When the surgery involves opening the thoracic cavity, preoperative and postoperative management are similar to the nurs-

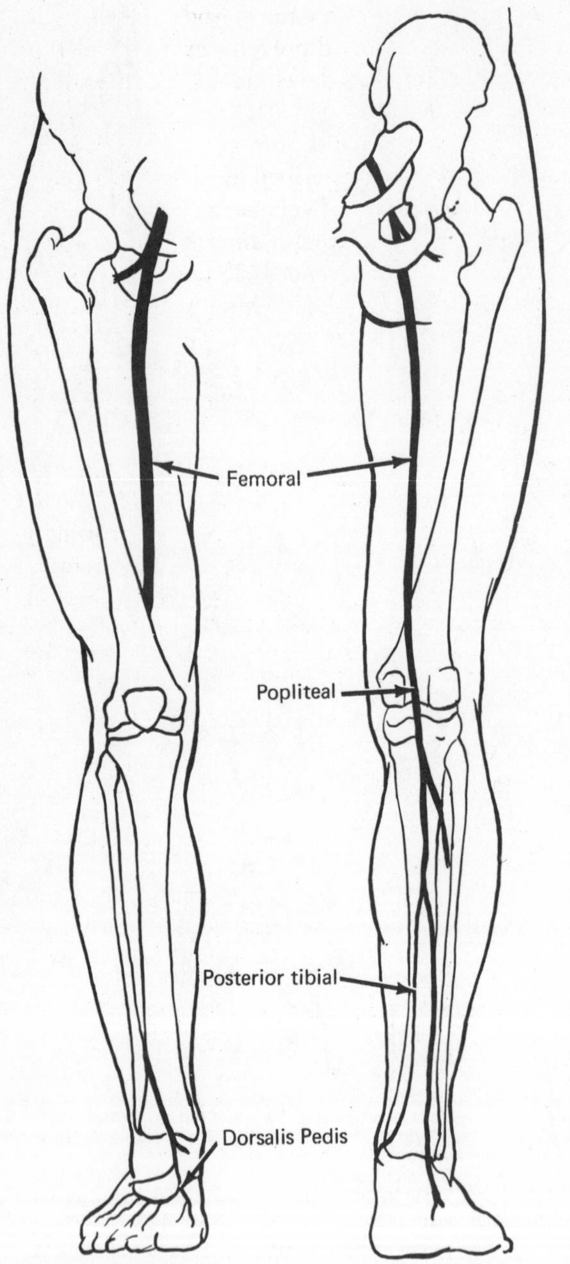

figure 27-5. Major arteries of the leg that can be palpated for pulsation where they come close to the surface, such as in the popliteal area and immediately below the ankle.

ing management of any patient who has had chest surgery (see Table 27-1).

The correction of an aneurysm, or other reconstructive vascular procedures, frequently necessitates a long incision. The abdominal aorta is reached through a midline abdominal incision, and the intestines are retracted to one side. To reach the thoracic aorta, the chest cavity must be entered. The aneurysm may not have been easily accessible, and the surgery may have been long and taxing. Consequently, the patient will have considerable incisional pain, which may interfere with his willingness to turn from side to side. The physician is consulted regarding the encouragement of coughing and the advisability of incision support with the hand or pillow when the patient coughs. An abdominal binder is applied when ordered, for an incision in that area. Vital signs may be taken frequently during the first 6 to 8 hours after surgery. The nurse should observe the pulses carefully (Fig. 27-5) especially during the first 24 hours. If the pulse cannot be detected, the surgeon is informed *immediately.* A thrombus may have formed. Sometimes a reflex spasm will prevent pulsation. The area where the pulse can be felt may be marked with ink preoperatively.

The patient is positioned flat in bed or with the head elevated, or the revascularized part may be ordered to be positioned above the level of the heart in order to improve venous and lymphatic drainage, reduce the formation of edema, and facilitate fresh arterial blood flow.

The patient's position is changed at least every two hours, and the patient is encouraged to move his legs

Table 27-1.
Nursing management of the patient following a revascularization procedure

Check blood pressure, pulse, respirations as ordered.
Check temperature q4h.
Check peripheral pulses below the area of surgery q½ to 1 h.
Check the color and temperature of the extremities q½ to 1 h.
Mark the area where the peripheral pulse has been palpated.
Monitor intake and output.
Change position and encourage leg exercises q2h or as ordered.
Support the incision when the patient coughs (if support is indicated by the physician).
Position the head or the foot of the bed as ordered.

frequently. Any pain or cramping in a leg should be reported immediately, as it may indicate the occlusion of an artery or a thrombosis in a vein.

When an abdominal aortic aneurysm has been repaired, the appearance of back pain may be serious. It may indicate a hemorrhage or a thrombosis at the graft site. Abdominal distention may be an uncomfortable complication, but it is less serious. Distention may occur, because the intestines were handled during surgery. A nasogastric tube may be passed and attached to suction apparatus.

Patients who have had successful surgery may look forward to complete or partial relief from symptoms. The return to full activity should be scheduled according to the physician's orders. The nursing measures for the protection of the extremity from tissue damage, including teaching the patient and family, are continued.

General nutritional considerations

- Since peripheral vascular disease is often only one manifestation of vascular disease affecting many different organs (e.g., myocardial infarction or diabetes may also be present), nutritional requirements for patients with concomitant disorders must be considered.
- Instruction concerning diet (e.g., low-cholesterol, reducing, or diabetic diets) is an important part of the teaching program and is an essential element in discharge teaching.

General pharmacological considerations

- Although patients with peripheral vascular disease usually have pain, narcotics are avoided. Non-narcotic analgesics such as salicylates may be used.
- Adrenergic blocking agents such as tolazoline (Priscoline) and phenoxybenzamine (Dibenzyline) have vasodilating action and may be used in the medical management of some peripheral vascular diseases (e.g., Raynaud's disease and Buerger's disease). Drug results may vary, with some patients obtaining more noticeable relief than others.
- When a vasodilating agent is given, the nurse should chart the patient's response or lack of response to drug therapy (i.e., the warmth and color of the extremities and relief, total or partial, of pain).
- Heparin therapy may be instituted for patients with a thrombotic episode. Heparin is an anticoagulant and prevents extension of the thrombus and the development of additional thrombi.
- Oral anticoagulants, for example, warfarin sodium, may be prescribed as part of the long-term management of venous thrombosis.
- Heparin is measured in *units* and the dosage regulated by such venous clotting time determinations as the Lee-White or the partial thromboplastin time (PTT). Optimum drug effect is reached when the Lee-White time is 2½ to 3 times normal and the PTT 1½ to 2 times the normal.
- Patients receiving *any* anticoagulant must be observed for signs of a tendency to bleed (e.g., blood in the urine or stool, easy bruising, bleeding gums, excessive bleeding from minor cuts or scratches).

Bibliography

ALEXANDER, M. M.: Physical examination, the lymph system, Part 4. Nurs. '73, 3:49, October, 1973.

BATES, B.: *A Guide To Physical Examination.* Philadelphia, Lippincott, 1974.

BEESON, P. B. and MCDERMOTT, W.: *Textbook of Medicine,* ed. 14. Philadelphia, Saunders, 1975.

BRAKL, M. J.: Help for the patient with problem veins. Patient Care 8:158, March 1, 1974.

BROWSE, N. L.: Ischaemic feet. Nurs. Mirror 138:68, May 31, 1974.

BRUNNER, L. S. and SUDDARTH, D. S.: *Textbook of Medical-Surgical Nursing,* ed. 3. Philadelphia, Lippincott, 1975.

COBEY, J. C. et al: Chronic leg ulcers . . . ongoing treatment (pictorial). Am. J. Nurs. 74:258, February, 1974.

EVANS, H. W.: Acute arterial occlusion in the leg. Consultant 14:26, June, 1974.

GOTH, A.: *Medical Pharmacology: Principles and Concepts,* ed. 7. St. Louis, Mosby, 1974.

GUYTON, A.: *Textbook of Medical Physiology,* ed. 4. Philadelphia, Saunders, 1971.

JACKSON, B. S.: Chronic peripheral arterial disease. Am. J. Nurs. 72:928, May, 1972.

RODMAN, M. J. and SMITH, D. W.: *Clinical Pharmacology in Nursing.* Philadelphia, Lippincott, 1974.

ROSE, M. A.: Home care after vascular surgery. Am. J. Nurs. 74:260, February, 1974.

SKILTON, J. S.: Lumbar sympathectomy. Nurs. Times 71:376, March 6, 1975.

SPARKS, C.: Peripheral pulses. Am. J. Nurs. 75:1132, July, 1975. The threat of thrombophlebitis. Nurs. '73, 3:38, November, 1973.

UNIT SEVEN

Disturbances of ingestion, digestion, absorption, and elimination

CHAPTER—28

Introduction, diagnostic tests, functional disorders

On completion of this chapter the student will:

- **Label the major organs and parts of a diagram of the gastrointestinal tract.**
- **Describe the diagnostic tests: gastric analysis, stool specimens, x-ray examinations, fluoroscopy, endoscopy.**
- **List the preparations for tests used to diagnose gastrointestinal disorders.**
- **Discuss the uses of gastrointestinal decompression and describe the types of tubes used for decompression procedures.**
- **Identify the major factors involved in nursing management of the patient undergoing gastrointestinal decompression.**
- **Describe the functional disorders of the gastrointestinal tract and define the treatment and nursing management of each of them.**

Introduction

Patients with gastrointestinal disorders have a wide variety of health problems involving disturbances in ingesting, digesting, and absorbing nutrients, and eliminating waste products from the gastrointestinal tract (Fig. 28-1).

Such problems may be caused predominantly by emotional factors, or by physical factors. There are many patients with gastrointestinal disturbances whose conditions cannot be neatly classified as emotional or physical in origin; their illnesses seem to have origins both in psychological and physiological malfunction, which tend to interact.

The functions of eating and eliminating are important in the emotional development of the child, and in his relationship with his parents. Food is usually associated with love; the infant nurses, and the child receives from his parents the food he needs and enjoys. Toilet training comes as a restraint or curbing of the young child's impulse to defecate when his rectum is full, regardless of time and place. The child learns to control defecation in order to please his parents. Later, it becomes a social expectation. The emotional significance of eating and eliminating does not cease when an individual has matured physically. Disturbance of these functions, from whatever cause, has important psychological as well as physiological repercussions. The patient who has a colostomy (opening of his colon onto the abdomen, for expulsion of feces) typically experiences considerable anxiety over the fecal soiling which occurs postoperatively, since one firm expectation adults have of themselves (and which others have of them) is ability to control bowel movements.

When working with patients with gastrointestinal disturbances, it is important to be sensitive to their emotional responses, as well as their physiological reactions. Both aspects require the nurse's expert management and observation. No matter how concretely "physical" the condition, it has an emotional component; no matter how obvious an association there is between emotional disturbance and physical symptoms, the patient's physical symptoms require care and relief. The patient who has a peptic ulcer needs his antacid on time, as well as a concerned "listening ear."

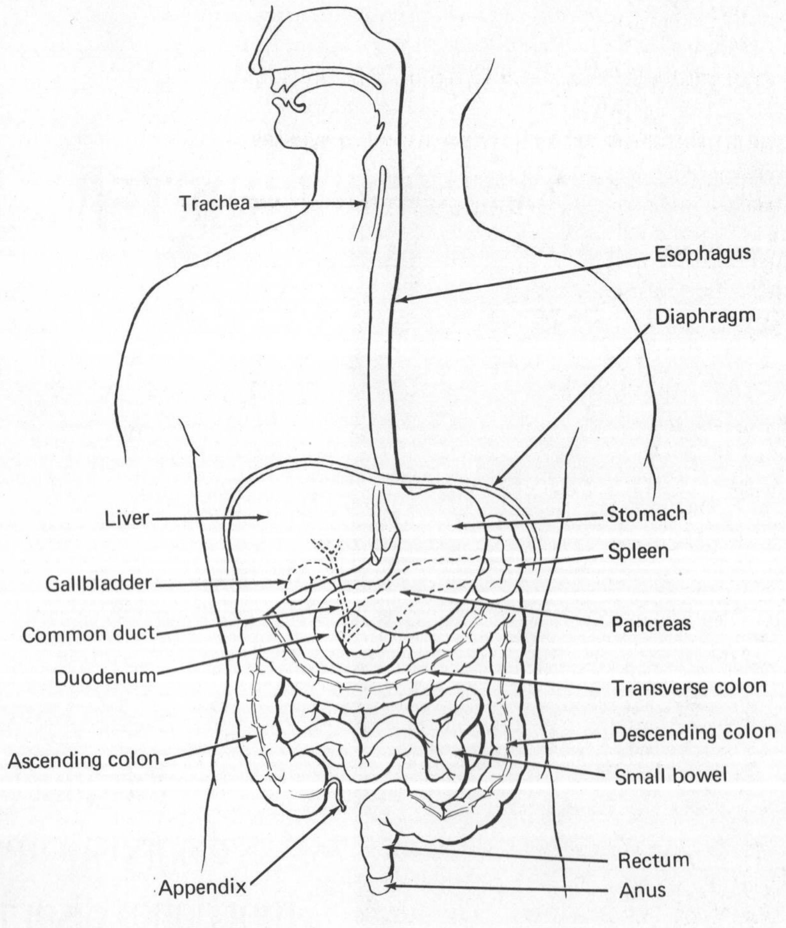

figure 28-1. Diagram of the gastrointestinal tract.

Another area of concern in management of patients with gastrointestinal problems is nutrition. The patient's nutrition may be affected only slightly, or so severely that he is in danger of death. Inadequate intake of foods by the patient (as in cancer of the esophagus and anorexia nervosa), and problems in absorption of nutrients (as in ulcerative colitis) can result in severe emaciation. A great deal of effort is necessary to provide nutrients in whatever form the patient can tolerate them. Observation of what nutrients the patient actually receives is essential.

Accurate observation of stools is also important. A tarry stool indicates bleeding into the intestinal tract, which may occur when the patient has a peptic ulcer. Bright red blood mixed with stool is indicative of bleeding near the rectum, as in hemorrhoids. Consistency of the stool, whether hard, formed, very soft, or liquid, is important, as is the color. The normal brown color may be replaced with a greyish color (the so-called "clay-colored stool") in various conditions affecting the liver and gallbladder.

Normally, the digestive tract contains many microorganisms. The food and fluids that we ingest are not sterile; the feces are laden with bacteria. This consideration is important when caring for patients with gastrointestinal disorders, because it is the rationale for using clean rather than sterile technique in certain nursing procedures. Nevertheless, the equipment for the procedures that do not require aseptic technique must be meticulously clean. Clean technique is not merely a careless way of using asepsis; it is a method of performing a procedure with a recognition of the characteristics of the part of the body that is being treated.

Normally, the walls of the digestive organs prevent the gastric and intestinal contents from escaping outside the lumen of the digestive tract. Since this material contains many microorganisms, any perforation that allows material to seep out of the digestive tract is a serious event because it will cause severe infection of surrounding tissues—particularly of the *peritoneum*, the sac that lines the abdominal cavity.

Knowledge of normal physiology and microbiology is essential in making judgments about how to proceed with nursing management.

Diagnostic tests

The diagnostic tests commonly used in disorders of the gastrointestinal tract include the collection of specimens, such as feces and gastric contents, endoscopy, and x-ray studies.

Gastric analysis

Specimens of gastric contents may be collected from vomitus or, more commonly, by passing a nasogastric tube and aspirating the stomach contents with a syringe.

Gastric analysis is useful to the physician in determining:

1. The patient's ability to secrete hydrochloric acid.
2. His level of secretory activity.
3. The possible presence of the Zollinger-Ellison syndrome in an ulcer patient. (In this syndrome, a pancreatic tumor produces a gastrin-like hormone that causes the stomach to secrete astronomical quantities of acid juice. The usual medical and surgical treatment of peptic ulcer fails and the patient requires a total gastrectomy.)
4. The completeness of a vagotomy. Impulses from the vagus nerve stimulate the parietal cells of the stomach to secrete hydrochloric acid. A vagotomy is a surgical procedure which will stop these impulses.
5. The effectiveness of therapy on secretory activity. Gastric analysis is of no value in the routine diagnosis of duodenal or gastric ulcer. It is helpful in conjunction with other tests in attempting to determine if a gastric ulcer is benign or malignant.

Food and fluids are withheld 8 hours before the test is done. Usually, the patient is instructed to take nothing by mouth after midnight, and the test is performed early the next morning. A nasogastric tube is passed, and specimens of gastric secretion are obtained by attaching a syringe with an adapter to the end of the tube and drawing back on the plunger. The number of specimens and the intervals at which they are withdrawn vary with different hospitals and physicians. Each specimen is placed in a separate bottle. The time the specimen is taken and the number of the specimens in the series are indicated on the label. (The first specimen is marked #1, the second #2, and so on.) The end of the tube is kept clamped between the withdrawal of specimens to prevent air from entering the stomach. The tube is taped to the patient's face.

There are two methods used at the present for gastric analysis: (1) The basal secretion method whereby specimens are collected for four 15-minute periods, and (2) the stimulated secretion method using histamine or betazole hydrochloride (Histalog). (One action of histamine is to stimulate gastric secretion.) This is called the Maximal Histamine Test. The insulin (Hollander) test is another stimulated secretion test used to determine the completeness of a vagotomy in inhibiting acid output of the stomach.

The physician should be asked if the part of the test requiring histamine is to be carried out. The use of histamine is not without danger, because some patients are sensitive to it. A sudden fall in blood pressure, weakness, pallor, sweating, rapid, weak pulse, and the clouding or loss of consciousness are indications of shock after the use of histamine. Emergency treatment of the shock includes the prompt administration of epinephrine. A fleeting sensation of warmth and a flushing of the skin commonly occur and are no cause for alarm.

The three most important points to remember in the use of histamine during gastric analysis are:

1. The drug is never given routinely; it is to be used only when specifically requested by the physician.
2. Although it is harmless to most people, histamine occasionally causes serious reactions. The patient should be carefully observed after an injection of histamine.
3. Epinephrine should be available for immediate use; the availability of this drug should be checked before the histamine is given.

Some physicians specifically order a dose of epinephrine (0.3 to 0.5 ml. of a 1:1000 solution is commonly used) to be given subcutaneously by the nurse in case a reaction occurs. The physician is notified promptly of the patient's condition, and of the fact that epinephrine has been given.

When the required number of specimens has been obtained, the nasogastric tube is withdrawn, mouth care is given, and, as soon as the patient feels hungry, breakfast is served.

Stool specimens

Stool specimens often are examined for occult blood (blood not visible to the naked eye), for fat, for intestinal parasites and eggs, and for various pathogens, as for example the typhoid bacillus. Usually, only a small piece of stool is needed. A tongue blade is used to place it in a disposable waxed container. Then it is labeled and sent to the laboratory. If the stool is being examined for occult blood, the patient is permitted to eat no red meat for 24 hours before the specimen is taken. If the stool is to be examined for parasites, it should be taken to the laboratory while it is warm and fresh, so that the motion of the parasites can be seen through a microscope.

Whether or not stool specimens are specifically ordered, it is important to save a sample of any fecal material that is unusual in appearance. For example, streaks of blood or large amounts of mucus may be noted. Sometimes, the nurse is the first to observe worms in the stool. When you are in doubt, it is best to save the specimen. If the material is not found to be significant, or if the physician already has observed it, no harm has been done, whereas discarding it may mean the loss of a valuable clue to the patient's diagnosis.

Sometimes, it is necessary to give an enema in order to obtain a stool specimen. The solution ordered is normal saline or tap water, so that no other substance, such as soap, will be mixed with the stool.

Roentgenography and fluoroscopy

The use of x-ray studies and fluoroscopy is very valuable in diagnosis, because they permit the visualization of the entire gastrointestinal tract. For example, tumors and ulcers may be noted by x-ray examination. The area to be examined should be as empty as possible, so that the contrast medium can outline clearly the entire area that is being studied. Barium sulfate is the contrast medium (radiopaque substance) used most often.

X-ray studies of the upper gastrointestinal tract often are called a "GI series." The patient swallows barium, and fluoroscopic and x-ray studies are made. The speed with which the barium passes through the tract and the appearance of the organs themselves are noted. Normally, the barium that the patient has swallowed leaves the stomach within 6 hours. Additional x-ray films may be taken 6 hours after the ingestion of barium to note whether any barium still remains in the stomach.

One discomfort caused by this test is hunger. The patient fasts after midnight, omits breakfast, and often has a late lunch. The x-ray department must be consulted to find out whether the series has been completed before the patient has anything to eat. Sometimes, he must return for additional films. When the series has been completed, the patient should promptly receive an appetizing meal. If lunch is delayed, cold foods should be kept in the refrigerator and hot ones reheated before the tray is served.

The taste of the barium is chalky and unpleasant. Some hospitals have barium that is flavored to make it more palatable. The series of x-ray examinations is quite tiring, especially for weak and aged patients. Besides fasting, they must assume various positions on the x-ray table while the series of films is being taken. Many of the patients return quite exhausted, and once they have eaten, they enjoy an opportunity for uninterrupted rest.

Roentgenography and fluoroscopy of the large intestine are carried out after barium has been introduced into the bowel by means of an enema. The procedure is usually referred to as a barium enema. The barium is administered in the x-ray department. The patient is asked to retain the barium while the films are taken. He then expels the barium, and additional films are taken. Air is instilled rectally as additional contrast when polyps are suspected.

A laxative and enemas are usually given by the nurse prior to the x-ray examination to cleanse the bowel of feces. The number of enemas, the type of solution, the times specified for their administration and the type of laxative vary in different hospitals.

Whenever barium is introduced into the gastrointestinal tract, provision must be made for its prompt elimination. Often, a cathartic is ordered after a GI series. Retained barium can become a hard mass that could cause an intestinal obstruction or an impaction in the anus or rectum. After barium has been used, it should always be noted whether the barium has been passed and whether the patient is having regular bowel movements.

Endoscopy

Endoscopy refers to the examination of organs through a hollow instrument passed through one of the body openings. The physician looks through the lumen of the instrument and, aided by the attached electric light, he is able to inspect the organ into which the scope has been passed. A significant advance in recent years has been the development of flexible fiberoptic endoscopes. These are more readily and comfortably passed than the former rigid instruments. Biopsies also may be performed through the lumen of the instrument. The following endoscopic procedures frequently are used in examination of the gastrointestinal tract:

- Esophagoscopy—visualization of the esophagus.
- Gastroscopy—visualization of the stomach.
- Sigmoidoscopy—visualization of the sigmoid colon, the rectum, and the anus.
- Proctoscopy—visualization of the rectum and the anus.
- Anoscopy—visualization of the anus.

The instruments used are named according to the procedures performed with them. All areas through which the scope passes are examined; therefore, sigmoidoscopy includes examination of the anus and the rectum, as well as the sigmoid colon. The area of the gastrointestinal tract being examined must be as empty as possible to permit effective visualization of the tissues.

Helping with Endoscopy. Passing an endoscope into any body cavity is uncomfortable, and sometimes quite painful. Use of the more flexible fiberoptic endoscopes has reduced the discomfort of this procedure. After the physician has discussed the need for the examination with the patient, the nurse can help to allay the patient's fears by explaining further what preparations will be necessary for the procedures.

Esophagoscopy and Gastroscopy. Nothing is given by mouth 8 hours prior to esophagoscopy and gastroscopy, so that the visualization of the organs will not be obscured by the presence of food, and the patient will not regurgitate as the gastroscope is being passed down his esophagus. Usually, this procedure is carried out in the operating room, or a special procedure room and the preparation is similar to that of any patient going to the operating room. For example:

- Morning care is completed before the patient leaves his room.
- Dentures, jewelry, and hairpins are removed.
- The patient is given the opportunity to void just before leaving his room, so that he will not be uncomfortable or embarrassed by this need during the procedure.
- The patient signs written permission for the examination.
- Sedation is given, as ordered by the physician. A barbiturate, such as phenobarbital, and meperidine (Demerol) often are ordered approximately 1 hour before the patient leaves his room. The physician may administer a tranquilizer such as diazepam (Valium) intravenously. Diazepam not only acts as a sedative but also has muscle-relaxing properties, thus facilitating the insertion of the endoscope.

If a tranquilizer is administered intravenously, the patient will be sleepy when he returns to his room. Once awake, he should be observed for any expecto-

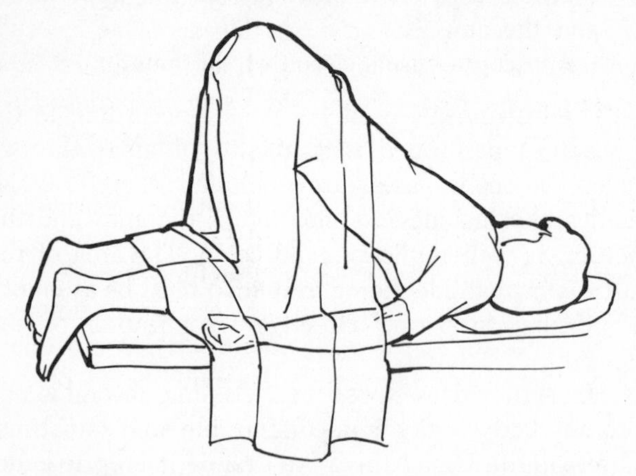

figure 28-2. Knee-chest position assumed for proctoscopy. Note that the patient is resting on her chest (not on her elbows) and her knees. Her feet are over the edge of the table, and her thighs are at right angles to the table. Because many people find the knee-chest position embarrassing, the nurse should be especially careful to drape the patient so that only the anus is exposed.

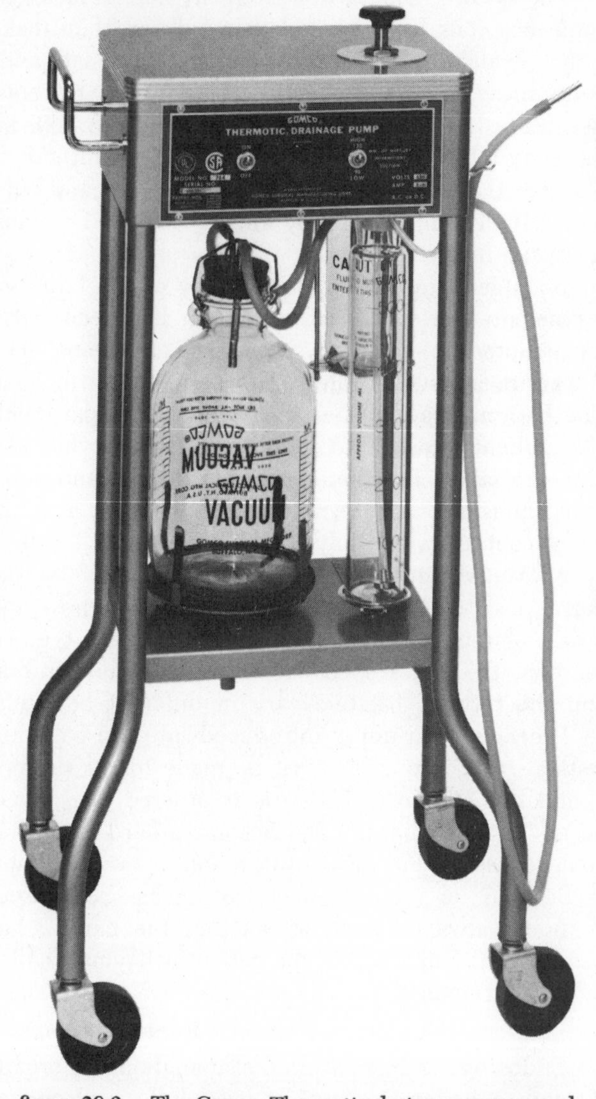

figure 28-3. The Gomco Thermotic drainage pump, used for gastric lavage, intestinal decompression, duodenal and fistula drainage, and drainage following prostatectomy, has two suction settings of 90 mm. (low) and 120 mm. (high) mercury. There is also a flushing device. Each stroke of the manually operated knob on the top of the stand delivers 35 to 50 ml. of solution through the drainage tube. (Gomco Surgical Manufacturing Corporation, Buffalo, N.Y.)

ration or vomiting of blood, since this may indicate injury to the esophagus. However, the expectoration of a small amount of blood-tinged mucus is not unusual. The patient's throat will usually feel sore. Assure him that this soreness will disappear gradually over a period of several days. Any severe pain should be reported to the doctor.

Sigmoidoscopy, Proctoscopy, and Anoscopy. Usually these are performed in a treatment room, clinic, or physician's office. Enemas are given, as ordered by the physician, before the examination is carried out, since the presence of feces in the lower bowel prevents adequate visualization during the examination. If the enemas are not effective, or if all the solution is not expelled, the physician should always be notified before the examination is begun. Disposable, commercially prepared enemas are often used in cleansing the lower bowel. Sometimes, the patient is instructed to limit his supper on the evening before the test to foods low in residue; for example, raw fruits and vegetables and whole-grain cereals would be excluded. Usually, the patient is permitted a light breakfast on the morning of the examination.

The patient is placed in the knee-chest position on the treatment table, and draped with a fenestrated sheet (Fig. 28-2). It is helpful to show the patient how to assume this position before the test is begun, since the position is awkward, and some patients make the mistake of resting on their elbows instead of the chest. Some physicians prefer that the patient lie on his left side with the head of the table elevated approximately 15°; the thighs are flexed on the abdomen, and the legs are extended. As the scope is advanced, the patient is asked to extend his thighs and legs to an almost straight position. It has been claimed that this position facilitates visualization of the rectum and low sigmoid and is more comfortable for the patient.

The physician first performs a digital examination

of the anus and the rectum, using rubber gloves and a lubricant. The scope is then lubricated and inserted. To facilitate the examination with the lighted instrument, the lights are turned off, and the shades are drawn. While the sigmoidoscope is in place, the physician uses long, cotton-tipped swabs to remove any particles of feces or mucus that may interfere with visualization. The swabs are passed through the scope and discarded immediately after use in a waste container. Also, a suction tip may be inserted through the scope to remove fluid. A suction machine should be available.

The details concerning the preparation of the equipment vary in different hospitals. For example, the physician may bring his own equipment with him, or it may belong to the hospital. In the latter case, the nurse is responsible for preparing the equipment ahead of time. The scope should be plugged in to make sure that the light goes on. Cotton swabs should be available, as well as biopsy forceps and a container for any tissue removed for biopsy. A wastebasket lined with a paper bag is needed for discarding soiled swabs.

The nurse's role in these tests involves the following preparative and supportive measures:

- Preparation of the patient—giving the enemas, explaining the procedure, and showing him how to assume the knee-chest position.
- Positioning and draping the patient for the test; observing and encouraging him during it.
- Preparing the equipment and assisting the physician (for example, turning the lights on and off, handing him swabs).
- Cleansing the anal region after the test is completed, and assisting the patient back to bed.
- Caring for used equipment; discarding waste, sending specimens to the laboratory, as ordered.

Gastrointestinal decompression

Gastrointestinal decompression refers to emptying or draining the contents of the stomach or the intestines. A tube is passed through the nose and down the esophagus to the stomach. If intestinal decompression is necessary, a special tube is used that is longer and has a device facilitating its passage along the intestinal tract.

The contents of the gastrointestinal tract are withdrawn by suction (Fig. 28-3). Because the suction usually must be continued for extended periods, a mechanical device is used that can be adjusted to provide continuously the amount of suction specified by the physician. An electric device, such as the Gomco suction machine, often is used. Wall suction outlets also are used, and this type of suction eliminates excess equipment at the patient's bedside. If the withdrawal of gastric contents is to be carried out over a brief period, such as specimens obtained for diagnostic purposes, the suction is applied by attaching a syringe to the end of the tube and drawing back on the plunger.

The indications for gastrointestinal decompresion will be discussed throughout this unit. Some of the more common of these follow:

- Withdrawal of specimens of gastric contents for diagnostic purposes.

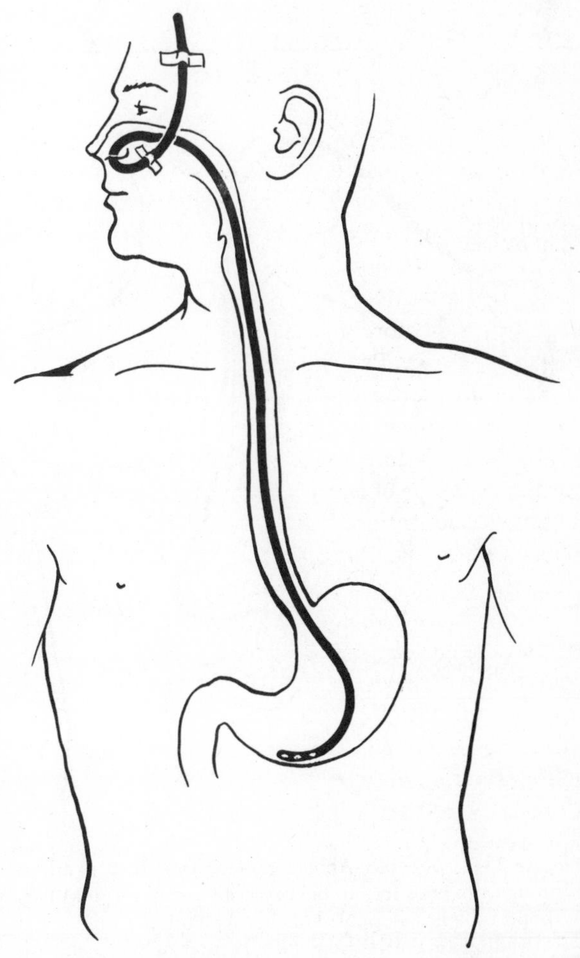

figure 28-4. A nasogastric tube in place. This tube is used to aspirate gastric contents or to convey liquids to the stomach.

- Prevention and treatment of postoperative distention, particularly after surgery on the gastrointestinal tract.
- Removal of accumulated contents of the gastrointestinal tract when there is obstruction in the tract.
- Emptying the stomach before emergency surgery or after the swallowing of poisons.

Kinds of tubes

Gastrointestinal decompression may be continued for several days. The type of tube most commonly used for gastric decompression is the *nasogastric tube,* also referred to as a *Levin tube* (Fig. 28-4, p. 375). The tube is usually plastic and has holes in several locations near its tip to permit withdrawal of stomach contents.

The Miller-Abbott and the Cantor tubes are often used for intestinal decompression. They are longer than the nasogastric tube, and contain devices that facilitate the passage of the tube along the intestinal tract.

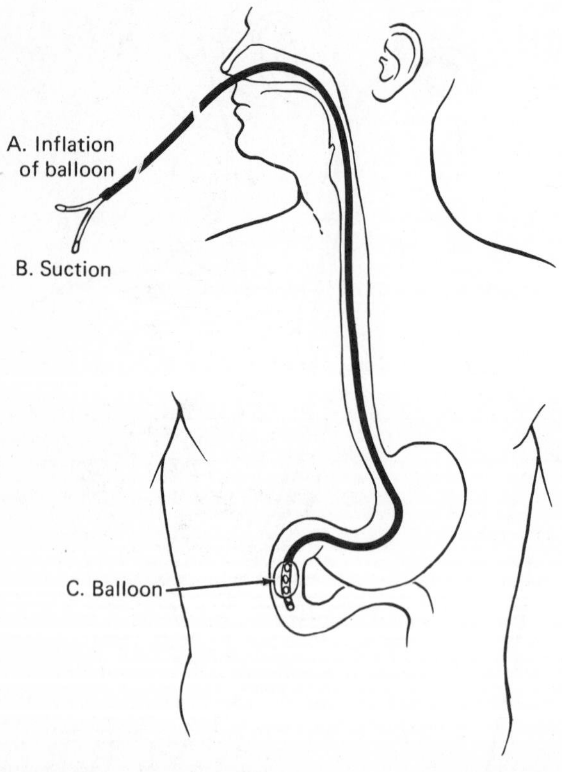

figure 28-5. A Miller-Abbott tube in place. It is advanced through the intestines to the prescribed point. The Miller-Abbott tube has a double lumen. (A) Portion of the metal tip leading to the balloon. (B) Portion of the metal tip leading to the lumen that can be suctioned. (C) Balloon inflated with air.

The *Miller-Abbott tube* has a double lumen (a tube within a tube) (Fig. 28-5). One tube connects with a rubber balloon at the tip. The other connects with the eyes, or holes, near the tip of the tube. When the tube has passed through the pylorus, the balloon is inflated with air, and then propelled along the intestinal tract by peristalsis, carrying the rest of the tube with it. The intestinal contents are sucked back through the holes.

Because the Miller-Abbott tube has two lumina, each with a separate opening, it is very important to correctly identify each lumen. The end of the tube that remains outside the patient's body has a metal adapter on it. The adapter has two openings—one for suction (it is marked "suction") and the other leading to the balloon. The latter is used by the physician for inflating the balloon. Labeling this opening will help everyone to remember its purpose and to understand that it should never be connected to suction or have irrigating solutions instilled into it.

The *Cantor tube* has just one lumen and a bag on the end, into which mercury is inserted (Fig. 28-6). The weight of the mercury helps to propel the tube along the intestinal tract. The mercury is injected directly into the bag with a needle and syringe before the patient is intubated. The mercury remains in the bag because the needle does not make an opening that is large enough to permit the escape of the mercury. The bag is elongated when the tube is inserted, so that it can be passed more easily and with less discomfort to the patient. Since the Cantor tube has only one lumen, there is only one opening at the end outside the patient's body, and therefore no confusion can result concerning which opening to use for suction and which for irrigation.

Nursing management

Positioning the Patient. After the physician has inserted a tube for intestinal decompression, he follows its course through the tract by x-ray films and fluoroscopy. The physician orders that the patient be placed in various positions to facilitate the passage of the tube through the pylorus and into the intestine. For example, he may request that the patient be placed in Trendelenburg's position on his right side, and then on his back in Fowler's position, and then on his left side with the bed flat. After the tube has passed through the pylorus, the physician may recommend that the patient walk about at his bedside to increase peristalsis and to help pass the tube along the intestinal tract. The specific time intervals and the desired positions are ordered by the physician in accordance with his observations of the position of the tube by x-ray and fluoroscopic examinations.

THE INTESTINAL TUBE is never taped to the patient's face or pinned to his bedding while it is being advanced through the intestinal tract, because these fastenings would prevent the tube from being carried along the tract. The extra length of tubing is left coiled on the bed. When the tube has reached the desired location in the intestinal tract (for example, when it has passed to the point just above an obstruction), it then may be taped to the face.

Sometimes, the physician asks the nurse to advance the tube through the patient's nose a specified distance (perhaps 3 inches) at stated times. If the peristalsis is not adequate to propel the tube, a condition that occurs in paralytic ileus, the weight of the mercury on the end of the Cantor tube helps it to pass through the intestines by gravity.

GIVING SUPPORT TO THE PATIENT. Gastrointestinal intubation is done so often that to the nurse it may seem commonplace. However, some patients describe the technique as the most upsetting and uncomfortable aspect of their entire hospital experience. The mere thought of swallowing a tube is repugnant to most people. Intestinal tubes that have a balloon on the end are especially uncomfortable to swallow. While the tube is in place, the patient is constantly aware of this foreign body that partially obstructs his nose and makes his nostril and his throat feel irritated and sore. Most patients treated by intubation are permitted nothing by mouth. This restriction, plus the mouth breathing to which the patient often resorts, make his mouth feel parched.

The patient's discomfort can be minimized in many ways. Before preparing the equipment, it is important to make certain that the patient understands what is to be done. Most patients respond much better if they know what to expect, and what is expected of them. The instruction should be carried out ahead of time. Merely repeating, "Swallow, now swallow," insistently while the tube is being passed is not adequate. The patient may become so tense that he is unable to swallow the tube, and he gags and vomits.

For this procedure, the patient is usually placed in a sitting position. Screening him is very important in preventing embarrassment, since some gagging and expectoration are likely to occur. A large towel or plastic apron should be used to protect the gown and the bedding, and tissues should be available for wiping the nose and the mouth. An emesis basin should be kept in readiness. Instruct the patient to relax as much as possible and to swallow when asked. Usually, the patient is allowed to have a few sips of water by mouth while the tube is being passed. Swallowing the water while the tube is being passed helps it to go down more easily. Those who are assisting in this procedure should try to stand and move in such a way

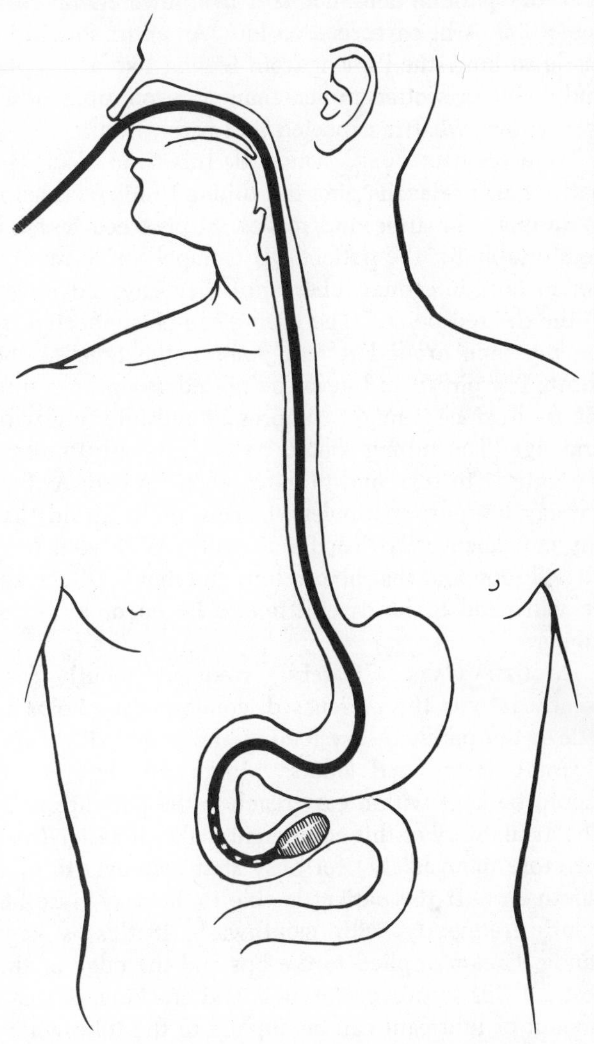

figure 28-6. A Cantor tube in place. This intestinal tube ends in a bag that is filled with mercury to help it to pass along the gastrointestinal tract to the point prescribed by the physician. Intestinal tubes are not taped in place until they have advanced fully. The holes for suctioning are behind the balloon.

that the patient does not feel overpowered or as if something is being forced on him. An effort should be made to keep the patient from feeling like a trapped and helpless victim rather than a responsible adult who knows what is expected and tries to do it.

CARE OF THE TUBE. Once the tube is in place, the patient may relax. Taping the tubing to his face helps to support the tube and makes its presence less uncomfortable for the patient. (It is important, however, not to tape intestinal tubes until they have advanced to the desired point.) The tubing can be supported by placing tape around it and pinning the tape to the sheet. The pin should never be placed around the tubing itself, since it might compress it and interfere with drainage. The tubing should be long enough to allow the patient to turn and to move about in bed. At first he may lie quite motionless, because he is afraid that any movement may dislodge the tube. With your help he will soon find that he can turn and move. Of course, he will need to be careful not to lie on or kink the tubing.

MOUTH CARE. Careful, frequent mouth care greatly lessens the patient's discomfort. This helps to relieve the parched, dry feeling and to get rid of unpleasant tastes and odors. Mouth-care equipment should be kept within easy reach in the patient's unit. The availability of this equipment makes it easier (and therefore more likely) for busy staff members to give mouth care. If the patient is able to, he may rinse his mouth frequently with mouthwash, if this is kept handy. Cream applied to the lips and the edge of the nostril helps to prevent dryness and cracking. A small amount of lubricant can be applied to the tube where it emerges from the nose, to prevent crusts of dried secretions from forming. Such crusts are very irritating to the nostril.

SUCTION; IRRIGATION; RECORDS. After the tube is in place and the desired amount of suction is achieved, it is the nurse's responsibility to make certain that the suction is continued. The tube is attached to suction by an adapter. The nurse should note whether fluids are being drawn out of the patient's gastrointestinal tract by watching the flow through the adapter to the drainage bottle. Also, drainage dripping into the collection bottle can be observed. If the suction does not seem to be operating satisfactorily, check the equipment for proper functioning. If there is still no suction, the physician should be notified. Distention caused by failure of the suction can have very serious consequences; for example, it may cause strain on the suture line in postoperative patients. Vigilance in noting suction is especially important during the night, when fewer personnel are observing the patient.

Often, the physician orders irrigations of the tube to keep it patent. Before you irrigate the tube, find out:

- Whether the physician has ordered the irrigations. They are not done routinely.
- How much solution is to be used, and how often the irrigation is to be done.
- What solution is to be used.
- Whether the procedure requires clean or aseptic technique.

Great harm can be done by improper irrigations. Injecting too much solution can cause distention, with strain on sutures. Normal saline, usually in the amount of 30 ml., is frequently ordered. The solution is injected with an Asepto syringe, or with a syringe that has been fitted with an adapter, so that it can be inserted tightly into the tube. After the fluid has been injected, it is aspirated with the syringe. The amount returned, as well as the amount injected, should be noted. The irrigating solution that is not aspirated will be suctioned into the drainage bottle. The amount of irrigating solution that is not removed immediately should be noted on a slip of paper at the patient's bedside. At the end of the day this amount is totaled and then substracted from the total amount of fluid in the drainage bottle.

Aseptic technique is usually advised for surgical patients during the immediate postoperative period. If the patient has not had surgery, clean technique is usually considered acceptable, because the fluid is entering an area that is not normally sterile.

The large quantities of fluids and electrolytes lost during gastrointestinal decompression must be replaced parenterally. The physician relies on nursing personnel to keep an accurate record of intake and output, so that the patient's needs for parenteral fluids can be accurately determined. The total amount of fluids administered, as well as the amount of urine output and the amount of drainage obtained by decompression, are recorded every 24 hours. The type of drainage should be noted and recorded, and specimens of any unusual drainage should be saved for the physician. For example, the drainage might be described as "greenish-yellow fluid containing shreds of mucus" or as "dark, brownish-red and granular, resembling coffee grounds." The drainage bottle must be washed thoroughly each time it is emptied.

WITHDRAWING THE TUBE. When the decompression is terminated, the tube is withdrawn gently.

Nasogastric tubes can be withdrawn quickly, while intestinal tubes are first deflated—the air or the mercury is removed *before* the tube is withdrawn. Intestinal tubes are removed gradually, several inches at a time; some resistance to removal of the tube is felt and removal should never be forced.

Usually, a great deal of mucus is secreted, due to the irritation caused by the tube. Tissues should be available so that the patient can blow his nose and expectorate. Mouth care is given after the tube has been removed. Soreness of the throat may persist for several days.

Functional disorders: interaction of the psychological and the physical

The functioning of the gastrointestinal tract is affected greatly by the autonomic nervous system, which in turn is affected by the patient's emotions. For instance, it has been demonstrated that frustration and repressed anger are associated with hyperemia and with increased secretion and motility of the stomach. A variety of social, psychological, and physiological factors cause the gastrointestinal tract to be a common area for functional disturbances. These disturbances can cause distressing symptoms, and yet they may not be accompanied by permanent pathological changes in the affected organs.

Almost everyone at one time or another has experienced some of these functional disorders—an attack of indigestion, a sudden loss of appetite, and constipation or diarrhea. Usually these disorders disappear promptly when tension and anxiety are relieved. Some people are chronically anxious, or they become involved in situations that make excessive demands on their emotional resources, and the symptoms continue unabated. These individuals need the help of a physician in differentiating the condition from organic disease, in gaining symptomatic relief, and in coping with their tensions.

Nausea and vomiting

Nausea and Anorexia. These are common problems, and if they continue long enough, may cause weakness, weight loss, and nutritional deficiency. Vomiting, particularly after breakfast, may occur.

Anorexia nervosa is a severe disorder in which the patient has an aversion to food. The condition is most often found in women, and usually it has its onset during young adulthood. It is believed that anorexia nervosa is related to profound emotional problems, and that it may be associated with difficulties in assuming the adult role. Emanciation is often extreme, and it is accompanied by a variety of symptoms, such as nausea, abdominal pain, and amenorrhea. The treatment of anorexia nervosa includes psychotherapy and painstaking help in restoring normal nutrition. Treatment often takes many years and is not always successful.

Here are some suggestions for working with patients who have functional anorexia, nausea, or vomiting:

- Emotional upsets should be avoided at mealtime. Painful or upsetting procedures should not be scheduled at this time.
- Minimal attention should be focused on how much the patient eats. What is eaten should be observed unobtrusively so that the physician may be informed, and yet the patient will not feel that someone is counting every mouthful.
- If the situation permits, the patient should eat with others who are up and about.
- The patient should not be made to feel guilt for not eating.
- The dietitian should be involved in seeing that the patient has the kind of foods that tempt the appetite. Food should be served attractively and in small portions.
- Negative comments about any particular kind of food should be avoided. In most cases it is not the food, but the patient's reaction to it that is causing the difficulty.

Heartburn and belching are also common. Regurgitation of gastric contents into the esophagus causes a burning sensation. It may follow too large a meal or emotional stress. The patient is often advised to eat smaller meals and to avoid hurry and anxiety. Physicians may recommend antacids, such as aluminum hydroxide gel or sodium bicarbonate, for symptomatic relief. Some people swallow large gulps of air when they become frightened or upset. Belching of air from the stomach follows. Nervous tension may cause excess gas to accumulate in the large bowel, causing pain, distention and flatulence. If the patient who swallows air is made aware of what he is doing, this awareness may help him avoid the habit.

Overeating. Just as some people lose their appetites when they are under emotional stress, others overeat.

Some people who feel nervous and jittery find that eating helps them to relax, and they often eat too much. Others, by overeating, may strive to make up for the lack of certain pleasures and satisfactions. Other people overeat from habit. Huge servings and frequent snacks may be customary in the family, and all its members may be overweight.

All too often, obese patients alternate between stringent, nutritionally inadequate reducing diets and overeating. One of the most difficult therapeutic problems is helping the patient to learn to eat only as much as his body requires and to realize that this type of diet will need to be followed for years rather than days.

Diarrhea and constipation

Diarrhea and constipation are often related to emotional stress. Although an individual may respond characteristically with one or the other of these symptoms, the same patient may alternately have diarrhea and constipation. The terms "diarrhea" and "constipation" may be used rather loosely by the patient, and it is important to have him describe just what he means by these words. Diarrhea to one patient may mean having two or three formed stools daily, whereas another may use the term to describe six to eight liquid bowel movements per day.

Individuals differ greatly in their bowel habits. Some people normally move their bowels every other day, whereas others have two or three movements a day. Differences in diet play a part, too. The ingestion of large quantities of fresh fruits and vegetables causes more stool. The terms "diarrhea" and "constipation," when they are used by physicians, are used to describe these symptoms:

- Diarrhea—loose, watery stools, usually occurring frequently.
- Constipation—hard, dry stools, usually occurring infrequently.

The material that moves down the large intestine is composed of food residues, microorganisms, digestive juices, and mucus, which is secreted in the large intestine and aids in moving the feces toward the anus. Water normally is absorbed from the stool while it is in the colon. When the feces are propelled unusually rapidly through the tract, less water is absorbed, and the stool is softer or even liquid. When the feces are retained in the sigmoid because of spasm, or in the rectum because of inattention to the defecation reflex, too much water is absorbed, and the stool is hard and dry. In differentiating normal from abnormal function, the consistency of stools is usually considered to be more reliable than their frequency.

Constipation may result from emotional stress or from poor diet or bowel habits. Frequently, the patient is not actually constipated; he just defecates less frequently than he believes is normal. Too much emphasis on the importance of moving the bowels once daily can lead the patient to develop dependence on laxatives. Instead of a normal movement every other day, he may induce a very loose stool with a laxative, which is followed the next day by no bowel movement, leading to another dose of a laxative. These patients need to be assured that a daily evacuation is not necessary, provided that the stool is not very hard and dry, and that avoiding laxatives will allow the bowels to function normally again.

The major emphasis is placed on helping the patient to maintain habits that foster normal elimination. Eating plenty of raw fruits and vegetables and whole grain bread and cereal, a high fluid intake, and regular rest and exercise are important. Allowing sufficient time for evacuation at a definite time each day is also very helpful in restoring normal function. The program of therapy is designed to help the patient return to normal patterns of elimination with the least possible use of enemas and cathartics.

Irritable Colon. This is one of the most common functional disorders of the gastrointestinal tract. It may also be called mucus colitis or spastic colitis. The patient has hypermotility of the large intestine, leading to diarrhea, cramps, and, if the condition continues for long, weight loss and dehydration. The stools are watery and may contain large amounts of mucus. Attacks may be mild and occur very infrequently in response to some unusual stress, or the condition may recur so frequently that the patient has few if any periods of normal bowel function. Sometimes, sudden, severe flatulence, accompanied by a feeling of churning and unrest in the abdomen, warns that an attack is starting. Some patients who have the condition are troubled alternately by constipation and diarrhea. Laxatives often further irritate the bowel and make the symptoms worse.

Treatment includes measures for symptomatic relief, as well as helping the patient gradually to recognize the relationship between the symptoms and the emotional states that precipitate them.

Many differences exist among physicians concerning the type of diet for these patients. Some restrict milk; others encourage it. Some advise the patient not to restrict his diet in any way, in the belief that he gradually will be able to tolerate all foods, and that the symptoms are not significantly affected by the type of food eaten.

Preparations, such as Kaopectate (kaolin and pectin) or bismuth and paregoric, are sometimes given for symptomatic relief. Antispasmodics, such as tincture of belladonna, sedatives, and tranquilizers, sometimes are prescribed.

In working with a patient who has irritable colon the nurse should:

- Avoid directing the patient's time and attention to counting and describing his bowel movements. Sometimes overemphasis on detailed reporting by the patient can make him concentrate too much on his elimination.
- Encourage the patient to establish one regular time for bowel movement (such as after breakfast) and to keep busy and diverted at other times.
- Encourage the patient to sit down after meals or during the morning rather than to stand or walk for prolonged periods. Since symptoms are most likely to appear at these times, being more quiet may help to relieve them.
- Help the patient to follow the diet recommended by his doctor.

Importance of medical treatment

Patients who have functional disorders of the gastrointestinal tract should seek medical advice. The symptom may indicate serious disease, such as cancer, and only the physician can carry out the necessary examinations in differentiating minor functional disturbances from early signs of organic disease.

General nutritional considerations

- Because patients undergoing upper gastrointestinal tract x-ray examinations, esophagoscopy, gastroscopy, or other studies which require fasting may experience hunger, the necessity for fasting should be explained to them. An appetizing lunch should be available for the patient as soon as the tests are completed.
- Special efforts must be made to avoid emotional upsets at mealtimes for patients suffering from anorexia nervosa.
- A diet plan based on a complete dietary history and a conference with the physician and dietitian is necessary for the patient with gastrointestinal problems.

General pharmacological considerations

- Patients undergoing the Maximal Histamine Test must be closely observed for side effects of histamine administration: sudden fall in blood pressure, weakness, pallor, sweating, rapid pulse, and the clouding or loss of consciousness. These side effects are indications of shock. Emergency treatment includes prompt administration of epinephrine. (Note: a fleeting sensation of warmth and flushing of the skin are common and are not a cause for alarm.)

Bibliography

French, R. M.: *Guide to Diagnostic Procedures,* ed. 4. New York, McGraw-Hill, 1975.

Fuerst, E. V., Wolff, L., and Weitzel, M. H.: *Fundamentals of Nursing: The Humanities and the Sciences in Nursing,* ed. 5. Philadelphia, Lippincott, 1974.

Given, B. A. and Simmons, S. J.: *Gastroenterology in Clinical Nursing.* St. Louis, Mosby, 1975.

———: *Nursing Care of the Patient with Gastrointestinal Disorders.* St. Louis, Mosby, 1971.

Gragg, S. H. and Rees, O. M.: *Scientific Principles in Nursing,* ed. 7. St. Louis, Mosby, 1974.

Guthrie, H. A.: *Introductory Nutrition,* ed. 3. St. Louis, Mosby, 1975.

Nordmark, M. T. and Rohweder, A. W.: *Scientific Foundations of Nursing,* ed. 3. Philadelphia, Lippincott, 1975.

Rodman, M. J. and Smith, D. W.: *Clinical Pharmacology in Nursing.* Philadelphia, Lippincott, 1974.

Skydell, B. and Crowder, A. S.: *Diagnostic Procedures. A Reference For Health Practitioners and a Guide for Patient Counseling.* Boston, Little, Brown, 1975.

Tilkian, S. M. and Conover, M. H.: *Clinical Implications of Laboratory Tests.* St. Louis, Mosby, 1975.

Wallach, J.: *Interpretation of Diagnostic Tests,* ed. 2. Boston, Little, Brown, 1974.

Willacker, J.: Bowel sounds. Am. J. Nurs. 73:2100, December, 1973.

CHAPTER—29

The patient with ulcerative colitis, peptic ulcer

On completion of this chapter the student will:

- **Describe the etiology and symptomatology of ulcerative colitis and peptic ulcer.**
- **Name the tests used in the diagnosis of ulcerative colitis and peptic ulcer.**
- **Describe the medical management of ulcerative colitis and peptic ulcer.**
- **Define the nurse's role in the management of ulcerative colitis and peptic ulcer.**
- **Formulate a nursing care plan and participate in the nursing management of patients with ulcerative colitis and peptic ulcer.**

Ulcerative colitis

The term *ulcerative colitis* refers to inflammation and ulceration of the colon. The mucosa of the colon becomes hyperemic, thickened, and edematous. The ulceration is sometimes so extensive that large areas of the colon are denuded of mucosa.

ETIOLOGY. The cause is obscure. Many who have studied this disease comment that it seems more prevalent in those who have certain kinds of emotional problems. Patients who develop the disease are sometimes described as being inwardly hostile and yet outwardly submissive and as having strong needs for dependence. Patients with this disease often exhibit a hopeless, helpless attitude. It has been suggested that an altered blood supply to the mucosa of the colon may occur in response to emotional influences and eventually lead to ulceration of the mucosa. Others point out that functional disorders, such as attacks of diarrhea when a patient is frightened, rarely progress to ulcerative colitis, and that emotional factors may have little to do with the disease. Usually, no pathogenic organisms or parasites can be demonstrated. The possibility that symptoms are caused by infection seems slight, although it has been suggested that organisms are present that cannot be demonstrated. Some physicians believe that ulcerative colitis is a disease of multiple causative factors, which may include infection, allergy, autoimmunity and emotional stress. The term *idiopathic* (no known cause) often is used to describe ulcerative colitis.

INCIDENCE. Ulcerative colitis is most common during young adulthood and middle life, but it can occur at any age. Both men and women are affected.

SYMPTOMS. The condition may have an abrupt or a gradual onset. The patient experiences severe diarrhea (12 to 20 or more bowel movements per day), and expels blood and mucus along with fecal matter. Weight loss, fever, severe electrolyte imbalance, dehydration, anemia, and cachexia may follow. Often diarrhea is accompanied by cramps, and the patient may experience anorexia, nausea, and vomiting, as well as extreme weakness. The urge to defecate may come so suddenly and with such urgency that the patient is incontinent of feces. Some patients have particular problems with incontinence while they are asleep; they are unaware that defecation has taken place until they awaken.

The condition may continue in fairly mild form for years, or it may run a rapid, fulminating course and cause death from hemorrhage, peritonitis, or profound debility. Some patients have sudden, dramatic recoveries. They may remain free of the disease for years or have a recurrence.

DIAGNOSIS. In addition to the history and the physical examination, x-ray examination, proctoscopy, sigmoidoscopy, and examination of the stool are carried out in diagnosing the disease. A careful search is made for other conditions that could be responsible for the symptoms, such as cancer, amebic dysentery, or diverticulitis. The nurse assists with diagnosis by preparing the patient for roentgenograms of the lower gastrointestinal tract, proctoscopy, and sigmoidoscopy and by giving the physician any necessary assistance. Cathartics are contraindicated in the preparation of colitis patients for a barium enema when the disease is acute. If the diagnosis can be made by sigmoidoscope, the physician may postpone the barium enema until the more acute phase is passed. Even then he may elect to have the patient on a liquid diet for a few days before, and give some gentle tap water enemas the morning of the x-ray examination.

TREATMENT

Medical treatment is supportive, and it is designed to provide rest for the bowel, opportunity for healing, and correction of anemia and malnutrition. About three fourths of patients can be managed medically and helped into remission. The remainder usually come to a total colectomy and permanent ileostomy when medical treatment fails or an acute complication such as perforation or severe hemorrhage occurs.

DIET AND SUPPLEMENTS. The patient usually is given a bland diet. Any substances that might further irritate the bowel, such as raw fruits and vegetables or highly seasoned foods, are usually eliminated. The patient is encouraged to eat as nourishing a diet as is possible. Protein foods, such as meat and eggs, are important. Often, small, frequent meals are necessary, because the patient feels too ill to eat large meals. The quantity and type of food that the patient eats are carefully noted, as are the fluid intake and output and the number and character of bowel movements. Some physicians advocate greater flexibility in the diet prescription for the patient who is not acutely ill, advising restriction only of those foods which the patient finds cause an increase of symptoms. The rationale behind this approach to diet therapy is that at present there is no clear evidence that certain categories of food make the condition worse.

Blood transfusions and iron are given to correct anemia. Parenteral fluids and electrolytes may also be needed. Because the patient's diet often lacks essential nutrients, such as vitamin C, found in raw fruits and vegetables, and because the disease itself may interfere with absorption of nutrients, supplementary vitamins are given.

REST in bed is important during the acute phases of the illness; it is continued until the severe symptoms subside, and the patient begins to gain weight and feel stronger. The prevention of pressure sores is important, particularly if the patient is very thin.

Drugs. A variety of drugs may be given. Although they do not cure the disease, they may lessen the symptoms and promote healing of the diseased bowel. Sedatives and tranquilizers often help the patient to relax and rest. Drugs that slow peristalsis, such as atropine or tincture of belladonna, or drugs used to coat and to soothe the mucosa, such as kaolin and pectin, may be ordered. Antispasmodics must be given with great caution as they may be precipitating factors in producing toxic megacolon—a marked dilatation of the colon sometimes leading to perforation and death. Any rather sudden onset of abdominal distention in a patient with acute ulcerative colitis is an ominous sign and should be reported at once.

Corticosteroid drugs may be given when the disease does not respond to other measures. A dramatic relief of symptoms often follows their use. In the acutely ill patient with severe diarrhea, fever, and abdominal pain, these drugs are often given intravenously until the patient can take them orally. To maintain a remission, the patient may remain on the drug for weeks or months in as low a dose as possible. The use of these potent drugs is not without hazard. The symptoms of peritonitis may be masked, and the patient may develop other undesirable reactions to the drug, such as moon face and edema. Although they are potentially dangerous, corticosteroids have helped many patients with this disease, as well as other diseases for which no certain cure is available, to live longer and more comfortably, and they have helped some to recover who otherwise might have succumbed to the disease. They have probably played a major role in reducing the operative mortality of elective colectomy by providing a better risk patient who is not as debilitated by his disease as those of the presteroid era. If a patient does not realize the drug's toxicity, he may not understand why he should not take a larger dose than the physician has prescribed, because the drug usually imparts a feeling of well-being. The patient should have ample opportunity to discuss his therapy with his physician. Because corticosteroids are not curative, they should be viewed as one aspect of treatment rather than as a replacement for other types of therapy.

Antibiotics are particularly apt to be used in preparing the patient for surgery in order to decrease the number of bacteria in the bowel and thus lessen the possibility of infection as a complication of surgery on the bowel.

Psychotherapy is often helpful when it is largely of a supportive nature. As symptoms improve, the patient may be helped to recognize some of the emotional problems that seem related to his illness. The understanding and the aid of the family are important, but members of the family will require a great deal of assistance from physician and nurse in understanding the patient's illness and their role in helping him.

Surgery is sometimes necessary when the disease does not respond to other treatment, or when complications occur. For example, perforation of the colon is an acute, surgical emergency, because it promptly leads to peritonitis. The surgical treatment of severe, intractable ulcerative colitis usually includes total colectomy (removal of the entire colon and rectum) and a permanent ileostomy (opening of the ileum onto the abdomen for the passage of fecal matter). Many patients adjust well, once the diseased colon has been removed. Others have considerable difficulty in adjusting to the ileostomy. The fecal matter is very liquid because it does not go through the colon where water normally is absorbed, and it is discharged immediately from the ileum.

Nursing management

Supportive care, both physical and emotional, can do a great deal to lessen symptoms and to assist the patient in overcoming the disease. Any illness that is associated with fecal incontinence is physically and emotionally distressing to the patient. Our culture emphasizes cleanliness in habits of elimination. The importance of not soiling oneself is stressed from earliest childhood, and finding that he has soiled his bedding or clothing can cause the patient a profound sense of shame and embarrassment.

Help the patient to minimize soiling by keeping a clean bedpan within easy reach, so that it is available if he needs it in a hurry. Assist him to clean himself and to wash his hands after using the bedpan. This care is important, not only for aesthetic reasons, but also because the skin around the rectum easily becomes excoriated. Applying petrolatum after the area has been cleansed helps to prevent irritation of the skin. If incontinence cannot be controlled (for example, if the patient defecates while he is sleeping), the use of perineal pads and disposable bed pads under the buttocks helps to control the extent of soiling and makes it easier to cleanse the patient.

When the patient is allowed up and about, he may at first need the extra protection and assurance provided by wearing a disposable pad; otherwise, he may be so afraid of having an accident that he refuses to go more than a few yards away from his bathroom.

Helping the patient to maintain an adequate dietary and fluid intake is essential. Small portions of food that the patient enjoys should be served in an environment that is clean and odor free. His appetite often improves when his morale does.

Some patients with ulcerative colitis appear to be both emotionally and physically ill. They may show this state by being excessively dependent on the nurse, by seeming apathetic, or by constantly criticizing whatever is done for them. The patient may become extremely frightened by symptoms that seem commonplace to the nurse. It is important to realize that emotional problems do not rule out physical illness. The patient has a serious, possibly fatal illness that may or may not be related to emotional disturbances.

The period of acute illness is not the time to expect the patient to conquer his emotional problems—even those that seem extreme, or those that present difficulties in relationships with the staff. Later, when the patient has improved physically, the combined efforts of the doctor, the nurse and the family may help him to deal more effectively with his emotional problems. Sometimes the physician refers the patient to a psychiatrist for treatment.

Peptic ulcer

PHYSIOLOGY. The opening between the stomach and the esophagus is called the *cardiac orifice;* that between the stomach and the duodenum is called the *pyloric orifice*. Both these openings are controlled by sphincters which, when contracted, close the orifice. When the sphincters relax, the orifice opens, permitting the contents to flow to the next organ.

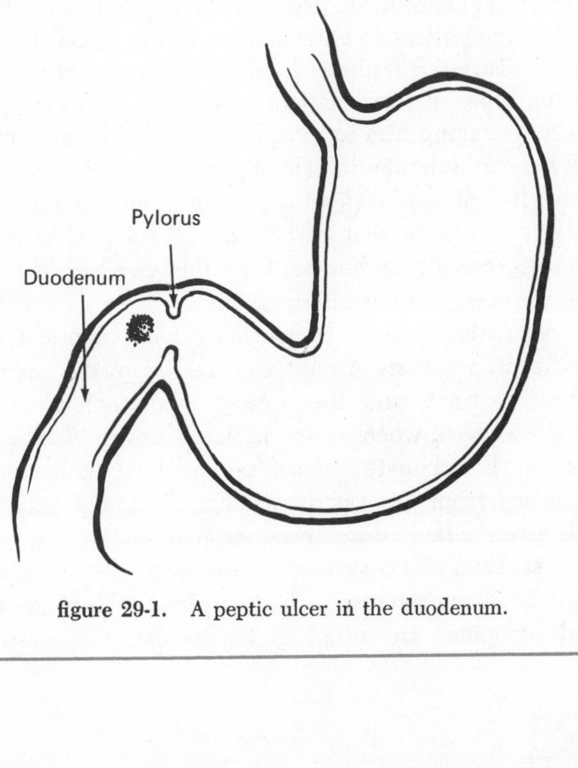

figure 29-1. A peptic ulcer in the duodenum.

The stomach stores food and prepares it by mechanical and chemical action to pass in semiliquid form into the small intestine. Gastric juice containing digestive enzymes is secreted continuously. However, the amount of secretion is increased when food is eaten. Gastric juice is acidic due to the presence of hydrochloric acid. The contractions of the stomach mix the food with the gastric juice and carry the mixture of semiliquid food and digestive juice to the small intestine. The length of time required for the stomach to empty depends on the amount and the composition of the food eaten. For example, fats tend to delay stomach emptying.

The small intestine is divided into three portions: the *duodenum,* the *jejunum* and the *ileum.* The duodenum is the first region, extending from the pylorus to the jejunum. The greatest amount of digestion and absorption of nutrients takes place in the small intestine.

A peptic ulcer is a circumscribed loss of tissue in an area of the gastrointestinal tract that is in contact with hydrochloric acid and pepsin. Most peptic ulcers occur in the duodenum (duodenal ulcers) (Fig. 29-1). However, they may occur at the lower end of the esophagus, in the stomach (gastric ulcer), or in the jejunum after the patient has had a surgical anastomosis between the stomach and the jejunum.

ETIOLOGY. The immediate cause of peptic ulcer is the digestive action of acid gastric juice and pepsin on the mucosa. The underlying cause, which would explain why some people develop the lesion and others do not, is unclear.

INCIDENCE. Peptic ulcer is a common disease among adults. Much has been written about the relationship of peptic ulcer to the stress and strain of modern life, and it is sometimes assumed that peptic ulcer occurs chiefly in executives, salespeople, and others who do competitive work in an industrial society. Actually, peptic ulcer occurs widely throughout the world and in all societies, ranging from the primitive to the highly industrialized. Men are affected more frequently than women. The highest incidence occurs during middle life, but the condition can occur at any age.

SYMPTOMS. The symptoms are due largely to the irritation of the ulcer by hydrochloric acid. Pain, which may be described as "burning" or "gnawing," occurs in the epigastric region. The pain has a definite relationship to eating. It usually occurs one to several hours after meals, and it is often relieved by the ingestion of protein foods, such as milk. Sometimes the pain is accompanied by nausea, and the patient may find that vomiting relieves it. Patients who are severe hypersecretors of acid may experience night pain, disturbing their sleep, and back pain, indicating pancreatic irritation by the ulcer. About 20 percent of patients may have bleeding as the first sign of the ulcer, and hematemesis and/or melena. Protracted vomiting secondary to scarring and resultant obstruction is also seen as the first symptom in patients who have ignored their "indigestion."

DIAGNOSIS. The diagnosis is usually suggested by the history with confirmation in the majority of patients by a G.I. series. In some patients the x-ray studies are not helpful, and a trial of therapy may help make a presumptive diagnosis. Duodenal ulcers are always benign, but gastric ulcers may be either benign or malignant. It is in the differentiation between benign and malignant ulcer that the combined use of roentgenography, gastric analysis, gastric washing for cytologic examination, and gastroscopy comes into play. Even if all these parameters indicate benignity, a trial of therapy in the hospital must be the next step. Failure to show significant healing by x-ray examination and gastroscopy after three weeks is usually reason to operate for suspicion of malignancy as is the occurrence of healing and then recurrence of the ulcer a few months after therapy.

MEDICAL TREATMENT AND NURSING MANAGEMENT

Medical treatment of peptic ulcer is designed to provide the optimum conditions for healing the lesion. The neutralization of acid, so that it does not further irritate the ulcer, and the reduction of hypermotility and secretion are objectives of therapy.

NEUTRALIZING THE ACID. Protein foods, which combine with acid, and alkalis are both useful in neutralizing acid. Frequent small feedings of such foods as milk, milk and cream, custard, and eggs are given. Cream is mixed with milk because the fat in cream is digested more slowly, thus delaying the emptying of the stomach. Cream is used sparingly, if at all, for patients in whom consumption of generous amounts of fat is contraindicated, such as in arteriosclerosis or obesity. Such patients often are given plain whole milk instead of milk and cream.

During acute illness a common regimen is to alternate a glass of half milk and half cream with hourly doses of a liquid antacid for about 24 hours.

As the patient's condition improves, soft foods, such as gelatin, custard, and soft cooked egg, are added to his diet. Hourly feedings of milk and cream may be continued, and in addition the patient gradually becomes able to tolerate six small meals daily. Substances that might irritate the ulcer, might cause excess secretion of acid, or are hard to digest or gas-forming usually are eliminated. The patient usually is not allowed any raw fruit and vegetables, highly seasoned foods, fried foods, meat broths or gravies, coffee, or alcoholic beverages. Smoking is usually prohibited, because it appears to irritate the ulcer. Diluted fruit juices may be permitted. The usual procedure is to give the small meals between 7 A.M. and 7 P.M. and to discontinue feedings during the night, to allow the patient to rest. If the patient has pain during the night, medications and hourly milk and cream may be continuous.

Hourly milk and cream feedings are discontinued when the patient's condition permits. Sometimes, he is able to return rather promptly to three or four meals daily, while he continues to eliminate irritating or hard-to-digest foods, or foods that cause increased gastric secretion. Some patients better tolerate smaller and more frequent meals; these patients may continue with a six-feeding schedule for several months or longer. Supplementary vitamins may be added. Constipation may be a problem, due to the lack of roughage in the diet, and gentle laxatives, such as bisacodyl (Dulcolax) suppositories, may be needed.

Some physicians now recommend a more liberal dietary regimen in the treatment of peptic ulcer. They advise the patient to eliminate foods that he has found cause distress. Emphasis is placed on more flexibility in the types of food that the patient is permitted and on encouraging him to return to a normal diet as soon as he can tolerate it. The rationale underlying the more liberal approach to diet is that there is no conclusive evidence that certain foods, such as coarse-grained cereals, either lead to the development of peptic ulcers or retard their healing.

Antacids are given to neutralize hydrochloric acid. These preparations are not absorbed from the gastrointestinal tract, and therefore they do not produce alkalosis even when given in large doses. Although sodium bicarbonate neutralizes acid, it is readily absorbed from the gastrointestinal tract, and may, if it is given in large doses, produce alkalosis.

REDUCING HYPERMOTILITY AND SECRETION. Cholinergic blocking agents, such as tincture of belladonna and atropine, are often given to decrease gastric motility and acid secretion. The side effects of these drugs include dryness of the mouth, dilation of the pupils, blurring of vision, and difficulty in voiding. The side effects of the synthetic cholinergic blocking agents such as isopropamide (Darbid) and mepenzolate (Cantil) are similar, but they may not be as marked.

These drugs are usually given 30 minutes before meals to suppress the increased acid secretion that follows food ingestion; they may be administered at bedtime. In patients with partial obstruction these drugs are contraindicated since they further decrease the motility of an atonic stomach and add to the obstructive symptoms.

Rest and relaxation are of prime importance in the treatment of peptic ulcer. In the absence of complications this aspect of treatment may not necessarily entail rest in bed. In most instances the patient may be permitted to use the bathroom and to relax in a chair as he reads or watches television. Sedatives may be prescribed to promote rest.

The long-term management of peptic ulcer includes avoiding fatigue and stress, and sometimes it involves maintaining a diet in which substances that might cause irritation and excess secretion of hydrochloric acid are eliminated. Patients are advised to avoid smoking and drinking alcoholic beverages, coffee and tea, and to take medications as they are ordered. Peptic ulcer tends to recur, and each recurrence brings the possibility of complications.

Table 29-1.
Postoperative nursing management of the patient undergoing gastric surgery

Check blood pressure, pulse, respirations q1-4h or as ordered.
Take temperature q4h.
Connect nasogastric tube to the type and amount (high, low) of suction ordered by the physician.
Have the patient turn, cough, deep breathe q2h.
IPPB as ordered.
Have the patient do leg exercises q2h.
Measure intake and output.
Check color and amount of gastric drainage hourly.
Report excessive bleeding immediately.
Check surgical dressing q2-4h and reinforce as needed. Report excessive drainage immediately.

Surgical treatment and nursing management

Peptic ulcer patients who do not respond to medical treatment, who have frequent recurrences, or who develop complications may require gastric surgery. Various surgical procedures are used in the treatment of peptic ulcer, depending on the location of the ulcer and the degree and location of the deformity that the ulcer may have caused.

Subtotal Gastrectomy; Gastroenterostomy; Vagotomy. Subtotal gastrectomy with gastroenterostomy is an operation in which the lower one half to two thirds of the stomach is removed, and the remaining portion of the stomach is joined to the jejunum. The surgical joining (anastomosis) of the stomach and the small bowel is called *gastroenterostomy*. The operation removes the ulcer and the portion of the stomach that stimulates the secretion of acid; the food passes directly from the upper portion of the stomach to the jejunum. (Sometimes the terms *subtotal gastric resection* and *hemigastrectomy* are used rather than *subtotal gastrectomy.*) The stomach may be joined to the duodenum (Billroth 1) or to the jejunum (Billroth 2). A patient whose duodenum is deformed due to a duodenal ulcer may have the remainder of his stomach joined to his jejunum, whereas a patient with a gastric ulcer whose duodenum is normal may have the remainder of his stomach joined to his duodenum.

Sometimes, in patients who are too infirm to tolerate such extensive surgery, a gastroenterostomy alone (without gastrectomy) is performed. The jejunum is drawn up close to the stomach, and an opening is made between the stomach and the jejunum. This opening allows the food to pass directly from the stomach to the jejunum, bypassing the duodenum, in which obstruction due to the ulcer may have developed.

Vagotomy (division of the vagus nerve) is sometimes performed in the treatment of peptic ulcer. When the impulses traveling down the vagus nerve are prevented from reaching the stomach, the secretion of hydrochloric acid and gastric motility are lessened. Vagotomy is always used in conjunction with a resection of part of the stomach or gastroenterostomy, because when it was formerly used as a sole procedure in the treatment of ulcer, there was a significant incidence of recurrent ulcer. There is good evidence that the nutritional problems that follow gastric resection are related to the amount of stomach removed. Consequently, the trend has been to lesser resections, e.g., hemigastrectomy, particularly in thin patients.

Preoperative and Postoperative Nursing Management (Table 29-1). Preoperatively, careful attention is given to water and electrolyte regulation. Whether fluids are given orally or parenterally, care is taken that the patient is well hydrated. Usually a nasogastric tube is inserted and connected to suction before surgery, to empty the stomach of food and secretions.

The patient returns from the operating room with a nasogastric tube in place. The tube is left in place as long as it is necessary—usually 2 or 3 days. Its purpose is to promote healing by keeping the operative area clean and free of pressure. Although at first a small amount of bright red blood may be mixed with drainage, this promptly disappears. If large amounts of bright red blood appear, or if the drainage should continue to be streaked with it, the doctor should be notified immediately. The drainage usually is dark red or brownish at first, indicating the presence of old blood, and then it changes to the normal greenish-yellow color of gastric secretion. The amount as well as the color of the drainage is carefully noted. Usually, the doctor orders irrigation of the nasogastric tube, so that it will remain clean and patent. The nasogastric tube should not be irrigated unless there is an order to do so. It is important to use only the *amount* and the *type* of solution specified by the physician, since it is being introduced into the operative area. Too much fluid could cause strain and pressure and might injure the incision.

Nothing is given by mouth until the physician orders oral fluids, as the operative area must have time to heal before food is introduced.

Mouth care greatly relieves the discomforts of dryness and unpleasant taste and odor from the anesthesia, inability to take oral fluids, and presence of the nasogastric tube. Usually, the patient is first given small sips of water or ice chips, followed by a clear liquid diet. The initiation of oral fluids depends on the extent of the surgery, the presence of peristalsis and the physician's preference. The patient gradually progresses to a soft diet and then, in most instances, to a normal diet. However, feedings are small and frequent.

The patient is observed carefully for any feeling of fullness or distention, and for vomiting. Repeated vomiting of small amounts of food usually indicates that the feedings are not progressing normally through the gastrointestinal tract. Sometimes this condition is due to edema near the incision. The nasogastric tube may have to be reinserted for 1 or 2 days, and oral feedings may be temporarily reduced or discontinued.

The patient is encouraged to breathe deeply and to cough up mucus. This is especially important, because the incision is high in the abdomen, and the patient tends to take shallow breaths to avoid pain. In most cases he is allowed to take a few steps and to sit in a chair for a short period on the day after surgery. This position change can be achieved without dislodging either the infusion needle or the nasogastric tube (both of which may still be in place), provided that the tubing is long enough and the patient is helped slowly and carefully. When these treatments have been discontinued, and the patient feels stronger, he is helped to walk about, and he is allowed to carry out more of his own personal hygiene.

By the time that the patient returns home, he is usually able to eat six small meals daily. Most patients who have had subtotal gastrectomy are gradually able to eat larger meals and to eat less frequently, because their bodies gradually adjust to the loss of a large portion of the stomach.

Dumping Syndrome. A few patients experience the "dumping syndrome," a complication of gastric surgery, which includes a sensation of weakness and faintness, frequently accompanied by profuse perspiration and palpitations. It is believed that these symptoms may be due to the rapid emptying of large amounts of food and fluid through the gastroenterostomy into the jejunum. (Normally, the food would pass through the entire stomach and the duodenum before reaching the jejunum.) The presence of this hypertonic solution in the gut draws fluid from the circulating blood volume into the intestine, thereby reducing the effective blood volume and producing a syncope-like syndrome.

Patients who experience the "dumping syndrome" are instructed to:

- Eat small, frequent meals.
- Avoid drinking fluids with meals. Fluids are taken later.
- Follow a low carbohydrate, high protein, moderate fat diet.
- Lie down for about a half-hour after eating.

Complications of peptic ulcer

Complications of a peptic ulcer are common, and their symptoms may be responsible for the patient's seeking medical care. The complications that are found most frequently are as follows:

Hemorrhage is the most frequent complication of peptic ulcer. Bleeding occurs when a blood vessel is eroded by the ulcer. If the vessel is large, massive hemorrhage results. If the vessel is small, even unnoticed blood loss occurs. (An examination of stool for occult blood is helpful in detecting this type of bleeding.) Continuous bleeding may be noted only when the loss of blood has been sufficient to cause faintness, weakness, and dizziness.

Vomiting of blood (hematemesis) or passing of tarry stools may occur. Blood that is vomited may appear bright red or as dark material that resembles coffee grounds. Although the tarry stool may not be as frightening to the patient as the vomiting of bright red blood, it is equally ominous, and treatment should be sought immediately. When bleeding occurs high in the gastrointestinal tract, the material passed looks black and sticky. Bleeding near the anus, such as that which may occur with hemorrhoids, causes bright red blood to be mixed with stool.

If the blood loss is severe, the symptoms of hemorrhage are acute: pallor, rapid, weak pulse, thirst, faintness, sweating, and collapse. Treatment includes complete rest, transfusions, and sometimes opiates or sedatives to relieve restlessness. Usually, nothing is given by mouth, and the patient is given intravenous fluids until the bleeding has stopped. Occasionally, small, frequent feedings of milk and cream are given while the patient is bleeding, provided that he is not vomiting.

When bleeding cannot be controlled by these measures, the patient is taken to the operating room, and the bleeding vessel is ligated; sometimes a subtotal gastrectomy is performed.

Usually every effort is made to control the bleeding without immediate surgical intervention, because it is preferable that patients who undergo surgery have supportive treatment beforehand, such as transfusions to replace lost blood. Often, surgery is necessary later to treat the underlying disease and to prevent future episodes of bleeding.

The patient is observed very carefully. Pulse, respiration, and blood pressure are taken at frequent intervals, as specified by the doctor. It is important to note restlessness, apprehension, and pallor, because they often indicate hemorrhage. The patient is kept as quiet as possible, and only the most essential aspects of personal hygiene are cared for until his condition has stabilized.

The patient is usually aware that he is bleeding and is very frightened. Assure him that measures are being promptly taken to control the bleeding and to replace the lost blood. Explain the importance of resting quietly in bed. Administer sedatives as ordered by the physician to control restlessness. Keep the environment as neat as possible; whenever possible, do not allow the patient to see the amount of blood lost. Remove soiled linen and utensils immediately. Nursing care should be carried out in a way that minimizes exertion and fatigue.

Obstruction. Edema, spasm, inflammation, and scar tissue surrounding the ulcer may interfere with the passage of food, causing retention of food in the stomach for longer than normal periods. Obstruction commonly occurs in the pyloric region. The degree of interference with the normal flow of gastric content varies. If it is slight, the patient may notice that after eating he has a feeling of fullness, distention, and nausea. If the obstruction is severe, the patient has nausea, vomiting, pain, and distention.

Physical examination, x-ray study of the gastrointestinal tract, and aspiration of the stomach contents help determine the location and severity of the obstruction. If obstruction is present, large amounts of food and secretion are obtained when a nasogastric tube is passed and the contents of the stomach are withdrawn by gentle suction.

Obstruction that is due to edema and inflammation often subsides when the patient has careful medical treatment for the ulcer. In addition to other forms of medical treatment, gastric intubation and decompression are used to drain retained food and secretions. Feedings of milk and cream are administered, sometimes by slow, continuous drip, to help neutralize gastric secretions as well as supply fluids and nourishment. The physician orders the amount and type of feeding and the length of time that it is to be administered. Sometimes, antacids are added to the feeding.

If the obstruction is treated surgically, preoperative and postoperative measures are similar to those discussed above for any patient having gastric surgery.

Perforation. The ulcer may penetrate the tissues so deeply that perforation occurs, allowing the contents of the gastrointestinal tract to seep out, causing peritonitis.

The symptoms of perforation and ensuing peritonitis are usually dramatic. The patient experiences sudden, excruciating pain in his abdomen, his face becomes ashen and drawn, and he perspires profusely. The temperature at this time may be normal or subnormal. The abdomen becomes rigid or "boardlike." It is extremely painful and tender, and the patient resists having it touched. Usually the patient lies with his knees flexed to lessen the pain. The extreme hardness of the abdomen is due to the rigidity of the abdominal muscles. Breathing is rapid and shallow. After an hour or two, the patient's face usually becomes flushed, and he develops fever. The abdomen becomes very distended and less rigid. Respirations become even more rapid and shallow. The pulse becomes rapid and weak, and the patient dies unless treatment is given promptly.

Perforation is an emergency condition. The treatment includes immediate surgical closure of the perforation, so that no further leakage can occur; suction during surgery to remove the gastric contents from the peritoneal cavity; and the administration of large doses of antibiotics. The longer the perforation goes untreated, the less likely is the patient's recovery.

When the patient returns from the operating room, he will have a nasogastric tube in place, which is connected to suction. After he has reacted from anesthesia, he is placed in low sitting position. Nothing is given by mouth, and parenteral fluids are administered. Antibiotics are given to combat the infection in the peritoneal cavity. The patient is observed carefully. Usually, his fever subsides, his abdomen becomes less distended, he breathes more easily and deeply, and his pulse is stronger and slower. Continued elevation of temperature, distention, weak, rapid pulse, and shallow, rapid breathing should be reported to the doctor, since they may indicate that peritonitis is not responding to treatment, or that the patient has developed an abscess. The patient should also be observed for symptoms of paralytic ileus, such as distention and failure to pass flatus or stool. When the patient recovers from surgery, the treatment of the underlying condition of peptic ulcer is continued.

General nutritional considerations

- The diet in the management of ulcerative colitis includes foods that are nonirritating to the bowel. Raw fruits and vegetables, highly seasoned foods, and foods high in roughage are to be avoided.
- If the patient with ulcerative colitis is a young person, it may be difficult for him to adhere to a diet that might exclude many favorite foods. Protein foods as well as a balanced nutritious diet are important.
- Neutralization of gastric acid (hydrochloric acid) by dietary measures may be employed in the treatment of gastric and duodenal ulcer. The dietary method used will vary and may be based on physician preference, the location of the ulcer, and the patient.
- Neutralizing the hydrochloric acid of the stomach promotes healing of the ulcer; thus diet becomes an extremely important part of the management of peptic ulcer.
- The diet may range from a milk and cream only regimen (Sippy diet) to a bland diet. Some authorities advocate frequent small feedings of *any* food that does not produce pain, burning, nausea, or vomiting.
- If a milk and cream regimen is ordered and the milk and cream are to be left at the bedside, they must be kept chilled to prevent souring. Placing them in a basin filled with ice or using insulated thermos-type containers will delay souring.
- Foods to be avoided by patients on a bland diet include:
  - all fried foods.
  - canned soups.
  - raw vegetables, gas-forming vegetables.
  - pork, meat gravies, smoked meats.
  - raw fruits (except bananas, orange juice).
  - coarse breads and cereals.
  - coffee, tea, alcoholic and carbonated beverages.
  - pastries, candy, nuts, raisins.
  - spicy foods, highly seasoned foods.

General pharmacological considerations

- Antacids (e.g., Maalox, Gelusil, Mylanta) are used to neutralize gastric hydrochloric acid. These drugs may be given every 1 to 2 hours up to 2 to 4 times per day. In some instances the antacid may be ordered left at the patient's bedside for self-administration.
- If the patient will be responsible for taking his own antacid, the nurse should (1) show him how to measure the drug in a medicine glass, (2) explain the importance of antacids in the treatment of peptic ulcer, (3) explain the time of day the drug is to be taken (every

hour, every 2 hours on the even hour, etc.), (4) be sure the patient has a clock or watch so he knows when to take his drug, (5) periodically check the supply of the drug and measuring cups, (6) periodically check to see if the patient is taking his medication.

■ Some patients may note that use of antacids may cause constipation or diarrhea.

■ Cholinergic blocking agents may be given to patients with a peptic ulcer to decrease gastric motility and secretions. These drugs may cause a variety of side effects the most notable of which are dry mouth, urinary retention, and blurred vision. Many patients experience only dry mouth. If combined with sedatives, these products may cause drowsiness; the patient should be cautioned about engaging in any activity (such as driving a car) requiring alertness.

■ Patients scheduled for bowel surgery may receive an antibiotic capable of reducing the number of bacteria in the colon. It is believed that the reduction in the number of bacteria lessens the chance of postoperative bowel or peritoneal infection. Examples of drugs used for this purpose are neomycin sulfate and kanamycin (Kantrex). When used for this purpose the drugs are given orally.

Bibliography

AMERICAN CANCER SOCIETY: *A Cancer Source Book for Nurses.* New York, American Cancer Society, 1975.

BALLINGER, W. F. et al: *Alexander's Care of the Patient in Surgery.* St. Louis, Mosby, 1973.

BARGEN, J. A.: Chronic ulcerative colitis (pictorial). Hosp. Med. 11:6, August, 1975.

CHERLOFSKY, N. et al: Dorothy B. Dx: ulcerative colitis (care st). Nurs. Care 8:10, January, 1975.

DELUCA, J. C.: The ulcerative colitis personality. Nurs. Clin. North Am. 5:23, March, 1970.

DONALDSON, R. M.: The puzzle of complicating peptic ulcer. Consultant 15:124, September, 1975.

EMMANUEL, S.: Basic surgery: Surgery for peptic ulcer, Part 4, (pictorial). RN 38:OR/ED 5, April, 1975.

HARDY, J. D. et al: *Rhoads' Textbook of Surgery,* ed. 5. Philadelphia, Lippincott, 1976.

NORDMARK, M. T. and ROHWEDER, A. W.: *Scientific Foundations of Nursing,* ed. 3. Philadelphia, Lippincott, 1975.

SCHWARTZ, S. et al: *Principles of Surgery,* ed. 2. New York, McGraw-Hill, 1974.

SHAFER, K. N. et al: *Medical-Surgical Nursing,* ed. 6. St. Louis, Mosby, 1975.

SLEISENGER, M. and FORDTRAN, J. S.: *Gastrointestinal Disease.* Philadelphia, Saunders, 1973.

WATKINSON, G.: Ulcerative colitis. Nurs. Mirror 142:50, July 24, 1975.

CHAPTER—30

The patient with cancer of the gastrointestinal tract

On completion of this chapter the student will:

- **Describe the early and late symptoms of cancer of the gastrointestinal tract.**
- **List the methods of diagnosis of gastrointestinal malignancies.**
- **Describe the treatment for cancer of the mouth, esophagus, stomach, colon, and rectum.**
- **Formulate a general postoperative nursing care plan for patients with surgery for gastrointestinal malignancies.**
- **Be able to participate in the nursing management of the patient with surgery for gastrointestinal malignancies, including preoperative as well as postoperative preparations and care.**

Cancer of the digestive tract is a major cause of illness and death. It occurs commonly in every major area of the gastrointestinal tract except the small intestine, where it is unusual. Cancer of the mouth, esophagus, stomach, or rectum is more common in men than in women, whereas cancer of the colon is slightly more common in women.

Symptoms

Cancer of the digestive tract causes the same general symptoms as cancer elsewhere in the body: for example, weakness, weight loss, fatigue, and anemia. As is the case with cancer of other organs, pain is often a late symptom. Cancer of the mouth and tongue has the advantage of usually being visible to the patient and his physician relatively early in the disease. Frequently, it appears as a lump, an ulcer, or a sore that persists.

Cancer of the esophagus, stomach, or colon causes few, if any, early symptoms, making the problem of prompt diagnosis difficult. Patients with cancer of the esophagus may notice a slight difficulty in swallowing solid food and a sensation of pressure or fullness under the sternum. Usually, these symptoms are so mild when they are first noted that they may be overlooked or attributed to "nerves" or indigestion. As the malignant tumor grows, the esophagus becomes obstructed gradually, and yet relentlessly. Inability to swallow solid food and prompt vomiting of food after it is eaten are typical. Pain may be severe late in the course of the illness. The patient becomes extremely emaciated, because food cannot pass beyond the obstruction.

Cancer of the stomach usually produces vague symptoms at the outset. Slight indigestion, loss of appetite, flatulence, and a distaste for certain foods that previously were enjoyed may occur. In other cases, the patient may experience no symptoms until late in the disease, when he may have severe pain, vomiting of blood, or passage of tarry stools.

A change in bowel habits is often the earliest warning of cancer of the large intestine. As the lumen of the bowel becomes gradually obstructed by the tumor, the patient may develop alternating constipation and diarrhea. Diarrhea results when the intestine attempts to push the material past the obstruction by very forceful peristalsis. General symptoms, such as anemia, may appear before any symptoms referable to the intestinal tract are noted. Later in the illness, the patient may have tarry stools, or if the lesion is near the anus, frank blood in the stool. Symptoms of intestinal obstruction appear when the tumor has become large enough to prevent the normal passage of intestinal contents through the colon.

The symptoms of rectal cancer may attract attention more promptly. The patient often passes bright red blood with his stool, or his stool may emerge pencil- or ribbon-shaped, due to passing through a narrowed opening. Constipation or diarrhea may occur. A feeling of fullness or discomfort in the rectum is sometimes noticed; however, severe pain is usually a late symptom.

Associated conditions

There are some benign conditions that are known to be predisposing to cancer. *Leukoplakia,* patches of white, thickened tissue in the mouth, is often considered to be a forerunner of cancer. Leukoplakia is most common among heavy smokers. If the white patches do not disappear when the patient stops smoking and gives careful attention to mouth hygiene, their surgical removal may be recommended to prevent the development of cancer.

Patients with *ulcerative colitis* have a higher incidence than the normal population of cancer of the colon.

People who have polyps in the bowel also may be predisposed to the development of cancer of the colon. The prompt and the effective treatment of conditions that often seem to precede cancer is important. The annual follow-up of patients with polyps found on sigmoidoscopy or by barium enema is important in detecting early malignancies which may supervene. Similar programs are followed in patients with ulcerative colitis despite inactivity of the colitis.

Diagnosis

Cancer of the digestive tract, like cancer elsewhere, is diagnosed by a careful history and physical examination, by special tests to reveal the presence of a tumor, and by biopsy. For example, an x-ray examination of the esophagus after the patient has swallowed barium may reveal a tumor that is obstructing the esophagus. Proctoscopy, sigmoidoscopy, and gastroscopy are also employed. Cytological examination of exfoliated cells (Papanicolaou's test) sometimes is performed. For example, a specimen of esophageal or gastric washings can be collected from the esophagus or the stomach by means of a saline lavage through a nasogastric tube; the cells in the specimen are examined for malignancy.

Although the appearance of a tumor may suggest cancer, the final diagnosis is established by microscopic examination of a piece of the tissue itself, to determine whether or not it is malignant. When the lesion is readily accessible, as in the mouth, biopsy may be performed very easily. Areas that are less accessible may have biopsies taken through the instrument used for visual examination. For instance, a biopsy of a rectal tumor may be performed through the proctoscope. Some tumors are so inaccessible that tissue for examination can be obtained only by surgery.

An awareness of danger signals is most important. If patients report even minor symptoms to the doctor, there is greater opportunity for early diagnosis, and cure is more likely.

Treatment

If the disease is discovered in time, malignant tissue may be removed surgically or destroyed by radiation. If the malignant tissue can be eradicated completely, the patient is cured. When the disease has metastasized, surgery, radiation, or chemotherapy may be used as palliative measures.

Supportive treatment includes the maintenance of nutrition, the use of drugs to relieve pain, and the correction of anemia by the use of transfusions.

Nursing management

In order to remove malignant tissue, it is often necessary to perform radical surgery that alters the appearance of the patient or the way in which his body functions. Extensive surgery of the mouth and the adjacent structures can be disfiguring. A patient who cannot swallow and cannot eat normally must be fed through a gastrostomy tube. The threat of cancer, the fear that all malignant tissue has not been removed, and the necessity for radical surgery have a tremendous emotional impact on the patient and his family. Preparation for surgery involves helping the patient to understand what it will entail, and how he can care for himself afterward. If complete recovery is not expected, the family may need to assume a large measure of responsibility for the patient's care when he returns home. Referral to the public health nurse is often very helpful in assisting the patient and his family with home care.

Regardless of the site of the primary lesion, the nursing needs of patients with cancer are in many respects similar.

Cancer of the mouth

The surgical excision of malignant tissue in the mouth may result in complete cure, provided that it is performed early (Fig. 30-1). Sometimes, surgery is extensive and may be disfiguring; it may interfere with normal breathing and swallowing as well. For instance, considerable edema may occur postoperatively, leading

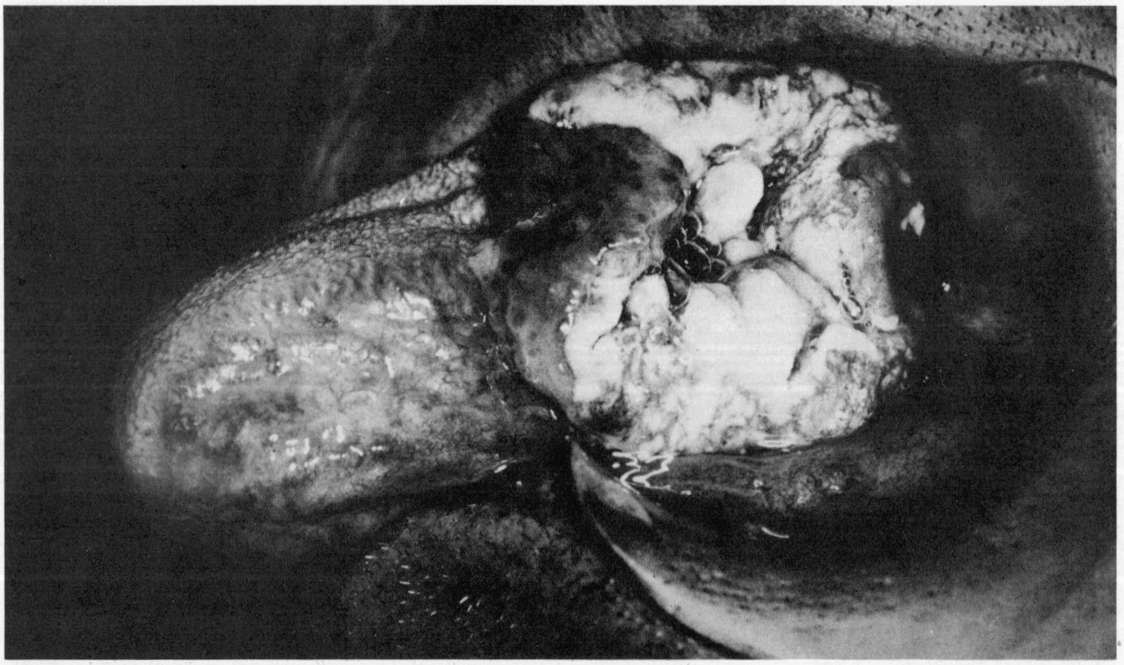

figure 30-1. Cancer of the tongue, advanced stage. (Photograph: Daniel P. Montayne)

to obstruction of the respiratory passages. A tracheostomy may be necessary during the postoperative period until edema subsides. The patient may have to be fed through a nasogastric tube until healing is sufficient to allow him to swallow.

Postoperative management

Ordinarily, when the patient returns from the operating room, he is positioned flat, either on his abdomen or on his side, with his head turned to the side to facilitate drainage from the mouth. Suction is carried out as necessary to prevent aspiration of secretions.

When the patient recovers from the effects of anesthesia, he is often more comfortable with the head of the bed elevated. This position usually makes it easier to breathe deeply and to cough up secretions, and it helps to control edema. Coughing and deep breathing are necessary in order to prevent postoperative pneumonia and atelectasis. Firm support of the patient's head and neck helps to lessen pain during coughing. At first the nurse provides this support for the patient; later he is taught to do it himself. The hands should be placed gently but firmly on either side of the patient's head, supporting his head to prevent excessive movement when he coughs.

Bleeding on the dressings, rapid pulse, a fall in blood pressure, or the coughing up of bright red blood should be noted and reported. Expectoration of some dark blood is to be expected in the immediate postoperative period. The patient's breathing should be observed and the physician notified immediately if the patient experiences respiratory difficulty or cyanosis. Equipment for suction, administration of oxygen, and care of, or performance of, a tracheostomy should be kept at the bedside during the immediate postoperative period.

Care and judgment are necessary in the administration of narcotics postoperatively, since they can cause respiratory depression.

Old blood and mucus tend to collect in the mouth during the postoperative period. Unless the mouth is kept scrupulously clean, infection is likely to occur, and very unpleasant odors and an offensive taste in the mouth are distressing to the patient and those who are near him. Cleansing must be done frequently, and precautions should be taken to prevent trauma or infection. Sterile technique is used in some hospitals; others use clean technique because the mouth normally harbors bacteria and cannot be kept sterile.

Usually, the mouth is gently irrigated to keep it clean. The frequency of irrigations and the type of solution to be used are ordered by the physician. Normal saline or hydrogen peroxide (H_2O_2) are commonly used. The patient's head should be turned to the side, to allow the solution to run in gently and flow out into the emesis basin. A soft rubber catheter is useful for this purpose, because it does not cause trauma. The mouth should not be irrigated until the patient regains consciousness after surgery, because he might aspirate the solution. Precautions should be taken to keep the dressings or the patient's bed or gown from getting wet during irrigations. The emesis basin should be placed carefully in position to catch the return, not allowing too much solution to run in at a time. Plastic material should be used to protect dressings and linen.

Because the postoperative patient is often unable to swallow, he is given parenteral fluids immediately, followed by feedings through the nasogastric tube. When the patient is able to swallow, he is first given small amounts of liquid, and gradually progresses from liquids to soft foods as tolerated. The patient should be observed carefully when he first attempts to swallow small amounts of liquid. If he coughs and

Table 30-1.
Postoperative nursing management of the patient with extensive oral surgery for cancer

Vital signs should be taken q1-4h or as ordered. The temperature is taken rectally.
The patient should be positioned in bed as ordered until he is awake and then the head of the bed should be elevated.
Signs of respiratory distress must be reported promptly.
The patient must be made to turn, cough, deep breathe, and do leg exercises q2h.
To lessen discomfort, the patient's head should be supported when he is coughing and moving.
Suction should be administered as necessary.
Special mouth care and irrigations are given as ordered.
Mouth and dressings must be checked for excessive bleeding.
A pad and pen or a Magic Slate should be supplied for patient-nurse communication.

has difficulty in swallowing, suction must be applied immediately. Further oral feedings should not be given without checking with the physician. Some patients have had such extensive surgery that they continue to require tube feedings. These patients are taught to carry out the feeding themselves.

Problems

Communication with others presents a real problem to patients who have had extensive oral surgery. The patient's ability to tell others about his discomfort, to express fears, to ask questions, or to call for help are impaired at the time when he most needs the opportunity to communicate with others. The Magic Slate is so useful that many nurses consider it standard equipment at the bedside of a patient who is unable to speak, yet able to write. Merely lifting the plastic cover erases the writing, and the slate is ready for reuse. Special care should be taken that the patient's call bell is within reach at all times, and that his call light is answered promptly.

The nurse may be helpful in minimizing the patient's distress over his appearance after oral surgery by:

- Providing privacy during his first attempts to swallow and to eat.
- Helping the patient to minimize the problem of drooling. He needs plenty of tissues, and must be directed to tilt his head at intervals, so that the saliva is directed back, where it can be swallowed. Sometimes a small catheter attached to low pressure suction is used to remove excess saliva from the mouth.
- Helping him to pay extra attention to personal cleanliness and grooming. Clean bedclothes, hair neatly combed, and attention to his appearance as soon as the physician permits, all help the patient to feel more presentable.

Complications

Hemorrhage. Large blood vessels, such as the carotid arteries, are near the oral cavity. Serious hemorrhage may result when an artery in invaded by cancer and becomes ulcerated, or when necrosis follows radiotherapy. The physician advises the nurse which patients are most likely to develop hemorrhage. These patients should be placed near the nurse's station, so that they can be observed frequently.

If hemorrhage should occur, the nurse applies direct digital pressure over the bleeding point until the physician arrives. Another nurse, or even a patient, should be asked to report the emergency, so that the nurse who first applies digital pressure can remain with the patient and continue to apply pressure until the physician arrives.

The physician usually orders a narcotic to relieve the patient's apprehension and transfusions to replace lost blood. Ligation of the bleeding vessel is often necessary. The nurse's role involves assisting the physician quickly with control of the bleeding and assuring the patient verbally and by means of swift, calm competent care that everything possible is being done to control the bleeding. After the bleeding has stopped, the patient is likely to be exhausted and apprehensive that it may recur. Visiting and observing him frequently are important in detecting any further bleeding and in assuring him that his condition is being checked carefully. The frequent observation of pulse and blood pressure is important.

Respiratory Obstruction. If respiratory obstruction should occur, it may necessitate an emergency tracheostomy. Labored breathing and cyanosis should be noted and reported promptly. Suction, avoiding oversedation and depression of the cough reflex, and encouraging the patient to cough up secretions are important in preventing pneumonia and atelectasis, which may be caused by aspiration of secretions or blood.

Cancer of the esophagus

Symptoms of cancer of the esophagus usually develop slowly. By the time the symptom of difficulty in swallowing (dysphagia) is noticeable, the cancer may have extended and invaded surrounding tissues and lymphatics. In the beginning, symptoms may be mild with vague feelings of discomfort and difficulty in swallowing some foods. As the disease progresses solid foods become almost impossible to swallow and the patient resorts to liquids. Along with this progressive dysphagia there is weight loss. Pain is a late symptom. Diagnosis is made by a barium swallow and esophagoscopy.

The patient who enters the hospital for the treatment of cancer of the esophagus often has become emaciated from inability to swallow and regurgitation of the food that he attempts to eat. Preoperative preparation involves improving his nutrition and restoring water and electrolyte regulation. The patient receives parenteral fluids as they are required, and if he is able to swallow liquids, he is given a high calorie, high protein liquid diet. Frequent opportunities to rinse his mouth help relieve unpleasant taste and odor.

Surgical treatment

Treatment of cancer of the esophagus usually depends on the extent of the lesion and evidence of metastasis. Radiation is used as a palliative measure for inoperable lesions but surgical resection of the esophagus is attempted if possible.

Several surgical approaches may be used, depending on the site of the lesion—whether it is in the upper, middle, or lower third of the esophagus. For tumors of the lower third, the esophagus is resected and the remaining two-thirds are anastomosed to the stomach. Lesions of the upper two-thirds of the esophagus are resected and the esophagus replaced with a section of jejunum or colon.

If the patient is too ill to withstand surgery, a gastrostomy may be performed, permitting food to be introduced directly into the stomach through an opening on the patient's abdomen. Sometimes the gastrostomy is a temporary measure that will be used until the patient's nutritional status has improved sufficiently to permit surgery. The gastrostomy opening is then closed.

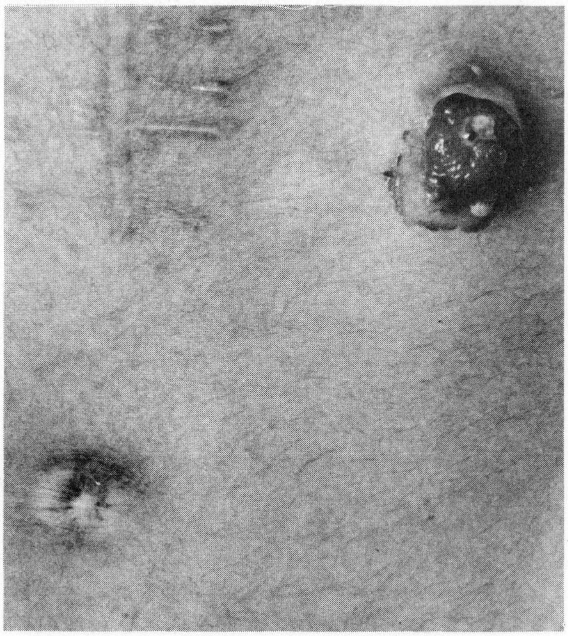

figure 30-2. A permanent gastrostomy may be performed when the patient cannot take food or fluids by the oral route. (Photograph—D. Atkinson)

Postoperative nursing management

After surgery for cancer of the esophagus, the patient is given intravenous feedings and nothing by mouth for several days to allow time for the healing of the tissues. The drainage from the nasogastric tube is carefully watched for any evidence of bleeding. Although a small amount of blood may drain through the tube when the patient first returns from the operating room, the drainage should return promptly to the yellow-green color of normal gastric secretions.

Measures that apply to the management of any patient who has had chest surgery include:

- Care of closed chest drainage.
- Particular emphasis on deep breathing and coughing.
- Administration of oxygen.

Often the patient is allowed to take a few steps and to sit in a chair the day after surgery to stimulate deep breathing and to improve circulation. Closed chest drainage and drainage from the nasogastric tube are continued even when the patient is out of bed. Special care is required to see that the tubing is long enough to permit the patient to move a step or two to his chair. Some patients are fed postoperatively through a temporary gastrostomy for 4 to 7 days. In these patients the gastrostomy tube rather than a nasogastric tube is used to decompress the stomach.

After several days the patient is permitted small amounts of water frequently. He is observed carefully for regurgitation of the fluid and for such symptoms as dyspnea and fever that might indicate seepage of the fluid through the operative area to the mediastinum. Sitting up during and just after the ingestion of water helps to prevent regurgitation.

The patient gradually progresses to swallowing other liquids, soft foods, and, finally, a normal diet. If the stomach has been drawn up into the thoracic cavity, the patient may have a feeling of pressure in his chest and dyspnea after eating. These symptoms can be minimized by frequent small meals and by not allowing the patient to lie down for several hours after eating.

Management of a patient with a gastrostomy

Cancer and stricture of the esophagus from swallowing chemicals are examples of conditions that cause obstruction of the esophagus, and that may necessitate either a temporary or a permanent gastrostomy (Fig. 30-2). Gastrostomy is a relatively minor procedure. It can be performed under local anesthesia, and it can be carried out even if the patient is very weak and debilitated.

Usually, it is very hard for the patient to face the prospect of gastrostomy. Eating is one of the very basic pleasures of life. Although the patient's nutrition can be maintained by gastrostomy, thereafter he is denied the physical satisfaction of taste and the emotional satisfaction of companionship during meals. The patient feeds himself by means of a funnel and a catheter inserted into his stomach through the gastrostomy.

When the gastrostomy is performed, a catheter is inserted into the opening and secured to the abdominal wall. To prevent the leakage of gastric contents, the end of the catheter is clamped except for the time that the patient is being fed. The leakage that may occur around the tube causes discomfort because the gastric contents are irritating to the skin. Dressings are applied to absorb any drainage that occurs around the tube; they must be changed frequently. The skin must be washed often with mild soap and water to prevent excoriation. Ointments such as zinc oxide may be applied to the skin to help prevent irritation.

Initial feedings through the tube usually consist of small amounts of tap water, which are gradually increased to larger amounts as tolerated. The amount of fluid and the frequency of its administration are specified by the surgeon. When the patient is able to take clear liquids through the tube, the feedings are begun.

After sufficient healing, the gastrostomy tube may be removed and inserted only for feedings. The patient learns to insert the catheter approximately 4 inches into the gastrostomy and to pour the feedings into a funnel that has been attached to the end of the catheter. Usually, about 300 to 500 ml. is given at a time. Some patients feel uncomfortably full and even nauseated unless the feedings are given in small amounts. Therefore, they must take their feedings more frequently to obtain the total amount ordered by the physician. The tube and the funnel are washed and rinsed thoroughly after each use. A permanent plastic "button," sutured to the abdominal wall, with a screw-in plug, keeps the stoma closed between feedings.

Many physicians recommend that the patient's normal diet be converted to a form suitable for tube feeding by the use of a blender. This method is considered desirable if tube feedings must be continued for a long period, since normal nutrition can be maintained, and the patient's family can prepare his meals readily at home.

Cancer of the stomach

Heredity and chronic inflammation of the stomach appear to be causative factors in cancer of the stomach. Early symptoms of gastric cancer are often vague. As the tumor enlarges, it usually begins to obstruct either the cardiac or pyloric openings, which gives rise to symptoms. The patient may notice a prolonged feeling of fullness after eating, anorexia, weight loss, and anemia. The stool usually contains occult blood. Pain is a late symptom.

Diagnosis is made by fluoroscopy, a barium swallow, and gastroscopy. A gastric analysis may show the absence of free hydrochloric acid.

The number of persons developing cancer of the stomach in the United States seems to be decreasing. The reason for this change is not understood.

The treatment of cancer of the stomach often involves total gastrectomy. The entire stomach is removed, and the continuity of the gastrointestinal tract is restored by joining the jejunum and the esophagus. Depending on the location and the size of the tumor, it may be possible to perform a subtotal rather than a total gastrectomy, thus preserving a more normal digestive function. The spleen is removed with all or part of the stomach in cases of cancer, since metastasis to the splenic lymph nodes is common.

Management of a patient after total gastrectomy differs from that of a patient after subtotal gastrectomy in that:

- The patient requires care similar to that of any patient who has had chest surgery since the thoracic cavity, as well as the abdominal cavity, must be entered to remove the entire stomach.
- Very little drainage should be expected to return through the nasogastric tube, because the stomach, which normally forms the secretions, has been removed.
- Oral feedings are begun several days postoperatively with small amounts of tap water given at frequent intervals. Gradually, the patient progresses to frequent, small feedings of bland foods.
- The patient continues to eat frequent small meals. Because of the removal of his entire stomach, he is unable to tolerate large meals, and often experiences difficulty in digesting food. He should be given easily digested foods and instructed to eat slowly and chew his food thoroughly.

■ Injections of vitamin B_{12} are sometimes necessary for the rest of the patient's life, because once the stomach has been removed, the intrinsic factor necessary for absorption of vitamin B_{12} is no longer produced. If therapy with vitamin B_{12} is not administered, the patient will develop symptoms of pernicious anemia.

Cancer of the colon

The chief symptoms of cancer of the colon (Fig. 30-3) are a change in bowel habits, blood in the stool, and anemia. If undetected and untreated, a bowel obstruction may result (Fig. 30-4). Treatment of cancer of the colon is primarily surgical. Sometimes a combination of surgery and radiotherapy is utilized. Depending on the location of the tumor and the time that treatment is instituted, it may be possible to completely remove the malignant tissue of the affected section of bowel and to restore the normal continuity of the tract by joining the remaining portions of the intestine. If this treatment is not possible because of the size and the spread of the tumor or because of the patient's general condition, a temporary or a permanent colostomy may have to be performed to relieve the obstruction caused by the tumor. Sometimes, a temporary colostomy is carried out to relieve obstruction, and more radical surgery, to remove the malignant growth and reestablish the continuity of the bowel, is performed when the patient's physical condition has improved. Discussion of the management of a patient with a colostomy is presented in Chapter 31.

Cancer of the rectum

Early signs of rectal cancer are a change in bowel habits, bright red blood in the stool, alternating constipation and diarrhea, and abdominal cramping.

The location of the tumor will help the surgeon to decide whether rectal cancer may be treated by an abdominoperineal resection or a "pull-through" operation that removes the diseased area of the rectum but preserves the anus. In some instances it has been found beneficial to give radiotherapy before undertaking surgical treatment.

Surgical treatment

In an abdominoperineal resection, the anus, the rectum, and part of the sigmoid colon are removed. The operation is a major and lengthy procedure. First,

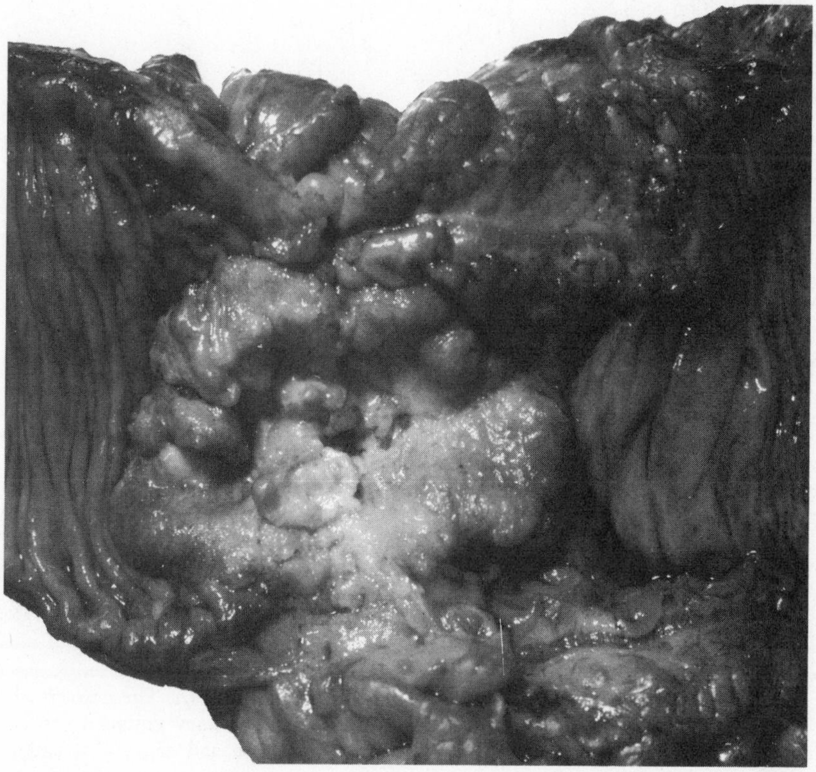

figure 30-3. Carcinoma of the transverse colon (Courtesy P. S. Milley, M.D.)

an abdominal incision is made; through it the sigmoid is divided, and the proximal portion of the sigmoid is brought out onto the abdomen to form a permanent colostomy. Then the patient is placed in lithotomy position, and the anus, the rectum, and the lower portion of the sigmoid are removed through the perineal incision.

When the tumor is located higher in the rectum near the sigmoid, it is sometimes possible to remove the tumor and the involved portion of the rectum, to leave the anal sphincter intact, and to pull the sigmoid colon down to the anus, thus enabling the patient to continue to evacuate through the anus.

Nursing management

After abdominoperineal resection, nursing management involves preparation of the patient and care following a permanent colostomy. In addition to the abdominal incision and the colostomy, the patient returns from the operating room with a perineal wound. Dressings over the perineal wound must be checked carefully for bleeding. Usually, there is profuse serosanguineous drainage, and sometimes the dressings must be reinforced a short time after surgery to prevent soiling. Placing small disposable bed pads under the patient's buttocks helps to protect the bedding. The pads can be changed easily and quickly whenever they become soiled. When sufficient healing has taken

Table 30-2.
Postoperative nursing management of the patient with an abdominoperineal resection

Vital signs should be taken frequently until stable. Then they may be taken q4h or as ordered. The oral or axillary method is used to determine temperature.
Urinary output should be checked via a Foley catheter hourly. The physician should be notified if output falls below 30 ml. per hour.
The rectal dressing must be observed hourly for excessive bleeding.
Pads beneath hips require changing when soiled with rectal drainage.
The patient's position should be changed q2h.
IPPB should be administered as ordered.
The patient should do deep breathing and leg exercises q2h while awake.
Medication for pain should be administered promptly.
The abdominal incision and colostomy dressing should be checked for drainage.
The nasogastric tube should be connected to suction. It is necessary to check hourly for effective suctioning of gastric contents.

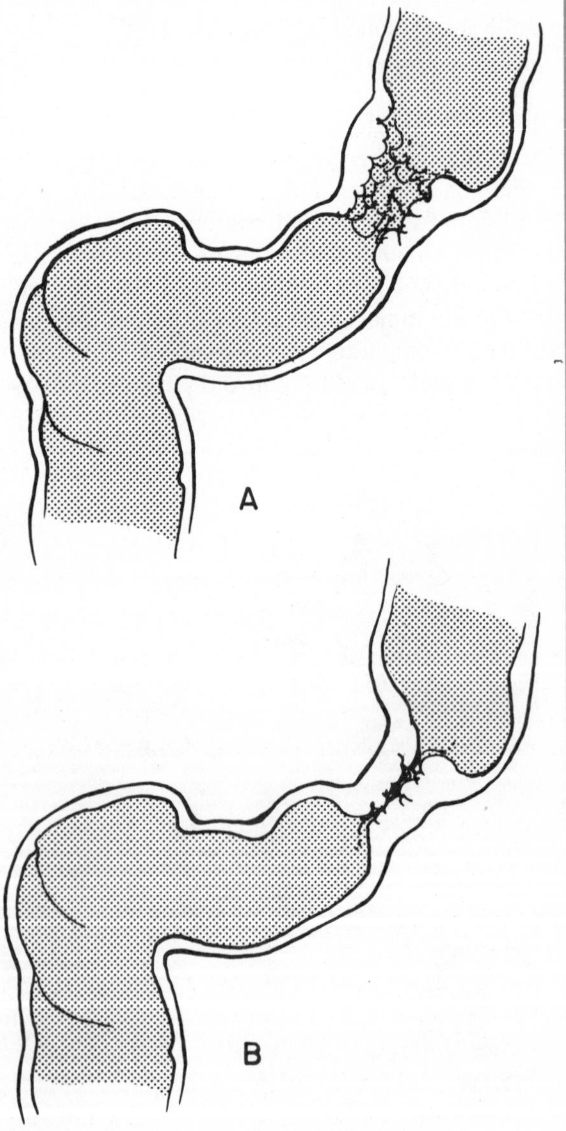

figure 30-4. Cancer of the colon. (A) The new growth proliferates. (B) As the malignancy grows, it can occlude the lumen of the colon and cause obstruction.

place, the physician may request that the entire rectal dressing be changed by the nurse whenever it becomes soiled.

Because abdominoperineal resection involves such extensive surgery, it is especially important to observe the patient for shock after he returns from the operating room. The physician's orders concerning the observation of pulse, respirations, and blood pressure must be followed carefully; an increased pulse rate and a fall in blood pressure must be reported immediately.

Patients who have undergone abdominoperineal resection usually are acutely uncomfortable during the first few days after surgery. Most surgical patients have one operative area to cause pain; these patients have two—one on the abdomen and one in the perineal region. As a result, they commonly require more frequent administration of narcotics than patients who have had less extensive surgery.

Measures that help to prevent respiratory complications and thrombophlebitis are especially important, because patients who have had abdominoperineal resection are usually kept in bed longer than most other surgical patients to permit the healing of the extensive perineal wound. If the patient stands and walks about before the pelvic floor has healed sufficiently, a hernia may develop in the perineal region.

Careful positioning helps to minimize pain. The patient is often most comfortable on his side, a position that avoids pressure on either of the operative areas. In the early postoperative period, he is turned frequently from one side to the other, and he is encouraged to breathe deeply, to cough, and to exercise his legs. When the most acute discomfort has subsided, the patient frequently finds that he can lie on his back as well as on either side. Supporting the perineal dressings firmly with a T-binder is important in encouraging the patient to move about in bed. Unless the dressings are held snugly in place, the patient is often reluctant to turn and move his legs for fear of dislodging the dressing.

Because a distended bladder is more subject to injury during operation, an indwelling catheter (Foley) is inserted just prior to surgery to keep the bladder empty. It is left in place for several days after the operation, since most patients have difficulty voiding immediately after abdominoperineal resection. The catheter also helps to prevent the soiling of perineal dressings with urine during the immediate postoperative period. When the catheter has been removed, the time and the amount of each voiding are carefully noted to determine whether the patient is able to empty his bladder satisfactorily. If the perineal dressings become soiled with urine, they should be changed promptly.

Gastrointestinal decompression ordinarily is carried out for several days postoperatively. Intravenous fluids and transfusions are given as necessary during this period. The patient then begins taking fluids orally, and he progresses gradually to a regular diet. Antibiotics are usually given to prevent infection.

The length of time that the patient must remain in bed varies. Often he is permitted out of bed 3 days after the operation. Because of the extensive surgery and the long period of bed rest, he is usually quite weak and needs considerable assistance. Placing a rubber ring or foam rubber pad on the seat of his chair helps to lessen discomfort while he is sitting.

If packing is left in the perineal wound, it is removed gradually. Some surgeons prefer the use of a drain or rubber dam rather than packing. Irrigation of the perineal wound with normal saline or hydrogen peroxide may be ordered. The surgeon may have to be consulted regarding his preference as to technique used in irrigating the area. Some surgeons prefer the insertion of a catheter; others order a superficial irrigation of the wound.

When the patient is allowed out of bed, sitz baths are often ordered to promote healing of the perineal wound. Because the patient is weak and may become faint, it is important not to leave him alone in the sitz bath the first few times that he has this treatment. Depending on the patient's condition and the distance between his bed and the sitz bath, it is often advisable to take him to the bathroom in a wheelchair. A rubber ring is placed in the bottom of the tub to lessen the discomfort caused by sitting in the hard tub and to permit the warm water to circulate freely around the operative area. Most patients find that sitz baths help in relieving discomfort, as well as in promoting healing.

Dressings are worn over the perineal wound until healing occurs, and drainage ceases. Later in the postoperative period, when healing has progressed and the patient is stronger, he learns to change the perineal dressings as well as the colostomy dressings or appliance. Perineal pads are often used instead of perineal dressings during convalescence. The patient is taught the procedure for taking sitz baths at home, using either the bathtub or a large basin.

General nutritional considerations

- Gastrostomy or nasogastric feedings may be necessary for the patient having surgery of the mouth and adjacent structures. Early in the postoperative period the patient is fed by the intravenous route until peristalsis returns.
- Patients with advanced cancer of the esophagus will require an intensive program prior to surgery to restore water and electrolytes and improve the nutritional state. While some may be able to take oral feedings, others may require gastrostomy feedings. A high calorie, high protein liquid diet is given. Hyperalimentation may be necessary in some cases.
- Gastrostomy feedings average 300 to 500 ml. per feeding. If the patient experiences discomfort or complains of nausea, the physician should be consulted regarding a reduction in the tube feeding volume.
- Patients going home with a permanent gastrostomy tube should be encouraged to purchase a blender for the preparation of gastrostomy tube feedings.

General pharmacological considerations

- Narcotics, which depress respirations, are administered with caution during the postoperative period to patients having surgery of the mouth and adjacent structures. If the patient has difficulty breathing, or if there appears to be excessive mucus or blood in the nose or mouth, the physician should be notified before a narcotic is administered. In some cases it may be necessary to give a smaller dose.
- The patient with a total gastrectomy will usually require injections of vitamin B_{12}. This drug is normally given on a monthly or bimonthly basis.
- Patients with an abdominoperineal resection usually require frequent administration of a narcotic analgesic. The nurse should observe these patients for signs of respiratory depression.

Bibliography

AMERICAN CANCER SOCIETY: *A Cancer Source Book for Nurses.* New York, American Cancer Society, 1975.

BOUCHARD, R. and OWENS, N. F.: *Nursing Care of the Cancer Patient,* ed. 2. St. Louis, Mosby, 1972.

GIVEN, B. A. and SIMMONS, S. J.: *Nursing Care of the Patient with Gastrointestinal Disorders.* St. Louis, Mosby, 1971.

GORMICAN, A. et al: Nasogastric tube feedings: Practical considerations in prescription and evaluation. Nurs. Dig. 2:59, January, 1974.

HARDY, JAMES D., ed.: *Rhoads' Textbook of Surgery,* ed. 5. Philadelphia, Lippincott, 1976.

HEIMLICH, H. J.: Esophagoplasty using the reversed gastric tube, (pictorial). Hosp. Pract. 10:80, July, 1975.

HENDRICKSON, F. R. et al: Radiotherapy treatment for cancer: Guidelines for nursing care. J. Prac. Nurs. 22:18, February, 1972.

MICHAELIS, L. L. et al: Bypass surgery: Nutritional palliation for alimentary tract cancer, (pictorial). RN 36:OR/ED 10, September, 1973.

RODMAN, M. J.: Anticancer chemotherapy, Part 1. RN 35:45, February, 1972.

———: Anticancer chemotherapy, Part 2. RN 35:61, March, 1972.

SHAFER, K. N. et al: *Medical-Surgical Nursing,* ed. 6. St. Louis, Mosby, 1975.

CHAPTER—31

The patient with an ileostomy or a colostomy

On completion of this chapter the student will:

- **Describe and define the methods used to divert the fecal stream and give the rationale for each.**
- **Formulate a nursing care plan and assist in the nursing management of a patient with an ostomy.**
- **Discuss the different methods of controlling gas and odor in the ostomy patient.**
- **Describe the signs and symptoms of intestinal obstruction and the methods used to relieve it.**
- **Recognize the impact of the change in body image in the new ostomate.**
- **Understand the influence of visitors from ostomy groups on the patient's acceptance of his stoma.**

Ostomy as used here refers to an opening of the bowel onto the skin. There are two main types: *ileostomy,* in which the ileum is opened onto the skin, and *colostomy,* in which the colon is opened onto the skin. Fecal material drains from both of these openings, which are called stomas.

Stomas are created in the treatment of such conditions as ulcerative colitis, multiple polyposis, cancer or other obstructive lesions, and injury. Other types of stomas may be created, for example, when a ureter is brought out onto the skin (ureterostomy). The patient need not be disabled; there is, however, a change in his body which he must learn to manage and control. Teaching him to achieve this control is an important nursing role. Equally important is the nurse's role in supporting the patient during his preoperative and postoperative experience, so that he is helped to accept the stoma.

The stoma may be temporary or permanent. At times it is not possible for the surgeon to determine the extent of surgery required. However, regardless of whether the ostomy is temporary or permanent, the patient requires assistance in learning to manage it.

The management of a patient with an ostomy should be patient-centered and living-oriented. It begins when the patient seeks care, and continues throughout the therapeutic phase and the period of recovery after discharge. The ostomate (one who has had ostomy surgery) continues to need medical and nursing care after hospitalization until he has gained security and competence in the management of the ostomy.

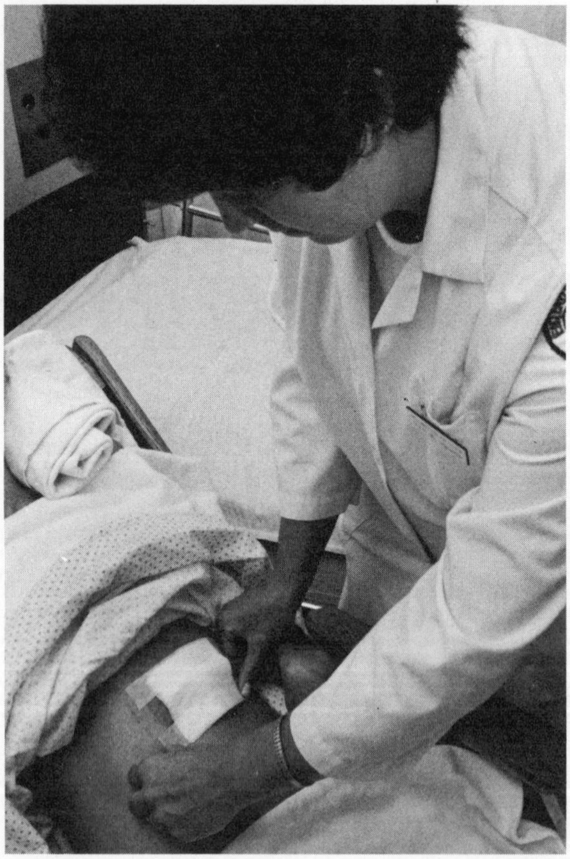

figure 31-1. An enterostomal therapist is a nurse trained in the care and teaching of ostomy patients. One of her important functions is helping the ostomate adjust to a temporary or permanent alteration in body image. (Photograph—D. Atkinson)

Planning nursing management

Each patient requires a care plan adapted to his individual requirements that considers not only his surgical experience, but also his preparation for surgery, his recovery from it, and his learning to live with the ostomy.

The patient may be given instruction about the ostomy and about equipment and general principles of care prior to surgery. Some patients are taught to apply the device even before surgery. Others, too ill or too bewildered to learn care of the ostomy preoperatively, are taught after surgery.

The overall plan for caring for the patient who has an ostomy is adapted to the individual. The plan includes instruction, but just how this instruction is carried out varies according to such factors as the patient's previous knowledge regarding ostomies and his emotional reaction.

A large selection of literature is available from ostomy groups as well as from manufacturers of ostomy supplies. Excellent visual aids such as slides, charts, mini-guides, and models are also available and are helpful in teaching the patient. A small plastic model of a stoma which has a belt attachment can be used for demonstration by the nurse, and the patient can also use these models in learning self-care techniques. Preparing the patient for the appearance of the stoma by use of models and diagrams can decrease his anxiety when he first looks at his own stoma. Some hospitals employ an enterostomal therapist—a nurse specially trained in the care and teaching of ostomy patients (Fig. 31-1). Even when such a therapist is available, the nurse may still be involved with teaching as well as with changing the surgical dressing or stoma bag.

The patient with a stoma has no sphincter, thus no sphincter control; he is left with the problem of incontinence for the rest of his life. Every effort is made to help the patient reach the stage of recovery in which he feels a mastery over the stoma.

Attitudes and reactions

The patient who for any reason is unable to control his bowel movement frequently experiences a great deal of anxiety concerning possible rejection by others. The patient looks upon those who care for him as a reflection of the world at large. The nurse's acceptance of the patient's stoma can help him to accept it. The reactions of friends and family also influence the degree of acceptance that can be expected from the patient. The family may be very upset, wondering whether the odor of fecal drainage will permeate the home, whether relationships with friends can be maintained, and whether or not they can successfully conceal their fear or repugnance from the patient. The nurse can help the family as well as the patient by maintaining a supportive attitude, by assisting the family to learn about the stoma and to deal with their feelings concerning it, and by serving as an example to both the patient and his family in her attitude toward the stoma and its care and in the care of the equipment being used.

It is essential to work with the patient at his stage of acceptance of the stoma, rather than to imply that he must meet certain inflexible standards set by others. For example, the nurse may set expectations for performance in the care of the stoma, such as not showing any change in facial expression or tone of voice. However, if the patient shows reluctance or distaste for carrying out care of his stoma, the nurse should convey patience and acceptance of his reaction rather than criticism of it. This approach usually helps the patient to deal with his own reactions and thus to resolve them.

The patient's reactions will be a guide to teaching him to change his own dressing. You may notice that he does not look at the stoma the first few times that the dressing is changed. Many patients look away, or they cover their eyes with an arm as they lie quietly in bed. It is better not to force a patient to look at his stoma by a comment like, "You'd better watch what I'm doing, because soon you'll be doing this yourself." Instead, carry out the dressing deftly and promptly, doing everything, such as controlling odors and disposing of waste, in a way that makes the procedure as smooth as possible. Be especially careful to insure privacy. Many patients dread having the stoma and drainage exposed, even to the nurse, and become very distressed if other patients or visitors see it. Make a special effort to show the patient that he is acceptable and clean. Keep everything in his unit spotlessly clean and neat so that visitors will not be repelled by odors or soiled equipment. Having members of the staff and convalescent patients drop by often for a chat helps the patient to feel that his stoma is not objectionable and that others do not avoid him.

Allow the patient an opportunity to express his feelings about the stoma. It is not unusual for a patient who appeared very brave and eager to learn before the surgery to become depressed and withdrawn afterward. If those who care for him show patience and support, the patient may soon begin to look at the stoma and to develop interest in its care. Sometimes a casual and yet factual comment like, "The drainage is more formed today," helps the patient to begin observing and taking part. If his avoidance continues, his physician should be consulted, so that further help with the emotional reaction can be planned. Sometimes the nurse's attention is focused quite narrowly on the stoma and its care. It is important for the nurse to spend some time with the patient to listen and allow the patient to verbalize his feelings about his surgery. If the patient is experiencing difficulty accepting his stoma, such periods can be of special importance in assisting him to cope with his feelings.

Explanation and assistance

As soon as the patient begins to observe and demonstrate interest in caring for his stoma, explain each step as you proceed. After several periods of observation, encourage him to help. Ask him to hold the equipment and hand you supplies as you need them. Give the patient an opportunity to wash his hands after he has helped with his bag or dressing change. Too often this important detail is forgotten even though it is taken for granted that the nurse will wash her hands.

Every patient needs to know that his nurse cares about him and understands some of his problems. He needs to know too that the nurse has the knowledge and ability to help him resolve these problems. The nurse demonstrates this concern and knowledge by the manner, skill, and attitude with which the care is given. Choice of words and tone of voice are important when the nurse discusses the ostomy with the patient.

When the patient has helped with his stoma care a few times and is regaining his strength, he is usually ready to begin to carry out the procedure himself.

Stay with him the first few times and help when needed. Sometimes the nurse thinks that the patient who carries out the procedure correctly for the first or second time needs no further help. This often gives the patient the feeling that the nurse is eager to be rid of the task of caring for his ostomy. Even though the patient can carry out the technique of his stoma care adequately, arrange to be with him sometimes when he changes the dressing. This will enable you to observe how he is applying what he has learned. It will also give you an opportunity to note the condition of the skin, and the type and amount of fecal drainage; it will also convey to the patient your continued interest and willingness to help.

For many patients this change in body function constitutes a loss and they will go through a grieving process. This cannot be hurried. It takes time and patience and a sincere sustained concern and interest in order to help such a patient at this time. The patient may experience a period of disbelief, denial, anger, discouragement, or despair before he finally accepts the situation. He may even be suicidal.

The nurse's and physician's presence, their concern, and their helpfulness are essential, not only in accepting the patient in his grief, but also in helping him to see what progress he has made (however slight). Recovered ostomates can also provide help and encouragement. Some patients require psychiatric help to progress through stages of grief and to begin to cope with the ostomy.

The nurse and the physician should discuss each patient and his care as it evolves. The nurse should initiate the instruction necessary after consultation with the physician. Decisions about who will teach the patient the various aspects of his care must be made promptly and definitely lest the patient be discharged before he is able to care for himself. The physician informs the patient what surgery is required and why and explains the pathology. The nurse reviews this with the patient as necessary. The plan of who teaches what must be definite and agreed upon by the nurse and physician. The nurse teaches what is necessary for self-care, appliance care, skin care, etc., as detailed elsewhere in this chapter. *The patient should receive the equipment and instruction in its use and care while hospitalized, and should have an opportunity to demonstrate his ability to manage the ostomy prior to discharge.* Referral to the visiting nurse service or a stoma clinic for nursing care should be made upon discharge.

Visitors from ostomy groups

It is often beneficial to have a member of the visiting committee of the local ostomy group visit the patient. A visit from a person who has successfully mastered the care of his stoma and who has resumed his work and family life can convey to the patient that it is possible to be well-groomed, attractive, and successful despite an ostomy.

The nurse or physician can find an ostomy visitor by contacting the local ostomy group (see listing in local telephone directory). Plans for the visit must first be discussed with the physician, since his agreement that the visit would be beneficial is necessary. It is helpful to give the person from the ostomy club who arranges visits the following information: type of visit (preoperative or postoperative), patient's age, occupation, language barrier, physical handicaps, or any other factor significant to rehabilitation.

The club's chairman of visiting arrangements will try to select a visitor with a background similar to that of the patient. The visitor may bring literature which will be left with the patient. The visitor checks with the nurse so that he can be introduced to the patient. This protocol provides the nurse with an opportunity to meet the visitor and discuss with him any special purposes in the visit.

The patient with an ileostomy

An ileostomy is a surgically formed opening into the ileum for the drainage of fecal matter. A loop of ileum is brought out on the lower right quadrant of the abdomen, slightly below the umbilicus, near the outer border of the rectus muscle, and a stoma is formed. The stoma is "matured" at the time of surgery by everting the bowel and suturing the cut end of the ileum to the skin. The rationale for maturing the stoma is that it provides a seal at the base of the stoma. This technique promotes healing and provides a smooth peristomal area, thus permitting the application of the permanent appliance much sooner than is permissible in the nonmatured stoma.

Fecal drainage from the ileostomy is of a liquid consistency since it is discharged before it passes through the colon where water absorption normally takes place. Therefore, an ileostomy requires the immediate application of a collecting appliance over the stoma. The surgeon applies a temporary disposable plastic pouch to the skin over the stoma at the time of the operation. This pouch should be of the drainable type and may have an adhesive facing or a karaya gum seal with or without an adhesive facing.

INDICATIONS FOR ILEOSTOMY. Ulcerative colitis is a common indication for ileostomy. It has been found that when a temporary ileostomy is performed, the disease process in the colon persists despite the diversion of the fecal stream. The removal of the diseased colon (colectomy) is necessary to halt the disease. When the colon has been removed, the ileostomy is permanent. The procedure may be done in one, two, or three stages.

IMMEDIATE POSTOPERATIVE MANAGEMENT

The principles of postoperative management are the same as those for any patient who has had surgery on the gastrointestinal tract. The use of a nasogastric tube and suction and the administration of parenteral fluids are usual in the immediate postoperative period. Within several days these treatments usually are discontinued, and oral feedings of easily digested foods are begun. The patient is encouraged gradually to resume a normal diet, excluding only those foods that cause gas.

Electrolyte imbalance due to large output of fluid through the ileum is a particular problem for the patient with an ileostomy. The patient is cautioned to observe for weakness, trembling, and confusion, especially when the ileal output is profuse. He may require administration of intravenous fluids for fluid electrolyte replacement; therefore, these symptoms should be reported to the physician when they occur. The nurse should have a *thorough understanding* of fluid requirements and fluid therapy replacement within the context of the nursing role.

The patient returns from the operating room with a stoma and a surgical incision through which the operation has been performed. The stoma is usually covered either with a plastic disposable pouch or with fluffy gauze dressings. Sometimes the proximity of the stoma to the surgical incision makes it especially difficult to avoid fecal contamination of the incision. The plastic pouch, which can be fitted snugly around the stoma and secured with adhesive, helps to prevent the fecal drainage from seeping into the surgical incision. Collodion may be used to seal the dressing over the incision, so that liquid feces cannot run in. Wide strips of adhesive may be applied tightly over the entire dressing covering the incision to protect it from fecal drainage.

Moving about in bed, coughing, and early ambulation may be made more difficult by the patient's fear of soiling his clothing and bedding. The dressing or disposable plastic pouch must be applied securely, so that the patient is more willing to move about. Above all, give him the feeling that some soiling is inevitable in the immediate postoperative period, and that the changing of dressings and even of bedding is both accepted and expected by the nursing staff. Promptness in changing the soiled dressings and proceeding in a matter-of-fact manner with a sure touch do more than words to assure the patient that his condition is accepted.

Nursing measures for deep breathing, coughing, turning, and exercising the toes and legs are carried out as for other surgical patients. Medication for relief of pain and discomfort should be given as required. Nursing care should be planned to provide the patient with adequate time to rest. Some surgeons advocate the use of elastic bandages or antiembolitic stockings to both legs to prevent thrombophlebitis until the patient is ambulating. If used, they should be removed and reapplied at least once each 8-hour period.

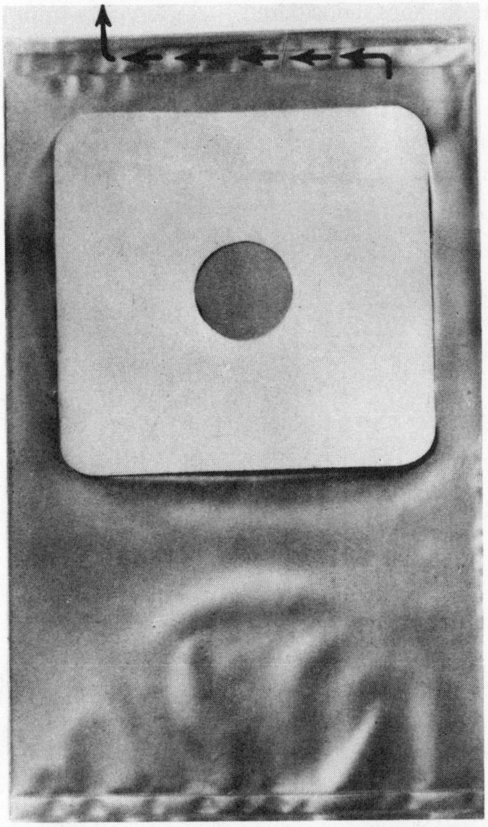

figure 31-2. The disposable Stomaplast pouch has an air vent on top (arrows) permitting only gas to escape when the pouch is gently pressed. (Marsan Manufacturing Company, Wausau, Wisc.)

A temporary bag or pouch is usually placed over the stoma during the immediate postoperative period. The stoma is measured and a hole is cut in the top of the pouch so that it will fit around the stoma. Some of the bags already have a hole in the top; however, this hole may have to be enlarged so that it will fit over the stoma. A commonly used type is made of plastic and has a square of double-faced adhesive at the top. One side of the adhesive sticks to the skin around the stoma; the other adheres to the plastic material. The lower end of the plastic pouch is folded securely and held closed with elastic bands. When the pouch is emptied, a large emesis basin is placed to catch the return, and the elastic bands are removed, allowing the drainage to flow out the bottom of the pouch into the emesis basin. The entire appliance is disposable, and a fresh one is used if leakage occurs.

The temporary plastic pouch is used for a variety of conditions in which drainage occurs from a stoma. Because of edema, the stoma is larger immediately after surgery than it will be later. The size of the stoma changes considerably during the initial postoperative period. The temporary appliance is especially useful because fresh ones can be cut to fit the stoma as often as necessary (Fig. 31-2, p. 407). After healing has occurred and the stoma has reached its permanent size and shape, a permanent appliance is fitted.

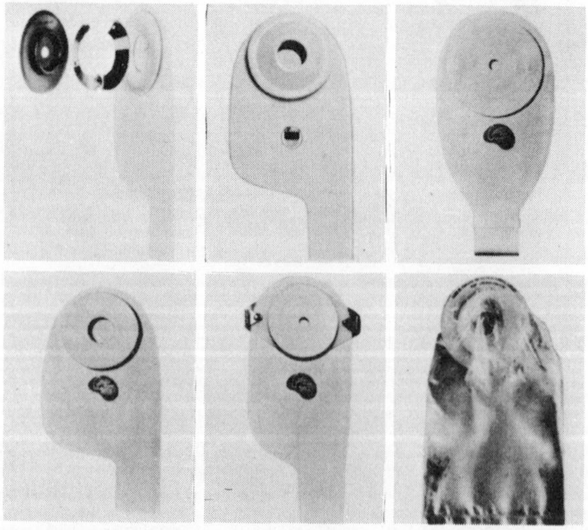

figure 31-3. The permanent ileostomy appliance. A variety of permanent ileostomy appliances are available from the manufacturer. The features of these appliances vary as to pouch size, pouch length, pouch shape, and faceplate (disc) design. (United Surgical Corp.)

Application of the Postoperative Appliance

Adhesive Type. Prepare the skin by cleansing with soap and water. Pat dry. Apply one or two coats of tincture of benzoin on wet skin and dust on karaya powder or apply surgical cement. Permit cement to dry five minutes if used. Tincture of benzoin should be tacky and dry before the appliance is applied. If temporary bag does not have exact size opening, measure stoma and add ⅛-inch clearance around stoma to allow for stomal size change. A karaya ring can be placed around base of stoma before applying bag. Secure end of bag with bands or barrette-type clamp.

Karaya Gum Ring with Adhesive Facing. Prepare skin as above. Peel off protective backing from adhesive facing and align carefully to guide over stoma evenly. Karaya gum ring should fit snugly around stoma. Secure closure as above.

Karaya Gum Ring. Prepare skin as above. Remove protective covering from karaya ring and guide over stoma. Secure closure as above. The karaya ring can fit snugly around base of stoma without injuring stoma. Care should be taken not to use hard surface rings close to stoma to avoid injury to stoma.

The three basic features of the *permanent* appliance are:

1. A disc (faceplate) which surrounds the stoma and usually adheres to the body;
2. A pouch for collecting the feces, usually oblong with a spout for emptying;
3. Accessories such as a belt, belt attachments, spout closures, bands, or clips.

The permanent appliance may be adhered with surgical cement, a karaya gum ring, or a double-faced adhesive disc.

Considerations for choosing a permanent appliance involve the disc and its design. Therefore, the location and characteristics of the stoma and the characteristics of abdominal contour and texture must be analyzed for each individual. The material and size of the disc will depend upon individual specifications and patient preferences.

The pouch is that part of the appliance which collects the feces. If there is no fitting problem, pouch size may be the deciding factor in choosing the appliance. Various types of plastic (Fig. 31-3) and qualities of rubber are used with respect to odor permeability. This may be the decisive factor for some patients. Allergy to rubber or other materials may be a factor.

Belts. The belt is an accessory to the appliance. However, it is usually worn for 24 hours just as is the appliance—bathing and sleeping are no exceptions. It may occasionally be omitted when a snugly fitted girdle is worn or if the disc edge is reinforced with adhesive. A rubber belt can be used during bathing or swimming as the elastic tends to stretch when wet.

The belt is used for several reasons. It holds the appliance in place when cement is not used, or it provides pressure for a good bond when cement is used. It may be used to support the weight of the appliance and filled pouch and thus prevent the disc from being pulled away from the abdomen by the weight of the liquid fecal material. It provides the new ostomate with the assurance that the appliance will not fall off.

Foam rubber, gauze, or flannel padding can be used under a belt which cuts into the flesh. Care should be taken to avoid upward or downward pull on the stoma. The belt should be placed at the level of the stoma, or double belts can be used to equalize pull on the top and bottom of the disc.

CEMENT is used to stick the appliance onto the body and must be applied to a clean, dry surface. Always apply cement in thin coats and permit each coat to dry thoroughly before applying the next one. This technique permits adequate evaporation of the solvent. Allow 5 minutes for drying of the cement and evaporation of the solvent. This prevents excoriation of the skin and permits the bond to form. Two thin coats of cement applied to the appliance and the skin will insure a complete covering of the area without excess cement building up. Finding the right cement is a trial and error procedure. The skin should be tested for sensitivity before a cement is used because sensitivity is common. It is not necessary to remove all paste from the disc each time the appliance is changed. Slight paste buildup provides for better adherence. However, the skin beneath the disc must be left as clean as possible.

Cement can be rolled off the skin and appliance after several days of wearing. If it does not roll off, a little solvent applied with a medicine dropper can be used *gently* with a gauze pad to rub off traces of cement. A *little* solvent is all that is necessary; wipe off the area with water after solvent has been used.

SOLVENT is a hydrocarbon which is highly inflammable. It is also very irritating and therefore should be applied sparingly between the body and the bag, using a medicine dropper. *Excessive* rubbing will cause skin irritation. *Never* use carbon tetrachloride in place of ileostomy solvent. Carbon tetrachloride is the most toxic of all commonly used solvents and is highly dangerous.

KARAYA GUM POWDER, KARAYA GUM RINGS. Karaya gum powder is made from the resin of the *Sterculia urens* tree in India. It is a useful product in that it protects the skin while it permits healing underneath; it also serves as an adherent for the ostomy appliance. Karaya gum is used by many in place of cement. Karaya gum powder becomes gelatinous when brought in contact with moisture and can be used in this gummy state. It can be resealed by applying pressure. Rings of karaya gum are also available commercially. One manufacturer supplies ostomy drainage bags with the karaya gum ring already attached. These rings can be cut, pulled or pushed into any shape desired and therefore can be used as a protection at the base of the stoma to correct the problems created by an ill-fitting appliance.

CHANGING THE APPLIANCE

The important factors in regard to changing the appliance are *time* and *frequency*.

There are two factors to remember. The first and cardinal rule for changing the appliance is that when there is a burning or itching sensation underneath the disc or pain around the stoma the appliance should be removed immediately. This should be done regardless of whether the appliance has been on 1 hour or several days. The stoma and skin should be examined carefully to determine the cause of the difficulty. Excoriation of the skin is to be avoided at all costs. Resorting to the use of a temporary postoperative appliance may be advisable until the cause is identified and eliminated. The most frequent cause is leakage of fecal drainage or reaction to solvent or cement. Stinging, tingling, or itching may be experienced immediately after an appliance change, and will subside quickly. If the sensation is prolonged or intensified, remove the appliance.

Second, the appliance should be changed at a time when the bowel is relatively quiet. For most ostomates this time is early in the morning, before eating, or 2 to 3 hours after mealtime. However, it is best to check the patient to note the times of least bowel activity. A record of these times should be made on the patient's chart in order to coordinate plans for management. At first, the patient will be very much aware of and concerned about the frequency of bowel activity. However, he should be assured that as the bowel adjusts to its new state, the activity lessens. Usually, the bowel is most active after eating and relatively quiet at other times. The patient should have quiet and privacy when making the appliance change.

Most surgeons advocate changing the appliance

ring when needed; that is, when the ring becomes separated from the skin. Too frequent changes are thought to be inadvisable, because in removing the appliance one may also remove the protective layers of epithelium and cause the skin to become raw and excoriated. The two-piece appliances permit inspection of the stoma by removing only the pouch while the disc remains cemented to the body.

Care of the skin

It is imperative that meticulous care be given to the area around the stoma to prevent excoriation and skin breakdown. Time and expense should not be spared, because ileal discharge contains digestive enzymes and acids which undermine the skin; the resulting excoriation may take weeks to heal. The nurse should be aware of such problems so that they may be prevented or treated early should they occur, and she should be especially careful to protect the circumstomal area from ileal drainage by placing a tissue cuff around the stoma or using something such as a small paper cup to collect the drainage while caring for the skin.

Control of odor and gas

Odor is an individual matter. There are two kinds of odor that the ostomy patient is concerned about: that which is present when the ileostomy pouch is emptied and that which occasionally envelops an ileostomate and follows him about. Personal cleanliness is essential; however, the ostomate must also cope with special problems, such as care of the pouch, to lessen odors.

The really serious odor problem is the particularly identifying smell that occasionally clings to the person. Leakage, the pouch, inadequate changing of the pouch, certain foods, or an impending complication may be responsible. Try to ascertain the cause so it can be remedied.

Many deodorants and deodorizers are on the market. These include tablets taken orally such as Derifil (water-soluble chlorophyll derivatives). Other methods of odor control include the use of deodorant tablets or liquids placed directly in the pouch. The powder of two crushed aspirin tablets is an effective deodorant.

To deter odor in warm weather, a plastic bag can be slipped over the appliance. Many patients prefer to use two pouches alternately. A *thorough* cleansing of the pouch is an absolute necessity for removing odors.

To control odor at its source, a restricted diet of tea, toast and marmalade and the addition of one food at a time may be tried. Foods containing condiments, fish, eggs, onions, and cheese should be omitted, as these frequently cause odors that linger. However, the patient must do this under medical supervision and work up to an adequate diet. Medications, especially antibiotics and antituberculous drugs, may cause particularly strong odors which cling to the appliance. The use of an old pouch or disposable pouches while these medications are taken is helpful.

Intestinal gas is often as much as 85 percent swallowed air. Sighing, chewing, gulping down food, and breathing with the mouth open all contribute to this component of intestinal gas. Eating slowly and chewing food well with the mouth closed help to reduce gas formation.

Some foods, such as cabbage, onions, pork, beans, and peppers, are gas producing and should be avoided. Later some individuals find they can add small amounts of these foods to the diet.

Charcoal tablets and simethicone (Mylicon) tablets or liquid may be prescribed to relieve distress due to gas. They break up the gas bubble at its source and reduce the discomfort of bloating.

Intestinal obstruction

Intestinal obstruction is a serious complication. It may be due to a twisted, strangulated, or incarcerated bowel, an internal hernia, or a bolus of poorly chewed, inadequately digested, stringy, pasty or fibrous food. Spare or absent ileal flow will signify an obstruction. *The physician should be notified.*

The permanent appliance should be removed and a temporary postoperative appliance with a larger disc opening than normally worn should be used to allow for stoma swelling and to permit observation of the stoma. The stoma may become edematous and cyanotic.

Careful irrigation by the physician may relieve an obstruction due to food. Surgical intervention may be necessary if the bowel is twisted or strangulated.

Stenosis, tightening, and narrowing of the stoma may eventually require surgical revision. The surgeon may wish to have the patient dilate the stoma daily for a while to prevent further difficulty. The patient inserts a well-lubricated index finger into the stoma for a few minutes. This should be done only on the surgeon's advice. The fingernail should be cut short to prevent injury to the bowel.

Prolapse or protrusion of the ileostomy is fairly common, and if it is of moderate degree (2 to 3 inches) it can be disregarded. Even longer prolapses might be symptomless and harmless. *However, should there be a sudden prolapse of the stoma, the permanent appliance should be removed immediately and a temporary appliance used, and the physician should be notified.* A prolapse should be treated by the physician as soon as possible. Edema may occur and lead to obstruction from restriction of blood supply; necrosis may result if the prolapse is not promptly and skillfully managed. Once prolapse of the stoma has occurred, recurrence is more likely.

The patient with a colostomy

A colostomy is an artificial opening of the large bowel brought out to the abdomen and fashioned into a stoma. The stoma is a small round structure which is pink in color and moist, velvety and smooth in texture. Changes in size and color of stoma vary with activity and emotional status. Anger or extreme annoyance may produce a very red or purplish color. Small beads of blood may ooze from the surface. Fright may cause blanching of the stoma. These are normal reactions and are insignificant in that the tissues will revert to their normal state when the cause is alleviated. It is important for the nurse to explain to the patient that these are normal reactions.

The presence of a cancerous lesion, an ulcerative inflammatory process, multiple polyposis, or injury can be indications for a colostomy.

Types of colostomies

A colostomy may be described in a number of ways depending upon its purpose, duration, or location. It may be temporary or permanent. If described by location, it may be ascending, transverse, descending, or sigmoid. It may have a single loop or a double loop (double-barreled). It may be described in terms of its therapeutic effect on the patient, i.e., either curative or palliative.

The type of colostomy the patient has will not only tell you the location of the stoma but also help you to anticipate the needs of the patient. A colostomy spoken of in general terms usually relates to a sigmoid location. Problems experienced by patients who have this procedure depend to a large extent upon the type of colostomy which has been created.

Single- and Double-Barreled Colostomies. Colostomies may be double-barreled or single-barreled. A double-barreled colostomy consists of two stomas, one of which connects with either the proximal or the distal portion of the bowel (Fig. 31-4). The portion of the bowel leading from the small intestine to the stoma, through which the feces pass to the outside, is called the *proximal portion,* and its opening is called the *proximal opening* or *loop* of the colostomy. The *distal portion* of the bowel leads from the stoma to the anus. Because the fecal drainage has been diverted, the distal portion of the bowel does not pass feces

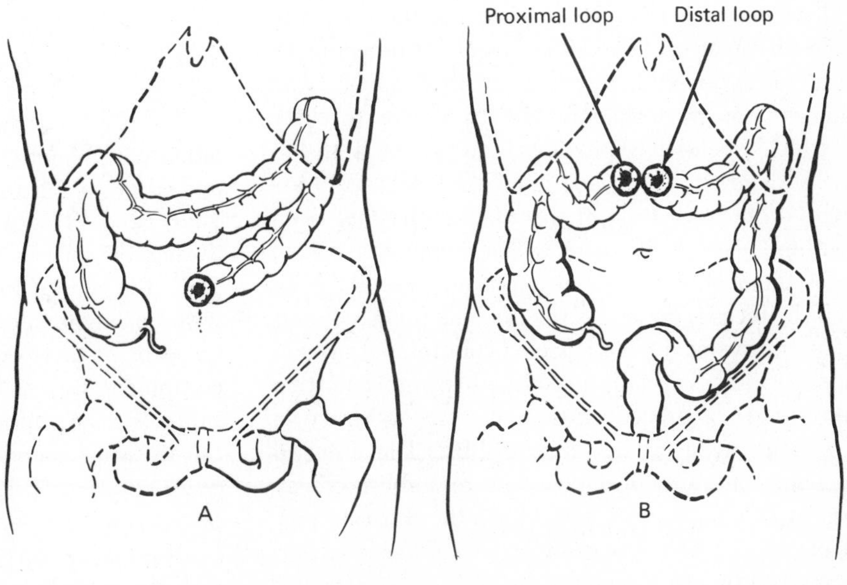

figure 31-4. Single- and double-barreled colostomy. (A) One type of single-barreled colostomy. The distal portion of the bowel has been removed, and the colostomy is permanent. (B) One type of double-barreled colostomy, showing proximal and distal loops. This type of colostomy may or may not be permanent.

by way of the anus. However, mucus often collects in this portion of bowel. Sometimes, the double-barreled colostomy is a temporary procedure and, after disease or injury in the distal portion has been treated, the continuity of the bowel is restored.

Often when a colostomy is performed, the stoma is matured at surgery. That is, the stoma is everted and sutured down, and thus is open. If the stoma is not matured at surgery, a loop of bowel is brought out onto the abdomen. About 24 to 36 hours after the operation, the loop of bowel is opened, by cutting or cautery, to form the stoma. In this way the initial healing of the incision takes place without danger of contamination. The latter procedure is not physically painful, since the bowel is not sensitive to pain as the skin is. The opening of the colostomy is usually carried out at the patient's bedside or in the treatment room. The bed should be well protected, and a temporary ostomy pouch rather than a basin is used to receive the initial flow of liquid feces. The initial gush of fecal material from the stoma can be upsetting to the patient even when he understands what to expect. The patient should be prepared for the pungent odor of the cauterized tissue, which will disappear shortly.

A single-barreled colostomy consists of one opening through which fecal matter is passed (Fig. 31-4). The opening is that of the proximal portion of the bowel. The distal portion of the bowel has usually been surgically removed, and the colostomy is permanent.

When a double-barreled colostomy is irrigated, it is important to distinguish between the proximal and the distal loops. Often the irrigation is ordered only for the proximal portion of the bowel. At other times, the doctor requests that both the proximal and the distal portions be irrigated. Ask the doctor to show you which opening is proximal and which is distal. Draw a diagram, and place it on the chart to guide all who do the irrigation. If this diagram has not been drawn and you are not sure which opening is which, inspect them both for a few minutes. The one from which the feces is flowing is the proximal loop.

The transverse double-barreled colostomy is usually temporary and is usually performed to rest a portion of the bowel, a procedure that may be necessary in the treatment of acute diverticulitis. The interval before the continuity of the bowel is reestablished may be up to 16 months or longer. When the diseased portion of the bowel is removed or healed the bowel is reconnected by anastomosis.

Keeping the patient clean

The content of the large bowel is liquid in the ascending colon, semiliquid to pasty in the transverse colon, semisolid in the descending colon, and solid in the sigmoid colon. The functions of the large bowel are to reabsorb water and to serve as a storage space for the feces until evacuation.

Control of fecal evacuation, therefore, is based upon the location of the stoma and the function of that portion of the bowel. An ascending-type colostomy will need a carefully applied temporary appliance or an ileostomy-type permanent pouch.

More frequent emptying of the appliance will be necessary. This should be done promptly to maintain the seal and to protect against soiling. Observe the patient to determine the frequency with which the appliance must be emptied.

At first, the stoma constantly exudes soft and liquid feces. Frequent emptying of the plastic pouch day and night is necessary to keep the patient as clean as possible, to control odors, and to prevent excoriation of the skin around the stoma from leakage.

The transverse colostomy will be more manageable if irrigated daily to reduce the number of movements and to help eliminate odor. Discuss the need for irrigation with the surgeon. The use of a temporary ostomy bag will protect the skin and prevent contamination of the surgical wound. The descending and sigmoid colostomies are easier to manage because the content of the bowel is semisolid to solid. Scheduled daily irrigation to establish regularity will help the patient achieve control more rapidly. When control is obtained on a once-a-day basis, the patient is ready to try an every-other-day schedule of irrigations.

Clean rather than sterile technique is used because the opening is into the bowel, which normally contains many bacteria, and because fecal drainage is laden with bacteria. Wash your hands carefully before and after caring for the stoma. If you have a cut on your hand, it is wise to wear a clean rubber glove during the procedure, and then it is essential to explain the reason for the glove to the patient. Otherwise he might interpret the use of the glove as reluctance or distaste on your part. Collect all the needed equipment first so that you will not have to obtain supplies from cupboards or dressing supply cart while the dressing change is in progress. If you should require additional supplies, wash your hands thoroughly before leaving the patient's unit.

It is convenient to keep all supplies at the patient's bedside, replenishing them as necessary. Supplies include newspapers or paper bags for wrapping soiled dressings, extra dressings or plastic pouches, and any medication that has been ordered for the patient's skin.

Remove the plastic pouch, empty it if necessary, and wrap it in newspaper. Gently wash the skin around the stoma with mild soap and water. Gauze fluffs or disposable washcloths are usually used for cleansing. If the skin is inflamed, use only water without any soap. Wash gently and yet thoroughly; avoid rubbing because the skin is very easily irritated.

Avoid leaving soiled articles within the patient's view. Wrapping the soiled dressings in newspaper as soon as they are removed helps to control odor as well as to make the entire procedure more acceptable to the patient. Provide adequate ventilation, but do not chill the patient. Room deodorizers may be helpful or a deodorant spray may be used.

Various preparations may be ordered by the physician to treat or to prevent excoriation of the skin. Whatever preparation is used, it is important to remove it periodically and to observe the condition of the skin underneath. Apply the dressings or the plastic pouch snugly to minimize leakage. The adhesive that holds the plastic pouch against the skin will not stick unless the skin is clean and dry. (If ointment is used, it is applied sparingly and the excess is wiped off.) Apply the bag smoothly to avoid wrinkles.

Change everything that is soiled including gowns or bedding as necessary.

Try to empty the pouch at least a half-hour or so before meals. Changing it close to mealtime or during the serving of trays interferes with the patient's appetite.

Methods of Colostomy Management. There are three popular methods of colostomy management—irrigation by standard method, irrigation by bulb syringe, and nonirrigation.

The most widely advocated method for irrigation is the standard method, which consists of a daily scheduled irrigation with 500 to 1500 ml. of water. The schedule gradually progresses to every other day, every third day, or even twice a week. Equipment used is an irrigating set: receptacle for solution (can or bag) attached to tubing and catheter, and irrigation sleeve or sheath for the fecal return. The patient may be free of spillage from 1 to 3 days with effective results.

The second method employs the use of a bulb syringe of soft rubber and a short rubber catheter. The equipment consists of the syringe, a quart container for solution, and an emesis basin or a plastic sheath or an apron. This method calls for several instillations of 250 to 500 ml. of solution at a time. Few patients have found this method effective for freedom of spillage for 24 hours or more. Some patients use two instillations a day. It may be an alternate choice when the standard method cannot be used.

With the nonirrigation or natural method, the patient may use a variety of devices to stimulate an evacuation. Prune or orange juice on arising or before bedtime, liquid breakfast, coffee, mild exercises, a mild laxative, or lemon juice in warm water are a few measures which have been effective. The patient usually does not know when the evacuation will occur.

Another device used by nonirrigators is the suppository—glycerine or bisacodyl (Dulcolax). It was found that at least 7 days elapsed before a pattern began to be established. The movements occurred three to four times daily. Each day the movements became fewer and fewer and the time lapse was greater until the patient had two movements a day—one in the morning and one in the evening, but neither at a scheduled time. Some patients use the suppository in addition to irrigation.

The irrigation procedure

It is essential that the colostomy patient be assisted with the irrigation procedure, because the effectiveness of the irrigation is the basis for establishing control. It can be easily and simply taught so that the patient can usually begin to do his own irrigation after it has been demonstrated by the nurse.

Once the equipment is assembled, irrigation solution prepared and air removed from tubing, the patient is seated on the toilet seat or on a chair in front of the toilet with the irrigation sheath directed into the toilet bowl. He is then ready to begin the irrigation. The bottom of the bag containing the irrigating solution is hung approximately at shoulder height. (The size of the catheter lumen and height of the bag determine the rate of flow. The catheter size may vary from size 18 to 28 Fr.)

The catheter is inserted through the plastic cup or through the irrigation sleeve, lubricated, and then inserted into the stomal opening. The belt can be secured after the catheter is inserted into the stoma. The catheter or irrigation tube should be inserted *slowly* and *gently* 2 to 3 inches by rotation. Difficulty inserting the catheter may be due to a hard piece of stool or to a fold of tissue. If there is difficulty inserting the catheter, withdraw and reinsert it or permit water to flow during insertion. *Never* force the catheter. Once the catheter is in place it can be advanced 4 to 10 inches as desired. However, it is necessary that the catheter be introduced only far enough for water to be retained in the bowel. Allow the water to enter the bowel slowly and gently because too rapid an instillation of fluid will result in painful cramping and an ineffective irrigation. If water returns as it is being introduced, clamp off the tubing until the flow ceases. Do not remove the catheter, because the return will flow around the catheter; also, difficulty may be encountered during reinsertion. Then release the clamp and continue irrigation until the desired amount of solution has been used. Remove the catheter and permit the return to flow into the irrigation sleeve. The patient may remain seated on the toilet seat or may close off the edge of the sleeve and walk about to help stimulate an evacuation. Shaving or other personal care can be done while awaiting a fecal return.

It usually requires 20 to 30 minutes for the return to be completed. This time varies from individual to individual and even in the same person at first. The patient will get to know when the irrigation is sufficiently effective and the bowel is clean of feces by a spurt of gas or just a feeling which he has learned indicates that sufficient evacuation has occurred. A clue to the effectiveness of the irrigation can be made by observing the return. If the return is watery and slightly colored and contains no stool, the bowel is probably clean. If the return is heavy with stool or thick, the bowel is not clean and an additional instillation of 500 to 1000 ml. of fluid may be necessary. Use as a guide the amount of water which returns. If what is instilled is returned, you can safely put in more. If what is instilled is not returned, you may need to siphon back the fluid or discontinue the irrigation at that point. Patients should be discouraged from using more than 2 quarts of water at a time lest water intoxication result. Soap is not recommended. Some surgeons may advise addition of salt or soda bicarbonate to the water for individual patients. As a general rule this is not necessary. Ordinary tepid tap water will suffice.

Cramping may be a problem to some patients during the irrigation. A slight cramp may simply be a signal that the bowel is ready to empty. Water which is too cold or introduced too rapidly or failure to release air from tubing before inserting the fluid may also cause cramping. If cramping occurs, merely pinch off the tubing and have the patient sit up straight, take a few deep breaths, and relax. Cramping will usually last about a minute. When the cramp is gone, release the tubing and continue the irrigation.

Failure of the water to return may occur occasionally, even in experienced individuals. This may result if the catheter is inserted too far and the water remains in the bowel temporarily; or water, trapped behind a hard stool, may be absorbed. To encourage the return of fluid material more promptly one or several of the following activities is suggested to the patient: gentle massage of the lower abdomen, tightening the abdominal muscles, taking several deep breaths and relaxing, gently twisting the body (at waist) from side to side, standing up, or sitting more erect. If these measures are not effective and the patient is uncomfortable or distressed, notify the physician.

Flushing the bag from below or through a small opening made near the top of the bag will help to eliminate odors from drainage. The irrigation set can be used to flush the bag. The opening at the top of the bag should be covered with a small piece of adhesive tape to prevent leakage.

After the irrigation is completed, remove the irrigation sheath, rinse in cool water to reduce odor, and discard, or clean in warm soapy water if it is to be reused.

It is the irrigation of the proximal loop that has been discussed above. If the distal loop is to be irrigated, the patient should sit on a bedpan or on the toilet seat because the solution will be expelled through the rectum. Usually mucus and, sometimes, necrotic tissue are expelled along with the solution. Examine the return carefully before discarding it.

There should be uninterrupted use of the bathroom for at least 1 hour for the irrigation. Select a time convenient to the patient to fit into his schedule of activities. Other members of the household should be considered when the time for irrigation is set.

Travel can be undertaken as soon as the patient receives his physician's permission. Upsets can be avoided by planning in advance and by sticking to established routine. Remember water that is not drinkable is not desirable for irrigation either. Boiled or bottled water can be used. The local public health service will advise about specific concerns regarding water or foods to avoid when the patient is traveling. The local ostomy society can give the names of physicians available in places to be visited. Any supplies or equipment which may be needed should be carried in a special bag or suitcase. Carrying this bag personally will prevent needless worry over possible loss of the bag during travel.

Stomal covering

The stoma may be covered with a gauze pad or temporary postoperative ostomy bag. If a gauze pad is worn, apply a small amount of lubricating jelly over the area which will come in contact with the stoma to prevent irritation of the stoma. An adhesive drainable bag or a karaya seal drainable bag is recommended for those individuals who continue to have drainage problems between irrigations.

Diet

Occasionally the physician may prescribe a special diet if there are irregular bowel movements or excessive gas. Otherwise a regular diet (unless there is a particular problem) can be taken with special attention to avoiding gas-forming foods such as dry beans, cabbage, uncooked onions, cheese, and fish. One new food should be introduced at a time to determine if it can be tolerated. At least one day should lapse between the addition of each new food.

Adjustment in the diet can be made if diarrhea or constipation is a problem. Elimination of distressing food items will help to control diarrhea. Increasing the amount of bulk, drinking water, or eating laxative-type foods will aid in correcting constipation. The physician should be consulted on these problems should they continue to persist after temporary measures have been used. Attention to eating slowly with mouth closed and chewing food well will reduce gas which is caused chiefly by swallowing air rather than by processes of digestion.

Clothing

With the exception of too tightly fitted items, no adjustment needs to be made regarding type of clothing worn. Girdles of light-weight expandable material such as lycra or spandex are suggested. It is *not* advisable to cut a hole in the garment for the protrusion of the stoma as this defeats the purpose of the garment. Those individuals who require a firm support (such as patients who have back problems and who wear braces) may find a stoma shield helpful in preventing undue pressure on or irritation of the stoma.

Cecostomy

An opening made in the cecum for the drainage of intestinal contents is called a cecostomy. Usually, this is a temporary measure performed to relieve intestinal obstruction. When the patient's physical condition has improved, further surgery may be carried out. The performance of the cecostomy is a relatively minor procedure, usually done under local anesthesia. An opening is made into the cecum through a small incision in the lower abdomen, and a large catheter is placed in the cecostomy to drain feces. The catheter is connected with a drainage bottle that collects the liquid feces and is sutured to the skin to prevent displacement.

Although the fecal material draining from the cecum is usually liquid, small clumps of formed stool may also be present and may clog the catheter. Irrigations of the catheter are usually ordered to prevent clogging. The frequency of the irrigations and the amount and the type of solution to be used are ordered by the physician. Normal saline is commonly used for the irrigation. It is allowed to run into the cecostomy tube by gravity, through an Asepto syringe. The glass portion of the syringe without the rubber bulb is used as a funnel through which the normal saline flows into the cecostomy tube. It is important not to exert any pressure (such as by using the rubber bulb) when doing the irrigation, because this might injure the bowel. If the fluid will not run into the tube by gravity, the physician should be consulted. The tube may be obstructed, and another tube may need to be inserted.

Fecal material may leak around the tube onto the skin. Disposable pouches are often preferred but dressings, if used, are applied to absorb the drainage and are changed frequently to control soiling and odor and to prevent excoriation of the skin. The principles of caring for any patient who has an opening of the bowel onto the skin are similar to those for a patient with a colostomy or an ileostomy.

General nutritional considerations

- The diet of the ostomy patient may have to be adjusted if excessive flatulence (gas) with or without cramping should occur. The colostomy patient may find it necessary to avoid certain foods that cause constipation or diarrhea.
- Fish, eggs, onions, and cheese are examples of foods that frequently cause lingering odors; it may be necessary to eliminate such foods.
- The formation of gas can be reduced or eliminated by eating slowly and chewing food well. Foods that cause gas, such as onions, cabbage, and beans should be avoided or eaten in limited amounts.
- Ostomates who note a persistent problem with gas or odor or who have severe constipation or diarrhea may find it necessary to eliminate almost all food from the diet and start a new diet with tea, toast, and marmalade. This is followed by adding one food at a time to

determine which food(s) may be causing the problem. A diet change such as this should not be attempted without the approval of the physician.

- The colostomy patient can usually avoid constipation by increasing the daily fluid intake or eating laxative-type foods such as bran cereal and prune juice.

General pharmacological considerations

- Some drugs, such as antibiotics, impart a lingering odor to the ostomy appliance. The patient taking these drugs should be warned of the odor and encouraged to use a plastic disposable pouch until the course of drug therapy is completed. Ostomy clubs as well as ostomy appliance manufacturers can usually supply a list of those drugs capable of imparting an odor to an ostomy appliance.
- Deodorizers for ostomy appliances include oral tablets such as Derifil and tablets or liquids placed directly in the pouch, e.g., the powder of two crushed aspirin tablets or oil of peppermint.
- Suppositories, such as glycerin, or bisacodyl (Dulcolax) may be inserted into the stoma, with physician approval, as a nonirrigating method of producing an evacuation.
- Antidiarrheal drugs should not be used by the colostomy patient unless the physician approves; overuse can result in fecal impaction. Use of laxatives should also be discussed with the physician.

Bibliography

American Cancer Society: *A Cancer Source Book for Nurses.* New York, American Cancer Society, 1975.

Bouchard, R. and Owens, N. F.: *Nursing Care of the Cancer Patient,* ed. 2. St. Louis, Mosby, 1972.

Brunner, L. and Suddarth, D. S.: *Lippincott Manual of Nursing Practice.* Philadelphia, Lippincott, 1974.

Carbary, L. J.: Cancer of the colon: Cure or crisis? Part 1. J. Prac. Nurs. 25:21, March, 1975.

Connors, M.: Ostomy care: A personal approach (pictorial). Am. J. Nurs. 74:1422, August, 1974.

Crary, W. G. et al: Depression. Am. J. Nurs. 73:472, March, 1973.

Davis, F. and Eardley, A.: Coping with a colostomy—the importance of the nurse. Nurs. Times 70:580, April, 1974.

Dericks, V. C.: The psychological hurdles of new ostomates: Helping them up . . . and over. Nurs. '74, 4:52, October, 1974.

Gallagher, A. M.: Body image changes in the patient with a colostomy. Nurs. Clin. North Am. 7:669, December, 1972.

Gibbs, G. and White, M.: Stomal care. Am. J. Nurs. 72:268, February, 1972.

Hardy, J. D., ed.: *Rhoads' Textbook of Surgery,* ed. 5. Philadelphia, Lippincott, 1976.

Jensen, V.: Better techniques for bagging stomas; Ileostomies. Part 3. Nurs. '74, 4:60, September, 1974.

Le Maitre, G. and Finnegan, J.: *The Patient in Surgery: A Guide for Nurses.* Philadelphia, Saunders, 1975.

Renkun, S.: Cancer of the colon and rectum: Cure or crisis? (pictorial). Part 2. J. Prac. Nurs. 25:18, April, 1975.

Schauder, M. R.: Ostomy care: Cone irrigations. Am. J. Nurs. 74:1424, August, 1974.

Sparberg, M.: *Ileostomy Care.* Springfield, Thomas, 1971.

CHAPTER 32

The patient with an intestinal or rectal disorder

On completion of this chapter the student will:

- **Describe the symptoms of appendicitis, peritonitis, hernia, diverticulitis, and pilonidal sinus.**
- **Develop a nursing care plan for, and participate in the nursing management of, patients with an intestinal or rectal disorder.**
- **List the various causes of intestinal obstruction, with their symptoms and management.**
- **Distinguish between diverticulitis and diverticulosis and describe the treatment and nursing management of each.**
- **Define malabsorption and describe the medical and nutritional management of this disorder.**

Appendicitis

Appendicitis is one of the most common surgical emergencies. The appendix—a narrow, blind tube located at the tip of the cecum—may become inflamed. While the rationale for inflammation is not clear, it is believed that obstruction occurs, making it difficult or impossible for the contents of the appendix to empty normally. Since the intestinal contents are laden with bacteria, an injury to the tissues in contact with the contents will often result in an infection. A hard mass of feces, called a *fecalith,* may obstruct and mechanically irritate the appendix. Inflammation and infection may quickly follow. The pressure from the fecalith and the edema of tissues that occurs during the inflammation may interfere with the blood supply, making the tissues more vulnerable to infection and leading sometimes to gangrene and perforation. Perforation is a dreaded complication, because if the intestinal contents flow into the peritoneal cavity, they can cause generalized peritonitis or, if the peritonitis is localized, an abscess.

Incidence and symptoms

Appendicitis can occur at any age but seems to be more common among adolescents and young adults. An attack of severe abdominal pain is the most common symptom of appendicitis. At first the pain is generalized throughout the abdomen or around the umbilicus. Later in the attack, the pain typically occurs in the right lower quadrant of the abdomen. *McBurney's* point, midway between the umbilicus and the right iliac crest, is usually the site of the most severe pain. Often, the pain is worst when manual pressure over McBurney's point is suddenly released. This is called *rebound tenderness.*

Slight or moderate fever and moderate leukocytosis are usually present. Nausea and vomiting may also be present. The symptoms among the very young and the very aged are often atypical.

Diagnosis

The physician performs a physical examination, noting especially the location of the pain and the tenderness in the abdomen. A white blood count is usually taken, and additional tests and examinations may be ordered as necessary to rule out other conditions that might be causing the symptoms.

Treatment

The appendix is removed surgically, resulting in complete cure. The appendix has no known function within the body, and its removal causes no change in body function. Parenteral fluids may be administered preoperatively or postoperatively. On the day after surgery the patient may be permitted food and fluids as tolerated, and is usually allowed out of bed. Convalescence may be rapid, but depends on the patient's age and general physical condition. A healthy young adult is usually able to return to his regular activities within 2 to 4 weeks. He is advised to avoid heavy lifting or unusual exertion for several months.

Nursing management

The nurse's role involves the early reporting of symptoms that may indicate appendicitis, the preparation of the patient for emergency surgery, and the postoperative nursing care required by any patient who has had abdominal surgery. Preparations for surgery and routine postoperative care are discussed in Chapter 9.

Prevention of Complications. Early diagnosis and modern surgical treatment have made death from appendicitis a rarity. Nevertheless, death can and does occur. Severe illness and death result all too often from a delay in seeking medical attention and from attempts to relieve the symptoms with home remedies.

The nurse can help to reduce complications and death from appendicitis by instructing families in what to do (and specially what *not* to do). When abdominal pain occurs:

- A physician should be consulted for any abdominal pain that is severe, or that does not disappear in a short period of time.
- Cathartics or enemas must be avoided. Either of these increases peristalsis, which may result in perforation of the inflamed appendix and in peritonitis.
- Nothing should be taken by mouth. Eating may aggravate the condition, and if surgery should be necessary, it is best that the stomach be empty.
- The patient must lie quietly in the position that is most comfortable until examined by a physician.

Peritonitis

The term *peritonitis* means inflammation of the *peritoneum,* a serous sac lining the abdominal cavity. The intestines, normally filled with bacteria, are among the organs enclosed in the peritoneum. Any break in the continuity of the intestines that causes a leakage of the intestinal contents can lead to inflammation and infection of the peritoneum. Two of the most common causes of peritonitis are perforation of the appendix and perforation of a duodenal ulcer. In both instances the intestinal contents escape into the peritoneal cavity, causing peritonitis. The infection may be widespread within the peritoneum (generalized peritonitis), or may be localized and lead to the formation of an abscess. Initial chemical inflammation of the peritoneum often follows the rupture of various organs; however, chemical inflammation is usually followed promptly by bacterial invasion.

Diagnosis

The most severe pain and tenderness usually occur over the area of the greatest peritoneal inflammation. The location of the pain helps the physician to determine, for example, whether the peritonitis is due to a perforation of the appendix or of the duodenum. A leukocyte count and an x-ray examination of the abdomen are other important aids in the diagnosis.

Symptoms

The symptoms of peritonitis include severe abdominal pain and tenderness, nausea, and vomiting. Fever may be absent initially, but the temperature rises as the infection becomes established. The pulse becomes rapid and weak, and the respirations are shallow. The patient avoids movement of the abdomen when he breathes, because such movement increases his pain. He often lies with his knees drawn up toward his abdomen, because this position seems to lessen the pain. *Paralytic ileus* (paralysis of the intestines), a condition in which peristalsis fails, and flatus and intestinal contents accumulate in the bowel, typically accompanies peritonitis. The patient's abdomen is rigid and boardlike. As the condition progresses, the abdomen becomes somewhat softer and very distended with the gas and the intestinal contents that cannot pass normally through the tract. Marked leukocytosis commonly occurs in peritonitis.

If the infection is uncontrolled, the patient becomes very weak; his pulse becomes more rapid and thready; his abdomen is distended further, leading to even more shallow breathing; and his temperature falls. The patient is moribund.

Prevention, treatment, and nursing management

The early diagnosis and treatment of such conditions as appendicitis have decreased the incidence of peritonitis. Strict surgical asepsis and the use of antibiotics before performing surgery on the intestines have diminished the number of patients who develop peritonitis as a complication of surgery.

Preventing further leakage of intestinal contents into the peritoneal cavity is an important measure in treatment. If the duodenum has perforated due to peptic ulcer, the area of perforation is closed surgically, so that no further escape of the intestinal contents can take place. If the intestinal contents are leaking from a ruptured appendix, the appendix is removed. Gastrointestinal decompression is used to drain the accumulated gas and the intestinal contents that are prevented by intestinal paralysis from passing normally through the tract.

The replacement of fluids and electrolytes is also important. The patient can take nothing by mouth, and water and electrolytes are being lost in vomitus and in the drainage from the gastrointestinal intubation. Large quantities of body fluids and electrolytes collect in the peritoneal cavity instead of circulating normally throughout the body, thus increasing the problem of water and electrolyte imbalance.

Large doses of antibiotics are given to combat infection. Analgesics, such as meperidine (Demerol), are often necessary to relieve pain and to promote rest. The head of the patient's bed is elevated to allow drainage to settle in the pelvic region, where, if abscesses occur, they may be drained more readily.

All of these measures are designed to aid the body in its fight against the infection, thereby providing favorable conditions for healing.

Nursing Management. The patient with peritonitis is very ill and requires detailed care and observation. His symptoms often change rapidly, and the nurse must be ready with answers to such questions as:

- Is his abdomen more distended? Is it softer, or more rigid?
- Is the pain growing less? Where does the patient feel the most severe pain?
- Is gas being passed rectally? Has the patient had a bowel movement?
- Is he vomiting? What is the character of the vomitus?
- Is the pulse weaker, more rapid? Is his temperature rising?
- How much has he voided? How much drainage has been returned through the tube which has been passed to the stomach or the intestines? How much parenteral fluid has he received?

Mouth care is very important. Often the patient is vomiting. The inability to take anything by mouth, the presence of a gastrointestinal tube, and fever make the patient's mouth feel dry and parched and cause an unpleasant taste and odor.

Cleanliness and an orderly environment help the patient to rest. Linen that has become wet with perspiration or soiled by vomitus should be changed.

Sometimes the patient becomes disoriented. Side rails on the bed are important to prevent him from harming himself, and he should be observed frequently.

The patient with peritonitis requires *gentleness* above all else. Every movement causes him added pain. If the patient must be removed from his bed to a stretcher for x-ray examination or surgery, the nurse will require assistance to lift him as gently and as smoothly as possible. Precautions should be taken to avoid placing any accidental pressure on the patient's tender abdomen.

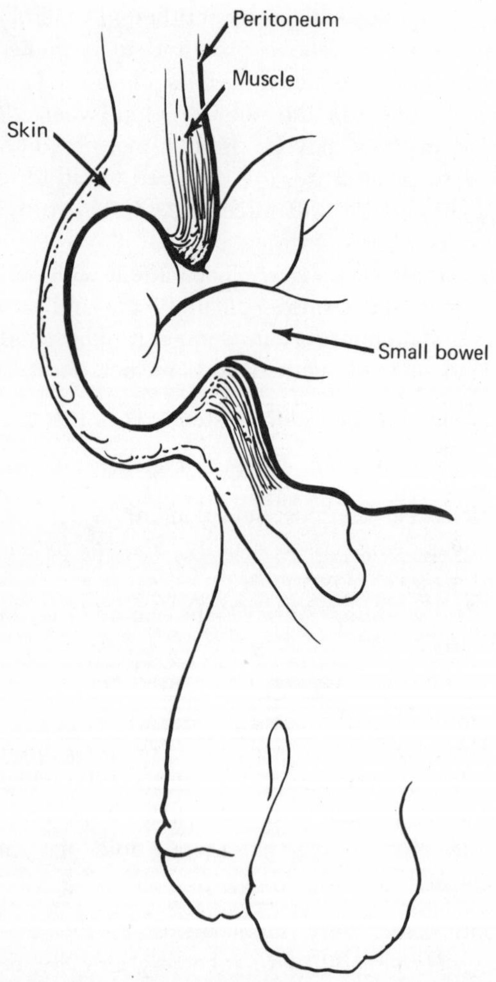

figure 32-1. Inguinal hernia, demonstrating how the small bowel can become caught in the herniated sac.

Hernia

Although the term *hernia* may be used in relation to the protrusion of any organ from the cavity that normally confines it, it is used most commonly to describe the protrusion of intestines through a defect in the abdominal wall. The word *rupture* is used sometimes by lay persons to describe this condition. When a hernia occurs, a lump or swelling appears on the abdomen underneath the skin. The swelling may be large or small, depending on how much of the viscera has protruded. Because hernia occurs frequently and sometimes causes no symptoms other than a swelling, its potential seriousness is often overlooked.

Types of Hernia. The most common types of abdominal hernia are inguinal (Fig. 32-1), umbilical, femoral, and incisional. Certain points on the abdominal wall are normally weaker than others, and they are more vulnerable to the development of hernia. These points are the *inguinal ring,* the point on the abdominal wall where the inguinal canal begins; the *femoral ring,* at the abdominal opening of the femoral canal; and the *umbilicus.*

Incisional hernias occur through the scar of a surgical incision when healing has been impaired. Incisional hernias can often be avoided by careful surgical technique, with particular emphasis on the prevention of wound infection. Obese or aged patients and those who suffer from malnutrition are especially prone to the development of an incisional hernia.

If the protruding structures can be replaced in the abdominal cavity, the hernia is said to be *reducible.* Lying down and applying manual pressure over the area often serves to reduce the hernia. An irreducible hernia is one that cannot be replaced in the abdominal cavity. Edema of the protruding structures and constriction of the opening through which they have emerged make it impossible for them to return to the abdominal cavity. This condition is called *incarceration.* If this process continues without treatment, the blood supply to the trapped viscera can be cut off, leading to gangrene of the trapped tissues. This condition is called a *strangulated hernia* and constitutes a surgical emergency.

Etiology. Congenital defects account for a large proportion of hernias, including those that appear after childhood. The hernia may be apparent in infancy, or it may appear in young adulthood in response to increased intra-abdominal pressure, such as that which occurs during heavy lifting, sneezing, coughing, or pregnancy. Obesity and the weakening of muscles may be responsible for the development of hernia in later middle life and old age.

INCIDENCE. Inguinal hernias are the type that occur most commonly. Men are more likely to develop an inguinal hernia, whereas umbilical and femoral hernias are more frequent among women.

DIAGNOSIS can usually be made by physical examination. Occasionally, x-ray films of the intestinal tract are ordered.

SYMPTOMS. Hernia may cause no symptoms other than the appearance of a swelling on the abdomen when the patient coughs, stands, or lifts something heavy. Sometimes the swelling is painful; the pain disappears when the hernia is reduced. Incarcerated hernias cause severe pain; as noted, if they are not treated, they may become strangulated. The symptoms of strangulated hernia are discussed under complications.

COMPLICATIONS OF HERNIA

When a hernia first occurs, the defect in the abdominal wall is usually small. However, as the hernia persists, and the organs continue to protrude, the defect grows larger, making surgical repair more difficult. The hernia may become incarcerated or even strangulated. *Strangulation is an acute emergency.* The patient suffers extreme abdominal pain, and the severe pressure on the loop of intestine that is protruding outside the abdominal cavity causes intestinal obstruction. Unless surgery is performed promptly, the patient may die. If a portion of the bowel has become gangrenous due to the curtailment of its blood supply, that part of the intestine must be excised, with anastomosis of the remaining portions of the intestine.

When a hernia is neglected for many years, the tissues in the area become weakened and do not heal as readily. Obese persons who have put off surgical repair of hernia for a prolonged period are especially prone to recurrence of the condition. Usually, the physician advises the obese patient to lose weight before the surgery is undertaken to lessen the possibility of recurrence.

HERNIA TREATMENT AND NURSING MANAGEMENT

Herniorrhaphy is an operation performed for the repair of a hernia. The protruding structures are replaced in the abdominal cavity, and the defect in the abdominal wall is repaired. Herniorrhaphy may be performed under spinal or general anesthesia.

IMPORTANCE OF EARLY TREATMENT. The nurse can help patients to appreciate the importance of seeking medical care for hernias that are not painful. It is hard to seek care (especially when one is quite sure an operation is needed) for something that causes little discomfort. It is so much easier to say, "It's not bothering me, so I won't bother it." But by the time the hernia does bother the patient, an operation that might have been relatively simple may be complicated by the poor condition of his tissues or even by strangulation. Therefore, most physicians advise patients to have hernias repaired promptly to avoid years of possible discomfort and the threat of complications.

NURSING MANAGEMENT. Usually, the patient is permitted out of bed on the day after the operation. If he has difficulty voiding, he may be permitted to stand at the bedside, with assistance, while he uses the urinal. If possible, an orderly or a male nurse should stay with the patient if it is necessary for him to stand to void on the day of surgery. If this is not possible, the nurse must evaluate by noting the patient's color and pulse, and whether or not he feels dizzy or faint, if it is safe to step outside the curtain for a moment to afford the patient some privacy.

Usually, the patient can tolerate food and fluids on the day after surgery. However, some patients, either because of the type and extent of the necessary surgery, or because of the existence of such complications as strangulation, are permitted nothing by mouth for several days postoperatively. These patients usually receive parenteral fluids until oral fluids are permitted.

Every effort is made to prevent conditions that might impair healing, since impairment of healing could lead to a recurrence of the hernia. Strict aseptic technique is important in preventing infection. An increase in intra-abdominal pressure, such as that which occurs when the patient is lifting or coughing, must be avoided. If the patient has a chronic cough, its cause should be investigated, and treatment given to relieve it before the herniorrhaphy is performed. The patient must be observed carefully postoperatively for the development of any sneezing or coughing. If these symptoms occur, they must be reported promptly to the physician. The patient should be shown how to splint the incision with his hand if he coughs or sneezes.

Walking about and breathing deeply are important in preventing postoperative complications. The patient should be encouraged to move, provided that he does not strain the operative area. Some patients are afraid to move or walk lest the hernia reappear. If the height

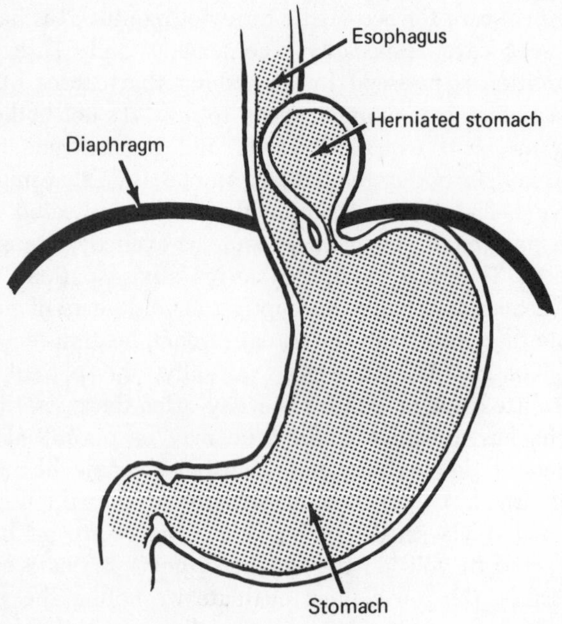

figure 32-2. Esophageal hiatus hernia—paraesophageal type. The herniated portion of the stomach protrudes through the diaphragm into the chest cavity.

of the bed is adjustable, it should be in the lowest position before the patient gets up, to avoid strain. If the bed is not adjustable, a footstool will help the patient to step easily from the high bed to the floor.

Male patients sometimes develop pain and swelling of the scrotum due to inflammation and edema after the repair of an inguinal hernia. Ice bags may be ordered for the relief of the pain and the swelling, and the scrotum may be supported with a suspensory. The male patient may find it easier to report pain, inflammation, and swelling of the scrotum to a male nurse or orderly. If the patient seems to be having unusual pain and is reluctant to move after the first 24 to 48 hours postoperatively, when the most severe pain near the incision has usually subsided, or if painful swelling of the scrotum has developed, the physician should be notified.

Because the operation is usually in the inguinal region, a man may feel embarrassed when the nurse checks the dressing postoperatively. Careful arranging of bedding, or giving the patient a towel to use as a drape will keep him from being exposed.

Restriction of Activities. Postoperative recovery for most patients is rapid. Patients who are in good health preoperatively often go home within a week. When the patient returns home, he is instructed to avoid strenuous exertion or heavy lifting until the physician feels this can be undertaken safely. Many factors determine the extent to which the patient's activities must be restricted: the location and size of the defect repaired, the condition of the patient's tissues, his age, and whether or not he is obese are examples. Patients who perform heavy physical labor may have to change occupations; those whose work is sedentary or light can usually return to full employment within a few weeks. Healthy young adults who have had repair of an uncomplicated hernia are likely to have no restrictions on activity.

Esophageal (diaphragmatic) hernia

An esophageal hernia is a protrusion, usually of a part of the stomach, through a defect in the diaphragm wall at the point where the esophagus passes through the diaphragm (Fig. 32-2). This is also called a diaphragmatic hernia. The condition may be caused by a congenital weakness in the diaphragm or by trauma. Factors which cause increased intra-abdominal pressure, such as multiple pregnancies, contribute to the development of hiatal hernia. The loss of muscle strength and tone that occurs with aging contributes to the condition; many persons who develop hiatal hernia are in older age groups, and the condition is especially common among older women.

The symptoms include heartburn, belching, and a feeling of substernal or epigastric pressure after eating. These symptoms are more severe when the patient lies down. The diagnosis is suggested by the history and confirmed by roentgenography. Most patients can be managed medically by weight reduction if obese, an ulcer-type diet, antacids, and elevation of the head bedpost on 6-inch blocks. This prevents the stomach acid from refluxing and chemically attacking the esophageal mucosa. Patients with reflex esophagitis secondary to hiatal hernia may bleed acutely, especially in the uncommon paraesophageal type. They may have melena or hematemesis. At times occult bleeding for long periods produces a typical iron deficiency anemia. Patients who do not respond to a rigid medical regimen are treated surgically.

Surgical treatment involves replacing the stomach or other protruding organs in the abdominal cavity and repairing the defect in the wall. The thoracic cavity is entered, so that postoperative care is similar to that of any patient who has chest surgery (see Chapter 21). Some repairs may be done with an abdominal rather than a thoracic surgical approach, in which case nursing management is similar to that of any general abdominal surgery. Continuous gastric suction usually is ordered postoperatively to prevent distention of the stomach and pressure on the surgical repair.

Mechanical intestinal obstruction

Cancer is the most common cause of intestinal obstruction, particularly in older persons. The tumor gradually becomes larger until it completely obstructs the bowel. Changes in bowel habits may be noted by the patient while an obstruction is partial. He may have alternating constipation and diarrhea. The diarrhea results from very forceful peristalsis, which is the body's way of pushing the intestinal contents through the narrowed lumen of the bowel. If the patient receives prompt diagnosis and treatment, complete obstruction may be averted.

Volvulus, a twisting or kinking of a portion of the intestines, is another condition causing a sudden obstruction of the intestine (Fig. 32-3). *Strangulated hernia* is a third common cause of acute intestinal obstruction.

Symptoms. The symptoms of severe intestinal obstruction may arise suddenly in a previously healthy individual. When the bowel is obstructed, the portion proximal to the obstruction becomes distended with intestinal contents, while the portion distal to the obstruction is empty. If the obstruction is complete, no gas or feces are expelled rectally. However, one or two bowel movements may occur soon after the obstruction has occurred, because the material already past the obstruction is being expelled. Peristalsis becomes very forceful in the proximal portion as the body attempts to propel the material beyond the point of the obstruction. These forceful peristaltic waves cause severe cramps, which tend to occur intermittently.

When an obstruction occurs high in the gastrointestinal tract, the patient usually vomits whatever contents are in the stomach and the small bowel. On the other hand, if the obstruction is low—for example, in the colon—vomiting usually does not occur.

The patient becomes dehydrated. He is unable to take oral fluids and loses water and electrolytes through vomiting. The failure of the mucosa to reabsorb the secretions that are poured into the intestine contributes to the water and the electrolyte imbalance.

Increasing pressure on the bowel due to severe distention and to edema often impairs circulation and leads to gangrene of a portion of the bowel. Perforation of the gangrenous bowel (which results from pressure against weakened tissue) causes the intestinal contents to seep into the peritoneal cavity, resulting in peritonitis. Intestinal obstruction is extremely dangerous and may prove fatal if prompt treatment is not instituted.

Diagnosis. The diagnosis is based on the patient's history and a careful physical examination. X-ray examination of the intestinal tract is usually necessary.

Treatment. Mechanical obstruction is most frequently treated surgically. The obstruction is relieved by a relatively minor surgical procedure, such as a temporary colostomy or cecostomy. After the patient's condition has improved as a result of relief of the obstruction and supportive therapy, more extensive surgery may be undertaken. Sometimes, because of the location and extent of a malignant process, a permanent colostomy is necessary.

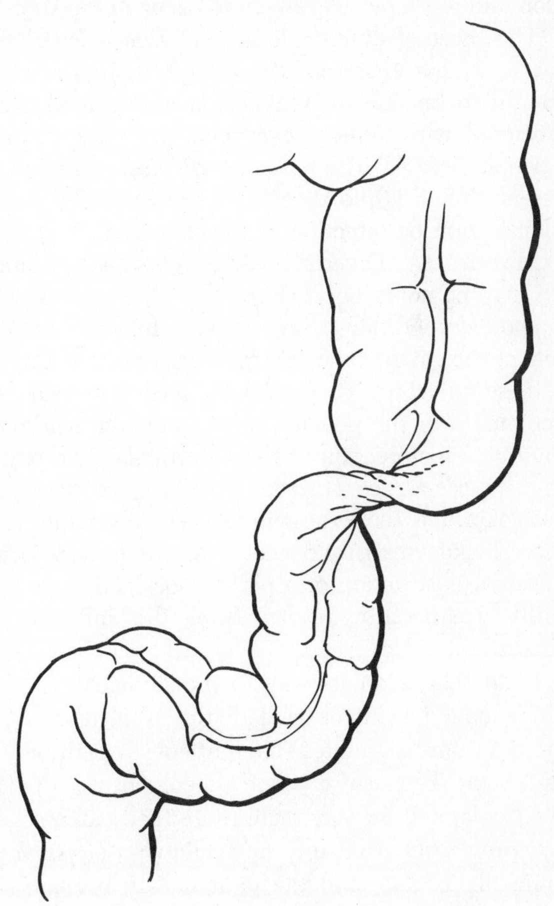

figure 32-3. Volvulus of the colon. The twisting can cause complete obstruction.

Intestinal decompression, parenteral therapy, and antibiotics, used preoperatively, help improve the patient's condition so that he can withstand surgery and make better progress during the postoperative period. Intestinal decompression is performed by passing a long tube, such as the Miller-Abbott tube, into the intestine. Large amounts of accumulated secretions and gas are drawn out through the tube by gentle suction, relieving distention and vomiting. Parenteral fluids and electrolytes are administered to correct fluid and electrolyte imbalance. Antibiotics may be ordered to combat infection.

Diverticulosis and diverticulitis

Diverticula are sacs or pouches caused by herniation of the mucosa through a weakened portion of the muscular coat of the intestine or other structure. Diverticula are common in the esophagus and the colon and are especially likely to occur in the sigmoid.

The cause of diverticula is unknown. It is believed that some diverticula are congenital, though most are thought to be due to weakness in the muscular coat associated with aging. Diverticula are most common in people over 50. The term *diverticulosis* refers to the presence of multiple diverticula; *diverticulitis* means inflammation or infection of the diverticula.

SYMPTOMS. Diverticulosis is often asymptomatic and may be noted only when x-ray films are taken for some other condition, or at autopsy. However, the contents of the gastrointestinal tract often become trapped in these pouches. For example, fecal material may accumulate in the pouches of the sigmoid, leading to irritation and infection of the diverticula. The patient may experience constipation, diarrhea or flatulence. Also, pain and tenderness in the left lower quadrant, fever, leukocytosis, and rectal bleeding may occur. Intestinal obstruction or a perforation leading to peritonitis occasionally results from the inflammatory process.

Food that is on its way to the stomach often becomes lodged in diverticula of the esophagus, where it remains and stagnates. The patient's breath may be unpleasant because of food decomposition in the diverticula, and he may regurgitate food eaten several days previously. Difficulty in swallowing (*dysphagia*) commonly occurs, and the patient may become seriously malnourished. Cough sometimes occurs because of irritation of the trachea.

TREATMENT. Diverticula noted during routine examination require no treatment if they do not cause symptoms. Diverticulitis with resultant stricture formation may be difficult to differentiate from carcinoma except at surgery.

Diverticulitis of the colon often responds to medical treatment. During a very acute episode with pain and local tenderness, the patient may be maintained on intravenous fluids for several days with no oral intake. As the inflammation subsides under antibiotic therapy, a low-residue diet is permitted. Constipation is to be avoided in these patients; good fluid intake and regular evacuation should be encouraged. Some physicians advocate the use of a stool softener or mineral oil to aid in normal evacuation. If the condition does not respond to medical treatment, or if complications such as perforation, intestinal obstruction, or severe bleeding occur, surgery is necessary. The portion of colon containing the diverticula is removed, and the continuity of the bowel is reestablished by joining the remaining portions of the colon. Depending on the location and extent of the disease and whether there is intestinal obstruction, a temporary colostomy must sometimes be performed. The continuity of the bowel is restored in a later operation, and the colostomy is closed.

Diverticula of the esophagus are usually excised if they are symptomatic. The resulting opening in the esophagus is closed, thus restoring normal function and giving complete relief of symptoms. If a diverticulum is located in the upper portion of the esophagus, the postoperative patient may take a liquid, followed by a bland diet, soon after surgery. General postoperative nursing management is required. If a diverticulum is lower in the esophagus, the operation must be performed through an incision into the thoracic cavity.

Regional enteritis

Regional enteritis (inflammation of the small intestine) is a disease of unknown cause occurring most commonly among young adults. The disease often has a patchy distribution throughout large portions of the duodenum, the ileum, and the jejunum.

The symptoms usually include pain in the right lower quadrant, fever, and diarrhea. The patient may also have leukocytosis and tenderness of the abdomen. The condition may be confused with acute appendicitis. Usually, the disease has an insidious onset and a variable course. Some patients have a gradual increase in symptoms, whereas others may have acute exacerbations alternating with remissions. Sometimes, the condition subsides spontaneously. Intestinal obstruction, perforation, or abscesses may occur, and fistulas may form between loops of the intestine.

Treatment is usually supportive. Rest, relief of emotional stress, and a bland diet high in proteins and calories often are prescribed. Parenteral therapy with fluids, electrolytes, and whole blood may be necessary to correct anemia and to restore the fluid and electrolyte balance. Supplementary vitamins, iron and corticosteroids may be prescribed. None of these treatments is curative.

Surgical treatment is usually reserved for complications such as intestinal obstruction or perforation. The affected sections of the small bowel may be removed or bypassed and anastomosis of the remaining segments performed. Surgical treatment is made more difficult because the disease tends to be widely scattered. An attempt may be made to divert the flow of the intestinal contents from the diseased area by joining the proximal healthy portion of the ileum with the colon (ileocolostomy), thus bypassing the diseased area of the ileum. Sometimes the diseased portion of the ileum is removed later. If the patient progresses satisfactorily, it is often considered unnecessary to remove the diseased segment. Regardless of the type of treatment used, a recurrence of the disease is common.

Malabsorption

Many conditions interfere with normal intestinal absorption of nutrients, water, and vitamins. Malabsorption results in general symptoms of weight loss, weakness, wasting, and the passage of abnormal stools. The stools are usually quite bulky, frothy, pale in color, and foul smelling due to the high content of fat, i.e., steatorrhea. The cause of malabsorption may be found in the wall of the small intestine itself as in adult celiac disease or may be secondary to deficiency of digestive enzymes as in pancreatic disease such as chronic pancreatitis. Symptoms are related to the particular type of malabsorption experienced by the patient. For example, deficient absorption of vitamin B complex can cause glossitis, tenderness of muscles, dermatitis, and peripheral neuritis. Vitamin K loss leads to hypoprothrombinemia and easy bleeding; loss of calcium causes tetany and bone demineralization.

Patients with adult celiac disease are unable to metabolize gluten, a protein which is contained in wheat, rye, and barley. In some way not fully understood, ingestion of gluten damages the intestinal mucosa, thus interfering with absorption of nutrients, vitamins, and water. Symptoms improve dramatically with administration of a gluten-free diet, which must be continued indefinitely; symptoms recur if the diet is discontinued. A marked familial tendency toward this disease has been noted.

Pancreatic insufficiency with secondary malabsorption is treated by ingestion of pancreatic extract with meals.

Malabsorption is not easily diagnosed in patients who do not have a severe form of the disease and are not malnourished. Therefore, the nurse's accurate description of the character of the stool seen in a patient with diarrhea may be critical in leading to a diagnosis of malabsorption.

Hemorrhoids

Hemorrhoids are varicose veins of the anus and the rectum. They may occur outside the anal sphincter (external hemorrhoids) or inside the sphincter (internal hemorrhoids) (Fig. 32-4). These sphincters keep the orifice closed except during defecation. External hemorrhoids appear as small, reddish-blue lumps at the edge of the anus.

Etiology. Pregnancy, intra-abdominal tumors, chronic constipation, and hereditary factors may foster the development of hemorrhoids.

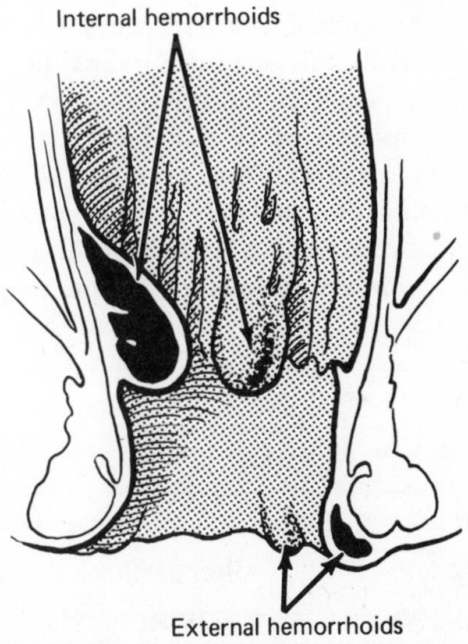

figure 32-4. Internal and external hemorrhoids.

Table 32-1.
Postoperative nursing management of the patient having rectal surgery

Vital signs should be taken as ordered or q4h. Body temperature should be taken orally.
The amount voided should be checked. If the physician allows it, the male patient may stand at the bedside to void and the female patient may use the bedside commode.
Sitz baths should be given as ordered.
The rectal area must be kept clean.
A rubber ring should be provided for the patient to sit on when he is allowed out of bed.

SYMPTOMS. Thrombosed external hemorrhoids are painful lumps appearing near the anus. One or two such swellings may appear and disappear spontaneously within a few days. The pain and swelling are caused by clotted blood within the vein. Thrombosed external hemorrhoids rarely cause bleeding. However, they may become large and more numerous, causing pain as well as itching. The pain is especially severe when the patient has a bowel movement, causing him to put off defecation as long as possible. Constipation results, or if already present, is aggravated. Constipation and straining at stool make the hemorrhoids worse.

Internal hemorrhoids often cause bleeding, but they are less likely to cause pain unless they protrude through the anus. The bleeding may vary from an occasional drop or two of blood on toilet tissue or underwear to a chronic loss of blood that leads to anemia. Internal hemorrhoids usually protrude each time the patient defecates. At first, he is able to push them back inside the sphincter with his finger. Gradually, as the masses grow larger, they remain permanently outside the sphincter and often cause a chronic discharge of blood and mucus.

DIAGNOSIS. The physician notes the presence of external hemorrhoids merely by inspection. Unless internal hemorrhoids protrude through the anus, an anoscope or proctoscope must be used to see them. Since the symptoms may be similar to those of cancer, a very thorough examination of the anal and rectal areas is necessary. The patient who experiences rectal bleeding may have hemorrhoids or cancer, or both.

Anyone who experiences pain, bleeding, or swelling in the anal region should be examined promptly, so that the cause of the condition can be determined.

TREATMENT AND NURSING MANAGEMENT

A small external hemorrhoid often disappears without treatment, or may be relieved by warm sitz baths. The physician may recommend an ointment containing a local anesthetic for the relief of discomfort. Ointments containing dibucaine (Nupercaine) are frequently used for this purpose. The correction of constipation is important both in relieving the condition and in preventing its recurrence. Mineral oil or a stool softener such as Surfak (dioctyl calcium sulfosuccinate) may be ordered.

Surgical excision of the dilated veins (*hemorrhoidectomy*) is frequently required. This procedure is the most common rectal surgery among adults.

The principles of caring for a patient after any type of rectal surgery are similar (Table 32-1). Although hemorrhoids are the most common indication for rectal surgery, the conditions listed in Table 32-2 are also encountered among adults.

Many patients have difficulty voiding after rectal surgery; thus it is important that voiding is checked for several days postoperatively. The first bowel movement will be painful. A stool softener may be ordered

Table 32-2.
Common rectal conditions

CONDITION	DESCRIPTION	TREATMENT
Anal fissure	Ulcer involving the skin of the anal wall	Sitz baths, local anesthetics, surgery
Anal abscess	Localized infection of tissues near the anus	Incision and drainage
Anal fistula	Abnormal tunnel or passageway within the tissues often caused by anal abscess	Fistulotomy

to relieve some of the discomfort. Sitz baths are used in postoperative management of patients having rectal surgery to increase circulation to the rectal area, thereby reducing congestion and swelling, and to relieve pain.

Pilonidal sinus

Pilonidal is a term which means "a nest of hair." The words *sinus* and *cyst* are both used to describe the condition. However, studies indicate that the lesion is not a cyst but a sinus. The condition typically occurs after puberty, when the hair in the anogenital region becomes thick and stiff. The skin deep in the cleft in the sacrococcygeal region becomes macerated. Persons with a deep cleft in this region and those who are hirsute are predisposed to the condition. Inadequate personal hygiene, obesity, and trauma to the area also contribute to the development of a pilonidal sinus. Stiff hairs in the sacrococcygeal region irritate and pierce the soft, macerated skin, becoming imbedded in it. The hairs then cause inflammation of the tissues. Infection readily follows, due to the break in the skin which permits the entrance of microorganisms. Several channels lead from the sinus to the skin; their openings on the skin are called *pilonidal openings.* Often, hair protrudes from them.

Usually, the patient is unaware that he has a pilonidal sinus until it becomes infected. Then he experiences pain and swelling at the base of his spine, and may note purulent drainage on his clothing.

The treatment of pilonidal sinus involves an operation in which the sinus and all its connecting channels are laid open; drainage of purulent material, removal of the hair, and cleaning facilitate healing with normal, healthy tissue. Antibiotics may be administered.

NURSING MANAGEMENT. In nursing management after the surgical treatment of a pilonidal sinus:

- Care must be taken to keep the dressings from being soiled.
- Mineral-oil and oil-retention enemas may be used before the first bowel movement.
- After the first few postoperative days the nurse may be asked to change the dressing.

During the immediate postoperative period the patient lies on his abdomen. He is kept in bed from 1 to several days. When permitted out of bed, he is instructed to take short steps and to avoid prolonged sitting, so that strain will not be placed on the incision. Also, the height of the bed should be adjusted, or a footstool used, when the patient gets in and out of bed to prevent strain on the operative area.

General nutritional considerations

- Patients with esophageal hiatal hernia may be treated medically with a soft bland diet. In the beginning the physician may order small portions and interval feedings in an attempt to prevent gastric distention.
- Patients with diverticulitis may be given a low-residue diet. On this diet fruits, sharp cheeses, milk, crackers, bread, whole grain cereals, pork, tough meats, pies, pastries, and vegetables are avoided.
- If the adult patient with malabsorption syndrome has adult celiac disease a gluten-free diet is necessary. On this diet wheat, rye, and barley and any foods made from these grains are avoided. Special dietary adjustments may be necessary and will usually depend on the severity of the disease.

General pharmacological considerations

- Anemia due to chronic blood loss from the gastrointestinal tract may be treated with oral or parenteral iron until corrected. Oral iron will color the stool black. Tarry stools due to bleeding in the gastrointestinal tract may have been present prior to therapy; therefore the patient should be warned about the color change of his stool due to iron therapy.
- Malabsorption may be treated with oral pancreatic enzymes which are taken *with* meals.
- Local anesthetic preparations may be used to treat external hemorrhoids. Examples of these are: Xylocaine suppositories, Anugesic suppositories, and Nupercainal ointment.
- Stool softeners such as Surfak (dioctyl calcium sulfosuccinate) may be used in patients who should avoid straining at stool. Mineral oil may also be ordered; however, consistent use of mineral oil has two disadvantages, (1) it prevents the absorption of oil soluble vitamins (A, D, E, K), and (2) with overuse and overdose it has a tendency to leak past the rectal sphincter, which may slow healing of anal tissue. Patients should be advised to check with their physician regarding the type of laxative to be used in rectal disorders.

Bibliography

AMERICAN COLLEGE OF SURGEONS, Kinney, J. M. et al, eds.: *Manual of Preoperative and Postoperative Care,* ed. 2. Philadelphia, Saunders, 1971.

BEHRINGER, G. E.: Diverticular disease of the colon (pictorial). Hosp. Med. 11:6, September, 1975.

BRUNNER, L. S. and SUDDARTH, D. S.: *Lippincott Manual of Nursing Practice.* Philadelphia, Lippincott, 1974.

EMMANUEL, S.: Basic surgery: Techniques of hiatal hernia repair (pictorial), Part 2. RN 37:OR/ED 1, September, 1974.

GELB, A. M. et al: Diverticulitis or colitis—or both? (pictorial). Consultant 15:139, March, 1975.

GIVEN, B. A. and SIMMONS, S. J.: *Nursing Care of the Patient with Gastrointestinal Disorders.* St. Louis, Mosby, 1971.

HARDISON, W. G. M.: Reflux—the real problem in hiatus hernia. Consultant 15:116, March, 1975.

PAINTER, N. S.: Diverticular disease. Emer. Med. 7:110, April, 1975.

REYNOLDS, W. J.: Sutureless hemorrhoidectomy (pictorial). RN 36:OR/ED 11, May, 1973.

RHOADS, J. E. et al: *Surgery: Principles and Practice,* ed. 4. Philadelphia, Lippincott, 1970.

SHAFER, K. N. et al: *Medical-Surgical Nursing,* ed. 6. St. Louis, Mosby, 1975.

SLEISENGER, M. and FORDTRAN, J.: *Gastrointestinal Disease: Pathophysiology, Diagnosis, Management.* Philadelphia, Saunders, 1973.

WILKES, E. T.: Straight talk about hemorrhoids. Family Health 6:48, October, 1974.

CHAPTER—33

The patient with disorder of the liver, gallbladder, or pancreas

On completion of this chapter the student will:

- Understand the general anatomy and physiology of the liver and its multiple and complex metabolic activities.
- Discuss the tests used in the diagnosis of liver disease and the related nursing management of the patient undergoing tests for the determination of liver function.
- Discuss overt symptoms, etiology, and nursing management of jaundice.
- List the types and causes of cirrhosis.
- Describe the signs, symptoms, and medical management of the patient with cirrhosis and hepatic coma.
- Participate in the formation of a nursing care plan and in the nursing management of a patient with cirrhosis or hepatic coma.
- Define esophageal varices and give the medical and surgical management of this disorder.
- Give the pathology, etiology, signs, symptoms and medical and nursing management of the patient with hepatitis.
- Understand the general anatomy and physiology of the biliary system.
- Discuss diseases of the biliary system—cholecystitis and cholelithiasis—and the medical and surgical management of each.

Behavioral objectives (continued)

- **Participate in the nursing management of a patient with biliary surgery.**
- **Discuss signs, symptoms, and medical management of pancreatitis.**
- **Participate in the formulation of a nursing care plan and in the nursing management of a patient with pancreatitis.**

The patient with liver disease

Management of patients with liver disease requires particular concern for nutrition, for health teaching over an extended period, and for meticulous physical care when the patient is acutely ill. Although some work is beginning to be done in relation to liver transplants, it is still in the very early stages. The emphasis in nursing management of patients with liver disease is, therefore, on measures to support the patient physiologically, so that his liver will have the best possible chance to regain adequate function, and to support the patient emotionally during a lengthy and often discouraging period of illness.

Anatomy and physiology

The liver is the largest glandular organ in the body, weighing between 1.0 and 1.5 kg. It is located in the right upper abdomen, just under the right diaphragm which separates it from the right lung. The liver has two major lobes, right and left, and two small lobes—the caudate and quadrate lobes—located on the under surface. The liver is supported in place by intra-abdominal pressure, as well as by various attachments called ligaments or mesenteries. These attachments connect the liver to adjacent intestines, abdominal wall, and diaphragm. Unless it is abnormally enlarged, the liver is not usually felt when the abdomen is palpated.

The liver receives arterial blood from the hepatic artery, an indirect branch of the aorta. The portal vein transports blood from the intestinal tract to the liver. After it has traversed vascular pathways inside the liver, the blood is collected by the hepatic veins and transported to the inferior vena cava, and then back to the heart.

Microscopically, the internal structure of the liver includes smaller ramifications of the hepatic artery, the hepatic and portal veins, lymphatics, and bile ducts. The cellular constituents of the liver are the hepatic parenchymal cells, which carry out most of the liver's metabolic functions, and the Kupffer or reticulo-endothelial cells, which engage in the immunologic, detoxifying, and blood-filtering actions of the liver.

The liver is involved in a multitude of vital, complex metabolic activities. Among the most important functions are the formation and excretion of bile; the utilization, transformation, and distribution of vitamins, proteins, fats, and carbohydrates; the storage of energy-yielding glycogen; the synthesis of factors needed for blood coagulation, including prothrombin and fibrinogen; the detoxification of endogenous and exogenous chemicals, bacteria, and foreign elements which may be harmful; and the formation of antibodies and immunizing substances, including gamma globulin.

Diagnosis of liver disease and related nursing management

Because different types of liver disease require extremely different kinds of treatment, great care is required in making the medical diagnosis, and many tests are often necessary. Sometimes the patient becomes weary or frightened by the diagnostic procedures, and it becomes especially important to help him understand the necessity for these tests.

Recognition of the importance of accurate diagnosis accents the necessity for nursing intervention which stresses emotional support of the patient during diagnostic tests and explanation to the patient of the procedure for the test. Nursing measures can diminish the patient's discomfort. For example, he is often kept fasting in the morning until blood samples are drawn. Promptly serving his tray as soon as the blood specimens have been taken and making sure that the food served is hot can lessen the patient's discouragement as well as promote adequate nutrition, so important in liver disease. Patients with liver disease frequently must have many venipunctures and sometimes become very tense about this procedure. While in most hospitals a technician draws the blood, it is essential for the nurse to remain during the procedure if the patient is frightened. Diverting the patient's attention from the venipuncture by asking him to look at you and to concentrate on squeezing your hand is a useful nursing measure. Helping the patient tolerate the procedure makes it easier for the technician to draw the blood, lessens the patient's discomfort, and minimizes trauma to the patient's veins.

Liver Function Tests. Most tests of liver function require samples of blood drawn while the patient is fasting. Ordinarily the blood specimens are taken in the morning, and the patient's breakfast is postponed until after the blood has been drawn. A technician from the laboratory is usually assigned the tasks of seeing that specimen bottles are accurately labeled and carefully transported to the chemistry laboratory and that tubes containing special additives are used when necessary (for prothrombin determination, for example, to avoid clot formation). Tests which employ dye, such as the BSP test, require calculation of the dose of dye based upon the patient's weight, as well as accurate timing of the period between dye injection and blood collection. Accuracy in carrying out these details is essential and is promoted by careful planning and coordination among all persons involved. In most hospitals the physician injects dye, such as for a BSP test, and collection of specimens is carefully timed after dye is administered. It is important to have an understanding ahead of time about which physician will administer the dye and when the dye will be given. Similar planning should occur with personnel from the laboratory. If telephone reminders are necessary during the test, the ward secretary should be given a list of persons to be called, indicating the times when the calls should be made.

Total Serum Bilirubin. The level is elevated in jaundice from bile duct obstruction or other causes. (See section on Jaundice.)

Urine bilirubin, urine urobilinogen, and fecal urobilinogen are other pigment tests given to assist in confirming findings indicated by serum bilirubin testing.

Alkaline phosphatase, serum glutamic oxaloacetic transaminase and glutamic pyruvic transaminase (SGOT and SGPT), and lactic dehydrogenase (LDH) are enzymes whose blood levels help in identification of hepatic neoplasms, obstruction, or infection. Liver cells have been found to be rich in enzymes such as transaminase. When the liver cells are damaged by viruses (as in hepatitis) or by alcohol (as in Laennec's cirrhosis), the enzyme is released into the bloodstream.

Both albumin and cholesterol are synthesized in the liver. In major liver dysfunction blood levels of both are depressed. Alkaline phosphatase of liver origin is elevated in obstructive jaundice whether of intra- or extrahepatic origin.

Prothrombin time measures the level of a coagulation factor, prothrombin, synthesized by the liver.

Bromsulphalein time (BSP), indocyanine green (ICG) and I^{131} rose bengal are dye-excretion tests which are useful determinants of liver damage. Because BSP is excreted by the liver in the same fashion as bilirubin, the BSP test has been used as a fine measure of excretory function when the level of serum bilirubin is still normal.

Serum albumin and globulin level, thymol turbidity and cephalin flocculation are tests of liver proteins and may reflect the nature and degree of hepatic disease.

Serum cholesterol level is reduced in severe liver damage, but usually elevated in biliary obstruction and liver cancers.

Serum ammonia level may be increased in a failing liver which cannot detoxify this endogenous waste product of intestinal protein metabolism.

Liver biopsy, one of the more complex tests used to define hepatic disorders, involves direct, microscopic analysis of liver tissue. This may be done percutaneously, by passing a special biopsy needle through the skin into the liver, or through a small abdominal incision under general or local anesthesia. Percutaneous needle biopsy is not performed if there is a bleeding tendency, obstructive jaundice which may result in hidden hemorrhage, or bile leakage from the biopsy site.

The patient is asked to sign an operative permit before the biopsy is performed. Preoperative prothrombin time is determined and the patient is usually kept fasting. Blood for transfusion will be ordered and kept in readiness in case it is needed. Postoperatively the patient is maintained at rest, and vital signs and the condition of the dressing are observed every hour. Fall in blood pressure, tachycardia, shoulder pain, abdominal pain or distention and staining of dressing with excessive blood or bile are indications of complications, and should be immediately reported to the physician.

Esophagoscopy, barium esophagogram, and upper gastrointestinal x-ray tests (GI series) may be ordered to help the physician assess the status of the esophagus and other parts of the upper gastrointestinal tract, because these organs are often affected by liver disease.

Portal venography and hepatic arteriography are methods by which contrast material is introduced into the hepatic circulation. Appropriate x-ray pictures will then define the character of the blood vessels as well as outline defects within the liver substance. Pressure in the portal venous system can also be determined in patients with portal hypertension and cirrhosis.

Liver scan following intravenous administration of radioactive substances such as $iodine^{131}$, labeled albumin, or rose bengal, and colloidal $gold^{198}$ can give a picture of liver size, shape and effects of space-occupying lesions such as tumors (primary or metastatic) or abscess. The pattern of radioisotope uptake may yield information as to the amount of liver damage and help to differentiate various types of disease. No special precautions are required in relation to radioactivity when the patient has received substances such as I^{131} intravenously.

Jaundice (icterus)

Jaundice is a greenish yellow discoloration of tissue due to staining by an abnormally high concentration of the pigment bilirubin in the blood. Normally, total bilirubin concentration is about 0.1 to 1.2 mg. per 100 ml. of blood. If this reaches over 3 mg. per 100 ml. of blood or higher, jaundice is visible, notably on the skin, mucous membrane of the mouth, and especially the sclera (white portion of eye).

Jaundice occurs in a multitude of diseases which directly or indirectly affect the liver. It is probably the most common sign of liver disorder. Important to the understanding of jaundice is a knowledge of bile formation and excretion.

When red blood cells are old or injured, they are picked up by the spleen and bone marrow where they are broken down by reticuloendothelial cells. Hemoglobin released from these red blood cells is then reduced to the compound known as "unconjugated" or "indirect" bilirubin. This type of bilirubin is then carried by the blood to the liver where further chemical processes transform it into "conjugated" or "direct" bilirubin. These two forms of bilirubin are distinct, can be differentiated chemically, and are important in the clinical discrimination between different diseases producing jaundice.

The "conjugated" bilirubin formed by the liver enters the bile ducts, reaches the intestine, and is there transformed into urobilinogen. Urobilinogen is then changed into urobilin, the brown pigment of stool. Urobilinogen enters the bloodstream and is carried back to the liver where it is changed into bilirubin for reexcretion in the bile. Another portion of urobilinogen is carried from the intestine to the kidney and is excreted in the urine.

In diseases causing jaundice, the laboratory determination of the type of pigments in blood, urine, and stool promotes a more accurate diagnosis and permits the most appropriate therapy.

For purposes of discussion, jaundice may be classified in three different forms: (1) hemolytic jaundice (due to the overabundance of breakdown products of blood); (2) hepatocellular jaundice (due to internal liver disease preventing normal transformation of bile by the liver cells); and (3) obstructive jaundice (due to the inability of normally formed liver bile to be passed into the intestine because of duct blockage).

Jaundice is both a sign and a symptom; it is not a separate disease.

Pruritus may be an extremely disquieting, difficult to control feature of obstructive jaundice. Soda or starch baths, calamine, and other soothing lotions may be helpful. Barbiturates and narcotics as well as any drug detoxified by the liver are contraindicated or are used with extreme caution in patients with liver disease.

In addition to the morning bath, sponge bathing with tepid water several times a day may be beneficial in lessening itching. Explain to the patient that scratching can lead to infection of the skin, and help him avoid this by such measures as:

- Keeping the nails short and clean.
- Avoiding too-warm bedding.
- Assisting him to find diversion, because concentrating on itching makes it worse.
- Giving him a supply of calamine lotion (if ordered) and cotton swabs with instruction to apply it to particularly itchy spots.
- Making special efforts to promote comfort at night by such methods as soothing backrubs, a starch bath (if ordered), and an evening snack. Itching tends to be worse at night, when the patient's attention is not diverted. If the patient scratches while asleep, have him wear white cotton gloves or mittens.

Bleeding. Because of associated blood coagulation defects, jaundiced patients may have bleeding tendencies such as rectal bleeding, tarry stool, blood in urine, bleeding gums, and black and blue marks (ecchymosis) from minor skin trauma. The nurse should observe for bleeding and perform procedures in a way which lessens the likelihood of bleeding. Intramuscular medicines should be given with small-gauge needles and the injection site firmly pressed and observed for hematoma formation. After an intravenous catheter is removed, immediate and prolonged pressure should be applied to prevent seepage which allows hematomas to form, making the vein unusable. These patients may require frequent blood tests or intravenous therapy so that every effort should be made to preserve integrity of the veins.

Cirrhosis

Pathology. There are several types of hepatic cirrhosis depending on etiology, pathology, and clinical manifestations. Basically it is a disease in which liver damage is followed by scarring with development of excessive fibrous connective tissue. This occurs as the liver attempts to repair itself and leads to considerable anatomical distortion, including partial or complete occlusion of blood channels within the liver.

TYPES OF CIRRHOSIS OF THE LIVER

- Laennec's portal cirrhosis (alcoholic; nutritional; toxic)
- Postnecrotic cirrhosis (posthepatitis)
- Parasitic cirrhosis (following schistosomiasis, malaria, etc.)
- Biliary cirrhosis (primary-idiopathic; obstructive)
- Congestive cirrhosis (cardiac cirrhosis)

LAENNEC'S CIRRHOSIS. Laennec's portal cirrhosis is associated with a heavy, chronic alcohol intake, usually coincident with poor nutrition. Laennec's-type cirrhosis can also follow chronic poisoning with carbon tetrachloride, a cleaning agent.

Incidence. Laennec's cirrhosis is most often seen in males between the ages of 45 and 65 with a history of alcoholism.

Signs and Symptoms. General manifestations of liver damage occur. There are disorders of protein, fat, carbohydrate and vitamin metabolism as well as defects of blood coagulation, fluid and electrolyte balance, and ability to combat infections and toxins.

Clinically, advanced findings include poor nutrition with tissue wasting; poor hemostasis and easy bleeding; vitamin deficiencies; water retention; sodium deficiency; weight loss; weakness, mental dullness; anorexia, nausea, vomiting; intra-abdominal fluid (ascites); low blood sugar (hypoglycemia); and low blood proteins (hypoproteinemia). The skin is thin with dilated veins especially noted over the abdomen. Nosebleeds (epistaxis), jaundice, ecchymosis, scant body hair, palmar erythema (bright pink palms) and cutaneous spider angiomata (tiny spider-like skin vessels of face and chest) also occur. Testicular atrophy is often seen in men and is probably due to the inability of the damaged liver to metabolize estrogenic factors produced from such organs as the adrenal gland.

A most important factor secondary to hepatic scarring in Laennec's cirrhosis is portal hypertension. The intrahepatic obstruction to the return of portal blood from the intestines leads to backup and diversion of blood through venous pathways in the stomach and esophagus. These engorged collateral vessels are called esophageal or gastric varices. As this obstructed backflow increases, pressure within the portal system also increases (portal hypertension). The gastric and esophageal veins distend and are then apt to rupture. Subsequent bleeding into the stomach and esophagus may be slow, but is often rapid and may result in massive hematemesis with exsanguination and death. This bleeding is aggravated by clotting disorders common to liver damage.

In addition to hemorrhage, another serious complication of advanced cirrhosis is infection due to lowering of natural resistance as liver function is reduced. Cirrhotic patients are to be protected from other patients with infection and visitors with colds or other contagious diseases.

Hepatic coma may occur in any form of liver failure; it frequently follows a bleeding episode, paracentesis, infection, surgery, or other stress. The patient becomes lethargic, drowsy, confused, irritable, and eventually stuporous, drifting into coma. Delirium tremens (DT's) may occur early in the development of hepatic coma. Elevation of the serum ammonia level may be a contributing toxic factor.

NURSING MANAGEMENT OF THE PATIENT WITH CIRRHOSIS. There is no specific cure or medicine for hepatic cirrhosis. The aim of therapy is to prevent further deterioration by abolishing underlying causes and to apply supportive measures while the liver attempts to reestablish its functional integrity.

If treatment begins in early phases when signs and symptoms are few and mild, satisfactory recuperation is frequent and long-term prognosis is good. To rescue patients with advanced disease who are jaundiced and hypoproteinemic and have ascites and other manifestations of severe injury is considerably more difficult.

General Supportive Measures. Encouraging the patient to eat is a major nursing task. Sustained, adequate nutrition is extremely important in the therapy of cirrhosis. The physician will usually prescribe a diet high in carbohydrates, proteins, and vitamins in the form of meat, fish, eggs, milk, fruit, and vegetables. Fats are sometimes deleted or included in amounts under ordinary daily requirements. Tobacco and especially alcohol are prohibited. If a high blood level of ammonia is present and impending liver coma is suspected, proteins (which are ammonia precursors) are omitted. When improvement occurs, proteins are added. The anorexia of severe cirrhosis may require frequent small semisolid or liquid meals rather than three full meals a day. Nausea and vomiting may require parenteral feedings. Vitamin B complex, vitamin K, and vitamin C, liver extract, and iron may be prescribed. Intravenous albumin may be given in severe hypoproteinemia, and blood transfusions may be necessary for anemia. Because of the tendency toward salt and water retention (which can lead to edema, circulatory congestion, and heart failure) the intake of these substances is carefully regulated and often restricted. Because salt makes food more palatable, its restriction poses a challenge to find other seasonings which the patient enjoys and is permitted to have.

Observation of daily weight, intake and output, vital signs, and the color, number, and consistency of bowel movements is important in care of the cirrhotic patient. Changes in any of these indicators of the patient's condition should be reported to the physician.

Bed rest is ordered if the patient has signs of liver failure such as mental or neurological disturbance, ascites, jaundice, and weakness. Thoughtful, attentive nursing care can make the difference between a relatively comfortable, really rested patient and an exceedingly uncomfortable, restless one. Helping the patient with bed baths and mouth care, applications of soothing lotions or powders, frequent turning to avoid pressure sores, and easy availability of urinal and bedpan are examples of measures which can increase the patient's comfort during the period of acute illness requiring bed rest.

As the patient's condition improves, helping him to walk and to find quiet diversion are important. Teaching the patient and his family assumes increasing importance as the patient recovers; this teaching requires the collaborative effort of the physician, nurse, and dietitian to help the patient learn how to adapt his way of life to provide the best possible chance of arresting the cirrhotic process. Emotional support is of particular importance. Sensitivity to the patient's concerns and willingness to listen can help him assess his own motivations and goals, and can assist him in accepting necessary restrictions.

Because immoderate use of alcohol is a significant factor in causing cirrhosis, the assumption is sometimes mistakenly made that cirrhotic patients are necessarily alcoholics. Some cirrhotic patients whose illness is not related to alcohol consumption are burdened by these assumptions and by rejection which, regardless of the etiological factors in the patient's illness, interfere with treatment and rehabilitation.

Alleviation of Fluid Retention. The increased fluid retention manifested as ascitic intra-abdominal fluid and tissue edema fluid involves several factors and relationships that are not entirely clear. Overproduction of the hormone aldosterone by the adrenal glands probably occurs in cirrhosis. This hormone causes intense sodium and water retention combined with potassium excretion. This, in addition to associated protein deficiency and factors affecting kidney function, allows abnormal fluid collections.

Ascites and edema may be partially alleviated by restricting sodium intake to 1.0 gm. or less per day and giving a diet rich in protein. The drug spironolactone (Aldactone) specifically antagonizes aldosterone, reversing the effects of this hormone so that sodium and water are excreted and potassium is retained.

When the abdomen is so tense with fluid that kidney function is impaired, a paracentesis may be required.

The rapid removal of abdominal fluid by paracentesis is achieved by carefully introducing a needle through the abdominal wall and allowing the ascites to drain. This may quickly relieve the severe discomfort of distention and difficulty in breathing secondary to a large volume of abdominal fluid pressing upon the diaphragm and lungs.

Only a few liters of fluid are removed, because removal of large quantities of fluid at once can cause drastic shifts between the vascular and extravascular compartments with resultant circulatory collapse (shock). Shock can occur immediately after the tap, due to the acute fluid, mineral, and protein shifts which act to replace the lost ascitic fluid. Other complications of paracentesis include perforation of intestine or bladder with peritonitis, and leakage of fluid from the needle site. To avoid perforation of the bladder, it is important to have the patient void before paracentesis. Prior to paracentesis an infusion is usually ordered and plasma is made available for rapid administration if necessary. Pulse, blood pressure, and breathing should be carefully observed before and after this procedure. Any changes in vital signs, abdominal pain, or fever should be reported.

Complications. *Hepatic Coma.* Coma may occur in any form of hepatic failure. Increased serum ammonia level seems to be related to the development or aggravation of hepatic coma, but is not the absolute cause. Therapy to reduce blood ammonia levels seems to ameliorate the comatose state. Ammonia formed in the intestine by bacterial action on ingested proteins is normally detoxified in the liver by conversion to urea which is then excreted by the kidneys. A failing liver, as in advanced cirrhosis, can no longer break down ammonia and allows it to accumulate in the blood. Also, with portal venous obstruction, ammonia-rich intestinal blood may be diverted from the liver, further reducing detoxification.

Therapy of coma includes reduction of protein intake to zero; avoidance of drugs and stress, and removal of residual protein or blood (if there has been recent hemorrhage) from the intestine by cathartics and enemas. Broad spectrum antibiotics such as neomycin may be ordered in the presence of hepatic encephalopathy. Because it is only poorly absorbed from the gastrointestinal tract, neomycin is frequently used for disinfecting the bowel, thereby lessening the production of ammonia by the intestinal flora. Cleansing enemas are often ordered to reduce the fecal bacterial substrate in the colon. Careful medical support of the comatose patient involves maintenance of fluid and electrolyte balance with parenteral nutrition. Multivitamins are often added to infusions.

Nursing management of a semicomatose or fully unresponsive patient involves observation of vital signs, frequent turning to avoid pressure sores, mouth care, endotracheal suction to prevent aspiration pneumonia, use of siderails and frequent observation to prevent falling, and similar commonsense measures. When it is impossible to reverse the pathological process, hepatic coma is a terminal state. In other instances, medical and nursing measures succeed and the patient recovers from coma.

Portal Hypertension and Bleeding Esophageal Varices. In the scarred cirrhotic liver the intrahepatic veins may be squeezed shut so that blood backs up

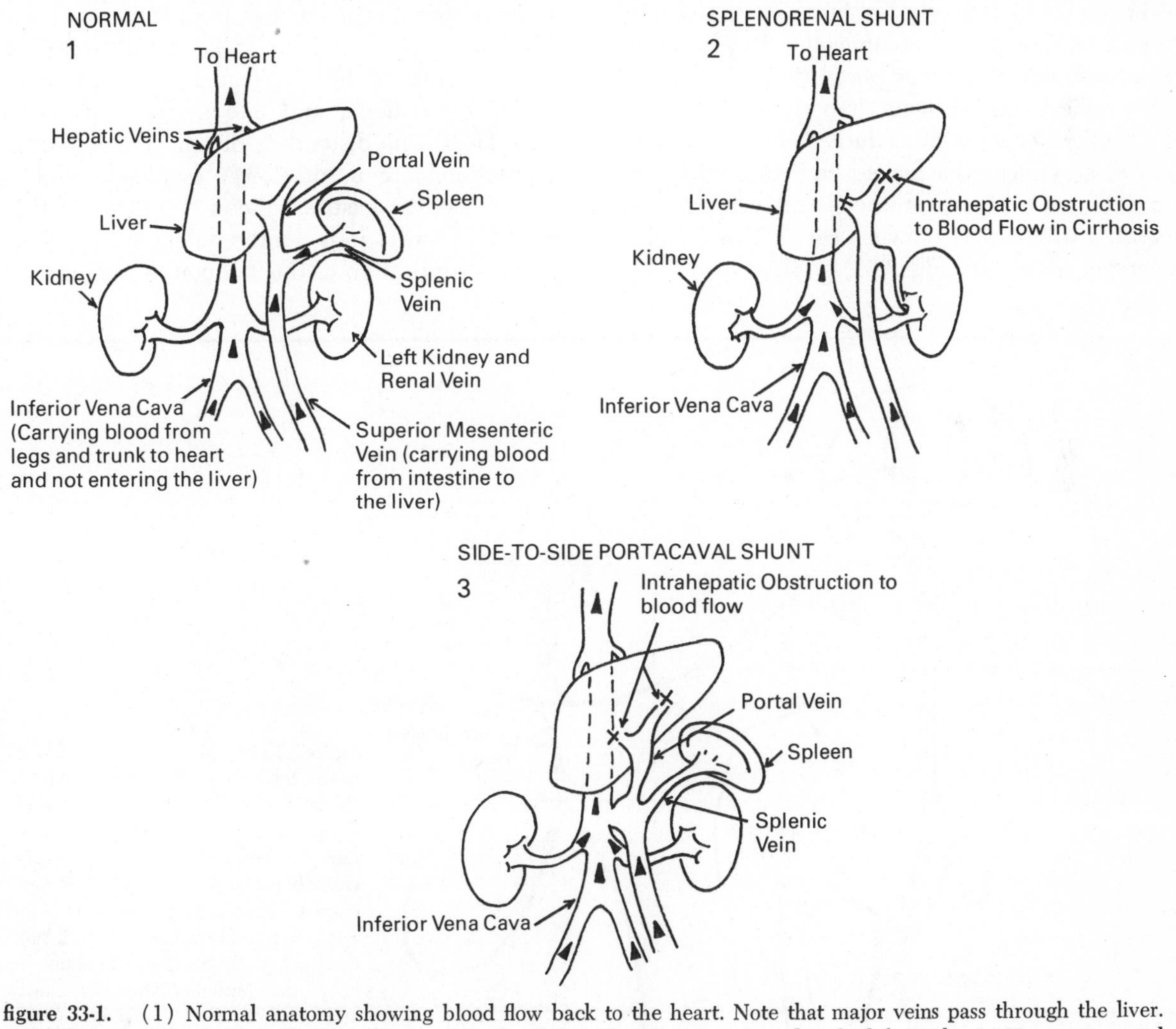

figure 33-1. (1) Normal anatomy showing blood flow back to the heart. Note that major veins pass through the liver. (2) Splenorenal shunt. The spleen has been removed and the splenic vein connected to the left renal vein. Now some portal blood can flow into the inferior vena cava by thus passing the liver. (3) Side-to-side portacaval shunt. The side of the portal vein is anastomosed to the side of the inferior vena cava. Now blood can flow from the portal circulation into the systemic circulation if there is significant intrahepatic obstruction.

into the portal vein and on into diverting channels around the esophagus and stomach. If the portal vein itself is obstructed (by tumor, clot, infection, or unknown cause), similar collateral diversion occurs. The buildup of pressure in the portal system is called portal hypertension. The most life-threatening complication for the cirrhotic patient is hemorrhage from esophageal varices. Patients with cirrhosis of the liver have a high incidence of duodenal ulcers, which may be another cause of gastrointestinal bleeding.

Portal hypertension can be relieved by surgically draining blood from the portal vein into an adjacent systemic vein. As less blood then goes through the portal system, the pressure drops and there is less chance that a collateral vessel will burst with resultant hemorrhage. The portal vein lies just next to the inferior vena cava. Surgically a connection can be made between these vessels so that portal blood is released into the vena cava, reducing hypertension. This is called a *portacaval shunt* procedure. Sometimes a similar beneficial effect is achieved by connecting the splenic vein (a tributary of the portal vein) to the renal vein (a tributary of the vena cava). This is called a *splenorenal shunt* (see Fig. 33-1, p. 435).

These are major operations. If done electively or prophylactically to prevent future hemorrhage, the patient should be in the very best possible condition preoperatively. The jaundiced, hypoproteinemic patient with electrolyte disorders and ascites is a poor risk and will frequently not tolerate this surgery. Such complications should be rectified before surgery.

Other emergency operations to stop bleeding from varices include direct division and ligation of varices in the stomach and esophagus. Both before and after surgery, physicians and nurses work as a team to carry out the intensive program of care and observation needed to pull these critically ill people through.

Sengstaken-Blakemore Esophageal-Gastric Balloon Tube. The use of this tube can be hazardous and requires *constant vigil by both physicians and nurses* in order to get the best effect. It has three separate openings. One inflates the esophageal balloon, one inflates the gastric balloon, and one aspirates the stomach (Fig. 33-2). The distended, bleeding varices of portal hypertension are in the lower esophagus and upper stomach. As the gastric balloon is inflated to the prescribed pressure, it is gently pulled up. In this way constant application of this balloon to the upper stom-

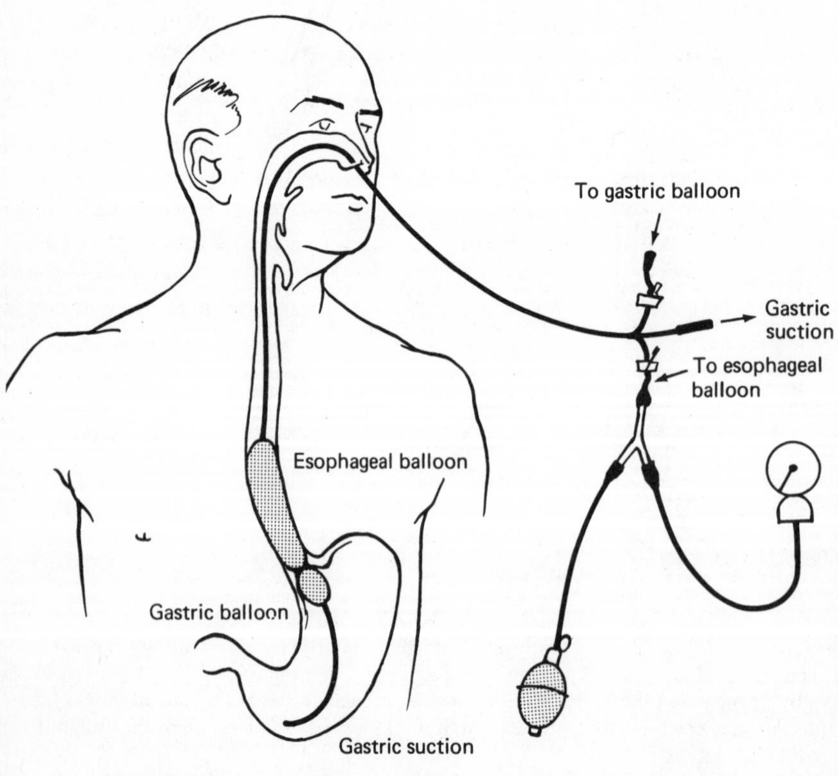

figure 33-2. A Sengstaken-Blakemore tube in place. The clamp on the tube that leads to the esophageal balloon is kept tightly closed to maintain the inflated balloon at the prescribed pressure. The clamp is loosened to check the pressure with the manometer. The gastric suction tube is attached to continuous suction to keep the patient's stomach empty and to prevent vomiting, which would dislodge the esophageal balloon. Irrigations of the gastric suction tube may be ordered to prevent clogging with blood.

ach wall squeezes any bleeding vessels shut. Similarly, as the esophageal balloon is inflated, it expands against the esophageal wall and ruptured bleeding varices are pressed closed. In this way bleeding can be controlled. Through the tube opening into the stomach, clots can be irrigated out (reducing protein by-products of digested blood which lead to ammonia production and possible hepatic coma).

Because patients who have this tube in place require continuous nursing care and observation, they are usually placed in the intensive care unit.

As the patient's condition stabilizes, the tube may be deflated, 24 to 48 hours later. It is hoped that bleeding will not recur. The tube is not removed, but kept in place so that rapid reinflation can be carried out if necessary. During this period the patient is observed for melena, further hematemesis, fall in blood pressure, fall in hematocrit, and tachycardia, which indicate further bleeding. If bleeding occurs or is uncontrolled, emergency shunt or ligation operations may be necessary. With this tube in place the patient may be restless, apprehensive, and uncomfortable, and will require frequent observation.

Viral hepatitis (infectious or serum hepatitis)

Pathology. Hepatitis is an infectious, contagious disease of the liver caused by a virus. The infection may cause simultaneous damage to the intestine and other organs, but the most significant damage is to liver cells, which may become necrotic and die. In fatal cases parenchymal damage is severe. Internal damage to the liver may prevent normal bile secretion or excretion, causing jaundice in addition to the metabolic dysfunction of parenchymal injury.

Etiology and Incidence. There are two types of hepatitis, both caused by viruses which, although similar in nature, produce slightly different clinical diseases: infectious hepatitis is caused by the IH virus, or virus A; serum hepatitis is caused by the SH virus, or virus B.

Both of these viruses resist drying, freezing, heating, and other physical and chemical treatment. They can be destroyed by heating at 60° C. for 10 hours. Albumin may be made virus-free, whereas whole blood and pooled plasma cannot be decontaminated and are frequent methods of transmission.

Infectious hepatitis is usually disseminated by contact with contagious virus in the stool of infected people. The virus may be transmitted by close contact with carriers and by contaminated food, water, or other items apt to be taken orally. Contaminated rectal thermometers, bedpans, and linen harbor the virus, which then reaches the fingers and may subsequently be ingested. Diseased food handlers, cooks, or waiters may create an epidemic, especially in the armed services, schools, and similar close community conditions. Virus A also occurs in the bloodstream of infected people, so that it can be transmitted by this route. The virus may be in the blood before, during, and after the period of infectivity. Duration of infectivity may be difficult to determine.

Serum hepatitis virus B is found only in blood and is transmitted by transfusions of blood or plasma and inoculation via contaminated syringes, needles, and surgical and dental equipment. Carriers are asymptomatic and may be infective for long periods. Incidence of this condition has risen markedly in areas where drug abuse is widespread. Drug addicts often use unsterile syringes and contract the disease in this way.

Signs and Symptoms. Serum hepatitis and infectious hepatitis are not clinically distinguishable. The incubation period of infectious hepatitis is from six days to six weeks whereas serum hepatitis takes 60 to 120 days to develop after infection occurs.

The disease pattern, except for the difference in incubation period, is basically the same. In the preicteric (early or prejaundice) phase, manifestations include fever, rash, joint pain, lymph-node enlargement, anorexia, nausea, vomiting, weakness, pain over the liver, and diarrhea. The liver may be enlarged and tender to percussion; there is often a distaste for smoking tobacco; fatigue may be profound. The spleen is often palpably enlarged.

All these manifestations may occur with varying speed of onset before jaundice is seen. Icterus may be evident from one to three weeks after onset of symptoms. Occasionally, a patient will die of massive liver failure even before becoming jaundiced. As jaundice appears, patients usually improve clinically and have an improved appetite, less pain, and increased strength. Jaundice usually persists 1 or 2 weeks. An important concern of the physician is to differentiate between jaundice due to hepatitis and jaundice due to obstruction.

Prognosis. A small number (fewer than 1 percent) of patients will proceed to hepatic coma and death. Most will recover, but they will be forever barred from being blood donors. A few patients will suffer from chronic active hepatitis, which usually progresses to cirrhosis and death unless corticosteroid treatment slows the active and inflammatory process.

Prevention. Gamma globulin has been used as a preventive against hepatitis with some small success. It may make the attack of hepatitis less severe. It does not give 100 percent protection; it probably gives no protection against serum hepatitis and is of no help if the patient has already contracted the disease.

With both types of hepatitis, extreme caution is required to avoid direct contact with the patient's blood. The nurse should use great care to see that she is not pricked accidentally by the needle that has been used to withdraw blood from a hepatitis patient. Disposable syringes and needles should be used for these patients.

Treatment. As there is no known drug or medical therapy that directly affects the hepatitis viruses, the treatment is directed at strengthening the body to withstand the insult of the infection. Rest is a cornerstone of treatment.

Bed rest and a nourishing diet, often one that is higher in protein and carbohydrate, are offered. Although the patient probably will be grateful for the rest, his poor appetite will make it difficult for him to accept the diet.

Nursing Management. Because the treatment is concerned mainly with improving the patient's resistance so that he can fight the virus, nursing management is of paramount importance. Bed rest should not be a mere twisting and turning in an uncomfortable tangle of sheets. Comfortable positioning, with pillows and changes of bed position, may help the patient to rest. The nurse also helps to protect the patient from disturbances by explaining the need for rest to visitors and by doing as much of what is necessary at one time so that he need not be bothered at frequent intervals.

His interest in food may be enlivened by an attractively served tray. A small quantity of food does not look as discouraging to the anorectic patient as does a full tray. Hot drinks that are really hot and cold drinks that are iced are more tempting than lukewarm ones. Any patient with jaundice (unless the presence of another disease contraindicates the rule) should drink a large quantity of fluid each day: 3,000 ml. is a desirable goal; dehydration can lead to hepatic coma. Color of skin, stool, and urine should be observed.

Although the mode of transmission of serum hepatitis and infectious hepatitis is different, the differential diagnosis between the two diseases may be difficult to make. Therefore all patients with hepatitis are usually placed in isolation. Linen is handled separately. Dishes and eating utensils are sterilized. When paper plates are used, they should be heat-retaining and able to contain food without becoming soaked. It is understandable that patients resent being served meals that arrive cold and on soggy plates.

Since the virus of infectious hepatitis lives in the gastrointestinal tract, stool precautions are required. The patient has his own thermometer, and, if it is a rectal thermometer, the nurse is especially careful to scrub her hands after handling it. The bedpan is kept for the hepatitis patient's sole use, and it is autoclaved or boiled for an hour when he leaves the hospital. The disposal of feces is carried out according to the hospital rules for stool precautions with strict attention to technique. The nurse is careful to wash her hands well after handling the bedpan. Rubber gloves should be used when she is giving the patient a rectal treatment.

Visitors should be given enough instruction in isolation precautions to enable them to protect themselves. They should be warned against close contact with the patient, sharing his food, and giving him the bedpan.

Viral hepatitis lowers the patient's resistance to secondary infection. Careful hand washing on entering the patient's unit protects him. No effort should be spared to keep the patient away from infective organisms.

Patients are generally kept in isolation until the fever has subsided and the jaundice begins to fade, usually for 1 or 2 weeks after the onset of symptoms. As the patient begins to feel well, he may have a tendency to overexert, causing a recurrence of symptoms. The nurse can help to prevent this relapse by encouraging a return to bed if he seems to be overexerting himself.

Noninfectious hepatitis (toxic or chemical)

Exposure to cleaning solutions with carbon tetrachloride, insecticides, and a variety of other drugs and chemicals can cause severe liver damage. Degree of damage, signs, and symptoms will vary with the amount of poisoning as well as associated damage to kidneys and other organs. The clinical picture may evolve gradually or abruptly and be indistinguishable from viral hepatitis. History of exposure, high WBC count, acute onset of jaundice, and hepatic failure with a rapidly enlarging tender liver are usually more indicative of toxic hepatitis.

Therapy involves removal of the toxic agent, a diet high in carbohydrates, proteins, and vitamins, and rest in bed. General supportive and convalescent management is similar to that prescribed for viral hepatitis.

Prophylaxis requires education of children, parents, industrial workers, and others by nurses, physicians and public health-minded individuals. The public should be advised to read labels carefully and observe precautions in use of cleaning solutions, insecticides, and other chemicals; provide adequate ventilation when using volatile chemicals; keep chemicals away from children; take no medicines unless specifically prescribed by the physician. Often patients will save unused portions of a prescribed medicine, then pass it on to a friend or relative, or even use it for a different condition without medical consultation in order to avoid expense.

Diseases of the biliary system

Anatomy and function

The gallbladder is attached to the midportion of the undersurface of the liver. Normally it has a thin wall and a capacity of about 60 ml. of bile. Bile formed in the liver enters the intrahepatic bile ducts and travels to the common hepatic duct. It usually then passes into the cystic duct and is stored in the gallbladder. When required, the gallbladder empties its bile, which now goes out of the cystic duct, into the common bile duct and on into the duodenum. Stones can be found in any portion of this bile system, most frequently in the gallbladder. Arteries, veins, and lymphatics are associated with all sections of the biliary tree, and along with the ducts themselves are subject to considerable variation.

The liver forms up to 1 liter of bile per day. Upon reaching the gallbladder, bile is altered by the absorption of water and minerals to form a more concentrated product. Upon reaching the intestine after gallbladder contraction (stimulated by ingested food, especially fats), this bile functions in the absorption of fats, fat-soluble vitamins, iron, and calcium. Bile also activates the pancreas to release its digestive enzymes as well as an alkaline fluid which may neutralize stomach acids reaching the duodenum.

Cholecystitis and cholelithiasis

These terms signify gallbladder inflammation and stones within the gallbladder. Gallstones (cholelithiasis) represent the most common abnormality of the biliary system, occurring in about 20 percent of people over 40 years (Fig. 33-3). There is progressive increased incidence with aging. They occur in women about four times more often than in men, particularly in women with a history of pregnancies, diabetes, and obesity. The etiology of gallbladder stones has not definitely been established. Bile stasis and infection have been generally implicated. Hemolytic anemias associated with excessive bilirubin formations are associated with development of pigment stones; hypercholesterolemia

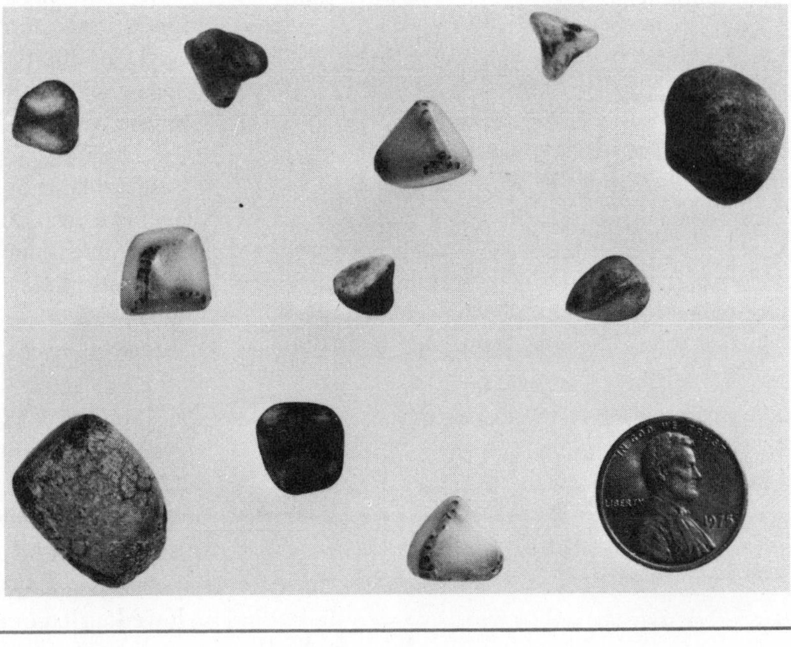

figure 33-3. Gallstones. The one-cent piece is for comparison. Note that the stones are of different colors, sizes, and shapes. (Photograph—D. Atkinson)

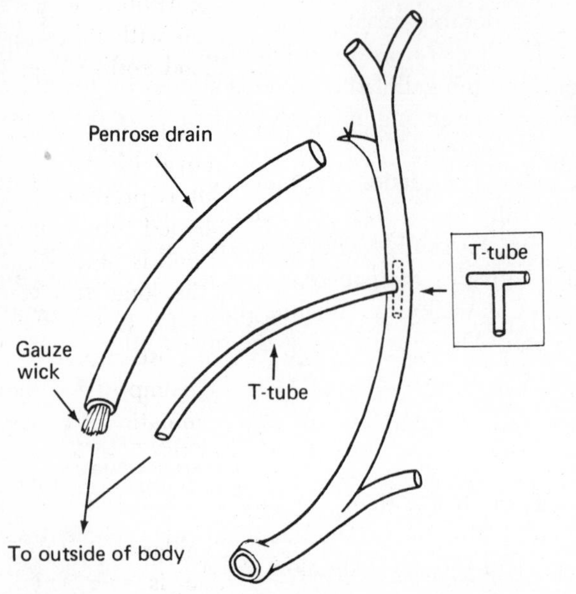

figure 33-4. After cholecystectomy the Penrose drain helps to remove exudate from the area formerly occupied by the gallbladder. The T-tube diverts bile to the outside.

is associated with the accumulation of cholesterol-type stones.

Chronic cholecystitis is rarely present without stones. Stones and infections are intimately related. Symptoms in this condition are probably secondary to transient blockage of the outflow of bile due to stones or spasms of the ductal system. Most usually, after a meal containing fried, greasy, spicy, or fatty foods the patient experiences belching, nausea, and right upper abdominal discomfort, with pain or cramps. Very severe pain is called "biliary colic." Pain may radiate to the back and shoulder. Vomiting may occur.

In simple, uncomplicated colic of chronic cholecystitis with stones, there is no jaundice, fever, chills, liver damage, leukocytosis, or evidence of peritonitis on abdominal examination. Many patients with stones in the gallbladder may never have significant symptomatology.

Diagnosis. In addition to suggestive signs and symptoms, definitive demonstration of cholelithiasis is by the cholecystogram (gallbladder series x-ray picture). The evening before x-ray examination, special dye-containing tablets are given the patient, after which he should fast until the time of testing. The nurse should be sure he gets and takes the tablets and remains fasting during the night. After ingestion, this dye reaches the liver, is excreted into the bile and passes into the gallbladder, making it radiographically visible.

Treatment. Because of the distress associated with this condition, removal of the gallbladder (cholecystectomy) is usually advised. Even in mild cases, because of the possibility of future distress and the complications of acute cholecystitis, cholecystectomy is still advised by many surgeons who prefer to operate electively rather than anticipate a more urgent situation.

Medical Management. Patients known to have cholelithiasis should be advised to avoid fried, greasy, spicy, and high cholesterol foods. These include eggs, pork products, rich dressings, cheese, cream and whole milk. A dietitian should instruct the patient and outline a palatable, wholesome diet also aimed to maintain a reasonable body weight.

During an attack of colic, therapy usually involves rest, a bland liquid diet, and sedation. If vomiting is a feature, hospitalization, nasogastric suction, and parenteral fluids may be needed. Meperidine (Demerol) and morphine may be used to reduce severe pain or colic. These drugs should be used sparingly and strictly if necessary because of their known capability to cause spasm of portions of the common duct.

Surgical Management. Patients whose attacks continue or grow worse are usually treated surgically. Cholecystectomy is performed under general anesthesia. After midnight the patient is placed on NPO; the morning of operation a nasogastric tube is usually put in place so that postoperative secretions and swallowed air can be removed from the stomach.

Table 33-1.
Postoperative nursing management of a patient with a cholecystectomy

Check vital signs q4h or as ordered.
Place bed in semi-Fowler's position.
Have patient turn, cough, deep breathe q2h. Support the incision during coughing and deep breathing.
Have patient do leg exercises q2h.
Measure intake and output.
If a T-tube has been inserted, connect to gravity drainage. Measure T-tube output q8h.
Check dressing q2-4h. Reinforce as necessary.

Postoperatively, emphasis is placed on deep-breathing and coughing. Because the incision is high on the abdomen, these patients find full expansion of the chest more painful than those with a lower incision.

Medication for relief of pain must be administered frequently enough so that the patient can rest and carry out his postoperative exercises, but not so frequently that activity is diminished and respirations become shallow or even depressed.

One or two soft rubber drains are placed in the area of the excised gallbladder to remove blood and bile which may accumulate after surgery. If the dressing is stained excessively with blood or bile, the physician should immediately be informed. A T-tube may also be used (Fig. 33-4) to drain bile from the common bile duct.

With a smooth course, the nasogastric tube is usually removed in 24 to 46 hours and liquid feedings are started with gradual progression to a general low-fat diet. The rubber drain is usually taken out by the third to fifth day. Patients are usually advised to keep to a low-fat diet indefinitely.

Nursing management is outlined in Table 33-1.

Acute cholecystitis is a progression of chronic cholecystitis in which a stone completely blocks off flow of bile from the gallbladder. If the stone impacted in the cystic duct does not dislodge spontaneously, the walls of the distended gallbladder may become gangrenous causing rupture and subsequent peritonitis. These patients are usually very sick with fever, vomiting, severe abdominal pain, and tenderness over the liver. The gallbladder may be so swollen that it becomes palpable; the WBC is high; slight jaundice due to associated hepatic inflammation may be evident.

Medical management, including antibiotics, parenteral fluids, and nasogastric suction, fails to relieve a significant number of patients. In these cases surgery may be lifesaving and consists either of cholecystectomy or cholecystostomy (opening of the gallbladder, removal of stones and placement of a tube for bile drainage to the exterior). If medical therapy is elected and is successful, cholecystectomy is carried out 2 to 3 months after inflammation has subsided.

Choledocholithiasis is the presence of stones anywhere in the ducts of the biliary system. The usual origin is the gallbladder. However, in a small number of people, stones form within the ductal system even after the gallbladder is removed.

Signs and symptoms are those of cholecystitis and cholelithiasis, and in addition jaundice is typical. If stones completely block the common duct, the stools will be clay-colored because no bilirubin reaches the intestine, and the urine will darken with bilirubin as this pigment backs up into the blood and reaches the kidney.

Treatment of choledocholithiasis is surgical exploration of the common duct, removal of stones, and cholecystectomy if the gallbladder is present. At the end of this operation, a small T-shaped tube is placed into the common duct. The small end is placed in the duct lumen aligned lengthwise; the long end comes out through the skin (see Fig. 33-4). If bile flow is temporarily obstructed because of postsurgical spasm of the duct, this tube will allow decompression by releasing bile externally. Before terminating the operation, dye may be introduced into the T-tube so that the ductal tree can be visualized, insuring that all stones have been removed.

Postoperative management is similar to that following cholecystectomy. The T-tube is connected to straight gravity drainage. The collection bag or bottle is attached to the bed below the level of the operation site. This is to prevent reflux of bile back into the duct as well as to avoid an excessive height against which bile would have to "climb" in order to drain. Furthermore, the receptacle must have a vent opening to prevent pressure buildup which would hinder bile drainage.

Usually the tube is constantly left open. Kinking must be avoided, as must occlusion of the lumen caused by the patient's rolling over. It should not be clamped without a physician's order. Drainage usually amounts to a few hundred milliliters of bile per day since most of the bile is expected to pass on into the intestine. However, if total obstruction is present in the common duct, up to 1 liter of bile may drain and the stool will be light-colored.

The T-tube is usually removed after the tenth postoperative day. Frequently a T-tube cholangiogram (in which dye is introduced into the tube and an x-ray picture is taken) is done prior to removal to be sure there is no residual obstruction.

The usual postoperative measures include early ambulation, nasogastric tube aspiration, observation of vital signs, and wound drainage for blood or bile.

The pancreas

The pancreas is a gland which has two major functions. As an endocrine organ it produces insulin. This hormone maintains the blood sugar level and is secreted directly into the bloodstream. As an exocrine organ it produces a variety of protein-, fat-, and carbohydrate-digesting enzymes. These do not enter the bloodstream directly, but instead enter the ducts of the pancreas and eventually are released into the lumen of the duodenum, where they act directly on arriving food. By a complex interplay of chemical and nervous stimuli, the pancreas is activated by ingested foods to release its enzymes at the appropriate time for most efficient digestion.

Acute pancreatitis

The exact etiology of pancreatitis is unknown. In simplest terms pancreatitis may be defined as an inflammatory disease characterized by the destruction of pancreatic tissue as well as functional capability. Pancreatitis may be acute and mild, or may occur abruptly with a fulminant, often quickly fatal course. Later it may occur as a chronic disease, with a long history of relapse and recurrent attacks. Mortality in acute cases may reach as high as 20 percent.

Pancreatitis is often noted to develop in people with a history of biliary tract disease, high alcohol intake and hyperparathyroidism. However, many persons who develop pancreatitis have no other illness.

Signs and Symptoms. In acute pancreatitis, the most common complaint is severe middle-upper abdominal pain, which may radiate to both sides and straight through to the back. Usually, nausea and vomiting are present. If the pancreatic inflammation is intense, with necrosis and hemorrhage of the gland, peritonitis, severe fluid and electrolyte imbalance, and shock may ensue. In fulminant cases the fatty tissue around the pancreas is digested by lipase, a fat-digesting enzyme. Calcium binds with the released fatty acids. In rare cases, this reduces the level of circulating calcium to a dangerous degree, resulting in tetany and convulsions. Also, in the more advanced circumstances of hemorrhagic pancreatitis, released blood may discolor the skin of the lateral abdominal wall.

In addition to the various radiological and blood tests that may be carried out in the diagnosis of pancreatitis, a serum amylase and lipase level are usually ordered. These two enzymes, normal secretions of the pancreas, will appear in elevated quantities in the bloodstream of most patients with significant pancreatitis.

Recurrent (relapsing) and chronic pancreatitis

Recurrent pancreatitis is the reappearance of intermittent attacks of pancreatic inflammation after an initial attack earlier in life. With chronicity, there may be partial to ultimate complete loss of function as pancreatic tissue is progressively destroyed.

With the late development of chronic recurrent pancreatitis, stones and strictures may obstruct the pancreatic ducts. Areas of pancreatic breakdown may disrupt to form "pseudocysts" which are fluid-filled pouches budding from the diseased pancreas. These cause symptoms by putting pressure upon adjacent organs or by rupturing. With the development of chronic pancreatitis, pain, weight loss, digestive disturbances, diabetes, malnutrition, and steatorrhea (excessive fat in the stool) occur, in addition to the usual signs and symptoms of acute pancreatitis. These problems are caused by the progressive loss of exocrine and endocrine actions of the gland.

Treatment. In acute pancreatitis measures are taken to relieve pain, reduce pancreatic secretion, restore fluid and electrolyte losses, and combat infection. The patient usually receives nothing by mouth and continuous nasogastric aspiration is applied. This will relieve nausea, distention, and vomiting as well as reduce stimulation of the pancreas by gastric contents entering the duodenum. Atropine or other anticholinergic drugs may be used to reduce the activity of the vagus nerve, which stimulates the pancreas.

Improvement usually occurs in about a week. The diet initially prescribed is extremely bland with slow progress to a low-fat diet. Alcohol, coffee, tea, and other irritants or rich foods are withheld. Since prolonged use of narcotics may lead to addiction, care and thought in their prescription and administration is essential.

There is no direct surgical therapy for acute pancreatitis. However, if pancreatic abscess is suspected, this must be drained surgically. Also, if acute cholecystitis or obstruction of the common duct is felt to be a coincident and/or inciting factor, drainage and simple stone removal may be necessary. Simple bile diversion by cholecystostomy or choledochostomy are felt by some authorities to give relief and hasten healing in acute pancreatitis.

The treatment of chronic, recurrent pancreatitis depends on the etiology and whether or not obstruction of the pancreatic duct is present. If pancreatic duct obstruction is not yet present, abstinence from alcohol, a bland fat-free diet, and correction of associated biliary tract disease or hyperparathyroidism may give good results. If there is scarring with stricture and stenosis of portions of the pancreatic duct, various complex surgical measures are available to attempt reconstitution of an unobstructed flow into the intestine.

Chronic pain may be relieved by severing the nerve fibers supplying the pancreas, as well as removal of part or all of the pancreas. The diabetes and digestive enzyme deficiency seen with advanced pancreatic destruction may be treated with insulin and exocrine enzyme replacement.

Nursing Management. Because severe pain is the outstanding symptom of pancreatitis, nursing intervention involves relief of pain by careful administration of prescribed analgesics, and by other measures such as changes of position.

During an acute attack the patient is kept NPO and a nasogastric tube is usually inserted. Both of these measures decrease pancreatic secretions. The patient will need mouth care, as does any patient with continuous nasogastric suction. His nasal passage also may feel dry and sore from the tube, and a small amount of glycerin may help.

The patient's urine should be checked 1 to 4 times a day for glucose and acetone as a method of detecting a decrease in insulin production by the pancreas. The presence of glucose should be brought to the physician's attention.

General nutritional considerations

- Patients with hepatic cirrhosis need a well-balanced diet. The physician may order a low-fat diet because of the inability of the liver to manufacture bile, which is necessary for the digestion of fats.
- If hepatic coma is present or impending, protein may be omitted from the diet.
- Patients with hepatic cirrhosis usually have poor appetites and may require frequent small feedings rather than three regular meals. If ascites or edema is present, a diet restricted in sodium and high in protein may be ordered.
- Patients with cholelithiasis may require a low-fat diet. Avoidance of greasy, fried, and spicy foods and foods high in cholesterol may also be necessary.

General pharmacological considerations

- Barbiturates, narcotics, and any drug detoxified by the liver are *contraindicated* or *used with caution* in individuals with liver disease.
- To reduce ascites and edema in the patient with cirrhosis, a diuretic may be ordered. One diuretic that is particularly useful is spironolactone, which antagonizes aldosterone. Reversing the effects of aldosterone increases water and sodium excretion while potassium is retained.
- Patients with acute pancreatitis have severe pain which often requires the use of narcotic analgesics. As the pain may persist for some time, care must be taken to avoid addiction.

Bibliography

American College of Surgeons, J. M. Kinney et al, eds.: *Manual of Preoperative and Postoperative Care,* ed. 2. Philadelphia, Saunders, 1971.

Anderson, L. et al: *Nutrition in Nursing.* Philadelphia, Lippincott, 1972.

Ballinger, W. F. et al: *Alexander's Care of the Patient in Surgery,* ed. 5. St. Louis, Mosby, 1973.

Bates, B.: *A Guide to Physical Examination.* Philadelphia, Lippincott, 1974.

Clinical features of pancreatitis. Hosp. Med. 11:19, July, 1975.

Curtis, S. J.: A guide to the practical use of liver function tests. Hosp. Med. 10:51, December, 1974.

Davidson, C. S.: Dietary management in hepatic diseases. Nurs. Dig. 2:90, March, 1974.

Elliott, D. W.: *Acute pancreatitis.* Emergency Med. 6:24, April, 1974.

Gallbladder surgery theories upheld. AORN J. 22:124, July, 1975.

Given, B. A. and Simmons, S. J.: *Nursing Care of the Patient with Gastrointestinal Disorders.* St. Louis, Mosby, 1971.

Gocke, D. J.: Current status of viral hepatitis (pictorial). Hosp. Med. 11:8, March, 1975.

Hepatic crisis (care st). Nurs. '74, 4:14, February, 1974.

Levine, M. E.: *Introduction to Clinical Nursing,* ed. 2. Philadelphia, Davis, 1973.

Luckman, J. and Sorenson, K. C.: *Medical-Surgical Nursing: A Psychophysiological Approach.* Philadelphia, Saunders, 1974.

MacBride, C. M. and Blacklow, R. S.: *Signs and Symptoms,* ed. 5. Philadelphia, Lippincott, 1970.

MAINGOT, R.: Gallstones—cholecystectomy. Nurs. Times 70: 1900, December 5, 1974.

MOIDEL, H. C. et al, eds.: *Nursing Care of the Patient with Medical-Surgical Disorders.* New York, McGraw-Hill, 1970.

PASTOREK, N.: "It's a mean disease! It's sneaky and malevolent." Today's Health 52:46, September, 1974.

Portacaval shunt effective in cirrhosis. AORN J. 22:412, September, 1975.

SCHERER, J. C.: *Introductory Clinical Pharmacology.* Philadelphia, Lippincott, 1975.

SLEISENGER, M. and FORDTRAN, J.: *Gastrointestinal Disease: Pathophysiology, Diagnosis, Management.* Philadelphia, Saunders, 1973.

WALLACH, J.: *Interpretation of Diagnostic Tests,* ed. 2. Boston, Little, Brown, 1974.

WILLIAMS, S. R.: *Nutrition and Diet Therapy,* ed. 2. St. Louis, Mosby, 1973.

WILSON, J. L., ed.: *Handbook of Surgery,* ed. 5. Los Altos, Lange, 1973.

CHAPTER—34

The urologic patient

On completion of this chapter the student will:

- Diagram and label the major parts of the urinary tract.
- Discuss the laboratory and x-ray tests and examinations used to diagnose urinary tract disease and identify the nursing management of the patient undergoing these tests.
- Understand the importance of aseptic technique in the care of the patient with a catheter in the urinary tract.
- Know basic techniques of catheter irrigations.
- Describe the nursing management of the patient with urinary incontinence.
- Discuss the etiology, symptoms, and diagnosis of urinary calculi, renal and bladder tumors, cystitis, and urethritis.
- Formulate a nursing care plan for and participate in the nursing management of the patient with urinary calculi, renal and bladder tumors, cystitis, and urethritis.
- Discuss the etiology and treatment of urethral strictures.
- Describe the nursing management of the patient who has had renal or ureteral surgery.
- Describe and discuss the postoperative management of the patient with a urinary diversion.

Behavioral objectives (continued)

- **Differentiate between acute and chronic glomerulonephritis with regard to etiology, symptoms, and treatment.**
- **Discuss the nursing management of the patient with acute or chronic glomerulonephritis.**

Patients with disorders of the urinary tract not only suffer from the accompanying physical discomfort, but often from embarrassment and anxiety as well. Because disclosure of genitourinary difficulties often involves the sharing of very personal information and

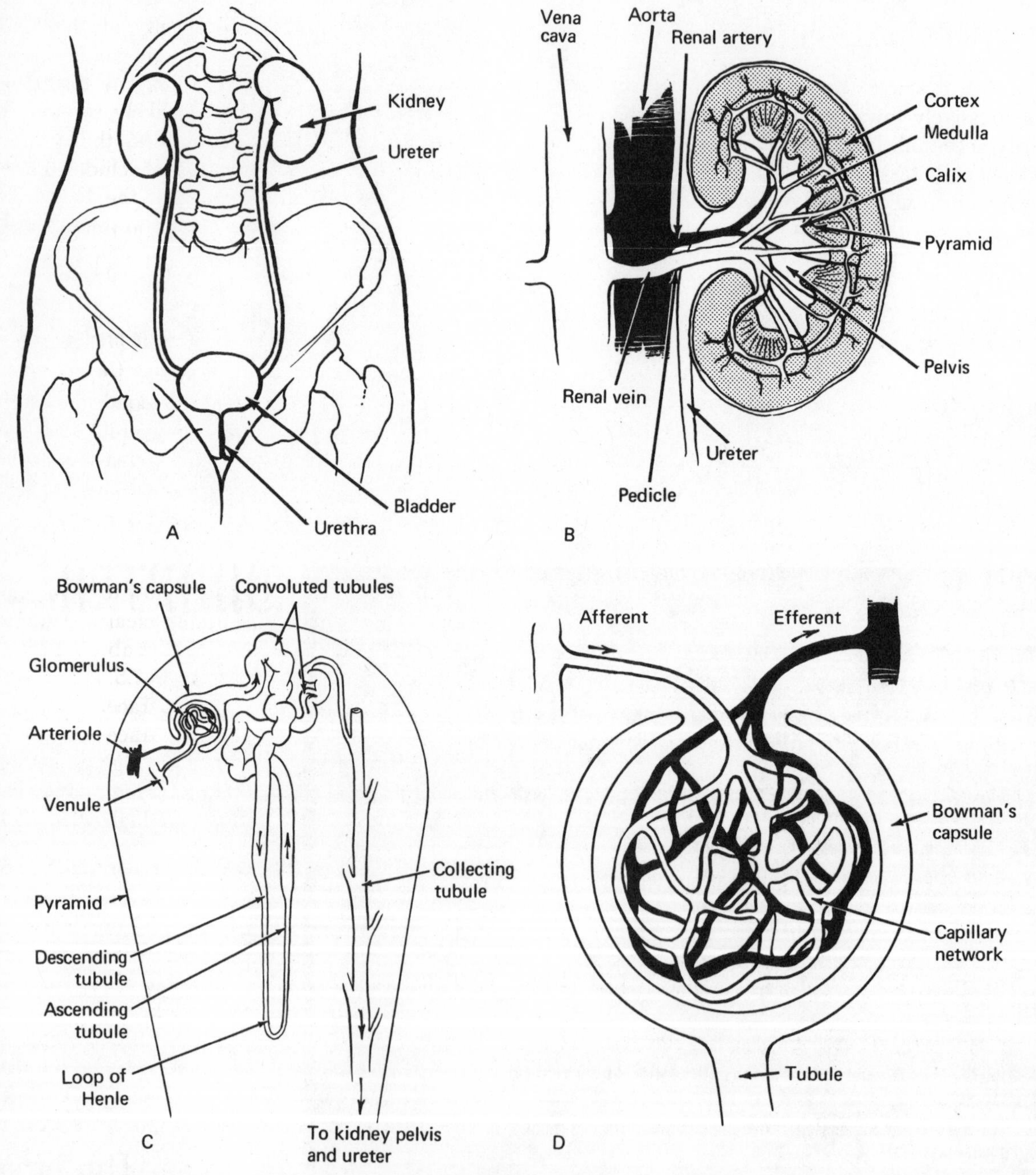

figure 34-1. Structures of the urinary system. (A) The urinary tract. (B) Interior of kidney. (C) A nephron. (D) Bowman's capsule.

the experience of an extensive physical inspection and examination of this part of the body, patients tend to delay seeking medical help. Since the sex organs and urinary tract are in close physical proximity, disturbances of urinary elimination may also pose the threat of sexual inadequacy. Every effort should be made to protect the patient's modesty and privacy and to deal matter-of-factly with the problem.

Urologic patients, like others, can express their anxiety in a variety of ways. The threatened male patient, for example, may behave more immodestly and aggressively toward the female nurse than is customarily accepted. It is important for the nurse to try to understand the reason for the patient's behavior. However, this does not imply accepting this behavior. Instead, it is necessary to set limits regarding behavior and to listen to and talk with the patient about his feelings and concerns. Overt sexual behavior of this type may be anxiety producing for the nurse, and she may react by withdrawing from the patient. The patient, in turn, becomes more threatened, and his self-esteem is lowered even more. Asking the patient to behave more appropriately shows a response to his overt behavior, respect for his capacity to change it, and paves the way for more appropriate anxiety-relief mechanisms such as talking with the nurse or physician about what is bothering him. Not only is it important to understand the patient's emotional response, but also the normal anatomy and physiology of the urinary tract and its alterations during disease.

The urinary tract is one of several waste disposal systems by which the body rids itself of the byproducts of metabolism. This system is also essential for the regulation of body fluids and their electrolyte content. When the kidneys are diseased or injured, and their function is impaired, or when there is an obstruction to the free flow of urine to the outside, serious illness is present or imminent. Often, conditions which develop require long-term management and treatment.

The urinary tract

The urinary tract consists of the *kidneys,* which secrete urine, and the various tubes and reservoirs necessary to discharge this fluid from the body (Fig. 34-1). The kidneys have at least three known functions. They excrete excess water and the nitrogenous waste products of protein metabolism; they play a significant role in maintaining the acid-base balance of the body and the equilibrium of plasma electrolytes. Finally, they produce enzymes, such as renin, which act on certain plasma constituents to form a compound that raises the blood pressure. The kidneys selectively filter over 50 gallons of plasma daily. All but a quart or so of this volume is resorbed back into the circulation every 24 hours.

The formed urine is excreted into the renal *pelvis* and carried down the *ureter* to the *bladder.* Here the urine is stored until the capacity of the bladder is reached at which time the patient voids the urine to the outside through the *urethra.* Any disorder which interferes with this process is likely to cause serious repercussions to the patient unless the situation can be corrected. These disorders include interference with the circulation of blood to the kidney, disease of the kidney itself, and obstruction to the drainage of the urinary tract.

Diagnostic procedures

Urinalysis

Much information about the condition of the kidneys, electrolyte balance, and overall health can be learned by studying the urine. Urinalysis is the most important diagnostic study of the urinary tract.

The characteristics of normal urine are:

Specific gravity	1.005 to 1.025
Color	Pale yellow to dark amber
Turbidity	Usually clear (cloudiness not always abnormal)
Acidity	pH 4.8 to 7.5
Protein	None to trace
Glucose	None to trace
Red blood cells	0 to 3 per high power field
White blood cells	0 to 4 per high power field
Casts	Rare per high power field

A red color to the urine may mean blood, but must be proved by microscopic examination. Certain metabolic disturbances, ingested dyes, or foodstuffs may impart a red color that is not blood. One fifth of patients admitted to the hospital with gross blood in the urine (hematuria) have cancer in the urinary tract and this finding requires a complete urologic investigation. Cloudiness of the urine may be due to phosphates (a normal finding) or to white cells, suggesting an infection or irritation of the tract. Proteinuria (usually albumin) may occasionally be normal. More often it implies disease of the system. Little of this material filters through the pores of the normal glomeruli. Casts are molds of the renal tubules and their size will vary with the size of the portion of the nephron whence they originate. They may be constituted of red cells, white cells, or precipitated protein.

The container in which the urine specimen is collected should be clean and dry; it should be sterile if a culture is to be taken. It is preferable to have the patient void directly into the container that is sent to the laboratory. Taking a urine specimen from a bedpan or a urinal that contains sediment from previous use may result in inaccurate results.

When infection is suspected, a specimen may be taken for culture. In men it is usually sufficient to cleanse the glans penis with an antiseptic and have the patient void about 60 ml., which are discarded, and then void into a sterile specimen bottle. The bottle is capped in such a way that it is not contaminated. In women, specimens for culture may be obtained by catheterization. However, because there is always the danger of introducing infection into the urinary tract with a catheter, the "sterile (or clean) catch" procedure is used in many hospitals. The labia are held apart, and the area is cleansed. The patient voids into a sterile container after the initial 60 ml. are discarded.

Since bacteria multiply in urine and to avoid decomposition of its contents, the specimen is delivered immediately to the laboratory or promptly refrigerated, until the specimen is taken to the laboratory.

Sometimes a specimen of all the urine excreted over a period of time, such as 24 hours, may be needed for examination of such constituents as tubercle bacilli and 17-ketosteroids. The patient empties his bladder immediately prior to the start of the time period, and this fluid is discarded. The entire specimen is refrigerated to prevent bacterial growth. To prevent any part of the specimen from being lost or contaminated, the patient is instructed to use separate receptacles for voiding and defecation.

Blood chemistry

When the nephrons fail to remove waste products efficiently from the body, the blood chemistry is altered. Deterioration in renal function is manifested chemically by rises in the blood urea nitrogen (BUN) and creatinine values, both of which are protein breakdown products. However, there must be a 50 to 75 percent decrease in function before these values rise. The normal BUN is 8 to 18 mg. per 100 ml., and creatinine 0.5 to 1.0 mg. per 100 ml. High blood levels of urea nitrogen can be accompanied by disorientation and convulsions. The patient with kidney disease should be observed for any abnormalities in blood chemistry reports. This information can serve as one guide to planning nursing management. For example, if the patient's BUN is high, he is observed particularly for disorientation and convulsions and necessary protective equipment is kept in readiness, such as side rails and a padded tongue blade.

Other useful determinations are the acid phosphatase, an enzyme produced by the prostate. In 75 percent of patients with prostatic cancer extending beyond the prostatic capsule, this figure is elevated. Alkaline phosphatase may be elevated with spread of cancer to the bones although other disorders may raise this value.

Blood calcium, phosphorus, and uric acid studies may be ordered when the physician is evaluating metabolic causes for certain types of urinary calculi (stones).

Concentration and Dilution Tests. Specific gravity shows the concentration of particles, such as electrolytes, in water. The specific gravity of distilled water is 1.000. Normally, the specific gravity of urine is responsive to the water and electrolyte situation in the body. On a hot day a person who is perspiring profusely and taking little fluid will have urine with a high specific gravity. Conversely, a person who has a high fluid intake and who is not losing excessive water from perspiration, diarrhea, or vomiting will have copious urine with a low specific gravity.

When the kidneys are damaged, this ability to concentrate or produce dilute urine is impaired: the specific gravity remains relatively constant, no matter what the water needs of the body are, or how much the patient drinks. It is often fixed low, 1.001 to 1.005. To test for the capacity to adjust the specific gravity of urine, the patient may be dehydrated by restricting fluids, and a specimen taken; then he is well hydrated by giving him a large amount to drink in a short time, and another specimen is taken. The specific gravity of each specimen is tested.

Phenolsulfonphthalein (PSP) Test. Phenolsulfonphthalein (PSP) is a red dye that the kidneys excrete after IV injection. The amount of dye excreted by the patient is compared with that excreted by a person with normal kidney function. In renal disease, particularly when the tubules are involved, there is a delay in excreting the dye.

The procedure of the test varies slightly from hospital to hospital. It is important that the directions be followed exactly. A few drops of urine lost or a specimen collected 4 minutes late may mean that test results are inaccurate, and the physician receives misleading diagnostic data.

INTRAVENOUS PYELOGRAM (IVP). This x-ray study is based on the ability of the kidneys to excrete radiopaque contrast media in the urine. Injected intravenously, the contrast medium shows up the outlines of the kidney pelvis, the ureters, and the bladder on x-ray film as the opaque medium passes along the urinary tract.

The medium contains iodine, to which the patient may be allergic. The physician may inject a very minute amount of medium intravenously and observe the patient for 5 or 10 minutes to determine if an allergy to iodine is present. Whenever radiopaque contrast media containing iodine are used, the nurse carefully observes the response of the patient and promptly reports to the physician any untoward effect, such as increasing anxiety, restlessness, wheezing, tachycardia, or signs of cardiovascular collapse. Oxygen, antihistamines, epinephrine (Adrenalin), corticosteroids and vasoconstrictor agents such as metaraminol (Aramine) as well as resuscitation equipment should be readily available.

If the patient is undergoing an extensive diagnostic work-up, the physician will probably delay barium studies of the gastrointestinal tract until urologic studies are completed. It may take several days for barium to be removed from the gastrointestinal tract and its presence in the gastrointestinal tract can distort IVP findings. The physician's orders before an intravenous pyelogram usually include the following:

1. Nothing by mouth for 12 hours before the pyelogram is scheduled. This fasting dehydrates the patient so that the urine (and, therefore, the contrast medium) will be at maximum concentration.
2. Cleansing of the bowel, so that its contents do not interfere with visualization of kidneys on the film. Usually, a cathartic is ordered the evening before the test and a rectal suppository or enema may be ordered early on the morning of the pyelogram. Because poor cleansing of the bowels may require that the test be repeated, it is a nursing responsibility to check that the bowel preparation has been effective, even if given by someone else.

Some patients have other conditions that make the usual preparation inadvisable. For example, in peptic ulcer there is the danger of intestinal perforation, and, therefore, the bowel-cleansing procedure must be modified. After the test, the patient is encouraged to rest and to take fluids liberally to overcome the dehydration and to flush any remaining dye from the urinary tract. Additional films may be taken as long as 24 hours later, in order to obtain additional information that helps the physician with diagnosis.

CYSTOURETHROGRAPHY. For this x-ray study, contrast material is instilled into the bladder through a urethral catheter.

ARTERIOGRAPHY

Renal arteriograms are used to evaluate blood vessels to the kidneys and delineate the nature of mass lesions. Using this x-ray study the surgeon can obtain accurate information as to the location and number of renal arteries especially since multiple vessels to the kidney are not unusual. The commonly used method is the percutaneous catheter technique. A catheter is passed up the femoral artery into the aorta to the level of the renal vessels. At this point, contrast medium is injected directly to produce an aortogram or the catheter may be manipulated into separate arteries individually. After the examination, a pressure dressing is applied to the femoral area for several hours and the pulses in the legs and feet are palpated for signs of interference with the circulation. The femoral area is observed for bleeding.

CYSTOSCOPY AND RETROGRADE PYELOGRAPHY

Cystoscopy is the visual examination of the inside of the bladder by the physician using a metal instrument known as a cystoscope. The cystoscope consists of a sheath with a light bulb for illumination at its tip. A telescope is inserted into the sheath for visualization. The cystoscope enables the physician to see the interior of the bladder clearly magnified. Inflow and outflow valves allow for irrigation. The size of the cystoscope is graded in the French (F.) scale; usually, 20 to 24 F. is used in adults.

Cystoscopy may be done for the following three purposes:

- Inspection. Prostate, urethra, bladder, and ureteral orifices can be seen. Cystoscopy is usually done in instances of bleeding of the urinary tract, since the bleeding may be a symptom of cancer. A catheter may be threaded into each ureter to gather separate specimens of urine from each kidney to indicate which one is affected by pus, cancer cells, tubercle bacilli, or other evidence of disease. Contrast media (about 3 to 5 ml.) can be injected into the catheters to outline the upper urinary tract and a *retrograde pyelogram* is thus obtained. Retrograde pyelograms are usually ordered only when there has been inadequate visualization by intravenous pyelography.

- Biopsy. Specimens of tissue may be taken from bladder or urethra through the cystoscope.
- Treatment. Tumors of urethra or bladder can be treated by electrosurgery (fulguration) with electrodes passed through the cystoscope. Small stones and other foreign bodies can be removed through the cystoscope. Sometimes, larger stones are crushed and then removed. A narrowed ureteral orifice can be incised, ureters dilated, the kidney pelvis drained and irrigated, and radon seeds implanted around or into malignant tumors.

Management of the Patient. Cystoscopy can be very frightening to the patient. The more tense he becomes, the more chance there is of increased pain due to spasm of the vesical sphincters. The procedure should be explained, including what the patient will actually feel during it. For example when the cystoscope passes the internal sphincter at the bladder neck and when the bladder is filled, the patient will feel the urge to void.

Additional preparation includes encouraging fluid intake so that adequate urine will be in the ureters for specimens. The patient should drink at least 400 ml. about one hour before the examination, or fluids may be given intravenously, especially if general anesthesia is to be used. Usually, food is withheld because the discomfort of the procedure may cause nausea. If x-ray films are to be taken during cystoscopy, the bowel is cleansed as for an intravenous pyelogram to remove gas and stool, which may throw confusing shadows on the x-ray film. A sedative may be given before cystoscopy. Signed permission must be obtained for this procedure. The examination can be performed without anesthesia or with local, spinal, or general anesthesia.

Postcystoscopy Management. When the examination is over, the patient's external genitalia are cleansed and he is helped to descend from the lithotomy position slowly. He is observed for dizziness and permitted to rest for a few minutes before proceeding back to his hospital room (via wheelchair or stretcher) or before getting dressed, if he is an outpatient.

The decision whether to perform these examinations on an ambulatory or inpatient basis and the type of anesthesia to be used will depend considerably on the physician's prior evaluation of the patient, an evaluation that includes emotional as well as physical considerations. Outpatients should rest for a half-hour before going home, and they should not travel unaccompanied. Not only has the patient just been through an uncomfortable procedure, but he may have had sedation. He should not plan to drive a car. Patients who have had spinal anesthesia are hospitalized at least overnight, and they are kept flat in bed for 6 hours or more after the procedure.

Fluids should be encouraged liberally to dilute the urine and to lessen the irritation of the lining of the urinary tract. The patient should be told that voiding will be painful for about a day. Mild hematuria is not unusual. Discoloration of the urine may be expected if dyes were used. Analgesics, several warm sitz baths, and explaining beforehand what to expect are ways that the patient's discomfort can be alleviated.

Underlying pathology may be aggravated by the instrumentation. For example, significant prostatic obstruction may culminate in complete urinary retention. If there is urinary infection, instrumentation may be followed by chills, fever, and possibly serious septicemia. The patient is observed for these symptoms, and they are promptly reported to the physician. He may order antibiotics. There may have been damage to the walls of the tract, even perforation (anuria and sharp abdominal pain often accompany perforation).

Many patients have a dull ache caused by distention of the renal pelvis with dye. The pain may be relieved by a hot bath or codeine. Outpatients should be instructed to return to the physician if there is frank bleeding, anuria, pain, or fever.

Observations

Because the function of the urinary tract is the elimination of metabolic products and electrolytes, and because it uses water as the vehicle for the movement of these substances, the nurse observes the patient for signs of electrolyte and water imbalance. An accurate measurement of the intake and output is *most important* in those with urologic disorders. The patient is observed for edema which may first become obvious as puffiness around the eyes (periorbital edema).

The physician correlates the laboratory findings with symptoms (Table 34-1). The nurse can help by being especially observant. If calcium is low, the patient is observed for signs of impending hypocalcemic tetany—muscle cramps and tingling of the fingers. The nurse should check to be sure there are ampules of calcium gluconate or chloride readily available. If the calcium is so low that the patient has had convulsions or is in danger of them, the side rails are padded and kept up, and a padded tongue blade or an oral airway is taped to the head of the bed. If serum potassium levels are elevated, the patient is observed for signs of mental confusion, listlessness, hypotension, and changes in pulse rhythm and rate. Whenever there is edema, the patient is usually weighed every day to keep track of possible loss or gain of fluids. Anemia and other blood changes may lead to a hemorrhagic disorder. The nurse observes for and reports to the physician any bleeding. For example, the stool is observed for unusual blackness, which may indicate the presence of old blood from gastrointestinal hemorrhage.

Observation of the urine can reveal a great deal. The daily amount is an important indication of the adequacy of renal function. Less than 500 ml. a day when the intake has been adequate means that there is serious trouble in the urinary tract that should be reported to the physician. The total intake and output for the 24- or the 8-hour period is checked to see whether the figures are approximately equal. Any wide discrepancy is reported to the physician.

Color and content of the patient's urine should also be observed for sediment, clots, and shreds of material; odor, color, and degree of opacity are also noted. If the patient has an indwelling catheter, the urine is observed as it passes through the glass or plastic connecting tube. This is a better index than the old urine in the drainage receptacle.

Blood pressure is another index of the course of the illness. The patient's usual blood pressure and what it was on admission are noted in the health history. These figures will give a standard against which to judge readings. Blood pressure is usually taken every 4 hours on patients with nephritis, all those with active kidney pathology, and those with uremia. If the blood pressure is not stable, it is taken more frequently. If the patient seems sluggish or complains of headache, the blood pressure should be taken more frequently. A progressive rise should be reported to the physician.

Fluids

Each day, the specific fluid-intake goal for each patient should be known. The amount of fluid he should drink in a 24-hour period is calculated, and then a schedule of fluid intake is planned for the patient's waking hours. One quarter of the total intake should be given at night. As a general rule, fluids are encouraged to keep the urine dilute. Dilute urine does not crystallize and form calculi as easily as concentrated urine; in cystitis, it burns less on urination; it rids the kidney quickly of noxious substances; and it washes away products of inflammation.

However, fluids may be limited (often to 600 to 800 ml.) when there is edema, and also when there is kidney failure. If the patient's body is unable to rid

Table 34-1.
Serum values

	Normal Serum Value	Changes in Pathology
Calcium	9–11 mg./100 ml. 4.5–5.5 mEq./L.	Lower in renal failure
Carbon dioxide combining power	21–28 mEq./L.	Higher in alkalosis
Potassium	3.5–5.5 mEq./L.	Higher in renal failure
Proteins, total		
Albumin	3.5–5.5 gm./100 ml.	
Globulin	1.5–3.0 gm./100 ml.	Lower in renal failure
Sodium	137–143 mEq./L.	Lower in renal failure
Urea nitrogen (BUN)	8–18 mg./100 ml.	Higher in renal failure

itself of water efficiently, damage results when large amounts of fluid are given.

When fluids are to be encouraged (often to 3,500 to 4,000 ml.), frequent, small offerings may be more palatable than large quantities presented less often. This is especially true of geriatric patients. Often, the patient himself takes responsibility for his intake. It is better for the patient to help himself as much as he can, because he will feel less helpless. It is essential that the patient understand how much he should drink, how to keep track of the amount, and why fluids are important.

The fluids available to him may take the form of fresh, iced water in his carafe, certain fruit juices, gelatin, fruit flavored drinks, ginger ale, cola, tea, or eggnog served at intervals in the day. When it is important to limit potassium intake, certain fruit juices, tea, coffee, and chocolate beverages, all of which have a high potassium content, are limited or omitted. Juices which are high in potassium include grapefruit, orange, prune, tangerine, and tomato. Juices which can be included in a 1,500 mg. potassium-restricted diet include apple, cranberry, pear, peach, and pineapple.

Because of the combination of a large intake of fluids with the symptom of frequency, the bedpan or urinal should be kept within easy reach, especially with an older patient for whom climbing in and out of bed may be tiring and dangerous.

When fluids are restricted, the patient should understand the reason for the restriction.

Thirst may be a problem, especially in hot weather. Fluids should be spaced throughout the day. Sucking on hard candy or ice may help; however, ice needs to be counted in total fluid intake. Mouth care can be carried out with a pleasant-tasting solution.

Records of intake and output should be scrupulously accurate; otherwise, the physician will base his treatment on incorrect information. Every person working with the patient should understand and agree to the method of keeping records and the amount of fluid that the cups and the glasses hold. If the aide believes that the glass holds 240 ml., and the nurse believes it to hold 200 ml., the physician will read erroneous figures on the chart. Each source of output should be recorded separately and then totaled. For example:

Vomitus	230 ml.
Cystotomy tube	560 ml.
Foley catheter	520 ml.
Total	1,310 ml.

All patients for whom fluids are encouraged are observed for overhydration (edema, wet breathing sounds), especially those who are elderly and those with a heart ailment or potential renal failure. Patients with edema have severe restriction of their sodium intake. Salt substitutes containing potassium for seasoning should not be used without the physician's approval.

Preventing infection

Every catheter or irrigating set presents a danger of introducing microorganisms into the urinary tract. Each time a catheter is irrigated or a closed urinary drainage system is used, aseptic technique must be used. If possible, the drainage system is not opened or disrupted, as once this occurs the tubing usually becomes contaminated with bacteria. Collection drainage bags that are emptied by opening and closing a valve at the bottom of the bag appear to be less likely to cause contamination of the drainage apparatus.

Comfort

Some causes of discomfort in the urologic patient and measures to relieve them include:

- Itching (pruritus). The physician may order an anesthetic ointment to relieve the itching. Cleanliness helps, too: perhaps this patient can have two baths instead of one a day. Although the skin is not efficient for the disposal of such waste chemicals as uric acid, it is all that the body has available when the kidneys are not functioning, and a clean skin is always more efficient and more comfortable.
- Other skin problems. Cream or lotion instead of alcohol is used on dry skin. The sheets under the swollen buttocks are kept taut. The patient should change his position frequently. Even lying on the strings of his gown can make a deep crease in the edematous back.
- Odor. Unless urine comes from a necrotic area, as in cancer, or is infected, it is almost odorless as it leaves the body. The characteristic odor of urine is caused by ammonia, which is formed from urea by bacterial action. The more stale the urine becomes, the more malodorous. It has been said that the quality of the nursing on a urologic ward can be judged by sniffing the air. In instances of infection and necrotic tissue, odor can be combated by ventilation, the use of sprays, and,

most important, prompt cleaning of the patient as he needs it.

Dryness of the mouth. Commercially prepared glycerine and lemon swabs can be applied to the lips to prevent cracking. Frequent mouth rinses help remove debris from the oral cavity.

Pain. Sitz baths, when they are allowed, may ease the discomfort of an inflamed urethra. The burning caused by cystitis is reduced by forcing fluids to dilute the urine.

Long-term bed rest. A consistently quiet position leads to, among other evils, urinary stasis, potassium imbalance, and infection. Without tiring the patient, the nurse has him do range-of-motion exercises regularly.

Embarrassment and fear. The nurse's matter-of-fact attitude and care in not exposing the urologic patient unduly will help him to accept the necessary treatments. A man may fear, with justification, that impotence will follow urologic surgery, or that he has cancer. If the patient expresses any of these fears he should be encouraged to talk to his physician.

Appearance. The patient with generalized edema may feel self-conscious about his appearance. The edema of nephrosis gives a bloated look that, in the extreme, is startling.

Management of patients who have catheters

If the patient has one or more catheters in place, it is imperative that the nurses know the function of each tube, and in what area of anatomical structure the end of each is placed. She should ask if she does not know. Each catheter should be labeled (this can be put on the drainage vessel, or on the catheter itself with a tag or a loop of adhesive tape), so that all nursing personnel can note and chart the material that comes from any drain.

Types of Catheters. There are several types of catheters (Fig. 34-2A), suited for different purposes:

For drainage of urine. This may be a Foley catheter (Fig. 34-2B) placed in the bladder, a retention catheter in the kidney pelvis, a ureteral catheter, or one for drainage through a suprapubic wound leading to the bladder.

For splinting. A tube used solely for splinting might be inserted after a plastic repair of the ureter. It is removed 2 to 3 weeks postoperatively.

Catheters are measured in the French system. An adult urethra usually takes a size 18 to 24 F. indwelling catheter.

Ureteral catheters are smaller. These catheters are irrigated by gravity, using a special ureteral syringe and adaptor or with a syringe and blunt needle. Ureteral catheters may become obstructed easily if there is purulent or bloody urine. The physician may order no more than 5 ml. of sterile normal saline to be instilled by gravity and returned by gravity. The physi-

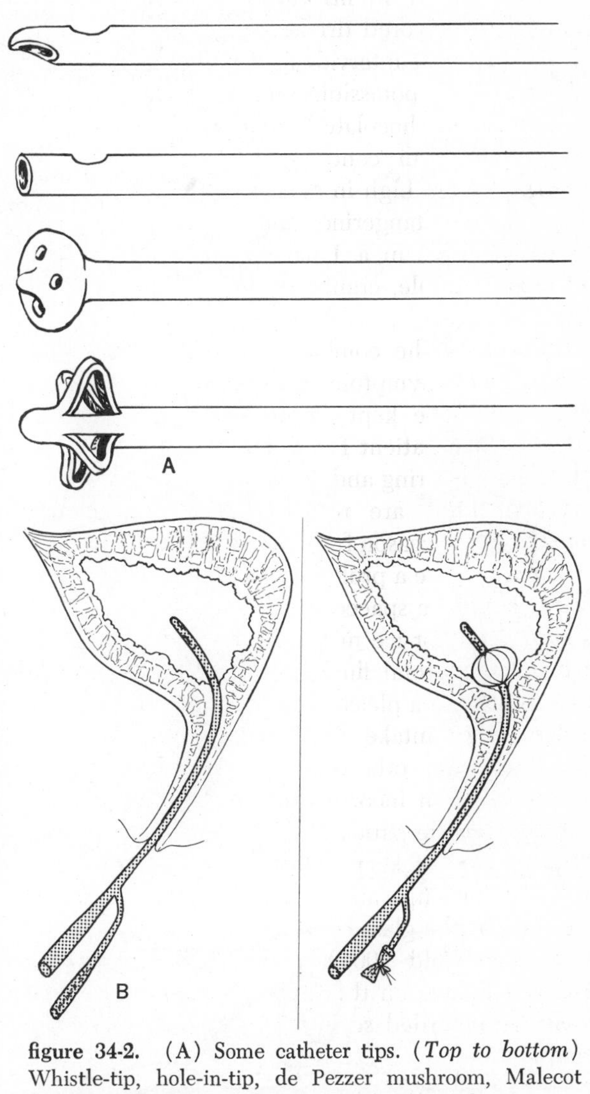

figure 34-2. (A) Some catheter tips. (*Top to bottom*) Whistle-tip, hole-in-tip, de Pezzer mushroom, Malecot 4-wing. (B) Foley catheter. (*Left*) The catheter is inserted into the bladder. (*Right*) The inflation of the bag prevents the catheter from leaving the bladder. The inner tube that leads to the balloon is tied.

cian is notified if patency of the catheter cannot be established by this type of irrigation.

One way to attach a ureteral catheter to drainage is to punch a small hole with a red-hot needle or pin in the rubber top of a sterile medicine dropper and thread the catheter through it. There are special adaptors available for connecting ureteral catheters to closed drainage systems. If there is a ureteral catheter in each ureter, they should be labeled "right" and "left."

Setting Up Drainage. As soon as the urologic patient with catheters is placed in bed, each urinary catheter is attached to the drainage vessel. If there is more than one catheter, *each* drainage bag is labeled according to the source of the catheter, for example, "suprapubic" and "urethral," or "left ureter" and "right ureter." The intake and output sheet is set up with a separate column for each source of urine. The drainage tube is secured to the sheet. Enough tubing is allowed between the pin and the patient so that there is no pull on the catheter when the patient turns, but not so much that the tubing will become tangled. A catheter must never be bent at right angles, as this will close the lumen of the tubing. The *entire* length of the tubing is inspected—from insertion into the patient to the drainage vessel—for kinks. Coiling excess tubing horizontally so that the urine does not have to flow uphill should keep it free of kinks. The kidney pelvis has a capacity of 5 to 8 ml. If a tube draining it is blocked for a half-hour (clot stuck in the lumen, patient lying on the tube, tube kinked), there will be backup of urine, perhaps strain on the suture line, and surely increased pain for the patient.

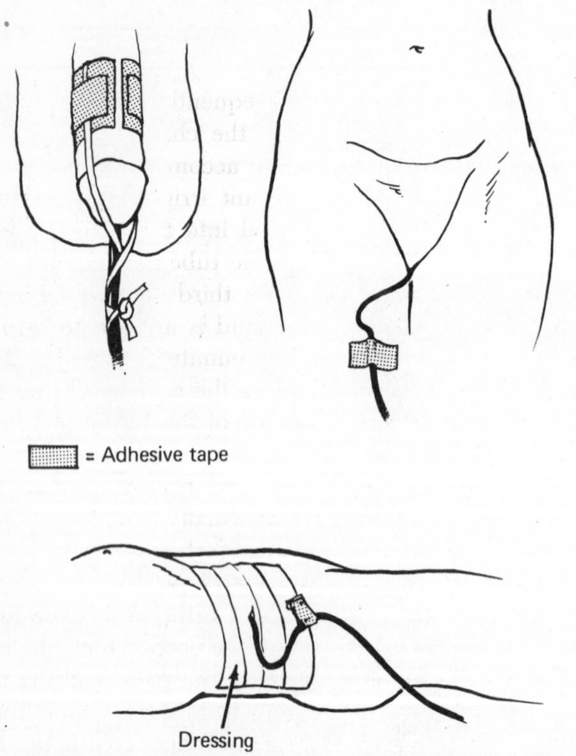

figure 34-3. Indwelling catheters should be anchored securely to prevent pull on them.

The end of the tube that drains the kidney pelvis should always be handled with aseptic precautions: a sterile drainage vessel is used, and the part of the tube near the opening is touched only with sterile forceps or the sterile gloved hand. The tubes that drain the ureter and the bladder are handled sometimes with clean and sometimes with sterile technique, depending on hospital policy. The drainage end of the tube should be kept above the level of the urine in the vessel.

Observations. When caring for urologic patients, the nurse first checks all urinary catheters for patency. Fresh catheters draining from the kidney pelvis or the ureter should be checked every half-hour, and others at least every 2 hours. If urine is appearing from a catheter that should not drain, the physician should be notified at once. If no urine appears from a catheter that should drain, the nurse should:

- Check the length of the tubing from the patient to the vessel for kinks, pressure, and other external compression of the tube that may be obstructing the lumen.
- Clamp the tube off near the patient and "milk" the remainder of the tube toward the drainage vessel. Feel for gravel (sediment made of phosphates and other mineral crystals). After milking, release the clamp and watch for urine.
- Disassemble the drainage system (without removing the catheter that goes into the patient) and flush it with sterile saline or water and a sterile syringe. Do not empty the fluid into the drainage vessel if a specimen of that urine is to be sent to the laboratory.
- If urine has not appeared, give the patient water to drink and notify the physician.

Changing the Catheters. The end of the catheter that goes into the patient should stay in place until the physician wishes it to come out. Some catheters going into wounds may be sutured in place; others should be firmly taped, except for Foley catheters, which usually maintain their position without outside anchorage. Taping a Foley catheter to the leg is done to prevent pull on the bag, which would cause pressure on the bladder outlet (Fig. 34-3). A catheter that accidentally becomes dislodged from the patient never should be reinserted. It should be replaced by a sterile one, which, depending on its location, may be inserted by the physician. Catheters that are positioned deep into the ureter or the kidney pelvis (Fig. 34-4) through a flank incision can, at times, be replaced only by reopening the wound. Thus it is extremely important that catheters are anchored properly and protected from accidental dislodging from the bladder or surgical wound.

Patients who go home with catheters in place learn to change them while they are still in the hospital. At home they may be helped by a visiting nurse, or a family member may be taught. Catheters or tubing for long-term use should be changed when sediment and debris obstruct the lumen. The glass or plastic connectors and tubing are changed whenever they become cloudy or plugged.

Drainage and Irrigation. Usually, drainage is accomplished by gravity, though occasionally, weak suction may be used. When the end of the catheter is in the kidney pelvis, only gravity drainage is used.

Catheters are irrigated with sterile saline or distilled water, but only when there is an order to do so. Generally, irrigation is done to keep the system of tubing open and not to rinse the cavity being drained. Because every irrigation carries with it the danger of infection, sterile technique always is employed. If fluid is instilled and does not return, very gentle suction may be used, *except* in recent postoperative patients and those whose catheters enter the kidney pelvis. If there is no return after suctioning once, the procedure is stopped and the tubing reattached to the drainage system and observed. If nothing has returned after an hour, the physician is notified. The amount of fluid that was instilled must be noted and subtracted from the total output.

The amount of fluid used for irrigations is ordered by the physician: a common amount for irrigating urethral tubing is 30 ml. of sterile saline. No more than 5 ml. at a time is used to irrigate tubing that goes into the kidney pelvis. Whenever a patient complains of pain during an irrigation, it should be momentarily stopped. Irrigations should be done slowly and gently.

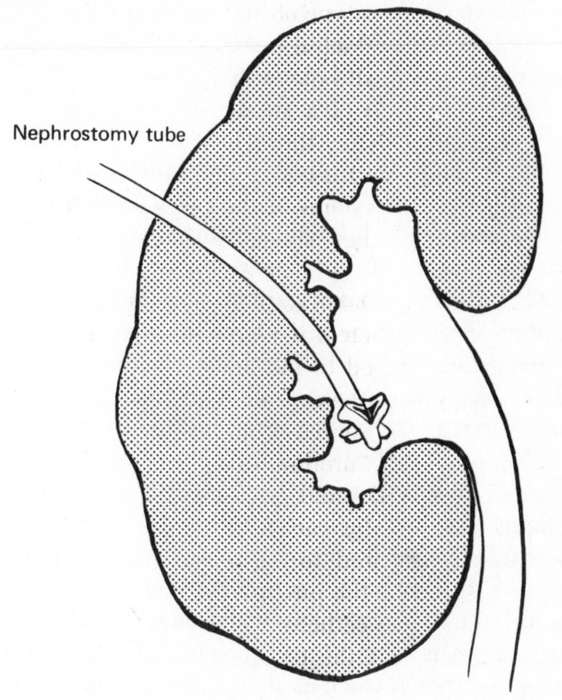

figure 34-4. A nephrostomy tube with a Malecot 4-wing tip draining the kidney pelvis.

If irrigation is required frequently, a closed system may be set up to decrease the chance of infection. Intermittent irrigation can be accomplished by releasing the clamp. When constant irrigation is ordered, a drip device is incorporated into the tubing, and a three-way Foley catheter (one tube admits fluid, one allows for drainage, and the third fills the balloon) may be used. Usually, the fluid is allowed to drip at a rate of 30 to 60 drops per minute. A closed system such as this is not used when the catheter is inserted into the kidney pelvis, because of the danger of admitting too much fluid.

After a catheter is removed from a wound, the closure of the surgical fistula usually is rapid, so rapid that if a catheter should inadvertently slip out of a wound, it may not be possible to replace it after a half-hour has elapsed. If a wound catheter inadvertently slips out, the physician should be notified immediately. After a catheter is removed by the physician, the site is observed. Urine may drain from it for a short time, but it should gradually stop. When a catheter has been removed from the urethra, the patient's voiding pattern is observed, and the time and amount of fluid recorded. Is he incontinent? If so, is he incontinent in all positions: lying down and standing up? How often does he void? What is the anticipated quantity? Does he void sufficient quantity each time and a sufficient quantity over a 24-hour period?

The patient with urinary incontinence

Ordinarily, the excretion of urine is controlled by two sphincters: the *internal sphincter,* which is close to the most dependent part of the bladder, and the *external sphincter,* which surrounds the urethra at a lower point. As the bladder fills, nerve endings are stimulated, giving rise to the sensation of needing to void.

The anesthetized, unconscious, or senile patient may not receive these stimuli, and in many of these patients the urinary sphincters relax involuntarily. Also, infection of the urinary system and accidental or surgical damage to either sphincter can cause loss of control. The sphincters may not function adequately when there is local tissue damage. Interference with the spinal nerves, such as that which occurs in tumors of the spinal cord, tabes dorsalis, herniated disc, post-operative edema of the cord, and cord injuries, can interfere with the conduction to the brain of the impulse to void, and result in a neurogenic bladder and incontinence. Many paraplegic patients do not know when they void because they have lost all sensation in the lower parts of their bodies. A neurogenic bladder may be spastic, preventing the retention of urine, or it may be flaccid, preventing the complete expulsion of urine. A tidal drainage system, with its periodic filling and emptying, simulates normal bladder functioning, thus preserving bladder capacity and muscle tone.

Nursing management

Nursing management is directed at establishing a voiding routine, when that is possible; and when it is not possible, at finding the most convenient way to collect the urine and to keep it off the skin.

Establishing a Schedule. The patient and the nurse working together may be able to set up a schedule, so that voiding is regular and predictable. Such a program takes great patience by all concerned. If it is successful, it gives the patient freedom from constant odor, wetness, and the embarrassment of accidents when he may be, for instance, at the movies or with company for dinner. The first step is observation of the patient's pattern of urination. If a pattern is observable, a bedpan or a commode should be made available (or the patient should be helped to the bathroom, if possible) just before it is believed his bladder will empty. As far as possible, any association with childhood experience should be avoided. This is not the same thing as toilet training in the child, and the patient's dignity should not be affronted.

Fluid intake can be spaced to help to establish a regular time of voiding. Spacing fluids will take experimentation. If the patient limits his fluids before going to bed or going out on a social occasion, it is essential that his intake is adequate at other times of the day. A patient with a neurogenic bladder may not completely empty his bladder when he voids. Because of the danger of infection and stone formation, it is doubly important that he drink sufficient fluids—at least 2,000 ml. per day. Increasing intra-abdominal pressure by gentle manual pressure just above the symphysis pubis may aid a patient with a neurogenic bladder to void.

Until a routine is well established, a record of the time and the amount voided should be kept. Such information can help the physician to see if there is overflow with retention of residual urine, and it can help the patient to regulate himself.

Rehabilitation. An indwelling catheter may be used to prevent retention of urine and incontinence. Initially, it may be allowed to drain constantly, but later, if the urologist determines that a reflex is present, a method of bladder training may be instituted. One method is an alternate clamping and unclamping of the catheter. The catheter is clamped for a specified length of time and then opened for a specified length of time. In the beginning the catheter is unclamped for 5 to 15 minutes every 1 to 2 hours. In this time the bladder is given a chance to hold urine and then to empty it, thus beginning to re-establish normal function. Gradually, the interval for releasing the catheter is lengthened to 3 to 4 hours, giving the bladder a chance to fill more completely. The patient can be taught to release the clamp on his own catheter at scheduled times. The retention catheter is changed once a week.

The catheter later is removed entirely, and the patient is instructed to void every hour. Usually he is not able to retain the urine longer, and frequent voiding is necessary to prevent incontinence. Gradually the interval is lengthened to 2, 3, or 4 hours. Since such frequent voiding would disturb the patient during the night, external drainage is used. A rubber sheath is placed over the penis and is connected by rubber tubing to a drainage bottle, or to a disposable urinary drainage bag (Fig. 34-5). Women wear absorbent pads and moistureproof pants. When the patient becomes able to retain urine longer, the voiding schedule is continued throughout the night.

The process takes a great deal of patience, and accidents do happen during the training period. The bed should have a full-length waterproof mattress cover. When an accident occurs, the linen should be changed promptly, and the patient assured that this is to be expected during the retraining process. He should not be made to feel that he has failed in his program.

At first many patients void in insufficient quantity, and they must be catheterized after voiding to remove residual urine. The patient should keep a careful record of his fluid intake and output.

Some incontinent patients never achieve complete freedom from catheters; others do. Success depends not only on the degree of injury, but on the motivation of the patient and the amount of skillful help and encouragement that he receives from the staff. Men patients usually do not achieve urinary control as readily as do women, probably because more convenient appliances are available for them than for women. A man can wear a catheter that is connected by means of rubber tubing to a rubber urinal. The urinal is strapped to the patient's lower leg. Each patient should have two urinals, one to wear and the other to wash thoroughly and to hang to dry. The man's trousers cover his urinal; no one need know that he uses it. Women use a less effective device, rubberized pants, plus an absorbent perineal pad.

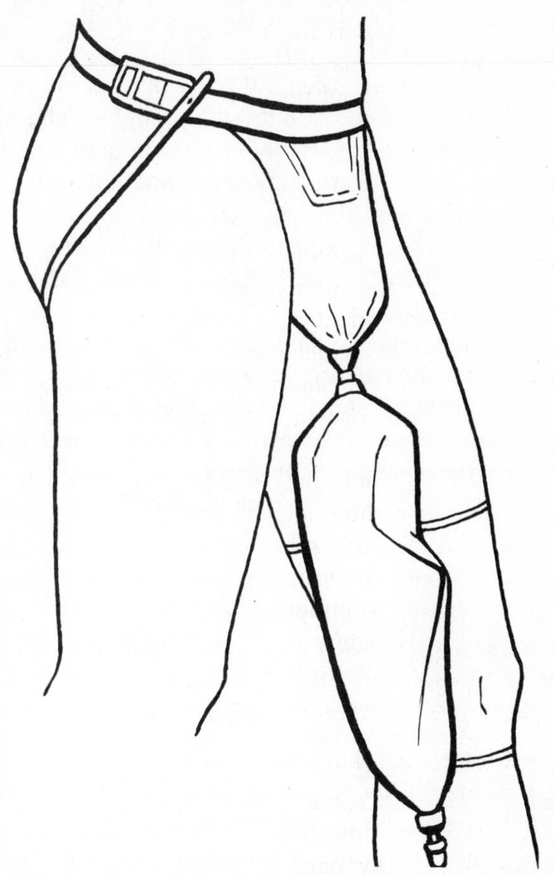

figure 34-5. A rubber leg urinal placed over the penis and held in place with a belt.

The bed patient

The male patient who is incontinent, bedridden, and unable to attend to his own needs can have a plastic or a rubber sheath with tubing (condom drainage) placed over the penis and attached to a drainage bottle.

The female patient is provided with a waterproof sheet covered with a drawsheet. The sheet under the buttocks should be large enough so that it does not roll into a wrinkled ball under the patient. The small sheet can be changed without disturbing the basic bedclothes. Pads that are placed under and on the patient may be disposable or washable. They should be arranged in proper order before the patient is disturbed. A pile of them ready for use can be kept nearby.

Urea-splitting organisms, among them *Micrococcus ureae,* cause the urea in urine to react with water. An end product of this reaction is ammonia, which causes both the odor of urine and the skin damage. One way to protect skin is to avoid any contact with urine. When this is not possible, an antiseptic, such as methylbenzethonium chloride (Diaparene Chloride), which kills the ammonia-forming organism in urine, may be used. The antiseptic, in ointment or powder, can (with the physician's approval) be applied to the skin of the incontinent ambulatory or bed patient. Light dusting with an absorbent powder, such as cornstarch, also helps to prevent ammonia dermatitis.

If powder, an antiseptic, liners, and protective pads are used, there should be no problem with odor or ammonia dermatitis, but these measures should not be a substitute for scrupulous cleanliness and the changing of padding as soon as it becomes wet. The buttocks and the genital area of the incontinent patient should be washed with soap and water several times a day. Unlike feces, urine on the skin is not visible. To prevent skin breakdown, the area actually must be free of urine; it is not sufficient that it appears to be clean. To avoid irritation, all soap must be removed from the skin and the skin dried thoroughly. The plastic or rubber sheet is washed with soap and water at least once a day. If an ammonia dermatitis is present, the affected area is kept clean, dry and exposed to the air. Exposure to an ordinary light bulb for 20 minutes several times a day, with the physician's approval, often helps.

The continuous vigilance and the care required by the incontinent patient who is unable to care for himself may seem tiresome. Having the necessary materials right at hand and a planned routine makes quick work of the changes. The reward is a healthy, unbroken skin and a comfortable patient.

The ambulatory patient

If it is not possible to establish a voiding routine, the nurse and the patient together should devise some system of collecting the urine. The objective is to provide for the urine an external reservoir that:

- Protects the skin from contact with urine.
- Is inexpensive to maintain.
- Is convenient for the patient.
- Can be worn under clothes.
- Does not leak.
- Is comfortable to wear.

The arrangement should be individualized. For example, if the patient is hemiplegic and cannot use one hand, he should be given a rubber or plastic urinal that he can manage one-handed. If the patient's skin is excoriated, the appliance should not irritate it further. A simple urinal for the ambulatory male patient can be made out of a disposable plastic bag that fits over the penis and is kept in place by taping it to a belt. There are commercially available rubber urinals for men that can be worn under a suit.

Women with incontinence may wear a perineal pad. There are also a number of protective pants on the market that have a rubberized or plastic outside layer and absorbent material inside. These pants can be pinned or snapped in place. (These pants should not be called "diapers.") Liners also are available and are worn next to the skin. Because they are nonabsorbent, the urine passes through them; and because they dry very quickly, they leave the skin dry and free of urine, even though the absorbent material is soaked.

Home care

Sometimes the decision concerning whether the patient can be cared for at home rests on management of the problem of incontinence—a condition which is embarrassing to the patient, and which the family may find very upsetting. Decisions about whether home care is feasible rest with the family, with the advice and support of the physicians and nurses. Often what appears to be a family's unwillingness to care for the patient at home actually is fear and uncertainty about the management of such care. A family can be shown that the ambulatory patient usually can care for himself without odor or fuss, or that the bed patient can be changed quickly, easily, and inexpensively. The nurse who finds a convenient way to keep the patient clean and dry, and who is able to teach the patient's family how to do this may be able to show the members of the family who wish to care for the patient, but who are uncertain of their skills, how home care can be carried out. The rehabilitation of the patient with a neurogenic bladder or with urinary incontinence from other causes is often a long-term complex nursing problem.

Urinary obstructions

An obstruction can occur anywhere in the urinary tract—from the kidney pelvis to the tip of the urethra. Obstruction may be caused by a tumor, a stone, a cyst, a kink in the ureter, stenosis or spasm of the ureters, or a diverticulum in the bladder wall that distends and blocks one or more of the three openings (two ureteral, one urethral) into the bladder. In older men an enlargement of the prostate gland is a common obstructing lesion. Congenital strictures are not infrequent, and some may not be discovered until the patient is an adult.

Acquired obstructions include surgical injuries to the ureters and urethral strictures from traumatic instrumentation. Neurogenic dysfunction of the bladder which causes stasis of urine is essentially an obstructive condition.

When urine cannot pass freely by the obstruction, it backs up. For example, if there is closure at the orifice that leads from the right ureter into the bladder, the ureter will become more and more distended as new urine passes into it from above. The back pressure moves into the kidney pelvis, which also becomes distended. Now the parenchyma of the kidney is squeezed between the pressure from the expanding pelvis and the internal pressure of the glomerulus and its continuous formation of urine. Likewise, the tiny blood vessels supplying the kidney tissue are being compressed, a dangerous condition because of the possibility of permanent kidney damage. Waste products accumulate in the bloodstream. When the kidney pelvis is swollen with backflow, the condition is called *hydronephrosis* (Fig. 34-6).

The lower the level in the tract that the obstruction occurs, the more slowly the kidney pelvis becomes distended with the backflow of urine. When the obstruction is in the urethra, the bladder distends, and finally diverticuli (outpouchings) of the muscular wall can form. Urine becomes trapped in these sacs, stagnates, and becomes a culture medium for bacteria. For this reason, infection goes hand in hand with obstruction. The infection may be blood-borne, such as that caused by streptococci, staphylococci, or pneumococci; or it may enter the urethra from the outside, such as that caused by *Escherichia coli.* Control of infection is extremely difficult until the underlying obstruction is corrected.

When the obstruction is minor, and the pressure from backed-up urine develops slowly, there may be no discomfort. However, infection is the rule rather than the exception, and with it come pain and fever. When the kidney pelvis becomes markedly distended, a mass may be palpated through the abdomen. Advanced hydronephrosis causes renal tenderness and pain. If there is a diverticulum of the bladder, the patient may find that he can pass more urine after emptying his bladder and waiting a few minutes. The final quantity of urine comes from the diverticulum sac and may be malodorous.

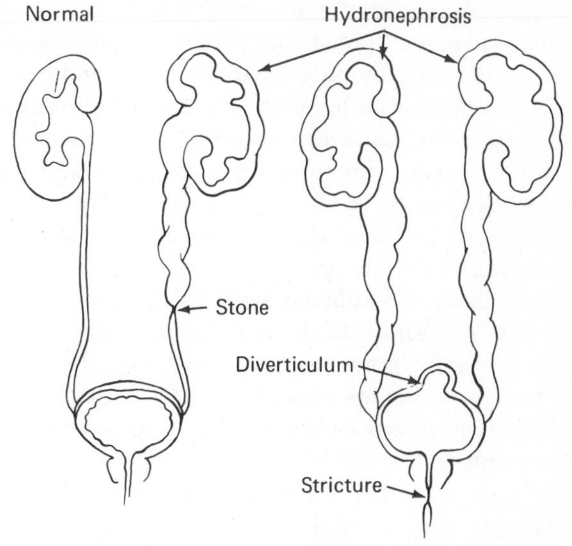

figure 34-6. Hydronephrosis caused by blockage of the urinary tract. Note how dilatation occurs above the point of obstruction.

The aim of treatment is to establish adequate drainage of urine. The first measure that the physician

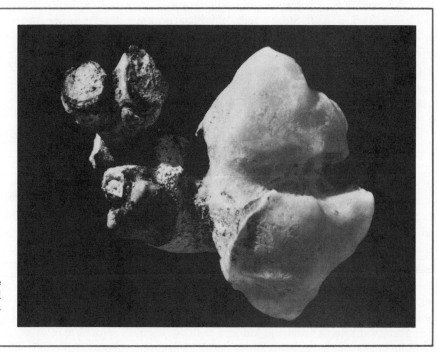

figure 34-7. Kidney stones can be very large. This stone was removed from the pelvis of the kidney. (Photograph—D. Atkinson)

takes may be temporary, designed to permit free flow of urine, to relieve the retention and to allow the edematous kidney to heal until it is sufficiently healthy to withstand surgery to correct the obstruction. For example, a patient with a ureteral calculus obstructing one kidney accompanied by severe infection may have chills, fever, and hypotension. Under these conditions the patient may be so ill that anesthesia and surgery to remove the calculus may be very risky. Therefore, the physician, during cystoscopy, may pass a ureteral catheter above the calculus with its tip draining the kidney pelvis. The catheter will not cure the pathology, but it will drain purulent urine from the pelvis and relieve hydronephrosis. When the patient's general condition improves, a more definite procedure can be performed.

As soon as a way for urine to leave the body is established, the patient should be encouraged to drink fluids.

If the obstruction is so complete that a catheter cannot be passed, temporary drainage may be accomplished by inserting a tube into the kidney pelvis through a skin incision (nephrostomy). When the acute process has subsided, surgery can remove the obstruction, repair the stricture, remove the stone, free the ureter from adhesions, or excise the tumor.

Calculi (stones, lithiasis)

Etiology. When the salts in urine precipitate instead of remaining in solution, they adhere and form stones (Fig. 34-7, p. 459). Stones, most of which form in the kidney, can plug the urinary tract, so that obstruction with stasis of urine is frequently found. The exact conditions that cause salts to precipitate are not fully understood. Excessive excretion of calcium, as occurs in patients with hyperparathyroid disease, appears to be one possible cause of stone formation.

Infection (particularly with Proteus species) and stones tend to coexist, but in a particular patient it may not always be clear which came first. Infection can make the urine alkaline, and the result may be the precipitation of calcium. On the other hand, when the pH of the urine becomes excessively acid, cystine and uric acid may precipitate. Patients with gout are likely to form uric acid stones. Osteoporosis (demineralization of bones) may also be a contributing factor.

Urinary stones frequently occur in patients on long-term bed rest, such as those with fractures or paraplegia. When urine flow is sluggish and there is poor gravity drainage from the kidneys as the patient lies on his back, there may be diffuse decalcification of bone, and stones may form. This hazard of immobility may be prevented by nursing action, such as active range-of-motion exercises practiced several times every day and encouraging liberal ingestion of fluids (when both of these are allowed).

Symptoms. Some small stones pass right through and cause no symptoms at all; others are troublesome, because they traumatize the walls of the urinary tract and irritate the lining, or because they obstruct the ureter or an orifice, preventing urine flow and inviting infection.

The following symptoms may occur:

- Hematuria, gross or microscopic, as the stone traumatizes the walls of the urinary tract.
- Pyuria (pus in the urine) due to infection behind the obstruction by the calculus. The patient may experience chills, fever, and can develop serious hypotension and other signs of a gram negative septicemia.
- Retention of urine or dysuria from blockage of the orifice between bladder and urethra. Some patients can void only in unnatural positions; others are unable to void at all.
- Flank pain.
- Acute renal or ureteral colic, due to violent contractions and spasms as the ureter tries to pass along a stone. The severity of pain is almost inversely proportional to the size of the calculus. Smaller stones frequently travel more rapidly down the ureter causing more forceful ureteral spasm and, therefore, greater colic.

The colicky pain is characteristic. It is agonizingly severe, coming in waves that may start in the kidney or the ureter and radiate to the inguinal ring, the inner aspect of the thigh or, in the male patient, to the testicle or the tip of the penis. In a female patient, the pain may go to the urinary meatus or the labia of the affected side. The patient may double up with pain and be unable to lie quietly in bed until it passes. The severity of the pain can cause nausea, vomiting, and shock. Often, morphine and antispasmodic drugs are given for relief. As the pain subsides, the patient should be made comfortable in bed. Fluids should be encouraged after nausea abates.

Until the kidneys and the ureters are free of stones, the colicky pains tend to recur. The violent spasm that causes the pain may move a stone along, and, sometimes after an attack of colic, the patient may pass "gravel" or the offending stone itself. On the other hand, a spastic ureter may clamp down on a stone and hold it in place.

In the hospital, the patient who is suspected of having stones should have all of his urine strained through gauze to catch any stones that he may have passed. The stones may be no larger than the head of a pin. At home the patient can void into a clear glass through a small kitchen strainer with cheesecloth lining it. Some stones will be sent to the laboratory for chemical analysis, for the composition of the stones will affect the treatment. All the stones should be saved and shown to the physician.

TREATMENT. Most ureteral calculi, 1 cm. or less in diameter, will pass into the bladder spontaneously. Unless there is an obstruction at the bladder outlet, such as an enlarged prostate or urethral stricture, they are voided spontaneously as well.

On admission, x-ray studies may be ordered to locate the stone. In some instances, an intravenous pyelogram is needed as some stones are not radiopaque and, therefore, will not show on routine films. When a radiopaque dye is injected, the stone is outlined by the dye and may be seen. The dye will also show if the stone is blocking the ureter. The patient may be observed for several days to see whether the stone will pass from his body. In some instances a large fluid intake is encouraged to reduce the concentration of crystalloids in the urine and to foster the passage of stones.

As soon as the acute colic subsides, the patient should be encouraged to walk as well as to drink. An active patient is more likely to pass a stone than a quiet one.

If the stone does not pass spontaneously, and there is continued colic, infection above the stone, or, in the opinion of the physician, little likelihood of spontaneous passage, surgery is generally performed. Calculi larger than 1 cm. in diameter in the renal pelvis are surgically removed.

For a stone in the renal pelvis, the surgeon may perform one of the following procedures:

- Pyelolithotomy. An incision is made into the renal pelvis, and the stone is removed.
- Nephrolithotomy. An incision is made into the parenchyma of the kidney from the outside to remove a stone in the calyx.
- Nephrectomy. The kidney is removed if the stone has so permanently and severely damaged it that kidney function is no longer possible. This operation is used when there has been unilateral kidney damage, with the other kidney retaining at least some healthy tissue.

Stones in the ureter may be removed surgically. This procedure is called a ureterolithotomy. In one method a small incision is made over the stone in the ureter. A drain of the Penrose type is placed at the site of the incision, and the urine is allowed to drain from the wound until the ureter heals. The physician may attempt extraction of lower ureteral calculi with a variety of stone baskets passed into the ureter by means of a cystoscope.

Occasionally, a ureteral stone can be crushed or grasped and pulled out with a special instrument during cystoscopy. Snaring the stone is an extremely delicate procedure because of the constant danger of rupturing the ureter. Usually, this cystoscopic procedure is performed under general anesthesia to avoid any sudden movement of the patient; and if any complications are encountered, open surgery is begun at once. If the procedure is uncomplicated and successful, the patient will have a ureteral catheter attached to straight drainage. The purpose of the catheter is to splint the ureter and to divert the urine past any possible tear in the ureteral wall. It is kept in place for 3 to 4 days. At times after a cystoscopy a ureteral catheter will be left in place for 24 hours to dilate the ureter in the hope that stones then will pass through it, or that the stone will be pulled into the bladder when the catheter is removed.

BLADDER STONES. Bladder stones may be removed through the transurethral route, using a stone-crushing instrument called a lithotrite. The procedure *(litholapaxy)* is suitable for small and soft stones. Larger, noncrushable stones must be removed through a suprapubic incision.

The surgery for renal calculi also includes correction of any anatomical obstructions which are thought to contribute to the development of stones. For example, a congenital ureteropelvic junction obstruction may require that the surgeon perform pyeloplasty along with removal of calculi, or stones will reform.

PREVENTION. Patients who have a tendency to form stones should always ingest adequate fluids (minimum 2,500 to 3,000 ml. daily) to help to prevent recurrence. Also, they should be instructed in the methods for straining urine and know that any stone should be brought to the doctor for examination.

The patient should be made aware of the importance of promptly reporting to the physician any hematuria, burning, or other signs of urinary tract infection, and infection anywhere in the body. An infection in another part of the body may set up a secondary focus of infection in the urinary tract that can help to recreate stones.

Patients with gout must limit their purine intake to prevent uric acid stones. Patients who have had stones of calcium may have to limit their intake of milk and milk products.

When it has been possible to determine the chemical composition of stones that have been passed or removed, dietary treatment then may be attempted to adjust the pH of the urine to keep the urinary salts in solution. However, these diets are not fully effective. Sometimes the desired pH of the urine can be achieved by relatively minor changes in the diet. To acidify the urine, the physician may suggest that the patient eliminate citrus fruits, fruit juices other than apple and cranberry, and carbonated beverages from his diet. Tomatoes may be eaten for vitamin C. An acidifying agent, such as sodium acid phosphate, may be given. To make the urine more alkaline, the physician may prescribe sodium bicarbonate or polycitrate solution, and 1 to 3 quarts of orange juice a day. Uric acid stones can sometimes be prevented by a low-purine diet and alkalinization of the urine by use of oral sodium bicarbonate. The patient is taught how to check his urinary acidity with litmus or nitrazine paper. Cystine stones can sometimes be prevented by using a vigorous fluid intake (up to 6 liters per day), and stringent alkalinization of the urine.

The most effective deterrent to calcium stones, particularly phosphatic ones, is the Shorr regimen. The patient is placed on a low-calcium, low-phosphorus diet to diminish the concentration of these substances in the urine. Basic aluminum hydroxide gel, 30 to 45 ml., is ingested after each meal and at bedtime to precipitate phosphorus as insoluble aluminum phosphates in the gastrointestinal tract, thus further decreasing urinary phosphate output. It is important that the patient understand and can fulfill the fluid requirement, and any dietary and drug or chemotherapy instructions, before he leaves the hospital.

Tumors of the kidney

The malignant hypernephroma (renal adenocarcinoma) is the most common tumor of the parenchyma of the adult kidney. Because the kidneys are deeply protected in the body, tumors can become quite large before they cause symptoms. An abdominal mass found on a routine physical examination or on x-ray examinations taken for other purposes may lead to the discovery. These tumors are dangerous because they usually metastasize early but may present distressing symptoms only late in the course of the disease. Hematuria may occur if the tumor invades the collecting system. It may be both intermittent and painless. Later, pain may be due to expansion of the kidney or colic-like discomfort from the passage of blood clots.

The symptoms of a malignant tumor may include weight loss, malaise, unexplained fever, and episodes of hematuria. Sometimes, the first symptom occurs at a secondary, metastatic site.

When kidney cancer is diagnosed, a complete removal of the kidney (nephrectomy) and its surrounding perinephric fat may be done. When the tumor arises from the collecting system or in the ureter a complete nephroureterectomy may be done. The kidney and ureter as well as a cuff of bladder tissue are removed because the recurrence rate in any stump of ureter left behind is very high.

Surgery may be followed by x-ray therapy while the patient is still in the hospital or on an outpatient basis. Follow-up cystoscopic examinations are imperative to find any early and newly metastasized areas in the bladder. If the unaffected kidney cannot adequately take over the function of excreting urine, or if extensive metastases are found, only palliative treatment can be given.

Urethral strictures

Since strictures are a form of obstruction, they are a danger to the upper urinary tract. The symptoms may include a slow stream of urine, hesitancy, burning, frequency, nocturia, and the retention of residual urine in the bladder, which may lead to bladder distention and infection. A voiding urethrogram aids in the diagnosis. If the patient is unable to void, a retrograde urethrogram may be done.

The urologist may treat urethral strictures by:

- Dilatation. This is done with specially designed instruments (bougies, sounds, filiforms and followers) passed very gently into the lumen of the urethra. Although this procedure is done gently, it is still painful. Taking deep breaths may help the patient to relax.

  Since forceful stretching of the urethra may cause bleeding and further stricture formation, the physician gently uses graduated size instruments. He may start with only a 6 or 8 F. and gradually increase the size until a 24 or 26 F. can be tolerated. Depending on the cause of the stricture and the patient's response to the therapy, the condition may subside after one or two treatments, but usually periodic dilatations are required indefinitely, or until the condition is corrected surgically. The nurse should help the patient to understand the importance of having these treatments regularly as prescribed and of not waiting until there has been too severe a reduction in the size of the urinary stream or other symptoms of obstruction. After a treatment, the patient may have slight hematuria and should be told about this in advance so that he will not become frightened. Of course, if a great amount of blood appears, or if bleeding persists, he should notify the physician immediately. Voiding will be painful for about 2 days after the procedure. Sitz baths help to relieve the discomfort.

▪ Urethroplasty. The urine is diverted from the urethra by way of a cystostomy tube or perineal urethrostomy tube attached to straight drainage until the urethra has been repaired. In one method of reconstructing the urethra, the constricted area is resected, and a mucosal graft (which may be taken from the bladder) is inserted to restore the continuity of the urethra. Postoperatively, the patient will have a splinting catheter in the urethra that will remain until healing has taken place. This operation may be performed in two stages: urinary diversion at the first operation and plastic repair at the second.

Nursing management

Preoperative management

The time that is spent waiting for surgery can be full of anxiety, especially if the operation that is planned is mutilating or changes vital functions. The nurse should follow the surgeon's explanation with opportunities for the patient to ask questions. Detailed preoperative explanations are important, and the patient must fully understand the extent of surgery and what physical changes (if any) will be temporary or permanent.

If a perineal approach is taken to any urologic surgery, the areas around the genitalia and the anus must be shaved. These are difficult areas to shave thoroughly. A good light and a sharp razor are essential.

Postoperative management

The three usual surgical approaches to the urinary tract are: (1) a flank incision just under the diaphragm to reach the ureter and the kidney on that side, (2) an incision in the lower abdomen above the symphysis pubis to reach the bladder (suprapubic), and (3) a perineal incision. Some procedures are done through the urethra. A transthoracic approach may be used for nephrectomy (excision of the kidney).

A flank incision is so close to the thoracic cavity that it is painful for the patient to cough and to breathe deeply. To counter this pain and to help to prevent hypostatic pneumonia, medications for the pain are used as ordered, and the wound site is supported with the hand when the patient coughs. Frequent turning, breathing deeply, and early ambulation are indicated.

After kidney surgery, patients may develop gastrointestinal discomfort, such as distention, due to pressure on the abdominal organs during the operation. A nasogastric tube attached to continuous suction may be used, and fluids may be given intravenously until the patient can take them by mouth. (For postoperative management of the patient with renal or ureteral surgery, see Table 34-2.)

Table 34-2.
Postoperative management of the patient with renal or ureteral surgery

Blood pressure, pulse, respirations should be checked every ½ to 1 hour for the first 4 to 24 hours.

Temperature should be taken every 4 hours.

Operative dressing should be checked for drainage and reinforced as needed.

Intake and output should be recorded. If a catheter(s) is left in the kidney or ureter and connected to a separate drainage system, the amount of urine collected from *each* catheter should be recorded, as well as from the Foley catheter (if used).

Color of urinary drainage should be charted.

Turn, cough, and deep breathing and leg exercises should be done every 2 hours. The surgeon should be consulted to see if the patient can turn on his operative side.

The incision should be gently splinted as the patient coughs or deep breathes.

Administer IPPB treatments as ordered.

The nurse should observe for the development of oliguria, and check the output from each catheter every ½ hour for the first 16 to 24 hours.

Danger Periods. The two periods when the patient is in the greatest danger from hemorrhage are immediately postoperatively, and the eighth to the tenth days after surgery, when tissue sloughing may occur. Ambulatory patients may be returned to bed rest for these 3 days. The nurse observes for hemorrhage the eighth to the tenth day after fulguration procedures. With the patient lying on his back or his side, blood may seep under him and not appear on the top of the dressing. Because of its position, this is especially true of a flank incision. The nurse checks frequently for hemorrhage by feeling beneath the patient for dampness, and depressing the bed at the point of bandage, so that she can observe for stains.

Detection of Bleeding. When there is a draining catheter left in place postoperatively, it will be easier to detect bleeding if the drainage apparatus is changed every 2 hours. Small bottles or large test tubes, which are easier to handle and easier to remember to change, are used, and each bottle is labeled with the time. The bottles can be lined up with a light source such as the window behind them, and their colors can be compared. Normally, the nurse should be able to see a progressive lightening from dark red to pink. If the urine remains the same color, or turns brighter red, the physician should be notified. After 48 hours the pink should give way to amber or, if the kidneys are working well, and the hydration is good, to yellow.

Protecting the Skin. Some wounds drain urine both through and around a catheter. To prevent skin excoriation and infection, the dressing must be kept dry. Because the dressing may need to be changed every half-hour, nurses often do the dressing changes early in the postoperative course, using aseptic technique. The moisture in the dressing and the frequency of the changes together invite infection, which can be prevented by employing rigid sterile technique and by never allowing the dressing to become saturated.

The skin can be protected in several ways. Zinc oxide can be applied carefully so that none enters the wound. Dressings previously soaked in an antiseptic to prevent the formation of ammonia in urine and then dried and sterilized can be used. A sheet of rubber may be prepared with a hole in the middle the size of the wound. It then is cemented in place over the operative site. Urine seeping from around the catheter runs over the rubber dam and does not come into contact with skin. However, dressing changes still must be frequent to prevent infection.

Positioning. Patients usually are not restricted in their position postoperatively. Variation of position and frequent change are encouraged to prevent pneumonia. The nurse should be sure that no tube is compressed by the patient's lying on it.

After a nephrectomy, a Penrose drain is left in place to catch the serous material that collects in the space left by the kidney. Of course, no urine comes from this drain. The amount and characteristics (color, consistency, odor, and contents) of this drainage, which may be blood-tinged in the beginning, should be charted. The drainage should stop after about 2 days. A sterile safety pin is usually placed on this drain by the physician so that it cannot disappear into the wound. Because the surgical area is close to the pleural cavity the patient is observed for a pneumothorax. In rare instances, the pleura is accidentally nicked during the operation, and air enters the pleural space from the lung and collapses the lung.

Positive pressure breathing treatments may be ordered. Splinting the incision with a binder, or manually, may help the patient to expand his rib cage. The patient may have a nasogastric tube for several days because paralytic ileus of reflex origin tends to develop. Fluids are encouraged when this tube is removed. The nurse observes for signs of hemorrhage especially during the immediate postoperative period and 8 to 12 days postoperatively when tissue sloughing is apt to occur.

If the hyperextended side-lying position was used for surgery, the patient may be troubled by muscular aches and pain. Pillow support and the use of prescribed muscle relaxants may give relief.

Tumors of the bladder

Bladder tumors may be benign or malignant. In malignant tumors, metastases have usually not occurred so long as the muscle is not penetrated.

The most common first symptom of malignant disease of the bladder is painless hematuria (another instance of the importance of immediately investigating hematuria). Diagnosis is made by cystoscopic examination and biopsy.

Treatment varies according to the type of tumor, and the grade and stage of malignant ones. Small, superficial tumors may be cut out through the transurethral resectoscope by means of an electric cutting instrument. Bleeding can be checked, or tumor tissue may be coagulated in the same manner. Fulguration may be used for small and benign tumors. Patients who have had papillomas removed should return for a cystoscopic examination every 3 months for the first year, and every 6 months for the next 4 years, so that recurrence of a benign tumor or a new malignant growth can be discovered early.

Some tumors may not be removable by the transurethral method because of their size or their location in the bladder. To remove these tumors a suprapubic incision is made, and the bladder is exposed and thoroughly explored. Part of the bladder may be removed (segmental resection) or all of it (cystectomy).

Bladder Surgery. When a portion of the bladder is removed (segmental resection), its capacity as a reservoir is decreased. Immediately postoperatively, the patient may be able to hold no more than 50 to 60 ml. of urine. This capacity should increase to 200 to 400 ml. within 1 or 2 months (depending on the amount of the bladder that was removed). Fluids should be encouraged during the immediate postoperative period, and the output from both the urethral and the suprapubic catheters shoud be watched and recorded. The patient becomes aware of being able to hold less urine when his catheters are first removed. Prior discussion of what to expect will help to lessen surprise and anxiety. The patient will need to adjust to the smaller reservoir capacity. For example, he should learn to restrict fluids before retiring or joining a gathering. However, it is important that his total fluid intake for the day be adequate.

After cystectomy (total removal of the bladder), the patient is usually quite ill. The bladder and large amounts of surrounding tissue have been removed. The patient is prone to surgical shock, thrombosis, cardiac decompensation, and other circulatory disturbances. Nursing management is similar to that of the patient with major abdominal surgery. In addition, permanent urinary diversion (see below) accompanies cystectomy. If the prostatic capsule has been removed, the male patient will be impotent.

Nursing management of patients with ureteral transplants

Some operations for urinary diversion are:

Ureterosigmoidostomy. The ureters are attached to the sigmoid colon. The lower colon becomes the reservoir for urine. The patient voids and defecates through the rectum.

The advantage of attaching ureters to the bowel is that the patient is not required to adjust to caring for a continuously draining opening in his abdominal wall. There are no appliances, and there is no need to care for the skin surrounding the orifices. The lower colon acts as a reservoir of sorts (holding about 200 ml.), and the anal sphincter controls the exit from the body of both urine and stool. The amount of urine that can be held is not so great as in the urinary bladder, and the urine liquifies the stool, but some patients learn to regulate themselves so that they can continue with daily activities. This operation is not performed if there is disease of the large bowel, such as diverticulitis, or if the anal sphincter is incompetent since the main advantage, voluntary urinary control, is lost.

If the ureters are to be attached to the bowel, microorganisms in the bowel will be minimized preoperatively with the use of a mechanical bowel preparation with cathartics and enemas and a drug such as kanamycin (Kantrex) or neomycin. The loss of the usual bacterial flora results in a soft, almost odorless stool. The nurse should observe the stool and chart its characteristics. Patients who have ureteral transplants to the bowel are given a low-residue diet both before and after the surgery, to minimize the formation of fecal material that would contaminate the operative area. The patient is placed on a low-residue diet about 3 days before surgery, then clear fluids 24 hours prior to operation.

Postoperatively, a sterile rectal tube is left in place for 5 to 10 days to keep the rectosigmoid empty and decrease the chance of urinary leakage through the anastomosis. Ureteral catheters may be brought out through the anus and anchored to the buttocks for about 10 days. During the first days after surgery note the hourly or two-hourly drainage. Later the rectal tube may be removed when necessary for defecation and reinserted. The stool at first will be liquid, but as the bowel adjusts to being a reservoir, stools become soft. A low-residue diet is usually ordered until the tubes are removed.

Sometimes the patient is taught in the hospital and discharged with instructions to insert a rectal tube each night, anchor it to the skin and attach it to straight drainage if there are problems with the resorption of urinary chloride and resultant hyperchloremic acidosis. The physician may also prescribe oral sodium bicarbonate. To minimize the absorption of waste products, the patient voids (rectally) every 2 to 4 hours. He should report symptoms of electrolyte imbalance such as nausea, vomiting, or lethargy.

The major disadvantage of ureterosigmoidostomy is that infection of the ureters and the kidney pelvis is very frequent. The urinary tract is unprotected from the organisms that normally inhabit the lower bowel. The patient should be taught to establish a regular routine of drinking 2,500 to 3,000 ml. of fluids daily, and to return to his physician on the first indication of pain, fever, or any other sign of infection. Some patients are placed on a small dose of a sulfonamide or an antibiotic and continue taking the drug for months or years in an attempt to prevent an infection of the urinary tract. Patients should tell hospital personnel on readmission that they void rectally. They do not need laxatives, and enemas would force fecal material into the ureters.

Cutaneous Ureterostomy. The ureters are brought to the skin surface. The patient wears one or two rubber collecting cups that drain the urine into a leg bag (an artificial bladder). The patient periodically empties the bag by releasing the stopper at the bottom. This operation is a relatively safe procedure and is often indicated in debilitated and older patients. Stricture of the ureter at the junction with skin or fascia is one complication of the procedure. Leakage and odor problems also can occur. After the cutaneous implantation of ureters, the patient returns from the operating room with splinting catheters inserted into the ureters. These catheters remain in place for at least 10 days. After that, studies are obtained to determine if the ureters will drain freely to the skin.

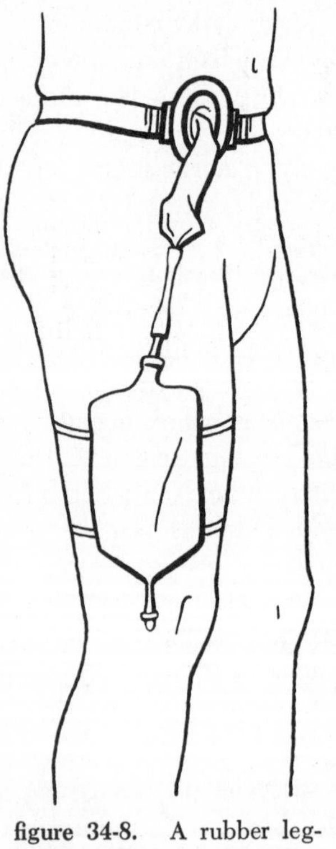

figure 34-8. A rubber leg-urinal collecting the urine draining from a ureter implanted into the skin. The end of the bag can be unplugged periodically during the day to empty the bag.

During surgery the ends of the ureters are everted and attached to the skin in such a way that a circle of mucosal lining is exposed to the air. It is like rolling the end of a tube back on itself. The purpose is to prevent the ureters from closing. These stoma are called ureteral buds. For about 5 days postoperatively, sterile wet saline compresses are kept over the exposed urethral mucosa. Saline can be added hourly with an Asepto syringe. Then the entire dressing is covered with several sterile combines to keep the rest of the patient's body from getting wet and to keep the underneath wet dressing sterile. Zinc oxide, aluminum paste, or petrolatum is used to protect the skin from maceration. The nurse observes for the color of the stoma and any edema that may occlude the opening.

After the catheters are removed, a collecting appliance is placed over the buds, and urine drains through it to a rubber or a plastic bag that can be attached to the leg with straps (Fig. 34-8). Care is taken that the straps are not too tight. The patient visits the bathroom at intervals during the day to release the stopper from the bottom of the bag, emptying it of urine. At night the bag is replaced by a drainage bottle at the side of the bed. The appliance is attached to the skin with bands that go around the patient's body, or with adhesive discs, or with cement. The cup is changed every 3 or 4 days, and while the patient is still in the hospital, he should learn to care for it himself. The skin is washed gently with warm water and bland soap and dried well, for the disc will not stick to wet skin. A sterile cotton ball can be placed over the orifices of the ureters while the cup is being changed, so that the urine will not flow over the skin. Signs of irritation of the skin should be observed. If it appears to be breaking down, exposure to dry heat and more frequent changing of the cup are indicated. The physician should be notified if the skin is becoming irritated. Until the skin becomes accustomed to the cups, tincture of benzoin may be ordered. It should dry on the skin over the area that the disc covers. Tincture of benzoin should not be applied directly to the stoma. To function properly, the disc must fit airtight. The patient may take a bath, since the cement is waterproof. The patient may be taught to dilate the stoma with a sterile catheter.

The cup, the tubing, and the urinal should be washed with soap and water, rinsed well, and allowed to air. Rinsing with a dilute white vinegar solution will help remove encrustations. At home, patients should have two sets, so that one may air while the other is being worn. The urinal should be washed and aired every night while the patient is using a drainage bottle. Referral to a visiting nurse agency is indicated if the patient needs help to care for himself at home.

If urinary drainage stops or if the patient complains of back pain, the physician should be notified immediately since an indwelling ureteral catheter may be necessary. If such catheters are required on a permanent basis (for example, if buds are not formed around the orifies), the patient is taught how to sterilize, irrigate and replace catheters.

Ileal Conduit. In this operation a small segment of ileum is resected from the intestines, with its nerve and blood supply kept intact. The proximal end of the segment is closed and the distal end brought out as a stoma in the lower right quadrant. The ureters are anastomosed to the pouch and drain through it. The ileal loop is no longer connected to the gastrointestinal tract. The term "ileal bladder" is a misnomer, since urine is not stored in the pouch; it only passes through it and out of the body via the stoma. The patient wears an ileostomy bag or special ileal conduit bag over the stoma of the pouch. An infrequent complication of this procedure is electrolyte imbalance.

Following construction of an ileal conduit, the patient may have some degree of paralytic ileus for as long as a week. Return of peristaltic activity in the isolated segment of conduit parallels that of the intestinal tract which was reanastomosed. For this reason, some surgeons will insert a multieyed catheter into the stoma at operation and it is not removed for 5 to 7 days. However, the catheter lumen readily becomes obstructed by intestinal mucus and may require frequent irrigations. An alternate approach is the application of a temporary clear plastic ostomy appliance connected to straight drainage. This has the advantage of less likelihood of urinary soilage of the surgical incision and the condition of the stoma can be observed through the plastic. The physician may decide to insert a catheter into the conduit at times to check for residual urine (normally the conduit is nearly empty since it does not have a reservoir function) or to provide for continued drainage should there be a leakage at one of the internal anastomoses.

Because the patient has also had an intestinal anastomosis, he will have a gastric tube in place for several days postoperatively to prevent distention and pressure on the suture line. The nurse observes for and reports promptly any symptoms of peritonitis (abdominal tenderness, fever, severe pain, distention) since the intestinal anastomosis can leak fecal material or the ileal conduit may leak urine into the peritoneal cavity. She also observes for any signs of distention of the conduit with urine, because this puts pressure on the suture line or back pressure on the kidneys, and promptly reports pain in the lower abdomen or decreased urinary output.

The mucosa of the ileum produces mucus, which may plug the orifice and prevent the drainage of urine. The mucus may be removed with sterile gauze. The physician may dilate the stoma daily during the early postoperative period. Until the patient is able to do it for himself, the nurse frequently checks the bag to see that the urine is draining adequately, empties it before it becomes full, and changes the temporary plastic ileostomy bag as needed. Each time the patient's position is changed, the nurse, and then the patient, check to make sure that the drainage system is not impeded in any way.

Additional Nursing Points. Nursing management of a patient with ureteral transplants is similar to that of a patient with a colostomy or an ileostomy. For example, in both instances the skin needs protection, the dressings should be changed promptly when they become soiled, the appliances need care and cleanliness, and the patient needs a nurse who can encourage the patient by her matter-of-factness and skill as she changes the dressing. But there are also differences. The drainage from a ureteral transplant is more liquid; hence, it is more difficult to manage. Infection is more prone to occur. This different way of voiding may be difficult for the patient. In the hospital, if he is on a urologic unit, he will see others who use the same method. However, the patient may worry about how he will get along outside the hospital. His own acceptance of the urinary diversion, the equipment, and its care can be helped by giving him the responsibility for it in the early postoperative period.

Early ambulation (taking the necessary equipment with him) demonstrates to the patient that he nevertheless can move about, and is not chained to a collecting apparatus at his bedside. If the patient wishes, he should be allowed to discuss his fears and misgivings about the surgery and its effect. By her manner and in discussion with him, the nurse shows the patient that she has confidence in his ability to handle the situation.

Preoperative explanation to the patient, the nurse's familiarity with various collection appliances, and an introduction to other patients who have successfully undergone urinary diversion will do much to allay the patient's fear. During the postoperative period, the patient is measured for his permanent appliance. Then he is thoroughly instructed, along with another member of his family, in its application, cleaning, and care. Teaching is continued until the patient can leave the hospital, confident in his ability to manage his own care alone or with the help of family members or the public health nurse.

Written instructions for the patient and family are helpful for home review. Anxiety in the hospital or on arrival at home may lead to memory gaps or misunderstanding.

Infection

A focus of infection elsewhere in the body—for example, a boil or an inflamed throat—may spread to the urinary tract, particularly the kidney, through the bloodstream or the lymphatics. An infection in the kidney can spread to the tissues of the rest of the urinary tract. An ascending infection (one that starts in the urethra and moves up) is caused commonly by *Escherichia coli.* In men the infection may extend to the tissue of the prostate, the seminal vesicles or the epididymis. The presence of foreign bodies, such as stones and catheters, predisposes to infection. The danger of introducing bacteria with a catheter or with irrigating solution is so great that only the strictest aseptic equipment and technique should be used.

When an indwelling catheter is necessary for a long period, it should be changed periodically, using sterile technique. In some hospitals it is the policy to change indwelling catheters once a week. Patients who have urinary procedures, such as dilatations, have samples of their urine tested at intervals for evidence of infection.

The treatment of all urinary tract infections includes surgical drainage of pus; identification and removal (when possible) of contributing factors, such as coexisting stones, obstructions or tumors; increasing the fluid intake (up to 1.5- to 2-liters of urine a day); and administering appropriate measures, such as antibiotics, to combat infection.

Tuberculosis

Since the advent of drug therapy, tubercular infections of the urinary tract are less common than they used to be. Tuberculosis of the urinary tract usually occurs secondarily to lesions in the lungs. The upper pole of the kidney is usually first involved, and the disease may eventually involve the ureters, bladder, prostate, and scrotal contents. A triple combination of the drugs isoniazid hydrazide (INH), para-aminosalicylic acid (PAS), and one other antitubercular agent such as cycloserine for at least 2 years is one mode of treatment.

If the renal tuberculosis does not respond to drug therapy and is unilateral, nephrectomy may be done. Rest in a hospital or at home is part of the treatment. While the pulmonary lesion may be no longer active, in the early stage of treatment the urine will contain the tubercle bacillus. Patients and nurses should wash their hands after contact with the urine; dressings soiled with it should be wrapped in protective coverings and burned, and soiled linen should be treated as contaminated.

Acute pyelonephritis

Pyelonephritis means infection of the renal parenchyma as well as the lining of the collecting system. In the acute form the patient is clinically quite ill. He experiences pain in the kidney, chills, fever, malaise, and nausea. The urinalysis will show pyuria. Frequency and burning on urination may be present if the bladder is also infected. It is often associated with pregnancy and with diabetes.

The patient is placed on bed rest, and liberal fluid intake to keep the urine dilute is urged. These patients are very sick and require attention to skin and mouth care, turning, and encouragement to eat. Every effort is expended to prevent both septicemia and the development of chronic pyelonephritis. When there are no complications, the prognosis for complete cure with adequate antibacterial therapy is excellent.

Chronic pyelonephritis

If the treatment of acute pyelonephritis is not permanently successful (for instance, if the infection is recurrent, or if urinary stasis continues due to an obstruction), the disease may enter a chronic stage. The kidney shows irreversible degenerative changes. It becomes small and atrophic, and the pelvic mucosa becomes pale and fibrotic. Many nephrons are destroyed. If enough nephrons become inoperative, the patient will develop uremia.

Although chronic pyelonephritis may be asymptomatic, the patient can have a low-grade fever, vague gastrointestinal complaints, and anemia. There may be acute attacks; some of the patients will develop hypertension due to renal ischemia. Sometimes stones form in the affected kidney.

Nothing known today can restore scarred kidney tissue. The aim of the treatment is to prevent further damage. Intensive therapy with antibiotics or chemotherapeutic agents is given. Any obstruction is relieved. An effort is made to improve the patient's overall health. A nephrectomy may be done if severe hypertension develops, and if the other kidney can support life. The fight against chronic pyelonephritis is a long one. Prolonged medication and constant attention to general health habits may be a dull and discouraging routine for patients.

In selected patients with chronic pyelonephritis the transplantation of a normal kidney to replace the diseased one offers a new lease on life.

Cystitis

Cystitis is inflammation of the urinary bladder. The contents of the bladder are normally sterile. Bacteria reach the bladder by way of infected kidneys, lymphatics and the urethra. Because the urethra is short in women, ascending infections are more common in women than men. Cystitis is prevented from being even more common than it is by a natural resistance of the bladder lining, which helps to prevent an inflammatory process from taking hold from the occasional invasion of the bladder by bacteria. This resistance cannot be relied on to counter the effects of the introduction of an unsterile catheter into the sterile environment of the bladder.

The symptoms include urgency (feeling a pressing need to void although the bladder is not full), frequency, dysuria (painful urination), perineal and suprapubic pain, and hematuria, especially at the termination of the stream (terminal hematuria). If bacteremia is present, the patient also may have chills and fever. Chronic cystitis causes similar symptoms, but usually they are less severe.

The diagnosis is made by the patient's history, the total physical examination, and urinalysis, including culture and sensitivity of the offending organisms to antibiotics or chemotherapeutic agents.

Medical care includes the location and the correction of contributing factors. If there is a partial obstruction, no cure of cystitis will be fully effective until adequate drainage of urine is restored by the removal of the obstruction. Treatment often is prolonged, and it may necessitate many return visits to the physician after the patient has been discharged from the hospital. For example, dilatation of a contracted bladder with normal saline instillations must be repeated many times.

If the patient has a fever or other systemic symptoms of infection, he may be put on bed rest. Even though he has urgency and frequency, he needs a great deal of encouragement to take large quantities of fluids. Warm sitz baths may provide some relief. Cranberry juice may be offered to the patient. This acidifies the urine and provides a less favorable climate for bacterial growth. The alert nurse finds out the patient's fluid preferences and provides for these so that the goal of a liberal fluid intake can be more readily met.

Urethritis

Inflammation of the urethra caused by organisms other than gonorrhea is called *nonspecific urethritis* (NSU). Urethritis also may be secondary to trichomonal and monilial infections in women.

The distal portion of the normal male urethra is not totally sterile. However, bacteria normally present there cause no difficulty unless these tissues are traumatized, usually following instrumentation such as catheterization or cystoscopic examination. Under such conditions, bacteria may gain a foothold to cause a nonspecific urethritis. The urethral mucosa becomes inflamed and pus forms in the tiny mucus-forming glands lining the urethra. Other causes for nonspecific urethritis include irritation during vigorous intercourse.

Gonorrhea, on the other hand, is a specific form of infection which can attack the mucous membrane of a normal urethra. Usually within 2 or 3 days after contact, the patient will notice a thick purulent discharge from the meatus.

The symptoms of infection of the urethra are discomfort on urination varying from a slight tickling sensation to burning or severe discomfort, and urinary frequency. Fever is not common and its appearance in the male implies further extension of the infection to such areas as the prostate, testes and epididymi. Treatment includes appropriate antibiotics, a liberal fluid intake, analgesics, warm sitz baths and improvement of the patient's resistance to infection by a good diet and plenty of rest.

The nurse should be gentle when catheterizing patients, so that the delicate wall of the urethra is not injured. The importance of avoiding the introduction of microorganisms with the catheter cannot be overemphasized. The patient is encouraged to drink copiously after all urethral procedures to flush out the lower urinary tract.

The periurethral area of any patient who cannot be placed in a tub should be washed daily with soap, water, and a clean washcloth. This should be done by the nurse for the patients who cannot wash themselves. Urethritis is commonly caused by irritation from indwelling catheters. If a patient has an indwelling catheter, the area should be washed more frequently, especially if the patient is incontinent of feces. It is not sufficient to wash only around anus and buttocks. Avoid wiping toward the urethra. If cotton pledgets are used, wipe from the urethral meatus to the anus in a single stroke and discard the pledget.

Nephritis (Bright's disease)

The term *nephritis* refers to a group of noninfectious diseases characterized by widespread kidney damage.

Acute glomerulonephritis

Etiology. Glomerulonephritis is a type of nephritis characterized by inflammation of the glomeruli. It has been repeatedly observed that the symptoms of acute glomerulonephritis appear approximately 2 weeks after an upper respiratory infection, usually one that has been caused by hemolytic streptococci. Recent influenza, scarlet fever, or chickenpox also may be given in the history. The exact relationship between the respiratory infection and the nephritis is not clearly understood. The organisms are not present in the kidney when the symptoms of nephritis appear. The disease may represent an altered tissue reaction to infection, a result of host response rather than damage from infection.

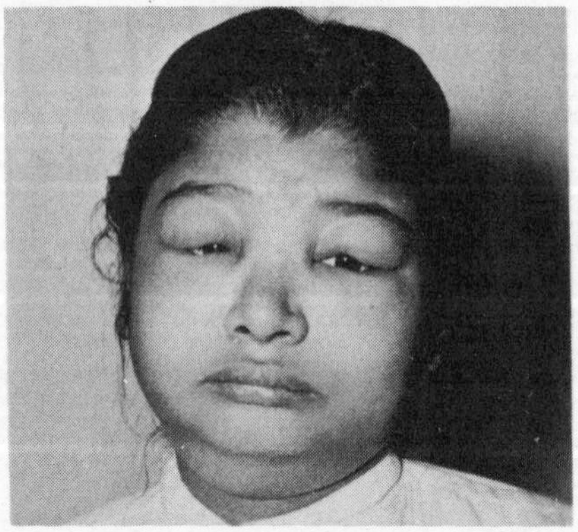

figure 34-9. This patient has acute nephritis. (Vakil, R. J., and Golwalla, A.: *Clinical Diagnosis*, Bombay, Asia Pub. House)

Acute glomerulonephritis occurs most frequently in children and young adults.

Symptoms. Early symptoms may be so slight that the patient does not seek medical attention, though occasionally the onset is sudden, with generalized edema (anasarca), fever, vomiting, anuria, hypertension, and dyspnea. There may be cerebral and cardiac involvement. Most patients survive the disease without sequelae, but death from uremia may follow delirium or convulsions, or the patient may die in congestive heart failure.

More often, the patient or his family notices that his face is pale and puffy (Fig. 34-9), and that he has slight ankle edema in the evening. His appetite is poor, and he is up frequently during the night to void (nocturia). He awakens with a headache (due to hypertension). His family and friends find him irritable, and he is out of breath after exertion. The patient may have only one symptom, such as a pitting, dependent edema. Visual disturbances, often due to papilledema or hemorrhage, are common. Nosebleeds may occur. As the condition progresses, he may develop hematuria, anemia, convulsions associated with hypertension, congestive heart failure, oliguria and perhaps anuria.

The laboratory findings may include a slightly elevated blood urea nitrogen and albuminuria. There will be gross or microscopic hematuria, giving the urine a dark, smoky or frankly bloody appearance.

Treatment. There is no specific treatment for acute glomerulonephritis. The therapy is guided by the symptoms and their underlying pathology. The following regimen is usual:

- Bed rest. While the blood pressure is elevated, and edema is present, bed rest may continue for several weeks. When progressive ambulation is slowly started, daily urine specimens are usually collected, and blood pressure is taken daily. Any increase in hematuria, albuminuria or blood pressure is an indication for a return to bed rest.
- Hydration. Fluids should be taken liberally. Since there is damage to the glomeruli, there is a filtration problem. To get rid of waste

products, the body needs ample fluids. However, fluids are limited to balance output in the presence of marked edema, oliguria or anuria.

- Diet. Sodium is restricted when edema is present. Carbohydrate intake is encouraged, especially when proteins are limited. Vitamins may be added to the diet to improve the patient's general resistance. Iron may be needed to counteract anemia.
- Medication. Antibiotics may be given to prevent a superimposed infection on the already inflamed kidney.

In the seriously ill patient a trial of corticosteroids may be given to attempt to alter the course of the disease. When the blood pressure climbs to high levels, antihypertensive drugs are usually given.

The patient is not considered to be cured until his urine is free of albumin and red blood cells for 6 months. Return to full activity usually is not permitted until the urine is free of protein for a month.

PROGNOSIS. Most patients with acute glomerulonephritis recover, usually completely. A few develop chronic glomerulonephritis. Subsequent infections with the same strain of hemolytic streptococci usually do not cause a second attack of acute glomerulonephritis. This is in sharp contrast with chronic glomerulonephritis, in which upper respiratory infections must be studiously avoided to prevent exacerbations of the disease.

CHRONIC GLOMERULONEPHRITIS

Chronic glomerulonephritis causes irremediable damage to the nephrons. Some disappear entirely. Bands of scar tissue contract the kidney and replace the functioning units. The cortex becomes distorted and shrunken.

SYMPTOMS. A small number of patients with chronic glomerulonephritis are known to have had acute glomerulonephritis, but most give no such history. The symptoms are similar to those of acute glomerulonephritis, but they may be even more individualized. There may be generalized edema, headache and hypertension, visual disturbances, nocturia, dyspnea, and albuminuria. Anemia, cardiac failure, and cerebral symptoms are not uncommon. The patient who develops anasarca (generalized edema) is said to be in the *nephrotic* stage. The generalized edema is due to the depletion of serum proteins, with loss of plasma osmotic pressure. These patients may remain markedly edematous for months or years. Quiescent periods occur between exacerbations. During this *latent stage* the patient is relatively free of symptoms and feels well, although his urine contains protein.

The course of the disease is highly variable. The patient may live for years, with only occasional acute episodes or none at all; or the disease may be rapidly fatal due to uremia.

COMPLICATIONS. Congestive heart failure, pulmonary edema, increased blood pressure that may lead to cerebral hemorrhage, and secondary infection are common and sometimes fatal complications. Blurring of vision and blindness may occur late in the disease. Anemia is usual. Increased capillary fragility causes nosebleeds, purpura, and gastrointestinal bleeding in many terminally ill patients. Bronchopneumonia is a serious danger in the nephrotic stage. High blood pressure over a period of months or years may lead to further renal insufficiency. (*Nephrosclerosis* is the term given to kidney disease caused by hypertension in its malignant phase. The resulting symptoms are those of chronic glomerulonephritis.)

TREATMENT. No treatment is given during the quiescent stages. Nurses are in a position to assist patients and their families to maintain a healthful regimen for the patient. Everything that can be done should be done to increase his resistance to infection, since even a mild infection may precipitate uremia. He should rest well and eat well and see his physician regularly. If the patient develops an infection, prompt medical treatment is imperative. Kidney function tests may be done annually. Death from uremia is the usual outcome of chronic glomerulonephritis, but it may be delayed for years with a regimen of healthful living.

When the disease becomes active, often evidenced initially by hematuria and edema, the patient is put to bed. Dietary considerations include low-sodium intake and regulation of protein intake. Mild analgesics may be given for headaches, hypertension, insomnia, and irritability. Diuretics containing mercury usually are not given, because they may increase the damage to the kidneys. Intravenous hypertonic solutions may be given to reduce intracranial pressure. If the patient has congestive heart failure, treatment of that condition, with such measures as digitalis, is necessary. Anemia, if it is severe, is treated with transfusions. The symptoms often subside in about 3 weeks, and very gradually the patient may return to normal activity. Because the restitution of renal function lags behind the patient's clinical improvement, his convalescence should be planned carefully to avoid intercurrent infection, marked exertion and the body stress that may, in turn, affect renal function.

The treatment in the nephrotic stage includes bed rest to decrease the work of the heart, diuretics, and regulation of the diet, including sodium and fluid restriction. During this phase the patient is especially prone to intercurrent infection, and he may die of bronchopneumonia. The patient needs to be protected against infection that is carried to him on the hands or in the throats of hospital personnel and visitors.

Nephrosis (the nephrotic syndrome)

The term *nephrosis* means a degenerative, noninflammatory disease of the renal tubules. The nephrotic syndrome is characterized by edema, albuminuria, decreased plasma proteins, and an increase of blood lipid and cholesterol. There may be degenerative and necrotic lesions of the distal tubules, and renal vasoconstriction. The decrease in blood flow to the kidneys may lead to anuria and uremia. If the damage has not been too severe, and the circulation has not been too greatly impaired, the tubules are capable of regeneration.

The aim of the treatment is to keep the patient alive until his kidneys repair themselves. When the administration of corticosteroids is effective, there is diuresis and lowering or cessation of the loss of protein in the urine. If the patient is not prostrated by the disease he is often treated at home. Bed rest may not be necessary, but he should engage only in moderate activity during the acute phase, and eat a high protein diet to replace the protein lost in the urine. Because of the edema, the diet probably will also be low in sodium content. In the hospital, if intravenous fluids are given (to supply electrolytes), special care must be taken to regulate the rate of the intravenous drip as it was ordered and to watch for signs of pulmonary edema. It is important to keep an account of the patient's weight; he may be retaining fluid.

The disease tends to be even more serious in adults than in children. Death may occur from renal failure, hypertension or intercurrent infection when the patient is on corticosteroid therapy. If the kidneys do not seem to be recovering, and death from uremia is impending, dialysis may be performed to give the kidneys more time to heal.

Other urinary tract conditions

Trauma

From the back and the sides, the urinary tract is encircled by the ribs, the spinal column and the pelvic girdle. Fracture of any of these bones should alert the nurse to watch for signs of damage to kidneys, ureters, or bladder. Any trauma to the lower portion of the body, such as a fall, automobile accident or a gunshot wound, may tear a portion of the urinary tract. The symptoms may not be immediately apparent while the more obvious wounds are being cared for. All patients with trauma to the area should be observed for anuria; perhaps the ureters are cut through, or the bladder may be ruptured. They should also be observed for symptoms of peritonitis; urine is a foreign substance in the abdominal cavity. Each urine specimen should be checked for gross or increasing hematuria. A sample can be left in a test tube for continuing comparison.

Polycystic disease of the kidney

This disease is a congenital familial disorder. It is characterized by multiple, bilateral kidney cysts and may not be diagnosed until middle life. As the cysts slowly enlarge, they squeeze the functioning parenchyma between them. The kidneys may become enormous and exert pressure on nearby abdominal and pelvic organs. Nephritis, calculi, infections, and hydronephrosis may result from and complicate the condition. The patient may have hematuria, pain, pyuria, anemia, and gastrointestinal symptoms from pressure caused by the expanding kidney. The patient usually is hypertensive. The treatment is the same as that for nephritis. Emergency surgery is required sometimes for hemorrhage. However, there is no cure for polycystic disease, and eventually uremia develops. Because the disease is bilateral, the prognosis is poor.

General nutritional considerations

- Fluid intake may be increased or decreased in patients with urologic disease or problems. When intake must be increased, the nurse should see that (1) the patient has a sufficient supply of fresh water at his bedside, (2) the patient is encouraged to drink extra fluids, (3) the patient understands *why* he must increase his fluid intake, (4) extra fluids are added to his meal trays.
- Offering *small* but *frequent* amounts of fluid often is easier to tolerate than a large amount of fluid consumed at one time.
- Kidney stone recurrence may be treated with diet. Calcium stones are treated with a diet low in calcium and phosphorus. Uric acid

stones may be treated with a low-purine diet and alkalinization of the urine.

- Foods generally avoided on a low calcium-low phosphorus diet are milk, cheese, liver, soybeans, whole grain breads and cereals, carbonated beverages. Foods generally avoided on a low-purine diet are liver, kidney, meat extracts, and sweetbreads (animal pancreas). Sea food, lentils, meat, poultry, dry peas, and beans are allowed in limited amounts.
- Cranberry juice to acidify the urine is often ordered for the patient with cystitis.
- Patients with acute and chronic glomerulonephritis may require a low-sodium diet in an attempt to control edema. Protein intake may be limited in patients with either acute or chronic glomerulonephritis in which case carbohydrates are encouraged. As these patients are often anorexic and the diet usually bland tasting (due to lack of sodium or salt), the dietary intake may be low.

General pharmacological considerations

- Patients scheduled for intravenous or retrograde pyelography or arteriography should have an allergy history because the contrast media used in these studies contain iodine. The physician may first inject a small amount of the dye and wait before giving the remainder to be sure the patient does not have a reaction to the dye. All patients having these studies should be observed for signs of iodine sensitivity: tachycardia, restlessness, cardiovascular collapse.
- Sodium bicarbonate (baking soda), usually in tablet form, may be used to alkalinize the urine in patients with kidney stones in an attempt to prevent stone recurrence.
- Patients scheduled for ureterosigmoidostomy will have the bowel prepared for surgery by the administration of an antibiotic, such as neomycin, to reduce the number of microorganisms in the large bowel. This reduces the chance of postoperative urinary tract and abdominal infection.
- Antibiotics and sulfonamides are drugs commonly used in treating urinary tract infections. Other drugs used are furan derivatives—nitrofurantoin microcrystals (Macrodantin) and nitrofurantoin (Furadantin), acids—methenamine mandelate (Mandelamine) and nalidixic acid (NegGram). An azo dye—phenazopyridine (Pyridium) may be ordered for its soothing effect on bladder mucosa and is often used in conjunction with urinary antibiotics.
- Other drugs used in kidney disease may include corticosteroids to control the inflammatory process of acute glomerulonephritis and diuretics to reduce edema in acute and chronic glomerulonephritis.
- Patients receiving drugs for urinary tract infections should be instructed to finish the course of therapy even though they may feel improved and be symptom-free after several days of therapy. A *completed* course of therapy is essential to be sure the infection is under control.
- Patients must be advised to follow the instructions of their physician regarding the medication(s) and any instructions specific to that medication, such as drinking excess fluids.

Bibliography

BEAUMONT, E.: Urinary drainage systems. Nurs. '74, 4:52, January, 1974.

CLARK, C.: Catheter care in the home. Am. J. Nurs. 72:922, May, 1972.

FENNEL, S. E.: Percutaneous renal biopsy. Am. J. Nurs. 75:1292, August, 1975.

FRYE, C.: Toxic nephropathy. Canad. Nurse 68:45, June, 1972.

HEKELMAN, F. P., et al: Symposium on care of the patient with renal disease. Nursing approaches to conservative management of renal disease. Nurs. Clin. North Am. 10:431, September, 1975.

KEUHNELIAN, J. G. and SAUNDERS, V. E.: *Urologic Nursing.* New York, Macmillan, 1970.

LUCKMAN, J. and SORENSEN, K. C.: *Medical-Surgical Nursing: A Pathophysiological Approach.* Philadelphia, Saunders, 1974.

MERCHANT, F.: Pyelolithotomy (care st). Nurs. Mirror 134:36, March 24, 1972.

PRILOOK, M. E.: Renal failure: what to do when the kidneys shut down. Patient Care 5:40, December 15, 1971.

RHOADS, J. E., et al: *Surgery: Principles and Practice,* ed. 4. Philadelphia, Lippincott, 1970.

SMITH, D. R.: *General Urology,* ed. 6. Los Altos, Lange, 1970.

TILKIAN, S. M. and CONOVER, M. H.: *Clinical Implications of Laboratory Tests.* St. Louis, Mosby, 1975.

WALLACH, J.: *Interpretation of Diagnostic Tests,* ed. 2. Boston, Little, Brown, 1974.

WHITEHEAD, S. L.: *Nursing Care of the Adult Urology Patient.* New York, Appleton-Century-Crofts, 1970.

WINTER, C. and BARKER, M. R.: *Nursing Care of Patients with Urologic Diseases,* ed. 3. St. Louis, Mosby, 1972.

UNIT EIGHT

Problems resulting from endocrine imbalance

- The patient with an endocrine disorder
- The patient with diabetes mellitus

CHAPTER—35

The patient with an endocrine disorder

On completion of this chapter the student will:

- **Locate and name the glands of the endocrine system.**
- **Give the etiology, symptoms, and treatment of hyperthyroidism.**
- **Describe the diagnostic tests of thyroid function.**
- **Formulate a nursing care plan for and participate in the pre- and postoperative nursing management of the patient with a thyroidectomy.**
- **Discuss the treatment and prevention of nontoxic goiter.**
- **Discuss the medical and surgical management of cancer of the thyroid.**
- **Give the etiology, symptoms, and treatment of hypothyroidism.**
- **Give the etiology, symptoms, treatment, and general nursing management of the patient with hypo- and hyperparathyroidism.**
- **Name the hormones of the adrenal gland and list the general functions of this gland and its hormones.**
- **Describe the etiology, symptoms, and treatment of Addison's disease and Cushing's syndrome.**
- **Formulate a nursing care plan for and participate in the nursing management of the patient with Addison's disease or Cushing's syndrome.**
- **Discuss the etiology and treatment of acromegaly and diabetes insipidus.**

The consequences of diseases of the ductless glands (Fig. 35-1) are usually due to overproduction or underproduction of the hormones that the glands secrete, causing a disturbance in the delicate balance that the hormones normally maintain, and often resulting in a widespread chain of pathological events within the body. Normally, many of the ductless glands respond to stimulation from the pituitary. If the glandular production is increased, the pituitary-stimulating factor is decreased as a counter-regulatory mechanism. This slows down the gland's activity. For example, an increase in the production of the thyroid hormones results in a decrease in the amount of the thyroid-stimulating hormone (thyrotropin or TSH) produced by the pituitary gland. Conversely, a decrease in the gland's output is countered by increased pituitary stimulation. In endocrine-disease states this relationship between the pituitary and a target gland may be lost.

The thyroid gland

This gland has the ability to concentrate iodine in the manufacture of thyroid hormones, which help to regulate the production and use of energy for the body's dynamic processes. The important active hormones that the thyroid gland releases are tetraiodothyronine (thyroxine or T_4) and triiodothyronine (T_3). Iodine is contained in these hormones.

Hyperthyroidism

In hyperthyroidism (also called Graves' disease, thyrotoxicosis, and exophthalmic goiter) the patient's metabolic rate is increased, due to an excessive secretion of thyroid hormones.

Etiology. The etiology is unknown. Apparently, any condition which demands that the thyroid produce a large amount of thyroid hormone can precipitate hyperthyroidism: emotional or physical stress, infection, adolescence, pregnancy. Women are afflicted more frequently than men.

Symptoms. Patients with well-developed hyperthyroidism are characteristically restless, highly excitable, and constantly agitated. They are emotionally labile, laughing one minute and crying the next. Often, they overreact to situations; they are incapable of resting. They may have fine tremors of the hands. Clumsiness, due to tremors, may cause them to drop things. Muscular weakness and fatigability are com-

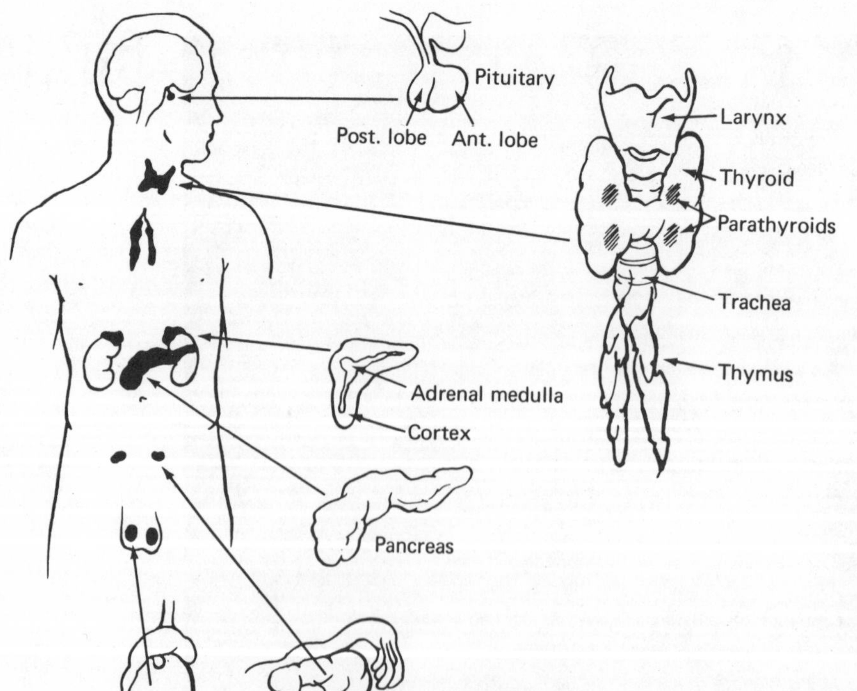

figure 35-1. Location of hormone-producing glands in the body.

mon. The pulse may be as high as 160. Characteristically, there is an increase in the systolic but not in the diastolic blood pressure. Patients may experience palpitations, and, if the condition is untreated, the continued excess activity may lead to cardiac decompensation.

The constant exercise and the high rate of metabolism cause the patient to lose weight, even though his appetite is usually great, and he consumes extra calories. It is important to satisfy the need for food of the patient with a severely overactive thyroid, and even the patient with less severe thyrotoxicosis should eat a high caloric, high carbohydrate diet.

The increased metabolic rate makes the patient intolerant of heat. This symptom can be troublesome, because in the hospital ventilation that is comfortable for the patient with Graves' disease chills the other patients.

Some patients with hyperthyroidism exhibit bulging eyes (*exophthalmos*) which give them a permanently startled expression (Fig. 35-2). Usually, there is a visible swelling of the neck due to the enlarged thyroid gland.

Other symptoms of thyrotoxicosis include characteristically fine and flushed skin, menstrual abnormalities, changed bowel habits, and excessive sweating. There may be hoarseness and difficulty in swallowing, due to the enlargement of the gland.

Diagnostic Tests. The following tests aid in the clinical diagnosis of hyperthyroidism:

Basal Metabolic Rate (BMR). This test determines the rate at which an individual consumes oxygen under standard resting conditions. The patient's temperature must be normal, since each increase in degree of body temperature increases the body's metabolic rate. Digestion and muscular activity also increase the body's consumption of oxygen, and so for this test the patient must have fasted for 8 to 10 hours, and he must have been lying quietly in bed in as near a state of complete rest as possible. Minus 11 to plus 11 is within normal limits. The BMR is not as accurate as some other diagnostic tests and is being used less often today.

The nursing management of a patient who is to receive a BMR test involves obtaining and maintaining basal conditions. The need for rest and quiet should be explained (even mild excitement or slight muscular exertion can result in large errors in the test results). If the patient knows what to expect, he will be able to help.

The morning of the test, the patient's room is kept dark or the curtains are pulled around his bed until the time of the test. The patient may be allowed to go to the bathroom, but he should return immediately to bed and rest. Or a drink of water, a bedpan, and equipment to wash his hands and face and brush his teeth may be brought to the bedside, if these measures will make him feel more comfortable and relaxed. Smoking is not permitted. If the test is not done at the bedside, the patient is transported in a wheelchair.

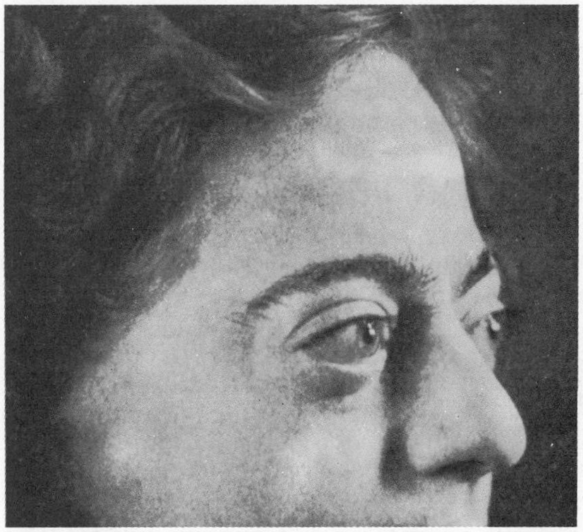

figure 35-2. Exophthalmos in Graves' disease. (Cecil, R. L. and Loeb, R. F. (eds.): *A Textbook of Medicine,* ed. 5. Philadelphia, Saunders)

Protein-bound Iodine (PBI). Triiodothyronine and tetraiodothyronine are bound to the blood proteins that transport them. Because iodine is contained in the hormones, measurement of the protein-bound iodine in a blood sample reflects the level of circulating thyroid hormone. Although the patient may be active and eat before blood is drawn for these tests, he should not have ingested any unusual amounts of iodine for several weeks beforehand. Substances containing iodine, such as some cough medicines and dyes administered for x-ray studies of the gallbladder, intravenous pyelograms, and bronchograms, will cause errors. Even antiseptic solutions of iodine on the skin should be avoided.

The normal concentration of protein-bound iodine varies with the laboratory method used, but it is usually 4 to 8 μg. per 100 ml. of plasma. Values below and above these figures usually indicate hypothyroidism and hyperthyroidism, respectively.

Serum T_3 and T_4 Determination. Serum triiodothyronine (T_3) determination and serum thyroxine (T_4) determination, also called T_4 (D) or T_4 by displacement, measure the two thyroid hormones without contamination by substances containing iodine.

Radioactive Iodine Uptake Test. The fasting patient is given sodium ^{131}radio-iodide either as a drink or in capsule form. Diluted in distilled water, the drug is odorless and tasteless. Then, 24 hours later, a *scintillator* (an instrument that measures radioactivity) is held over the thyroid gland to measure the amount of ^{131}iodine that the thyroid has taken up. The normal thyroid will remove 15 to 50 percent of the radioactive iodine from the bloodstream. The thyroid gland of a patient with hyperthyroidism may remove as much as 90 percent.

Thyroid Scanning. The patient ingests sodium ^{131}radio-iodide. Then a scintillator (Fig. 35-3) is passed back and forth across the throat, and a picture of radioactivity is recorded. The pattern of the scan indicates the concentration of the iodine in the thyroid and other tissues and helps the physician to differentiate between noncancerous and malignant tissue of the thyroid when this test is used with other clinical findings.

^{131}I Urine Excretion Test. This test measures the amount of ^{131}I excreted in 24 or 48 hours. Normally, 40 to 80 percent is excreted, but a patient with hyperthyroidism excretes less than 40 percent of the amount ingested. The nurse should be careful to save all the urine specimens during the test period; none should be discarded. The dose is not large enough to warrant isolation precautions for radioactivity. If the patient appears worried, he can be told that the amount of radiation in the tracer dose is minute and harmless.

Blood Cholesterol. In this diagnostic test, 5 cc. of blood are taken from the fasting patient. The normal values are 150 to 250 mg. per 100 cc. of blood. In hyperthyroidism, the patient's blood cholesterol is often lower than normal, but the results of this test vary greatly. The serum cholesterol is elevated in myxedema and can be followed during treatment of this condition.

TREATMENT AND NURSING MANAGEMENT. The treatment for hyperthyroidism may be medical or surgical. The nurse has important responsibilities in both kinds of therapy.

Antithyroid Drugs. These agents block the production of thyroid hormone. Propylthiouracil, methimazole, or another drug of the thiouracil group may be given as medical treatment of hyperthyroidism or as preparation for surgery. The effects of the drug do not become evident until the excess thyroid hormone stored in the thyroid gland has been secreted into the bloodstream. This process may take several weeks.

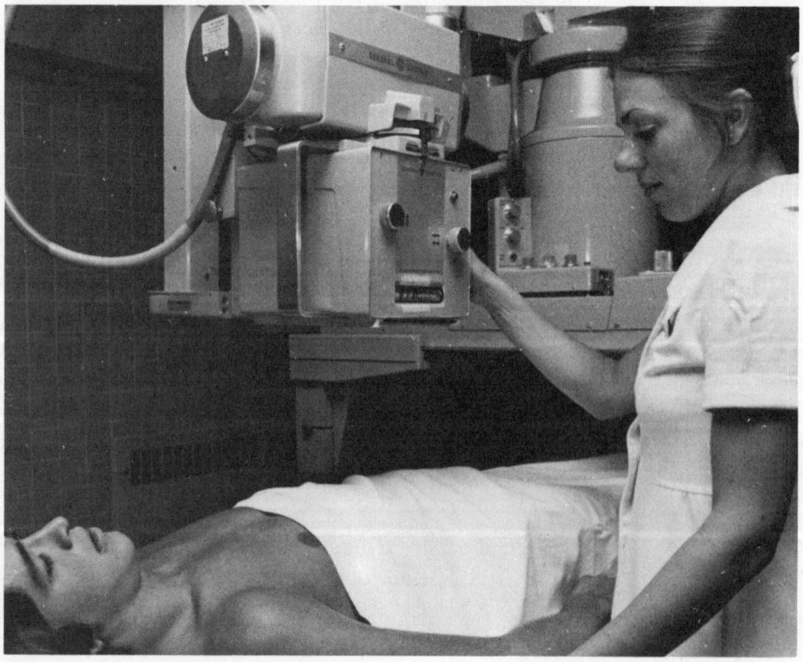

figure 35-3. A patient having a thyroid scan after ingesting ^{131}radio-iodide. The test is not painful. (Photograph—D. Atkinson)

The nurse should instruct the patient to follow the physician's directions about the number of tablets to take and the intervals at which the drug should be taken. The patient who is treated without surgery usually takes the antithyroid drug for at least a year, and during that time must see his physician frequently.

Radioactive iodine (^{131}I) may be given to a patient with thyrotoxicosis to destroy the hyperplastic thyroid tissue by radiation. Because the thyroid gland is quick to pick up iodine from the bloodstream, the radioactive iodine is taken up and stored in that gland, and for this reason it is currently believed that the usual therapeutic dose does not seriously affect any other tissues of the body. No increase in the incidence of leukemia, cancer of the thyroid, or fetal abnormalities has been noted after the use of radioactive iodine in adults. However, as a precautionary measure, young patients and pregnant women are usually treated with surgery or antithyroid drugs. The dosage of radioactive iodine is based on the estimated weight of the thyroid gland, the patient's age, his clinical symptoms, and the emanations from the gland as shown on a scintillator or Geiger counter. The drug is given once, and the patient is watched for several months. If there is no remission of symptoms, a second dose may be given, and perhaps a third. The internal irradiation allows a dose to be given without endangering the skin. There may be transient symptoms of radiation sickness (nausea, vomiting, malaise, fever), and the gland may feel tender. These reactions are rare. A more common unfortunate sequela of radioactive iodine is hypothyroidism (discussed later in this chapter). It has been reported that as many as 43 percent of patients treated with ^{131}I develop hypothyroidism when they are followed for longer than 10 years. Because this complication may not occur until long after the administration of ^{131}I, patients must remain under medical supervision for many years.

In about 6 to 8 weeks after the initial dose of ^{131}I, the patient often notices the beginning of remission of symptoms. The length of time required before the patient notices improvement is one of the disadvantages of this treatment. The patient should be instructed to avoid strenuous activity and to eat a nutritious diet.

^{131}I emits gamma and beta rays. Even though gamma rays penetrate tissue (beta rays travel only a few millimeters) the dose administered in the treatment of hyperthyroidism is not large enough to constitute a radiation hazard to others. The patient may be worried about this and also about the effects in his body. The nurse can supplement the physician's teaching and assure the patient that the medication is not a radiation danger.

A third antithyroid drug, Lugol's solution, contains 5 percent iodine and 10 percent potassium iodide in water. Iodine causes the gland to involute and become less vascular. To decrease bleeding during surgery, patients who are scheduled for a thyroidectomy will often have a short course of iodine treatment for at least two weeks before surgery. The drug is diluted in milk or fruit juice to prevent burning from the iodine and to make it more palatable. Drinking it through a straw will prevent staining of the teeth by the iodine. The maximum effect is expected in 10 to 14 days.

Surgery of the Thyroid. Subtotal thyroidectomy is an effective treatment for hyperthyroidism. About seven eighths of the glandular tissue is removed. Total thyroidectomy may be performed if malignancy is present. Because of the effectiveness of treatment with ^{131}I, surgery is more commonly performed when malignancy is suspected, in patients under 35 years of age, and in pregnant women for whom the physician is reluctant to use irradiation.

Preoperatively, the patient is given a course of antithyroid drugs; a high caloric and high vitamin diet and rest are also part of the preoperative regimen. Usually, surgery is delayed until the patient is euthyroid clinically as well as by laboratory tests. If the hyperthyroidism is not controlled before surgery, there is increased risk of postoperative thyroid crisis. The patient may take antithyroid medications at home or he may spend several days in the hospital and then go home until he is ready for surgery. The preoperative period may be as long as several months, and the suspense is especially trying for the patient, who usually feels jittery anyway because of the increased metabolic rate.

The patient should be helped by the nurse not to feel ashamed of his restlessness and irritability. The nurse can point out the temporary nature of the highly emotional state and explain that it is related to the disease. The patient with hyperthyroidism often talks too excitedly and too much, and so the nurse should avoid garrulity. The patient's environment should be as calming as possible. The nurse may help the patient to find diversion, such as reading, that is both restful and enjoyable. Talking quietly with the nurse may help the patient to relax and rest.

The patient's visitors should help him to rest. Visitors are encouraged to keep their visits short, calm, and pleasant. To help the patient to sleep at night, the nurse might give him a back rub and straighten the

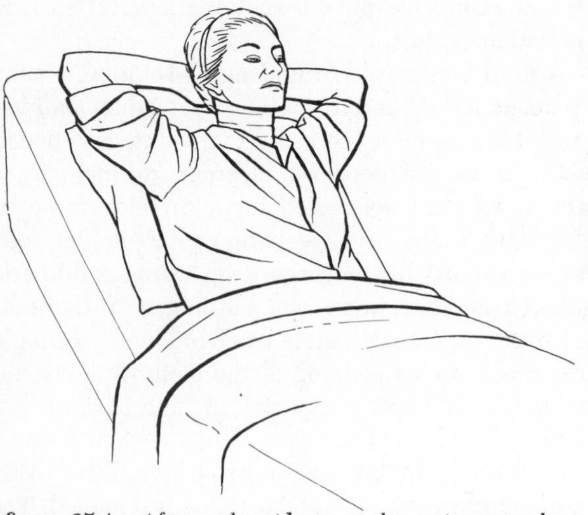

figure 35-4. After a thyroidectomy the patient uses her hands to support her head while she raises herself to a sitting position. This support helps to avoid strain on the neck muscles.

bed just before the lights go out. These measures help to relieve the feeling of warmth and irritability so common among patients with hyperthyroidism.

In preparation for surgery, the patient should be encouraged to eat as much as possible. Orange juice or eggnog should always be available for snacks. The patient is weighed and his blood pressure recorded every day. When taking the patient's pulse, the nurse will watch for irregularities as well as count the rate. If the patient's heart has been affected by the thyrotoxicosis, he probably will be placed on bed rest. Helping the patient to rest during this period is a great challenge. He will need help in getting comfortable, in settling down to something that interests him, and in not feeling lonely.

Postoperative Nursing Management. The patient is usually placed on his back, with small, firm pillows holding his head still, thus preventing excess tension on the incision. The patient needs constant observation for mucus and frequent, prompt suctioning. When he has reacted, the head of his bed may be moderately elevated. Pillows are positioned under head, neck, and shoulders, with firm support being the objective. The patient should not move his head up and down until the wound has healed considerably. When the patient is helped to move in bed, his head should be supported, so that it does not fall back or place any strain on the neck muscles. When the patient is alone, his beverage, tissues, and whatever else he might need should be placed on the overbed table in front of him, so that he does not have to reach over to the stand.

The patient usually is allowed out of bed the day after the operation. His head should be well supported while he gets into position to dangle his feet (Fig. 35-4). He should hold his head still with his hands while he takes a step or two, and it should be supported with firm pillows while he sits up in a chair.

Immediately after surgery the nurse will watch for symptoms of respiratory obstruction. Edema or bleeding can compress the trachea, causing an inability to breathe. This catastrophe must be treated within minutes by the insertion of an endotracheal tube or by a tracheostomy. A sterile tracheostomy set is kept in the patient's room or at the nurse's station ready for immediate use if needed.

Aspiration is a danger, since there will be depression of laryngeal and tracheal reflexes. Suction is applied as necessary. When swallowing and coughing reflexes have returned, the patient is encouraged to breathe deeply every 2 hours the first day.

The nurse will watch for bleeding, because a small amount of blood in the wound can obstruct respirations. Attention should be given to the patient's complaints of a sense of fullness in the wound. Blood may not be evident on the front of the bandage, but it may ooze around to the back of the patient's neck. Periodically during the first 12 hours postoperatively, a hand should be passed behind the patient's neck to see whether it feels damp. When the patient is turned to his side, the dressing is checked for blood. If the bandage encircling the neck becomes too tight, it is loosened but not removed, and the surgeon is called. Restlessness, apprehension, respiratory distress, increased pulse or temperature, decreased blood pressure, and cyanosis may occur. Neck swelling may be due to bleeding and accumulation of blood in the wound, distending the tissues.

Infrequently, the recurrent laryngeal nerve is injured during the operation. The patient is hoarse or may be unable to speak due to vocal cord paralysis. Respiratory obstruction may result. Hoarseness or any voice change is reported to the physician. Keep talking to a minimum the first 2 postoperative days. Steam inhalations may be ordered.

Another infrequent postoperative complication is tetany (muscular hypertonia with spasm and tremor), due to a low concentration of calcium from the inadvertent removal of the parathyroid glands during the thyroidectomy. The patient complains of numbness and tingling of the extremities and muscle cramps.

Tetany also can cause laryngeal spasm. The treatment is intravenous or oral calcium.

Thyroid crisis or storm, now a rare complication of thyroid surgery, may occur within the first 12 hours postoperatively. All the symptoms of hyperthyroidism are exaggerated. The patient's temperature may be as high as 106° F., the pulse becomes very rapid, and cardiac arrhythmias are common. There may be persistent vomiting and extreme restlessness with delirium. The patient becomes exhausted and not infrequently dies from cardiac failure. The treatment is intravenous sodium iodide, intravenous corticosteroids, oxygen, and cooling by the application of ice, cool enemas, or a controlled thermoblanket.

Since the incision for a thyroidectomy is made in a crease of the neck, the healed scar is barely visible; it is merely a thin line. If a patient seems concerned about it, clothing that covers the neck, such as high-necked dresses and scarves, can be worn until the scar contracts to its final tiny size.

Table 35-1.
Postoperative management of the patient with a thyroidectomy

Check blood pressure, pulse, respirations q1-4h or as ordered.
Place a small pillow under the patient's head to prevent tension on suture line.
Check dressing and bedding behind the neck for drainage q1-3h. Reinforce as necessary.
Check voice quality q1-2h; otherwise keep talking to a minimum.
Have the patient deep breathe, turn q2h. Check with the physician regarding coughing exercises; i.e., should the patient be asked to cough?
Support the patient's head when he is changing positions.
Keep the call light within easy reach.
Be alert for early signs of tetany: tingling of toes, fingers or around the mouth, apprehension, muscle twitching.
Keep suctioning equipment at the bedside and tracheostomy set readily available.

Postoperative management is outlined in Table 35-1.

Nontoxic goiter

The word *goiter* refers to an enlargement of the thyroid gland. Simple goiter is an enlargement without the symptoms of thyrotoxicosis. The enlargement may be caused by a deficiency of iodine in the diet, or by the inability of the thyroid to utilize iodine, or by relative iodine lack owing to increasing body demands for thyroid hormones. Iodine is essential to the production of thyroid hormones. As the gland tries to meet the body's need for thyroid hormones in spite of the relative or absolute deficiency of iodine available to it, it enlarges and becomes more vascular.

The condition occurs in areas where the soil and the drinking water are deficient in iodine, such as parts of the Alps, the Himalayas, and other mountain regions. In the United States, endemic goiter areas are the Great Lakes area, Minnesota, Ohio, and the Pacific Northwest.

Nontoxic goiter is more frequent in women than in men. It appears (sometimes only temporarily) when there is an increase in the need for thyroid hormone and thus for the iodine to make it—at times of stress, during infection, in adolescence, and in pregnancy. In some areas of the world, a large percentage of adolescent girls have nontoxic goiters.

Symptoms. The thyroid gland gradually grows larger. There may be a sense of fullness in the throat. Eventually, the hypertrophy can cause difficulty in swallowing and breathing if the thyroid begins to press on the trachea; otherwise, the general health is usually not affected.

Treatment and Prevention. Oral administration of iodide may reduce the goiter if deficiency is present and treatment is started before irreversible cellular changes have occurred in the thyroid tissue. Many months of treatment may be required. Thyroid hormone may be given instead of iodide. If there is pressure on the trachea or considerable disfigurement, the goiter can be removed surgically.

The body needs very little iodine to satisfy the requirements of the thyroid gland. For the normal adult, 25 to 50 mg. of inorganic iodine a year is sufficient. In the United States, state boards of health have asked salt manufacturers to add iodine to common table salt—about 0.01 percent of potassium iodide—in order to prevent iodine-deficient goiters. Most grocery stores carry iodized table salt, and as a result iodine deficiency goiters are less common than they used to be.

Thyroid cancer

Thyroid cancer is suspected when there is an enlarged lump which is hard to the touch, when there is invasion of other local structures, and when the area of the thyroid containing the lump does not concentrate ^{131}I as well as the surrounding normal thyroid tissue. Biopsy may be performed by making an incision (open biopsy), or by inserting a needle through which a small amount of tissue is withdrawn (closed biopsy). Most physicians object to the closed procedure, since the needle may miss the cancer; and if it contacts the tumor, it may spread it.

Considerable difference of opinion exists concerning the surgical treatment of carcinoma of the thyroid. If the tumor is accessible, the treatment is surgical and most often radical (total thyroidectomy with removal of the local lymph glands in the neck). Some surgeons advocate the less extensive procedure of thyroid lobectomy.

After the operation, thyroid replacement therapy is given in order to supply those hormones that can no longer be produced due to the absence of the thyroid gland and to suppress pituitary TSH so that it will not stimulate the growth of any residual malignant thyroid tissue.

If thyroid cancer, either local or metastatic, is inaccessible and can take up iodine, radioactive iodine may be given. The malignancy will take it up and be destroyed. This effect can be enhanced by administering TSH, because it stimulates increased uptake of the radioactive iodine by the thyroid.

The cure rate of thyroid cancer depends on the type of tumor present. Papillary carcinoma, the most common thyroid carcinoma, does not grow rapidly, whereas undifferentiated cancer grows more rapidly and is more difficult to control. Since most thyroid cancers are papillary carcinomas, the physician often can convey optimism to the patient.

Hypothyroidism

This disease is due to a deficiency of thyroid hormones, causing a lowered rate of all metabolic processes. It results in a set of symptoms called *myxedema* in the adult. The condition may originate within the thyroid (primary hypothyroidism) or within the pituitary, manifested by TSH lack (secondary hypothyroidism).

Diagnosis. Laboratory tests such as the T_3, T_4, ^{131}I uptake and Thyroid-Stimulating Hormone (TSH) test are decreased. The patient's history may reveal one or more of the general signs of hypothyroidism.

A problem in the early recognition of hypothyroidism is that many of the symptoms are nonspecific and may not be sufficiently dramatic to bring the patient to the physician. This condition can go untreated for years. The nurse who notices such symptoms as puffiness of the face, chronic fatigue, or intolerance to cold should suggest a visit to the physician.

Etiology. Atrophy of the thyroid gland may occur after pneumonia, typhoid fever, and influenza. Thyroid inflammation and surgery or irradiation for hyperthyroidism also can cause hypothyroidism. Or, the deficiency may be due to an autoimmune process, in which the patient develops antibodies against his own thyroid tissue. Very often the cause is unknown. Women are affected more often than men.

Symptoms. The symptoms of hypothyroidism are opposite in many respects to those of hyperthyroidism. The metabolic rate and both the physical and the mental activity are slowed. The hypothyroid patient feels lethargic and lacking in energy, dozes frequently during the day, is forgetful, and has chronic headaches. The face takes on a masklike, stolid, unemotional expression, yet the patient is often irritable. The tongue may be enlarged, the lips may be swollen, and there is nonpitting edema of the eyelids. The temperature and pulse are decreased, and there is intolerance to cold. The patient gains weight easily. Skin is dry, and hair characteristically is coarse and sparse, tending to fall out. Menstrual disorders are frequent. Constipation may be severe enough to require daily enemas. The voice of the myxedema patient is low-pitched, slow, and hoarse. Hearing may be impaired. There may be numbness or tingling in the arms or legs, unrelieved by change of position. Hypothyroidism may lead to enlargement of the heart due to pericardial effusion and an increased tendency toward atherosclerosis and heart strain. Anemia may also be present.

Treatment and Nursing Management. Because metabolic processes are depressed, the patient may feel chilled in a room that is comfortable for others; he may need extra blankets or a robe while he is in bed. Even though his appetite is poor, he has a tendency to gain weight. The diet is usually low calorie and may be high in roughage and protein. The nurse should check daily as to whether or not he has had a bowel movement. Too many days without one may lead to an impaction. Lotions or creams will keep the skin soft and relieve dryness.

Patients with hypothyroidism are inordinately susceptible to sedative and hypnotic drugs. If any are ordered (a rare circumstance), the patient is watched carefully for extreme drowsiness and diminished respirations.

Hypothyroidism is treated by replacement therapy. The patient is supplied with thyroid hormone in the form of desiccated thyroid extract or with one of the synthetic products, such as crystalline thyroxin or triiodothyronine. Thyroid extract is very slow to act; and the dose, given by mouth, can be taken once a day. Patients may be started on 15 mg. of thyroid extract and maintained on the dose found most appropriate. The side effects of replacement therapy may include dyspnea, rapid pulse, palpitations, precordial pain, hyperactivity, insomnia, dizziness, and gastrointestinal disorders, in other word signs of *hyper*thyroidism. Occasionally, a skin rash may be seen.

Once the replacement therapy has begun, a dramatic change may be seen in a few weeks. The patient feels a new interest in life. His hair again becomes soft and attractive, and he can stay awake for 16 hours in one stretch. His mental and physical activities are quickened.

Because these changes may be rapid and profound, the patient may be hospitalized during the early days of treatment. The nurse has an important responsibility to observe carefully for changes in the symptoms. If the heart or blood vessels have been affected by the hypothyroidism, the sudden improvement in his metabolic rate may impose an additional strain on the cardiovascular system. For instance, if the coronary arteries are sclerotic, they may not be able to supply the heart with sufficient blood for its sudden increase in activity. The nurse should be alert to changes in the pulse rate and complaints of precordial pain and dyspnea. Any complaints that may indicate cardiac involvement are reported to the physician.

These patients usually have to take thyroid extract for the remainder of their lives. A patient who is treated early and is well-regulated should continue to feel well. However, periodic visits to the physician are necessary to ensure continuation of the proper dosage. The nurse should emphasize to the patient the importance of keeping his appointments.

The parathyroid glands

The parathyroid glands are tiny bodies, shaped like beans, imbedded on either side of the thyroid gland. The parathyroid glands are usually four in number, although there may be more. The upper parathyroid is usually found posteriorly, at the junction of the upper and middle third of the thyroid. The lower parathyroids are more variable in location, but usually lie among the branches of the inferior thyroid artery. They may also be found in the chest. They secrete the parathyroid hormone—parathormone—which regulates the concentration of calcium and phosphorus in the blood and influences the passage of calcium and phosphorus between bloodstream, bones, and urine.

Hyperparathyroidism

Pathology and Symptoms. In hyperparathyroidism, an overproduction of parathyroid hormone (parathormone) results in increased urinary excretion of phosphorus and loss of calcium from the bones. The bones become demineralized as the calcium leaves them and enters the bloodstream. The excess serum calcium that has been taken from the tissues is lost in the urine. The large amounts of calicum and phosphorus passing through the kidneys may lead to stones, pyelonephritis, and uremia; thus, renal disease is a serious outcome. The amount of serum phosphorus is decreased. The shift of calcium to the blood from the tissues leads to a chain of events including muscle weakness, fatigue, apathy, nausea and vomiting, constipation, and cardiac arrhythmias. Excessive blood calcium depresses the responsiveness of the peripheral nerves, accounting for the fatigue and the muscle weakness. The muscles become hypotonic, and this hypotonia is the basis for constipation. Metastatic calcifications can occur, due to the excess of calcium in the bloodstream. Because the bones have lost calcium, there is skeletal tenderness and pain on bearing weight; the bones may become so demineralized that they break with little or no trauma (pathologic fractures).

Diagnosis. The diagnosis is made on the basis of an elevated serum calcium and a low serum phosphorus in the absence of other causes of hypercalcemia. A 3-day low-calcium diet may be given; and the amount of calcium excreted in the urine may be measured to help to establish the diagnosis and to determine the severity of the disease.

Treatment and Nursing Management. The treatment of hyperparathyroidism is the surgical removal of hypertrophied gland tissue or of an individual tumor. Postoperative nursing management is similar to management of the patient with a thyroidectomy, as the surgical approach is similar. Also included is observation of the patient for the symptoms of hypoparathyroidism, especially for tetany. Intravenous 10 percent calcium lactate should be kept at the bedside for the first few postoperative days in case the patient does develop tetany. Usually, it is given in an infusion of normal saline. Until the phosphorus-calcium balance is restored, the patient may be prone to pathologic fractures, and it is important to keep this in mind during administration of nursing care.

Hypoparathyroidism

Pathology and Symptoms. The underproduction of parathyroid hormone causes a decrease of calcium and an increase of phosphorus in the blood, with a decrease of both in the urine. The main symptom of hypoparathyroidism is tetany. The patient may feel numbness and tingling in the fingers or toes or around the lips. A voluntary movement may be followed by an involuntary, jerking spasm. Tonic (continuous contraction) flexion of an arm or a finger may occur. If the facial nerve (immediately in front of the ear) is tapped, the patient's mouth twitches and his jaw tightens (Chvostek's sign). A spasm may occur in the larynx, causing the patient to become dyspneic, with long, crowing respirations as he tries to get air past the constriction. He may become cyanotic and in danger of asphyxia. He may have generalized convulsions or gastric distress. Nails become brittle and break easily. Skin is coarse and dry and hair is patchy and thin.

Diagnosis. The diagnosis is made on the basis of a low serum calcium and an elevated serum phosphorus in the absence of other causes of hypocalcemia.

Treatment and Nursing Management. The treatment for hypoparathyroidism includes the administration of vitamin D or vitamin D_2 (calciferol). These drugs increase the blood level of calcium. The dosage is related to the degree of hypocalcemia, which is determined by frequent measurements of the blood calcium. The urine calcium levels also may be checked.

The treatment of hypoparathyroid tetany also includes the administration of calcium salts, and occasionally of parathyroid extract. Calcium gluconate may be given first intravenously, 10 to 50 ml. of a 10 percent solution in 1,000 ml. of normal saline. Intravenous calcium causes vasodilation; the patient feels hot and nauseated. Calcium is never given intramuscularly, since it causes tissue sloughing. When a patient is receiving calcium intravenously, special care must be taken that the needle does not slip out of the vein, spilling the solution into the tissues. If the intravenous solution extravasates into surrounding tissues, it must immediately be discontinued.

Because estimation of the correct doses of these drugs may be difficult, the nurse should observe the patient frequently for *hyper*calcemia, which may occur with the administration of any of these preparations. Vomiting, usually one of the earliest symptoms, should immediately be reported to the physician. It may be followed by fever, listlessness, and coma.

The adrenal glands

The adrenal (suprarenal) glands are located above the kidneys. The outer portion of the gland is called the cortex and the inner portion the medulla. The adrenal *cortex* manufactures and secretes glucocorticoids, mineralocorticoids, and small amounts of sex hormones. Collectively these hormones are called corticosteroids. The adrenal *medulla* produces two neurohormones: epinephrine and norepinephrine.

Glucocorticoids and mineralocorticoids are essential to life and influence many organs and structures of the body. Glucocorticoids affect body metabolism, suppress inflammation, and help the body withstand stress. Mineralocorticoids are concerned with the maintenance of water and electrolyte (sodium, potassium, chlorides) balance.

Addison's disease
(adrenal cortex hypofunction)

Etiology. Addison's disease can result from destruction of adrenal cortical tissue by tuberculosis or by idiopathic atrophy. It is suspected that excessive stress (overwhelming infection, surgery, or prolonged drain of the body's emergency resources) plays some role in causing insufficient steroids to be secreted. Cancer may invade the adernal cortex. This disease can also result from long-term use of large doses of steroids that cause adrenal atrophy by suppressing adrenocorticotropic hormone (ACTH). Of course, bilateral adrenalectomy causes an absence of the hormones secreted by the adrenal gland. Addison's disease is comparatively rare.

Pathology and Symptoms. Certain corticosteroids regulate absorption, distribution, and excretion of body salts and water; a decrease in these hormones leads to increased urinary excretion of sodium and retention of potassium. Dehydration, with reduction of blood plasma volume, results. The patient feels weak and tires easily. His blood pressure, BMR, and temperature are low. Because he develops hypotension from sudden changes of position, such as from lying down or sitting up too quickly, he may faint. He is prone to vascular collapse due to poor myocardial tonus, decreased cardiac output, and lowered blood pressure. He loses weight, is anemic, and may become cachectic.

His appetite is poor, and he may suffer from a variety of gastrointestinal symptoms. He feels nervous and has periods of depression. Patients with Addison's disease have an abnormally dark pigmentation, especially of exposed areas of the skin and the mucous membranes, and a decrease in hair growth. Because the body is deficient in those hormones that facilitate the conversion of protein into glucose, the patient suffers episodes of hypoglycemia, which may develop 5 to 6 hours after eating; the early morning before breakfast is an especially dangerous time. The symptoms of hypoglycemia are hunger, headache, sweating, weakness, trembling, emotional instability, visual disturbances and, finally, disorientation, coma, and convulsions.

Acute Adrenal Crisis. Because the hormones of the cortex of the adrenal glands are prominent in effecting the body's adaptive reactions to stress, patients with Addison's disease collapse when they are faced with excess stress. Even uncomplicated surgery, such as an appendectomy, requires more physiological adaptive ability than a patient with Addison's disease usually possesses. Salt deprivation, infection, trauma, exposure to cold, overexertion—any abnormal stress—can cause adrenal crisis. The crisis may start with anorexia, nausea, vomiting, diarrhea, abdominal pain, headache, intensification of hypotension, restlessness, or a high temperature. Unless given corticosteroids, the patient will experience acute adrenal crisis, which is a severe flare-up of Addison's disease. His blood pressure becomes markedly depressed, perhaps so low as to be unobtainable. The patient is in *adrenal shock*, which is primarily due to lack of adrenal hormones.

Adrenal (Addison's) crisis is an emergency; death may occur from hypotension and vasomotor collapse. Corticosteroids are given intravenously in solutions of normal saline and glucose. Antibiotics may be ordered because of the patient's extremely low resistance to infection. Vital signs are taken frequently. The patient is kept warm and as quiet as possible. He should not be permitted to do anything for himself until the emergency is over. Fluids are also important aspects of therapy.

Diagnostic Tests. The pituitary gland secretes ACTH (adrenocorticotropic hormone), which stimulates the adrenal cortex to secrete its own hormones. A test used to diagnose Addison's disease is the determination of the adrenal cortical response to ACTH. The excretion of adrenal cortical hormones is measured after the administration of ACTH in an intravenous solution. Normal persons have an increased excretion of 17-hydroxycorticoids and 17-ketosteroids, whereas patients with Addison's disease show little or no increase. Also, eosinophils in the patient's blood are measured. Normally, a drop of 60 to 90 percent in the eosinophil count occurs after the ACTH is given, but there is less change in Addison's disease.

Laboratory tests in Addison's disease show a low blood sodium and a high potassium; the BMR is minus 10 to minus 20. A glucose tolerance test may be done. In Addison's disease the glucose in the bloodstream does not rise as high as normal, and it returns to its fasting level more quickly than it would under normal conditions.

Treatment and Nursing Management. Addison's disease is treated by replacement of the missing hormones. Fludrocortisone (Florinef), a synthetic corticosteroid preparation that possesses glucocorticoid and mineralocorticoid properties, is often selected for corticosteroid replacement therapy. The dosage of the hormones may be stabilized during the patient's stay in the hospital and continued on a maintenance basis after he is discharged.

It is imperative that the patient take the hormones as prescribed, and that he see his physician regularly. If the patient does not have active tuberculosis, and if he follows his prescribed drug regimen carefully, the outlook for his well-being is good (a prognosis that could not have been made before the availability of these hormones as drugs). As in diabetes, the patient's understanding of his condition can mean the difference between disability and an active life. The patient himself must be aware of his body's inability to handle stress of any sort and of the importance of seeking medical attention for the readjustment of dosage whenever he is threatened by stress of any kind: an infection, a car accident (even if he is not noticeably hurt), exposure to cold, an insoluble family crisis, or an excessive work load. *No patient with Addison's disease should receive insulin by error; he may die from hypoglycemia.* He is also extremely sensitive to opiates and barbiturates.

Part of the nurse's responsibility to the Addisonian patient is to teach him and his family about the disease, how to protect his health by avoiding stressful situations when possible, and to obtain medical adjustment of his drugs when this is indicated. The patient with Addison's disease should not be made to feel that his condition should keep him out of the mainstream of everyday life. The patient should be encouraged to wear identification, such as a Medic-Alert tag, stating that he is suffering from adrenal cortical insufficiency.

Because of recurrent hypoglycemia, the patient

may do better on five or six small meals than on three big ones. If sodium chloride is ordered, it may be tolerated best if taken with meals. Salt intake may need to be increased during hot weather. The patient can be instructed to add extra salt to his food if he has perspired more than usual.

When hypoglycemia occurs, it is treated by giving glucose, orally or intravenously. To prevent recurring episodes of hypoglycemia, between-meal snacks of milk and crackers are preferable to candy and other rapidly absorbed sugars. If the patient's meal is delayed because of diagnostic tests, the fasting period should be kept to a minimum, and during the fast, his activities should be limited; he should be kept in bed and quiet. If he has to leave the unit, a stretcher or wheelchair should be used.

Because of hypotension and muscle weakness, a patient with this condition is subject to falling. Side rails are used unless he is well-regulated and knowledgeable. Importance of getting out of bed slowly is emphasized. If he is dizzy on sitting up, he should lie down again. Blood pressure is taken if there are any symptoms, such as weakness or faintness, which indicate that it is lower than usual. A change from previous readings is more important than any one reading.

Cushing's syndrome (adrenal cortex hyperfunction)

This condition is the opposite of Addison's disease. An overproduction of adrenal cortical hormones may result (1) from overstimulation by the pituitary gland, with resultant hyperplasia of the adrenal cortex, and (2) from benign or malignant tumors of the adrenal cortex. In a very few patients, Cushing's syndrome is caused by extra-adrenal carcinoma, which produces an ACTH-like substance that causes adrenal hyperfunction and hyperplasia. In Cushing's syndrome, extensive protein depletion occurs, leading to muscle wasting and weakness. Carbohydrate tolerance is lowered, and diabetes may result. There is a redistribution of fat, leading eventually to the typical moon face and buffalo hump seen in patients who have had long-term corticosteroid therapy, which can lead to the symptoms of Cushing's syndrome. The skin is thin, and the face is ruddy. The patient becomes progressively weaker, and the symptoms of infection are masked—perhaps dangerously. Therefore, the nurse should be especially alert for minor signs, such as a slight sore throat or a small rise in temperature, that may indicate the presence of a more severe infectious process. The blood vessels are extremely fragile, the patient bruises easily, and striae may form over extensive skin areas. The bones become so demineralized that the patient may have backache, kyphosis, and collapse of the vertebral bodies. Sodium and water are retained; the patient suffers peripheral edema and hypertension. In women, Cushing's syndrome usually produces masculinization with hirsutism and amenorrhea.

Diagnosis. The urine may be examined for 17-hydroxycorticoids (17-OH) and 17-ketosteroids. The former are almost always increased, and the latter are increased or decreased, depending on the nature of the lesion. As is done in the diagnosis of hypofunction, ACTH may be given intravenously and the 17-hydroxycorticoid excretion measured. Patients with bilateral adrenal cortex hyperplasia have a marked urinary increase in both 17-hydroxycorticoids and 17-ketosteroids, while patients with carcinoma of the adrenal cortex may show no such increase. Twenty-four hour urines may be collected for the measurement of urinary hydrocortisone and its major metabolites. Sometimes fractional urines are ordered because normally there is an increase in the excretion of hydrocortisone and its metabolites during the early morning, but this diurnal variation is not seen in Cushing's disease.

Another test is the urinary 17-hydroxycorticoid suppression test, in which a steroid such as dexamethasone is given to suppress ACTH from the pituitary. If, on a low dosage, urinary 17-hydroxycorticoid is not suppressed, the patient probably has hyperplasia of the adrenal cortex. If, on a high dosage of dexamethasone, there is no suppression of urinary 17-hydroxycorticoids, the patient probably has a carcinoma or an adenoma of the adrenal cortex. Hyperplasia and carcinoma may also be differentiated by giving a pituitary stimulant such as metyrapone (Metopirone). Normally and in hyperplasia, 17-hydroxycorticoid in the urine is increased when metyrapone is given, but this is not seen in carcinoma.

Occasionally, an abdominal x-ray film may show an adrenal mass, and an intravenous pyelogram may show changes in the renal shadow caused by an abnormally large adrenal gland.

Treatment and Nursing Management. Treatment depends on whether the disease is due to a tumor or to hyperplasia, and on the views of the physician. X-ray therapy to the pituitary may be used if there is hyperplasia. An adrenalectomy may be preferred; the operation may be total or subtotal, unilateral or bilateral. If an adrenalectomy is to be done, adrenal cortical hormone therapy may be started preoperatively in anticipation of the time when the body will be unable to produce its own hormones. However, considerable difference of medical opinion exists concerning the advisability of administering adrenal cortical steroids preoperatively when an adrenalectomy is to be performed.

After the operation the patient is treated as if he had Addison's disease—which, indeed, he now has. A postadrenalectomy syndrome of nausea, vomiting, diarrhea, muscle tenderness, and aching should be called to the physician's attention. Hypotension may be a problem, and the nurse should watch for signs of it. Also, she should observe for such complications as hemorrhage, atelectasis, and pneumothorax, since the adrenals are located close to the diaphragm and the inferior vena cava. Patients who had a unilateral tumor may now have an atrophy of the cortex of the unaffected adrenal gland, and probably they will be given adrenal cortical hormones in slowly decreasing amounts until they produce enough of their own.

Because the adrenal glands and the body water and electrolyte regulation are closely related, both preoperatively and postoperatively, the nurse should keep careful records of fluid intake and urinary output. Preoperatively, the patient is often placed on a low-sodium, high-potassium diet. Because depression is common in Cushing's syndrome, the nurse must be alert for changes in mood and for any suicidal tendencies. The patient needs protection from upsetting situations.

Hyperaldosteronism

Aldosterone is one of the hormones secreted by the adrenal cortex. Primary hyperaldosteronism is a rare disease in which this hormone is produced in excess, resulting in hypertension and renal loss of potassium. The hypokalemia causes muscle weakness, which may progress to paralysis and polyuria. The disease can be caused by carcinoma, adenoma, or hyperplasia of the adrenal cortex. Hyperaldosteronism characteristically occurs in early middle life.

The treatment is removal of the adrenal tumor. Preoperative preparation includes potassium replacement for 5 to 7 days and restriction of sodium intake. Postoperatively, intake and output are measured and the patient is observed for any signs of urinary dysfunction.

Pheochromocytoma

This term refers to a tumor, usually of the adrenal medulla, which causes increased secretion of epinephrine and norepinephrine. The symptoms are hypertension (intermittent or, more frequently, persistent), tremor, nervousness, sweating, headache, nausea and vomiting, hyperglycemia, polyuria (increased urination), and vertigo. A diagnostic test for pheochromocytoma is the phentolamine (Regitine) test. If the administration of phentolamine results in a drop in blood pressure, pheochromocytoma is suspected. Another diagnostic test involves measuring the urinary excretion of catecholamines and their breakdown products; this diagnostic measure is both reliable and safe.

The treatment is the surgical removal of the tumor. The operation has been dangerous, especially in the past, because of the wide fluctuation of blood pressure that may occur during and after surgery, due to a sudden liberation or an abrupt stoppage of epinephrine or norepinephrine. Surgery is less dangerous now than in the past, because it is now possible to control these fluctuations preoperatively and during surgery by the use of phentolamine (Regitine).

The pituitary gland (hypophysis)

Although the pituitary gland weighs only about 600 mg., it is a key organ. No system or structure of the body is exempt from its influence. There are two secretory parts of the pituitary, the anterior and the posterior lobes. At least nine hormones are secreted by the pituitary gland, only a few of which will be discussed here. Hyperfunction and hypofunction of the gland may be manifested in many ways, depending on which glandular cells are involved.

The anterior lobe

Acromegaly. Hyperplasia or tumors of the anterior pituitary can cause overproduction of the growth hormone (somatotropin). When there is excess of this hormone in a youngster before the ends of the long bones are fully united (epiphyseal union), gigantism results. Overproduction of somatotropin during adulthood brings about a condition called *acromegaly,* in which the overgrowth of many tissues, including the skeleton, results in a characteristic appearance of coarse features, huge lower jaw, thick lips, bulging forehead, bulbous nose, and large hands and feet. Headache resulting from pressure on the sella turcica, when the overgrowth is due to a tumor, is common. The patients may become partially blind from pressure on the optic nerve. Heart, liver, and spleen may enlarge. In spite of the patient's enlarged tissues, muscle weakness is a symptom. The joints are hypertrophied and may become painful and stiff. Men often become impotent, and women may have amenorrhea, increased facial hair, and deepened voices.

Acromegaly is sometimes treated surgically and sometimes by radiation. The tendency now is to treat these patients surgically. Unfortunately, the growth changes due to acromegaly are irreversible, even if the disease is arrested successfully.

SIMMONDS' DISEASE. Simmonds' disease, or panhypopituitarism, a rare disorder, results from the destruction of the pituitary gland by postpartum emboli, surgery, tumor, or tuberculosis. There is a gradual atrophy of the gonads and the genitalia. Because of the impairment of pituitary stimulus, thyroid and adrenals fail to secrete adequate amounts of their hormones. The patient ages prematurely and may become extremely cachectic.

Tumors that threaten pituitary tissue may be irradiated. Surgery is difficult and dangerous because of the location of the gland. Medical treatment includes the administration of substitute hormones of the glands dependent on the pituitary for stimulation.

THE POSTERIOR LOBE

DIABETES INSIPIDUS. The hormone vasopressin, also called antidiuretic hormone (ADH), regulates the reabsorption of water in the kidney tubules. In this rare disease there is a reduction in the secretion of ADH, leading to an outpouring of water through the kidneys. The urine is so copious that the patient does not have an unbroken night's sleep. From 15 to 20 liters of urine may be passed in a 24-hour period. The urine is very dilute with a specific gravity of 1.002 or less. The excretion of urine cannot be controlled by limiting the intake of fluids. Thirst is excessive and constant. The need for drinking and emptying the bladder embarrasses the patient and limits his social and work activities; he can never be too far from a bathroom. The patient is weak and anorectic, and he loses weight.

The treatment is the administration of vasopressin (Pitressin) subcutaneously or by inhalation. The objective is to reduce the patient's urine output to 2 to 3 liters during 24 hours.

General nutritional considerations

- The patient with hyperthyroidism may require a diet high in calories. Some hospitalized patients require between-meal feedings in addition to regular meals.
- Some thyroid function studies are affected by the ingestion of iodine prior to the test. The patient should be asked if he has eaten health foods or health food products containing iodine, seaweed, or kelp. If these products have been used in the past 6 months, the physician should be informed *before* any thyroid studies or tests are performed.
- The hypothyroid patient usually requires a low-calorie diet and may need an explanation of this diet before discharge from the hospital.
- The patient with Addison's disease and recurrent hypoglycemia may require five to six small meals rather than three regular meals. The nurse should check to see that the food is served at regular intervals.
- The patient with Cushing's disease may be placed on a low-sodium, high-potassium diet. Limiting the amount of salt and foods containing sodium is important in controlling the edema accompanying this disease.

General pharmacological considerations

- Antithyroid drugs may be used in the treatment of *hyper*thyroidism. Some patients respond well to these drugs and attain a euthyroid (normal) state; others respond with only fair results and surgery may be necessary.
- Agranulocytosis is the most serious side effect of antithyroid therapy with thiouracils and methimazole (Tapazole), and requires termination of therapy. Agranulocytosis is manifested by susceptibility to infections: fever, sore throat, ulcerations in the mouth.
- Iodine, as well as other antithyroid preparations, may be prescribed for the patient who is scheduled for a thyroidectomy. These drugs reduce the vascularity of the gland, thus reducing the risk of bleeding during surgery.
- Radioactive iodine (^{131}I) may be used as an antithyroid drug with results (i.e., decrease in the symptoms of hyperthyroidism) in approximately 6 to 8 weeks. Some patients develop hypothyroidism after treatment with radioactive iodine and will require thyroid drugs for the remainder of their lives.
- Intravenous calcium gluconate may be administered to the *hypo*thyroid patient as an emergency measure to correct hypocalcemia

(low serum calcium). If the intravenous solution extravasates into surrounding tissues, the administration is stopped immediately, as the drug is extremely irritating to soft tissue.

- Fludrocortisone (Florinef) along with a glucocorticoid such as hydrocortisone is administered to patients with Addison's disease. Patients must *thoroughly* understand their drug therapy: (1) the dosage is *never* increased or decreased except by order of the physician, (2) a dose is not omitted or the medication stopped *for any reason,* (3) if ill and unable to take the drug orally, the patient must go to the hospital (preferably the one where his physician is on staff and/or his records are kept), (4) identification such as Medic-Alert is to be carried at all times, (5) any signs of illness or infection are to be reported to the physician immediately.
- Diabetes insipidus is treated with the administration of vasopressin (Pitressin) subcutaneously or by inhalation nasal spray.

Bibliography

BEESON, P. B. and McDERMOTT, W.: *Textbook of Medicine,* ed. 14. Philadelphia, Saunders, 1975.

BENNETT, A. H. et al: Tumors of the adrenal gland (pictorial). Hosp. Med. 9:108, October, 1973.

BLALOCK, J. B.: Surgical treatment of parathyroid disease. AORN J. 20:696, October, 1974.

DANOWSKI, T. S.: Cushing's syndrome (pictorial). Hosp. Med. 10:90, February, 1974.

DILLON, R. S.: *Handbook of Endocrinology: Diagnosis and Management of Endocrine and Metabolic Disorders.* Philadelphia, Lea & Febiger, 1973.

EMMANUEL, S.: Surgery of the thyroid and parathyroid glands, Part 3. RN 37:OR/ED 1, November, 1974.

KASTRUP, E., ed.: *Facts and Comparisons.* St. Louis, Facts and Comparisons, Inc. Updated monthly.

LEMAITRE, G. and FINNEGAN, J.: *The Patient in Surgery: A Guide for Nurses.* Philadelphia, Saunders, 1975.

LUCKMAN, J., and SORENSON, K. C.: *Medical-Surgical Nursing: A Psychophysiological Approach.* Philadelphia, Saunders, 1974.

McCONAHEY, W. M.: Hypothyroidism (pictorial). Hosp. Med. 11:98, April, 1975.

McGANN, M.: Cushing's syndrome: Its complexities and care (pictorial). RN 38:40, August, 1975.

———: Treatment and care of the patient with hyperparathyroidism (pictorial). RN 37:48, November, 1974.

RATCLIFF, J. D.: I am Joe's thyroid. Reader's Digest 102:74, March, 1973.

SCHERER, J. C.: *Introductory Clinical Pharmacology.* Philadelphia, Lippincott, 1975.

SPENCER, R. T.: *Patient Care in Endocrine Problems.* Saunders Monographs in Clinical Nursing, 4. Philadelphia, Saunders, 1973.

WILLIAMS, R. H.: *Textbook of Endocrinology.* Philadelphia, Saunders, 1974.

CHAPTER 36

On completion of this chapter the student will:

- Discuss the pathology and symptoms of diabetes mellitus.
- Describe the symptoms and medical management of diabetic ketosis and coma.
- Name the tests performed in the diagnosis of diabetes.
- Discuss the place of diet therapy in the medical management of diabetes mellitus.
- Formulate a nursing care plan for and participate in the nursing management of a diabetic patient.
- Name the various types of insulin and oral hypoglycemic agents used in the treatment of diabetes mellitus.
- List the points that should be covered in a diabetic teaching program.
- Recognize a hypoglycemic reaction and describe symptoms observed and emergency actions taken to terminate the reaction.
- Describe the physical problems that may be encountered by the diabetic patient: vascular disturbances, visual problems, neuropathy, nephropathy, infection.

The patient with diabetes mellitus

Diabetes mellitus is a metabolic disease in which there is some degree of insulin insufficiency, resulting in an impairment of the body's ability to metabolize carbohydrate and also fat and protein. Because of the lack of insulin or inadequate insulin action, abnormal amounts of glucose accumulate in the bloodstream and subsequently are excreted in the urine. As the condition worsens, excessive ketone bodies are found in the blood and urine. Every cell in the body is affected by the metabolic derangement.

Incidence

No age group is exempt, but diabetes is most frequent between the ages of 40 and 60. The incidence is rising, probably partly because the case-finding methods are better and because people are living longer and have time to develop diabetes.

Pathology and symptoms

A normal person has a fasting level of 80 to 120 mg. of glucose in each 100 ml. of venous blood. Within half an hour after he has eaten, some of the ingested carbohydrate is digested and absorbed into the blood. The blood glucose rises to about 150 mg. per 100 ml. Two hours after eating, the blood glucose has returned to its fasting level. In liver and in muscle, glucose is converted to glycogen and stored. As the body needs fuel, the liver changes glycogen back to glucose and passes it out to the bloodstream, where it becomes available to muscle and other body tissues as fuel for energy. Insulin is an important link in this process; it promotes the storage of glycogen in the liver, it aids in the utilization of glucose by the tissues, and it influences the metabolism of fats and proteins.

Insulin is secreted into the bloodstream by the beta cells of the islets of Langerhans in the pancreas. Diabetics have less insulin available than their metabolic processes require, or, according to some theories, the insulin they produce cannot be utilized effectively. Because of the inadequate insulin activity, the ability of the liver to convert glucose to glycogen and the use of glucose by the tissues are impaired.

In diabetes the fasting blood-glucose content may be normal or elevated, but after eating it may rise to high levels (exceeding 150 mg. per 100 ml. of blood.)

The condition of excess glucose in the blood is called *hyperglycemia.* With so much additional glucose in the blood, some of it is excreted by the kidneys. Glucose is usually found in the urine when it rises over 180 mg. per 100 ml. in the blood. This is called the renal threshold for glucose. The presence of glucose in the urine is called *glycosuria.*

To eliminate glucose, water also must be excreted. Therefore, one of the symptoms of untreated diabetes is *polyuria* (excessive urine). The patient complains of needing to urinate frequently and of passing a large amount each time. Because so much water has been lost in the urine, the patient feels thirsty (*polydipsia*). Often, the amount that he drinks is not enough to compensate for water loss and he becomes dehydrated.

While the needed glucose is being wasted, the body's requirement for fuel continues. The patient feels hungry, and he increases his intake of food (*polyphagia*). He becomes hungrier and weaker, and he loses weight, literally starving while he is overeating. To meet the rising need for energy, additional amounts of fats and proteins are metabolized.

Diabetic ketosis and coma

Normally, when fat is metabolized, ketone bodies are formed in the liver and transported to muscle and other tissue, where they serve as a source of energy. (Ketone bodies are chemical intermediate products in the metabolism of fat.) In the process of serving as a source of energy, ketone bodies are oxidized to carbon dioxide and water. The more fat is metabolized, the more ketone bodies are formed. The ketone bodies are beta-hydroxybutyric acid, acetoacetic acid, and acetone (note that two of them are acids). All three are toxic if they accumulate in the body.

If ketone bodies are produced faster than they can be oxidized in the tissues, they accumulate in tissues and body fluids. Ketone bodies are buffered by the bicarbonate buffer system. Thus, ketonemia causes a decrease of plasma sodium, potassium, and alkali reserve. The loss of sodium and potassium salts in the urine further contributes to the development of acidosis. The CO_2 combining power of the blood is reduced, and the alkali reserve of the body is lowered, leading to further electrolyte imbalance. Chloride, particularly, is lost in the vomiting that accompanies acidosis, and sodium, potassium, and calcium are also wasted. The increased diuresis causes dehydration, which leads to diminution of the circulating blood volume and fall of the blood pressure. Air hunger (Kussmaul breathing) is common in acidosis. Acetone, being volatile, can be detected on the breath by its characteristic odor. If treatment is not given, the outcome is circulatory collapse, renal shutdown, and death. This complex is known as *diabetic coma* (though severe ketosis can be present without the patient's being comatose).

Anything that causes glycogen depletion in the liver and that therefore increases the need for oxidation of fat (for instance, insulin deprivation, infection, surgery, anesthesia, vomiting) may result in an excess of ketone bodies. Infection and surgery invite ketosis and diabetic coma, because they increase the demand for insulin that the diabetic's pancreas cannot deliver.

The metabolic situation is further complicated by overactivity of the anterior pituitary, the thyroid, and the adrenal cortex. The secretory activities of these glands may stimulate the formation of glucose, reduce the utilization of glucose, and therefore elevate blood-glucose levels. Although these hormonal interrelations as they affect carbohydrate metabolism are not yet fully understood, there are indications that diabetes is not an uncomplicated disease of merely the islets of Langerhans.

Diagnostic tests

Although diabetes is a highly complex disease, a diagnostic test for its detection is extremely simple. Normally, there is no easily detectable glucose or acetone in urine. In diabetes there may be both. Since glucose is not adequately utilized by the body, it is excreted in urine. If fats are metabolized faster than the body can utilize the ketone bodies, acetone will appear in the urine. The relative ease of these urinary tests helps to facilitate case-finding programs for the early detection of diabetes. Because glucose in the urine is not always an indication of diabetes, and because not all diabetics excrete glucose in the urine, blood glucose and glucose tolerance tests may be necessary to establish the diagnosis.

Urine tests

Collection of Urine Specimen. It is important to test the *second voided specimen.* The first specimen voided may contain urine collected in the bladder for 7 to 8 hours (as, for example, the first voided specimen in the morning). In testing urine for glucose, it is essential that the test reflect the presence of glucose and acetone *currently*—not for 8 hours past. The patient voids and the first specimen is saved in case he is unable to produce a second specimen; then, a half hour later, he voids again, and the second specimen is tested. This procedure is essential if the dosage of insulin is to be based on the results of the test.

When a patient has an indwelling catheter, it is essential *not* to take a specimen for testing from the collection bag, as this urine may have been collected over a 6- to an 8-hour period. Instead, the end of the tubing is removed from the collection bag and some fresh urine is allowed to run into a clean container for testing.

While the patient is still in the hospital, the nurse teaches him to test his own urine for glucose and acetone, because once he is at home, he will need to do it himself. By the time of discharge he should have done it so many times and be so proficient that he thinks no more of performing the procedure than he does of washing his hands. The patient should be taught not only the technique of urine testing but also the significance of the findings.

Glucose. *Benedict's Test:* Put 5 ml. of Benedict's solution in a test tube. Add 8 drops of urine. Mix. Place in a hot-water bath or, more simply, hold over a direct flame until the mixture has boiled (not so vigorously as to spatter) for 5 minutes. The opening of the test tube should be held away from the face. Allow it to cool, and compare it with the color chart that should be nearby.

- Clear blue—no sugar
- Pale green—trace of glucose
- Yellow—up to 0.5% glucose
- Orange—0.5% to 1.5% glucose
- Brick red—1.5% and over glucose

This test is the least expensive of the urine tests for glucose.

Tes-Tape: Dip a strip of Tes-Tape into urine. If glucose is present, the tape will turn green or blue. Only the end of the tape that is not touched by fingers or previously exposed to light or air should be used.

Clinitest: Put 10 drops of water in a test tube. Add 5 drops of urine. Add 1 tablet of Clinitest. Grade the resulting color in accordance with the Clinitest color chart.

Clinistix: Dip the test end in urine and read against the color chart.

An advantage of the last three tests is that the materials are convenient to carry. If necessary, a patient can test his urine with these methods in the restroom of an airplane or while he is at a hotel. Because they are quick and easy, these tests are more commonly used than Benedict's test.

Acetone. Although there are several tests for urinary acetone, the most common are Acetest tablets and acetone test strips. Put 2 drops of urine on the tablet and compare with the color chart to show the amount of acetone present. A positive test turns the tablet purple. The test strip is dipped into the urine.

Be sure to replace the cap on the bottle, because tablets and testing strips that have absorbed moisture from the air become useless. These testing materials can be bought in drugstores.

This test becomes especially important when the patient has a fever, is vomiting, or consistently has glucose in his urine. In these situations the chances for formation of ketone bodies are the greatest.

Blood tests

Glucose Tolerance Test. As mentioned previously, normal blood glucose in the fasting person is 80 to 120 mg. per 100 ml. of venous blood. When the nondiabetic is given glucose orally, his blood-glucose level will return to normal in about 2 hours (when glucose is given intravenously, the level returns to normal in about an hour). If the patient is diabetic, his fasting blood-glucose level may be high, and stay higher for over 2 hours after ingesting glucose.

The usual procedure for the standard oral glucose tolerance test is:

The patient receives a high carbohydrate diet for 3 to 5 days before the test. The diet contains at least 150 gm. of carbohydrate per day. This preparation for the test is important, because, without the preliminary diet, blood glucose values may be high.

Blood and urine samples are taken before breakfast (fasting control).

The patient drinks glucose in water. The dosage is determined by the patient's weight.

Blood and urine specimens are taken at intervals of a half-hour, 1 hour, 2 hours, and 3 hours after the patient has had the glucose. If desired, specimens are also taken at the fourth and fifth hours.

CO_2 Combining Power. The CO_2 combining power is a general measure of the acidity or alkalinity of the blood. Alkalosis is manifested by an increase above normal, while acidosis is manifested by a decrease in CO_2 combining power.

Treatment

Treatment of diabetes must continue for the rest of the patient's life; therefore the patient (or in some instances, a family member) has the responsibility for carrying out treatment prescribed by the physician, except during periods of illness (such as during complications of diabetes or some other illness) when physicians and nurses temporarily carry out treatment until the patient can again assume this responsibility. Before the patient can be expected to learn to carry out his treatment, he requires assistance in accepting the fact that he has diabetes and in dealing with his own feelings about having the disease. The nurse has an important role in helping the patient gradually to accept the condition and begin to understand his feelings about it, and in teaching the patient how to carry out his treatment.

Before beginning to teach the patient it is important to assess how accepting he is of the illness, and how realistically he is viewing it. The patient should be given time to talk about his reaction to the diagnosis and to absorb what it means to him, before starting to learn to carry out his treatment.

As the necessity for treatment is explained, an unrealistically glib approach should be avoided. The patient has a potentially serious illness, and most patients know this. An approach which implies, "This is really nothing—all you have to do is spend a few extra moments each morning testing your urine and giving yourself insulin," serves more to relieve staff of their responsibilities than to help the patient learn about his illness and deal with his feelings concerning it. It is important to avoid implying a promise that if the patient carries out his treatment faithfully, he will never experience complications. This is not true, and it can form a basis for later resentment. The nurse might explain that treatment will help the patient feel well and avoid complications, but she should not say or imply, "If you follow your treatment, you will not have complications."

Coordination between physician and nurse in developing a plan for teaching is essential. However, it is not appropriate for the nurse to wait for a physician's order before considering the patient's need for instruction. Often the nurse assumes that the physician is teaching the patient, and the physician assumes the nurse is teaching him.

Diabetes is especially prevalent among the elderly. Many older diabetics can learn to care for themselves if they are given sufficient time, instruction, and help in overcoming disabilities of age (using a magnifying glass to see the markings on a syringe clearly or to read the label on a medicine bottle, for example). Although it is useful for a family member to learn how to care for the elderly person, excluding the patient from instruction and concentrating on teaching a family member should be avoided unless it is clear that the patient cannot assume responsibility for his own treatment.

Diet

What the patient eats is one of the most pertinent factors in controlling diabetes. If his intake of carbohydrate is more than he can use or store, eventually he will go into ketosis. If he eats too little food, he ultimately will not only become malnourished but also, if he is taking insulin, be in danger of *hyper*-insulinism with resultant *hypo*glycemia. Prevention of hypoglycemia involves following the diet, both in *quantity* and *quality*, that is prescribed.

The Prescribed Diet. When a physician is calculating a diabetic diet, he takes into account the sex, the age, the height and weight, the activity, the state of health, the former dietary habits and the cultural background of the patient. A professional tennis or hockey player needs a different diet than would a secretary or writer. Having diabetes does not obviate the patient's need for a well-balanced diet adapted to his individual life situation.

Exchange Lists. The American Diabetes Association, the American Dietetic Association, and the Public Health Service have jointly prepared exchange lists which assist the patient with meal planning. There are several lists of foods, with each item measured by cup or spoon. On any one list the patient can exchange one item for any other and still obtain approximately the same food value. Thus, if the diet allows one meat exchange for lunch, the person can check a list and see that he can have an ounce of meat or chicken, an egg, a slice of cheese, ¼ cup of canned fish, or a frankfurter. Without deviating from the diet, he can choose freely from the list of unrestricted vegetables.

The following foods are usually excluded from a diabetic diet: sugar, candy, honey, jam, jelly, marmalade, preserves, syrup, molasses, pie, cake, cookies, condensed milk, chewing gum and soft drinks.

The patient should be told that alcohol has a high caloric value. Any alcohol consumed should be counted in the total diet. A large intake of alcohol is not advised, because the high caloric value adds greatly to the amount of calories in the prescribed diet, thus reducing the permissible intake of foods necessary for adequate nutrition.

The following foods are usually unrestricted: unsweetened gelatin, clear and fat-free broth, unsweetened pickles, cranberries, rhubarb, coffee and tea, and certain salads.

Dietetic Products. A number of sugarless products are on the market today. The physician's approval should be sought before they are used. There are two precautions: first, the fats, proteins, and carbohydrates in such foods still have to be counted within the framework of the patient's diet; second, it is important for diabetic patients who wish to buy these commercially produced foods to *read the label.* The sugar, fat, and protein contents should be listed. "Low calorie" and "dietetic" are not synonymous with "no sugar."

Teaching the Patient. As is the case with anyone going on a diet, the patient may need help in understanding why it is necessary and in not feeling discouraged. It is important that diabetics eat at prescribed intervals throughout the day to provide a steady supply of carbohydrate in relation to the amount and the kind of medication that they take. This requirement is especially applicable to patients on insulin. A midafternoon slice of toast and a snack before retiring are often calculated in the diet plan for patients taking insulin.

Before leaving the hospital, the patient should know how to realistically plan menus for meals and snacks according to the prescribed diet. Ideally, the patient should be allowed gradually to select and to plan his own diet, with help, before going home.

Some diabetics can be controlled on diet alone. These patients have the disease in a mild form; usually, its onset is later in life. The diabetic who is overweight may be placed on a weight-reduction diet by the physician. It is never healthy for a diabetic (or anyone else, for that matter) to become fat. Diabetes is aggravated by excess weight. If a patient is following his diet and is hungry, he must neither suffer in silence nor adjust his diet or insulin by himself; instead, he should tell his physician. If he is unable to eat at all, the physician must be notified immediately. A gastrointestinal upset that is minor for the nondiabetic is a medical emergency for the diabetic if it prevents him from eating the proper foods, or if it causes vomiting or diarrhea.

The better informed the patient is, the more effective will be the control that he will have of his disorder, and, therefore, the healthier he may stay.

Insulin

Insulin is medicine, but it is not a substance foreign to the body. New patients may be relieved to hear that what they are taking is a hormone that is a normal element of the body. Unfortunately, insulin is inactivated by gastrointestinal juices, and therefore it must be injected. Table 36-1 lists insulin preparations.

It is the nurse's responsibility to safeguard the hospitalized patient by insuring the correct timing of insulin injection and meals. This is one medication that should always be given on time. If the patient is fasting for a blood-glucose or glucose tolerance test, or for any other reason he does not eat, he should not be given insulin until 15 to 30 minutes before he takes his regular meal. Exact timing is most important with the quick-acting insulins.

Insulin should be kept in a cool place but does not need to be refrigerated. Insulin must not be placed near heat (radiators, etc.) or on a windowsill. In very hot weather it may be necessary to place insulin in the lower part of the refrigerator and then allow it to warm to room temperature before administration. On trips, the insulin can be placed in an insulated bag.

Insulin bottles carry an expiration date; the patient should be shown where the dates are stamped and instructed to check these dates periodically. Outdated insulin should *not* be used.

Injecting Insulin. Insulin comes in units. Units are clearly marked on the bottle and on the insulin

Table 36-1.
Insulin preparations

Insulin	Onset	Peak	Duration
Rapid-Acting Insulins			
Insulin injection USP (regular insulin, regular Iletin)	½–1 hour	2–6 hours	5–8 hours
Prompt insulin zinc suspension (Semilente Iletin, Semilente Insulin)	½–1 hour	3–9 hours	12–16 hours
Intermediate-Acting Insulins			
Globin zinc insulin	1–4 hours	6–16 hours	16–24 hours
Insulin zinc suspension (Lente Insulin, Lente Iletin)	1–4 hours	7–12 hours	24–36 hours
Isophane insulin suspension (NPH Insulin, NPH Iletin)	1–2 hours	7–12 hours	24–30 hours
Long-Acting Insulins			
Extended insulin zinc suspension (Ultralente Iletin, Ultralente Insulin)	4–8 hours	10–30 hours	34–46 hours
Protamine zinc insulin suspension (Protamine, Zinc and Iletin)	1–8 hours	12–24 hours	30–36 hours

Note: References may vary slightly on these figures.

syringe. U40 means that 1 ml. contains 40 units; U80 means that 1 ml. contains 80 units, and so on. The physician usually specifies both the *dose* and the *type* of insulin to be used, such as "Regular Insulin, 10U." When picking up the syringe, the first thing to do is to match the correct scale to the bottle and the patient's ordered dose.

Teaching the Patient. The patient should be taught to vary the site of the injection, so that no two injections are closer than 1 inch to each other within a 2-week period. Repeatedly using the same site might cause tissue damage. Insulin lipoatrophy, which is atrophy of subcutaneous fat, is an all too common reaction to repeated insulin injections into the same area. It causes deep depressions of the skin and gives an undesirable cosmetic appearance. Lipohypertrophy, which is spongy, painless swelling, also is unsightly. Insulin is poorly absorbed when injected into such damaged tissue.

Almost all diabetics who need insulin can and should be taught to inject it themselves. Because injection is a daily procedure, it is important that the patient be independent and have control over his own regimen. Teaching can start with the new diabetic in the hospital as soon as he has experienced relief of symptoms and a treatment regimen has been established by his physician. First, he needs to know the essentials of sterile technique: how to pick up, put down, and hold the syringe without contaminating the needle or the plunger; to wash his hands, and to scrub the vial top with alcohol or another antiseptic. He is shown how to withdraw the insulin; to clean the injection site; to insert the needle, to pull back on the plunger, and to shift his fingers to push the plunger in.

Teaching is done in steps with each step of the program presented clearly and in logical order (Table 36-2). One of the easiest tasks to learn is urine testing, and this is often taught first. It is not easy to learn to insert a needle into the flesh of another person. For many people it is even harder, initially, to give an injection to themselves. It may help some patients to get the feel of the resistance of skin if they first inject solution into an orange. For the first injection into his own skin, the nurse may wish to guide the patient's hands. Remember that although injections have become commonplace to the nurse, they are not so to the majority of others.

For safety's sake, one other member of the family

Table 36-2.
Points to be covered in a diabetic teaching program

Urine Testing
When to test urine
How to test urine
Materials used to test urine
Insulin
Type(s) of insulin to be used by the patient
How to buy insulin: checking labels regarding the correct type of insulin, expiration dates—before leaving the drugstore
How to store insulin
How to measure insulin in the syringe to be used
Principles of aseptic technique
How to withdraw insulin from the bottle
Administration of insulin and rotation sites
Signs of hypoglycemia; what to do if hypoglycemia occurs
Wearing of identification tags or bracelets such as Medic-Alert

should learn to give insulin in case the patient cannot do it for himself. The relative can be taught in the hospital, at home, or in the clinic. The clinic is an ideal place for group teaching. Informal classes in diet, foot care, insulin, and urine testing can lead to group discussions concerning the problems that diabetes causes. One patient may help others.

The necessity for periodic evaluation of the way the patient is caring for himself cannot be overemphasized. Too often a brief program of instruction is given to the newly diagnosed diabetic without necessary follow-up. Often the patient is uncertain about aspects of his self-care, and soon makes mistakes.

When the patient's ability to carry out his own care is evaluated, it is more effective to ask him to explain what he does and to demonstrate how he does it, than merely to repeat to him the instructions which he may have heard many times, but which he may misunderstand or apply incorrectly.

Oral hypoglycemic agents

There are two groups of oral hypoglycemic agents: the sulfonylureas, which act by stimulating the beta cells of the pancreas to secrete more insulin; and the biguanides, whose action is not clearly understood.

In the first group are such drugs as tolbutamide (Orinase), chlorpropamide (Diabinese) and acetohexamide (Dymelor). These agents cannot lower blood sugar in a patient who has no pancreas, or in a patient whose pancreas cannot be stimulated to release more insulin. Undesirable side effects include liver damage (the patient should be observed for jaundice), especially with chlorpropamide; allergy (skin manifestations seem most common); gastrointestinal disturbances; and, rarely, bone-marrow depression. When alcohol is ingested, there may be flushing and headache. Hypoglycemia may occur; this is more frequent with chlorpropamide and acetohexamide than with tolbutamide.

Phenformin (DBI, Meltrol) is in the biguanide group of oral hypoglycemic agents. There are two types of phenformin: regular tablets and timed-disintegration tablets. Side effects include gastrointestinal symptoms, a metallic taste and, rarely, ketonuria and lactic-acid acidosis, which may occur with little or no glycosuria. Side effects are especially likely to occur in patients with hepatic and renal disease. It is important that patients receiving phenformin routinely test their urine for ketone bodies as well as for glucose, and that they have periodic determinations of the plasma bicarbonate level.

A danger of these oral medications is that the patient may underestimate the danger in the progression of his disease; he may fail to remain under medical supervision, or he may neglect his diet, his feet, or testing his urine. He may erroneously believe that his disease can be ignored, because taking a pill is so much simpler than the injections taken by others with the same diagnosis. In talking with the patient the nurse should help him to recognize the need for care, but to lessen anxiety which can interfere with his ability to care for himself.

Exercise

Exercise is good for diabetes. It improves the circulation, which frequently is rather poor, and it helps to metabolize carbohydrate, thus decreasing the insulin requirement. Of course, if a patient sits at his desk all day Friday and plays touch football Saturday, he will have wide fluctuations in his blood sugar. If his schedule calls for such differences in activity, he should consult his physician, who may regulate his food and insulin requirements accordingly, and advise him to revise his schedule. During exercise it is especially important for the patient who takes insulin to carry some food or other physician-approved form of glucose with him, which he can eat if he feels any of the symptoms of hypoglycemia. (Diabetics should always have some form of easy-to-eat carbohydrate in their pockets or purses, in case hypoglycemia occurs in such inconvenient places as a subway or a concert hall.)

Complications

Diabetic ketosis and coma

The early symptoms of ketosis may be vague, but they become more definite—and serious—as more and more ketone bodies accumulate in the bloodstream unchecked. The patient may have weakness, thirst, anorexia, vomiting, drowsiness, and abdominal pain. The cheeks may be flushed, and the skin and mouth may be dry. There may be an odor of acetone on the breath. Kussmaul breathing, fast, deep and labored, may be evident. The pulse often is rapid and weak, and the blood pressure is low. If the patient is unconscious, he probably will be restless.

Diabetic coma now occurs less often than formerly, due to more effective regulation of the disease and greater emphasis on teaching patients and families. However, it still occurs. In some instances the patient develops coma in spite of having carefully followed his physician's recommendations. Such patients may be in the group of severe diabetics whose disease is hard to control. On occasion a patient is admitted to the hospital in diabetic coma who had not known previously that he was a diabetic. Diabetic coma also occurs with greater frequency among persons who have inadequate medical care. One of the most common causes of diabetic coma is infection.

Diagnosis. Only nonspecific treatment (such as intravenous fluids to help to correct the circulatory collapse and the electrolyte imbalance) is instituted when diabetes is known or suspected, until blood and urine samples are taken for the determination of glucose and ketone bodies, electrolytes, and CO_2 combining power to confirm the presence and degree of diabetic coma.

If the patient is comatose, he is catheterized, and a retention urinary catheter may be left in place for future specimens. Some hospitals have a coma cart on which the necessary equipment for diagnosis and treatment of this emergency is assembled, so that it is readily available when a patient in coma is admitted. The cart contains urine specimen bottles, test tubes, tubes for blood-glucose and CO_2 combining power tests, intravenous fluids, gastric lavage, and catheterization sets.

Treatment and Nursing Management. Treatment for coma includes the administration of regular insulin. Insulin lessens the production of ketones by making carbohydrate available for oxidation by the tissues and restoring the liver's supply of glycogen. Regular, rather than long-acting, insulin is given for rapid effect.

The nurse observes for a patent airway and suctions mucus away when necessary, keeps the patient flat in bed, and notes changes in the patient's condition that indicate deepening of the coma or response to therapy. The nurse keeps the intake and output record, writes down the results of the urine testing each time a test is performed, and charts the insulin given and her own observations of the patient's symptoms, so that the most current information is always immediately and easily available to the physician.

Insulin may be given every half-hour, and the urine may be tested as often. The nurse should watch for signs of muscular weakness and difficulty in breathing. The patient may be suffering from potassium depletion. Supplementary potassium may be ordered. An enema or gastric aspiration may be necessary, since patients may have gastric dilatation. The gastric contents of a dilated stomach may be vomited and aspirated by the partially comatose patient. In severe circulatory collapse epinephrine or caffeine and a blood transfusion may be needed.

As the patient recovers and is able to take fluids by mouth, the physician may order milk, salty broth, orange juice, or oatmeal gruel, approximately 120 ml. every hour. Until the patient is well out of danger, the nurse stays with him, taking vital signs, collecting urine specimens when called for, and giving insulin as ordered. Specimens of blood and urine continue to be tested for glucose at frequent intervals; and treatment with insulin and carbohydrate feedings (to prevent episodes of *hypo*glycemia), fluids, and electrolytes continues until the diabetes is regulated. Long-term management with diet and insulin resumes.

Hypoglycemic reaction (hyperinsulinism)

When there is too much insulin in the bloodstream in relation to the amount of available glucose—in other words, when blood glucose goes below about 60 mg. per 100 ml. of blood—hypoglycemia results.

Symptoms. The pattern of symptoms varies somewhat from patient to patient, depending on the degree of hypoglycemia, the patient's individual reaction, and the type of insulin taken. For example, the symptoms of overdose may be headache, nausea, drowsiness, and a feeling of malaise. Many patients who are having an insulin reaction initially experience weakness, nervousness, hunger, tremors, and excessive perspiration.

Some patients have characteristic personality changes. One may become negativistic; another, weepy. Confusion, aphasia, delirium, and vertigo may occur. If the hypoglycemia is not relieved, the symptoms may progress to difficulty with coordination, and the patient may see double. If he still is untreated, he may have convulsions and become unconscious; if he is neglected further, he may suffer permanent brain damage, and in very rare cases he may die. The symptoms are variable, but they have a tendency to be repeated in the same person whenever he has too much insulin and too little food. The sequence may be extremely rapid, with the patient convulsing or dropping into unconsciousness before any other symptoms are noticed.

When a diabetic patient is found unconscious, he may be suffering from diabetic coma or insulin reaction. Although it is the physician who makes the diagnosis and prescribes the treatment, nurses and patients should be familiar with the symptoms of both coma and hypoglycemia, so that these can be noticed in their early stages (Table 36-3).

TREATMENT AND NURSING MANAGEMENT. The treatment for insulin reaction is carbohydrate. If the patient is conscious and able to swallow, he is given orange juice, candy, warm tea or coffee with sugar, honey or a dextrose solution. If the patient is unconscious, dextrose will be given intravenously. Whenever there is a diabetic on the unit, there should always be some orange juice in the refrigerator, some sugar in the sugar bowl, and some intravenous dextrose. In a severe reaction the patient may need repeated feedings before the symptoms of insulin reaction are relieved. The physician may order glucagon to increase the patient's alertness and to stimulate the liver to release some of its store of glycogen.

Patients who develop personality reactions are often not able to treat themselves with sugar, so someone else must do it. While the patient who feels faint and weak often is viewed as sick, the one who becomes obstinate or aggressive may not be treated as promptly. Asking such a patient, "Would you like to have some sugar?" usually evokes the response, "No!" Instead, the nurse should hand him the sugar or the glass of orange juice, see that he takes it, observe his response, and notify the physician. It is important to teach nursing aides, the family, and anyone else who may be with the patient that personality change may represent a hypoglycemic reaction and should be treated as such.

Insulin reaction is as much a medical emergency as is diabetic coma. The nurse stays with the patient, observing him, and participating in therapeutic measures. After such an episode the regulation of the patient's metabolism is very difficult for about 24 hours, and he should be closely observed for further symptoms of imbalance.

Table 36-3.
Symptoms of hyper- and hypoinsulinism

	HYPOINSULINISM (DIABETIC COMA)	HYPERINSULINISM
History	Insufficient or omitted insulin Intercurrent infection Dietary indiscretion Gastrointestinal upset	Excessive insulin Unusual exercise Too little food
Onset	Slow, hours to days	Sudden, minutes
Skin	Flushed, dry, hot	Pale, moist, cool
Behavior	Drowsy	Excited
Breath	Acetone	Normal
Respirations	Rapid, weak	Normal to rapid, shallow
Pulse	Air hunger	Normal or slow; full, bounding
Blood pressure	Low	Normal
Vomiting	Present	May be absent
Hunger	Absent	Often present
Thirst	Present	Absent
Urinary sugar	Large amounts	Absent in 2nd specimen
Response to treatment	Slow	Rapid

Adapted from Lilly Research Laboratories: *Diabetes Mellitus.*

Poor regulation of carbohydrate metabolism, with the dangers of diabetic coma, on the one hand, and of hypoglycemia, on the other, may be brought about by ignorance of or carelessness by the patient, by an infection, or by extreme emotional stress. A patient who has been well-regulated may become depressed and not care any longer; may fail to keep his diet or refuse to test his urine and to take insulin. A gastrointestinal upset with vomiting may force him to eat less. He may then reason that he needs less insulin, and cut down on his daily dose. This is a dangerous fallacy, and it may lead to ketosis, because illness often increases the need for insulin. Nurses should teach diabetic patients that any slight illness, such as a head cold, is an indication for more frequent testing of the urine, and for particularly careful adherence to the regimen of diet and insulin or oral hypoglycemic agent. If ketonuria is present, or if the slight illness persists or grows worse, the patient should see his physician.

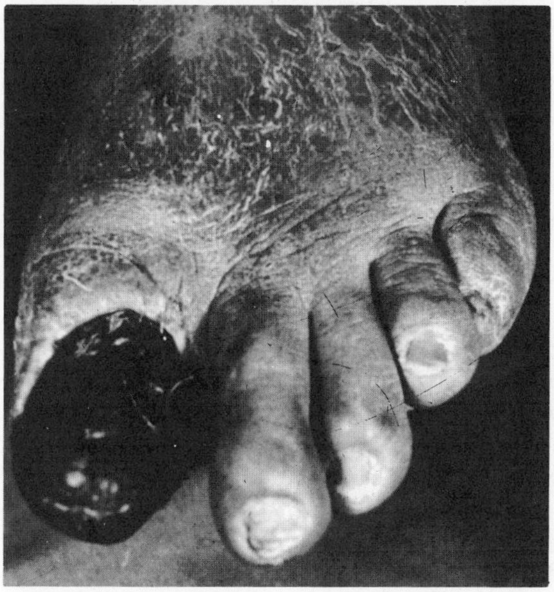

figure 36-1. Gangrene of toe. (Dr. W. L. Lowrie, Detroit)

Vascular disturbances

Diabetics are particularly prone to circulatory disturbances. The incidence of arteriosclerosis in diabetics is higher than in nondiabetics. Why this is so is not known. In addition, there are many vascular changes in the diabetic, some of which are not seen in nondiabetics, and some of which become more severe when the metabolic aspects of the disorder are poorly controlled. For example, an almost consistent finding in diabetic patients is thickening of the walls of some capillaries, arterioles, and venules. It is suspected that these pathologic changes start before there are any symptoms of diabetes, and this is one reason that attention is turned to the identification of prediabetic people.

Any part of the body can be affected by vascular disturbances, but nerves, eyes, kidneys, and legs are particularly likely to be affected. The lower extremities are especially vulnerable to changes brought about by decreased blood supply to the tissues. Because of lessened blood supply, cramps may occur; infection is not fought effectively and may lead to ulcer formation and eventually to gangrene (Fig. 36-1), which may necessitate amputation. Surgery is an added strain on the body, and the surgeon and internist must work closely together to regulate the patient's diabetes during the period of extra stress. Uncontrolled diabetes frequently retards wound healing.

Visual problems

In diabetics the retinal capillaries tend to develop multiple tiny aneurysms, accompanied by small points of hemorrhage and by exudates. The scarring resulting from repeated hemorrhages may eventually cause blindness.

The partially sighted diabetic may have difficulty seeing the tiny markings on a syringe. A thin strip of tape on the syringe can underline the point at which he should stop the plunger when pulling back. There are also magnifying attachments for insulin syringes.

Neuropathy

Any nerve tissue can be affected. There may be facial paralysis, atony of urinary bladder, diarrhea, or constipation. However, the legs are most frequently affected. The patient may experience itching, numbness, tingling, and pain, which often is aggravated at night. There also may be a loss of sensation, so that the patient does not feel intense heat and can be burned without realizing it.

Nephropathy

Nodular glomerulosclerosis is frequent among diabetics. The symptoms include albuminuria, edema, and hypertension. Renal failure may be the outcome.

Infection

In patients with diabetes, infections heal slowly, and the diabetes itself becomes more severe while the infection persists. Tuberculosis is more frequent in diabetics than in nondiabetics. Carbuncles and furuncles can be a major problem. A cardinal rule for diabetics is: call the physician at the *first* sign of any illness. The patient with a common cold should go to bed, drink copious fluids, test his urine, and call the physician. Any skin eruption should be brought to the physician's attention.

Prognosis

Although diabetics do not have as long a life expectancy as nondiabetics, there has been significant increase in life expectancy as a result of modern therapy, and, in part, probably as a result of other health measures, such as emphasis among the population as a whole on the hazards of obesity. Patients whose disease is treated within the first year of its discovery outlive those whose treatment is delayed. The patient who understands the disease and whose morale is high is better able to keep diabetes under control than is the ignorant or depressed patient.

Social aspects

Prejudice against hiring diabetics is common. Some employers fear that insulin reaction or coma will occur on the job, or that time will be lost due to illness. The prejudice seems unjustified. Well-regulated diabetics can enter a variety of occupations, such as teaching, nursing, medicine, and carpentry. However, employers should know that a person is diabetic, just in case he should need care while he is on the job. The prejudice against employing diabetics leads to concealment of the fact that diabetes is present.

Diabetics need not be conspicuous socially. A diabetic can eat in restaurants by estimating portions and sticking to foods of known composition. He can pack his own box lunch for picnics.

Travelers can carry their syringes and needles in metal cases that are specially designed to maintain sterility. Or they can boil the syringe and the needle, using a commercial plug with metal prongs that fits into a cup and boils water in 2 minutes. Disposable insulin syringes and needles are also available.

Helping the patient to acknowledge the condition and to adapt his way of life accordingly, is a challenge for the nurse. Assisting the patient to recognize the choices open to him (for instance, the choice between learning to follow a diet and becoming ill from unregulated diabetes) and helping him to learn from his own experiences are measures which can assist the patient to deal effectively with his condition. Too often threats and dire warnings are used in an attempt to frighten the patient into following instructions. Sometimes the nurse adopts a "policeman" role, searching the patient's bedside stand periodically for forbidden food. Such measures are largely ineffective. The decisions about self-care and the will to abide by them must be fostered within the patient since in most instances he carries the responsibility for his own care.

General nutritional considerations

- Diet is as much a part of the treatment of diabetes as is drug therapy with insulin and oral hypoglycemic agents. The patient must understand the importance of diet and that the use of drugs to treat diabetes does *not* allow him to eat any foods he desires.
- The diabetic diet is prescribed in calories (usually 30 to 35 calories per kilogram of body weight), and the amounts of allowed fat, carbohydrate, and protein is expressed in *grams.*
- The daily intake (in grams) of fat, carbohydrate, and protein is divided according to the type of insulin the patient is receiving. Thus the patient receiving intermediate-acting insulin will eat the greatest amount of food during the peak hours of the insulin's action and only a small snack at night before retiring. The patient on long-acting insulin will usually have a larger evening meal and a snack before retiring. The diabetic controlled only by diet will have a different distribution of food than the patient on an oral hypoglycemic agent or insulin.
- The dietary plan for the diabetic will also be based on his physical activities, type of work, age, food preferences and eating habits.
- The diet is prescribed by the physician, for example: 1800 calories, 80 grams protein, 80 grams fat, 180 grams carbohydrate. The dietitian will then plan a diet that includes foods that can be eaten; for example, breakfast might be composed of:
  1 fruit exchange
  2 bread exchanges
  1 meat exchange
  1 milk exchange
  2 fat exchanges
- The patient will have a list of foods that can be used for the exchanges. In the breakfast above, 2 bread exchanges for this patient

might be 2 slices of bread, and 1 milk exchange might be 8 ounces of milk.

■ The patient will require time to understand what to eat and how to substitute and use exchanges. The dietitian can also supply literature, exchange lists, sample menus, lists of foods to be avoided, etc.

General pharmacological considerations

■ There are three types of insulin: (1) rapid-acting insulin, (2) intermediate-acting insulin, and (3) long-acting insulin.

■ Three properties of insulin—onset, peak, and duration—are of importance. Onset is *when* the insulin first begins to act in the body; peak is the time when insulin is exerting *maximum action,* and duration is the length of time the insulin remains *in effect.*

■ Insulin is used to treat juvenile-onset diabetes and maturity-onset diabetes that cannot be controlled with oral hypoglycemic agents and diet.

■ Oral hypoglycemic agents are used to treat maturity-onset diabetes, usually of the patient who can be controlled on 40 or fewer units of insulin per day.

■ Hospital policy dictates the action(s) to be taken when a patient taking insulin or one of the sulfonylurea group of oral hypoglycemic agents experiences hypoglycemia. Most hospitals approve of the administration of oral glucose (fruit juice, Karo syrup and water, ginger ale, etc.) if the patient can safely swallow. The unconscious or semiconscious patient will require intravenous administration of 50 percent dextrose or glucagon.

■ Insulin is measured in *units* and is available in various strengths: U40, U80, U100. U40 means there are 40 units in each milliliter of solution. The insulin is measured in a syringe calculated to measure *units* of insulin. Various types of insulin syringes are available, e.g., a syringe to measure one specific strength of insulin such as a U40 syringe, or a syringe with two scales such as a U40/U80 syringe.

■ The measurement of insulin *must* be accurate as patients may be sensitive to minute dose changes. The patient should be checked for signs of hypoglycemia after the insulin is given, at the expected onset, and again at the peak of action.

■ Oral hypoglycemic drugs also must be given at the time of day ordered. The patient receiving one of the sulfonylureas is also observed for signs of hypoglycemia; however, the time the reaction might occur is not predictable and could be from 30 to 60 minutes to many hours after the drug is given.

Bibliography

BRUNNER, L. S. and SUDDARTH, D. S.: *Textbook of Medical-Surgical Nursing,* ed. 3. Philadelphia, Lippincott, 1975.

The diabetic foot: Ischemic or neuropathic? Patient Care 5:38, January 30, 1971.

Diabetic ketoacidosis. Emergency Med. 5:103, February, 1973.

FULTON, M. et al: Helping diabetics adapt to failing vision. Am. J. Nurs. 74:54, January, 1974.

GRANCIO, S. D.: Nursing care of the adult diabetic patient. Nurs. Clin. North Am. 8:605, December, 1973.

GUTHRIE, D. and GUTHRIE, R.: Coping with diabetic ketoacidosis. Nurs. '73, 3:14, November, 1973.

KIMBLE, M. A.: Diabetes. Nurs. Dig. 2:113, November/December, 1974.

KINTZEL, K. C. et al, eds.: *Advanced Concepts in Clinical Nursing.* Philadelphia, Lippincott, 1971.

MALONE, J. I.: Diabetic ketoacidosis: Dangerous but preventable. Consultant 15:39, September, 1975.

MITCHELL, H. S. et al: *Nutrition in Health and Disease,* ed. 16. Philadelphia, Lippincott, 1976.

NICKERSON, D.: Teaching the hospitalized diabetic. Am. J. Nurs. 72:935, May, 1972.

O'CONNOR, M. L.: Glucose tolerance test. Nurs. '75, 5:10, July, 1975.

SCHERER, J. C.: *Introductory Clinical Pharmacology.* Philadelphia, Lippincott, 1975.

SCHUMANN, D.: Assessing the diabetic. Nurs. '76, 6:62, March, 1976.

TRAYSER, L. M.: A teaching program for diabetics. Am. J. Nurs. 73:92, January, 1973.

Understanding diabetes. Patient Care 9:34, June 1, 1975.

WILLIAMS, S. R.: *Nutrition and Diet Therapy,* ed. 2. St. Louis, Mosby, 1973.

UNIT NINE

Disturbances of sexual structures or reproductive function

CHAPTER 37

Introduction: the female reproductive pattern

On completion of this chapter the student will:

- **Discuss the emotional support given to the patient who has a gynecological problem.**
- **Label a drawing of the anatomy of the female reproductive system.**
- **Describe and discuss the normal physiology of the menstrual cycle and hormonal regulation during the cycle.**
- **Discuss the physiology, occurrence, symptoms of and the emotional reactions to menopause.**
- **Name the disorders of menstruation and describe the symptoms of each.**
- **Discuss fertility and infertility and the tests used to determine the possible cause(s) of infertility.**

The nurse and the gynecological patient

Emotional support

Besides the basic determination of a patient's physical needs, one of the fundamental requirements of effective nursing management of the gynecological patient is an ability to hear the patient's requests for reassurance and information and to recognize manifestations of anxiety. This ability demands sensitive listening because many patients, ashamed of their ignorance, will pose questions in anecdotal form or attribute them to friends and relatives. A nurse who is listening for such subtleties can often discover the nature of a patient's anxiety and can help by allowing the patient to verbalize her fears and by supplying facts and advice when necessary. It is well for the nurse to remember that patient whose gynecological symptoms are sufficient to require hospitalization is almost certain to be anxious. Many patients fear cancer. This fear is not confined to any one age group, although it usually increases with age, just as the likelihood of developing cancer becomes greater among women during and after menopause. If the patient asks the nurse if she has cancer, the nurse can explain that this is an appropriate question to ask the physician and encourage the patient to ask it. If the patient is afraid of the possibility of cancer, the nurse cannot remove this fear. But by listening supportively the nurse may be able to lessen it and help the patient think through just what it is that she fears.

In addition to cancer, fear of impairment or loss of reproductive capacity and reproductive organs may cause anxiety in a woman of child-bearing age. Many women fear that the capacity to respond sexually may be impaired or lost. Worry about how to support another child if the patient is pregnant is another concern. The possibility of abortion, natural or therapeutic, the relative merits of various birth control methods, and the ability to carry a fetus to term are other concerns a patient may wish to discuss with the nurse. It is important to create an atmosphere in which the patient feels free to broach these topics if she wishes. The nurse is one of the persons in whom the patient may confide, and, in confiding, the patient may gain confidence to discuss some of her anxieties with others, such as her physician, husband or clergyman.

Although her ability to listen may help the patient to define her fears, the nurse cannot supply answers to all of the patients' questions. It is often wise for the nurse to encourage the patient to discuss her fears with the physician. For example, a seemingly simple operation, such as a dilatation and curettage (D and C), may be performed for diagnostic purposes, the outcome of which will most certainly be of concern to

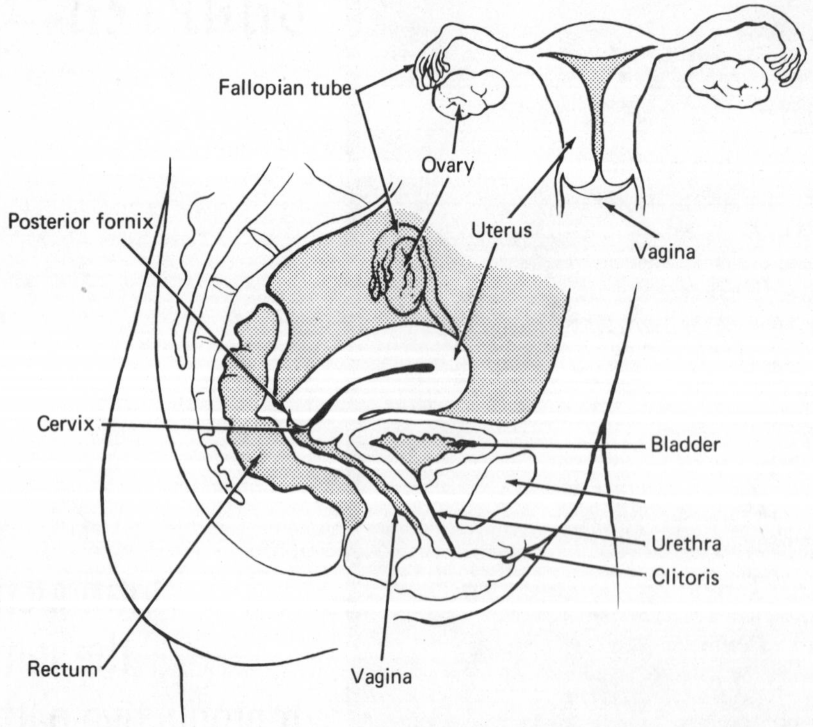

figure 37-1. Anatomy of female reproductive organs.

the patient. Or, a D and C may be performed on a patient who has aborted to remove products of conception that, if left in the uterus, would cause vaginal bleeding. Such patients require sensitive emphatic nursing care, and, because their hospitalizations are brief, they need nurses who can quickly "tune in" to them as women undergoing stress.

Teaching the patient

Community health is the rightful concern of every member of the health team. The nurse in the gynecological unit has the opportunity to counteract misguided notions about personal hygiene, menstruation, sexual intercourse, birth control, and venereal disease. Many women have little understanding of their own body processes. Some women may have received information about female reproductive functions from mothers and sisters who themselves were ill-informed and superstitious. How many gynecological patients believe that bathing is harmful during menstruation? How many take douches daily, using strong and potentially harmful solutions? With the nurse's help, admission to a gynecological service can provide women an opportunity to learn desirable health practices while they are treated for a particular gynecological disturbance. Responsible nursing practice means that the nurse takes every opportunity to correct her patient's misunderstandings regarding her own physiology and care.

Anatomy and physiology applied

When catheterizing female patients, remember that the urethral opening is between the clitoris and the vagina (Figs. 37-1 and 37-2). A good light is necessary in order to find these landmarks prior to insertion of the catheter tip. If the tip enters the vagina accidentally, a new catheter should be used, since the vagina is not sterile. In this event, the used catheter should be discarded in the area set aside for contaminated supplies. Because the clitoris is a very sensitive organ, poking it with the catheter may cause the patient discomfort. The nurse spreads the labia first, by placing her fingers carefully so that she does not have to change their position during the procedure, thereby contaminating the area.

Since the vagina is not sterile, and the bladder is sterile, vaginal irrigations are usually done with clean technique, whereas catheterization is always a sterile procedure. Douching usually is contraindicated during late pregnancy and postoperatively. Although the perineal area is not sterile, some situations may require sterile technique in perineal care when clean technique would normally be used. The area is always wiped anteriorly to posteriorly, and a new cotton ball or sponge is used for each stroke to avoid bringing any organisms from the anal area to the vagina or the urethra.

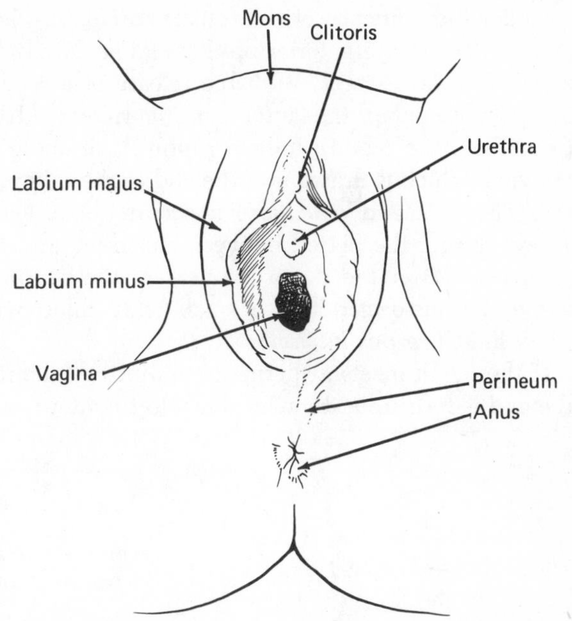

figure 37-2. Diagram of female external genitalia.

Because the urethral opening is so close to the vagina, postoperative care of surgical perineal wounds is often complicated by voiding problems. Dressings should be changed whenever they become wet. After gynecological surgery, patients may have a catheter in place, and catheterization may be ordered preoperatively to empty the bladder and to avoid accidental trauma to the bladder during surgery.

The menstrual cycle

Menarche, the start of menstruation, usually occurs between ages 10 and 14. If menses, even if irregular, have not begun by the time a girl is 15 or 16, the parents should be advised to take her to a gynecologist who will look for endocrine imbalance, an imperforate hymen, and congenital anomalies. The hymen normally contains an opening adequate to allow the menstrual flow to occur. Occasionally there is no opening in the hymen, and the menstrual flow is held back.

Physiology

Under the influence of the follicle-stimulating hormone (FSH) of the anterior pituitary (Fig. 37-3), the ovarian follicle matures. With the release of a second pituitary hormone, the luteinizing hormone (LH) (Fig. 37-3), the mature follicle ruptures, discharging the ovum, which is drawn into the end of the fallopian tube. This is called *ovulation*; it occurs about every 28 days during the period between menarche and the menopause. After the ovum is released, the ruptured follicle is transformed into a small body filled with yellow fluid (*corpus luteum*).

If the ovum meets a spermatozoon in the fallopian tube and is fertilized, it moves down to the uterus and implants itself in the endometrium, which is prepared to receive it. If fertilization does not occur, the ovum passes through the uterus and vagina and is expelled from the body.

Whether the ovum is fertilized or not, the *endometrium*, a highly vascular glandular tissue lining the inside of the uterus, prepares itself for a possible pregnancy. The development of the uterine endometrium is governed by the hormone estrogen, produced by the maturing ovarian follicle. The follicle is under the influence of FSH. Estrogen production is in turn probably regulated by LH. After the follicle has ruptured, the corpus luteum produces another hormone, progesterone. This stimulates a change in the endometrium,

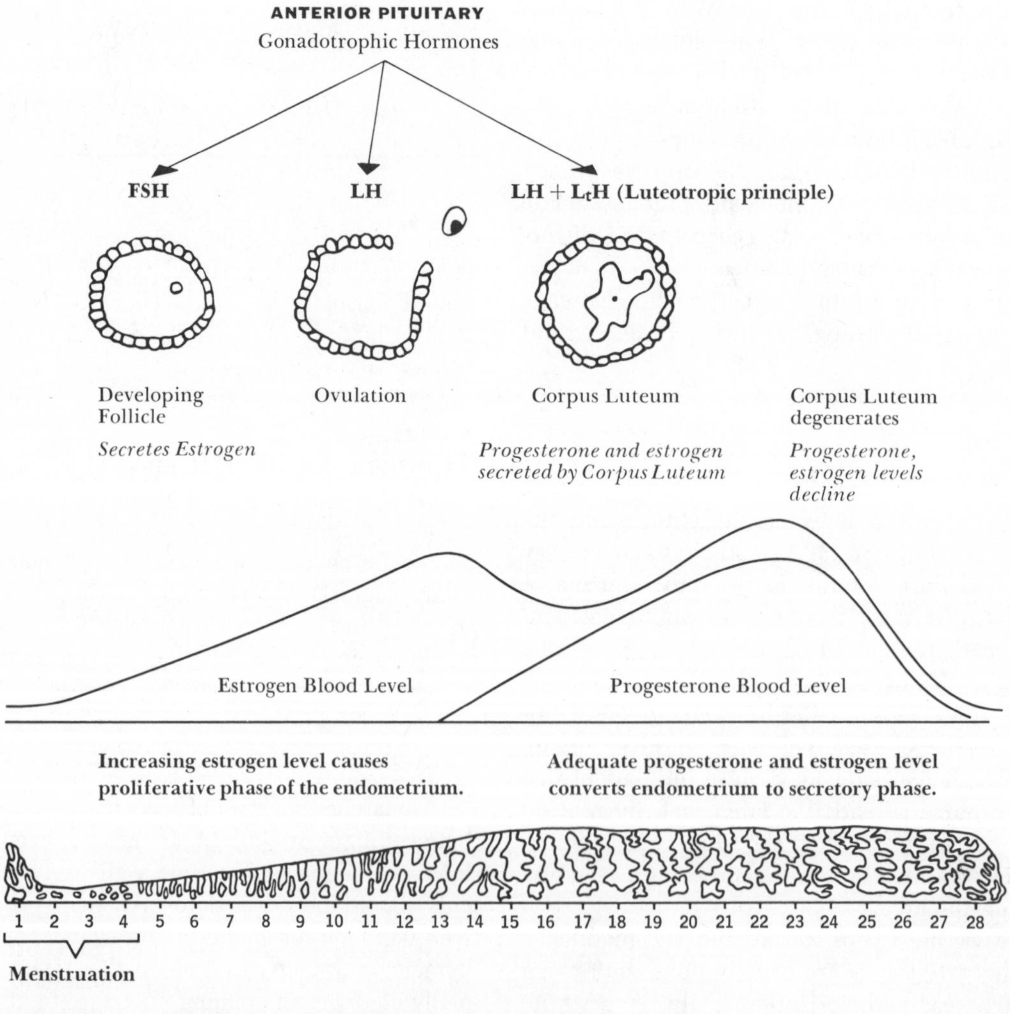

figure 37-3. Simplied version of the normal menstrual cycle. (The Upjohn Company, Kalamazoo, Mich.)

making it richer and thicker in preparation for a possible fertilized ovum. The production of FSH is now inhibited.

If the ovum is not fertilized, the prepared endometrium degenerates, and the menstrual flow begins about 2 weeks after ovulation. After menstruation, the endometrium again begins to grow thicker and more vascular. Because of these cyclical, hormone-dependent changes, the microscopic picture of the uterus is almost constantly changing. Thus it is important that each gynecological specimen sent to the laboratory, such as vaginal smears or curettings obtained by scraping the uterus, be marked with the date of the beginning of the patient's last menstrual period.

When conception occurs, the corpus luteum persists during early pregnancy. When conception does not occur, the corpus luteum degenerates and shrinks, and the thickened endometrium sheds its outer layers with some bleeding. Menstrual flow usually lasts 4 to 5 days, with a loss of 30 to 180 ml. of blood.

Helping the adolescent to understand

The onset of puberty is characterized by breast development, redistribution of body fat, the growth of pubic and axillary hair, and the beginnings of menstruation. The young girl experiencing these changes in herself and in her peers may be very confused and ill prepared to cope with them. The nurse may be called upon to give advice and information.

Since puberty proceeds at different rates for different individuals, many young girls feel embarrassed or ashamed either because they have developed these secondary sex characteristics or because they have not. It helps these young people to know that they will have caught up with one another before they graduate from high school. The nurse can explain this when girls express concern about it. A girl may wonder, but not ask, about the normal vaginal secretion that occurs between menses. If she knows that most women have this discharge, she may be saved some worry.

The amount of discomfort experienced during menses is significantly related to attitudes toward menstruation and femininity. This, of course, does not rule out the possibility of disease or abnormality, and any woman, regardless of age who experiences severe dysmenorrhea should be advised to have a gynecological examination. Actually, the 4 or 5 days of discharge should be accompanied by little or no discomfort. Most physicians believe that there is no reason to curtail activities during menstruation.

The menopause

The term *menopause* means the cessation of the menstrual cycle. The term *climacteric* is the long period during which ovarian activity gradually ceases. The terms are often used interchangeably, and this period of time is also called the "change of life." The menopause normally occurs between the ages of about 45 and 55.

Physiology

Ovulation gradually ceases and with it the menstrual cycle and the reproductive capacity. The change usually is not sudden; rather, the menses are scanty, or sometimes unusually copious, and irregular for a time before they stop permanently. The uterus, the vagina, and the vulva decrease in size. As ovarian function diminishes, so does the production of estrogen and progesterone. The resulting endocrine imbalance may lead to fatigability, nervousness, sweating, palpitation, severe headaches, vasomotor disturbance, and especially, hot flashes which may be so mild and so transitory that they almost escape notice, or which may last as long as two minutes and occur every ten to thirty minutes around the clock. In some instances the hot flashes are disturbing enough to interfere with sleep. Since normal and abnormal changes may readily be confused, it is especially important for women to have regular gynecological examinations during this period.

Emotional reactions

To many women the climacteric objectifies the relentlessness of the aging process. The reasons that women often interpret menopause in this way are many, and all centered around the experience of loss. But menopause need not signal the end of useful life to a woman unless she so chooses. Some examples of the fears that have been expressed by women undergoing menopause are:

- Loss of role. ("My children don't need me any more.") It is clear that this reaction has more to do with the age of the children than the physiological processes of the mother. Nevertheless, many women equate the two phenomena. The woman who has gradually sought experiences and satisfactions in addition to those of caring for her home and family is in a better position to continue this development during the climacteric than is the woman whose interests and satisfactions have been focused almost exclusively on her home and children.

- Concern for loss of marital relationship. ("Maybe my husband won't want me.") It may be that the woman who voices this fear is actually more afraid of some of the more general concerns of women in that age group; continued sexual satisfaction, wrinkles and grey hair, or perhaps her husband's response to his own aging.
- Loss of attractiveness and femininity. A regular program of enjoyable exercise (not just more housework if the woman is already bored by it), can counteract the tendency to weight gain and muscle flabbiness and provide stimulation and pleasure. Does the woman skate or just take her children to the rink? Does she swim or sit on the beach and watch? Branching out in her tastes, activities, and style of dress can help the woman look and feel more attractive. A new hair style, some new clothes, or learning a new skill can help her feel more confident and energetic.
- Fear of physical or mental disability. (Getting cancer or having a nervous breakdown.) Instead of just worrying that she might have cancer, the woman can go to the clinic twice yearly for a Pap smear and breast examination. Instead of withdrawing from her husband and wondering what his attitudes are about change of life she can talk with him about it, voicing some of her concerns and listening to his. The views of others who are significant to her, such as her husband and children, have important effects upon the woman who is going through the menopause.

Verbalizing such fears does not remove them, but can help the woman to begin to deal with her fears and can help her realize that others have similar concerns. The nurse can help the patient to consider what her own attitudes are toward menopause and aging. Often the woman has not sufficiently delineated her own views on this matter. If her adolescent children think it silly for their mother to return to college or to a job, does she have to agree with them?

Alertness for symptoms of depression among menopausal women is essential for nurses who work with these patients in hospitals or in the community. Depression can be so incapacitating that the patient may be unable to carry on any of her usual activities, or it can lead to suicide. The nurse should be especially observant for such communication from the patient as:

- Feelings of worthlessness and uselessness.
- Feelings of emptiness and hopelessness.
- Lack of interest in others and in usual activities.

If such indications of serious depression are observed, they should be reported immediately, so that the patient can be referred promptly for psychiatric treatment. It is difficult to relate to depressed and withdrawn persons. Therefore, the nurse should make a particular effort to make contact with the depressed patient and to show concern for her while the process of referral is going on and until she is receiving treatment for depression. Such concerned contact can help prevent further deepening of depression and can help prevent suicide.

Treatment

There has been considerable discussion, and some disagreement still exists among physicians, concerning the use of supplementary estrogens for menopausal and postmenopausal women. Some physicians consider the postmenopausal state virtually a deficiency condition and believe that supplementary estrogens should be prescribed. Those who subscribe to this view believe that the woman's overall health will be improved by estrogen administration and that the incidence and severity of some diseases of later life, such as osteoporosis, can be lessened by long-term estrogen therapy.

A more widely held view is that decisions concerning estrogen therapy must be individualized. One question the physician considers is whether the administration of estrogens may stimulate the growth of cancer in the uterus or breast. A patient with a history of uterine or breast cancer is not treated with supplementary estrogen, and patients who receive estrogen supplements are examined regularly for any sign of cancer of the uterus or breast. Some patients experience little discomfort at this period and do not require estrogen therapy. The primary consideration in therapy of menopause, according to physicians who advocate highly individualized treatment, is helping the woman to feel physically and emotionaly well. Estrogens, sedatives, tranquilizers, or mood elevating drugs may sometimes be prescribed to alleviate symptoms.

The climacteric can be precipitated by the surgical removal of the ovaries or by the radiological destruction of the ovarian function. Because of the suddeness of the artificially induced menopause, replacement therapy sometimes is given to supply the hormones of which the patient's body has been so abruptly deprived.

Disorders of menstruation

DYSMENORRHEA. Painful menstruation usually is idiopathic (primary dysmenorrhea) and no pathology is found. Mild symptoms are made more severe by fatigue, cold, and tension. Premenstrual tension is common. Edema may be present and is sometimes treated by diuretics and a low-sodium diet. In some women, discomfort is intensified by an emotional need for more satisfying human contacts. Others fear menstruation or are convinced that they really are sick during this time. Menstruation, by its regular occurrence, calls attention to one's femininity. One way of helping some women who have dysmenorrhea is to help them think through and accept the physiological phenomena as part of their physical selves, a part that will be with them for more than 20 years.

The patient who suffers from dysmenorrhea should visit the physician to uncover any possible pathology. If none is found, symptomatic relief can be given by the application of heat to the lower abdomen, a hot beverage, rest and, when ordered, aspirin. Primary dysmenorrhea is generally believed to be peculiar to ovulating women, and, therefore, appears to be related to progesterone in the second half of the menstrual cycle.

Dysmenorrhea may be secondary to other pathology, such as endometriosis, displacement of the uterus, or narrowing of the cervical canal. For some conditions, exercises may be suggested by the physician. For example, if dysmenorrhea is related to retroversion of the uterus (the uterus tilts backward), the knee-chest position may be prescribed. Surgery may sometimes be necessary, as, for example, in severe endometriosis. However, every effort is made to preserve child-bearing function. The main consideration in therapy of dysmenorrhea is to help the woman feel well throughout her menstrual cycle so that she can continue her accustomed activities. For women in whom emotional difficulties seem to play a prominent part in causing the painful menses, psychotherapy may be helpful.

AMENORRHEA, absense of menstrual flow, occurs normally before menarche, during pregnancy, after menopause, and sometimes throughout lactation if the new mother is breast-feeding her baby. The term oligomenorrhea means infrequent menses. Oligomenorrhea and amenorrhea may be caused by endocrine imbalance, some tumors of the endocrine glands, wasting chronic disease (such as tuberculosis or starvation), and psychogenic factors. There are variations in the extent to which emotional reactions affect the menses. The woman who misses periods should see a gynecologist to determine the cause.

MENORRHAGIA, excessive bleeding at the time of normal menstruation, may be caused by endocrine imbalance, fibroid tumors, emotional upsets, abnormalities of blood coagulation, ovarian cysts, uterine polyps, and a variety of other pelvic abnormalities. Unchecked menorrhagia can lead to anemia. Because the amount of blood loss is difficult to describe, a rough estimate can be made by asking the patient how many pads or tampons she uses a day. Menorrhagia is a symptom that should bring the patient to a gynecologist.

METRORRHAGIC, bleeding at a time other than a menstrual period, may consist of a slight pink or brownish spotting, or it may be frank bleeding. It can be caused by the same abnormalities that cause menorrhagia, or by various abnormalities in the vagina or cervix. Spotting may also occur in early pregnancy, and sometimes it is a warning symptom that abortion is imminent. Some women spot for a day or two midway between menstrual periods. This functional bleeding is thought to be at the time of ovulation and does not indicate pathology. However, metrorrhagia should always be brought to a physician's attention, because it may be an early indication of cancer. Postcoital bleeding may be an early symptom of cancer of the cervix. It is not the amount of blood that is important; it is the fact that it occurred when no bleeding was expected. Nurses should explain the necessity for a visit to the physician, stressing the importance of an examination but making every effort not to frighten the patient. The nurse who shows concern for the patient and who is supportive in her approach is more likely to persuade the patient to visit the physician than a nurse who uses scare techniques. Metrorrhagia may be difficult for the menopausal woman to identify if her periods have become irregular. Is the spotting a scanty menstrual flow or an abnormal symptom? When she is in doubt, she should consult a gynecologist, because intermenstrual bleeding is not a normal characteristic of the climacteric.

Fertility and infertility

Sperm are manufactured in the testes, pass in tubules through the epididymis into the vas deferens and are discharged into the urethra and out of the body by rhythmic contraction of the muscles of the vas deferens and the penis during the sexual climax. The accumulated fluid carrying the spermatozoa is called *semen.* It is alkaline; spermatozoa are rapidly immobilized in an acid environment. In human males, spermatozoa are produced continuously, even though they leave the body only periodically.

High in the fundus of the uterus are two openings for the fallopian tubes, along which ova travel from the ovaries to the uterus, and which sperm enter from the uterus. The tubes are about 4 inches long. After the ovum is shed from the ovary, movement of the cilia at the fimbriated end of the fallopian tube, and muscular contractions of the tube itself draw the ovum down toward the uterus. If the ovum is not fertilized it degenerates and is shed.

The volume of the normal semen ejaculate is 2.5 to 3.5 ml., in which there is an average of 100 million spermatozoa. For conception to occur, it is necessary for a spermatozoon to make its way, by movement of its taillike portion (Fig. 37-4), up the entire length of the uterus and into the fallopian tube, to find an ovum, and to insert its head into the ovum by piercing the outer coat (zona pellucida). Although the actual fertilization is by one spermatozoon, it is probably necessary for more than one sperm to be present in order to dissolve the zona pellucida sufficiently to allow one spermatozoon to enter. Usually, there is only one ovum as a result of ovulation; it is probable that many spermatozoa find their way into the fallopian tubes.

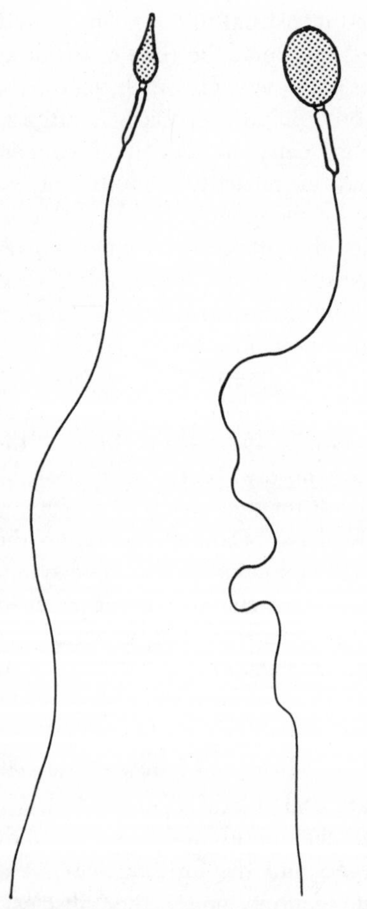

figure 37-4. Two normal spermatozoa. The long tails give the sperm motility.

Ovulation apparently occurs midway between menstrual periods, but in individuals there probably is variation in ovulation from month to month. Women are fertile, capable of becoming pregnant, soon after ovulation. Couples wishing to have a baby may be advised by their physician to have intercourse every other day, from the 10th through the 16th day after the first day of the woman's menstrual period. Alternating days allows for sperm buildup. Couples wanting a baby may not know about ovulation, and they may limit sexual intercourse to the times just before and after menses, when conception is least likely to take place, thus inadvertently practicing rhythm control of conception.

Basal body temperature (BBT) is a useful but far from infallible indication of when ovulation occurs. To determine BBT a woman takes her temperature when she first wakes up in the morning, before she drinks anything, smokes, or arises. Near ovulation there is a slight drop from normal body temperature, followed by a rise of 0.3 to 0.5 of a degree within the first 24 hours after ovulation.

In about one half of the couples the reproductive difficulty lies with the male. The causes of sterility in men can be general debility, hypopituitarism, hypothyroidism, obesity, infection, absence of a genital organ, undescended testicles (even when they are corrected), orchitis after mumps, irradiation of the testes, and mental stress. Conception can occur when the sperm count is as low as 2,250,000 spermatozoa per ml. of semen, but the chance of a sperm contacting an ovum is less than when the count is higher. In normal semen, 15 percent or less are nonmotile, and 20 percent or less are formed abnormally. When these percentages rise above 15 and 20 percent respectively, the chance of conception decreases.

Women, like men, may be infertile from systemic causes, or they may have problems interfering with normal ovulation such as a variety of endocrine disorders. Occluded tubes are a significant cause; gonorrheal, streptococcal or other infections can cause tubal strictures that prevent the ova from traveling down and the sperm cells from traveling up the tubes. Endometriosis is a common cause of infertility in women. In both men and women, psychological factors sometimes play an important part in causing infertility.

Diagnosis

When a woman is unable to conceive after several years of married life, she and her husband should be examined by the physician. He probably will give them a complete physical examination to rule out a possible systemic cause. Studies may be ordered to determine thyroid function, and the urine may be examined for pituitary gland function. The husband may be examined first, because his examination can be made more readily (Table 37-1).

Treatment

If a systemic disorder, such as endocrine imbalance or infection, is causing the infertility, the physician will treat the underlying disorder. Tubal strictures may be treated by surgery, though the operation is rarely successful. Uterine displacement may be treated by the use of a pessary and exercise or by surgery.

In some infertile couples, no physiological defect can be found. There is a psychic factor in fertility that is poorly understood. Sometimes a pregnancy occurs only after the couple has given up hope of conceiving and have adopted a child.

Nurses can help the couple by making sure that each partner knows how and when the ovum is fertilized so that intercourse is not avoided at the midpoint between menses. Does the woman douche immediately after intercourse? The woman whose physician has advised her to douche, for whatever reason, or who feels that she must douche, should wait until the next morning to do it.

Summary of teaching points

Some women may be reluctant to ask questions of a man, even a physician, whereas they may feel more comfortable approaching a female nurse. The nurse

Table 37-1.
Infertility tests

Test	Description	Comment
Male		
Semen examination	The number, motility and shape of sperm cells from a fresh semen collection is examined under microscope.	(1) Absence of sperm cells in *repeated* exams suggests infertility. (2) A low sperm count decreases the possibility of conception.
Testicular biopsy	Tissue is examined to see if sperm cells are being produced.	If sperm are being produced but are not present in the semen, the problem may be an obstructive lesion.
Female		
Rubin test	Carbon dioxide is forced through the uterus, the fallopian tubes and into the peritoneal cavity to check for occluded tubes.	In some instances the gas may blow out the obstruction resulting in fertility.
Sims-Huhner (postcoital)	Vaginal and cervical secretions are aspirated 6 to 12 hrs. after intercourse and examined microscopically.	The interreactions of the wife's secretions and the husband's sperm can be observed.
Hysterosalpingography	X-ray study of the uterus and fallopian tubes with radiopaque dye.	Bowel cleansing before the X-ray study is usually ordered.
Endometrial biopsy	Microscopic examination of tissue shows whether or not the endometrium has been prepared for surgery.	Frequently done premenstrually or on first day of period. Also used to help diagnose cause of dysmenorrhea and amenorrhea.

should keep herself approachable, but be gentle and tentative, especially if she meets resistance.

If the physician has recommended taking a douche, the patient may not know how to do it and may be too shy to ask. The normal processes of menstruation or the menopause may not be understood. A woman may not know how conception takes place, or even how a baby is born. "Where does it come out?" is a question few would ask for fear of being laughed at. A woman who is ignorant may fear to ask questions that are important to her. The nurse must be prepared with the correct information, and make it easy for the patient to talk to her in privacy. She should encourage the patient to express her ideas and to voice her questions.

A woman may believe that cleanliness demands that she take a douche after sexual relations and after menstruation. The normal healthy vagina ordinarily requires no vaginal irrigation; unnecessary douching may lead to irritation or infection, and it should not be encouraged. A patient should consult her physician about this. If douching is desirable, he will tell her so and advise what solution to use. In general douching is being used less and less in the treatment of various gynecological disorders. If douching is recommended, the following are significant teaching points to remember:

- Douching at home is done best while the patient is lying down in the bathtub, since sitting on the toilet does not allow the solution to go up in the vagina. The back of the tub is padded with a towel for comfort.
- The patient is taught to insert the nozzle gently upward and backward, and to rotate it when the solution starts to flow.
- The distance should be measured, so that the receptacle of fluid hangs at a height of 12 to 18 inches and not from the top of the door or shower curtain.
- If the patient has an infectious disease, the nozzle should be boiled between irrigations.
- The patient is taught to regulate the temperature carefully (105° F.) to avoid burning herself and to mix the solution correctly.
- As some solution may drip out after the patient stands up, she may wish to wait a half hour before getting dressed, to wear a pad for a few minutes, or to sit where she is for 5 or 6 minutes.

Two other common situations which require teaching among gynecological patients are perineal care and sitz baths. Patients who have had surgery in the perineal region should have careful demonstrations of how to cleanse the area, particularly in relation to cleansing after a bowel movement. This teaching should begin as soon as the patient becomes ambulatory in the hospital, thus insuring that the patient uses acceptable technique while in the hospital, and later when she goes home. The patient is shown how to cleanse from front to back, using disposable cotton pledgets or a disposable washcloth. Although this technique is essential after any perineal surgery, it is an important hygienic measure for all women.

The sitz bath is recommended by the physician as an aid to comfort, healing, and cleanliness. A helpful modification of the usual procedure is the use of plastic disposable basins for the sitz bath. The patient can take the basin home with her, making it easier for her to carry out the treatment at home.

Bibliography

See bibliography at the end of Chapter 38.

CHAPTER 38

The woman with a disorder of the reproductive system

On completion of the chapter the student will:

- Recognize the importance of a regular gynecological examination for all age groups.
- Describe patient preparation for the gynecological examination and the nurse's role in patient preparation.
- Describe the purpose of the Papanicolaou test and the cervical biopsy and how each test is carried out.
- Discuss the preoperative and postoperative management of a patient with a D and C.
- Describe the types of abortion and list the treatment and nursing management of the patient who has had or may have a termination of pregnancy.
- Identify the types of infections occurring in the female reproductive system and the treatment and nursing management of the patient with an infection.
- Define endometriosis and discuss the treatment of this disorder.
- Discuss the treatment and nursing management of malignant and benign tumors of the uterus and malignant lesions of the vulva.
- Formulate a nursing care plan for and participate in the nursing management of the patient who has had gynecological surgery.

Treatment of the gynecological patient is undertaken with two objectives: to preserve or restore the woman's health, and to preserve her child-bearing capacity, insofar as possible. The first objective is operative throughout the patient's life span; the second, until the woman has passed through the menopause.

Regardless of when pathology occurs, early diagnosis and medical attention are essential. The nurse familiar with normal function can often help to educate women about the importance of regular gynecological examinations and the time to seek medical help.

It is very important to recognize that feelings are involved. A permissive atmosphere should be provided for the patient, so that she can cope with her own emotions. This kind of atmosphere is not achieved by ignoring the patient's feelings. Rather, the nurse must be sensitive to expressions of anxiety (clear or subtle), and be calm and efficient, so that the patient can feel the security of being among professional people who know what they are doing. If a patient becomes agitated over some minor procedure, the nurse should not cut her off. Perhaps this is the patient's way of communicating the presence of different and more significant fears.

The patient should be told what to expect. A hysterectomy (without oophorectomy) will not cause a sudden menopause, although it is a common belief that it will. Patients may worry about this even though they do not discuss it, and many will be grateful for an explanation of the terms they hear but cannot interpret.

Common operations for gynecological disorders include:

1. Salpingectomy, unilateral, removal of one fallopian tube. It does not cause sterility, but bilateral salpingectomy does. Menses continue.
2. Hysterectomy, removal of the uterus. Menses stop; but because the ovaries are not removed, hysterectomy does not cause an artificial menopause.
3. Oophorectomy, unilateral, removal of one ovary. It does not cause sterility. Bilateral oophorectomy causes sterility and induces an artificial (or surgical) menopause.

In many gynecological diseases, sexual relations must be suspended; in some conditions, such as very radical surgery for cancer, they must be terminated. This necessity may have a profound effect on the relationship between husband and wife. In either instance, it may help if the physician discusses this problem with the husband as well as the patient in order to aid them in resolving it together. Sometimes the nurse can help by suggesting that patient, husband, and physician discuss the matter together.

A patient in her early adolescent years may be admitted to the gynecological service of a hospital, perhaps for a dilatation and curettage to diagnose the cause of a delayed menarche. Because she is at an age when she is still forming attitudes about her bodily changes, she may be embarrassed and upset over her hospitalization and the types of examinations she may have. The procedures must be explained to the adolescent patient. It is bad enough to be embarrassed by what the physician does. To fail to understand the reason for the examination or the procedure adds an unnecessary burden.

Diagnostic procedures

The gynecological examination

Most women dread having a gynecological examination because they are embarrassed about being examined. They fear not only exposure, but also what the physician may find. The patient usually feels less embarrassed when the nurse acts in a matter-of-fact fashion. It may help if the nurse answers an apprehensive patient who has said that she is frightened or embarrassed by asking what she is frightened or embarrassed of, and by finding ways, if possible, to alleviate these feelings. For example, if the patient says she fears the pain of the examination, the nurse can explain to her, and have her practice before the examination, the deep-breathing and muscle-relaxing measures which will lessen discomfort during the examination.

Preparing the Patient. The nurse tells the patient that she will stay with her during the procedure. A nurse *always* remains in the room the *entire* time that a patient is being examined. All the needed equipment should be on hand so that the nurse does not have to leave the room during the examination. A speculum of the correct size for each patient should be available. If in doubt, the nurse should ask the physician before the examination begins. The nurse also informs the patient that the physician will ask questions about her menses: when it started, how frequently it occurs, and how heavy the flow is. He will ask her about any pregnancies and perhaps about any vaginal discharge that she may have. The patient should be encouraged to give a full and honest history.

The patient is instructed to remove her underclothes from her waist down and to loosen anything tight around her waist. She is given a sheet to wrap around her until she is positioned on the examining table. The patient is asked to void, for a full bladder may interfere with the examination. For example, a distended bladder may lead to confusion as to the presence or absence of an ovarian cyst or tumor.

The most common position for the gynecological examination is the lithotomy position (Fig. 38-1). It is uncomfortable for anyone to maintain. With a sheet around her, the patient sits at the edge of the examining table and lies back. The nurse helps the patient to lift both legs at the same time, and places the feet in the stirrups. If the stirrups are metal, the patient wears her shoes for a better grip and more even distribution of pressure on the soles of her feet. Now the nurse places her hands under the patient's buttocks or around the patient's thighs and helps her slide right to the edge of the table. By draping the patient securely, the nurse does more to reassure her that her modesty will be protected than is possible with words.

Although the vagina is not a sterile cavity, equipment is sterilized each time it is used, to prevent any introduction of pathogens. In addition, it is important, both for preventing infection and for aesthetic considerations, that the patient have a fresh sheet to lie on and that the physician and the nurse wash their hands after examining a patient and before handling equipment in preparation for the next patient. The necessary equipment is listed in the hospital procedure manual. A bright spotlight is set up behind the physician's stool. On occasion, a flashlight held by an assistant will be used.

THE PHYSICIAN'S EXAMINATION. The order in which the physician performs various aspects of the pelvic examination varies. It is considered preferable for the physician to begin the examination by observation, first of the external genitalia and adjacent structures, and then of the vaginal walls and the cervix of the uterus through the bivalve speculum (Fig. 38-2).

After examining the external genitalia and performing the visual examination of the vaginal walls and cervix through the speculum, the physician places one or two fingers of his gloved hand into the vagina. By palpation, he examines the structures beyond the orifice. Then, the physician performs the vaginal-abdominal examination. Without removing his gloved fingers from the vagina, he places the fingers of his other hand on the patient's lower abdomen. Between his two hands he can palpate the position, the size, and the contour of the uterus, the ovaries, and other pelvic structures. At the end of the examination, the physi-

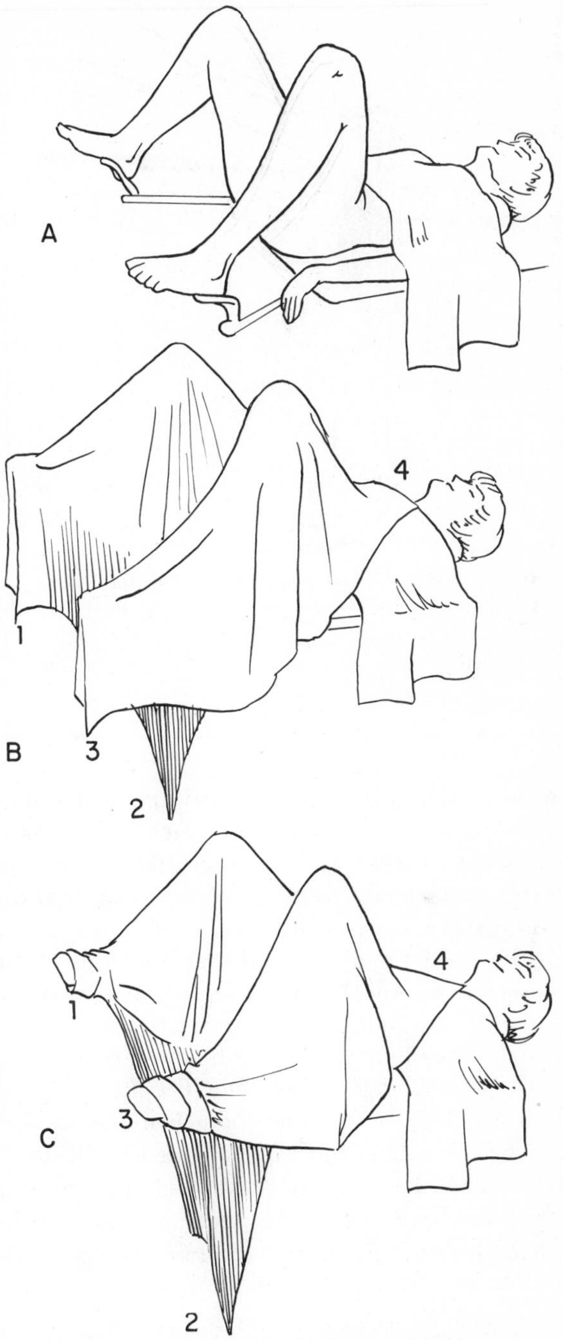

figure 38-1. Draping a patient in the lithotomy position. (A) The patient is placed in this position while she is under a sheet (which was removed for this picture). Note that the patient's hips are right at the edge of the table. (B) The sheet is turned on the diagonal. One corner (4) is placed under the chin, the opposite corner (2) hangs down between the legs, and the other corners (1 and 3) go over each foot. (C) Corners (1) and (3) are wrapped around the feet. When the physician is ready for the examination, corner (2) is folded up, and only the patient's vulva is exposed.

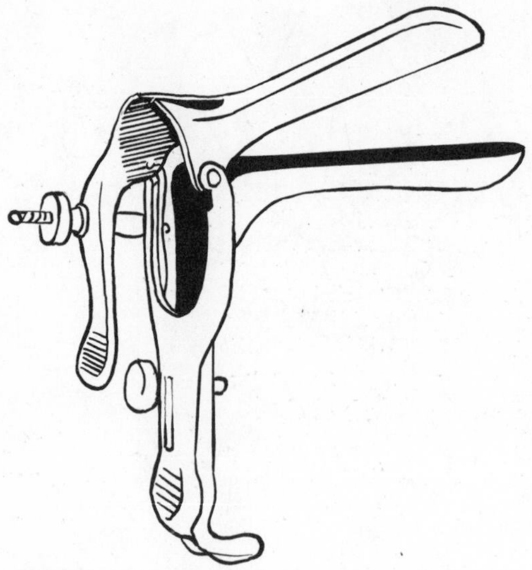

figure 38-2. A bivalve speculum. With the mouth of the speculum closed and well lubricated, the speculum is passed into the vagina. Then it is opened to give the physician a clear view of the cervix. Specula come in various sizes.

cian may place a gloved and lubricated index finger into the patient's rectum; he can reach as high as the level of the posterior surface of the uterus. The presence of hemorrhoids, fistulas, and fissures can also be noted.

Although the gynecological examination is uncomfortable, the patient should not feel pain unless disease is present. The more relaxed the patient's lower abdominal muscles are, the better the physician can palpate the internal organs. Breathing deeply through the mouth may help to relax the abdominal muscles. During the examination, the nurse's place is with the patient—helping her to relax, preventing her from wriggling to the head of the table, talking to her, holding her hand if that seems to give comfort—and not beside the physician peering through the speculum.

Nursing Management After the Examination. The nurse cleans the perineum of any lubricating jelly. She helps the patient to slide her hips back from the edge of the table, removing both feet from the stirrups at the same time to prevent strain, and helps her off the table. After the patient has been in the lithotomy position, she may wish to rest for a few moments on the stool or a chair before she gets dressed. The nurse gives her a tissue or gauze to wipe off the remaining lubricating jelly, and sees that she gets a moment of privacy. Although the nurse wipes the perineum after the examination, the patient may prefer to finish the job. The nurse provides her with a fresh sanitary pad, if she needs one, and the wrappings in which to dispose of the old one. She shows patient where to dispose of it, and where she may wash her hands. If the physician used gentian violet, the patient will need a pad to prevent the dye from staining her underclothing. Considerations such as these smooth the way and convey acceptance and caring.

The nurse rinses the used equipment in cold water to prevent secretions from sticking, scrubs the equipment with soap and water, and resterilizes it. The nurse washes her hands after cleaning the perineum or touching used equipment. She keeps her hands away from her face, especially, to protect her eyes from infectious organisms such as the gonococcus.

If the patient has a discharge, she should not douche before the examination. The physician may want to see the discharge and to take a specimen for more detailed study.

Cytologic test for cancer (Papanicolaou test)

This test provides a means by which cells that exfoliate may be examined for malignancy (Fig. 38-3). Secretions from various body parts are studied microscopically to determine the presence of malignant cells. In gynecology, the test is used mainly to detect early cancer of the cervix, which is the most common form of malignancy of the reproductive tract in women.

The diagnosis of endometrial carcinoma is best achieved by dilatation of the cervix and curettage of the uterus (D and C). Endometrial smears are another diagnostic measure used to determine the presence of carcinoma. A malleable cannula is placed in the uterine cavity and attached to a syringe to aspirate the secretions. As is always the case, the slides are labeled with the source of the smear, the date, and the patient's name, and sent to the laboratory. After this test, the patient may have a cramped feeling that can usually be relieved by heat over the uterine area or by a mild analgesic. The patient should not bathe for at least 2 hours, or douche for 2 or 3 days before the test, because irrigation may remove the exfoliated cells.

Patients can be taught to obtain their own vaginal smears. Having patients take their own specimens and mail them to a laboratory for examination can increase the number of patients who benefit from this diagnostic test. Some physicians prescribe the test every 6 months; some, yearly.

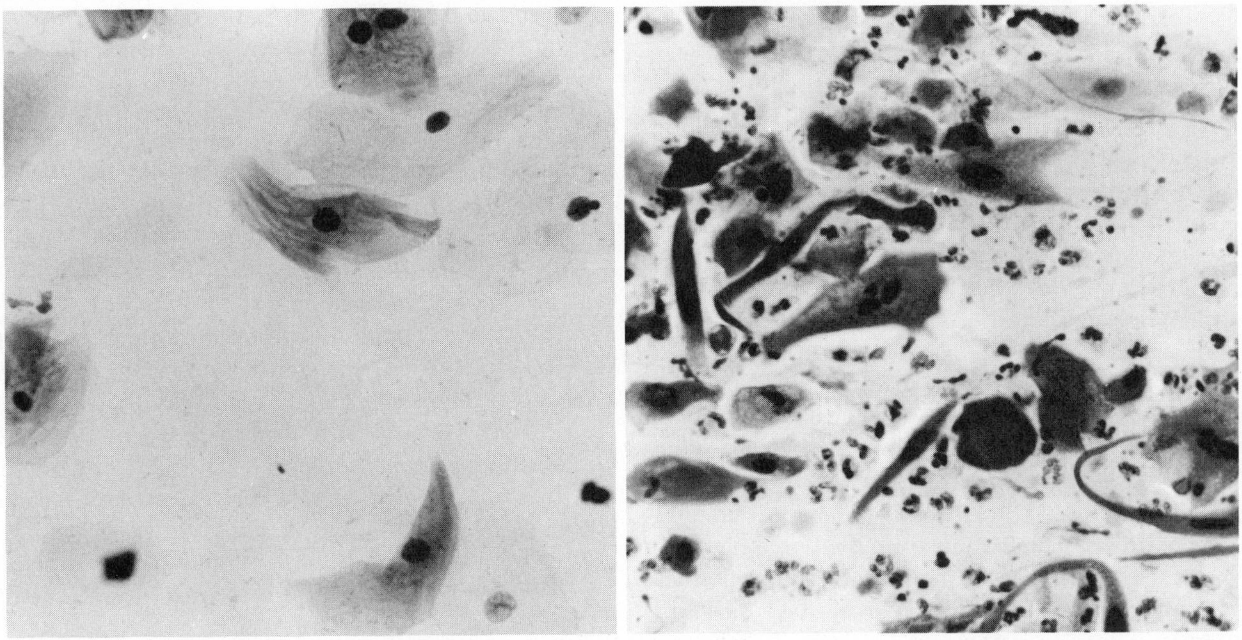

figure 38-3. Papanicolaou smears from the vagina. (*Left*) Normal cells. (*Right*) Malignant cells. (Photograph—D. Atkinson)

Cervical biopsy

Cervical biopsy is the usual follow-up when a cytologic test is positive or questionable. When the physician suspects cancer, he may take a tiny piece of the cervix for laboratory examination. This procedure may be conducted in the physician's office or in the clinic. Thus, preferably, it should be scheduled approximately one week after the cessation of the patient's monthly menstrual flow, when the cervix is least vascular. The patient may have some discomfort, but the procedure is not painful, since the cervix does not have pain receptors. A biopsy forceps is used to obtain the specimen. After the biopsy has been taken, bleeding may require additional treatment, such as use of packing. The patient should rest before she leaves for home. If packing was inserted into the vagina, the patient should be instructed not to remove it until the prescribed number of hours has passed (usually 24). She is instructed to avoid unusual physical strain and heavy lifting for the remainder of the day.

Most patients have slight bleeding for a day. The patient is instructed to call the physician or to return to the clinic if there is serious bleeding. Because of the danger of bleeding and infection, the patient should be instructed not to douche, have sexual intercourse, or use tampons until the physician says that she may.

Dilatation of the cervix and curettage of the uterus (D and C)

Dilatation here refers to expansion of the mouth of the cervix; *curettage* means scraping the lining of a cavity (in this instance the endometrium). This common gynecological operation often is performed to find the cause of abnormal bleeding and, also, to examine the patient for the presence of malignancy and fibroid tumors. The scrapings are sent to the laboratory for investigation.

If the D and C is done as part of an investigation of the cause of sterility, it is performed before menstruation. When the scrapings, which are sent to the laboratory along with the date of the last menstrual period, are examined microscopically, the physician can determine whether ovulation occurred during this menstrual cycle, the adequacy of the endometrial lining, and the state of hormonal balance. Cervical dilatation is performed initially to permit uterine curettage, though it is done also to relieve stricture or stenosis of the cervical orifice, to permit tubal insufflation, and, in selected instances, to relieve dysmenorrhea. It is done in the operating room, under a general anesthetic, with the patient in the lithotomy position. Curettage is usually avoided when vagina, cervix, or fallopian tubes are infected, because of the danger of spreading the infection.

Preoperative and postoperative care (D and C)

Preparation for a dilatation and curettage includes care similar to that of any patient about to receive general anesthesia: food and fluids are withheld for 12 hours prior to surgery; rest, skin cleansing, and safety precautions are important. Opinions concerning whether the patient's vulva and perineum should be shaved prior to D and C vary among gynecologists.

An enema is usually ordered. Because of their proximity to the operative area, special care is taken to make sure that bladder and lower bowel are empty on the morning of surgery. If the patient has lost a significant amount of blood—for example, during an incomplete abortion—a transfusion will be started.

When the patient returns from the operating room or the recovery room, she may be wearing a perineal pad, but probably she will not have a belt to hold it in place. The nurse provides her with a belt or a T-binder to keep the pad in place for comfort and to prevent the sheets from being soiled. There will be a serosanguineous discharge for several days. Postoperatively, the nurse should investigate the perineal site and note the drainage on the perineal pad. Immediately after surgery the pad should be observed every 15 or 20 minutes for the first 2 or 3 hours. Perineal pads should be used while the packing is in place. Packing is infrequently used now after D and C; when used, it is removed after one or two days.

The nurse checks for voiding and charts the time and amount of the first voiding. However, voiding problems are usually minimal following D and C. Patients allowed to be out of bed the day of surgery usually void without any difficulty.

Because the cervix is dilated, sexual relations, douching, and tub baths should be avoided until the physician says they may be resumed. The patient should know that her menstrual period may be delayed and that a vaginal discharge may be present during her convalescent period.

Perineal Care. As long as there is sufficient vaginal discharge to warrant a perineal pad, perineal care should be given. The technique will vary from hospital to hospital, but the principles remain the same: the area is kept clean and the patient is kept comfortable. Before going ahead with perineal care or teaching the patient to do it, the nurse finds out which technique is required. Many hospitals use a disposable washcloth, especially for ambulatory patients.

In some hospitals perineal care is given as a warm sitz or tub bath. The tub bath, relaxing in itself, is often preferred by the patients. Of course, the tub is scrupulously cleaned between patients. In some hospitals individual disposable basins are used for sitz baths. To many patients, perineal irrigation is particularly comfortable. Sterile or clean water, 100° to 105° F., is poured over the vulva from a pitcher no higher than 6 inches over the patient. The perineum can be dried with sterile cotton balls or a clean washcloth, depending on the technique used.

The nurse should give perineal care during the first 48 postoperative hours. Giving perineal care affords the nurse an excellent opportunity to observe the surgical area. Perineal care always should be done after a bowel movement and after voiding. No patient with sutures should give herself perineal care. She cannot see the area, and a piece of cotton or washcloth might catch on a suture and pull it, or stay there and induce infection. Also, the perineal area with sutures deserves the nurse's direct observation several times a day. Likewise, when packing is in the vagina, the nurse should give perineal care, being especially careful not to dislodge the packing. Embarrassment of the patient can often be minimized by draping, ensuring privacy, and by sure movements.

Abortion

Abortion is the termination of a pregnancy before the fetus is viable. The term *abortion* is used to designate interruption of pregnancy before the fetus weighs more than 500 gm. (about 20 weeks of gestation). Between this time and a full-term delivery, the expulsion of the fetus is called a *premature birth.*

Types of abortion

Spontaneous Abortion. About 10 percent of all pregnancies result in spontaneous abortion ("miscarriage" is the layman's term), usually before the 12th week. (The nurse might remember when talking to patients that some people associate the word *abortion* only with an intentional termination of the pregnancy, and, for them, "miscarriage" may be more acceptable.) Abnormalities of the fertilized ovum or the placenta, inconsistent with life, are believed to be the most frequent cause. Maternal disease, such as a severe acute infection, endocrine imbalance, or a chronic wasting disease, may also be a cause of an abortion. Physical trauma rarely causes abortion.

Abnormal uterine bleeding in any woman during her childbearing years may indicate an abortion in the early weeks of gestation—so early in her pregnancy that she is unaware that she was pregnant. Pain and bleeding are common symptoms. The pain may be so mild that it is disregarded or as severe as labor pains. Bleeding may range from spotting to hemorrhage. Generally, spontaneous abortion occurs approximately 6 weeks after the fetus has died.

Threatened Abortion. Bleeding or spotting may indicate that abortion is threatened. Other signs may be cramps or backache. Some may lose the child; in others the pregnancy may proceed entirely normally.

Incomplete Abortion. Some of the products of the pregnancy are expelled, and some (usually a portion of the placenta) are retained. Incomplete separation of the placenta from the uterine wall causes hemorrhage. In a *complete abortion* all of the products of conception are expelled.

Missed Abortion. The fetus dies, but is not expelled. It may be retained 2 months or longer.

Habitual Abortions. Such abortions occur repeatedly without apparent cause. Bed rest and hormonal therapy have helped some women to carry a fetus to term. Emotional support can be an important factor in helping the patient carry the baby to term. If abortion occurs, support from the physician and nurse can assist the patient to deal with the loss of her baby. The fear of being unable to carry a baby to term is very common among women who have once suffered a spontaneous abortion.

Treatment

A pregnant woman should report the first signs of a vaginal discharge, bleeding, or cramps to her physician. He probably will advise bed rest and a light diet, and warn her against any straining, such as when she moves her bowels. She should save all formed vaginal discharges for the physician to examine. If the bleeding stops, he may allow her out of bed in several days, but only for quiet activity. If abdominal pain becomes severe or uterine bleeding increases, abortion may be imminent, and the physician will probably hospitalize the patient. An incomplete abortion is treated by curettage. The patient may enter the hospital bleeding profusely. Typing and cross matching are done, and an infusion is started. Sometimes a transfusion is necessary. In missed abortion, the uterus usually is allowed to empty itself. Occasionally it is necessary to remove the dead fetus. In incomplete abortion, drugs such as oxytocin and ergonovine are frequently used to make the uterus contract and to control bleeding.

Nursing management

Nursing management after an abortion is similar to that given after a D and C or that given any time after the cervix has been dilated. Perineal care is given as long as there is a discharge; because the cervix is dilated, the patient should not have douches or sexual intercourse.

If abortion is threatening, there is the possibility that a quiet stay in bed will save the baby. If abortion is imminent, or incomplete, bed rest will prevent the increase of bleeding caused by activity. The patient should be observed carefully and repeatedly for hemorrhage. All large clots and tissue are saved for the physician to examine. The patient should not use the toilet; instead, she should use the bedpan to avoid passing the fetus or the placenta unnoticed. If the patient begins to have cramps, the physician is informed immediately.

A patient with a threatened abortion may remain on bed rest for a long period of time. A few women spend the major part of the 9 months in bed, although they may not be in the hospital for the entire time. Many of these women carry the infant to term, but the husband or a relative has to take care of the household. For the woman who wants a baby, the suspense of a threatened abortion is very difficult, but she is usually motivated to follow the prescribed treatment, including bed rest, if necessary. She may be resentful that other women are able to carry a baby without having to stay in bed. She may feel guilty because she has to be waited on and cannot contribute to the work of the household. Because she has little exercise in bed, her diet should be light but nutritionally sound.

A woman who has aborted may grieve over the lost baby. Her emotional reaction will be governed by many factors; for example, it will make a great difference whether the patient is 20 years old or nearing the end of her childbearing period. If she seems bitter over losing the baby, she should be encouraged to recognize this emotion. She will still be angry, but being listened to will give her some relief. If there is likelihood that the patient can again become pregnant, the physician explains this to her. Although knowledge that she is likely to conceive again does not take away the loss of the fetus, it can help the patient deal with her grief and begin to look forward to becoming pregnant again.

Ectopic pregnancy

This term refers to the implantation of the fertilized ovum outside the uterus. The fallopian tubes are the most common ectopic site, but implantation may occur elsewhere, such as in the abdominal cavity. The fetus starts to develop just as it would in the uterus. In most cases the patient has all the classic signs of pregnancy. In addition, she may complain of spotting and pain in the lower abdomen.

Because there is so little room for expansion in the fallopian tube, the enlarging fetus and the placenta will rupture it. The diagnosis of a tubal pregnancy is rare until rupture occurs. The patient has a sudden, sharp pain, and often she is admitted to the hospital in severe shock from hemorrhage. Profuse bleeding occurs both vaginally and into the abdominal cavity. The patient is taken immediately to the operating room, and a salpingectomy is usually performed. Preparing the patient for the operating room has to be accomplished with speed. Treatment for shock and hemorrhage is started immediately. Blood transfusions are given as soon as blood typing and cross matching are done.

Postoperatively, careful and frequent observation of vital signs is imperative, until both are well stabilized. The nature and the quantity of the vaginal discharge should be noted and perineal care given as long as there is vaginal discharge. Preoperative bleeding into the abdominal cavity may cause peritonitis postoperatively; therefore, abdominal pain, nausea, and vomiting should be reported to the physician. The rupture of a tubal pregnancy is a sudden and shocking event not only for the patient, but also for the family. The patient will probably need time postoperatively to assimilate the experience and to accept the fact that she has lost the baby.

Infections

Vaginitis

The normal acidity of the vaginal secretion at maturity (pH 3.5 to 4.5) is a natural defense against infection. Nevertheless, a variety of pathogenic organisms can invade and infect the vagina—most commonly the protozoon *Trichomonas vaginalis* and the fungus *Candida albicans,* and certain bacterial species.

An abnormal vaginal discharge is a prominent symptom of vaginal infection. It may be copious and malodorous, and often it is irritating, causing itching and redness of the perineum and the anus. If the mouth of the urethra is affected, the patient may have urinary symptoms, such as burning on urination and the feeling that she has to void frequently. Also, there may be some discomfort in the lower abdominal region. In contrast with an abnormal discharge, a normal vaginal discharge has little odor and is colorless.

Normal vaginal discharge changes in character and amount during the menstrual cycle, usually becoming more noticeable at ovulation and before menses. It varies from clear to cloudy.

Trichomonas vaginitis can cause a white, frothy, highly irritating leukorrhea, and candida infection can cause a leukorrhea that has the consistency of cottage cheese and itches intensely.

The patient is often treated as an outpatient. Diagnosis of trichomonas vaginitis is made upon microscopic examination of the vaginal secretions. The patient should not douche before the examination, since washing away the secretions will prevent the physician from noting their characteristics and from taking an adequate smear. After determining the cause of the infection the physician may swab the infected area with a cleansing solution. A vaginal jelly or suppository may then be inserted, or tampons prescribed to absorb the discharge. A sulfonamide cream may be given intravaginally to combat streptococcal or staphylococcal infection. Douches are sometimes ordered for cleansing and esthetic reasons. By favoring the production of lactic acid, Döderlein's bacillus serves to maintain an acid medium as a natural defense mechanism. Trichomonas prefers an alkaline climate. Intravaginal creams may also be employed. When a vaginal cream is prescribed, its use is continued through the menstrual period, because this is a time when the secretions become more alkaline.

Monilial vaginitis, caused by the fungus *Candida albicans,* is a common infection during pregnancy and after antibiotic treatment because the antibiotics destroy the normal vaginal flora. It also is frequent in diabetics whose urine contains glucose (the monilial fungus is supported by carbohydrates), and occasionally this infection is seen after long-term corticosteroid therapy.

Nystatin (Mycostatin), an antibiotic fungicide, may be given orally and in suppositories, at bedtime. When the perineum is badly irritated, Mycostatin ointment may be prescribed to be applied locally three times a day. If the patient has diabetes, the elimination of glycosuria through the control of the diabetes is an aspect of the treatment. Gentian violet may be painted onto the vaginal mucosa several times a week. After the medication is applied, the physician may insufflate the vagina with cornstarch or other drying powders, since the infecting organisms thrive better in a moist environment than a dry one.

Teaching a Patient the Aspects of Treatment and Self-Care. Before the patient leaves for home, she must understand every detail of what she needs to do. In most instances, the treatment will be performed by the patient at home. Does she know that she should wash her hands before inserting a vaginal suppository? Does she know that she should be in the dorsal recumbent position, use her longest finger, and aim up and back toward the posterior fornix? Some suppositories and creams come with long applicators that the patient may not know how to insert. She needs to learn how to hold the applicator, to lie down on a bed with her hips elevated on a pillow, how to insert the applicator and to stay in this position for 10 to 15 minutes when cream or suppository is used so that it will melt and the dissolving medication will cover the vaginal vault. A good way to use a vaginal suppository is to have the patient insert it while she is in bed just prior to retiring. It probably will not dislodge and will melt during the night. The next morning a perineal pad may be worn, or a tampon inserted instead if the pad is irritating to the already infected perineum. When douches are part of the treatment, they should be used before insertion of the suppository.

Vaginitis can be stubborn and discouraging. Vigorous early treatment may overcome its tendency to become chronic. At best, the patient can expect at least 6 weeks of treatment before she is cured. At worst, vaginitis persists for years, recurring at the very moment when it appears to be cured. Patients with long-term vaginitis are understandably discouraged. They are tired of the malodorous discharge, of wearing perineal pads every day of the month, of going to the physician for treatment.

The nurse should be available if the patient needs someone to talk to about her vaginitis, or if she needs to talk with someone who is not a family member or friend about how to set up a more healthful regimen for herself. Having a discharge is in itself upsetting, and to many it suggests uncleanliness. An infection of the genital area is often linked with venereal disease, even if it is not venereal. The patient may ask whether or not vaginitis is infectious and a hazard to her family; and if it is not a venereal disease, what is it? The patient may ask whether she should use the same toilet seat as the rest of the family. Most infections are not transmitted this way. Of course, if some discharge drops on the seat, she should wash it off with soap, water, and some antiseptic cleansing agent.

Perineal pruritus (itching)

Itching of the perineum can be caused by a deficiency of vitamin A (especially in older women who do not eat enough butter, milk, and yellow vegetables); an irritating vaginal discharge; glucose in the urine of those with uncontrolled diabetes mellitus (diabetic vulvovaginitis); uncleanliness; leukoplakia; urinary incontinence; an inflammatory skin disease or local skin infection such as moniliasis, scabies, and pediculosis pubis. Allergic reactions to fabric or dye can produce or contribute to the pruritus, which is a symptom, not a specific disease. It is seen in many genital conditions, both in the presence and in the absence of a vaginal discharge.

The treatment is directed at the underlying cause. Obese patients often suffer pruritus because, as they walk, the skin surfaces rub against each other. In such cases a light dusting with cornstarch may help to decrease the friction. Itching may be severe. If the patient must scratch, the chance of infection can be minimized by keeping the hands clean and not using the nails. The physician may approve of cold or hot compresses or applications of calamine lotion to help to relieve the itching. Clothing should be light and nonrestrictive. Girdles or pants with long legs keep the skin surfaces separated and are a great comfort, especially in hot weather.

Cervicitis

Cervicitis (inflammation of the cervix) may be caused by a number of infectious organisms. Streptococcal and staphylococcal infections are common, especially after childbirth, when the organisms are able to enter the cervical tissue through small lacerations. Gonorrhea is a frequent cause of cervicitis, and cases from this cause have increased alarmingly in recent years. Cervicitis also may be caused by a change in the pH of the cervical secretions (which are normally alkaline pH 7.5 to 8). Cervicitis may also be due to cancer, and it is thought that the constant irritation of chronic cervicitis from any cause can lead to cancer.

Inflammation can cause erosion of cervical tissue, which may cause spotting or bleeding. Leukorrhea is the prominent symptom. There may be *dyspareunia* (painful sexual intercourse) or slight staining after sexual intercourse. Early cervicitis may fail to show any symptoms at all. A severe cervicitis may cause a sensation of weight in the pelvis. Unless acute cervicitis is treated promptly, it has a tendency to become chronic and difficult to cure. Examination of the cervix 6 weeks after giving birth, in addition to regular gynecological examination for all women, is important in discovering the condition before it becomes chronic.

Treatment and Nursing Management. Acute cervicitis may be treated with douches and local and/or systemic antibiotics. Chronic cervicitis may be treated with electrocautery. The procedure is usually done in the physician's office or the clinic 5 to 8 days after the end of the menstrual period. The patient is placed in lithotomy position, a vaginal speculum inserted, and the cervix painted with an antiseptic. The nurse should be sure that the physician has a good light. He may first take a biopsy for a microscopic examination for cancer cells. The eroded tissue is touched with a thin electrical rod, burning strips around the mouth of the cervix, destroying any cysts present. Usually no anesthesia is used, since there is no pain. If the cautery blade is inserted into the cervical canal, there may be a momentary cramping sensation.

For a day or two after electrocautery the patient should rest more than usual. No straining or heavy lifting should be undertaken. If slight bleeding occurs, the physician may advise bed rest. Frank bleeding should bring the patient back to the physician. Cervical or vaginal packing, or electric coagulation of the bleeding vessel, may be necessary. The nurse should be sure that the patient knows to expect a gray-green slough (discharge) for about 3 weeks after cautery. The discharge is watery at first; then as the burned tissues become necrotic, the discharge becomes malodorous. Slight bleeding may occur about the 11th day. The physician will wish to re-examine the cervix 2 to 4 weeks later. Dilatation is done if there is cervical stenosis. Sexual relations should not be resumed until the physician gives his approval. Healing takes 6 to 8 weeks.

Severe chronic cervicitis may be treated by *conization* (removal of the diseased portion of the cervical mucosa). The procedure is done with an electric instrument that simultaneously cuts tissue and coagulates the bleeding area. The patient usually is hospitalized, but not always, and anesthesia may or may not be given.

As with cautery, approximately 6 to 8 weeks are required for healing. The follow-up visits (usually about every 2 weeks) to the physician are most important, so that he may observe the patency of the cervix. Successful treatment eliminates the distressing leukorrhea, may aid fertility, and eliminates the constant irritation.

Pelvic inflammatory disease (PID)

Pelvic inflammatory disease is an inflammatory disorder of the pelvic organs (except the uterus). There may be inflammation of the ovaries (oophoritis) or of the fallopian tubes (salpingitis); pus in the fallopian tubes (pyosalpinx); inflammation of the pelvic vascular system or of any of the pelvic supporting structures.

Infection may enter these structures through the vagina, the peritoneum, the lymphatics, or the bloodstream. The most frequent cause is the gonococcus, although other organisms, such as streptococci and staphylococci, may also cause PID.

Pelvic inflammatory disease caused by the tubercle bacillus spreads most frequently by the bloodstream, and it may occur years after the primary lesion in the lungs has become inactive. The patient with tuberculous PID may have night sweats, weight loss, and an afternoon rise in temperature. Antituberculosis drugs are usually ordered. Tuberculosis is not often found now in these organs, since chemotherapy helps to control the primary pulmonary infection.

Symptoms of PID may include a malodorous discharge that is infectious and should be handled with care by both patient and nurse to prevent spread of the disease. There may be backache, severe or aching abdominal and pelvic pain, a bearing-down feeling, fever, nausea and vomiting, menorrhagia, and dysmenorrhea. Pain may be felt during sexual intercourse or a pelvic examination. Severe infection may cause urinary symptoms or constipation.

The patient with acute pelvic inflammatory disease is usually hospitalized and kept in bed. Often the bed is adjusted to a semisitting position to facilitate pelvic drainage and to help prevent the extension of the infection upward. Antibiotics usually are administered, and warm lower abdominal applications may be ordered. Heat improves the circulation to the area. Warm sitz baths may be given. The tub should be well scrubbed afterward to prevent the spread of infectious organisms. Douching is usually avoided because there is danger that the infection will be spread by it.

If there is leukorrhea, the perineal pad should be changed frequently. The pad is wrapped in paper before discarding it, or the patient is provided with bags in which to deposit it. The patient, and any auxiliary personnel who care for her, must wash their hands well after changing the perineal pad. When there is copious discharge, perineal care should be given each time that the pad is changed, and after the patient uses the bedpan. When the causative organism is particularly infectious, as in gonorrhea, the patient is placed on isolation precautions, and whoever gives the patient perineal care should wear gloves. Amount, color, odor, and appearance of the discharge should be recorded daily on the nurse's notes. Tampons should not be used, because they may obstruct the flow of discharge. If the infectious process of PID is not treated early, it may localize and form an abscess.

One way of preventing PID is early medical attention to such symptoms of infection in the genital or urinary tracts as a feeling of pressure in the pelvic area, burning on urination, and leukorrhea. Early treatment may prevent the infection from moving up the genital tract. When early treatment of acute PID is delayed or inadequate, the infection may become chronic.

After discharge from the hospital the patient should refrain from sexual intercourse as long as leukorrhea or any other abnormality exists, since intercourse tends to extend the infection and may also infect the husband's genitourinary tract.

Puerperal infection

Puerperal infection is the term given to an infection, usually streptococcal or staphylococcal, which follows childbirth. The infection often centers in the endometrium, but it may spread anywhere in the pelvic and peritoneal cavities. It can cause generalized sepsis after entry of the organisms into the bloodstream. Puerperal infection is a grave danger of criminal abortion during which unsterile instruments are used. The retention of bits of the placenta after a normal delivery provides a good culture medium for pathogenic organisms. Also, rupture of the membranes several days before delivery, postpartum thrombophlebitis, and delivery of a baby under unsterile conditions may lead to puerperal infection. Careful technique to prevent infection is extremely important once the patient's membranes have ruptured.

The patient with a puerperal infection is febrile and, if the endometrium is involved, she will have tenderness in the area and a vaginal discharge. Antibiotics or sulfonamides are given to combat the infection. If there is retention of placental fragments, a D and C is performed. The patient on bed rest is placed in a semisitting position. Change of position is encouraged to facilitate pelvic drainage and to help to prevent thrombophlebitis in the legs. The patient is usually given a supportive, high-vitamin diet. Thorough handwashing by the personnel caring for the patient is necessary before and after any procedure in which the genital area is touched. Frequent perineal care and change of the vaginal pad provide some comfort to the patient and help to prevent extension of the infection.

Endometriosis

In this condition, tissue that histologically and functionally resembles that of the endometrium is found outside of the uterus—most frequently on the ovaries, commonly elsewhere in the pelvic cavity, and occasionally in the abdominal cavity. Endometrial tissue has been reported even in the thigh and the forearm. The ectopic tissue apparently responds to estrogen, and perhaps also to progesterone, stimulation. It menstruates when the uterus does, and it shrivels after menopause and may regress during pregnancy. Endometriosis is serious, since the tissue bleeds into spaces that have no outlets. The free blood causes pain and adhesions. During menstruation, dysmenorrhea may be severe and bleeding copious. The fallopian tubes may be occluded, causing sterility. If the endometrial tissue is enclosed in an ovarian cyst (chocolate cyst) there is no outlet for the monthly bleeding. Occasionally the cyst ruptures, spilling its old blood and endometrial cells into the pelvic or the abdominal cavity. There may be menorrhagia, metrorrhagia, dyspareunia, and pain on defecation.

This condition is relieved by menopause: natural, surgical, or radiological. However, because it is a disease of women in their childbearing years, an artificially-induced menopause raises many problems. Surgical treatment often is designed to remove the cysts and as much of the ectopic tissue as possible, and to free the adhesions caused by bleeding, without destroying the childbearing function. Endometriosis that is widespread throughout the pelvic organs may necessitate extensive surgery, such as panhysterectomy (removal of the uterus, both fallopian tubes and ovaries). Sterility of course results. One aspect of medical management is to give the patient hormones to keep her in a nonbleeding phase of her menstrual cycle for a prolonged time, such as nine months. Sometimes this therapy controls the ectopic tissue, so that the patient is symptom-free for several years. Small doses of testosterone may relieve the symptoms without making the patient infertile. Synthetic oral progestins prevent ovulation while the patient is taking the hormone, but pregnancy can occur when the drug is discontinued. Large doses are required to prevent breakthrough bleeding. Norethynodrel and norethindrone are two such synthetic hormones. Patients taking these drugs may experience nausea, vomiting, and diarrhea. Taking the tablets with food may reduce the nausea. Breasts may become tender, and there may be dizziness, weight gain, and stomach cramps. Patients should be taught good leg care (such as not using round garters, not sitting for long periods with legs crossed, and using supportive stockings if there are varicosities), because these synthetic hormones may cause thrombo-embolic phenomena. If the patient notices vaginal bleeding during hormonal therapy, she should notify the doctor. The dosage may need to be increased.

Benign tumors of the uterus

Myomas (fibroids) growing in the uterine wall are the most common tumor of the female pelvis (Fig. 38-4). The development of these tumors is believed to be stimulated by estrogen. They may be small or large, single, or multiple. Growth is usually slow except during pregnancy. Fibroid tumors can occur in various locations in the uterus: subserous, intramural, and submucous. The latter are most frequently associated with excessive menstrual bleeding (Table 38-1).

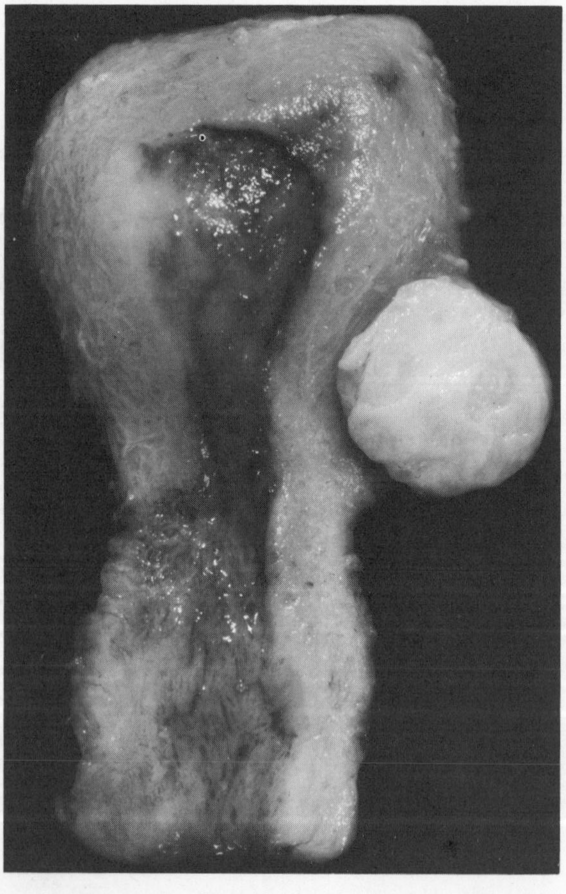

figure 38-4. Fibroid tumor of the uterus. (Courtesy P. S. Milley, M.D.)

Sometimes, this benign tumor causes no symptoms, and the woman is unaware of its existence. When there are symptoms, menorrhagia is the most common. Also, the patient may have a feeling of pressure in the pelvic region, dysmenorrhea, anemia (from loss of blood), and malaise.

The treatment of benign uterine tumors is governed by a number of factors. An asymptomatic tumor in a woman who wishes to have children is usually watched closely by her gynecologist, but it is not treated. The patient is re-examined every 3 to 6 months. A Papanicolaou smear is taken at least once a year.

When the patient has had abnormal bleeding, she may be admitted to the hospital, and a D and C performed to determine the cause of the bleeding, which may be a coexisting condition, unrelated to the fibroid. Sometimes, a curettage is performed to control the bleeding. Although it does not remove the tumor, it preserves the uterus, and it may make immediate, more extensive surgery unnecessary. Surgical removal of the tumor (myomectomy), which also preserves the uterus, may be performed. These operations are done only when the physician is certain that the tumor is benign. Further surgery in the future is often required—if possible, after the patient's family is complete. A hysterectomy is performed when the symptoms are severe and incapacitating. Myomectomy or hysterectomy may be done through a vaginal or an abdominal approach. If the patient is a poor operative risk, and the symptoms are extreme, the tumor may be treated by radiation. The disadvantage of irradiation is that it brings about an artificial menopause, which surgery does not cause, since it does not affect the ovaries.

Cancer of the uterus

Cervical Cancer. The most common malignancy of the female reproductive tract is cancer of the cervix. Only cancer of the breast exceeds it in frequency. Routine inspection of the cervix, with Papanicolaou smears and biopsy of suspicious tissue, is imperative for early diagnosis. When cancer is suspected or diagnosed, the physician may do a Schiller's test. The cervix is painted with an iodine preparation. Biopsies are taken of all unstained tissues, since cancerous tissues are among those that remain unstained.

Cure is possible if the disease is discovered before it has spread. When the cellular change is still confined to the mucosal layer of the cervix, it is called *carcinoma in situ*. Invasion of surrounding tissue may not occur for 5 or more years after the pre-invasion

Table 38-1.
Ovarian cysts and tumors

Ovarian Cysts	Comments	Treatment
Follicular cysts	Caused by retention of fluid, they are often symptomless and may disappear.	Usually no treatment is required; needle aspiration or surgical excision may be required.
Corpus luteum cysts	These cysts form when the corpus luteum fails to regress after the discharge of the ovum.	Surgical excision of the corpus luteum may be necessary; the rest of the ovary can usually be saved.
Ovarian Tumors	**Comments**	**Treatment**
Benign: Serous pseudomucinous Fibroma Cystic teratoma (dermoid)	May cause cessation of menstruation, hirsutism, atrophy of the breasts, sterility.	Surgical removal of tumor, occasionally oophorectomy; reversal of sexual changes follows.
Malignant	May cause (1) pressure on the bladder leading to frequency and urgency or (2) pressure on the portal blood vessel leading to ascites. In the late stages there is weight loss, severe pain, and GI symptoms.	Panhysterectomy Deep x-ray therapy Chemotherapy

period. In this early stage there are no symptoms. Even when the cancer has begun to invade the cervix, there still may be no symptoms. Bleeding is the most prominent symptom.

At first, there is spotting, especially after slight trauma, such as douching or intercourse. Later, if the condition is still untreated, the discharge continues, growing bloody and malodorous as the cancerous tissue becomes necrotic. There may be pain, symptoms of pressure on bladder or bowel, and the generalized wasting of advanced cancer.

If the patient wants children, and the disease is still *in situ,* it may be treated by a cone-shaped amputation of the cervix, leaving the fundus in place for childbearing. Postoperatively the patient is monitored with frequent Papanicolaou smears. Usually, however, a hysterectomy is performed if the cancer has not spread. If the cancer is invasive, it is treated by radical surgery, such as hysterectomy with pelvic node dissection and radium inserts, x-ray or radioactive cobalt therapy, or drug perfusion.

Theoretically, all cancer of the cervix begins *in situ.* It may take 10 to 15 years to become invasive. Therefore, regular Papanicolaou smears are very important for women in their 20s. The means are theoretically available for completely eliminating cancer of the cervix as a cause of death.

Cancer of the Fundus. Carcinoma of the fundus occurs most frequently, and yet not exclusively, in menopausal and postmenopausal women. Bleeding is the earliest and commonest symptom. Before the menopause it may appear as menorrhagia. All vaginal bleeding after the menopause must be investigated.

When cancer is suspected after a gynecological examination and a Papanicolaou smear, the patient may be admitted to the hospital for a diagnostic curettage. This procedure is not without danger, because the scraping may spread the cancer cells.

If malignancy is revealed, the treatment is directed at removing the tumor. A hysterectomy may be done; radium, in a rigid applicator or interstitial needles, may be inserted into the uterine cavity, or deep x-ray therapy may be given to the pelvis. If the tumor is large, it may be irradiated before surgery to reduce its size. Radiation may follow surgery if metastases are suspected.

Cancer of the vulva

This is a relatively rare malignancy usually occurring in women past their 60s. Pruritus is the most frequent early symptom. Later, there may be a bloody discharge, enlarged nodules (as the adjacent lymph nodes become involved), ulceration, edema and a visible mass; finally, there is severe pain. As the cancer ulcerates, there may be a bloody, perhaps a purulent, discharge from the vulva.

Diagnosis is confirmed by biopsy. Vulvectomy with removal of the inguinal lymph nodes (radical vulvectomy) is the treatment of choice. After 5 years, 60 to 75 percent of the patients are alive and considered to be cured. When the disease has spread to an inoperable stage, radiation therapy may be used. There then may be exaggerated tissue reaction, causing the patient to have considerable discomfort.

In view of the patients' average age, the operation may be done in two stages: first the vulvectomy and later the groin dissection. The patient usually is very uncomfortable after vulvectomy, and she probably will need frequent administration of analgesics for at least 2 weeks. Because the urethra is involved in the operation, the patient will return from surgery with a Foley catheter inserted into her bladder. A record should be kept of urinary output. Placing the patient in a semirecumbent position may relieve some of the pressure on the sutures, which will probably be taut. However, she should not remain in one position, even if a comfortable one is found. When she is on her side, the upper leg should be bent and supported with pillows to prevent pull on the operative area. She should do leg exercises frequently—at least once an hour during the early postoperative period. She should be assisted with passive movements until she can move her legs herself. Straining at stool should be avoided. The patient will be given enemas preoperatively and a low-residue diet postoperatively. After she does have a bowel movement, the nurse should avoid contaminating the wound when cleaning the anal region.

The initial pressure dressing is held in place with a T-binder. After this dressing is removed, give frequent perineal care (sterile technique, usually). Sterile saline, peroxide, or an antiseptic solution may be ordered for cleaning the surgical area. If drains are inserted, they should not be disturbed. The nurse notes and records drainage from the drains. Heat-lamp treatments are used to dry the area after perineal care and also to improve the circulation, thus promoting healing. After the sutures have been removed, warm sitz baths may be given. Also, these may help the patient to urinate after the Foley catheter has been removed. The patient's privacy should be insured during perineal care, the heat-lamp treatments, and the sitz baths.

When cancer of the vulva is inoperable, wet dressings and perineal irrigations with a deodorizing solution may help to control the odor and the infection that so often occurs in the ulcerating neoplasm.

Table 38-2.
Postoperative nursing management of the patient with a hysterectomy

Check blood pressure, pulse, respirations every 4 hours or as ordered.
Connect indwelling catheter to closed drainage.
Measure intake and output. Report signs of oliguria or anuria immediately.
Remove and reapply anti-embolitic stockings every 8 hours.
Institute passive leg exercises every 2 to 4 hours or as ordered.
Assist the patient to turn, cough, and deep breathe every 2 hours. Support the incision when coughing.
Check dressing for drainage and reinforce as necessary if the surgical approach was abdominal.
Check for vaginal drainage; use perineal pads as needed.
If surgical approach was vaginal, check for vaginal drainage every 2 hours. Check vaginal packing.

General nursing management of patients with gynecological tumors

Because gynecological tumors can be a threat to both life and reproductive power, the patient should receive as much emotional support as possible from the nurse. The desire for children, the fear of returning to the physician for observation of a fibroid, the fear of cancer, the dread of mutilation, and of the loss of femininity are emotions that lie deep. Sterility, resulting from some gynecological surgery and usually from gynecological irradiation, often requires severe adjustments by the patient. Postoperative tearfulness may be based on hormonal changes as well as a feeling of depression. If it seems helpful, the nurse should discuss the patient's reactions with the family, so that they, too, can support her while she makes her difficult adjustment. The husband should be carefully listened to, since his wife's condition has a special meaning to him as well. Perhaps the nurse can help him to help her.

Preoperative preparation may include catheterization or the insertion of an indwelling catheter to minimize the chance of damaging the bladder. The patient is usually given an enema. Perineal preparation of the skin usually is done with the patient first in the lithotomy position and then in Sims's position to shave the anal region. A hysterectomy or the removal of a large tumor causes sudden shifts in the body spaces, and distention is a frequent and uncomfortable complication.

A patient with a vaginal hysterectomy will wear perineal pads. In some hospitals, sterile pads are used. The nurse changes the pads frequently, and makes sure that the patient has a T-binder or sanitary belt to hold them in place. There will be some serosanguinous drainage, particularly if a radical operation was done. The patient should have frequent perineal care, including after each use of the bedpan. The ambulatory patient who gives herself perineal care still needs the nurse to observe the operative area at least once every 8 hours. The nurse also observes for hemorrhage. With both a vaginal and an abdominal hysterectomy, there should be no more bleeding than is seen in a normal menstrual period. The nurse checks the perineal pad every 10 to 15 minutes during the first few postoperative hours, and then every hour for the rest of the day. There will be a moderate to a slight amount of drainage for the first one or two days, and some spotting for about two weeks. Frank bleeding is not expected. Bleeding may, of course, be internal.

Patients who have had perineal surgery may have discomfort from perineal stitches. Heat in the form of a lamp, sitz baths, or warm perineal irrigations may be ordered.

Inability to void is a frequent postoperative complaint because the urinary tract is in the operative vicinity. There may be edema, inflammation, and loss of muscle tone of bladder and urethra. A Foley catheter usually is inserted preoperatively, and removed on about the 4th postoperative day. After removal, the patient often is catheterized immediately after each spontaneous voiding to note the amount of residual urine, until there is no more than 50 to 80 ml. residual. The nurse observes and records the fluid the first few times that the patient voids spontaneously. Is the amount adequate? Is it bloody? Occasionally, surgical injury to the ureter or the bladder occurs during gynecological surgery. Decreased urinary output and a low backache may indicate that a ureter has been ligated.

Thrombophlebitis is a common complication of hysterectomy. The surgery itself, or the position of the patient during surgery (the lithotomy position is used for vaginal hysterectomy) may interfere with circulation. Frequent turning and active exercises of the legs are in order. To avoid the pooling of blood in the pelvis and pressure on leg veins, the patient should be helped to exercise, and the head of the bed should not be raised higher than midsitting position. The patient should lie flat for short periods during the day. She probably will be out of bed, with help, the day after surgery.

Occasionally, a patient will have the entire contents of her pelvis removed (*pelvic exenteration*). This operation includes a panhysterectomy, a cystectomy, removal of the rectum, and an abdominal-perineal resection. A colostomy is done and the ureters are transplanted into the skin or into the ileum. Both the physical and the emotional trauma resulting from this extensive surgery can well be imagined, considering the radical alterations in physiology and the extensive adjustments in activities of daily living. If the patient is not already past the menopause, she will have a surgical menopause. Because of the severity of the operation, the water and electrolyte regulation will be upset. After vaginectomy the patient will be unable to have sexual intercourse, unless there is sufficient remaining vagina to permit it. Weakness and fatigue will be all-consuming for some time after surgery. In addition, the patient has to adjust physically and emotionally to both a colostomy and a ureterostomy.

On returning home after any kind of gynecological surgery, the patient should know that heavy lifting, straining, or active sport should not be undertaken for several months. Any constrictive clothing, such as a panty girdle, which binds in the area of the groin, should not be worn.

Management of the Patient with Inoperable Malignancy. Death from cancer of the reproductive tract is often prolonged. It may be caused by uremia, as the ureters slowly are shut off by the growth. The patient frequently has severe pain and is emaciated. In addition, there is a thick, foul-smelling vaginal discharge, which is extremely distressing to the patient. She needs frequent perineal care and cleansing douches. Chlorine solutions may help to control the odor. Sensory nerve connections may be severed to relieve intractable pain. A chordotomy destroys the pain tract at a specific level in the spinal cord, and

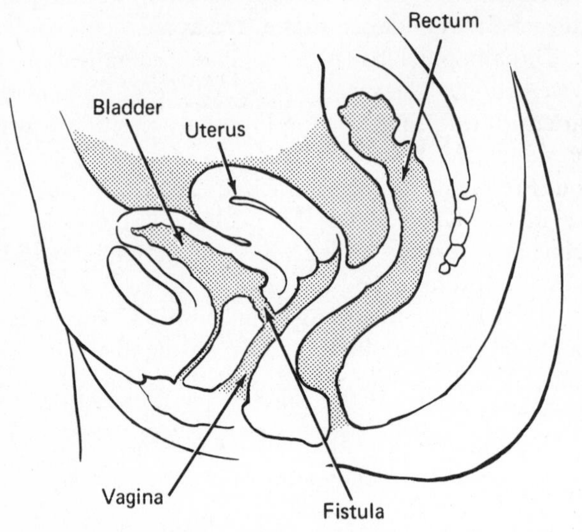

figure 38-5. A fistula between bladder and vagina (vesicovaginal fistula).

may be considered when the pain is difficult to control with narcotics.

Vaginal fistulas

Fistulas may be congenital or a result of obstetric or surgical injury, but the most frequent cause in adults is a breakdown of tissue due to cancer or irradiation. The opening may be between a ureter and the vagina (*ureterovaginal* fistula); between the bladder and the vagina (*vesicovaginal* fistula) (Fig. 38-5); or between the rectum and the vagina (*rectovaginal* fistula).

A large fistula causes the patient endless distress. An opening between the urinary tract and the vagina means that there is continuous leakage of urine from the vagina. The vaginal wall and the external genitalia become excoriated, and often become infected. The patient may not void at all through the urethra, since there may be no accumulation of urine in the bladder. Rectovaginal fistulas cause fecal incontinence and discharge of flatus through the vagina. The feces, added to the leukorrhea that is already present or is initiated by the passage of stool over the vaginal mucosa, are so distressingly odorous that the patient easily withdraws from social contacts. Frequently, the tissues are in such poor condition that surgical repair is not possible.

Treatment and nursing management

Surgery is only performed under as close to optimum conditions as possible: when inflammation and edema have disappeared, and this may mean months of waiting. Unfortunately, surgery for a rectovaginal fistula is frequently unsuccessful.

When surgery is done for a rectovaginal fistula, both preoperatively and postoperatively the patient is placed on neomycin or kanamycin to clean the bowel of colon bacilli. She is given a light, low-residue diet preoperatively, to keep the stool soft, and an enema and a cleansing vaginal irrigation the morning of surgery. Postoperatively, the patient may be kept on clear fluids for several days to inhibit bowel activity, and then graduated first to a light, low-residue diet and then to a general diet. The genitalia may be kept clean and warm perineal irrigations, and perineal heat-lamp treatments ordered to promote healing and to lessen discomfort. Because patients with vaginal fistulas are often debilitated, they need attention to overall health measures, such as an adequate diet, fluids, and rest.

After repair of a vesicovaginal fistula, an indwelling catheter will be inserted. Its drainage should be noted carefully. If the tube becomes blocked, and the bladder is allowed to fill, the pressure may break down the surgical repair and cause the fistula to reappear. If irrigations are ordered, they are done very gently, so that no pressure is applied to the suture line. Vaginal serosanguinous drainage is expected. The absence of urine in the vagina indicates healing of the fistula. If douches are ordered, the pressure should be kept to a minimum.

When the fistula cannot be repaired, as in advanced cancer, frequent sitz baths and deodorizing douches help to control infection and odor and make the patient feel cleaner. A perineal pad or rubber underpants will be needed. Before she joins a social gathering, a woman with a rectovaginal fistula may give herself a low, gentle cleansing enema. If the enema is to be effective, the tube must be inserted above the point of the fistula, and directed away from the opening.

The patient with a fistula usually is discouraged and uncomfortable. It is difficult for her to feel clean. She is always wet with urine, which perhaps is mixed with feces. Not only does she feel the opposite of fastidious, but her skin becomes raw and irritated.

Although the problems remain serious as long as the patient has the fistula, certain measures may help to make her more comfortable. She may wear an absorbent material, such as a perineal pad. Frequent changes of the pad and sitz baths help to reduce odors and lessen the irritation of the skin. Wearing a liner next to her skin helps to keep the urine off the skin. Some patients are soothed by a light dusting of cornstarch. Waterproof underpants are sometimes worn to protect clothing and furniture.

Relaxed pelvic muscles

When the muscles and the fascia that support a structure relax, the structure sags. After unrepaired postpartum tears, childbirth, multiple births, or sometimes without apparent cause (perhaps from a slight congenital weakness), the floor of the pelvis relaxes, and uterus, rectum or bladder may herniate downward. The bulging of the bladder into the vagina is called a *cystocele,* the most common type of poor pelvic support. Herniation of the rectum into the vagina is called a *rectocele.* Downward displacement of the uterus is called *prolapse.* A cystocele and a rectocele usually accompany uterine prolapse. The presence of the uterus low in the vaginal vault is a *first-degree prolapse*; a *second-degree prolapse* is the extension of the cervix beyond the vaginal os; and when the entire uterus hangs outside the body, a *third-degree* or *complete prolapse* (procidentia uteri) is present. The improved obstetrical care now available to many women before, during, and after delivery has greatly reduced the incidence of postpartum pelvic relaxation as a result of childbirth.

Symptoms may include backache, pelvic pain, fatigue, and a feeling that "something is dropping out," especially when lifting a heavy object, coughing, or with prolonged standing. A cystocele may cause difficulty in emptying the bladder, resulting in stagnation of the urine and possible cystitis. There may be stress incontinence: a little urine seeps out every time that the woman coughs, bears down, or strains. A rectocele can cause difficulty in evacuation; constipation can result. In some instances, the patient may need to put her finger into her vagina and apply pressure to the posterior vaginal wall to reduce the herniation before she is able to evacuate the stool collected in the pocket.

Any tissue that protrudes below the vaginal orifice is subject to irritation from clothing or rubbing against the thighs in walking. This is especially seen in second- and third-degree prolapse. Ulceration and infection frequently follow. These symptoms are annoying and they may be incapacitating. They may forbid standing for a long time, walking with ease, or lifting and other activities that are difficult to avoid.

Treatment and nursing management

The surgical repair of a cystocele is called *anterior colporrhaphy.* Repair of a rectocele is called *posterior colporrhaphy.* Repair of the tears (usually old obstetric tears) of the perineal floor is called *perineorrhaphy.* The operations are done by the vaginal route and occasionally under local anesthesia. A vaginal hysterectomy may be done to remove a completely prolapsed uterus.

The patient may be kept on bed rest for one or two days before surgery to decrease any edema of the area. The bed should not be placed in a high-sitting position, which would increase congestion in the pelvic region. Before posterior colporrhaphy an enema is given to empty the bowel.

Postoperatively, perineal dressings are not commonly used; rather, perineal care is given several times a day, and always after the patient has urinated or defecated. A heat lamp is sometimes ordered to dry the area and to promote healing. Every effort is made to prevent pelvic pressure and stress on the suture line. An ice pack may be ordered to relieve edema and pain, and this should be placed so that the weight of the pack lies on the bed and not on the patient. If sitz baths are given, a rubber ring should be placed in the bathtub. Until healing has taken place, the patient may be more comfortable sitting on a pillow placed over a rubber ring. About the 3rd or 4th postoperative day, the patient may be given a suppository or an oral cathartic to prevent strain when having a bowel movement.

After an anterior colporrhaphy, a Foley catheter usually is inserted to keep the bladder empty, since overdistention of the bladder could weaken the repair. The catheter is attached to straight drainage while the patient is in bed. When the patient is ambulatory, the nurse finds out whether the catheter is to be clamped, or whether straight drainage is to be continued. Clamping may be ordered to allow the bladder to fill to increase its muscle tone. However, it should be released every 4 hours to prevent overdistention. If the patient does this herself, the nurse checks to be sure that the patient remembers to release the clamp. No more than 150 ml. should accumulate in the bladder.

After the catheter is removed (2 to 7 days postoperatively), the nurse observes for adequate voiding. The patient should urinate every 4 hours, but may have frequency without adequately emptying the bladder. Catheterization for residual urine may be ordered. Urinary output should be measured for the first day or two after the catheter is removed.

Because these conditions are most frequently found in older women, sometimes there are complicating diseases that make surgery too great a risk. Under such circumstances the displacement may be reduced by inserting a pessary, which repositions the uterus. The pessary should be kept as clean as possible to avoid infection. A sterile lubricant should be applied to it before it is inserted. Once the pessary is in place, the patient should feel nothing. Discomfort may indicate that it is placed incorrectly, or that it is causing irritation. The appearance of leukorrhea may indicate an infection, in which case the patient should see the physician immediately. The pessary usually is kept in place for 6 weeks at a time. The patient should return to the physician one week after its insertion and then about every 2 months. Hard rubber or plastic pessaries have less tendency to become soggy than soft rubber ones. Assuming the knee-chest position for a few minutes once or twice a day helps to keep the genital organs and the pessary in good position. Modern surgical techniques, and concern over the possible harmful effects of chronic irritation from the pessary, have made the use of pessaries infrequent.

Pelvic relaxation happens over the years. It is not uncommon for a woman to tolerate the increasing discomfort until a more "convenient" time for surgery. She may wait until cystitis is well developed. All nurses, and particularly those in community health and industry, are in a position to urge early medical attention before complications become severe, and the condition is incapacitating.

Uterine displacement

In some women the position of the uterus is abnormal. Displacement usually is congenital; sometimes backward displacement is due to childbearing. *Anteflexion* is the term given to a uterus that is bent forward at an acute angle. In *retroversion* the uterus tilts backward. In *retroflexion* the fundus is bent backward on the cervix (the opposite of anteflexion).

Displacement may be asymptomatic, or it may cause backache, dysmenorrhea or sterility. The condition may be treated by the insertion of a pessary and the assumption of the knee-chest position several times a day. If the displacement causes severe discomfort, or if there is a chance for sterility to be corrected, surgery may be attempted, during which the uterus is moved to a more natural position.

Bibliography

ANTHONY, C. P.: *Structure and Function of the Body,* ed. 4. St. Louis, Mosby, 1972.

AVERY, W. et al.: Vulvectomy . . . women who have this surgery require physical and psychological care (pictorial). Am. J. Nurs. 74:453, March, 1974.

BARTER, R. H.: Vaginal hysterectomy with anterior-posterior colporrhaphy (pictorial). Hosp. Prac. 9:71, October, 1974.

CARBARY, L. J.: Vaginitis: the common female complaint. Nurs. Care 7:29, September, 1974.

CREIGHTON, H.: The new abortion ruling. Super. Nurse 4:8, July, 1973.

DI MAURO, J.: The threat of hysterectomy. J. Prac. Nurs. 23:28, April, 1973.

Explaining hysterectomy. Nurs. '73, 3:36, September, 1973.

GREEN, T. H.: *Gynecology.* Boston, Little, Brown, 1971.

Hysterectomy . . . helping patients adjust. Nurs. '73, 3:8, February, 1973.

MATTHEWS, A. E. B.: Endometriosis. Nurs. Mirror 139:65, July 5, 1974.

MEMMLER, R. L. and RADA, R. B.: *The Human Body in Health and Disease,* ed. 4. Philadelphia, Lippincott, 1977.

NEWTON, M.: Essentials of the gynecologic examination. Consultant 13:72, December, 1973.

SCHERER, J. C.: *Introductory Clinical Pharmacology.* Philadelphia, Lippincott, 1975.

SHANKLIN, D. R.: Endometrial cancer: a worsening problem. Consultant 14:94, September, 1974.

SOIKA, C. V.: Gynecologic cytology. Am. J. Nurs. 73:2092, December, 1973.

CHAPTER—39

The man with a disorder of the reproductive system

On completion of this chapter the student will:

- **Label a diagram of the male reproductive tract.**
- **Discuss the medical and surgical management of the patient with benign prostatic hypertrophy.**
- **Formulate a nursing care plan for and participate in the nursing management of the patient with benign prostatic hypertrophy.**
- **Name the four operative approaches used for the removal of the prostate.**
- **Formulate a nursing care plan for and participate in the nursing management of the patient having a prostatectomy.**
- **Describe disorders of the testes and adjacent structures—cryptorchidism, epididymo-orchitis, spermatic cord torsion, hydrocele, varicocele, and prostatic and testicular malignancy—and medical or surgical management of each disorder.**

Embarrassment, fears of impotence, and the feeling of loss of self-esteem frequently make a disorder of a reproductive organ hard for the patient to bear. It is important to realize that although the patient may more readily discuss his concerns with

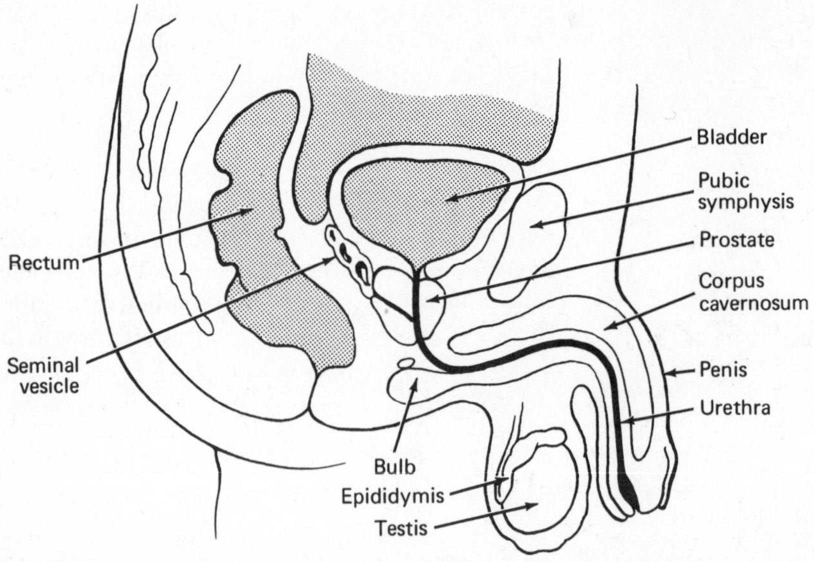

figure 39-1. Male genitourinary tract.

the physician, the nurse should also show a willingness to listen. If the patient appears worried about his illness or an impending operation, a knowledgeable nurse can let him know that his fears are neither strange nor unexpected, and that he may discuss any matters that he wishes. If he seems unduly shy or hesitant, the nurse might mention these observations to the physician so that he may open the subject. The patient himself decides how he wishes to proceed.

In the male, the lower urinary tract and reproductive system are so closely associated that disorders in this area frequently affect both systems. This is in contrast to the female where, although close together, these systems are somewhat more separate. The male genital system consists of the testes which produce sperm and the epididymides and vas deferens which deliver the sperm to the seminal vesicles and prostate (Fig. 39-1). The bladder urine and seminal fluid are both discharged, although separately, to the outside through the urethra, which traverses the penis.

Benign prostatic hypertrophy

The prostate gland is an accessory sex organ which produces most of the seminal fluid. This fluid contains zinc, invert sugars, and other substances necessary for nutrition of the sperm. The prostate is located just below the urinary bladder. The urinary stream travels through the center of the gland in the prostatic urethra. With advancing age and seemingly under the influence of male sex hormones, the periurethral glandular tissue undergoes hyperplasia, with gradual enlargement of the gland. This outward expansion is not of any clinical importance. However, inward encroachment of this tissue which diminishes the diameter of the prostatic urethra certainly is.

The symptoms of "prostate trouble" are all secondary to an increasing impediment to urinary flow. Symptoms appear gradually. At first the patient may notice that it takes more effort to void and there is decreasing force and narrowing of the urinary stream. As the residual urine remaining in his bladder accumulates, the bladder fills more quickly, and the patient finds that he has the urge to void more and more frequently. Urgency, to the point of incontinence, is common. At night he awakens for trips to the bathroom. There may be difficulty in starting the stream, and hematuria when it does start. Residual urine is a good culture medium for bacteria, and if infection results, symptoms of cystitis will also be present. The combination of hesitancy, narrowed stream, straining to void, frequency, urgency, and nocturia is known as prostatism. Any obstruction in the lower urinary tract can cause these symptoms, but the most common is prostatic enlargement.

Diagnosis

If the patient has prostatic hypertrophy, examination will demonstrate that the gland is enlarged and elastic. Cystoscopy will reveal the extent of the infringement on the urethra and the effects on the bladder. Pyelography will give information about the possible damage to the upper urinary tract due to the backup of urine. Blood chemistry tests are done to reveal kidney malfunction. Measurement of significant quantities of residual urine (usually at least 60 ml.) adds to the data confirming the diagnosis.

Treatment and nursing management

Symptomatic benign prostatic hypertrophy is treated by surgically removing part of the prostate gland. Unless the patient has marked symptoms or is totally unable to void, a urethral catheter is not inserted preoperatively. The history will indicate whether the patient has had an acute episode of urine retention, or whether larger and larger residual amounts have been building up over a long period of time. In cases involving sudden acute retention, a urethral catheter is inserted and connected to straight drainage. If, on the other hand, the history suggests a gradual worsening of chronic retention, complete relief of the obstruction and rapid complete emptying of the bladder may have dire consequences, including profound hematuria due to rupture of the numerous stretched mucosal blood vessels and postobstructive diuresis with loss of large amounts of sodium in the urine. If unnoticed and unreplaced, the salt and water loss may be serious enough to cause the patient to go into shock. Consequently, if the retention is chronic, the bladder will be decompressed slowly (over a period of hours).

Preoperative Regimen. During the preoperative period, the patient is put on a healthful regimen, with emphasis on copious fluids, a good diet, and rest. Other illnesses are treated, such as regulation of diabetes and digitalization for heart failure.

If catheter drainage is not provided, the patient is taught to measure his urine and keep a record of the time and the amount voided each 24 hours. The chart may reveal an abnormal pattern that will be fairly consistent from day to day.

If during the preoperative evaluation period the physician finds significant damage to the upper urinary tract, he may elect to perform a suprapubic cystostomy (a small suprapubic incision into the bladder through which a catheter is inserted). This type of urinary drainage bypasses the prostate until there is adequate recovery of renal function so that a definitive operation on the prostate can be performed safely. The use of the suprapubic catheter for long-term drainage prevents epididymitis and other serious infections associated with prolonged use of a urethral catheter. The patient may be sent home with this drainage for several months. He and a family member need instruction in the care of the catheter and skin before discharge from the hospital.

Types of surgery

As benign prostatic hypertrophy develops, the hyperplasia of the periurethral glands forms an adenoma which comprises the bulk of the prostate. The adenoma thins and compresses the surrounding true capsule of the gland. Between the adenoma and capsule there is a plane of cleavage which can be developed easily by the surgeon. The aim of all surgical procedures for benign prostatic hypertrophy is removal of the adenoma, leaving the true capsule behind. Subsequently, the patient urinates through this fossa. Healing, by re-epithelialization, occurs over a 2- to 3-month period.

The four operative approaches used for the removal of the prostate are: (1) suprapubic prostatectomy, (2) retropubic prostatectomy, (3) perineal prostatectomy, and (4) transurethral resection of the prostate (TURP). At open operations (retropubic, perineal, and suprapubic prostatectomy), the surgeon develops the cleavage plane between the adenoma and capsule by either finger or sharp dissection. The adenoma is removed along with the mucosa of the prostatic urethra. The transurethral method accomplishes the same objective except that the adenoma is removed piece by piece through an instrument inserted through the urethra.

Transurethral prostatectomy is the easiest of the four operations for the patient, since there is no external wound. It is performed most frequently on patients with complicating conditions, such as heart disease and advanced age, and those with a small amount of prostatic hypertrophy. Hemorrhage can result around the eighth to tenth day when tissue sloughing may occur.

The surgeon's preference, his experience with various techniques, the size of the adenoma, and the general condition of the patient play a part in the type of operation performed. If the patient is very obese, the transurethral or perineal approach may be preferable to an abdominal one.

One patient may become discouraged if he observes another patient who entered at the same time with the same complaints going home 1 week after a transurethral resection. Such a patient should be helped to understand that the transurethral approach would not have been the best procedure for him, and that results,

Table 39-1.
Nursing management of a patient following a prostatectomy

Take blood pressure, pulse, respirations q1-4h or as ordered.
Take *oral* temperature q4h.
Connect catheter(s) to closed drainage system. Label the source of each container (for example, "urethra").
Measure intake and output. Record the output of each catheter.
Apply traction to urethral catheter if ordered.
Note and record the color and description of drainage from each catheter.
Check surgical dressing q2h. Reinforce as needed. Report any excessive drainage.
Help patient turn, cough, deep breathe, and do leg exercises q2h. Initiate IPPB if ordered.
Irrigate catheters only if ordered. Use the type and amount of irrigating solution ordered by the physician.

even with the same operation, differ from patient to patient.

Although the majority of patients retain potency following operations for benign prostatic hypertrophy, there is a significant percentage in whom it is impaired following perineal surgery. Consequently, the perineal approach is reserved either for the elderly or for patients in whom there is a strong suspicion of cancer and a radical prostatectomy may be planned. There is also some danger of injury to the rectum resulting in incontinence and possible fistula formation. Following simple perineal prostatectomy, patients generally do not require catheter drainage for longer than 1 week.

Preoperatively, many surgeons will order a bowel prep to decrease postoperative fecal wound contamination.

Nursing management after prostatectomy

No matter which surgical approach is used, there are general principles of care applicable to all post-prostatectomy patients (Table 39-1).

When the patient returns to his room, the catheter or catheters are attached to the prescribed type of drainage. Output of each is separately recorded.

The patient may also return to his bed with a Penrose drain inserted into the tissues of the operative site. This drain, which does not enter the urinary tract, removes blood and urine that have leaked into the area. The Penrose drain is removed when all drainage has ceased.

The following are matters of considerable import following prostatectomy:

Bleeding. Clear urinary drainage following any type of prostatectomy is rare. Hematuria is generally present. However, frank bleeding is a serious emergency and a potential complication for several days after surgery. Color of the urine and the presence of any clots must be noted. Bright red blood indicates an arterial bleeding source while a deep black red suggests venous oozing. Clots can obstruct the catheter causing spasm, pain, and further bleeding. Therefore, the catheter must remain patent at all times. The bladder is checked for fullness and tenderness. If these are present, the bladder could be distended with clots and the physician should be promptly notified.

To control arterial bleeding, the surgeon may put traction on the urethral catheter. One method used is that of taping the inflated catheter to the thigh. The traction may be maintained for 6 hours, but after this there is danger of damage to the bladder sphincter causing temporary incontinence. The physician may order the tension to be decreased gradually or may reapply more gentle traction overnight. The patient has a sensation of having a full bladder even though the bladder is empty. If he tries to void around the catheter the bladder muscles contract causing a painful spasm. The nurse can explain to the patient that the bladder is kept empty by the catheter and that trying to void causes irritation to the bladder mucosa. Encouraging fluid intake (if permitted) helps to decrease bladder mucosal irritation because there is a constant passage of fluid over the irritation. Explaining to the patient why he feels this need to urinate may help him not to worry about it.

Drainage and Irrigation. The doctor usually orders straight drainage without irrigation. Overzealous irrigation may induce further bleeding and cause frequent and uncomfortable bladder spasms. The nurse follows the doctor's orders regarding *when* to irrigate and *how much* and *what kind* of solution to use.

In selected patients, continuous irrigation is ordered. The continuous gentle flow of fluid helps to prevent clots from forming in the bladder and plugging the catheters. The drip is regulated to maintain the drainage at a light pink. When this through-and-through irrigation is ordered, the urethral catheter is usually used for inflow and the cystostomy tube for outflow. The danger of bleeding is increased if the irrigating fluid is continued when the outflow is obstructed by clots.

Normal saline is preferred for irrigation, especially if a large volume of irrigant is necessary, to prevent dilution of blood as a result of absorption of the irrigating solution.

When the urethral catheter is removed, the time and amount of each voiding should be recorded for several days. The patient may be instructed to do this. Occasionally, if urinary function does not progress satisfactorily, reinsertion of the catheter may be necessary.

Bladder Spasms. It is important that the nurse distinguish between catheter obstruction and bladder spasm. Usually with catheter and, consequently, bladder obstruction there is gradual and increasing discomfort with absence of urinary output. The bladder becomes distended and is tender on palpation. Relief of the obstruction is urgent. If there is an order for catheter irrigation by the nurse she should do this gently. If patency is not achieved, or there is no order for irrigation, the urologist should be notified.

When bladder spasm without catheter obstruction is present, the patient will have a urinary output, but pain may be constant or intermittent. Some bladder spasms are extremely painful, but fortunately each spasm lasts only a few seconds. Narcotics do not seem to lessen the spasms, but they will help to decrease pain from the operative area. An antispasmodic drug such as propantheline (Pro-Banthine) may be ordered.

Dressings and Wounds. The nurse changes the cystostomy and perineal dressings as frequently as necessary to keep the patient clean and dry. Care must be taken not to disturb any tissue drains placed by the surgeon. Montgomery straps simplify frequent dressing changes. Strict aseptic technique is essential to prevent wound infection.

After a cystostomy tube is removed, the suprapubic wound frequently leaks urine for a few days. A saturated, wet dressing, the odor of urine, and wet bed clothes can be very uncomfortable and embarrassing to the patient. If his dressings are not changed promptly when necessary, he may attempt to keep dry by restricting his fluid intake. The nurse encourages liberal fluid intake (when the patient's medical status permits) by demonstrating to the patient that he will have his dressings changed promptly and by attempting to provide the type of liquid which is most appealing to him. An ample supply of dressings is kept at the bedside and replenished as needed.

The nurse will observe and chart the amount of urine that comes from the wound and the condition of the skin surrounding it. To prevent irritation, the skin should be washed frequently. A medicated powder or ointment may be prescribed if irritation develops. The wound heals slowly, depending to a great extent on the general health of the patient. If it becomes infected, healing is even slower.

Although a perineal wound may not be as painful as an abdominal incision, the patient may experience some discomfort when sitting for the first week or two. A male T-binder is used to support the dressing. In some instances, beginning on the second or third postoperative day, special wound care consisting of cleansing the incision with surgical soap and water followed by exposure to a heat lamp is performed three times daily. The procedure is completed by applying an antiseptic and a dry sterile dressing. Sitz baths may be ordered after removal of the drains. By 10 days after operation, perineal wounds are usually well on their way to healing. Early postoperative patients should have help in cleansing after a bowel movement to avoid contaminating the wound. Much of the nursing care following a perineal prostatectomy is the same as that for any perineal or rectal procedure: for example, sitz baths and the maintenance of extreme cleanliness.

Rectal Precautions. Generally, the use of rectal tubes, rectal thermometers, and enemas is not resumed until at least a week following prostatectomy to avoid perforation or hemorrhage. This precaution is observed especially for patients having perineal surgery.

Bowel Hygiene. After prostate surgery the patient should be cautioned to avoid straining to have a bowel movement because this can cause prostatic hemorrhage. Stool softeners may be ordered daily, or a mild cathartic may be ordered after the third day. Copious fluids and dietary roughage, as permitted, help to prevent constipation.

Convalescence. Since most patients having prostatic surgery are in the older age group, surgery can be a severe strain and one more contributory factor to pre-existing depression. Personality change as a result of increased emotional and metabolic stress should be anticipated after surgery. Following removal of the urethral catheter, the patient may notice some dribbling of urine requiring frequent changes of clothing. This problem may disappear after a few days but in some cases may become persistent.

After discharge from the hospital, the patient should continue to maintain established fluid and bowel routines and follow his physician's orders for physical activity. Generally, no lifting or straining is permitted for several weeks. A referral to a visiting nurse agency and other community resources may be indicated.

Cancer of the prostate

Prostatic carcinoma is most common in men over the age of 50. As life expectancy increases, more and more men live to the age group of highest incidence of this disease. Along with cancer of the lung and gastrointestinal tract, it is among the more common malignancies of older men.

Symptoms

At first there are no symptoms, and none may occur for years. The disease usually starts as a nodule in the posterior lobe of the gland which is farthest away from the urethra. If the tumor grows large enough, it will obstruct urinary flow and cause frequency, nocturia, and dysuria. Thus, a patient with cancer of the prostate who has urinary symptoms is usually in the more advanced stage of the disease. Many patients who have prostatic cancer also have benign prostatic hypertrophy, and the symptoms of urinary obstruction may be due to the latter condition. Spread of the cancer is by way of the bloodstream and lymphatics to the pelvic lymph glands and skeleton, particularly the lumbar vertebrae, pelvis, and hips. The first symptoms may be back pain or sciatica due to metastases to the nerve sheaths. In 75 percent of patients with prostatic cancer extending beyond the prostatic capsule, the acid phosphatase, an enzyme produced by the prostate, is elevated in the blood. Because early cancer of the prostate is asymptomatic, and because cure is possible only when the disease is discovered early, regular annual or biannual rectal examinations of all men over 50 are as important as are regular gynecologic and breast examinations for women.

Treatment and nursing management

In the presence of a solitary nodule, an open perineal biopsy with frozen section may be suggested. The surgical approach is as for simple perineal prostatectomy. If the nodule is benign and the patient has symptoms of prostatic obstruction, a simple prostatectomy can be performed at that time. If the nodule is seemingly localized cancer, a radical perineal prostatectomy can be performed. In contrast to prostatectomy for benign disease, the so-called radical operation involves en bloc removal of the entire prostate with its capsule and the seminal vesicles. The bladder neck is sutured to the membranous urethra over a Foley catheter which is left indwelling for 10 to 14 days. Disadvantages of the operation include virtually guaranteed impotence (versus a chance to be cured of cancer) and some serious difficulty with urinary control in 5 to 10 percent of patients.

Preoperative Management. If the patient is to have radical surgery through a perineal approach, bowel preparation usually includes enemas and a liquid diet the day before the operation. After surgery the patient is kept on a low-residue diet until healing occurs, so that he does not strain at stool.

Postoperative Management. The patient returns to his unit with a Foley catheter placed so that the balloon supports the urethral anastomosis to the bladder neck. Care must be taken that the tube is not displaced from this position. The nurse remains watchful for hemorrhage. She notes and records the color of the urine. The Foley catheter is removed in 10 to 14 days. The patient will have a tissue drain. Initially, there may be seepage of urine through the wound, but this should stop in about 2 days.

Perineal irrigations may be ordered to help to keep the wound clean and to decrease pain and inflammation. After the sterile dressing is removed, the nurse irrigates very gently with the solution that is ordered, often a mild antiseptic, such as hydrogen peroxide. This treatment gives the nurse an excellent opportunity to observe progress in healing and signs of disturbance in the healing process. Additional wound care and nursing measures are similar to those carried out for the patient following rectal or perineal surgery.

The perineal dressing is very close to the rectum, and should not be allowed to remain soiled with fecal matter. Since a fistula easily develops in the fragile tissue of the operative site, nothing is inserted into the rectum—no rectal thermometers, no rectal tubes, no enemas—unless specifically ordered by the surgeon. Fluids should be encouraged to 3,000 ml. a day, unless there are orders to the contrary.

Often, patients are assisted out of bed the second postoperative day. They should sit on a firm, even surface. They should never sit on a rubber ring or an air mattress, either of which could cause compression of or congestion in a portion of the operative site.

If urinary or fecal incontinence results, some patients may be helped to regain fecal control by doing perineal exercises to improve muscle tone and by regulating their diet. Perineal exercises may be done by contracting and relaxing the gluteal muscles. The patient can be taught to observe the effects of various foods. He should avoid only particular foods that cause diarrhea, and not any important food groups. Dietitian, physician, and nurse work with the patient to help him to establish a dietary regimen that results in good nutrition and regular, formed bowel movements.

The thought of incontinence for the rest of his life may be very depressing to the patient. He should be taught how to keep himself dry and odor-free, so that he will not feel shy about mixing with other people. Teaching the patient to care for himself should start while he is in the hospital and has the support of the staff. One object of this teaching is to make self-care as simple and routine as possible, so that the patient will be relatively free to concentrate on matters other than his condition.

Prognosis

The outlook for most patients with prostate cancer is relatively good in that many men who are obviously incurable may experience prolonged palliation on conservative therapy. Manipulation of the patient's hormones may give surprising, if temporary, relief of symptoms. Where there had been severe pain, there may be none; where there was bladder neck obstruction, urine may flow freely. Many tumors will progress under the influence of androgens and regress on estrogens. Following the decrease in androgens by castration (bilateral orchiectomy) and treatment with estrogens, 50 percent of men with "incurable prostate cancer" will be reasonably comfortable and well 5 years later. Because of fluid retention problems associated with estrogen therapy, the patient with congestive heart failure must be very carefully observed. A low salt intake is recommended.

As androgens are decreased and estrogens are given, the patient's voice may become higher, hair and fat distribution may change, and breasts may become tender and enlarged; gastrointestinal disturbances may also occur. When estrogens are used in lower doses, the patient may not experience these feminizing changes.

If, even after drug therapy, the tumor obstructs the bladder neck, a transurethral prostatectomy may be necessary to establish urinary drainage. Occasionally, permanent suprapubic drainage will have to be established.

In the late stage of the disease, there may be severe pain which may be treated by chordotomy. Radiation therapy may give some relief from painful metastases.

Disorders of the testes and their adjacent structures

Cryptorchidism (undescended testicle)

Failure of the testicle to lie in the scrotum is known as cryptorchidism (or undescended testicle). At least one testis (plural, *testes*) must be in its normal position in the scrotum for the patient to have reproductive function. The undescended testis may lie in the inguinal canal, in the abdominal cavity, or rarely in the perineum or femoral canal. If undescended testes are not placed in the scrotum by age 5 or 6, the likelihood of their being good sperm producers diminishes markedly. Undescended testes have a significantly higher incidence of malignant degeneration whether or not they are placed in the scrotum, but the overall incidence of tumors of undescended testes is low. In some individuals, undescended testicles find their way into the scrotum without treatment during childhood or at puberty.

Some physicians advocate a short (1 week) trial of hormone (androgen) therapy. If there is no response within 3 weeks, surgery may be performed (orchiopexy). Other physicians feel that surgery should be performed in all those with undescended testes, preferably before puberty. After orchiopexy the patient may have three wounds: inner thigh, scrotal, and inguinal. The surgeon makes an inguinal incision and locates the testis. It is held in the scrotum on tension to a taped rubber band attached to a suture through the lower pole of the testis and to the skin of the upper thigh. The suture is usually removed in 5 to 7 days. Often there is an associated congenital hernia which is repaired at the time of orchiopexy. The patient can move his leg, but, of course, undue pressure should not be placed on this traction. The nurse should inspect the traction, which will be outside the dressings, several times a day to make sure that it is functioning well.

Adolescent boys who have this operation may be particularly embarrassed to have a female nurse present during dressing changes or to have her inspect the dressings. If there is a male on the nursing team, the patient may feel more comfortable in his care. Some young people in their embarrassment will joke excessively. A matter-of-fact but friendly and accepting manner on the nurse's part may help them to regain their poise.

Epididymo-orchitis

Infection and inflammation of the testis and epididymis usually occur simultaneously. The most common cause is infection ascending via the vas deferens and its surrounding lymphatics from a prostatitis. A less common cause of acute epididymitis is untreated gonorrhea.

The symptoms are chills, fever, scrotal pain, and tenderness. The scrotal skin may be erythematous and tense. A markedly swollen testis and epididymis can be palpated. Elevation of the scrotum with a 4-tail bandage or adhesive taped across the upper thighs (Bellevue bridge) relieves the pain considerably by lessening the weight of the testes.

Strict bed rest is usually ordered during the early stage. An ice bag may be ordered to help to relieve the pain. It should be placed under the tender scrotum; not on top of it or leaning against it. The cold bag should not be kept constantly next to the skin, because it may damage tissue. On an hour, off a half-hour is one routine that may be followed. Heat is not applied to the scrotal area, because spermatozoa are damaged by heat that is even a few degrees above body temperature. (The normal temperature of the scrotum is lower than that of the rest of the body.) As with any infection, copious fluid intake is encouraged. Antibiotics may be ordered.

Orchitis without epididymal involvement is most often caused by mumps occurring after puberty. This viral orchitis may result in testicular atrophy and sterility. For this reason men who have not had mumps as children and who are exposed to it are advised to receive immediate medical attention. The administration of gamma globulin may have the effect of lessening the severity of mumps if it develops. Commonly, there will be a sudden onset of chills, fever, and testicular swelling 1 or 2 weeks after the parotid swelling. Urethritis may also be present. Besides local treatment, corticosteroids may be prescribed.

Bilateral epididymitis frequently leads to permanent azoospermia (absence of sperm), especially when the infection recurs frequently, or when it becomes chronic. Vasectomy (removal of a section of the vas deferens) prevents recurrent attacks, but it causes sterility if it is performed bilaterally.

Torsion (twisting of the spermatic cord)

This condition occurs in prepubescent boys and men whose spermatic cords are (congenitally) unusually unsupported in the vaginal sac and are freely movable. Torsion may follow severe exercise, but it also may occur during sleep or following such a simple maneuver as crossing the legs. There is a sudden, sharp testicular pain and local swelling. The pain may be so severe that nausea, vomiting, chills, and fever occur. The testis is extremely tender and the usually posterior epididymis may be located anteriorly. In contrast to inflammatory conditions, elevation of the scrotum will increase the pain by increasing the degree of twist.

Treatment consists of immediate surgery to prevent atrophy of the spermatic cord and to preserve fertility. The torsion is reduced, excess *tunica vaginalis* (the membrane surrounding the testis) is excised, and the testis is anchored with sutures in the scrotum. A similar prophylactic procedure may be performed on the opposite side.

Hydrocele

Normally, there is a small amount of fluid in the space between the testis and the tunica vaginalis. A large accumulation of fluid in that space is known as *hydrocele*. This common cause of scrotal enlargement may be due to an infection, commonly epididymitis or orchitis, or trauma; the majority occur without known cause. When the accumulation of fluid is slow (chronic hydrocele), there is usually no pain, even when the scrotum becomes as large as a grapefruit. A hydrocele causes few symptoms in most instances except for its weight and unsightly bulk. Acute hydrocele is accompanied by both pain and swelling and may follow trauma or local infection.

Treatment, if indicated, consists of surgical excision of the sac. Aspiration is rarely done, particularly since the fluid will reaccumulate and there is a real danger of introducing infection. Postoperatively, the patient has a drain and a pressure dressing. A snug support is required for some weeks afterward.

Varicocele

This condition usually occurs on the left side of the scrotum and consists of dilation and tortuous clumping of tributaries of the spermatic vein. Swelling and pain are the major symptoms. Very rarely does a varicocele per se cause enough symptoms to warrant surgery. In certain instances of infertility, correction of a varicocele has resulted in significant improvement in the semen specimens, for unknown reasons. The surgery involves an inguinal exploration of the spermatic cord with ligature and division of the major spermatic vein tributaries in this region.

Cancer of the testes

Malignancy can occur anywhere in the male reproductive system but is not common in the testes. Testicular tumors tend to metastasize early, and the first symptoms may be related to the secondary site of growth. The symptoms may be abdominal pain, general weakness, and aching in the testes. Gradual or sudden swelling of the scrotum should always receive medical attention.

The diagnosis is most often made when the physician discovers a hard, nontender scrotal swelling. If testis cancer is suspected, the operation suggested is an orchiectomy performed through an inguinal incision. Biopsy risks spilling tumor cells; these tumors are highly malignant.

Depending on the pathology, further treatment may be radiotherapy to the lymph glands (para-aortic nodes), surgical removal of these glands followed by radiotherapy, or chemotherapy. When radical lymph node dissection through a thoracoabdominal incision is done bilaterally, the procedure involves extensive surgery, and the patient is very uncomfortable postoperatively. Because the tissue supporting the kidneys may have been removed, he may be kept in a Trendelenburg position for a week or two to help to maintain the kidneys in good position. In this position it is difficult to eat, read, urinate, and defecate. X-ray therapy is usually begun immediately after surgery.

Pharmacological considerations

- The patient with prostatic carcinoma may be treated with estrogens. Depending on the dose used, the patient may or may not experience feminizing changes: enlargement and tenderness of the breasts, change in fat distribution in which the hips and thighs often increase in size, voice changes (rise in pitch). Since these changes may be distressing to the patient, their occurrence should be explained before therapy is begun.
- Some physicians may elect to treat cryptorchidism with a trial of hormone (androgen) therapy. Other physicians feel that the administration of the male hormone only produces a precocious puberty and that the reason for the cryptorchidism is a defect in the inguinal canal, requiring surgical correction.
- Chemotherapy for testicular cancer is often intensive, as the tumor metastasizes rapidly. The patient often becomes acutely ill from the drug(s), and hospitalization is often recommended during drug therapy.

Bibliography

ANTHONY, C. P.: *Structure and Function of the Body,* ed. 4. St. Louis, Mosby, 1972.

BALLINGER, W. F., et al.: *Alexander's Care of the Patient in Surgery,* ed. 5. St. Louis, Mosby, 1973.

CARBARY, L. J.: Problems of the prostate. Nurs. Care 8:12, August, 1975.

KEUHNELIAN, J. and SAUNDERS, V.: *Urologic Nursing.* New York, Macmillan, 1970.

Kidney and Urinary Tract Infections. Indianapolis, Lilly Research Laboratories, 1971.

LE MAITRE, G. and FINNEGAN, J.: *The Patient in Surgery: A Guide for Nurses.* Philadelphia, Saunders, 1975.

RODMAN, M. J.: Anticancer chemotherapy. Against solid malignant tumors, Part 2. RN 35:61, March, 1972.

RODMAN, M. J. and SMITH, D. W.: *Clinical Pharmacology in Nursing.* Philadelphia, Lippincott, 1974.

WINTER, C. and BARKER, M. R.: *Nursing Care of Patients with Urologic Diseases,* ed. 3. St. Louis, Mosby, 1972.

CHAPTER 40

The patient with breast disease

On completion of this chapter the student will:

- Describe the normal physiological functions of the female breast.
- Discuss the incidence of breast disease.
- Name the signs and symptoms of breast disease.
- Describe the method of self-examination of the breasts.
- Recognize the emotional trauma experienced by the woman undergoing breast surgery.
- Describe the preoperative management of the patient having breast surgery.
- Differentiate between simple and radical mastectomy with regard to structures removed and extent of the surgery.
- Formulate a nursing care plan for and participate in the nursing management of a patient having breast surgery.
- List the complications of breast surgery.
- Name the various methods of treatment of metastatic breast cancer.
- Discuss the surgical, medical, and nursing management of a breast abscess.

Physiology of the breast

The breast is a complicated glandular organ that produces milk after pregnancy. Considerable space in the breast is devoted to a network of ducts that carry milk to the nipple. The lymphatic and blood supplies are rich.

The breast manufactures milk from elements in the blood. The transformation of amino acids and glucose in the blood to the proteins and lactose in milk is a chemical process not yet fully understood. To make 30 ml. of milk, it has been estimated that the breast must process 12,000 ml. of blood.

Although the most dramatic changes occur in the breast during its preparation for its primary function —lactation—the mammary glands are a part of the female reproductive system, and thus they respond to the hormonal cycle associated with menstruation. Estrogen, secreted by the ovaries, brings about the growth and development of the duct systems and suppresses lactation. Progesterone, secreted by the corpus luteum of the ovary, stimulates lactation, as does prolactin, an anterior pituitary hormone.

Incidence of breast disease

The most common breast disorder is cystic disease. Although frequent, benign tumors such as fibroadenoma are less common than cystic disease.

In American women the breast is the most common site of cancer. It is estimated that 1 of every 25 women in the United States today will develop breast cancer. When the disease is discovered and treated early, the 5-year level of cure for small lesions is about 80 percent. After 20 years it drops to 60 percent. More than half survive at least 5 years after diagnosis.

This disease can occur at any age, but it is most common during and after the menopause. The longer a woman lives, the greater is her chance of developing breast cancer. The disease is more common in women who have a relative who has had the disease, and it is less common in those who have nursed babies. Each year more than 50,000 women in the United States have a *mastectomy* (removal of a breast). These patients may be helped by knowing that it is not they alone who have lost a breast. Though it primarily affects women, men, too, can develop breast cancer.

Diagnosis

Although cysts and tumors start microscopically, when they grow larger, they sometimes cause physical changes in the breast that may occur before there is any discomfort or pain. Because women have a better chance for cure when cancer is detected early, every lump and every change in the appearance of the breast should be brought immediately to medical attention. The earlier cancer is diagnosed, the less chance that it has spread. Axillary lymph nodes and the internal mammary lymph nodes drain the breasts. Enlarged nodes occur in breast abscess and cancer. The rate of survival is not as great if the lymph nodes are involved. The 5-year 80 percent survival figure applies to small lesions—less than 3 cm. in diameter and with negative nodes.

Signs and symptoms of breast disease

Pain. At times breast pain may be normal. It is not uncommon for the breasts to become enlarged and tender during the period immediately before menstruation. These physical changes are probably associated with the hormonal changes of the reproductive cycle, and they may be due to an increase in extracellular fluid tension, but the mechanism is not fully understood. Women with cystic disease also frequently experience fullness, tenderness to the touch, and some pain in the breast immediately before they menstruate.

Lumps. This is one of the prime symptoms of a breast disorder. The chief importance of self-examination lies in the discovery of lumps, as a lump may be a cyst, a benign tumor, or a malignancy. Many lumps disappear at the time of menses and only those present postmenstrually are significant. Characteristically, malignant lumps are painless in their early stages. The differential diagnosis can be made by a physician, but only if it is brought to his attention. Rarely in malignancy, a lump in the axilla is the first sign that is noticed. In those women who do not regularly have breast examinations, most lumps are discovered by accident. For example, a woman receives a sharp blow to her breast. That night the area is still tender, and she puts a hand up to it. She discovers a lump. The lump was not caused by the blow, but its discovery was.

Nipple Discharge. A discharge that spots the brassiere or drips out without being elicited requires medical attention immediately. Cheesy and milky discharges are usually of no significance. Bloody, brown, or clear fluid discharges should be checked immediately.

Change in Appearance. A breast with an adhering lump near the surface may *dimple* the skin outside, or it may cause the nipple to *retract*.

A deep-adhering cancer may fix the breast tissue

to the underlying pectoral muscle. There may be a change in *firmness, redness, chapping* of the areolar area, *erosion,* or *edema.*

Examination

Self-Examination. In order to discover carcinoma of the breast early enough so that its excision may be life-saving, regular examination of their breasts by all women is advocated. The best protection against cancer is *effective early action.*

The following technique is suggested for self-examination of the breasts:

- Sit or stand in front of a mirror, with arms relaxed at sides, and examine breasts carefully for any changes in size and shape. Look for any puckering or dimpling of the skin, and for any discharge or change in the nipples.
- Raise both arms over head, and look for exactly the same things. See if there's been any change since breasts were last examined.
- Lie down on the bed, put a pillow or a bath towel under left shoulder, and left hand under head. With the fingers of the right hand held together flat, press gently to feel the inner, upper quarter of the left breast, starting at the breast bone and going outward toward the nipple line. Also feel the area around the nipple.
- With the same gentle pressure feel the lower inner part of the breast. Incidentally, in this area, a ridge of firm tissue or flesh will be felt. Do not be alarmed. This is perfectly normal.
- Now bring left arm down to side, and still using the flat part of fingers, feel under armpit.
- Use the same gentle pressure to feel the upper, outer quarter of breast from the nipple line to where the arm is resting.
- And, finally, feel the lower outer section of the breast, going from the outer part to the nipple.
- Repeat the entire procedure on the right breast.
- Examine the breasts every month right after menstruation. Be sure to continue these check-ups after menopause.
- If a lump or a thickening is found, leave it alone and see the doctor. Most breast lumps or changes are not cancer, but only the doctor can tell.

In spite of the excellent educational program of the American Cancer Society, there has not been a significant drop in the death rate due to cancer of the breast. Many women are not aware of what they themselves can do to discover early disease. Some women have not been exposed to the idea of self-examination. Others have, but fail to attend to it. Small early cancers can only be found by regular examinations.

Emotional Factors. In the education of women for protecting themselves from death from cancer of the breast, the imparting of knowledge is not enough. The educator also must understand why there is resistance to action, and how people may be helped to overcome their apparent indifference. Apathy, fear, and the magical belief that cancer will happen to the other person and not to oneself leads to resistance to regular examinations of the breasts.

The knowledge that two thirds of all breast operations are for benign lesions is not necessarily reassuring. The patient knows that she may be in the other third. Those who have seen a close relative die of cancer of the breast may find self-examination especially difficult.

Some women fear the cure as much as the disease. Breast amputation is mutilating; irrevocably it alters a woman's body, and particularly significant is the fact that it affects a part of her body intimately associated with sexual fulfillment and childbearing. Concern with appearance after surgery may be mitigated only partly by the use of prosthetic devices. The change in her body is one that the woman herself must learn to accept and cope with, regardless of what measures she may use to conceal the disfigurement from others.

These are deep and significant feelings, not to be ignored. Nurses should help women to come to grips with these feelings by listening to them. Without prying, the nurse can help the woman to identify exactly what it is that troubles her. She can be encouraged to talk to her physician without feeling embarrassed, and provided with the factual information that she needs. The patient needs a great deal of support from the physician, nurse, office secretary, friends, and family.

Fear of cancer is not limited to those outside the medical and the nursing professions. The United States culture is one which places high value on the female breast as a primary source of identification with the feminine role. Since most nurses are women, some may find the care of patients with breast cancer threatening and anxiety producing because of their vulnerability to this disease. Unwittingly, they may avoid the patient except for highly structured activities such as teaching exercises. If the nurse is to be supportive of patients, she must have the opportunity to become aware of her own feelings and reactions.

Some women seem to survive the surgery without damage to their self-concepts. One woman who had had a bilateral mastectomy said, "My breasts weren't *me*. The *me* is still there." This woman suffered no depression postoperatively and says that when she is dressed she does not feel that her appearance is markedly altered.

EXAMINATION BY A PHYSICIAN. All women should have their breasts examined by a physician at least once a year. Those over 30, those with cysts, and those who have a relative who has had cancer should be examined every 6 months. Women should go immediately to a physician when a lump in the breast is discovered.

To investigate a breast lump the physician completely palpates the breasts and nodes. Palpation of adjacent (such as axillary) lymph nodes helps to determine evidence of cancer that has spread. The spread to lymph nodes is sometimes diagnosed by biopsy. The breasts are inspected from every angle with the patient sitting, standing, and bending. *Mammography,* or soft tissue x-ray examination of the breast without the injection of a contrast medium, may be ordered. On these films it is possible for the radiologist and the surgeon to distinguish with considerable accuracy a benign from a malignant lump, and also to discover lesions that are still too small to palpate. When a malignancy is suspected, the surgeon usually takes a biopsy to confirm the diagnosis.

Malignancy in the breast seems to be somewhat more common in patients with cystic disease than in women with normal breasts. The most important point in the nursing management of these patients is to encourage them to have regular examinations. The search for new lumps is complicated by the already existing ones caused by the cysts, but the woman who becomes familiar with her own breasts by periodic examination often can identify new growths.

Incisional biopsy is performed in the operating room. The microscopic frozen section is examined by the pathologist while the patient is anesthetized. The surgeon is guided in his treatment by the pathologist's report. X-ray pictures may be taken to determine whether or not there are metastases to bone.

Cystic disease

Chronic cystic mastitis is not inflammatory (as the word *mastitis* would imply). In this disorder normal breast tissue proliferates and forms many masses throughout the breasts. The masses become fibrotic and block the ducts, causing cysts to form.

Cystic disease of the breast may cause no symptoms other than lumps, or the breast may be tender, especially premenstrually. There may be shooting pains 1 or 2 days before menstruation. A well-fitted brassiere may be advised by the physician. During periods when the breasts are tender, the patient may feel more comfortable if she wears a brassiere during the night as well as the day. Multiple cystic disease sometimes is treated by simple mastectomy. The areola may be saved, and reconstruction surgery may be done with fat and fascia or a plastic insert to preserve the appearance of the breast (augmentation mammoplasty).

A single breast cyst may develop, frequently with a bluish color, which has prompted the name *blue-domed.* Cysts are usually movable in the surrounding breast tissue. They have far less tendency to adhere and to cause retraction than does cancer.

Breast surgery

PREOPERATIVE MANAGEMENT

A benign tumor usually is excised and the incision closed. When there is malignancy, the surgeon usually removes the pectoralis major, the pectoralis minor, and the entire breast along with the adjacent lymph nodes in an attempt to remove all of the cancer cells from the patient's body: this is a *radical mastectomy.* A *simple mastectomy* is removal of a breast without lymph node dissection.

Other procedures for malignancy include simple mastectomy with axillary dissection, extended radical mastectomy with chest wall resection, and superradical mastectomy in which the sternum is split and the lymph nodes are dissected from the mediastinum. Since the latter two procedures involve opening the thoracic cavity, additional postoperative care is required.

In surgery for a lump in the breast, the preparation of the patient for operation is for the more extensive operation, because until the doctor sees the pathology report he does not know whether the lesion is benign or malignant.

The spread of cancer is capricious and inconstant. It may begin early or late. At first it is microscopic, and is not detectable grossly. A very small lump in the breast may have sent some cells along the lymphatics to the axillary nodes. Cancer spreads through the lymphatics and blood vessels.

Before surgery the patient should be told by the surgeon that a radical mastectomy may be necessary. Skin preparation includes the axilla. Blood typing and cross matching are done. The operative permission includes radical mastectomy.

This is a time of tension and suspense for the patient. She does not know whether she will awaken from the anesthesia with only a lump removed or an entire breast removed and a diagnosis of cancer. She must be helped in every way possible to face the impending operation.

It may be easier for her to talk to a woman about her fears than to a man. The nurse should be sure to know what the surgeon has told the patient. She may not know that cancer is the disease in question (although that would be rare today); the word should not be used first by the nurse, who can let the patient talk without adding to her anxiety. Some patients prefer not to mention the word "cancer," even though they are aware that it is a possible diagnosis. The patient can be assured that her breast will not be removed unless the physicians know that this operation will be necessary for her health. If she has doubts about this subject, either preoperatively or postoperatively, she should have the opportunity to express them, but the idea that the operation is necessary must be conveyed. When the patient seems unable to accept the surgery, this should be discussed with the surgeon before the operation is performed. This is essential in order to help to lessen serious postoperative sequelae, such as severe depression or the patient's inability to recognize and to acknowledge that a breast has been removed.

When there is no doubt that a radical mastectomy must be done, a short visit from a recovered patient may assist the patient to accept the surgery more readily.

The operation

The patient is prepared for a radical mastectomy and is kept under general anesthesia while the biopsy specimen is being examined. The pathologist requires about 15 minutes to make his diagnosis of the tiny piece of tissue. If the diagnosis is of a benign tumor, the surgeon may simply excise it and close the wound.

The excision of a benign breast tumor is minor surgery. If it were not for the possibility of performing a radical mastectomy, many benign tumors could be removed under local rather than general anesthesia. The surgery is over quickly, and the incision is small; the patient usually goes home after 2 or 3 days in the hospital.

If at operation the pathologist's report shows that the lesion is malignant, the surgical drapes are changed and the operating team rescrubs and proceeds with a radical mastectomy.

A drain is often inserted to prevent the accumulation of fluid in the wound. A skin graft (often from the anterior thigh) may be required to close the resulting wound. When there is a graft, a drain may be left in the axilla to drain fluid that may form under the graft and prevent its "take." Pressure dressings are applied on both the donor and the recipient sites.

If the cancer is so far advanced that there are metastases to other portions of the body, the removal of the breast will not cure the disease, and a mastectomy may not be done. A simple mastectomy may be performed to remove a grossly enlarged, draining breast to make the patient more comfortable.

The combined operations—breast amputation and bilateral oophorectomy for node metastases from breast cancer—are performed in premenopausal women by some surgeons. Because the ovaries are removed to eliminate the source of estrogen from the body, no replacement estrogens are given to help to relieve the distressing symptoms of the surgical menopause. The suddenness of the lack of estrogen supply frequently causes these patients more severe menopausal symptoms than those associated with natural menopause.

The two operations, singly or in combination, are threatening to a woman's image of herself, especially for women of childbearing age. One operation prevents a woman from having children, and the other mutilates her appearance.

Postoperative management

Patients who have had a radical mastectomy frequently discover the diagnosis for themselves when they are beginning to recover from anesthesia. Unlike many other types of surgery, this operation makes the diagnosis evident to the patient. The doctor and the family have no time to talk over how, if, and when to break the news. The patient, whose emotional and physical resources have been lowered by anesthesia, surgery, drugs, and suspense, needs a nurse to be there to help her at the time of the anguish of discovery.

Arm Position. Because in radical surgery the incision is extensive, disturbing the integrity of a large area of skin and muscle, immediately after the surgery the upper arm on the affected side is prevented from excessive motion, especially abduction. That arm may be bandaged to the body, with the elbow bent at a right angle, especially if grafting has been done. Motion might pull the graft free of its attachments. Whether the arm is bandaged or not, abduction of the arm on the affected side should be prevented. The arm must be kept especially still when grafting has been done. A pillow may be placed under the arm to help to support it and to elevate it above breast level at least for the first day. This aids in preventing lymphedema that commonly develops postoperatively from interference with the circulatory and lymphatic systems. If the arm is bound to the body, the hands should be checked for signs of impaired circulation (swelling, cyanosis, coldness, tingling). If such signs are noted, the surgeon is called.

THE DRESSING. Drains may be inserted at the time of surgery to remove the serous fluid that collects under the skin, thereby delaying healing and predisposing to infection. A drainage tube may be attached to low-pressure suction such as the Hemo-Vac which enables the patient to be easily up and about and eliminates the need for constantly reinforcing dressings. Drainage tubes are irrigated daily by the physician in order to free any clots.

Some wounds drain copiously. Color, amount, odor, and consistency of any drainage, whether from a drain or on the dressing, are noted and charted. The dressing is checked for drainage and oozing, any evidence of these is reported to the physician. The nurse will feel with her hand under the patient's side, since fluid seeping from the wound may not be visible on the front of the bandage, but it may flow underneath the patient. Immediately after the operation, the dressing should be checked at least every 15 minutes. On the second and the third postoperative days it is checked at least three times a day, but not disturbed. The dressing, which is bulky to hold the skin flaps down, is usually left in place until the fifth to the ninth day after the operation, depending on whether a graft was used and the preference of the surgeon. At that time the dressing is changed.

Table 40-1.
Postoperative nursing management of the patient with a radical mastectomy

Take blood pressure, pulse, respirations q1-4h or as ordered. Do not take blood pressure on the arm on the affected side.
Take temperature q4h.
Elevate head of bed.
Elevate arm on operative side on pillows.
Measure intake and output. Empty Hemo-Vac q8h or as ordered. Do not allow Hemo-Vac to become too full as suction will be lost.
Check surgical dressing q2h. Reinforce as necessary. Report any excessive drainage.
Help the patient turn, cough, deep breathe, and do leg exercises q2h. Institute IPPB as ordered.
If a skin graft has been done, check donor site. Reinforce dressing as needed. Report excessive drainage.
Do not draw blood from or administer intravenous fluids in the arm on the affected side.

Every effort should be made to assist the patient to look at the incision before going home, but she should not be pushed into this at the time of the first dressing change. In addition to the incisions, stab wounds for drains are also present and the overall appearance can greatly upset the patient who may react with hysteria, anger, crying, depression, or withdrawal. Helping the patient involves anticipation of and sensitivity to her reaction. Timing the encouragement for the patient to look requires an assessment of the patient's state of readiness. Sometimes, having the husband, daughter, or other person who will help the patient at home come to the hospital for the dressing change is beneficial. The nurse can offer support and answer questions.

The patient needs to know that in time, redness, swelling, and irregularity disappear, the scar becomes less prominent, and tissues become more normal in color. The healing period for the wound is 4 to 8 weeks for most patients. Pressure dressings may be continued after the initial dressing change, and dressings are changed daily until healing occurs.

Since dressings tend to constrict the chest, the patient needs to be assisted to cough deeply and take deep breaths. Pain is considerable and narcotics are given liberally as ordered by the physician. Because the movement of the chest is painful and opiates depress respirations, the patient is helped to take full breaths after medication for pain has had its effect.

AMBULATION. The patient may be helped out of bed for the first time on the operative night or the next day. Patients who have had radical surgery, with or without drainage, are helped to walk as soon after surgery as patients who have had a simple mastectomy. If the patient needs assistance as she walks, support her on the *unaffected* side. She will have a tendency to splint the operative site and to balance herself by hunching that shoulder. Encourage her to keep the shoulder level and the muscles relaxed. For approximately 2 weeks (the length of time varies with the surgeon's preference) the arm on the affected side usually is supported in a sling whenever the patient is out of bed.

ENCOURAGING SELF-SUFFICIENCY. Immediately postoperatively, the patient will need help with those activities that she cannot do for herself, such as cutting meat. To avoid placing her in the dependent and embarrassing position of having to ask for such services, they should be performed before it is necessary for her to request them. However, as soon as it is possible, she should be encouraged to be independent and to do everything for herself that she can; this should be done without conveying the impression that the nurse does not want to be bothered with her.

Postoperative nursing management is summarized in Table 40-1.

EXERCISES of the affected arm will be ordered by the physician and may begin on the third or fourth postoperative day. With grafting, no exercise is used without definite written orders from the surgeon. In patients who do not have grafts, exercises are frequently preceded from the first postoperative day by such activities of daily living as brushing the teeth, washing the face, and combing the hair with the affected hand. Squeezing a rubber ball stimulates circulation and helps restore function. Exercises prevent shortening of muscles, contractures of joints, and loss of muscle tone.

Active exercises are always more effective than passive ones. As soon as the physician has given permission, the patient starts on a regular program that can enable her to perform all the activities in which she used her arm preoperatively. The first exercises may be opening and closing the hand, flexing and extending the fingers, and bending the wrist forward and backward. In some hospitals no order is needed to commence these exercises, and they are started on the first postoperative day. There is a psychological as well as a physiological point to starting active exercises soon after surgery. This is something that the patient herself can do to aid in her recovery. When the drains are removed and the first dressing is changed, the surgeon may consider that the wound has healed sufficiently so that the patient can abduct her arm. Raising the elbow away from the body may be started. If fluid collects in the wound, exercises are delayed.

Whenever the exercises start, it is important for the return of full function that they be practiced regularly. The removal of the pectoral muscle causes some temporary loss of strength, but no loss of arm function. Though the arm on the affected side will present the most difficulty, exercises should be bilateral to avoid pain and postural change resulting from inconsistent development and consequent structural change.

Some hospitals have group classes for postmastectomy patients. Doing exercises with other women who have the same difficulties can help a patient to feel that she is not odd or clumsy, and that she is one among others who share a common problem and have common goals. A mimeographed pamphlet that can be given to the patient, illustrating the exercises, may help her to practice those ordered for her. *Help Yourself to Recovery*, a pamphlet written for patients, describes postmastectomy exercises. Published by the American Cancer Society, it is available from your local Cancer Society chapter.

The teaching of exercises is important but it should not be the focus of the nurse-patient relationship. The feelings and reaction of the patient afford the framework in which the nurse teaches. A perfect teaching plan can be a failure if the patient is not ready to learn or is so anxious that her perception is distorted. Because patients vary in their grief reactions, some may be too depressed to be able to meet the nurse's expectations for participation in self-care activities. The normal healing processes of grieving cannot be accelerated and some patients need more time, artful listening, gentle suggestion, and passive performance by the nurse before they are able to accept the changes in themselves and be ready to learn. As the patient's mourning and depression lessen, she will be able to be more aware of how the exercises are helping her and become a more active participant in the learning process.

SKIN CARE. After the bandage has been removed, the nurse can help the patient to care for the skin area herself. She should wash it gently with a soft washcloth and soap. Complete healing of the wound takes considerable time and varies with the patient's state of health and complicating factors, such as wound infection. Whereas some wounds heal in 2 months, others may require 6 to 8 months for complete healing. It is not unusual for patients to have some discomfort in the operative site for several months. One described the discomfort thus: "It pinches and pulls and feels as if it is bandaged with sandpaper." Cold cream, pure lanolin or any emollient may be applied to the scar. Talcum powder may relieve itching.

ATTITUDES. The emotional significance of a mastectomy varies from patient to patient. To some it is but a surgical experience, and life continues as before.

To others it means the first signal of the death process. Many women are occupied with thoughts of death, but find no one with whom to discuss it freely. Family and friends understandably tend to avoid conversations about death, and the patient is expected to carry on as before. Not only are these individuals emotionally involved with the patient, but a conversation about another's impending death is a reminder that one, too, will die.

The postmastectomy patient often feels isolated, with no one to help her face the annoying problem of the healing incision and the larger problems of social acceptance and worry about death. How effectively the patient maintains her contacts with family and friends when she returns home is determined by her prior relationship with them and by her attitude, and theirs, to the surgery. The nurse can encourage the patient to maintain her ties with friends and family during hospitalization by showing courtesy to the patient's visitors and by assisting the patient, if she needs help, when she wishes to write letters or to make telephone calls. Perhaps the greatest help that the nurse can render in aiding the patient to maintain her ties with others after discharge lies in showing acceptance of the patient and willingness to help her come to grips with the impact of the surgery.

If the patient learns to care for her skin while still in the hospital and has your support and interest, she may have less tendency to shun the scar once she gets home. If she is repelled by the sight of it, allow her to tell you. Show interest in its progress of healing, and help her to become used to it. You can tell her that the scar will become less noticeable in time. For example, the married patient who can begin to accept her scar before she leaves the hospital can help her husband to feel less shy or embarrassed about it, and then in turn he can help her to feel more comfortable about it.

A Prosthesis. On discharge from the hospital the patient is seldom ready to wear a commercial prosthesis because the wound is not healed. When the surgeon tells the patient that she is ready for a commercial prosthesis, she has her choice of several different types (Fig. 40-1). Some are made of foam rubber; others are inflated with air or filled with fluid. Sponge rubber is light and easily washable. Excessive heat and careless handling should be avoided. If a rubber prosthesis is worn under a bathing suit, it can be squeezed dry unobtrusively with the forearm while the woman dries her face with a towel. The prostheses that are filled with water assume natural contours in keeping with those of the other breast as the woman changes position. These prostheses feel more like a normal breast and even assume body warmth.

It is especially important for nurses to know where to refer their postmastectomy patients, since it is frequently the nurse to whom the patient will turn for help.

Some surgical supply houses and corsetieres who sell breast prostheses have an experienced female prosthetist who can give the patient a correct fit and instruct her in the care of the prosthesis. Some companies have excellent pamphlets prepared for postmastectomy patients. Be sure that the physician approves of the literature, the prosthesis, and the store before suggesting any of these resources to the patient. The addresses of several stores can be given to the patient. Some hospi-

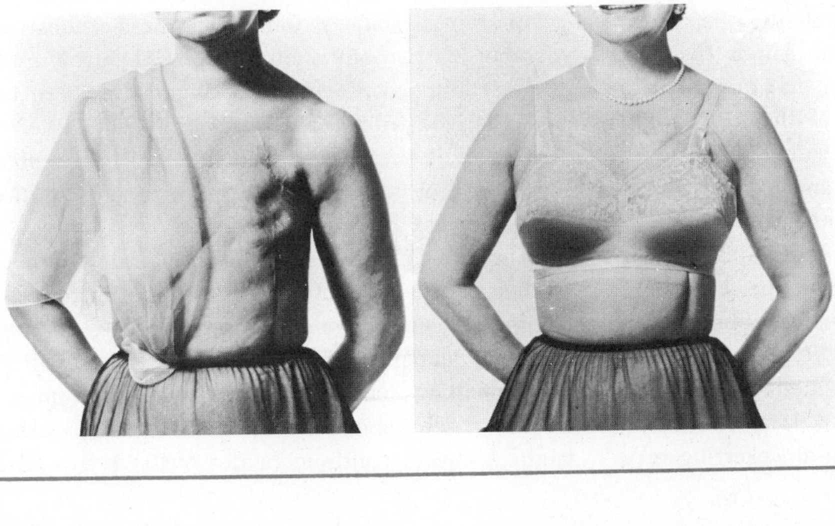

figure 40-1. (*Left*) Radical mastectomy scar. The slight irregularity is typical. (*Right*) Same patient fitted with a prosthesis. (Identical Form, Inc., New York, N.Y.)

tals keep samples of different types of breast forms to show to the patients.

Complications of breast surgery

Some postmastectomy patients develop sympathetic pain in the other breast. Encourage such a patient to call this symptom to the attention of her physician. It usually does not represent organic disease. At times the remaining breast becomes larger. The amputation site may become infected, or serous fluid may collect beneath the incision. When changing the dressing, and after the dressing is no longer necessary, the nurse will inspect the wound daily, looking for pockets of swelling, redness, discharge, odor, and breaks in the suture line.

Slight and transitory swelling of the arm is usually relieved as soon as the arm regains function. However, in some postmastectomy patients lymphedema is disabling. It may develop shortly after the operation or years later. The cause is unknown, but it is believed that an infection that obstructs lymphatic flow may be involved. Radiation may aggravate lymphedema. Because infection may play a role in its etiology, and because the complication may occur years later, women who have had a mastectomy should be told to treat as serious even slight infections of that arm and that hand. Any symptoms of infection of the hand or cellulitis of the arm (fever, pain, red streaks, on the arm) should bring the patient immediately to her physician. Cutting the cuticles should be avoided, because it may lead to infection. The patient should exercise care not to break the skin when she cuts her nails, and hangnails should be cut, if at all, by a physician. Most women are understandably reluctant to go to a doctor to have a hangnail cut, but they must be warned not to pull at it or to bite it, to keep it very clean, and to report to the physician at the slightest sign of soreness or infection. The healthy, unbroken skin is the best protection against a minor infection that may lead to the major complication of edema of the arm. Night creams may help to keep the skin soft. Patients with lymphedema should not be given any form of injections or vaccinations in the affected arm.

Edema of the arm is treated by antibiotics to abolish the underlying infection; however, this treatment is effective only if it is applied before fibrosis has blocked lymphatic outflow. Often the patient is hospitalized, and her arm is kept elevated on a pillow. An air pressure machine may be used. It automatically fills the segments of the sleeve with air, exerting progressive cumulative pressure on the arm. The most distal portion of the sleeve fills first, then the next, and so on, forcing fluid past incompetent lymphatic valves toward the heart. After all the segments are filled, the air is released, and the cycle starts over again. The machine is set approximately 5 mm. below the diastolic blood pressure. This treatment must be used several times a day to be effective. Significant arm edema can be controlled in some cases with the use of an elastic sleeve or bandage. Patients who are obese will need help in losing weight, as obesity complicates the reduction of the edema. Low sodium diets and diuretics are sometimes prescribed.

Treatment of metastatic cancer

It is estimated that slightly over two thirds of the individuals affected with mammary cancer will sometime during their lifetime have disseminated mammary cancer. Metastases often cause pain in the new site. Lymph nodes are most commonly involved in metastasis with bone and pulmonary involvement following in order. Many organs and systems can be affected before death. When bone becomes involved, there is danger of pathologic fracture (fracture after slight or no trauma). The patient is taught to take precautions against falling and to avoid bumps. Without frightening her, the nurse will encourage her to keep regular appointments with her physician.

Treatment varies with the physician and specific type of metastasis and is aimed at providing the greatest period of palliation for the patient. All forms of treatment carry the possibility of unpleasant side effects and complications.

Hormonal Therapy. Normal function of the mammary gland is dependent on the action of several stimulating hormones. Changing the hormonal environment of the body should inhibit the growth of the primary tumor or metastatic tissue elsewhere in the body derived from the primary tumor. The hormonal environment of the body can be changed by *ablation* (removal) of an endocrine organ or by *addition* of exogenous sex hormones.

Endocrine ablative procedures include prophylactic or therapeutic destruction of the ovaries or testes (castration) by surgery or radiotherapy. Also, the adrenal gland is capable of producing estrogen. Bilateral adrenalectomy sometimes is performed in women who have estrogen-dependent metastatic cancer, and whose vaginal smears continue to demonstrate a high level of estrogen activity. This operation may cause the cancer to regress and the patient to feel less distress. Lifetime replacement of cortisone with adjustment of dosage in times of stress is necessary after adrenalectomy.

The removal of the pituitary gland (hypophysectomy) may be done in the treatment of estrogen-dependent tumors to suppress both the adrenal glands and the ovaries. Other endocrine glands will be suppressed as well, and the patient may require adrenal and thyroid replacement therapy. After both adrenalectomy and hypophysectomy the nurse should watch the patient for polyuria and other water and electrolyte balance disturbances. Stress may bring about symptoms of adrenal or pituitary insufficiency. (See Chapter 35 for a more detailed discussion of observations to be made and nursing management in these conditions of endocrine imbalance.)

Additive hormonal therapy to change the internal environment includes the use of androgens, estrogens, progesterone, and cortisone.

Large doses of estrogen and testosterone are used sometimes to help to alleviate the pain, weight loss, and malaise of metastatic cancer. Estrogen is contraindicated in premenopausal women, for whom large doses of testosterone may be ordered for its antagonistic effect. Hormonal treatment does not cure cancer that has spread, but it may increase the life span by months or even years, and it makes some patients more comfortable during much of this time. Why the hormones have this effect is unexplained.

Estrogen therapy can cause nausea and vomiting, pigmentation of the nipple and areola, and uterine bleeding. Stress incontinence is frequent. Sodium may be retained, leading to excessive storage of intercellular fluid and edema. To help to relieve this situation, diuretics and a low-sodium diet may be ordered. Large doses of estrogen sometimes cause the mobilization of calcium into the bloodstream. When this happens, the kidney may be damaged in excreting the excess calcium.

Intramuscular androgen (testosterone) therapy is used especially when there are metastases to bone. Patients may have increased bone pain after the first few injections, but as therapy continues, pain is frequently lessened, there is some recalcification of bone, and the patient has an increased appetite and gains weight. Androgen therapy may cause fluid retention and distressing symptoms of virilization, such as deeper voice, hirsutism, and increased libido.

The results of therapy aimed at decreasing the amount of estrogen in the patient's body may be observed by vaginal smears and studies of the urinary excretion of estrogen and calcium.

RADIOTHERAPY may be given preoperatively or postoperatively. If the surgeon finds that the axillary nodes contain cancer cells, a series of x-ray treatments may be ordered prophylactically, even though the nodes have been removed. Postmastectomy exercises should continue during the x-ray treatments. For palliation purposes, radiotherapy may be directed to treatment of primary tumors, regional or distant metastases especially to bone, or local recurrence to the chest wall.

CHEMOTHERAPY. Metastases to soft tissue and bone are most responsive to chemotherapeutic agents. Use of antineoplastic drugs may cause bone marrow depression, granulocytopenia, anemia, nausea and vomiting, hypotension, dermatitis, malaise, diarrhea, and stomatitis.

The use of any of the above measures may prolong the patient's life and make her more comfortable. Many patients eventually will succumb to the disease, but some will die from other causes. Some patients are symptom-free for long periods and lead relatively comfortable and fruitful lives. Unfortunately, others, like the young woman with galloping metastases, may die quickly. Still more might have to endure long periods of suffering before they succumb. The victims of breast cancer offer to nursing unlimited challenge.

Breast abscess

Abscesses occur most frequently as a postpartum complication (Fig. 40-2). Fissures and cracks in the nipple provide an entry for organisms, especially staphylococci, which thrive in milk. The patient is usually hospitalized, placed on isolation precautions, and treated with antibiotics. A localized lesion may be incised, drained, and packed. Because the soiled dressings are highly infectious, the nurse should keep a separate dressing tray at the patient's bedside.

Montgomery straps are applied so that the frequent removal of adhesive tape will not irritate the skin. If warm soaks are ordered, zinc oxide is applied to the surrounding skin to avoid maceration. A massage of the neck and shoulder muscles on the affected side may help to decrease the pain by relaxing those muscles. The arm and shoulder are supported with pillows. The patient is instructed not to shave axillary hair on that side until healing is complete. A postpartum patient admitted to the hospital with a breast abscess is often worried about the new baby she had to leave in someone else's care at home, and about the added expense of a second, unexpected hospitalization.

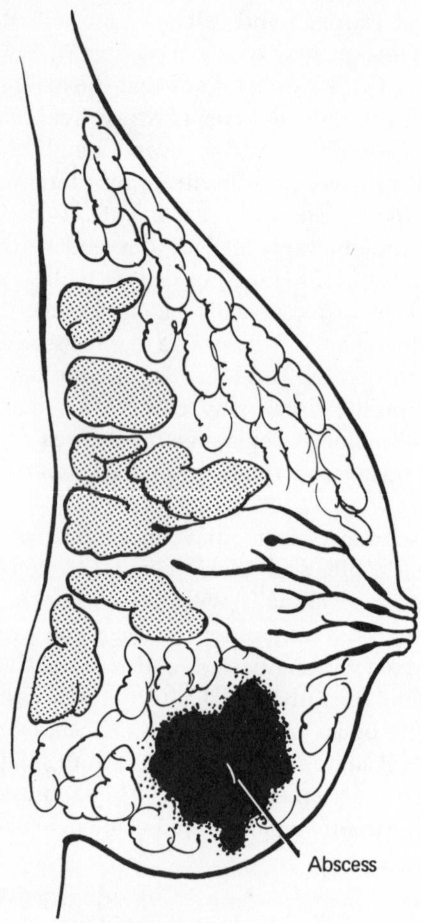

figure 40-2. A breast abscess.

Pharmacological considerations

- Testosterone may be used in the treatment of metastatic breast cancer in the female. Use of this drug may result in some noticeable body changes, namely a development of masculine characteristics such as deepening of the voice and appearance of facial hair. Hypercalcemia and sodium and water retention may also occur. When the patient is given testosterone, the body changes should be explained *before* therapy is begun.
- The diabetic patient receiving testosterone should have her urine checked more frequently, as she may require an adjustment of insulin or oral hypoglycemic drugs.
- Estrogen is also used in the treatment of metastatic breast cancer but *only in those women 5 or more years past menopause.* As with testosterone, sodium and fluid retention may occur, and the diabetic patient should have her urine checked more frequently.
- Various antineoplastic agents may be used in the treatment of breast cancer. Drug package inserts or reliable references should be consulted regarding the wide variety of side effects that may occur.

References

BOUCHARD, R. and OWENS, N. F.: *Nursing Care of the Cancer Patient.* St. Louis, Mosby, 1972.

BRUNNER, L. S. and SUDDARTH, D. S.: *Lippincott Manual of Nursing Practice.* Philadelphia, Lippincott, 1974.

FITZPATRICK, G.: Care for the patient with cancer of the breast, Part 2. Nurs. Care 9:8, February, 1976.

FOSS, G.: Postmastectomy exercises: How to make them painless, more effective (pictorial). Nurs. '74, 4:23, June, 1974.

GREEN, T. H.: *Gynecology.* Boston, Little, Brown, 1971.

GRIBBONS, C. A. et al: Treatment for advanced breast carcinoma. Am. J. Nurs. 72:678, April, 1972.

LE MAITRE, G. and FINNEGAN, J.: *The Patient in Surgery: A Guide for Nurses.* Philadelphia, Saunders, 1975.

LICHTENDORF, S. S.: How to do the most for your mastectomy patient. J. Prac. Nurs. 25:18, March, 1975.

MAMARIL, M. P.: Preventing complications after radical mastectomy (pictorial). Am. J. Nurs. 74:2000, November, 1974.

ROBERTS, M. M. et al: Simple versus radical mastectomy. Nurs. Dig. 2:85, January, 1974.

RODMAN, M. J. and SMITH, D. W.: *Clinical Pharmacology in Nursing.* Philadelphia, Lippincott, 1974.

CHAPTER—41

The patient with venereal infection

On completion of this chapter the student will:

- **Name the common venereal diseases and give the causative organism of each.**
- **Describe the symptoms and treatment of gonorrhea, syphilis (primary stage), lymphogranuloma inguinale and chancroid.**
- **Name and describe the stages of syphilis.**
- **Discuss the nursing management of patients with venereal diseases.**
- **Discuss the emotional and social repercussions that may result from a venereal infection.**
- **Understand the importance of early detection and treatment of venereal disease.**

A venereal disease can be described as one that is communicated through sexual intercourse with an infected person. The major part of this chapter deals with gonorrhea and syphilis, the two most common venereal diseases.

Gonorrhea

Gonorrhea is a bacterial infection. The primary site of infection is the genital tract, from which the disease can spread to other parts of the body.

Incidence

Gonorrhea is the most common of the venereal diseases. It is worldwide, but no country has accurate statistics on its incidence. The reluctance of physicians to report the disease, due to the social stigma associated with it, interferes with accurate reporting of cases. In the United States, as well as in many other countries, there has been an increase in the number of cases of gonorrhea over recent years, so that it is now one of our foremost health problems. The problem of spread of the disease is intensified by the fact that infected persons may be asymptomatic. The person who has no symptoms but who harbors the infection may unknowingly spread the disease.

Etiology

The organism responsible for gonorrhea is the *Neisseria gonorrhoeae* (also called the *gonococcus*), named for Neisser, who first described it in 1897. The bacterium is gram-negative. The gonococcus does not live long on a dry surface, and the likelihood of adults contracting the disease by ways other than sexual intercourse is minimal, and perhaps not possible. However, newborn infants may contract the infection from the mother's birth canal, and infants and young children may contract it from contamination by fingers or articles. Natural immunity is not acquired after having an infection.

Symptoms

The usual incubation period is 3 days to 2 weeks after intercourse with an infected person. In men, the infection first settles around the mouth of the urethra, so that the first symptom is usually burning and pain on urination, followed by a yellowish discharge containing pus. In women the organisms frequently invade Skene's or Bartholin's glands, sometimes causing abscesses at these sites. However, many infections in women are asymptomatic for long periods of time.

If the disease is not treated, the infection may move up into the uterus and the fallopian tubes in women, and into the epididymis in men. The thick pus can completely clog both fallopian tubes, bind them with strictures, and render a woman sterile. The adhesions may cause pain, disturb menstruation, or cause ectopic pregnancy. If the infection spreads still further it can cause a generalized infection of the abdominal cavity (peritonitis). Intercourse, douches, and menstruation may spread the infection upward. Men may develop prostatitis, epididymitis, and infection of the seminal vessels. Adhesions of the urethra can result in urinary symptoms, and adhesions of the tract along which spermatozoa travel can result in sterility.

The infection, if it still is untreated, may enter the bloodstream, causing the patient to have typical symptoms of septicemia: fever, chills, and malaise. Once the organisms are in the bloodstream, they have access to every part of the body. They may cause arthritis, or more rarely meningitis or endocarditis. All these complications are quite rare, considering the tremendous number of cases of gonorrhea.

Laboratory diagnosis

In men a stained smear of the urethral discharge demonstrates the gonococcus. In women, however, smears are not reliable, and cultures should be obtained using a special medium in conditions which promote the growth of the delicate gonococcus.

Treatment

The recommended therapy is antibiotic therapy. Spectinomycin (Trobicin), penicillin, tetracycline, and ampicillin are some of the antibiotics that may be used. Many penicillin-resistant strains of gonococci are emerging. If the patient is allergic to penicillin, or if the organism is resistant, another antibiotic, such as one in the tetracycline family, can be equally effective.

Syphilis

Syphilis (lues) is a venereal disease that can result in widespread destructive lesions in the body. Syphilis exists throughout the world, and it is the second most prevalent venereal disease in the United States. As is the case with gonorrhea, the hope that availability of antibiotics would markedly decrease the incidence of syphilis has proven unfounded.

Etiology

The cause of syphilis is a thin spirochete known as *Treponema pallidum.* A most significant fact about this spirochete is that it must stay wet to live. It is also sensitive to cold, and soap kills it. Transmission is by sexual intercourse, although theoretically other types of intimate contact might also transmit syphilis. (Syphilis can also be transmitted via the placenta from mother to infant. Congenital syphilis will be discussed later.) Persons with untreated syphilis are infectious for about 1 year; they are rarely infectious during the later latent period. Persons with primary syphilis who are successfully treated rapidly become noninfectious: the organisms usually disappear from the lesions within 24 hours of the start of therapy.

Laboratory diagnosis

A definite diagnosis of syphilis is made when the spirochetes are identified microscopically by dark-field examination of a smear taken from a lesion. This is the only way to make a definite diagnosis in the early stage of the disease. After the disease is well established in the body (about 3 weeks after infection), a positive blood test can be obtained. Many serologic tests for syphilis have been devised since the original Wassermann test. These tests have frequently been named after their inventor and fall into two general classes: the nontreponemal tests and the treponemal tests. The VDRL (Venereal Disease Research Laboratory) is the most common of the nontreponemal tests. The FTA-ABS (Fluorescent Treponemal Antibody-Absorption) is the most common of the treponemal tests.

Treponemal tests are more specific than nontreponemal tests. However, because the VDRL is relatively simple and inexpensive, it has become the standard screening test. Treponemal tests are reserved for special cases, to rule out false positive reactions, which are sometimes seen in patients who have collagen diseases, or who have recently been inoculated. A positive serologic test, like a positive tuberculin, may remain so throughout the patient's life and does not necessarily indicate active disease. The presence of lesions and the adequacy of any past therapy are the usual criteria for determining the need for treatment.

A majority of the states require a serology test for syphilis before a marriage license is issued. In the Armed Forces and some industries, blood tests for syphilis are done for routine screening. In many hospitals a serology test for syphilis is routine for all newly admitted patients.

Symptoms

After direct contact with a mucous membrane, as in kissing or sexual intercourse, the spirochetes in the syphilitic lesion enter the mucous membrane through tiny cracks and immediately establish a colony there. They also spread through the circulation almost immediately; in about 3 weeks the patient may notice a chancre, the first lesion of syphilis (Fig. 41-1). This is the *primary* stage. A chancre is a painless, round lesion on the genitalia, inside the wall of the vagina, on the nipple, or perhaps in a crack in the side of the mouth. The untreated chancre is alive with millions of spirochetes. It disappears entirely within 2 to 5 weeks. During this period some people have headaches, and most have enlarged lymph nodes near the chancre, but in general feel well. A person who is ignorant of the disease is given little hint of the dangers that lie ahead if he fails to obtain treatment.

The *secondary* stage of the disease starts about 6 weeks after the initial infection. Many persons (but not all) with untreated syphilis have a skin rash during this period. The rash can take any form; frequently, it is diffuse, and it leaves as suddenly as it appeared. On mucous membrane surfaces, such as about the anus or in the mouth, luetic plaques (condylomas) may develop. These tend to crack and to ulcerate, and they are highly infectious. Sometimes the patient loses hair in patches, giving the head a characteristic moth-eaten appearance. Fever, headache, malaise and a sore throat may occur; or, on the other hand, the infected person may still feel well.

By now the serology test will be positive. During this stage there is generalized enlargement of the lymph nodes. Cutaneous and lymph node changes are the most prominent features of secondary syphilis. Other manifestations, such as iritis, arthritis, or even meningitis may occur, but are rare. After a few weeks it is usual for the symptoms to disappear. Although they come back, to disappear again, the untreated and unsuspecting patient may still be unaware of the seriousness of his illness.

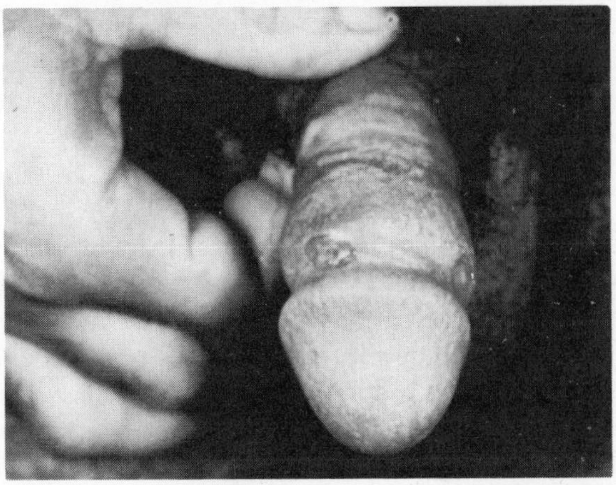

figure 41-1. Chancre, the primary lesion of syphilis. (Medichrome—Clay-Adams, Inc., New York, N.Y.)

The disease now enters a latent period. The patient feels well, and he has no symptoms related to syphilis. Some of the untreated infected persons will be troubled by the disease no longer. Others are not so fortunate. This disease is quiescent, perhaps for a year, often 4 or 5 years, and perhaps for 20 or 30 years.

Complications

At the tertiary stage, symptoms of the serious, damaging late complications begin to appear. Because the spirochete has had access through the bloodstream to all the tissues of the body, any organ now can be stricken with syphilis. Most commonly affected are the aorta, the eyes, and the central nervous system. Spirochetes may cause either widespread or local disease with a fibrous reaction. These well-defined local lesions are called *gummas.* They have fewer syphilis organisms than the earlier chancre, but they do contain a certain number. Gummas may develop anywhere in any tissue, but they appear most frequently in skin, bones, liver, larynx, and (in men) testes. Wherever these lesions occur, they may give rise to symptoms of dysfunction of the infected organ.

Even though the effects of the organisms on the internal organs may be devastating, the patient with tertiary syphilis generally is not a hazard to others. The elderly patient, for example, who is admitted to the hospital with a late cardiovascular disease due to lues has no discharging lesion and there is no reason to use special precautions for preventing spread of disease.

Complications to Pregnancy. Pregnant women with untreated syphilis commonly have a miscarriage; if the baby is carried to term, it may be stillborn, or it may be viable with congenital syphilis. In congenital syphilis, the fetus contracts the infection through the placenta. Congenital syphilis may cause severe damage to practically any organ, including those of the central nervous system.

Cardiovascular Complications. A manifestation of late syphilis that is dangerous to life is the involvement of the cardiovascular system. Patches of necrosis produced by the disease in the walls of blood vessels weaken that area of the wall, leading to aneurysms, which commonly develop in the aortic arch. The pulsing aneurysm can balloon out, pushing all other structures—lungs, nerves, even vertebrae—out of its way. It can grow larger and larger, with its wall becoming thinner and thinner, until it ruptures, and the patient bleeds to death.

In the heart the spirochetes may invade the aortic ring or the aortic valves, causing narrowing of the coronary vessels and coronary insufficiency, or valvular damage and aortic insufficiency.

Neural Complications. Syphilitic lesions of the nervous system occasionally cause meningitis, which responds to antiluetic treatment. Another manifestation of central nervous system involvement is general paresis, a chronic syphilitic meningoencephalitis. At first the patient exhibits slight changes in personality, which may start 10 or 20 years after his original infection. Memory and judgment become impaired. The mental state varies from euphoria to depression to paranoia. Optic atrophy with blindness may occur. If the disease progresses, the patient becomes totally helpless, both physically and mentally, and eventually expires.

In tabes dorsalis (also called *locomotor ataxia* or *syphilitic posterior spinal sclerosis*), the posterior spinal nerve roots, the posterior columns of the spinal cord, and the posterior root ganglia become infected and degenerate. The syndrome may appear 5 to 20 years after the original infection. Because the kinesthetic fibers are the first ones to be affected, the first symptoms are pain and a loss of position sense. Pain, frequently in the legs (although it also may occur in the arms or the trunk) is severe, knifelike and burning. Tabetic crisis is an acute attack of severe abdominal pain with vomiting.

The patient with tabes dorsalis has eye involvement. For example, his eyes accommodate to near and far vision, but his pupils do not react to light (Argyll Robertson sign). Optic atrophy with blindness may occur.

Charcot Joint. A further complication that is found most often in patients with tabes dorsalis is the Charcot joint. The joint atrophies due to syphilitic involvement of its innervation. It becomes hypermotile, and it will not support weight. The knee and the spine are most frequently involved.

Treatment

Early. A single injection of 2.4 million units of long-acting penicillin or daily injections of procaine penicillin (600,000 units for 10 days) cures early syphilis. Unlike *Neisseria gonorrhoeae,* there is no evidence that *Treponema pallidum* becomes penicillin-resistant. Periodic follow-up is indicated, and serologic tests should be repeated every 3 months for 1 or 2 years. Infection does not give natural immunity. Reinfections do occur, but not so commonly as with gonorrhea.

If the patient cannot tolerate penicillin, he may be treated with tetracycline or erythromycin.

LATE. In the later stages of syphilis, penicillin or another antibiotic is given but the spirochetes may be less susceptible to the drugs than they are in early syphilis. Damaged organs cannot be restored to complete function. Therapy is also directed at the treatment of any damaged structures of the body, with specific measures dictated by the pathology and symptoms. For example, the treatment and nursing management of the patient with cardiac symptoms caused by syphilis is similar to that given any patient with heart disease, and the patient with an aortic aneurysm due to syphilis may undergo surgical treatment.

Lymphogranuloma inguinale (lymphopathia venereum)

This disease is caused by one of the large viruses. It starts with a fleeting, asymptomatic ulcer. The disappearance of this lesion is followed by an enlargement of the inguinal lymph nodes. Abscesses form, which become necrotic and may suppurate through the skin. These lesions are called *buboes.* The patient feels weak and has fever, chills, and anorexia. If untreated, late persistent edema (elephantiasis) of the genitals and rectal stricture may result.

Diagnosis is made by the Frei test, in which antigen is injected intradermally. The test is read in 48 to 72 hours. Broad spectrum antibiotics such as tetracycline are the treatment of choice. Lymph nodes may be aspirated, but should not be incised.

Chancroid

Chancroid is an acute disease characterized by large multiple ulcerations of the genitals. Regional lymph nodes are also involved with abscess formation. The causative organism is *Hemophilus ducreyi.* This bacterium is difficult to isolate, and diagnosis is made on the basis of the clinical findings, and exclusion of other venereal diseases, such as syphilis. Of course, the two diseases may occur concurrently in the same patient. Sulfonamides and tetracyclines are effective therapy for chancroid.

Granuloma inguinale

Granuloma inguinale is a slowly progressive disease of the skin and mucous membranes, with some involvement of the lymph nodes. Ulcerative, nodular, and scarring forms occur, with gradual extension over the genital and inguinal areas. Severe, mutilating effects occur in untreated patients, who have an increased likelihood of developing carcinoma in the involved areas. The causative organism is *Donovania granulomatosis,* a bacterium which can be demonstrated by biopsy. Antibiotics of the tetracycline type are effective therapy.

Nursing management of patients with venereal diseases

PHYSICAL MEASURES

Venereal disease is usually treated on an outpatient basis. "Routine" isolation precautions are unnecessary for patients with syphilis or gonorrhea. The unnecessary use of such precautions as gowns and masks can lead the patient to feel rejected. Because of the stigma associated with venereal disease, it is especially important to convey acceptance to the patient, and to avoid measures which are likely to cause him to feel isolated.

Contact with discharges while they are still wet is avoided. For example, the nurse would wear gloves if she gives an enema, patients should wash their hands after going to the bathroom and after changing a perineal pad. Because the gonococcus has a special predilection for the eye (gonorrhea used to cause a large percentage of the world's blindness, infecting the newborn baby when it passed through the vagina), both the nurse and the patient should be especially careful to wash their hands before touching the face, after coming in contact with the discharge. In some hospitals the linen is considered contaminated for the first 1 or 2 days after treatment for gonorrhea is started. However, this organism dies so quickly on drying that the danger of spread of the disease by any means except direct contact with the still-wet discharge on a mucous membrane or an open cut is practically nonexistent.

If a patient known to have untreated primary syphilis is admitted to the hospital, precautionary measures are applied to avoid direct contact with the lesion during the brief period that the spirochetes are still alive in it after treatment has been instituted. For example, the nurse would wear gloves if she were giving care which required touching the chancre.

ATTITUDES

Attitudes of patients toward their illness are especially important in control of venereal disease. Some patients report to a venereal disease clinic with trivial symptoms, while others whose symptoms are acute require all the persuasion of a skilled nurse or other public health worker to convince them that they need medical attention. Between these two extremes are patients who come to the clinic with a realistic appreciation of their need for treatment, either because a sexual partner has named them as contacts, or because of the symptoms they are experiencing.

One of the major problems in venereal disease control is its prevalence among young people.

The nurse can do a great deal to bring young people with venereal disease to treatment, by being approachable and nonjudgmental, and by participating in programs which educate young people about various health problems, including venereal disease. Some cities have a VD Hotline, a telephone information service run by teen-agers and young adults. Young people who believe they have contracted a venereal disease should be encouraged to use this service if it is available in their city.

The problems created by venereal disease are added to those already faced by adolescents and young adults. For older patients, the problems may be slightly different, but they are no less severe. A man may have to tell his wife that he has been unfaithful to her, because the wife must be examined to determine if she is infected; or a woman may become terrified of infecting her children.

Venereal disease is not limited to any socioeconomic group, although the wealthier patient will probably be treated by his own physician, rather than in the clinic. Such a patient is probably less likely to have his disease reported to health authorities than is one who seeks care at a clinic. Attitudes toward the diseases may vary according to the socioeconomic level. In some groups the acquisition of gonorrhea is considered halfway between a joke and a sign of virility. This attitude may not be so acceptable to the nurse with a middle-class background, yet this patient also will need her teaching and understanding. This patient will also require help in realizing that gonorrhea is a serious disease which can cause severe illness and disability.

The increasing transmission of venereal disease, both syphilis and gonorrhea, through homosexual intercourse poses a difficult problem. Contact-tracing is especially difficult and is often impossible under these circumstances, because of the social stigma of homosexuality. Another difficult problem is posed by transmission of venereal disease from infected adults to children. Because of the stigma involved, treatment may not be sought. It is especially important for all who work in the field of venereal disease—prevention, detection, and treatment—to deal with their own feelings about sexual practices in a way which does not impede reporting and treatment.

In working with patients who have venereal disease the nurse is especially careful always to respect the patient's privacy, and to avoid condescension.

It is not safe to have the attitude that "a single injection of penicillin cures venereal disease, so why be afraid of it?" The security given by the knowledge that venereal disease is cleared up by a single injection leads some people to be careless in attending to the early symptoms. Because they are sure of a cure, they may delay seeking it until the disease has spread. A careless attitude about reinfecting oneself or others may develop.

The entire disappearance of venereal disease was optimistically predicted after the discovery of the effectiveness of antibiotics. Less money was appropriated for case finding, and less attention paid to public education. It has now become clear that efforts to control venereal disease must be intensified. The development of penicillin-resistant strains of the gonococcus has intensified the urgency of the problem by contributing to more frequent treatment failures. It remains to be seen whether a program of medical and epidemiologic measures can effectively check the spread of venereal disease.

Pharmacological considerations

- Patients with venereal disease will require antibiotics. They must be warned that a *complete course* of therapy (when more than one dose is required) is necessary in order to ensure *complete* control of the disease. Also important, in many instances, is a follow-up examination to be sure the infection has been controlled.
- Patients should be instructed to avoid sexual contact until the physician determines the disease to be under control and no longer infectious.
- Patients with venereal disease are usually treated as outpatients; therefore they should thoroughly understand what therapy entails (such as the number of visits required). Those receiving oral medications should thoroughly understand when the medication is taken (i.e., every day, twice a day 12 hours apart, and so on).

■ Drugs used to treat venereal disease include penicillin, spectinomycin, tetracycline, demeclocycline (Declomycin), minocycline (Minocin), cephaloridine (Loradine), erythromycin, streptomycin, and the sulfonamides.

Bibliography

Ahern, C.: "I think I have VD." Nurs. Clin. North Am. 8:77, March, 1973.

Baker, R.: VD: The old enemy within. Nurs. Care 7:16, August, 1974.

Benenson, A. S., ed.: *Control of Communicable Disease in Man.* Washington, D.C., American Public Health Association, 1970.

Brown, M. A.: Adolescents and VD. Nurs. Outlook, 21:99, February, 1973.

Hoeprich, P. D.: *Infectious Diseases.* Hagerstown, Harper and Row, 1972.

Huxall, L. K.: The "social diseases": gonorrhea and syphilis, Part 2. J. OGN Nurs. 4:16, January/February, 1975.

Major sexually transmitted diseases. World Health, May, 1975, p. 18.

McInnes, M. E.: *Johnston's Essentials of Communicable Disease,* ed. 2. St. Louis, Mosby, 1975.

Rodman, M. J. and Smith, D. W.: *Clinical Pharmacology in Nursing.* Philadelphia, Lippincott, 1974.

Scherer, J. C.: *Introductory Clinical Pharmacology.* Philadelphia, Lippincott, 1975.

She may look clean, but . . . Emergency Med. 3:98, March, 1971.

UNIT TEN
Common problems involving disfigurement

- The patient with a dermatological condition
- The patient undergoing plastic surgery

CHAPTER 42

The patient with a dermatological condition

On completion of this chapter the student will:

- **Discuss the importance of the skin and the impact, both physical and emotional, of skin disorders.**
- **Name the more common dermatological conditions and give the basic treatment of each.**
- **Discuss the nursing management of the patient with a dermatological condition.**
- **Describe the techniques used in the application of dressings in dermatological conditions.**
- **Recognize the patient's emotional responses to his physical appearance.**

Since the skin is in constant contact with the environment, it is unusually subject to injury and irritation. Nurses are in a strategic position to help others to maintain a normal, healthy skin. In bathing a hospitalized patient or in teaching patients in outpatient departments, industry, or their homes sound practices in skin care, the nurse can help others to avoid abusing the skin and subjecting it to disease or injury.

Probably no other organ in the body is so subject to the application of remedies without medical advice. The accessibility of the skin makes self-treatment commonplace. Although most people recognize the importance of healthy skin as an asset to personal appearance, those who unhesitatingly seek medical advice for other symptoms may try a variety of nostrums on skin lesions, often making the condition worse. The idea that skin disease is never serious and therefore can be trifled with is far from the truth.

Cleanliness. Our culture values cleanliness, beauty, and the avoidance of body odors. Skin diseases of all sorts are often attributed to poor personal hygiene, and a vigorous program of scrubbing and cleansing is sometimes undertaken to "clear the condition up." Popular advertising reinforces these ideas, and emphasizes the wonderful properties of various soaps and cleansers. How clean does skin have to be to be healthy? If one bath is good, are two better?

Thorough scrubbing with soap and water or a detergent does temporarily reduce the number of bacteria, but this number rapidly returns to previous levels. Countless bacteria, most of them nonpathogenic, normally exist on the skin. Because most skin disorders of adults in this country cannot be traced to germs and dirt, vigorous cleansing is not a cure-all. In fact, many conditions, such as those related to excessive dryness or to allergy, are made worse by preparations that increase skin dryness by removing natural oils, or that further irritate a sensitive skin with a variety of perfumes and colorings. People with oily skin need to bathe more frequently than those with dry skin. Older people, especially women, tend to have dry skin. Often, they cannot tolerate the drying effect of a hot tub bath daily. Instead, they may sponge-bathe the hands and the face, the axillae, the genital region, and the feet daily and take a tub bath or a shower two or three times a week. Lukewarm water is less drying than hot water. Bathing quickly rather than luxuriating in a leisurely bath is also less drying, becaue it avoids prolonged contact with soapy water. Adding a little oil to the bath water also lessens the drying effect.

Sweat glands are present over the entire body, but they are especially abundant in axillae, forehead, palms, and soles. In adults perspiration in the axillary region has an odor that is considered unpleasant. Deodorants are commonly used by both men and women to banish it. When bathing a patient, the nurse should apply the patient's deodorant if he desires it and is unable to do so.

Preventing Dryness. The sebaceous glands, which surround the hair follicles, secrete sebum, an oily substance that protects the hair and skin from becoming excessively dry. However, some persons produce less sebum than is desirable for keeping the skin soft. This is particularly common during later life.

Heredity is important in determining the type of skin that a person will have. It is often noted that very dry or oily skins are most common among persons who have a family history of these conditions.

Creams help to keep the skin soft and smooth by reducing the loss of moisture from the skin. Creams and creamy lotions help to prevent dryness and chapping, particularly during cold weather, when moisture is lost more quickly. Products containing hormones cannot "restore youthful beauty." Their value lies primarily in the cream, rather than the hormones. Most people, as they grow older, find that creams and lotions applied to face, hands, elbows, and feet help to keep the skin smooth and soft. Wearing rubber gloves during the use of soaps and detergents for laundry and dishwashing also is helpful in preventing dryness. Such simple measures can greatly reduce chapping and cracking, which make the skin not only unattractive and uncomfortable but also vulnerable to infection and rashes.

Dandruff. People who have oily scalps need to shampoo the hair more frequently than those with dry scalps. Pronounced oiliness and the shedding of greasy scales (commonly described as dandruff) may require treatment by a dermatologist. This condition is quite common, and many people either neglect it entirely or indulge in self-medication. If neglected, dandruff can be a factor in the thinning and the loss of hair. Regular brushing and shampooing and the avoidance of such constricting apparel as tight hat bands are important in preserving a healthy scalp.

Sunlight. Tanning in response to exposure to sunlight helps to protect the skin against the damaging effects of excessive ultraviolet light. But exposure to sunlight can be either a bane or a blessing, depending on the condition of the patient's skin and on the length of the exposure. For example, acne usually is improved by exposure to sunlight, but a prolonged exposure, particularly of fair-skinned persons who tend not to tan effectively, can cause a painful sunburn. Adolescents and young adults tolerate exposure to sunlight better than older persons do, because the skin becomes thinner, drier, and less protective with increasing age. Prolonged exposure to sun eventually causes the skin of farmers, sailors, and other outdoor workers to become coarse and leathery. Skin cancer is more common among those whose skins have had excessive exposure to sun and wind. People who work outdoors can avoid unnecessary exposure by wearing wide-brimmed hats and by covering the skin (wearing a T-shirt as well as slacks).

The condition of the skin is indicative of one's general health. Good health habits help to keep the skin, as well as the rest of the body, in good condition. Plenty of sleep, relief from worry and tension, regular exercise, and an optimum diet are important.

Nursing considerations

Particular dermatological problems are often encountered by the hospitalized patient, and the nurse can help to prevent them in these ways:

- The alkalinity of ordinary soaps sometimes causes irritation, especially in older, bedridden patients. The nurse can have the physician suggest a soap substitute of neutral pH, such as Lowila.
- When giving a bed bath, the nurse should rinse the soap off with clear water. The cake of soap should be removed from the bath water, because it makes the water soapy and also wastes soap. The water in the basin needs to be changed frequently, so that the process of rinsing is not actually a reapplication of soap.
- The method that provides the best possible rinsing compatible with the degree of activity permitted the patient should be used. A patient who can have a tub or a shower with assistance should not be restricted to a bed bath.
- Instead of "routine baths," especially for long-term patients, it is better to plan ahead and allow time for shampoos and care of the nails.
- The patient's elbows should be kept covered by the sleeves of his gown or pajama top. Creams and lotions applied to the elbows and the knees help relieve dryness.
- If skin lesions appear, the nurse should avoid washing them with soap and water and should not try to clean off any scales or exudate, since the appearance of the lesions is important to the physician in making a diagnosis. Removal of the scales or exudate may also cause bleeding. The nurse should report the symptom to the physician promptly, and be ready to answer questions concerning the medicines that the patient is receiving. Drugs are a frequent cause of skin lesions in hospitalized patients.

Nurses can apply these measures to safeguard the health of their own skin, and, in addition, they can take the following special precautions against specific occupational hazards:

- Unnecessary contact with medications should be avoided; many of them can cause allergic skin reactions. Careful handling of syringes, needles, and of the medicines themselves can greatly reduce physical contact. If a medicine spills on the hands, it must be washed off promptly.
- Thorough hand washing is important in preventing the spread of infection. Because nurses must wash their hands often, hand cream or lotion should be applied liberally, and hands dried well after washing. These precautions will help to prevent chapping and cracking of the skin.
- If a patient has a contagious skin disease, the necessary medical aseptic technique or isolation procedure should be followed. (This rule applies, of course, to any contagious condition, dermatological or otherwise.)

Injury and disease of the skin

By adulthood, almost everyone has experienced some of the common disorders of the skin. The following are some causes of skin disorders with examples of the resulting conditions:

- Allergy—urticaria (hives)
- Congenital lesions—nevus (mole)
- Emotional disturbances—neurodermatitis (a form of eczema)
- Hormonal imbalance—acne
- Infection—furuncle (boil)
- Malignant growth—malignant melanoma
- Trauma—accidents: burns, lacerations; radical surgery, such as that for cancer of the head and neck

Disorders of the skin may be classified also according to the degree of involvement of the entire body.

For example, a burn may be small and produce only local symptoms; or it may cover a large area of the body and produce systemic as well as local symptoms, because of the marked physiological disturbance accompanying it. Some diseases of the skin produce only local manifestations—acne, for example. On the other hand, many systemic diseases produce dermatological symptoms (Tables 42-1 and 42-2); measles and syphilis are examples. Systemic lupus erythematosus and scleroderma are diseases that are manifested in many systems of the body, including the skin. Both of these diseases affect collagen, a connective tissue widely distributed in the body.

The problem of disfigurement

The condition of the skin determines to a great extent the appearance that an individual presents to others. Our society places a high premium on youthful beauty, and advertising continues to hammer home an ideal which, though patently unrealistic, is nonetheless highly persuasive. What effect has this on the person whose skin is disfigured from disease or trauma? Skin diseases have long been associated with immorality, uncleanliness, and contagion. Despite the lack of justification for these associations, an inflamed and pimply skin just does not convey the look of fresh cleanliness that a clear skin does. Some skin lesions exude serum that has an unpleasant odor, further adding to the impression of uncleanliness. Only a very few skin diseases are contagious; nevertheless, many persons have a fear of touching the person with skin disease, or even of being near him. People whose faces have been scarred by burns or cuts may be severely disfigured, and may even have their facial expressions changed.

It is not difficult to understand why people who suffer severe facial disfigurement often undergo per-

Table 42-1.
Systemic conditions with dermatological symptoms

Condition	Cause	Description and Course	Treatment
Erysipelas	Hemolytic streptococcus	Chills, fever, headache, and a raised, reddened area of the skin which spreads rapidly and is sometimes accompanied by blistering.	Antibiotic therapy.
Erythema nodosum	Believed to be an allergic reaction to drugs or to viral or bacterial infections	Red, tender nodules in cutaneous and subcutaneous tissues. Shins, thighs, and forearms are commonly involved. Possibly fever and malaise.	Identify and, if possible, remove the cause. Salicylates, bed rest, and corticosteroids used for symptomatic relief.
Polyarteritis (Periarteritis nodosa)	Unknown	Nodules appear along the course of arteries. There may be muscle and joint pain, nausea, vomiting, diarrhea, abdominal pain, fever, and weight loss.	Symptomatic; use of analgesics, rest and corticosteroids.
Erythema multiforme	Undetermined; may be secondary to drug reaction or infection	Eruption of red macules, papules, vesicles, and bullae affecting the wrists, hands, elbows, knees, feet, and face. Systemic symptoms may involve muscles, and GI, urinary, respiratory, and nervous systems.	Treatment of any underlying conditions. Soothing lotions Antihistamines Symptomatic therapy

Table 42-2.
Systemic conditions with grave prognoses

<table>
<tr><th>Condition</th><th>Cause</th><th>Description</th><th>Treatment</th><th>Nursing Considerations</th></tr>
<tr><td>Pemphigus</td><td>Unknown; may be hereditary</td><td>Bullae (large blisters) appear and rupture, leaving a raw lesion with an offensive odor and intense itching.</td><td>Baths or wet dressings with mild antiseptic solutions.
High protein diet to compensate for protein lost through weeping lesions.
Chemotherapy.</td><td rowspan="3">1. Observe for toxicity to drug therapy, which may be prolonged.
2. Foster independence for as long as possible.
3. Provide meticulous care to improve patient's comfort.
4. Be available to lend emotional and physical support when necessary.</td></tr>
<tr><td>Systemic lupus erythematosus</td><td>Believed to be auto-immune disorder; affects collagen</td><td>Red butterfly pattern over the cheeks and bridge of the nose; painful joints; edema; fever, and anemia. Kidneys, heart, and lungs may be affected.</td><td>Corticosteroids plus local symptomatic therapy.</td></tr>
<tr><td>Scleroderma (Progressive systemic sclerosis)</td><td>Unknown; some evidence suggests autoimmune cause</td><td>Hardening of collagen in many organs. Skin becomes tight and smooth; movement becomes difficult. The heart and lungs may be affected causing dyspnea, cyanosis, and edema. The esophagus and intestines are often involved.</td><td>Symptomatic treatment including ointments, massage, heat, physiotherapy, and hydrotherapy. Cortisone may be used.</td></tr>
</table>

sonality changes. They become acutely and painfully aware of the stares, the avoidance, and even the revulsion of other people, and they tend to withdraw from social and business contacts. Many occupations are closed to those who are disfigured, particularly jobs that place heavy emphasis on personal attractiveness, such as receptionist, airline stewardess, or salesman.

More instances of disfigurement are seen nowadays. Cancer of the head and neck is treated more often by radical surgery, as new advances in surgical techniques are developed. Although the malignant cells may be removed successfully, the problem of disfigurement remains. People with severe injuries of the face and the neck have a better chance of survival, because of such treatments as antibiotics and parenteral fluids. Plastic surgery has worked successfully for many of these patients—an ear may be reconstructed so skillfully that it can scarcely be distinguished from the normal ear. Nevertheless, some patients are so severely mutilated that they remain disfigured despite all that plastic surgeons can do for them. Rehabilitation must emphasize function, but appearance is important, too.

Learning to accept those who are disfigured is a big challenge. Often, the nurse is the one who is with the patient when he becomes aware of the change in his appearance. It is easy to preach acceptance, but it is not always easy to act on it, because nurses, too, are not immune to prejudice. The points listed below may seem commonplace but perhaps because care of disfigured patients is often difficult, they will spell out some ways to help the patient feel accepted. The patient will be an amazingly sensitive observer of the nurse's reactions, because they serve as a foretaste of what is to come.

- When dressings or treatments are required, the nurse must not hesitate to touch the part as she ministers to the patient. Only the logical and necessary protective techniques should be used. For example, gloves should be worn only if the skin disease is contagious, and their purpose should be explained to the patient. Even if the patient is physically able to carry out his own treatments, the nurse should arrange to do some part of the care of the lesions as a way of demonstrating acceptance of the patient and his condition. Understanding the disease will help the nurse feel confident enough to use a firm rather than a gingerly touch.

- It is important to neither stare at the patient's disfigurement nor avoid the sight of it. The nurse should try to look at the patient—at all of him, including his rash or his scar—as if he were any other patient.

First experiences with severely disfigured persons can be trying, stimulating shock, pity, or revulsion. Recognizing this will help the nurse control the expression of such feelings to the patient. Gradually, in working repeatedly with the same patient, or with others who have a similar disability, the nurse will find that the changed appearance can be accepted more easily.

Treatment of skin disease

Both local and systemic treatment may be used in skin disease. Lotions, powders, and ointments may be applied to soothe and to soften the skin (*emollients*), to relieve itching (*antipruritics*), and to protect the lesions. In addition, local preparations may be keratolytic (dissolving thickened or horny skin), antiseptic, or antiparasitic. Here is an example of each of these types of preparation:

- Emollient—lanolin
- Antipruritic—calamine lotion
- Protection—zinc oxide ointment
- Keratolytic—salicylic acid plaster (contained in many corn plasters)
- Antiseptic—potassium permanganate solution
- Antiparasitic—Desenex powder

Local preparations for the skin often are combinations of several ingredients carefully chosen by the dermatologist for their specific effect. Even patients who have similar skin disorders may respond very differently to a particular preparation. It is always unwise to recommend any local preparation for the treatment of a disease of the skin, even though the nurse has observed that it has helped patients with apparently similar conditions.

Systemic treatment usually forms part of the patient's management. Most skin disorders grow worse when the patient is tired or under emotional stress. Therefore, rest and sleep are an important part of treatment.

Diet also may be an important part of treatment, as certain foods may cause a rash or skin eruption in some individuals. For example, a patient may develop hives (*urticaria*) from eating fish, and therefore he may have to eliminate it from his diet.

Since some skin diseases are manifestations of systemic disorders, the variety of drugs given is as broad as the study of pharmacology itself. These are some commonly used preparations:

- Corticosteroids help to relieve many severe skin diseases. They do not effect a cure, but often relieve the symptoms. As is true of their use in other diseases, these drugs can have serious toxic effects. Therefore, they are used primarily to relieve acute attacks. Continued use in long-term conditions brings greater risk, and it is justified only when the disease itself is very serious and cannot be relieved by other treatments.
- Antihistamines are frequently prescribed when allergy is a factor in causing the disease, and for the relief of itching.
- Sedatives and tranquilizers are used to help the patient to relax and rest.
- Antibiotics are used to treat infection.

Sunlight is important in the treatment of some dermatological problems. For example, its effects—bacteriostasis, drying, and mild peeling of the skin—are helpful in acne. Exposure to ultraviolet light can produce a similar effect in much less time, and ultraviolet treatments are often given by dermatologists. Usually, only the part being treated is exposed to the light. Any type of heavy cloth or opaque paper can be used to protect the other parts of the body from exposure.

X-ray therapy provides relief from the symptoms of a variety of skin diseases. The dosage is measured carefully, and the number of treatments that can be given safely to any one area of the body is limited. Excessive use can cause loss or thinning of hair, dryness and wrinkling of the skin; it may even predispose to malignant changes in the skin. When very large doses are given, deep burns may result. Sometimes, when a dose of radiation is given to treat cancer of other organs, the skin becomes pink and dry as an unavoidable consequence. However, because of mounting concern over the hazards of radiation therapy, this form of treatment is now used less commonly for benign conditions.

Nursing management of patients with skin disease

The physician may wish to examine the skin of the patient's entire body, including the scalp and the perineal region, even though the patient may state that the condition is limited to only one part. The nurse should adjust the light to facilitate the examination and to drape the patient carefully. Only those areas being examined at that time need be exposed. The examination may not be limited to the skin. Some skin diseases are related to systemic illness, and the physician may request laboratory studies such as urinalysis and CBC. A biopsy of the skin lesion may be necessary. The necessity for the tests must be carefully explained to the patient, who may see no connection between them and the lesions on his skin.

Itching

Although itching (*pruritus*) is a common and very distressing symptom of many skin diseases, the mechanism of itching is still somewhat obscure. The itch impulse probably has a lower frequency and intensity than the pain impulse, thus differentiating the feeling of pain from the sensation of itching. Certain factors tend to make itching worse: excessive warmth (as from too many blankets); rough, prickly fabrics; emotional stress; and idleness. Itching uually is worse at night, probably because the patient's attention is not occupied, and he is therefore more aware of the sensation.

Severe itching is agony. Scratching leads to trauma and excoriation, and often to infection. Helping the patient with severe pruritus to obtain some degree of comfort and to avoid scratching is a challenge to all who care for him. Reminders not to scratch are little help; usually, all that is accomplished is that the patient grows tired of being scolded, and the nurse is irked, because he does not stop scratching. Instead of scolding the patient, the nurse should:

- Provide enough clothing and bedding for comfortable warmth, but avoid having the patient become overheated. Carefully check the temperature of the room to prevent chilling or excessive warmth.
- Encourage the patient to keep his nails short and very clean. This will minimize trauma and infection from scratching.
- Have the patient wear white cotton gloves if he scratches at night.
- Help the patient to avoid emotional upsets.
- When the sensation of itching is acute, and the patient cannot resist the impulse to touch his skin, have him press his finger or hand against it, without scratching.
- Help the patient to sleep. Note carefully any bedtime treatment or medications ordered to relieve the itching or to promote sleep.

A variety of treatments may be ordered to alleviate itching. The treatment of the disease itself, thus eliminating the cause of the symptom, is, of course, the most effective. However, in waiting for curative treatment to take effect, or in treating conditions in which complete cure is unlikely, much relief of itching can be achieved by symptomatic treatment. Wet dressings or starch baths often help. The relief of emotional tension helps to reduce itching; sedatives and tranquilizers often are ordered for this purpose. Soothing lotions, such as calamine, often give temporary relief. When allergy is a factor, antihistamines may provide considerable relief.

Dressings

If dressings are needed, apply them so that they fit snugly and yet do not bind. Dressings applied to open, denuded areas should be sterile. Cotton should not be placed next to the skin, because of its tendency to stick to moist surfaces. Gauze or cotton cloth may be used. Applying adhesive tape directly to the skin should be avoided, because it can cause trauma and irritation.

Wet Dressings. When a wet dressing is applied, it should be determined whether the procedure is to be clean or sterile. The nature of the lesion (acute or chronic; open, weeping, or dry) helps to determine whether sterile techniques must be used. In either case, scrupulous cleanliness is important.

Wet dressings have a cooling and soothing effect, produced by the evaporation of the moisture from the dressing. To avoid chilling, the nurse should make certain that the rest of the patient's body is kept warm.

Wet dressings may be applied by either the open or the closed method:

Closed

Moist compresses are applied and then covered with waterproof material, such as plastic sheeting or waxed paper.

Open

Moist compresses are applied and left open to air. The affected part should not be covered with bedclothes. The foundation of the bed is protected by laying a rubber or a plastic sheet, covered by a cotton draw sheet under the part.

Several points must be considered in keeping the dressing wet:

- A dressing should not be allowed to become completely dry. The nurse may be the first to discover a dressing that needs attention and should never moisten it by pouring solution over the dry, outer layers of the gauze. The solution may not even penetrate to the gauze next to the patient's skin, and can carry dirt inward from the surface of the dressings. The dressings must be completely removed, and the treatment resumed. Fresh dressings should be immersed in a bowl of solution and applied as ordered.
- An open dressing that is changed frequently enough to prevent soiling and is not allowed to dry out may usually be remoistened at intervals, using an Asepto syringe.
- If the dressing is dry and stuck to the skin, it is necessary to first remove the outer layers of gauze, then moisten the inner layer with solution, using an Asepto syringe. A dressing that is stuck must never be pulled at roughly, because this will cause pain and trauma.
- A closed dressing that is protected by outer wrappings may usually be remoistened by the use of an Asepto syringe to squirt solution on it, provided that the dressing has not dried out.

Often, the patient can assist in keeping the dressing moist if sterile technique is not necessary; the area is one that he can reach; his physical condition permits; he is shown how to do it; and the necessary supplies are provided for him. The nurse is always responsible for seeing that the treatment is carried out, whether or not she performs every aspect of it.

STARCH BATHS. Starch baths (colloid baths) are useful in relieving itching. Usually, they are ordered at bedtime to help the patient sleep. The patient may be able to carry out the treatment with only a little help, as long as he is physically able. He should be carefully instructed, and there must be an effective call system in the bathroom, so that he may signal for help if he needs it.

The bathtub should be filled with lukewarm water. One pound of cornstarch or laundry starch is added, and the water stirred so that the starch is mixed through it. The patient immerses his whole body by stretching out full length in the tub. A washcloth or a compress may be used to apply the solution to the face and any other parts not covered by the solution. The cloth or compress should be applied gently, without rubbing the skin. Soap is not used with the starch bath. Although the primary purpose of the bath is soothing, it also helps to cleanse the skin. Unless this fact is explained to the patient, he may reach for the soap, and its use could irritate his skin. The bath is often ordered for 20 to 30 minutes at a time. The bathroom should be comfortably warm, and more hot water should be added occasionally to prevent the patient from becoming chilled. When the treatment is over, the skin should be patted dry, never rubbed, since rubbing would cause irritation.

At this point the patient needs the nurse's assistance most. Whatever local medication is ordered should be taken to the bathroom and applied immediately after the patient's skin has been dried. Irritation and increased itching may result if the application of the local medication is delayed after the bath. Often, patients with a skin disease are susceptible to chilling, particularly after a bath. Therefore, it is important that the patient wears his bathrobe and slippers to and from the bathroom.

Common dermatological conditions

ACNE VULGARIS

Acne vulgaris is one of the most widespread skin conditions. The cause is not fully understood, but acne characteristically occurs during adolescence, and it is believed related to the hormone changes during that period of life when the secondary sex characteristics are developing. Other factors may aggravate the condition, although they alone do not appear to cause it.

The skin of the affected areas (usually face, chest and back) is excessively oily. The lesions consist of comedones (blackheads), papules (pimples), and pustules (pimples filled with pus). In severe cases, cysts sometimes occur, appearing as large, reddish swellings. The severity of the condition ranges all the way from an occasional pimple, which during adolescence is so common that it is considered to be almost normal at this age, to a face that is covered with bright red pimples and peppered with blackheads. Severe acne, if neglected, can lead to the formation of deep, pitted scars that leave the skin permanently pock-marked. Oiliness of the scalp and the shedding of greasy scales (seborrhea) often accompany acne. Infection and the formation of pustules are fostered by picking and squeezing the lesions.

The possibility of scarring from severe acne is too often overlooked. These scars are *not* outgrown, and they can spoil a complexion for life. But probably the emotional scars are just as important. For some young people these matters mean just temporary distress, but for others who feel less secure, who already have difficulty in making friends, severe or unusually prolonged acne can interfere seriously with their developing into poised, confident adults. Acne that is in any way pronounced or unsightly should be treated—the more prompt the treatment, the less likelihood of scars, physical or emotional.

TREATMENT. Despite the fact that there is as yet no certain cure, much can be done to relieve the symptoms and, in time, to help them disappear. Instruction in personal hygiene from a person whom the patient considers to be an authority on health matters is heeded more often than the advice of parents.

The physician can remove the blackheads and drain the pustules with special instruments. This process should never be attempted by the patient or by family and friends, because infection and scarring can be caused by unskilled manipulation. "Hands off" is an ironclad but difficult rule that the patient must learn to follow. The patient is instructed to keep his fingernails short and clean, since this helps to prevent infection of the skin lesions. He should wash his hands thoroughly before applying medication or carrying out any other treatment of the lesions. Mild soaps that do not irritate are preferable to hard or highly perfumed varieties. Medicated preparations should be used only with the physician's advice. Some physicians recommend washing the skin with an antibacterial soap to keep the number of staphylococci on the skin to a minimum. Sometimes, an abrasive soap, rubbed in gently, helps in peeling the skin. The diet should exclude any foods that make the condition worse. The hands should be kept away from the face. Some physicians strongly recommend keeping the hair away from the face. This can be distressing to the young adult who may have to modify his or her hair style.

Exposure to sunlight is beneficial, because it lessens oiliness, reduces the number of infection-causing bacteria, and causes peeling of affected skin. The combination of increased exercise, relaxation, and sunlight often makes acne improve during the summer. Exposure to the sun should do no more than produce slight pinkness and peeling; a painful sunburn is not beneficial. Short treatments with ultraviolet light, administered by the physician, provide benefits similar to exposure to direct sunlight, and they have the added advantage of year-around application and controlled dosage to prevent burning.

SEBORRHEIC DERMATITIS

The common term for mild seborrheic dermatitis is *dandruff*. The symptoms are familiar: oily scalp, formation of greasy scales, itching, and irritation. Severe cases have inflammation with redness, swelling, and, sometimes, exudation and infection. Seborrheic dermatitis frequently accompanies acne, but unlike acne is not limited typically to adolescence. Often, it persists throughout adulthood. It primarily affects the scalp, but it may spread to the eyebrows, the skin around the ears, the sides of the nose, and the forehead near the hairline, causing the skin in these areas, as well as the scalp, to be red, oily, and scaly.

Normally, new cells are constantly being formed and pushed to the outside of the skin, where they die and are gradually and imperceptibly shed (*keratinization*). In the presence of certain diseases, such as seborrheic dermatitis, keratinization is speeded up, and scaling becomes visible.

Prompt and persistent treatment often results in great improvement, to the degree that only good scalp hygiene is required to avoid a return of the condition. However, many people are not so fortunate and continue to require regular medical treatment to control the symptoms. These individuals have chronically overactive sebaceous glands; the condition may be related to heredity, emotional tension, a diet too high in fat, or endocrine imbalance.

TREATMENT. The treatment includes regular cleansing, application of local medication between shampoos, and a regimen of healthful living. When the oiliness is severe, daily shampoos may be needed. Although the scales are removed by washing, they promptly accumulate again until the condition is controlled. The physician rather than the hairdresser should be consulted about the selection of a shampoo. The physician will advise the use of an antiseborrheic shampoo such as Selsun, or Fostex cream. When the condition is unresponsive, mildly antiseptic lotions or medicated ointments may be prescribed for use between shampoos. The lotions should be applied directly to the scalp rather than to the hair. The patient must understand the importance of systematically applying medication to his entire scalp by parting the hair frequently and reaching all areas of the scalp.

ALLERGIC REACTIONS OF THE SKIN

The skin is one of the organs most frequently affected by allergy. The allergic response of the skin is characterized by dilation of the blood vessels, causing redness and swelling, and sometimes by vesiculation (blister formation) and oozing. Itching is a prominent symptom.

Allergic reactions of the skin are commonly caused

by substances in contact with the skin, such as cosmetics, fabrics, or chemicals. The resulting disorder is called *contact dermatitis.* The condition also may be caused by drugs (dermatitis medicamentosa) and foods. Penicillin frequently causes urticaria.

Irritants are differentiated from contact allergens in that an irritant, if it is used in sufficient quantity, causes skin inflammation in almost everyone, whereas an allergen provokes a reaction only in the small proportion of people who are hypersensitive to that particular substance.

Patch tests, which place small amounts of various substances in direct contact with the skin, may be helpful in identifying the causes of the reaction. A careful history is very important in any allergic condition, as the reason for the allergy may be obscure. Through careful questioning also the cause of the allergy may be identified.

Urticaria (hives); angioneurotic edema

The round red wheals seen in those patients with urticaria are a result of localized edema, due to increased capillary permeability. Urticaria is usually an allergic response, although sometimes emotional stress seems to cause the condition.

Treatment includes avoidance of the allergen and the use of antihistamines and epinephrine and, in severe cases, corticosteroids. Cold compresses applied to the affected areas help provide relief.

In *angioneurotic edema* the affected part shows an all-over swelling rather than the patchy swellings of hives. The lips may be swollen to three times their normal size, or the tissues around the eyes may be so edematous that the patient cannot open them. Angioneurotic edema is a serious and sometimes emergency event. Patients with allergic reactions must be observed for the symptoms of respiratory obstruction, because edema of the larynx may interfere with respiration. Mild forms of angioneurotic edema are usually treated with antihistamines. When the edema is severe, the patient will require close observation for respiratory difficulty. Should breathing become difficult, treatment must begin immediately. Oxygen and drugs such as antihistamines, epinephrine, and corticosteroids may be administered. If respiratory distress becomes acute, a tracheostomy may be necessary.

Eczema

The term *eczema* refers to a group of skin diseases that tend to be chronic and are related to heredity, allergy, emotional stress, and, possibly, endocrine disorder. The lesions consist of tiny vesicles (blisters) on reddened, itchy skin. The vesicles sometimes burst, causing the area to weep and later to form crusts from the dried fluid. The skin of the affected area is red, dry, and scaly. Leathery thickening (lichenification) and darkening of the skin result from continued irritation and scratching. A form of eczema called *infantile eczema* occurs in children under the age of two. The chronic type of eczema frequently seen in adults is called *atopic eczema* or *neurodermatitis.*

Eczema typically occurs in the folds of the elbows and the knees and on the neck and the face. During acute attacks it may spread to other part of the body. The symptoms tend to come and go. The patient may have a severe flare-up that necessitates absence from work or school. Several months later he may have no symptoms of the disease, and he may remain symptom-free for months or even years. However, the condition tends to recur. Frequently, an exacerbation of eczema can be traced to an emotional upset. At other times the immediate cause of the attack is obscure. People with chronic eczema frequently have patches of thickened, dark skin in the bends of their elbows and knees or on their necks. These patches persist long after the acute attack subsides. During an acute attack these areas become red, scaly, oozing and crusted, and later they revert to their darkened leathery appearance. A form of eczema occurs in the perineal region, causing itching and inflammation.

Treatment. Caring for the patient with eczema demands the utmost skill and understanding. Medical treatment includes local creams and ointments that are soothing and antipruritic, such as hydrocortisone cream. If the skin is very inflamed, wet dressings or starch baths may be ordered. Antihistamines may help to relieve the symptoms. Sedatives and tranquilizers may be necessary to calm a tense, restless patient. Corticosteroids are sometimes administered orally when the symptoms are very severe. Rest and sleep are essential treatments, and yet are difficult to provide because of severe itching and discomfort. Sedation can help to break the cycle of insomnia, tension, itching, and scratching. X-ray therapy is occasionally used in controlling acute attacks.

The patient should understand the importance of giving a complete account of his previous treatment if he consults a new doctor. This directive is especially important in relation to x-ray therapy, because there is a limit to the number of treatments that may safely be administered to any one part of the patient's body.

The nurse can play an important role in helping the patient learn to manage his condition by:

- Trying to understand some of the social and emotional pressures that may affect the patient beside his physical discomforts.

- Helping the patient to feel less tense. The nurse should allow him to talk; help him to find diversion and to obtain adequate sleep.
- Not giving the patient the impression that you think he could snap out of it, or that he has purposely brought it on himself, if emotional tension seems to play a large part in causing the condition.
- Remembering that eczema is not contagious and not being afraid to go near the patient.
- Learning specifically what, if any, allergens the patient must avoid, keeping them away from him when he is in the hospital, and teaching him to recognize and avoid them when he goes home.

Some suggestions the nurse can pass on to the patient in terms of self-care follow:

- Ointments should be applied sparingly; otherwise, they will be wasted and cause clothing to become unnecessarily soiled.
- Some soiling of underwear is inevitable while the condition is acute. White cotton underwear helps to protect clothes. (Cotton is more absorbent than nylon or elasticized fabric.)
- Toilet tissue, especially if it is rough or highly colored, may be irritating to an already inflamed skin. After a bowel movement, soft cotton pledgets and plain water may be used for cleaning. The small pieces of cotton can be flushed down the toilet after use.
- Soap should not be used, because it irritates the lesions.
- For aesthetic reasons, cleaning and drying should be carried out with some soft disposable material like cotton. All that is necessary is the observance of good practices of personal hygiene since the condition is not contagious.

Other common dermatologic conditions

Psoriasis. Both men and women are affected by psoriasis, usually during young adulthood and middle life; men are affected more often than women. The cause is unknown. It may be related to metabolic disorder, heredity, or emotional conflict.

The disease is characterized by patches of erythema (redness) covered with silvery scales, usually on the extensor surfaces of the elbows and the knees, the lower back, and the scalp. Itching is usually absent or slight, but occasionally it is severe. The lesions are obvious and unsightly; the scales tend to shed.

There is no cure for psoriasis; therefore, treatment is aimed at the control of scaling and itching. Some factors which apparently cause a flare-up of the disorder are: stress, alcoholism, obesity, infection, trauma; these should be prevented or controlled. The patient must understand that treatment is usually for a lifetime and the plan of therapy must be followed.

Treatment is individualized and may include the use of topical ointments, drugs, and ultraviolet light. Topical agents may be corticosteroids or tar ointments, the latter staining the clothing. Anthralin (Anthra-Derm), a form of tar, may be used on thick plaques but may irritate the unaffected skin areas. Corticosteroids, applied topically or injected intradermally into the plaque, have proved beneficial. Methotrexate, an antimetabolite used in the treatment of cancer, may be prescribed in cases that are severe and do not respond to other forms of therapy. This drug inhibits the production of cells that divide rapidly (cancer cells, cells comprising the skin and mucous membranes, and so on) and is capable of decreasing plaque formation. Dosage must be carefully regulated as such drugs can cause serious side effects.

The prognosis for psoriasis is guarded. Some patients respond very well to treatment. However, the condition tends to recur. Those who obtain little relief from therapy may be easy prey for a variety of widely advertised remedies promising quick relief.

Contact Dermatitis (Dermatitis Venenata). Exposure to or skin contact with substances the individual is sensitive or allergic to can result in contact dermatitis. Drugs, cosmetics, poison ivy, chemicals, dyes, and ultraviolet light are some of the many causes of this skin disorder. Although the exact mechanism is not fully understood, it is thought that the molecules of certain substances may be absorbed through the skin and in some individuals create an antigen-antibody response. The individual then becomes sensitized to the substance and develops a dermatitis when future contact with it occurs.

Contact dermatitis is characterized by erythema, edema, vesicles, and itching. The area of contact may be outlined as, for example, skin manifestations appearing under a leather watch strap when the individual is sensitive to leather.

Treatment involves removing the cause if known; however, finding the cause may involve extensive history-taking to determine the substance(s) responsible. Location of the dermatitis may give early clues in some cases, but often there may be hundreds of possible substances that could be offending agents. Other treatment includes wet compresses or soaks, medicated baths, ointments, systemic corticosteroids, and antihistamines.

Impetigo Contagiosa. More common in children than adults, impetigo is caused by a streptococcal or a staphylococcal infection of the skin. The symptoms include erythema and vesicles that rupture and are covered with a sticky yellow crust (Fig. 42-1). Face and hands are common sites.

Impetigo is highly contagious and contact by other persons with the lesions or the exudate should be avoided carefully. The patient should never share his towel or bed linen. Meticulous hand washing after applying any medication is important. The patient himself should avoid touching the lesions unnecessarily. Because the condition can be spread from one part of his body to another, as well as to other people, he should wash his hands immediately after touching the lesions.

The crusts should be removed with soap and water, or with mineral oil, before any local medications are applied. Remember that applicators or gauze used for this purpose must be wrapped carefully and immediately discarded. Various preparations may be ordered, such as neomycin-bacitracin ointment, ammoniated mercury ointment, or gentian violet.

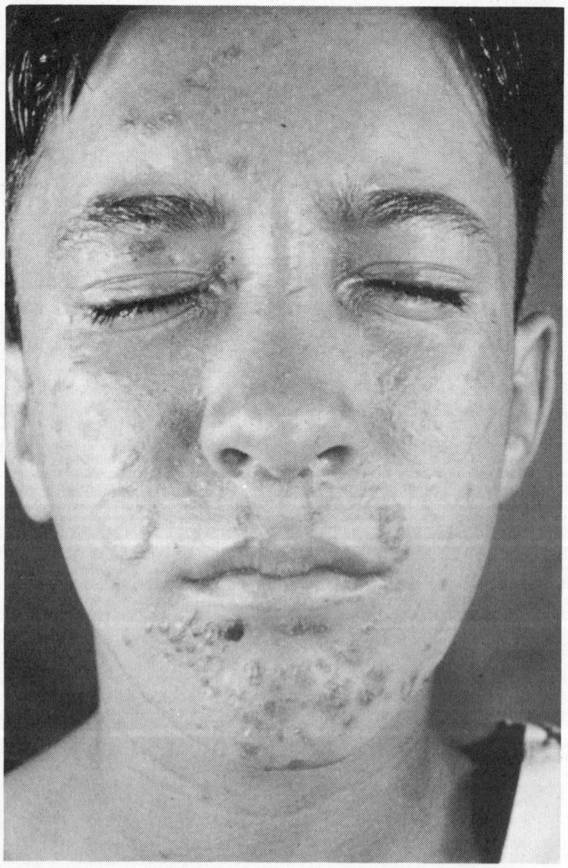

figure 42-1. Impetigo. Note crusts that form over lesions. (Medichrome—Clay-Adams, Inc., New York, N.Y.)

Usually, the condition is cured in a week. However, it can be especially severe in the newborn, and it can even cause death.

Herpes Simplex (Cold Sore). Herpes simplex is caused by a virus. It is believed that many people harbor the virus, and that a variety of factors, including colds, fever, emotional upsets, and menses may precipitate the appearance of herpes simplex.

A group of blisters occurs on reddened, inflamed skin, usually near the mouth, or on the genitals. Usually, pain and burning accompany the lesion. Herpes simplex is often called a cold sore or a fever blister. The lesions subside in about a week. Some people are especially susceptible to herpes simplex, and they have frequent recurrence of the lesions.

Usually, the symptoms are mild, and the condition subsides without treatment. No specific treatment is available that can shorten the duration of the lesion. Sometimes smallpox vaccine is administered in an effort to control recurrent eruptions of herpes simplex.

Herpes Zoster (Shingles). Herpes zoster is caused by a virus. The virus is the same one that causes chickenpox. The cutaneous lesions of this disease usually follow the course of a sensory nerve.

Before skin lesions appear, the patient may experience fever and malaise. Erythema and vesicles then appear, usually on the trunk or the face, along the course of a sensory nerve. Neurological pains occur, and may be severe, particularly in elderly persons. The condition subsides in about three weeks; however, the neuralgia may persist for months or even longer.

No specific treatment is available. Analgesics are ordered for the relief of pain. Local applications like calamine lotion are used to soothe the lesions. In older people systemic corticosteroids may be given. Clothing should be loose and nonirritating.

Furuncle, Carbuncle, Furunculosis. Streptococci, staphylococci, and other pathogenic organisms sometimes exist harmlessly on the surface of the skin, but when the normal protective functions of the skin are impaired, these pathogens may cause infection. For example, dryness and chapping of the skin may result in cracking, which allows microorganisms to enter and cause infection. These lesions are usually caused by staphylococcal infection. Often, an injury such as that caused by squeezing a pimple is the immediate cause, since it allows infection to enter through a break in the skin. Furunculosis is frequently due to lowered resistance, poor general health, and poor diet. Sometimes virulent strains of hospital-type staphylococci are the cause.

The descriptive symptoms of these conditions are:

- Furuncle: A whitish, raised, painful lesion, surrounded by erythema. The area feels hard to the touch. After a few days the lesion exudes pus, and later a core. It heals, leaving a tiny scar. Neglect or mismanagement can cause a larger, obvious scar.
- Carbuncle. A large swollen lesion, often on the back of the neck, surrounded by erythema. It is acutely painful; it has several openings through which pus drains.
- Furunculosis. In addition to multiple boils, the patient may have fever, anorexia, weakness and malaise.

Hot wet soaks are used to localize the infection. Often, for a single boil, this is the only treatment necessary. Antibiotics may be ordered to control the infection. Often, large doses are prescribed when fever is present, or if the lesion is a carbuncle. Incision and drainage may be necessary. Measures to improve general health are important in treating furunculosis.

The patient should never pick or squeeze a boil, as this practice favors spread of the infection to surrounding tissues or even to the bloodstream, causing septicemia. The exudate should be allowed to escape through the opening without the patient's squeezing the lesion or picking the top off. Drainage from a boil is infectious; strict medical aseptic technique is essential to prevent the spread of the infection to other parts of the patient's body or to other persons.

SEBACEOUS CYSTS. Sebaceous cysts are caused by obstruction of the duct of a sebaceous gland. The gland continues to secrete sebum despite the obstruction, thus causing accumulation of an oily secretion in the blocked duct. A swelling appears which at first is small, but which can grow large and unsightly. Treatment of the condition is surgical excision of the cyst, or cysts. If the lesion is small it may be removed outside the hospital; larger cysts must be dealt with in a hospital operating room.

DERMATOPHYTOSIS (ATHLETE'S FOOT). Dermatophytosis is a fungus infection most common in young adults. Usually, dermatophytosis first affects the toes, and particularly the skin between them. The affected skin becomes red, scaly, cracked and sore. Sometimes, the condition also affects the sides of the toes and the soles of the feet. It may spread to hands, axillae and groin. The nails may also become involved and are characteristically yellow, friable, and opaque.

The treatment includes benzoic and salicylic acid ointment (Whitfield's ointment), undecylenic acid (Desenex powder and ointment), and tolnaftate (Tinactin). Griseofulvin (Grifulvin) is useful in treatment; it is given orally. The drug may be required for many weeks in order to eradicate the infection. In severe cases corticosteroids may be administered for a limited time (e.g., one week) to lessen inflammation.

The disease may be transmitted from person to person through towels, locker rooms and bathroom floors. Towels and slippers should not be shared, and those using locker rooms or "community" bathrooms in dormitories should avoid going barefoot. Early diagnosis and treatment are important in preventing spread. Keeping the feet (particularly the area between the toes) dry increases resistance to the infection. People whose feet perspire freely often find that powdering between the toes helps to keep the area dry. Washing and drying the feet, and putting on clean, dry socks and a different pair of shoes after coming home from work is another aspect of personal hygiene that helps to keep the skin of the feet healthy.

Because the fungus can survive in shoes, slippers, and socks and these can constitute a source of reinfection, socks should be boiled after each use; slippers and shoes may have to be discarded. The fewer articles that come in contact with the patient's feet, the less the problem of disinfection, and the fewer chances of reinfection. For example, it is preferable for the patient to wear clean socks at all times, even at night, rather than place his bare feet in contact with slippers and bedding. Shared bath mats can be a source of infection for others. If the patient uses a separate towel as his bath mat, it can be more easily boiled and laundered than a heavy bath mat or rug—and is therefore less likely to spread infection. The patient should clean the tub or the shower floor with a disinfectant, such as creosol (Lysol), after each use.

INFESTATION AND BITES. An infestation with pediculi (lice) results in *pediculosis*. The following terms are used to describe pediculosis:

- Pediculous capitis—infestation of the hair or the scalp.
- Pediculous corporis—infestation of the body surfaces with a louse larger than the one that affects the scalp and the hair. This parasite and its eggs may be found also in the patient's clothing—particularly within cuffs and seams.
- Pediculous pubis—infestation of the pubic area with a very tiny louse shaped like a crab —hence the lay term, *crabs*. Although this condition occurs primarily in the pubic area, it may occur in the hairy areas of the axilla.

The symptoms of pediculosis include itching, scratching, and irritation of the skin. Scratching denudes the skin, making it susceptible to infection. Eggs are deposited on the hair near the scalp, and may be confused with dandruff. These eggs, often called *nits,* cannot be brushed out as dandruff can, but are attached firmly to the hair. The lice are tiny, grayish-brown creatures that may be seen when they move on the scalp.

Benzyl benzoate and benzine hexachloride are contained in a variety of onitments, powders, and lotions that are effective in killing pediculi. Kwell lotion and shampoo are commonly used preparations. Although the pediculi can be promptly killed by these modern remedies, repeated infestations are likely if the individual continues to have close contact with others who harbor the parasites, and if personal hygiene is poor. Pediculosis capitis can be spread by shared toilet articles, like combs, and by close personal contact, such as that occurring in crowded places. Pediculosis pubis can be transmitted by sexual intercourse.

Scabies is caused by infestation with the itch mite (*Sarcoptes scabiei*). The symptoms include intense itching, which is usually worse at night, accompanied by excoriation and burrows (the lesion caused when the female itch mite invades the skin, burrowing underneath, leaving a dark line). The lesions occur most often between the fingers and on the forearms, the axilla, the waistline, women's nipples, men's genitals, the umbilicus, and the lower back.

Benzyl benzoate in lotions and ointments is highly effective in treating scabies. Thorough bathing, clean clothing, and the avoidance of contact with others who have scabies are essential in preventing recurrence. Before any treatment is started, the patient should have a thorough bath. After medication has been applied, he should have a complete change of clothing.

The itch mite can be transmitted readily from one person to another by close personal contact and by sharing towels and clothing.

Bedbug bites are caused by tiny, dark-brown insects that infest mattresses and wooden bed frames. In heavily infested dwellings, bedbugs may live in crevices of the woodwork or in upholstered furniture. Although they are more common in crowded, unsanitary homes, bedbugs may be brought into any home on clothing or even on newspapers. The symptoms of bedbug bites include the appearance of wheals (hives) with central points or dots. These lesions may appear on any part of the body, but they are most commonly found on the wrists, the ankles, and the buttocks. Usually, the bites require little local treatment. Sometimes, calamine lotion or witch hazel is applied to soothe the lesions. The services of an exterminator are frequently required to get rid of the bugs.

Social and Emotional Implications. The diagnosis of pediculosis or scabies or bedbug bites often causes embarrassment and is difficult for many people to accept. This is true whether the patient comes from a clean home in a good neighborhood, or whether he lives in a slum. To the person who lives in a crowded, dirty environment the condition may be viewed as further evidence of economic and social disadvantages. Whether or not it is common in his neighborhood, he will be sensitive to the attitudes of those who care for him. Indications of disgust and distaste will serve to make the patient less willing to seek treatment the next time he needs health care.

The nurse who recognizes the interdependence of social, economic, and health factors, will understand the degree to which people can be the victims of poverty and lack of opportunity. The nurse who can accept the patient—even the one with pediculosis—has taken the biggest and most important step in helping that patient recover from the condition and learn to prevent its recurrence. Instruction must be handled with great tact.

Premalignant and malignant skin lesions

Skin lesions are usually readily observable, thus facilitating prompt diagnosis and treatment. Nurses have a responsibility to teach people to seek medical advice for any lesion that persists. If it is malignant, prompt treatment often can prevent spread and cure the condition.

Several factors predispose to malignant changes in the skin:

- Prolonged, repeated exposure to ultraviolet rays. Sailors, farmers, overzealous sun bathers, and others who are exposed to a great deal of sunlight are particularly vulnerable.
- Exposure to radiation.
- Ulcerations of long duration and scar tissue. Both are prone to malignant changes.

PRECANCEROUS LESIONS. Some lesions are considered precancerous. *Leukoplakia* is characterized by shiny white patches that usually occur on the mucous membrane of the mouth or the female genitalia. If leukoplakia occurs in the mouth, smoking is definitely contraindicated, because it makes the condition worse. Rough, jagged teeth should be replaced, so that they do not irritate the lesion. Surgical excision of the lesions is often recommended because of the danger of cancer. The lesions also may be removed by electrodesiccation.

Birthmarks (*nevi*) are of various kinds, including vascular nevi (*angiomas*), brown moles and black moles. The lesion may not be visible at birth; however, the beginnings of the lesion are present at birth and may appear later. Black, smooth moles are the most likely to become cancerous. However, any mole that becomes irritated, bleeds, or begins to grow larger should have prompt medical attention. Surgical removal usually is recommended. Light brown moles that are not located where irritation from clothing is a problem usually do not have to be removed unless it is desirable for cosmetic reasons.

Senile keratoses are brownish, scaly spots appearing on the skin of older persons. They are most likely to occur on exposed portions of the skin, such as the face, the ears, or the hands. Patients who develop senile keratoses should be advised to seek medical attention. Because the lesions are common and seem to be insignificant, they are often disregarded. However, they may become malignant, and their removal is usually recommended.

MALIGNANT LESIONS. Malignant growths of the skin are usually primary lesions. The spread to other parts of the body may be prevented by prompt removal of the malignant tissue. *Epithelioma* is a common type of skin cancer. It arises from the surface layers of the skin. If immediately treated by surgical excision, electrodesiccation, or x-ray therapy, these lesions may be controlled promptly. On the other hand, *malignant melanoma* is a highly malignant, rapidly spreading lesion. Usually it is coal-black (Fig. 42-2). Wide surgical excision may be attempted to save the patient's life; however, because of the rapid spread, the prognosis is poor. *Squamous cell carcinoma* is another dangerous type of lesion because it tends to metastasize to internal organs. This type of cancer often occurs on the tongue or the lower lip. (Chronic irritation from pipe smoking is a common causative factor in lesions involving the lower lip.) Depending on the size and the location of the lesion, the treatment may involve electrodesiccation, surgical excision, or x-ray therapy.

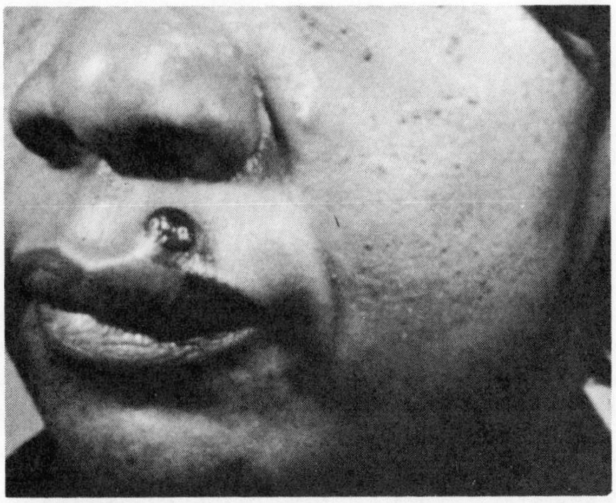

figure 42-2. Melanoma. (Medichrome—Clay-Adams, Inc., New York, N.Y.)

General pharmacological considerations

- Ointments, creams, and lotions prescribed for dermatological disorders are to be applied *exactly* as the physician directs—e.g., sparingly, thick, thin coat covering the lesion, etc. The patient should also be reminded that unless the drug is applied exactly as ordered it may not be of therapeutic value, or if excess is used, it will constitute a waste of the drug.
- Various drugs, both local (such as ointments) and systemic may be prescribed for itching. These drugs are not effective in all cases and other nursing measures—for example, the wearing of protective gloves at night—may have to be employed.
- Drugs prescribed for dermatological conditions may relieve symptoms but do not necessarily cure the disease. Skin disorders may require long-term therapy, often with a periodic change in prescriptions. This can be discouraging to the patient. The nurse should encourage persistence in following the dictates of the physician.

Bibliography

BOWDEN, L.: Current trends in treating malignant melanoma. AORN J. 17:84, March, 1973.

DEGRANCIANSKY, P., and BOULLE, S.: *Color Atlas of Dermatology*. Vols. 1-5. Chicago, Year Book Medical Publishers, 1965.

DERBES, V. J.: Rashes: Recognition and management (pictorial). Nurs. '73, 3:44, March, 1973.

MITCHELL, D. M.: Eczema (pictorial). Nurs. Mirror 136:37, March 2, 1973.

MOHS, F. E. et al: Chemosurgery and skin cancer. AORN J. 13:89, February, 1971.

PARRISH, J. A.: *Dermatology and Skin Care*. New York, McGraw-Hill, 1975.

ROACH, L. B.: Assessing skin changes: The subtle and the obvious. Nurs. '74, 4:64, March, 1974.

ROBINS, P.: Skin cancer from cause to cure. RN 37:29, March, 1974.

STEWART, W. D. et al: *Synopsis of Dermatology*. St. Louis, Mosby, 1970.

CHAPTER—43

The patient undergoing plastic surgery

On completion of this chapter the student will:

- **Discuss the conditions treated by plastic surgery and give examples of cosmetic surgery.**
- **Differentiate between autographs and homographs.**
- **Name the various types of skin grafts and briefly describe each.**
- **Discuss the nursing management of patients having plastic surgery.**

The terms *plastic surgery* and *reconstructive surgery* are often used interchangeably to refer to the repair of defects that may be congenital or acquired through injury or radical surgery. The repair surgery may have been performed for cosmetic purposes or to improve function. For example, a crooked nose may be straightened, or contracted scar tissue in the axilla may be freed to restore normal motion to the arm. A deformed hand may be totally reconstructed by repair of tendon, bone, nerve, or skin. An eyelid that has been damaged by trauma may be repaired by means of a pedicle graft or advancement flaps.

The four main kinds of conditions treated by plastic surgery are:

1. Congenital deformities, such as harelip and protruding ears;
2. Deformities resulting from trauma, such as burns and automobile accidents;
3. Conditions for which the patient seeks cosmetic surgery, such as face-lifting;
4. Disfigurement resulting from malignant disease, such as cancer of the mouth.

This highly specialized treatment combines art and medicine. In cosmetic surgery the aim is not to produce beauty as such, but beauty in the sense that the changed appearance is appropriate for the particular patient and blends unnoticeably into his features, producing a natural appearance.

Cosmetic surgery and functional improvement

Plastic surgery holds the promise of a more normal appearance and improved function for many patients. Both appearance and function are important considerations; however, their relative importance varies with the part of the body involved. For instance, function is a prime consideration in reconstructive surgery on the hand (Fig. 43-1), and appearance is of particular significance in surgery involving the face. Surgical treatment that produces the greatest functional improvement may not be the same as that which leads to the most satisfactory cosmetic result.

When we think of cosmetic surgery, we usually think only of the face and the neck. Although these areas are frequently involved in plastic surgery, it is by no means limited to them. The degree of disfigurement can range from slight to marked; however, it may not be a reliable indicator of the patient's reaction to his condition. A very tiny flaw may seem like a huge blemish to a person who is very sensitive about his appearance. Cosmetic surgery may bring great relief to patients who are very conscious of, for example, a hooked nose; straightening the nose may bring the person a new feeling of poise and assurance.

However, people who tend to blame all their failures and disappointments on what may seem to others a barely noticeable blemish have unrealistic expectations of what plastic surgery can accomplish. Sometimes, plastic surgery is contraindicated if the patient's

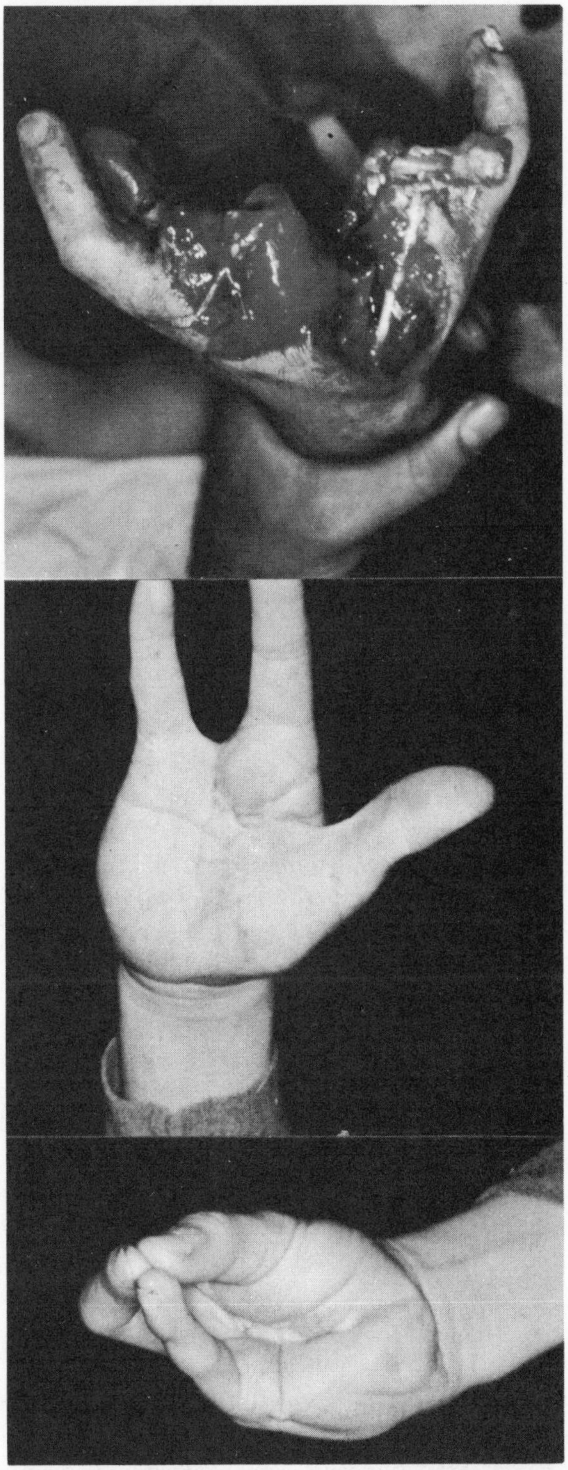

figure 43-1. (*Top*) Hand mangled in an accident. (*Center*) After plastic reconstruction. (*Bottom*) There is good function in this hand. (Dr. Alvin Mancusi-Ungaro, Montclair, N.J.)

dissatisfaction with his appearance seems to be an expression of a deeper emotional problem.

Examples of plastic surgery performed for cosmetic purposes include:

- *"Face-lifting" and blepharoplasty.* Most of the incision for face-lifting is made in the hairline. Wrinkles are removed by tightening the fascia and skin and removing excess skin. Most of the fine scar resulting from surgery is concealed by the hair. Modern face-lifting techniques produce results that are longer lasting than was the case formerly. Although more time is necessary to evaluate how long the results of these newer procedures last, it is believed that one face-lifting procedure will suffice for many years.

  Frequently blepharoplasty (eyelid reconstruction) is carried out as part of the surgical procedure, in an effort to remove the aged appearance which frequently sets in at about the age of 50, when the elastic fibers of the dermis relax, and some of the subcutaneous fat that produces a youthful look becomes absorbed. In eyelid reconstruction, incisions are made which are hidden in normal crease-lines. The excessive eyelid skin and orbital fat (if necessary) are removed.
- *Rhinoplasty.* Since the nose is the most exposed part of the face, it is frequently injured, often without the individual's remembering the accident. Reconstruction of the tissues is now a fine art. Usually within 2 to 3 weeks after the surgery, improvements in appearance, breathing, and senses of smell and taste are apparent, as well as improvements in poise, assurance, and morale.
- *Dermabrasion* is a technique for removing surface layers of scarred skin. It is useful in lessening such scars as the pitting from severe acne. The outermost layers of the skin are removed by sandpaper, a rotating wire brush, or a diamond wheel. A local anesthetic, such as an ethyl chloride-freon mixture may be used during the procedure. Afterward, the skin feels raw and sore, and some crusting from serous exudate occurs. Patients frequently say that the discomfort is much like that from a burn. The patient is instructed not to wash the area for 5 or 6 days, until sufficient healing has occurred. Picking and touching the area must be avoided, since this contact might cause infection or produce marking of the tissues.
- *Tattooing* is used to change the color of the skin. Pigments are blended to just the right shade for the patient's skin and then are implanted into it. The treatment is useful in covering up dark red birthmarks (port wine stains), and in matching the color of grafted skin to the surrounding skin more exactly. However, the pigments may shift position beneath the skin so that they are no longer effective in covering up the blemish. Also, the pigments sometimes look different in environments of various temperatures. For example, a tattoo that is not noticeable at room temperature may become noticeable, due to color change, when the patient goes out into the cold.

  Tattooing and dermabrasion are usually carried out in the physician's office or in a clinic.
- *Artificial parts* may be used to camouflage defects. For instance, part of a nose or an ear may be made of plastic to match the patient's features so exactly that it is hard to tell which is the prosthetic part, and which is natural. Plastic materials are also used as framework or supporting structures over which the patient's tissues grow. For instance, a plastic material, such as silicone rubber, may be used beneath the skin to correct an underdeveloped chin.
- *Mammoplasty* may be performed to change the size and shape of the breasts. Very large breasts may make a woman self-conscious, contribute to poor posture, and interfere with breathing. Excess tissue is removed surgically under general anesthesia. Afterward, the patient must wear a firm supporting brassiere for several months until healing is complete and the tissues are firm. Surgery is sometimes undertaken to enlarge small breasts (augmentation mammoplasty). Tissues from the patient's own body, such as a buttock, or plastic materials, such as silicone gel within a Silastic bag, are used as an implant between the chest wall and the breast. Placing the material here, rather than inside the breast, has two advantages: (1) the function of the breast is unimpaired: the woman can lactate normally; and (2) the possibility of carcinogenesis from introduction of foreign materials in breast tissue is obviated.

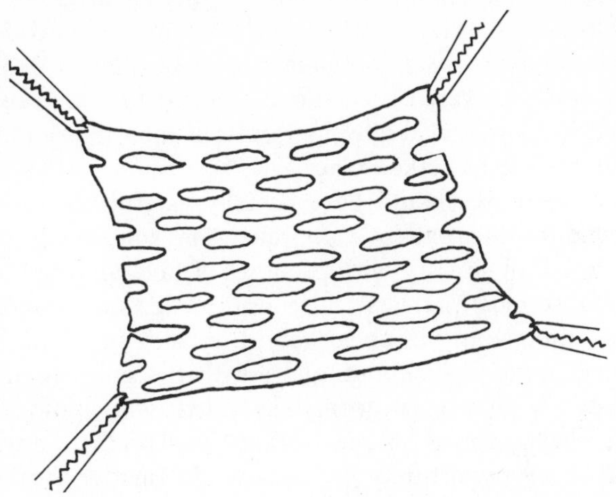

figure 43-2. The slit or lace graft. The slits allow for stretching of the graft.

Skin grafts

Skin grafts may consist of *autografts* (skin transplanted from one part of the patient's body to another) or of *homografts* (skin transplanted from one person to another). Only autografts or skin transplanted from one identical twin to another can become a permanent part of the patient's own skin. However, homografts are useful in temporarily closing large defects, thus preventing further loss of tissue fluid. Although the homografts slough away after 1 or more weeks and must be replaced by autografts, they tide the patient over the critical period of illness and help him to recover enough to permit the use of autografts. Other body tissues, such as bone and cartilage, may also be used as grafts. Skin grafting is done in surgery, under general anesthesia.

In order for grafts to "take," there must be a sufficient blood supply to the part and an absence of infection. The graft must stick close to the tissues on which it is to grow; excess blood or serous fluid can cause the graft to become separated from the tissues and to fail to grow. Sometimes warm, moist saline compresses are placed on pedicle grafts. The skin being transplanted by a pedicle has blood supplied from the donor site. The warmth transmitted to the recipient bed through the graft is believed to favor the development of blood circulation in the graft.

Types of skin grafts

Split-thickness and *full-thickness* grafts are the two basic types of skin grafts. Split-thickness autografts vary in thickness—0.008 inch to 0.024 inch—size, and shape, and are usually obtained from the buttocks or thighs. The skin is removed from the donor site by use of a dermatome, a scalpel, or another special instrument. A *pinch graft* is a small piece of skin cut from the donor site and placed on the recipient site. A *postage stamp graft* is a piece of skin about the size of a stamp and like the pinch graft is cut from the donor site and placed on the recipient site. A *full cover graft* is a large piece of skin removed by means of a dermatome or another special instrument. Sutures are usually necessary to anchor this type of graft in place. A *slit graft* (also called a lace or an expansile graft) is used when the area available as a donor site is limited, as in patients with extensive burns. The skin is removed from the donor site and passed through an instrument that puts slits in it; thus a smaller piece of skin is stretched (Fig. 43-2) to cover a larger area.

Full-thickness grafts are usually used to restore function to and improve cosmetic appearance of a burned area. When the recipient site is the face or neck, the skin from the donor site is matched, as closely as possible, to the skin of the recipient site. While split-thickness grafts cover the area, they do not give as good a cosmetic appearance as full-thickness grafts.

Free full-thickness grafts, which may be 0.035 inch thick, are skin grafts that include subcutaneous tissue. This type of graft may be used in burns during the management stage when the burned area is fairly small or when the hands, face, and neck are involved. *Pedicle flaps* are full-thickness grafts that include skin and subcutaneous fat with a tube formed from the piece of skin. This tube is then moved to another site and anchored.

Surgeons use various methods of grafting, much depending on the size and location of the recipient site, the available areas of donor sites, the condition of donor sites, and the patient's age. When grafts are planned during the treatment and rehabilitation stages, the surgeon carefully evaluates present and future needs. Serious problems that may occur after skin grafting involve infection or failure of the graft to "take" properly; repeated grafts may be necessary if the autograft is rejected. Such factors, as well as those pertinent to a specific patient, must be taken into account when plans are made for skin grafting.

Nursing management of patients who have plastic surgery

Classifying surgery as *minor* or *major* has many pitfalls. A great deal of plastic surgery is referred to as minor, because the areas involved are usually superficial and readily accessible. Nevertheless, the success or the failure of the surgery has grave consequences *for the patient.* Permanent grafts must be obtained from the patient's own skin; yet, when large areas of the skin have been destroyed by trauma, such as a severe burn, the amount of healthy skin available for grafting is limited. The failure of the graft to grow can mean that another operation is necessary, or that the procedure cannot be repeated because of the scarcity of healthy skin. Most patients who undergo plastic surgery already have suffered a great deal.

The nurse has an important part to play in insuring the success of a plastic-surgery procedure. For instance, care must be taken to avoid excessive pressure that might impair circulation. (A bandage that is too tight can interfere with circulation.) The part must be protected from injury. The patient should not be allowed to lie on or bump the area. The most meticulous aseptic technique is necessary to prevent infection. If a warm, moist dressing is ordered, the solution must be sterile, poured into a sterile basin, and wrung out and applied with sterile forceps. A dressing that is too hot could damage the tissues rather than help them to grow. Dressings should never be changed unless the physician specifically requests it; removing the dressing may take the graft with it. Any evidence of bleeding or of pus on the dressing should be reported to the physician.

Patients with skin grafts have two sites to be cared for before and after the surgery—the donor site and the recipient site. Usually, the skin of the donor site is shaved before the patient goes to the operating room. The surgeon will specify which area (often the upper thigh) is to be prepared. The recipient site is the wound or the defect to which the grafts will be applied. The surgeon will specify the particular care needed for this area, too. Postoperatively, the nurse must observe both the donor area and the recipient area. For instance, a sheet or a slice of skin may have been removed from the anterior thigh by a dermatome, leaving a raw, weeping surface. Often, petrolatum gauze is placed over the wound and covered by a dry dressing. The nurse must observe this area for any sign of infection or bleeding, and she must protect it from injury until it has healed.

Whether the patient has skin grafting or reconstructive surgery of some feature, such as the nose, it is important for him to understand what to expect from the surgery. The surgeon will discuss the operation with the patient in advance, but there may be many times during his recovery when the patient will turn to the nurse for repeated explanation and reassurance. For instance, immediately after plastic repair of the nose (rhinoplasty), the nose may be swollen and bruised. His first thought may be that he looks worse than ever. He should be helped to understand that he cannot evaluate the results of the surgery until the healing has taken place.

The nurse should be especially careful not to respond to the patient's apprehension concerning the outcome of surgery with promises of favorable results. Because most patients feel considerable tension about the outcome of plastic surgery, they may question the nurse repeatedly about matters that should be discussed with the surgeon. The nurse will allow the patient to express his concerns and explain that he will have the opportunity to discuss the matter further with his physician. Because some patients are hesitant to voice some of their worries to the physician, it is important for the nurse to mention to the physician the questions which the patient has raised, so that he can talk further with the patient about them.

The patient's reaction to the change in his appearance may sometimes seem baffling—particularly when the surgery results in a considerably improved appearance. Instead of immediately showing pleasure and gratitude, the patient may cry. (Even when a change in his body is a cosmetic improvement, some loss of the "old self" is inevitable, and grief can occur over the loss, even of a deformity.) Ordinarily, grieving is short-lived when the surgery results in improved appearance. It is important during this period to help the patient to realize that his reactions are acceptable and not unusual. The patient should be given the opportunity to talk about his feelings concerning his changed appearance. Another possible reaction after plastic surgery is hostility, which the child may show by tantrums and fighting with neighborhood children, but which in an adult is more likely to be expressed as crankiness, impatience, and general dissatisfaction. Reasons for such behavior are individual, and each patient must discover these and deal with them himself. An accepting, concerned listener can help him to do so. Possibly he has stored up anger as a result of many years of humiliation over a deformity, and once it is removed, so too is the muzzle he has placed on the expression of his anger.

Sensitivity is required in helping the patient to resume his contacts with others after surgery. This is especially problematic if the patient's appearance has been altered for the worse. For example, the disfigurement of a patient who has been badly burned may only partially be alleviated by plastic surgery, and this improvement may be the result of numerous operations over a period of many months. The patient may dread being seen by family and friends but also be badly in need of the encouragement and support their visits can bring. Often the nurse can help in such situations, by gently preparing visitors before they enter the room for the first time.

Tactfully encouraging the patient's contact with other patients on the unit can also help lessen his isolation. Careful assessment of the patient's readiness, and that of other patients, is important. A patient who is painfully self-conscious about his appearance may tolerate and then begin to enjoy the visits of a quiet person who comes to offer some brief service, such as sharing a newspaper, but be overwhelmed by being wheeled to a solarium where a group of patients are gathered.

Bibliography

Clery, A. B.: Treatment of burns by split skin grafting. Nurs. Times 70:1893, December 5, 1974.

David, D. J.: Skin grafting. Nurs. Times 68:1437, November 23, 1972.

Gill, S. A.: Nursing the plastic surgery patient. AORN J. 17:66, May, 1973.

Hurwitz, A.: About faces. Am. J. Nurs. 71:2168, November, 1971.

Isler, C.: The world of transplants. The tissue banks. Part 2. RN 35:40, December, 1972.

Krause, C. J. et al: The aging face (pictorial). RN 38:OR/ED 1, February, 1975.

Reichenbacher, F. W.: The use of porcine skin in burn treatment. AORN J. 21:652, March, 1975.

Trowbridge, J. E.: Caring for patients with facial or intra-oral reconstruction. Am. J. Nurs. 73:1930, November, 1973.

Wehner, R. J.: Therapeutic, cosmetic effects of oral surgery (pictorial). AORN J. 22:52, July, 1975.

UNIT ELEVEN

Intensive care nursing

- **Introduction**
- **The patient in shock**
- **Respiratory insufficiency and failure**
- **The patient with heart disease: cardiac arrhythmias**
- **The patient with acute myocardial infarction**
- **Cardiac surgical nursing**
- **The patient in renal failure**
- **The burned patient**
- **The patient with neurological disease**

CHAPTER 44

Introduction

On completion of this chapter the student will:

- **Recognize the importance of the intensive care unit and the need for skillful and intelligent nursing management of the patient in this unit.**

The concept of intensive care involves a concentration of medical and nursing staff and allied health personnel specially prepared to observe, assess, and treat critically ill patients with the assistance of various kinds of technology. The patients may have the same diagnosis, such as acute myocardial infarction. Or, in a mixed intensive care unit, there may be patients in acute renal or respiratory failure, patients after cardiac surgery or severe trauma, patients with third-degree burns, septicemia, postsurgical complications, or metabolic crises, such as diabetic ketoacidosis, among other diagnoses.

Because of the need for close and constant observation and the potential for deterioration of the patient's condition, the ratio of nurses to patients is high. But a high nurse-patient ratio is not the essence of intensive care nursing. Skilled intensive nursing care is a blend of expertise in the technical-judgmental skills and the interpersonal skills exercised in behalf of the patient and family caught in a life-death crisis, many for the first time.

The importance of performing technical tasks in a knowledgeable, precise, and manually dexterous manner with necessary adjustments to the individual patient cannot be overestimated. The nurse who traumatizes a patient because of an unskilled attempt at nasal or oropharyngeal suctioning can cause the patient to resist or refuse to be suctioned again, despite his need.

The patient admitted to an intensive care unit has special problems different from the patient admitted electively. His illness is most often acutely disruptive of his work or home life. The nature of his admission by ambulance with siren screeching, the rush of personnel, and the emergency therapies, serve to reinforce the message which his pain, or dyspnea, or bleeding, or vomiting has already conveyed to him—that he is gravely ill and may even die. The sights, sounds, and smells which surround his small living space in the intensive care unit are foreign and threatening to him. It is hard to distinguish night from day when lights are on all the time and activity is constant. Restrained from moving by intravenous lines, monitoring electrodes, and various kinds of other devices, and separated from family and friends, the acutely ill patient faces a fearsome burden. Nursing assists the patient to cope with all of these strange and threatening conditions so that his major efforts can be directed toward the work of healing.

Providing emotional support for the patient is as much a part of sound physiological management as is the overtly technical procedure. The patient's psychological response to an acute physical problem stresses his cardiovascular, respiratory, and endocrine systems. Increase or decrease in heart rate, cardiac arrhythmias, hyperventilation with subsequent shift in pH, and the outpouring of catecholamines from the adrenal gland are examples of physiological responses to stress. These responses are also experienced at times of crisis by members of the staff, as well as by the patient's family or associates in the waiting room. Just as one needs specialized education to deal with newer technical aspects of care, so do the members of the intensive care staff need continuing assistance to deal with their own emotional responses so that they can be more supportive of patients and visitors.

There is considerable challenge and satisfaction in intensive care nursing. Many lives are saved by a caring, competent team. Newer treatment modalities offer new opportunities for sharing and collaboration between physicians and nurses in the interest of quality patient care (Figs. 44-1 and 44-2).

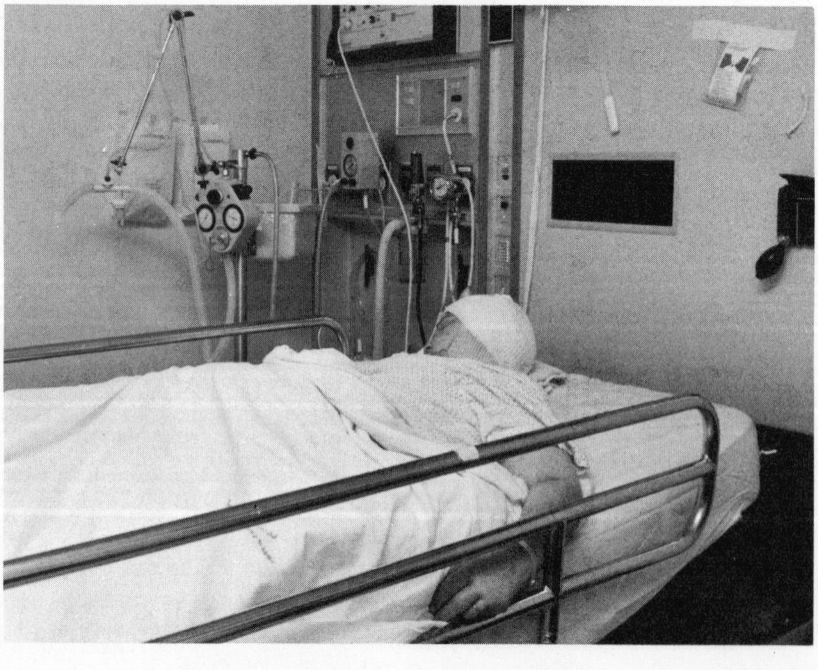

figure 44-1. The concept of intensive care involves the observation, assessment and treatment of critically ill patients. (Photograph—D. Atkinson)

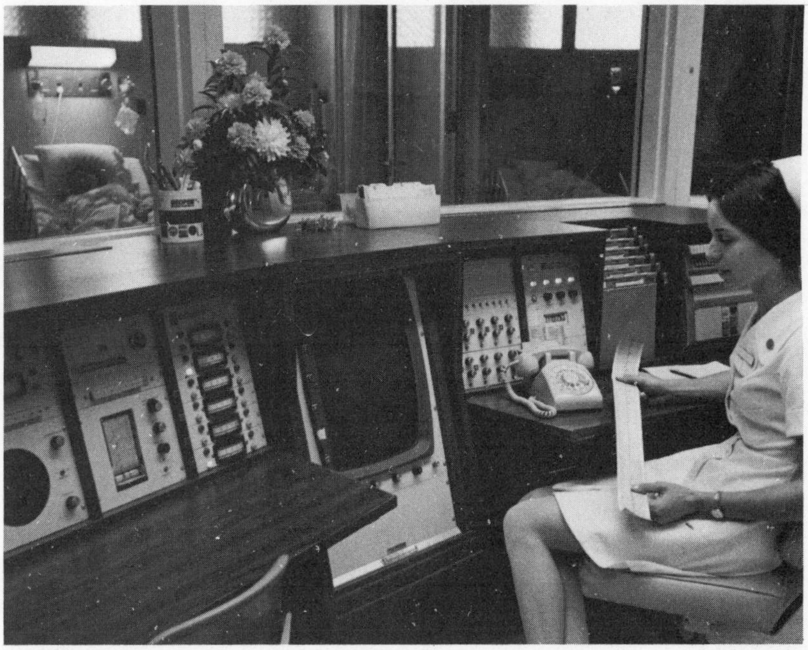

figure 44-2. The Coronary Care Unit, Phase I, at Sisters Hospital, Buffalo, New York. The console monitors the electrocardiogram of each patient in the unit. (Photograph—D. Atkinson)

Inevitably, some patients will die. They and their families need as much support and dignity as the situation permits. Sudden death means that the patient and his family have had no time to prepare for it; the news may overwhelm them. In their shock and sorrow they may feel aggressive against the hospital staff. The nurse should understand the family members' reaction, even though it may be difficult for her to listen to them, and explain that everything possible was done for the patient.

The patient's stay in the intensive or coronary care unit is generally a short one, and he is transferred out as soon as possible to a general hospital area. Patients who are not prepared for this transfer through early anticipation of the time of transfer, discussion of the meaning of the move, weaning the patient from equipment such as a cardiac monitor on which he may have developed a degree of dependence, and acceptance by a knowledgeable new nursing staff, may experience sufficient stress to cause a major setback. In addition to patient preparation, the staff on the general nursing unit needs a full nursing history and well-developed written nursing care plan so that nursing management can continue without disruption.

CHAPTER—45

The patient in shock

On completion of this chapter the student will:

- **List and describe the classifications of shock.**
- **Discuss how shock can be prevented in some cases.**
- **List the signs and symptoms of shock.**
- **Name and give the relevance of the observations made by the nurse when a patient is in shock.**
- **Describe and discuss the treatment and nursing management of the patient in shock.**

Why blood vessels occasionally fail to maintain the balanced constriction that maintains normal pressure is not completely understood. It is known that master adjustment centers in the brain can be impaired by drugs, by hypoxia, by anesthesia, and by trauma, among many examples, and that poor vascular tone can result. Despite much investigation, agreement on the exact pathophysiological disturbances involved in shock or on modes of treatment has not been reached. It is agreed that shock is a complicated series of interwoven events—vascular, hormonal, neural, metabolic, and hemodynamic.

Shock is a clinical syndrome indicating inadequate circulation that results from a variety of causes. Inadequate circulation leads to tissue hypoxia. Regardless of the cause, prolonged shock is incompatible with life. The faster the shock state can be reversed, the greater the chance of uncomplicated recovery. There are few instances in the care of patients where careful attention to nursing practices and principles is as important to recovery as in the management of the patient in impending or actual shock.

Shock can be classified according to etiology:

HEMATOGENIC SHOCK, in which there is a reduction in the volume of circulating blood (hypovolemic shock). This type of shock may be caused by hemorrhage, in which blood is spilled from the usually closed system of arteries and veins. Other causes include severe burns, in which a large amount of fluid seeps from the circulatory system into the injured area; and the loss of large amounts of fluid in vomitus and diarrhea. Hemorrhage into a cavity, such as thoracic or abdominal, may be hidden from sight, but it is just as deadly as the hemorrhage one can see from an external wound.

CARDIOGENIC SHOCK, in which the circulatory failure involves faulty pumping of the heart. A common cause of cardiogenic shock is acute myocardial infarction.

VASOGENIC SHOCK, in which there is diffuse vasodilation, resulting in an increase in the size of the vascular bed. When blood becomes trapped in small vessels and in the viscera, it is lost temporarily to the mainstream of circulating fluid. The skeletal muscles and the viscera may become engorged with blood, while the volume of circulating blood is reduced dangerously. This type of shock is *normovolemic*. That is, the amount of fluid in the circulatory system is not reduced, but it is not circulating in such a way that permits effective perfusion of the tissues. Anaphylaxis is an example of vasogenic shock.

NEUROGENIC SHOCK, which results from an insult to the nervous system. Intracranial damage and certain drugs can cause neurogenic shock. Vasodilation is a prominent feature.

PSYCHIC SHOCK, in which pain, severe fright or other strong emotion interferes with normal vascular control. *A frightened patient makes a poor surgical risk.*

BACTEREMIC SHOCK, which may be seen in any overwhelming bacterial infection, usually occurs in the patient who is succumbing to the infection. Bacteremic shock is more common in patients in whom bacteremia is caused by gram-negative organisms. Endotoxins released by the organisms are probably a major cause.

Prevention

The ability of an individual to avoid shock cannot be predicted. The patient who has undergone a known cause of shock is safer when cared for as if shock might develop. For example, all accident victims and patients with acute myocardial infarction should be treated as if shock were imminent. To maintain an appraisal of the circulatory state, frequent observations of the patient's vital signs are ordered until the occurrence of shock is no longer considered probable. All postoperative patients belong in this category. Even if the surgical procedure involves practically no blood loss, the stress of going to surgery, the anesthetic, and the necessary trauma of the surgical incision are influences that can contribute to shock.

Careful preoperative preparation, both physical and psychological, is important in preventing shock. However, hypovolemia is more significant as a cause of shock than such factors as anesthetic agents and psychic stress.

Nurses should become expert at estimating fluid loss. How many ml. are in a puddle of vomitus on the floor? How many ml. are soaked into the bed linen after a severe nosebleed? How much fluid can a saturated 4-inch square sponge hold? One way to train the eye is to take a known amount of fluid and pour it on the floor, in a sheet, or on a sponge, and see what it looks like. Another way to estimate fluid loss is by weight. For example, in the operating room weigh a dry sponge. Then weigh a blood-soaked one and subtract. A healthy adult can lose up to approximately 500 ml. of blood without need for replacement. The ill, the elderly, and the poorly nourished need replacement therapy for less blood loss. Central venous pressure monitoring is being used more frequently prophylactically in order to better evaluate volume replacement needs.

Signs, symptoms and observations

The nurse must watch for signs that the body is being forced to call on major defenses to maintain blood pressure. Although deep shock can develop in minutes, more often there is a warning period. In hypovolemic shock the rate of volume loss is most directly related to the speed with which the symptoms of shock appear. For example, the patient whose aorta ruptures progresses almost instantaneously to profound circulatory collapse, whereas the patient sustaining a venous hemorrhage will go into shock in a more orderly, step-by-step fashion through the sequence of symptoms indicating impending circulatory collapse.

Every nurse should be thoroughly familiar with the signs and the symptoms of shock. The signs and symptoms are not difficult to remember once they are correlated with the pathological changes that cause them.

Skin

Peripheral blood vessels constrict to direct blood from the skin to more vital organs, such as the kidney and brain. Ischemia renders the skin pale and cold. It is clammy due to activation of the sweat glands. There may be cyanosis, especially of the fingernail beds, lips, and earlobes. Cyanosis indicates severe tissue hypoxia. Its absence, however, does not prove the absence of hypoxia. Recognition of cyanosis may be obscured by deep skin pigmentation, anemia, and poor lighting conditions.

Arterial blood pressure

Blood pressure is a valuable but not an infallible index of shock. Organ blood flow and tissue perfusion, not blood pressure, are the critical determinants.

The blood pressure falls because cardiac output is reduced. For the average adult, the following may be used as comparative figures:

	Systolic Blood Pressure
Average, normal	100–130 mm. Hg
Impending shock	90–100 mm. Hg
Shock	Below 80 mm. Hg

In order to determine if shock is present, the patient's usual blood pressure should be known. Regardless of the numerical figure, the consistent progressive fall of blood pressure with a rapid, thready pulse is a serious sign. In the early stages of shock the blood pressure may not yet have fallen. A rapid pulse, apprehension, or air hunger may be the only indication of impending shock. The physician should be made aware of any fall in systolic blood pressure below 100 mm. Hg or any fall of 20 mm. Hg below the patient's usual blood pressure when this is an unexpected occurrence.

Blood pressure measurement may be difficult or even impossible to obtain or may give falsely low readings. This is particularly true of those patients with peripheral vessel arteriosclerosis compounded by the effects of vasopressor drugs. Intra-arterial blood pressure monitoring is becoming more commonplace because it is more accurate than the usual indirect auscultatory method.

The systolic blood pressure level may be ascertained by palpation, using a sphygmomanometer with the fingertips on the radial pulse. After the cuff has been inflated sufficiently to obliterate the pulse, the column of mercury is reduced sufficiently for blood to begin flowing through the radial artery. The systolic blood pressure is recorded as the point at which the radial artery is palpable. When peripheral arterioles are constricted in shock, diastolic pressure rises initially because blood has to be at an increased pressure to flow through the constricted vessels.

Pulse

Cardiac output is depressed in shock. A compensatory tachycardia occurs in an attempt to raise the output.

Pulse pressure is the difference between the systolic and diastolic blood pressures. In shock, a fall in systolic blood pressure with a rise in diastolic pressure results in a narrowed pulse pressure. The small spurts of blood passing in the artery feel more like a quiver than the thump of a full pulse. It is often described as a "rapid, thready pulse." In the later stages of shock, the pulse is imperceptible.

Respiration

In shock, the tissues are receiving less oxygen. In response, the patient tries to gain more oxygen by breathing faster (tachypnea). Rapid respirations are helpful in moving blood along in the large veins toward the heart. The respirations are shallow and there may be grunting. In earlier stages the patient is hungry for air, but in profound shock the respiratory rate decreases to two or three a minute. To treat hypoxia, humidified oxygen is given.

Temperature

Heat-regulating mechanisms are depressed in shock and heat loss is increased by added diaphoresis. With the possible exception of bacteremic shock, subnormal temperature is characteristic. Since there is a definite temperature range for cellular function and enzyme activity, the patient should be kept comfortably warm through control of environmental temperature and light covers. Direct heat to the skin should not be used since it causes vasodilation, further increasing heat loss and reducing the flow to critical organs. Heat also raises the metabolic rate, which raises the tissue requirement for oxygen.

Restlessness and pain

Restlessness in shock is caused more often by hypoxia than by pain and may be relieved by oxygen administration. Pain can cause or enhance shock and it lessens the patient's adaptive response.

Narcotics cause further respiratory and circulatory depression. Opiates administered subcutaneously or intramuscularly to patients already in shock often are not absorbed effectively from the tissues because of the diminished circulation. If several injections of narcotics are given during shock, a double or triple dose may be absorbed when the patient's circulation improves, causing serious toxic effects. This result can happen with any drug given by an intramuscular or subcutaneous route. When symptoms of shock are present, the nurse should call the physician and in the meantime withhold all previously ordered drugs. Narcotics should be given very judiciously to a postoperative patient whose blood pressure is falling, or to a patient who shows other symptoms that may indicate the approach of shock. The physician may give the drug in such situations intravenously in a diluted bolus dose administered slowly and titrated to the patient's response.

pH and blood gases

The measurement of hydrogen ion concentration (pH), oxygen tension (PaO_2) and carbon dioxide tension ($PaCO_2$) in arterial blood is an effective way to evaluate lung function, lung adequacy, and tissue perfusion.

Arterial blood gas specimens may be drawn from a direct arterial puncture and may be serially or continually monitored with an indwelling arterial catheter. Venous samples are taken through a central venous catheter, not from a peripheral vein.

Central venous pressure

Central venous pressure (CVP) is the pressure of the blood in the right atrium or venae cavae. It serves to distinguish relationships among the hemodynamic variables in shock—the venous return, the quality of the pump, and vascular tone. Thus it is a critical guide in the management of the patient in shock. Normal central venous pressure is 3 to 10 cm. of water.

An isolated CVP reading is of little value unless it is unusually high or low. Central venous pressure is best used by obtaining a baseline value and then taking frequent readings. The response of the patient to drug therapy or to volume expansion or contraction can then be evaluated. To be accurate, the zero level on the manometer must always be at the same height in relation to the patient's right atrium.

Effects on vital organs

Kidney. Vasoconstriction, the body's physiological response to shock, contributes to a marked reduction in renal blood flow. Many physicians believe that the rate of urine formation is the most important indicator of the status of the patient in shock. The patient in shock or impending shock needs an indwelling urethral catheter and hourly measurement of urine output. The physician should be notified of urinary output below 30 ml. per hour so that therapy may be initiated promptly to promote adequate renal perfusion.

With rapid reversal of the shock, urine output usually returns to normal. Continued oliguria indicates renal damage which is thought to be due to a reduced blood flow to the kidney.

Brain. Alteration in cerebral function is often the first sign of impaired oxygen delivery to the tissues. Mild anxiety, increasing restlessness, agitation, or other change in behavior can be clues in advance of the more obvious signs of shock. As the condition deteriorates, the patient becomes listless, stuporous, and finally unconscious.

Heart. Minimal essential myocardial perfusion pressure to maintain coronary artery blood flow is considered to correspond to a systolic pressure of about 80 mm. Hg. Below this the myocardium becomes increasingly hypoxic. The force of myocardial contraction decreases and the potential for dangerous cardiac arrhythmias, including ventricular fibrillation, increases.

Treatment and nursing management implications

The nurse who is alert and has recognized the early warnings can begin to improve the situation while the body's defenses are still in control. If a patient shows early warning signs of shock, the physician should be notified. While waiting for him, the nurse will monitor the vital signs and administer oxygen. An intravenous line should be opened for drug therapy. Obvious causes of shock, such as external hemorrhage, should be controlled. A nurse should remain with the patient to observe and reassure him.

The treatment of shock depends on the clinical assessment of the patient and the complex hemodynamic variables involved. Treatment of hypoxia, pain, and cardiac arrhythmias proceeds concurrently with treatment of the shock state.

Replacement therapy

Hypovolemic shock is best treated with the type of fluid that is being lost. In hemorrhage, this is whole blood; in burn shock, plasma; in extreme vomiting and diarrhea, solutions containing electrolytes. When blood is given, the physician usually orders that the transfusion run rapidly while the blood pressure is low, and that the rate of administration be slowed to the usual 40 drops a minute when the blood pressure rises. At times, in order to keep pace with blood loss, several simultaneous transfusions may be given. Blood may be forced by pressure into a vein to achieve more rapid introduction into the circulation than could be accomplished by free flow of the blood. When whole blood is desired but not available, the intravenous infusion may be started with plasma, concentrated albumin, low molecular weight dextran, or saline, until blood can be obtained.

Infusing measured increments of fluid while observing CVP response serves two purposes:

1. It establishes a true CVP. Initial low or normal levels are meaningless unless the response to an additional fluid load is observed.
2. As a therapeutic measure it serves to increase the effective circulating blood volume and increase cardiac output.

When the CVP is initially elevated or rapidly rises to high levels with volume increments of fluid, intravenous fluids are deferred. Efforts to improve the pumping effectiveness of the heart are then made with drug therapy.

The nurse remains alert for symptoms of overdose of fluids into the vascular system. CVP rise above 15 cm. H_2O indicates the inability of the right heart to accept a further fluid load. If more fluid arrives at the heart than the left side of the heart can hold and move forward, blood accumulates in the lungs. Its rising pressure in the pulmonary vessels squeezes some fluid from the vessels into alveoli. This condition is called pulmonary edema; the fluid collecting in the alveoli can drown the patient. During hypovolemic shock, when an inadequate volume of blood is reaching the heart, the infusion of blood or other replacement therapy is providing the heart with something to pump. As the blood pressure improves, and as the fluid of the infusions, plus the body's own blood supply, reach the heart effectively, an overload may develop. The nurse will notice that the patient feels as if he cannot breathe well, and his respiration will be rapid and may sound moist. Frothy pink sputum may be coughed up. All these signs point to the complication of pulmonary edema, and without immediate help this can be as serious as the shock state. The infusion should be stopped and the physician notified.

Drugs

It is postulated that the effects of the sympathetic nervous system are mediated by receptors located throughout the body called adrenergic receptors. Adrenergic receptors are classified as alpha and beta on the basis of their characteristic responses.

When stimulated, alpha receptors cause constriction of the smooth muscle of blood vessels supplying skeletal muscle, the splanchnic vascular bed, skin and mucosa.

Beta adrenergic stimulation results in excitation of the S-A node resulting in increased heart rate, increased cardiac conduction (positive chronotropic effect), and increased myocardial contractility (positive inotropic effect). The smooth muscles of the arteries, veins, and bronchi are relaxed, resulting in dilation of the bronchi.

Administration of adrenergic drugs such as levarterenol (Levophed) or metaraminol (Aramine) for hypotension will require close observation and constant evaluation of the patient's blood pressure, pulse, and overall response to drug therapy.

Position

Unless the physician specifically orders otherwise, the patient in shock is kept supine with the legs elevated 20 to 30 degrees. A *small* pillow may be placed beneath the head; use of a large pillow will flex the head forward and interfere with breathing.

Patients in shock from conditions resulting in increased intracranial pressure (after brain surgery, for example) are positioned flat in bed, or even in a low sitting position. Patients in cardiogenic shock may benefit from a low Fowler's position. A slight elevation of the head of the bed prevents the abdominal organs from pushing up against the diaphragm and thus decreasing lung expansion.

Activity limitations

The metabolic activity of the patient in shock must be kept to a minimum without introducing further hazards of immobility. Physical and emotional activity increase cellular needs for oxygen and nutrients and increase the formation of metabolites. Positioning, lifting, and turning are done gently by the nurse. The patient must be protected from unnecessary and controllable stimulation. Visitors are limited. Understandably, they are distressed and need to be approached periodically and informed of the patient's condition.

Prognosis and complications

When shock has progressed too far before treatment is started, or when, despite prompt treatment, the patient fails to respond, or when the underlying condition, such as a huge infarction of the myocardium, cannot be effectively treated, death follows.

Fortunately, when shock is treated adequately and promptly, the patient usually recovers. As vital signs return to normal, careful withdrawal of therapeutic measures can be made gradually.

A grave complication is failure of the kidneys to resume work after blood pressure improves. The nurse records both the amount of urine and the time of voiding and should inform the physician if no urine is excreted and blood pressure has been satisfactory for 2 hours, or if less than 30 ml. per hour is being put out.

Other complications that are not always observable may occur until the patient has recovered from shock. Even in uncomplicated recovery the patient requires a period of convalescence to end the effects of the changes the body commanded when it called out its defensive reactions to fight shock.

General pharmacological considerations

- Shock demands intensive treatment. Drugs used in the treatment of shock include:

  Adrenergic drugs having profound vasopressor action, such as epinephrine (Adrenalin), levarterenol (Levophed), metaraminol (Aramine), and phenylephrine (Neo-Synephrine).

  Norepinephrine precursor: dopamine (Intropin).

  Whole blood, blood products (plasma, albumin, etc.) and plasma expanders (e.g., dextran-40).

- Other drugs relevant to the patient's physical problems and possibly the cause, in whole or in part, of shock in an individual patient are often concurrently administered. Drugs in this category might include cardiovascular preparations (digoxin, lidocaine, procainamide), diuretics, and corticosteroids.
- Administration of powerful vasopressors demands constant nursing supervision. The patient's blood pressure must be monitored every 2 to 5 minutes if he is receiving levarterenol (Levophed) and every 3 to 8 minutes for other vasopressors (circumstances may change these intervals). The rate of drug administration by intravenous infusion is adjusted according to the patient's blood pressure. The site of intravenous infusion and surrounding areas are frequently inspected for signs of extravasation.
- If extravasation should occur, the infusion will have to be discontinued, especially if levarterenol (Levophed) is being administered (this drug causes severe tissue necrosis). *Before* the infusion is discontinued, an identical infusion is started in another extremity. Failure to keep the intravenous solution infusing (even though some is extravasating into tissue) may result in circulatory collapse. If the intravenous needle is totally displaced from the vein, the infusion can be discontinued *as* or *before* another is started. In the latter case, speed in restarting the infusion is of the utmost importance.
- The patient in shock is observed for signs of fluid overload. If this should occur while a vasopressor is still required, the drug may be given in more concentrated form; that is, less fluid is utilized as a vehicle for the administration of the drug.

Bibliography

Boyd, J. M. L.: Understanding and treating cardiogenic shock. RN 38:53, April, 1975.

Carey, L. C.: Pathophysiology of shock. AORN J. 18:311, August, 1973.

———: Shock: Differential diagnosis and immediate treatment (pictorial). Hosp. Med. 11:68, May, 1975.

Cosgriff, J. H. and Anderson, D. L.: *The Practice of Emergency Nursing.* Philadelphia, Lippincott, 1975.

Door, K. S.: The intra-aortic balloon pump (pictorial). Am. J. Nurs. 75:52, January, 1975.

Kepner, S.: They wait without. J. Prac. Nurs. 75:30, August, 1975.

Life in the balance (pictorial). Emergency Med. 5:24, October, 1973.

Mitty, W. F. J. et al: Treating shock in the emergency department. RN 36:OR/ED 1, August, 1973.

Moyer, J. H. et al: Vasopressor agents in shock. Am. J. Nurs. 75:620, April, 1975.

Rodman, M. J. and Smith, D. W.: *Clinical Pharmacology in Nursing.* Philadelphia, Lippincott, 1974.

Royce, J. A.: Shock: Emergency nursing implications. Nurs. Clin. North Am. 8:377, September, 1973.

Tharp, G. D.: Shock: The overall mechanism (pictorial). Am. J. Nurs. 74:2208, December, 1974.

Wiley, L. ed.: Staying ahead of shock (pictorial). Part 1. Nurs. '74, 4:18, April, 1974.

CHAPTER 46

Respiratory insufficiency and failure

On completion of this chapter the student will:

- Recognize the seriousness of respiratory insufficiency and the need for immediate medical intervention.
- Define terms used to describe abnormalities in ventilation.
- Discuss the role of various body systems in the maintenance of normal arterial pH.
- Recognize early and late signs of acute respiratory failure.
- Discuss the treatment modalities for patients with respiratory insufficiency and failure.
- Discuss the use of endotracheal intubation and tracheostomy as a means of relieving respiratory insufficiency or failure.
- Discuss the use of respirators and ventilators in respiratory insufficiency and failure.
- Describe the nursing observations and management of the patient on a ventilator or respirator.

The acute disruption of breathing and increasing anxiety go hand in hand. Regardless of the cause, survival is threatened and the human organism reacts swiftly and strongly to respiratory failure with emergency neural adaptive mechanisms. As breathing is facilitated, anxiety is reduced, and as anxiety lessens, breathing improves. The patient with continued respiratory distress has the double task of dealing with the underlying disease process and the anxiety generated by it. The major objectives of nursing management for the patient in respiratory distress are to facilitate ventilation (O_2 intake and CO_2 removal) and to reduce the work of breathing. Competent observation, judgment, technical ministration, and emotional support of the patient are the ingredients of nursing management of the patient in respiratory distress. The nurse's supportive presence is a powerful factor in relieving apprehension.

Because life processes depend on the continuing availability of oxygen to each body cell, all intensive care patients can be considered to be respiratory patients as well. Some will have respiratory disease as their major problem; all require nursing action which prevents respiratory complications. The encouragement of periodic coughing and deep-breathing exercises and correct positioning with a regular routine of turning become part of the care plan for each patient in the intensive care unit.

Lung function

The main function of the respiratory system is to exchange oxygen and carbon dioxide between ambient (atmospheric) air and the blood. Usually it has sufficient reserves to maintain normal partial pressures or tension of these gases in the blood during times of stress. If, however, there is too much interference with the following aspects of lung function, respiratory insufficiency develops.

- *Ventilation* is the movement of air in and out of the lungs in volumes sufficient to maintain normal *arterial* oxygen and carbon dioxide tensions.
- *Perfusion* of the lungs is the filling of the pulmonary capillaries with venous blood returning from the systemic circulation via the right ventricle.
- *Diffusion* is the process by which oxygen and carbon dioxide are exchanged across the alveolar-capillary membrane.
- *Distribution* is the delivery of ambient (atmospheric) air to the separate gas exchange units in the lung.

Results of lung dysfunction

Abnormalities in ventilation, perfusion, diffusion, or distribution lead to the following conditions:

- *Hypoxia,* or the diminished availability of oxygen to the cells of the body.
- *Hypoxemia,* or reduced oxygen in the body fluids (refers particularly to oxygen in arterial blood).
- *Hypercapnia,* or excess carbon dioxide in the body fluids.
- *Hypocapnia,* or lessened carbon dioxide in body fluids.

The patient who is hypoxemic but normocapnic (without hypocapnia) has a low arterial oxygen tension. He is not receiving sufficient oxygen into the pulmonary capillaries. A frequent cause of this is atelectasis and veno-arterial shunting. This patient is restless, anxious, and has tachypnea (rapid respirations) and tachycardia. As the condition progresses, the patient shows other signs, such as duskiness, cyanosis, sweating, cardiac arrhythmias, and he might be restless and confused. The physician directs therapy toward improving oxygenation by such means as vigorous suctioning, supplemental oxygen, humidification, or bronchoscopy to remove mucus plugs.

The patient who is hypoxemic and hypercapnic has a low arterial oxygen tension and elevated carbon dioxide tension. This is a result of alveolar hypoventilation. As carbon dioxide accumulates in the blood, the patient develops headache and becomes successively drowsy and then comatose. The hypoxia is the last remaining stimulus to respiration since the respiratory center becomes narcotized or "anesthetized" from excessive carbon dioxide. The patient is in a state of respiratory acidosis. To give the patient oxygen only, despite his bluish appearance, would take away his last stimulus to respiration and, though his color might improve temporarily, he could die from respiratory arrest. The physician would order assisted or controlled ventilation with intubation and a mechanical respirator. Evacuating carbon dioxide allows adequate oxygenation to take place. Because mechanical ventilators are very powerful, the physician will want the reduction of carbon dioxide to take place slowly over several hours rather than several minutes. If there is a precipitous rise in pH by ventilatory removal of carbon dioxide, there can be dangerous fluctuations in myocardial potassium with serious cardiac arrhythmias. What had been the state of respiratory acidosis could swiftly become metabolic alkalosis.

The patient who is both hypoxemic and hypocapnic would be one, for example, in serious shock where all body processes are depressed. The physician would attempt to control the patient's respiration and maintain alveolar ventilation with a volume-limited respirator.

Acidosis and alkalosis

The kidneys and the lung, together with the body fluids and electrolytes and several buffer systems, act and react to keep the arterial pH (hydrogen ion concentration) within the normal limits of 7.35 to 7.45. Since normal pH is essential for correct enzyme action and cellular metabolism, the body's ability to make adjustments is of critical importance.

Alveolar ventilation determines the amount of carbon dioxide in the body. An increase in carbon dioxide, present in body fluids primarily as carbonic acid, decreases the pH below the normal of 7.4; a decrease in carbon dioxide increases the pH above 7.4. The hydrogen ion concentration, or pH, affects the rate of alveolar ventilation by a direct action of hydrogen ions on the respiratory center in the medulla oblongata. The kidneys contribute to the normal pH by maintaining serum bicarbonate between 21 to 30 mEq. per liter and excreting excess hydrogen ions.

The lung and kidneys combine to maintain the carbonic acid to bicarbonate ratio at 1:20, fixing the pH at about 7.4.

In the critically ill patient, various homeostatic mechanisms operate to compensate for altered physiology. Buffer ratios shift, the lung can "blow off" carbonic acid as carbon dioxide, or the kidneys can excrete more bicarbonate in an attempt to maintain normal pH. Compensatory mechanisms, however, can become overstressed and fail, and dangerous clinical conditions develop, which, in the intensive care patient, are generally superimposed on an already serious underlying condition. The patient's condition is said to be compensated as long as the ratio of carbonic acid to bicarbonate remains 1:20.

By convention, disturbances in pH which involve the lung and carbonic acid levels which result from dissolved carbon dioxide are termed respiratory; the other disturbances are termed metabolic. At times, metabolic and respiratory derangements coexist. Blood gas studies done on a sample of arterial blood enable the physician to assess the acid-base balance dependably and rapidly. The blood may be withdrawn by single arterial puncture or repeated samples may be drawn from an indwelling arterial catheter. A heparinized syringe is used and is carefully filled to avoid bubbles. If delay in analysis is anticipated, the syringe is immediately immersed in ice. This decreases the metabolic activity of the blood cells and prevents oxygen consumption in the syringe.

Some laboratory values of importance in the care of the respiratory patient or other patients requiring assessment of acid-base balance are:

Arterial Blood

pH	7.35–7.45
PaO_2	80–100 mm. Hg
$PaCO_2$	38–42 mm. Hg
SaO_2 saturation	95%
Bicarbonate ion concentration	22–26 mEq./L.

Because of the numerous ways in which individuals can vary in their response to illness, laboratory tests serve as guides, but are not black and white indicators of the overall clinical condition of the patient. It must be remembered that laboratory values may vary from hospital to hospital as well as in various references that may be consulted.

Laboratory reports of blood gases require prompt decision making; they cannot be relegated to a spindle for the physician to look at the following morning. In many hospitals an intern or resident maintains a close check on the patient's condition. In some hospitals, specially prepared nurses review the laboratory and clinical data and make adjustments in therapy according to previously written physician's orders or following telephone communication with him. Close observation of the patient, including his general behavior, state of consciousness, skin turgor, urinary output, rate and depth of respiration, muscle function, intestinal function, and abdominal distention, is an essential nursing activity.

Acute respiratory failure

Acute respiratory failure, or acute ventilatory failure, is a life-threatening complication in which alveolar ventilation becomes inadequate to maintain the body's vital need for oxygen supply and carbon dioxide removal. Though the signs are not specific, the patient initially may be restless, agitated, confused, and diaphoretic.

The most frequent circumstance of acute respiratory failure is that in which a patient with moderate to severe chronic obstructive lung disease develops an acute bronchopulmonary infection, is oversedated, undergoes general anesthesia, has chest trauma, or incurs some other type of insult to his already embarrassed pulmonary reserve. Other patients with neurological disorders, acute poisoning, or surgical intervention (especially abdominal operations) are susceptible to respiratory failure.

At first the patient may be alert, but he is apprehensive, dyspneic, wheezing, and perhaps cyanotic. There is marked use of the accessory muscles of respiration. Though the patient often looks as if he would benefit from sedation, because of his apprehension, the physician prescribes therapy aimed at relieving the patient's symptoms by improving ventilation. Sedation, alone, can further depress respiratory effort. In the presence of continued hypoventilation, cardiac arrhythmias, hypotension, and congestive heart failure can develop.

If carbon dioxide retention develops slowly, there is time for the kidneys to excrete chlorides and reabsorb bicarbonate and sodium ions, thus maintaining the pH within normal limits. If the renal mechanisms fail to compensate for rapidly accumulating carbon dioxide, the pH falls below the normal 7.35 and respiratory acidosis develops.

Treatment modalities

The physician plans a program of care for the patient which encompasses the following aspects of management:

- Clearing the airways.
- Combating bronchospasm.
- Giving oxygen for hypoxemia while assisting or controlling ventilation.
- Humidification.
- Combating infection.
- Monitoring clinical and laboratory values.
- Treating cardiac and circulatory status.
- Maintaining fluid and electrolyte balance.

Essential to nursing management of the patient is an understanding of the aims of therapy, an explanation of these to the patient as they are about to involve him, skilled observation and judgment, technical expertise with various forms of equipment utilized by the respiratory care team, and effective communication with the patient so that he knows what is expected of him and knows what he can expect of others. The patient's fear is lessened when he is assisted to remain in control of his situation for as long as possible. When he can no longer do so, he must have the confidence that he can temporarily relinquish the control to others who are concerned and competent to do the job for him.

Airway maintenance

Cough is the major mechanism for clearing the tracheobronchial tree of abundant, tenacious mucus. Effective coughing requires that the patient be assisted to a sitting position, that he take a deep breath prior to coughing, and that he use his abdominal and accessory respiratory muscles to forcefully exhale and cough. In the event that the patient's cough is ineffective but he is conscious and cooperative, the physician may wish to stimulate coughing by tracheal irritation with a catheter. The use of the intermittent positive pressure respirator serves to inflate the lungs and enhance the ejecting mechanism of the cough by driving air past mucus secretions.

Simply giving the patient an intermittent positive pressure breathing (IPPB) treatment is not enough. After the treatment, the patient must be assisted to cough or the treatment will be ineffective. Thus, he requires nursing attention even if another member of the respiratory care team, such as the inhalation therapist, actually turns on his machine.

Encouraging fluid intake within the maximum limits of the patient's treatment regimen aids in preventing the drying of secretions. Turning and positioning the patient every hour aids in directing mucus to the main airway whence it can be expelled. Humidification of the surrounding air also helps liquefy secretions.

Secretions often must be thinned to be expectorated. To be most effective, sterile solutions or medications must be delivered to the mucus-covered surface. Nebulization therapy is the least traumatic and most effective method of accomplishing this.

When the patient cannot cough effectively despite therapy, the physician may utilize nasal-tracheal suction. Passage of the suction catheter is facilitated if the patient is sitting upright and leaning slightly forward with his jaw extended. An assistant can grasp the patient's tongue. A 16-inch, 18-24 F. catheter, lubricated with a water-soluble substance, is inserted gently, without suction, into the nostril. As the patient coughs or pants repeatedly, the glottis opens and permits the catheter to be passed between the vocal cords and into the trachea. The catheter is attached to a suction apparatus with a "Y" connection. As the opening of the "Y" is occluded, gentle suction (40 ml. of water) is applied. The catheter is rotated between the left thumb and forefinger to sweep the walls. Suction is applied for no longer than 15 seconds at a time. The catheter can be guided into either main bronchus by turning the patient's head to the side opposite that to be catheterized. Sterile normal saline, 5 to 10 ml., can be inserted into the trachea through the catheter once it is in place. The catheter can be left in place between periods of suctioning, but oxygen is given during these intervals. As the catheter is withdrawn, suction is applied to clear the oropharynx of secretions.

ENDOTRACHEAL INTUBATION. Suctioning can also be accomplished through an endotracheal tube which the physician inserts through the patient's nose or mouth. It can remain in place for several days, and, when its cuff is inflated to provide a tight connection, it can be attached to a respirator for controlled ventilation. The patient, however, cannot speak. Suctioning is not as effective as a tracheostomy, but the time delay, surgical trauma, and complications of tracheostomy are avoided. Once the patient is intubated with an endotracheal tube, the following points are important considerations:

Placement of the Tube. If the tube is not anchored securely to the exterior, it can slip into the right main stem bronchus. As a result, the left lung would not be ventilated and is actually completely obstructed from the flow of air. When the patient is intubated, both sides of the thorax should rise evenly during inspiration. Because this is not always a reliable sign, both sides of the lung should be auscultated with a stethoscope to hear the flow of air. The physician or nurse can do this.

The tube can also be misplaced and pass into the esophagus. If the patient is still breathing spontaneously, breath sounds will still be heard in both lung fields. The physician can check correct placement of the tube by attaching it to an Ambu bag or other type of anesthesia bag, and, while squeezing the bag, simultaneously auscultate the thorax.

Because of dangers of tube displacement, it is not generally considered advisable to turn this patient from side to side. Suctioning is used to prevent airway obstruction.

Obstruction of the Tube. Absence of breath sounds in either lung can indicate obstruction of the tube. The tube can become obstructed by: (1) secretions; suctioning and liquefying secretions are required; (2) kinking of the tube; (3) biting down on the tube by the patient; this can be prevented by the use of a bite block or an oropharyngeal airway; (4) the cuff, which, when inflated, provides a tight seal between the tube and the trachea, can slip down and occlude the orifice; and (5) the distal end of the tube, which may press on the wall of the trachea. All of the above situations demand emergency action because of the immediate danger of asphyxiation.

Removal of the Tube.

- Accidental removal by the patient must be guarded against as this can result in laryngeal edema or spasm and predispose to respiratory arrest.
- The physician makes the decision to remove the tube when the patient's vital capacity, measured with a ventilometer, is adequate. Blood gas values are also used as a guideline for tube removal.
- The endotracheal tube should be removed only by a person who can replace it if necessary. The necessary emergency equipment should remain at the bedside.
- Before the cuff is deflated, the pharynx is aspirated so that secretions do not gravitate downward. The tube is usually removed with the patient in semi-Fowler's position. Laryngospasm can occur. If so, the physician gives air by positive pressure, or he may re-intubate the patient.

Postextubation Care.

- High or semi-Fowler's position promotes chest expansion and optimal alveolar ventilation.
- The patient's posterior pharynx may be dry and he may be hoarse. Humidification aids in preventing further complications. Hard candy may be comforting.
- The patient should be observed carefully for signs of laryngeal edema or increased respiratory distress.

TRACHEOSTOMY

An opening into the trachea with insertion of a cuffed tracheostomy tube provides a portal for suctioning and the tube can serve as a connection for a respirator (Figs. 46-1 and 46-2). Complications of tracheostomy include infection, bleeding, tracheal trauma, and pneumothorax. Humidification is necessary to prevent drying and incrustation of the mucous membrane in the trachea and the main stem bronchus.

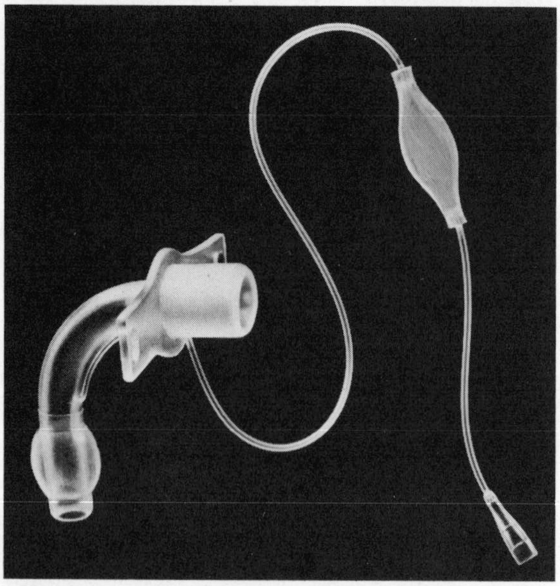

figure 46-1. Bassett cuffed tracheostomy tube. (Portex, Ltd., Hythe, Kent, England)

Crusts can break off, obstruct the lower airway, and cause asphyxiation.

Ideally, a new disposable suction catheter and disposable sterile glove should be used each time the patient is suctioned, and then discarded. The frequency of suctioning depends on the amount of secretions present.

Because of the danger of necrosis of the tracheal wall, the cuff of the tracheostomy tube should be deflated on a regular basis. Physicians have their own preferences regarding deflation routine. These vary, for example, from 15 minutes of deflation every two hours to five minutes of deflation every hour. The amount of air injected into the cuff should be just enough to prevent an air leak around the tube or through the mouth. For the average patient, 5 to 7 ml. of air is sufficient.

Oxygen

Compensatory responses to hypoxia, such as increased cardiac output with hypertension and tachycardia, peripheral sympathetic overactivity, tachypnea (rapid breathing), and hyperventilation can reach a maximum of usefulness after which the patient's condition deteriorates.

The exact oxygen tension (or partial pressure of oxygen in the arterial blood) at which observable signs of lack of oxygen develop varies among patients. When the partial pressure of oxygen (PaO_2) decreases below the normal, the patient may become tachypneic with a rate of about 25, breathe with his mouth open, and be short of breath on walking. With further decrease, the patient breathes faster, speaks in short, broken sentences, uses his facial muscles with expiration, and may appear dusky. As oxygen tension decreases to dangerous levels, cyanosis, restlessness, hypotension, diaphoresis, and combativeness are likely to be present. Serious cardiac arrhythmias and cardiac arrest can develop quickly.

There is medical controversy regarding optimum and safe levels of oxygen tension. Generally, optimum arterial oxygen tension is maintained between 80 and 120 mm. Hg. An oxygen tension of 70 is of concern and an oxygen level below 60 is dangerous. Recently it has been noted that oxygen toxicity can be as great a problem as hypoxia. Levels of oxygen tension over 120 mm. Hg are unnecessary and may lead

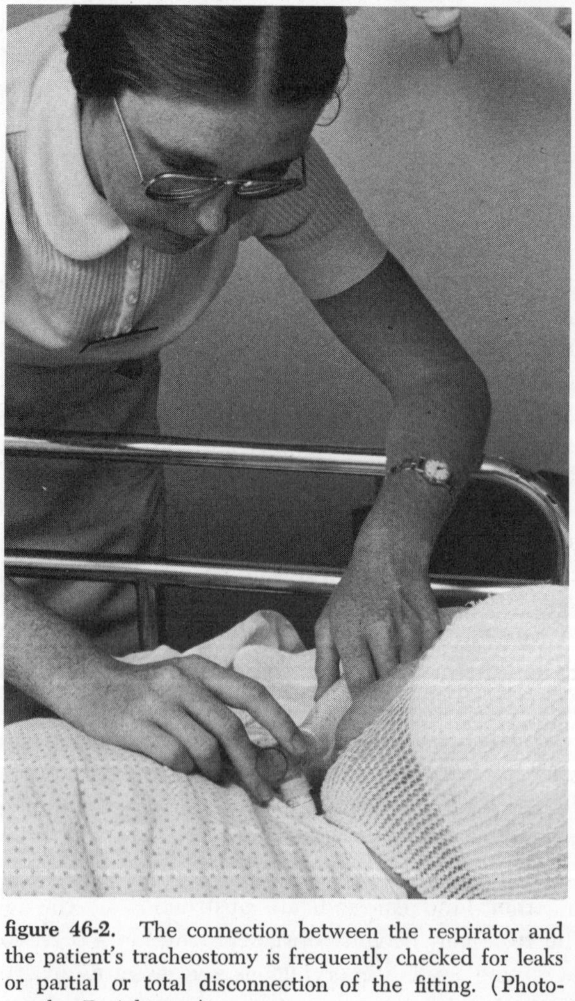

figure 46-2. The connection between the respirator and the patient's tracheostomy is frequently checked for leaks or partial or total disconnection of the fitting. (Photograph—D. Atkinson)

to oxygen toxicity. High levels of oxygen depress respiration and also damage the surface membrane of the lung and lead to progressive atelectasis.

If airway clearance and conventional oxygen therapy are not sufficient to maintain adequate oxygenation above 60 mm. Hg and removal of carbon dioxide, a respirator (ventilator) attached to a cuffed endotracheal or tracheostomy tube may be ordered.

THE PATIENT ON A RESPIRATOR (VENTILATOR). Ventilators are used to do the work of breathing. Air is forced into the lung to give the patient adequate tidal volume (adequate-sized breaths). Small bedside units have replaced the body or tank type respirator, the so-called iron lung, which was widely used for the respiratory failure of acute poliomyelitis. The patient's respiration can be either assisted (patient-cycled) or controlled (machine-cycled).

Ventilators are either pressure-cycled (pressure-limited) or volume-cycled (volume-limited). Pressure-cycled ventilators can be used intermittently for deep breathing exercises or for the delivery of aerosols; they also can be used for continuous cycling of the patient's respirations. For respiratory assist, a valve near the patient connection opens in response to the patient's spontaneous effort. His respiration is then boosted by the machine until a preset inspiratory pressure is exceeded. The inflow valve closes and expiration is into the atmosphere. In many types of machines, after a set period of delay, the machine will trigger a breath if the patient's own effort fails to trigger the machine. For respiratory control, inspiratory flow can be automatically triggered and the machine is used in conjunction with the cuffed tracheostomy or endotracheal tube. Pressure-limited ventilators are small, are driven by compressed air or air-oxygen mixtures rather than electric power, are reasonable in price, but require frequent maintenance. The physician determines inspiratory flow, sensitivity, rate, and expiratory pressure.

In the volume-cycled respirator, a motor-driven piston pumps air or air-oxygen mixture. The rate of respiration and the volume of air per respiration or stroke (tidal volume) can be varied and are determined by the physician according to the patient's blood gases and predicted tidal volume needs. Volume-cycled machines are always used with a cuffed endotracheal tube for short-term treatment, or with the tracheostomy tube, for longer periods of treatment. They deliver the predetermined volume regardless of resistance of the lungs. They are more reliable and more expensive than pressure-cycled units.

In controlled ventilation, the inspiration is initiated by the machine at a preset rate. The patient's spontaneous respiratory effort, if any, must be synchronized with the machine. Fighting the respirator, or the patient becoming asynchronous with the respirator, is usually caused by inadequate alveolar ventilation, by hypoxemia, or by low-cardiac output. The patient who is struggling to breathe on his own has to be convinced that the respiratory care team is concerned and competent to take over, temporarily, the work of breathing for him.

Airway pressure depends on the amount of air delivered and the resistance of the lung to inflation. A safety or "pop-off" valve prevents excessive pressure. Increases or decreases in pressure can be signaled by an alarm built into or attached to the system. An elevation of pressure is an indication of obstruction usually due to retained secretions. A decrease in pressure usually indicates lack of a closed, or airtight, system. The inflation of the cuff of the endotracheal or tracheostomy tube should be checked. Fall in pressure can also indicate a decrease in bronchoconstriction and mean progress for the patient. Supplemental oxygen and humidification can be provided with volume-cycled respirators. As with all types of mechanical equipment, precise knowledge of the principles of the instrument and the manufacturer's instructions are essential for all members of the team who will be involved in its use.

NURSING MANAGEMENT. Some important nursing considerations for management of the patient on a respirator are:

- One of the major problems leading to intubation and intensive respiratory care is retained secretions. Positive pressure breathing does not adequately ventilate the entire lung parenchyma unless secretions are moved from the distal air passages to the main stem bronchi and carina, where they can be cleared by suctioning or coughing. This is a nursing responsibility and is accomplished by frequent position changes and deep-breathing and coughing exercises. In cases of excessive respiratory secretions, pulmonary physical therapy techniques, such as gentle vibration and percussion over the lung fields, may be employed. This latter maneuver may be performed by the nurse trained in this technique or by the physical therapist.
- The patient must be in synchrony with the ventilator or else he is not getting the proper rate or volume. The physician or therapist is notified if the patient is out of phase.

■ Gastric dilatation and paralytic ileus are not uncommon problems of patients on respirator therapy. Gastrointestinal bleeding from a stress ulcer can also occur. Abdominal distention is reported promptly to the physician, who can initiate early use of gastric decompression. Vomiting with aspiration spells disaster for these patients. The patient's stools and gastric secretions should be checked for blood, and a fall in the hematocrit should be promptly reported.

■ It is convenient to suction the patient at the fixed intervals when the cuff is routinely deflated to avoid necrosis of the tracheal mucosa. Before the cuff is deflated, the upper airway is suctioned so that secretions do not gravitate downward. Suction is done more frequently if necessary. The color, consistency, and odor of secretions are noted. The cuff inflation *should not exceed* the quantity of air which is just sufficient to prevent the patient from talking or to prevent air escaping from the patient's mouth.

■ Respiratory alkalosis from hyperventilation can occur in patients on respirators. The patient might complain of chest pain, numbness or tingling of the extremities, vertigo, or lightheadedness, muscle spasm, and may even develop tetany. This can sometimes be avoided in the susceptible patient if the respiratory rate is periodically decreased.

■ To keep average intrathoracic pressure close to atmospheric pressure and to avoid fall in cardiac output for the patient on controlled ventilation, the physician may order that inspiration comprise one third of each respiration and expiration be twice as long as inspiration, or some other proportion in which the duration of expiration exceeds that of inspiration. Settings on the machines are used to make this kind of adjustment.

■ Patients with tracheostomies may be on oral feedings, but patients with endotracheal tubes receive nothing by mouth.

■ Vital signs including blood pressure, pulse, and respiratory rate should be checked hourly or at more frequent intervals if the patient's condition warrants it.

■ Temperature is recorded every four hours.

■ The patient on a ventilator *should not be left alone*.

■ The patient's level of consciousness, color of lips and nailbeds, pupils, and muscle strength are checked every hour.

■ It should be remembered that the patient cannot talk, but can hear, and can usually write. A bell should be left with him at all times and a Magic Slate or pad and pencil should be left at the bedside within easy reach. The patient's dominant hand is left free of intravenous needles, if possible, so that he can write more easily. Frightening aspects of the patient's condition should not be discussed where he may overhear the conversation and become more alarmed.

■ Many respirator patients are conscious and alert during the major part of their illness. All are apprehensive; many are depressed, especially if they are victims of recurrent episodes of respiratory failure and between hospitalizations constantly have to fight the battle of breathlessness. Some patients may be bitter, having become acutely ill despite adhering closely to the home regimen prescribed for them. The patient becomes easily frustrated because of his inability to communicate verbally with physicians, nurses, inhalation therapists, and family. Explanations to the patient must continue, however.

The patient knows that his life is dependent on the competence of people and the mechanics of machines. Accidental disconnection from the respirator, kinking of the tubes, or occlusion of them with a mucus plug can mean rapid asphyxiation. Once an accident occurs, fear of its recurrence can plague a patient and he will expend tremendous energy trying to guard his own life. A manual device, such as an Ambu bag, must be at the bedside of each patient in the event of mechanical breakdown of the ventilator or asynchrony creating an emergency. The patient must have the reassurance that he is under constant, competent supervision.

Weaning the Patient. Considerations employed by the physician to determine that the patient can be gradually removed from respirator support are his vital capacity and blood gas values. Weaning is initiated as soon as possible so that the patient's respiratory muscles can be restored to normal tone more quickly and also because the patient psychologically benefits from control of his own life processes and signs of improvement. Generally, the longer the patient has received artificial ventilation, the slower will be the weaning process. Also, how successfully the patient is weaned from the respirator depends to a large extent on the quality of nursing management he received during the intensive treatment process. Weaning is best initiated early in the morning, the patient's responses should be closely watched, and the time intervals increased during the day. Patients who were receiving volume-controlled assistance may be switched to a pressure-cycled respirator before weaning is attempted. The sensitivity can be gradually decreased on the pressure-cycled respirator so that more burden is put on the patient to initiate respiration himself.

While off the ventilator, the patient receives humidified oxygen. Some patients may require mild sedation to allay their anxiety. Team efforts are directed toward early mobilization of the patient by having him sit in a chair as soon as possible. All patients require the constant presence of the nurse who observes their tolerance, gives constant support to their efforts, and is prepared to assist them back to respirator support if they are not able to breathe on their own.

Even when weaning appears complete, the patient should be observed for several days by the specially prepared respiratory staff. This is especially true for the older, debilitated patient.

General pharmacological considerations

■ Patients with respiratory insufficiency and failure are not given narcotics, barbiturates, and tranquilizers unless absolutely necessary because of the potential of these drugs to depress respiratory rate and depth. If a narcotic analgesic or sedative is necessary, the drug is given in a lower than normal dose and the respiratory *rate* and *depth* checked frequently for 2 to 4 hours after the drug is given. Various drugs may be used in patients with respiratory insufficiency and failure: bronchodilators such as aminophylline and isoproterenol, cardiovascular drugs to treat an accompanying cardiac problem (when present), drugs to liquefy thickened secretions (mucolytics) such as Alevaire or potassium iodide.

Bibliography

ALEXANDER, M. M. et al: Physical examination. Chest and lungs (pictorial), Part 12. Nurs. '75, 5:44, January, 1975.

BATES, B.: *A Guide to Physical Examination.* Philadelphia, Lippincott, 1974.

BURRELL, L. O. and BURRELL, Z. L.: *Intensive Nursing Care,* ed. 2. St. Louis, Mosby, 1973.

CODD, J. et al: Postoperative pulmonary complications. Nurs. Clin. North Am. 10:5, March, 1975.

EGAN, D. F.: *Fundamentals of Respiratory Therapy.* St. Louis, Mosby, 1973.

GREISHEIMER, E. M. and WEIDEMAN, M. P.: *Physiology and Anatomy,* ed. 9. Philadelphia, Lippincott, 1970.

HUDSON, L. D.: The acute management of the chronic airway obstruction patient. Heart Lung 3:93, January/February, 1974.

METHENY, N. M. and SNIVELY, W. D.: *Nurses' Handbook of Fluid Balance,* ed. 2. Philadelphia, Lippincott, 1974.

NETT, L.: The use of mechanical ventilators (pictorial). Nurs. Clin. North Am. 9:123, March, 1974.

SECOR, J.: *Patient Care in Respiratory Problems.* Saunders Monographs in Clinical Nursing, No. 1. Philadelphia, Saunders, 1969.

WALLACH, J.: *Interpretation of Diagnostic Tests,* ed. 2. Boston, Little, Brown, 1974.

CHAPTER 47

The patient with heart disease: cardiac arrhythmias

On completion of this chapter the student will:

- **Understand basic cardiac rhythmicity and its regulation.**
- **Name and describe the major cardiac arrhythmias.**
- **Identify the basic parts of a normal electrocardiographic tracing.**
- **Describe the three methods of treatment of cardiac arrhythmias: mechanical, chemical, and electrical modalities.**
- **Discuss the types and uses of cardiac pacemakers (pulse generators).**
- **Describe the nursing management of the patient with bradycardia who requires a pacemaker.**
- **Define cardiac arrest and describe the steps taken when it occurs.**

Cardiac rhythmicity and its regulation

In order to pump blood, the heart must alternately relax and contract, allowing blood to enter its chambers during the relaxation phase and forcing it out during the contraction phase.

The alternate contraction and relaxation is provided by an inherent rhythmicity of cardiac muscle.

In the posterior wall of the right atrium, there is a small area known as the sino-atrial (S-A) node. This node has a rhythmic rate of contraction of muscle fibers at about 72 beats per minute. As one considers the muscle mass of the heart from atria to venticles, one finds that the tissue retains its capacity to contract rhythmically, but the lower down the pacemaker site, the slower the inherent rate of the pacemaking tissue. An A-V node pacemaker functions at a rate of 40 to 60 times per minute, while a ventricular pacemaker functions around 20 to 40 times per minute. Because the sinus node has a faster inherent rate than the other portions of the heart, impulses originating in the S-A node spread into the atria and ventricles, stimulating these areas so rapidly that they cannot slow down to their natural rates of rhythm. As a result, in health the rhythm of the S-A node is called the pacemaker of the heart.

Cardiac muscle fibers are joined together in a kind of lattice-work formation. An electrical impulse arising in any single fiber eventually spreads over the membranes of all of the fibers. The normal muscle cell has more negative than positive ions inside the cell membrane, and the electrical cardiac impulse is caused by sudden transfer of some of these ions through the membrane so that more positive than negative ions then appear on the inside. This process is called *depolarization*. Once depolarization has occurred, another normal cardiac impulse cannot be carried until the ions realign themselves to their original condition. This is called *repolarization*. During this period the cell is said to be *refractory*.

Depolarization and repolarization produce an electrical field. Because of the ease with which body tissues conduct current, this electrical potential can be detected by electrodes placed on the external surface of the body and recorded by a machine known as the electrocardiograph.

A special conduction route known as the *Purkinje* system exists in the ventricles to transmit the cardiac impulses throughout the ventricles as rapidly as possible causing all portions to contract simultaneously and exert a coordinated pumping effort.

Sequentially, the cardiac impulse originates in the S-A node and travels through the atria causing them to contract. A few hundredths of a second after leaving the S-A node the impulse reaches the A-V node where it is delayed a few hundredths of a second while the ventricles fill with blood. The Purkinje system fibers begin in the A-V node, extend through the bundle of His into the ventricular septum, where they divide into major branches: a right bundle branch and anterior and posterior divisions of a left bundle branch. After the delay at the A-V node, the cardiac impulse spreads rapidly through the Purkinje system, thence to the ventricular musculature, causing both ventricles to contract in full force within the next few hundredths of a second.

Normal heart rhythm can be disturbed in a variety of ways. Some of these are the result of disease. Others are harmless adaptations in normal function. When arrhythmias occur in the absence of heart disease and are noted by the physician in the course of his examination, he usually does not mention them to the patient.

Each of us has had the sensation of a pounding heart, perhaps in a moment of fright when we are dodging an oncoming car. Most of the time we are not aware that our hearts are beating. Without our conscious awareness, the heart adjusts its work to the changing needs of the body. It can increase the amount of blood that it pumps in two ways: by beating more rapidly and by increasing the volume of blood pumped with each beat. Sudden fright often causes the heart to beat faster and more forcefully, and we become aware of our heartbeat.

These adjustments in heart action are beyond conscious control. The stimulation of the sympathetic nervous system quickens the heart; the stimulation of the parasympathetic nervous system slows it. Both systems constantly affect the heart. In fright the stimulation of the sympathetic nervous system causes a temporarily greater effect and, consequently, a faster and a fuller heartbeat.

In some very frightened or shocked people, however, vagal reflexes predominate and heart rate slows, cardiac output falls, and the person becomes weak or faint (vasovagal syncope). Such patients should be assisted to a supine position to encourage cerebral blood flow until equilibrium is restored.

Cardiac arrhythmias

In disease, the pacemaker of the heart can be too fast or too slow. The myocardial cells can become overly excitable or develop a shortened refractory period; the Purkinje system can be damaged, or blocks can develop in the conduction system. The cardiac arrhythmias that result can be major, that is, imminently life threatening, or relatively minor. Because of their irregularity, all cardiac arrthymias affect the rhythmic pumping action of the heart to some degree.

Many ambulatory patients receive treatment for cardiac arrhythmias and are able to live essentially normal lives. When their cardiac reserve, however, becomes overtaxed by coexisting illness, they become subject to more dangerous arrhythmias or more serious consequences of their underlying hemodynamic disturbance.

In recent years it has become evident that "sudden" cardiac arrest is really not so sudden, but is very often heralded by less dangerous warning arrhythmias. In the critically ill patient or the patient with heart disease, even "minor" arrhythmic changes can compromise cardiac function by causing a fall in cardiac output, thereby reducing coronary artery blood flow. Arrhythmias also increase myocardial oxygen need, lead to more dangerous arrhythmic complications, and make treatment of the patient's underlying disease more difficult and complex.

Many clinical states predispose to cardiac arrhythmias. Myocardial ischemia following infarction, disturbances in pH, inadequate ventilation, electrolyte imbalance, anxiety, and pain can disturb heart rate, rhythm, and conduction.

Though an arrhythmia can be diagnosed from an electrocardiogram rhythm strip, the effect of the arrhythmia on cardiac output is the crucial factor. A person with a normal heart who develops a sinus tachycardia (rate over 100) after running up a flight of stairs is showing a normal physiological response. The patient with an acute myocardial infarction, however, who has a continued sinus tachycardia on bed rest, can add an intolerable work load to his already damaged heart.

A cardiac monitor attached to a patient is useless unless accurate observations are made, interpreted correctly, and acted on appropriately. For example, the nurse may administer a p.r.n. medication, notify the physician, or institute emergency measures required in the interim until the physician arrives.

The development of nursing skill in arrhythmia detection takes considerable study, supervised practice, and time. Only one lead of the ECG is generally necessary to accomplish nursing goals in arrhythmia analysis. The cardiologist reviews the entire 12-lead ECG and in addition to arrhythmia interpretation makes other cardiac diagnoses such as heart enlargement, electrolyte disturbance, ischemic tissue damage, necrosis, and intraventicular conduction delay.

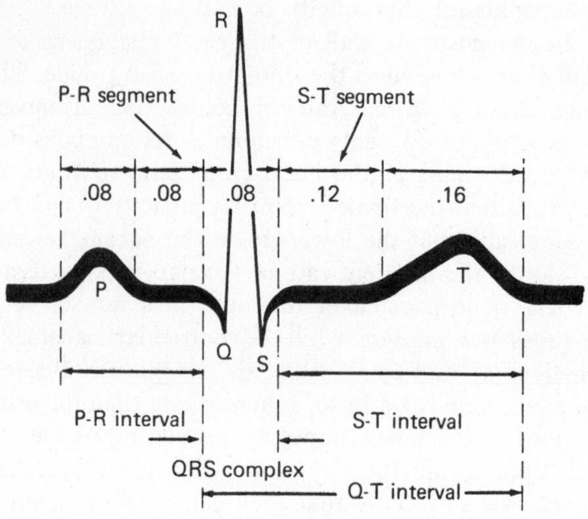

figure 47-1. Basic electrocardiographic trace. (Hewlett-Packard Co., Medical Electronic Division, Palo Alto, Calif.)

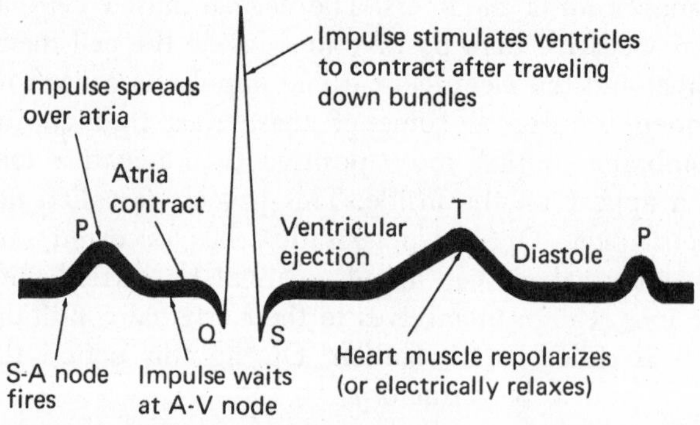

figure 47-2. Electrical and mechanical events of basic ECG tracing. (Hewlett-Packard Co., Medical Electronic Division, Palo Alto, Calif.)

ARRHYTHMIA ELECTROCARDIOGRAPHY*

The electrocardiographic display of the heart's electrical events (Lead II) is shown in Figures 47-1 and 47-2.

A systematic approach to arrhythmia detection includes knowing certain norms, gathering data, comparing this data with a set of facts characteristic of

* The arrhythmia ECG tracings which follow are from the Magnetic Tape Recording Library of Physiological Training Company, San Marino, Calif., reproduced on the Brush Instruments Recorder.

certain arrhythmias, and then gathering data regarding the clinical state of the patient. For example, change in cardiac output can be reflected in blood pressure, pulse volume, skin color and degree of moisture, appearance and orientation, urinary output, chest pain, and dyspnea.

The following are illustrations of the normal heart rhythm and some arrhythmias with possible hemodynamic consequences:

NORMAL SINUS RHYTHM (NSR) or regular sinus rhythm (RSR). The S-A node is the pacemaker and impulses are conducted normally through the conduction system (Fig. 47-3).

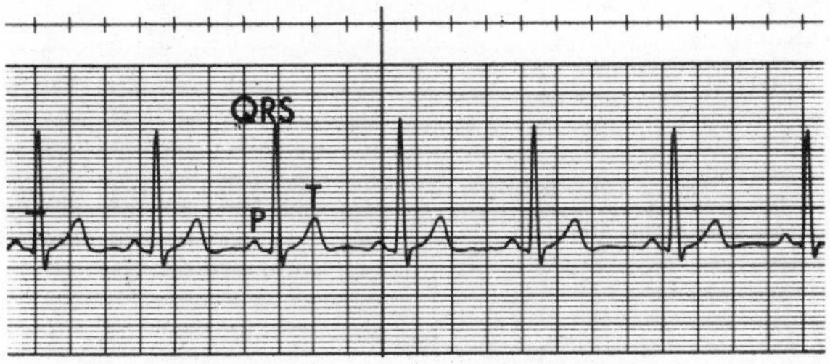

figure 47-3. Normal sinus rhythm.

RATE: 60 to 100
P WAVES: Each has the same configuration and precedes the QRS.
P-R INTERVAL: 0.12 to 0.20 second
QRS: 0.07 to 0.10 second
SIGNIFICANCE: Normal
TREATMENT: None

SINUS BRADYCARDIA. The pacemaker site is the S-A node but the rate is below 60 (Fig. 47-4). The rhythm is regular. The heart can be slow normally in athletes and laborers who have normally enlarged hearts from regular strenuous exercise and greater than normal stroke volume. Emotional states, such as fear or shock, can result in increased vagal tone and slowing of the heart which can result in syncope. Bradycardia is sometimes seen in patients with increased intracranial pressure, hypothyroidism, or digitalis toxicity. Carotid sinus pressure, the Valsalva maneuver, and eyeball pressure result in vagal stimulation and slowing of the heart. Bradycardia can occur during anesthesia or following administration of morphine.

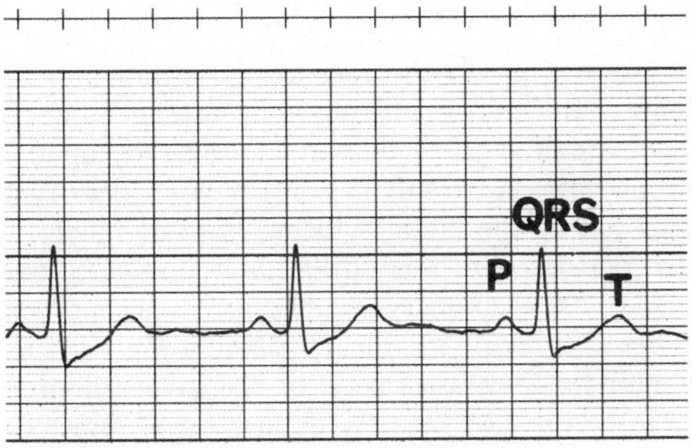

figure 47-4. Sinus bradycardia.

RATE: Below 60; a relative bradycardia may exist at a faster rate if it is insufficient to maintain cardiac output.
RHYTHM: Regular
P WAVES: Normal and precede each QRS
P-R INTERVAL: Normal
QRS: Normal
SIGNIFICANCE: Since cardiac output equals stroke volume times heart rate (c.o. = s.v. × h.r.), slow rate may not be sufficient for adequate cardiac output.
TREATMENT: Atropine sulfate 0.4 mg. IV may be ordered to override the vagal stimulus and increase sinus heart rate, thereby suppressing postbradycardia idioventricular beats. Isoproterenol (Isuprel) may be ordered to increase the heart rate by stimulation of the S-A node. An artificial pacemaker may be inserted to keep the heart beating at a minimum rate to maintain cardiac output.

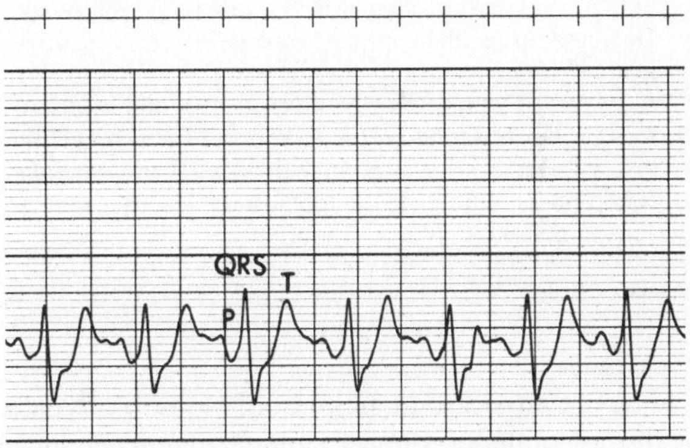

figure 47-5. Sinus tachycardia.

RATE: 100 to 160
RHYTHM: Regular
P WAVES: Normal, but may be obscured in T wave of previous cycle if rate is very fast.
P-R INTERVAL: Normal
QRS: Normal
SIGNIFICANCE: Can increase the work of the heart to the point of decompensation
TREATMENT: The underlying disease or the cause of the tachycardia must be treated. For example, anxiety is alleviated, fever is reduced, oxygen is given for hypoxia, or digitalis may be ordered for congestive heart failure. Keep the patient to minimum activity until rate decreases to compensated level.

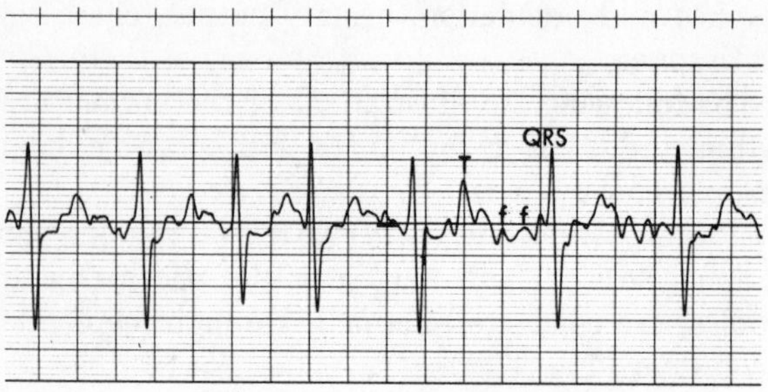

figure 47-6. Atrial fibrillation.

RATE: 350 to 800 (atrial) Ventricular rate varies but is irregular unless there is also a complete block at the A-V node in which case no atrial impulses are conducted and the lower pacemaker site produces a regular rhythm. In atrial fibrillation which is considered "controlled" either physiologically or by drugs, the ventricular rate is between 60 to 75 per minute. In uncontrolled atrial fibrillation, the ventricular rate is much faster.

RHYTHM: Irregular

P WAVES: There are no P waves; there is an irregular rapid undulation of the baseline of the ECG; the atrial twitchings are called f waves.

P-R INTERVAL: Since there are no P waves, the P-R interval is not measurable.

QRS: Normal

SIGNIFICANCE: Loss of atrial contraction diminishes cardiac output by about 15 per cent. Irregular ventricular filling and rhythm diminish the pumping efficiency. Decrease in cardiac output can result in congestive heart failure.

TREATMENT: Digitalis may be given to slow the ventricular rate by its action on the A-V node; then, quinidine to convert the atria to normal rhythm. If the patient's condition is potentially deteriorating, electric cardioversion is used.

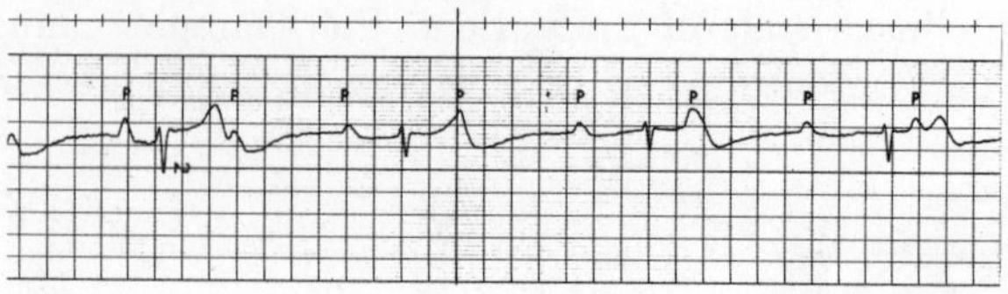

figure 47-7. Third degree A-V block (complete heart block).

RATE: Atrial rate is normal; the ventricular rate is 20 to 40 beats per minute.

RHYTHM: Atrial and ventricular rhythms are regular.

P WAVES: Normal

QRS: Configuration is normal if pacemaker site is in A-V node below block, but widened if pacemaker site is in ventricle.

SIGNIFICANCE: The slow ventricular rate is usually ineffective in maintaining adequate cardiac output; angina, congestive failure, or Stokes-Adams syndrome from cerebral hypoxia can occur; ventricular standstill or ventricular fibrillation may ensue.

TREATMENT: Withhold digitalis; isoproterenol (Isuprel) may be ordered. Pacemaker is considered essential; adequate ventilation to correct hypoxia and treatment of other associated clinical conditions is needed.

In acute myocardial infarction, sinus bradycardia is often an ominous sign of reflex vagal mechanisms. The slow rate may not be sufficient to maintain cardiac output in an already damaged heart. In addition, escape ectopic beats or rhythms such as idioventricular rhythm may take over as the primary pacemaker if their inherent rate is faster. This can increase ventricular irritability which is dangerous in myocardial infarction.

SINUS TACHYCARDIA. Impulses are initiated by the S-A node and the rate is regular, but above 100 beats per minute (Fig. 47-5). Sinus tachycardia occurs in persons with normal hearts as a physiological response to strenuous exercise or strong emotion, pain, fever, hyperthyroidism, hemorrhage, shock, or anemia. Cardiac output, coronary blood flow, and blood pressure can increase up to the rate of about 150 beats per minute. After that cardiac decompensation can occur. A decrease in vagal tone or an increase in sympathetic tone or both can result in sinus tachycardia. Tachycardia can be the initial evidence of heart failure.

In persons with myocardial infarction or coronary artery disease, coronary insufficiency with chest pain can develop because coronary blood flow cannot keep up with the increased need of the myocardium imposed by the fast rate. With fast rates, disastole is shortened and the heart does not have sufficient time to fill. Congestive heart failure, chest pain, or other symptoms of reduced cardiac output can occur.

ATRIAL FIBRILLATION. There is totally disorganized rapid atrial activity and the atria quiver rather than contract normally (Fig. 47-6). The ventricles respond to the atrial stimulus in an irregular fashion depending upon the sensitivity of the A-V node and the conduction system. Some of the ventricular beats are so weak that they are ineffective in opening the aortic valve and propelling blood, and a pulse deficit exists. An apical-radial pulse should be taken.

COMPLETE HEART BLOCK. The atria and ventricles function without any relationship to each other; therefore P waves have no sequential relationship to QRS's though the rhythm of each is usually regular (Fig. 47-7). The S-A node functions normally; the

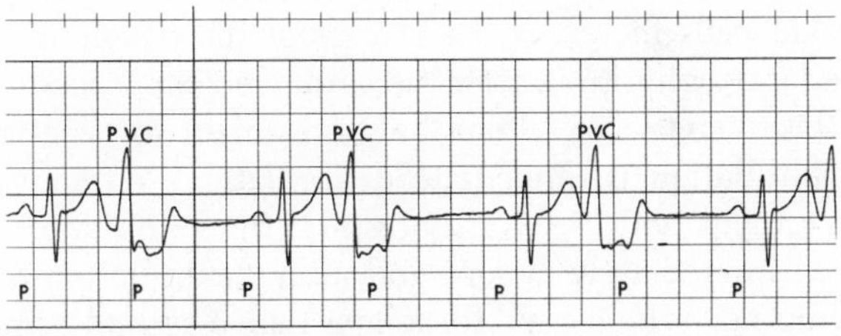

figure 47-8. Premature ventricular contractions (ventricular bigeminy).

RATE: Normal dominant rhythm
RHYTHM: Irregular
P WAVES: Normal, but absent in idioventricular complexes
QRS: Bizarre in configuration; widened above 0.12 second in idioventricular complexes; T wave following PVC usually is opposite in direction to its QRS.
TREATMENT: Notify physician promptly. Digitalis may be withheld; myocardial depressant drug such as lidocaine is begun promptly if the patient has myocardial infarction, to prevent ventricular fibrillation.

main pacemaker in the heart is below the block in the A-V node. What might appear to be a P-R interval changes with each complex. However, there is really no P-R interval due to the complete interruption in conduction from atria to ventricles.

PREMATURE VENTRICULAR CONTRACTIONS (PVC's). A PVC is a ventricular ectopic beat which occurs before depolarization of the ventricles by an atrial impulse is due (see Fig. 47-8). Therefore it is not preceded by an atrial impulse and, since it is not dependent on an impulse from above, it is also called an idioventricular beat. A PVC is usually followed by a long pause known as a "compensatory pause." This occurs because the normally occurring atrial impulse finds the ventricle refractory when it arrives because it has not recovered from its depolarization by the PVC. The next normally occurring atrial impulse succeeds in depolarizing the ventricle. If the heart rate is very slow, the ventricles can repolarize after a PVC in sufficient time to receive the atrial stimulus precisely when it is due and there is an extra beat, but the basic rhythm is not interrupted. This is called an *interpolated* PVC.

PVC's are very common; many people experience them at one time or another. It often causes a "flip-flop" sensation in the chest. Some people describe it as a "fluttering of the heart." The symptoms may be associated with pallor, nervousness, sweating, and faintness.

PVC's are usually harmless. Some people have them in response to anxiety and stress, and, as it so often happens, the symptoms then make them even more tense and fearful. Also, PVC's may be associated with fatigue or excessive use of alcohol or tobacco. Although PVC's are usually unassociated with organic heart disease, the person who is frequently troubled by them should consult his physician. A thorough examination is important in making certain that no organic heart disease exists and in assuring the patient that his heart is normal. Once the patient has received his physician's assurance that nothing is seriously wrong, he will find it easier to ignore the symptoms. This in itself often causes them to occur less frequently and to disappear more quickly.

In the presence of acute heart injury such as after surgery or in acute myocardial infarction, PVC's that occur in certain patterns are indicative of myocardial irritability and are precursors of lethal arrhythmias. These patterns or types are:

- More than six unifocal PVC's per minute. A run of ventricular bigeminy (a normal beat followed by a PVC) could also meet this criterion.
- Runs, bursts, or salvos of PVC's, that is, two or more in a row.
- Multifocal PVC's, that is, from more than one location in the ventricle.
- A PVC whose R wave falls on the T wave of the preceding complex.

Treatment of cardiac arrhythmias

Methods of treatment for cardiac arrhythmias are aimed at:

1. Cardioversion (reversion) of the disturbed conduction to normal sinus rhythm, if possible.
2. Where reversion to sinus rhythm is not possible, achievement of maximum physiological improvement.
3. Reduction of the number or severity of arrhythmic episodes and prevention of acute life-threatening attacks.

Treatment for cardiac arrhythmias includes mechanical, chemical (pharmacological), and electrical modalities. Mechanical means include use of carotid sinus pressure, eyeball pressure, or the Valsalva maneuver, which slow the heart, and external cardiac compression. These treatments are administered or instituted by the physician.

Drug therapy

Drugs used in the treatment of cardiac arrhythmias include the following classifications:

1. Drugs acting primarily on tissues within the heart:
   - Myocardial depressants such as lidocaine (Xylocaine), procainamide HCl (Pronestyl) quinidine sulfate, propranolol (Inderal), and phenytoin (Dilantin).
   - Drugs that increase cardiac rhythmicity and contraction such as epinephrine and isoproterenol (Isuprel).
   - Drugs which depress conduction but increase contractile force, such as digitalis preparations.
2. Drugs acting on the autonomic nervous system:
   - Cholinergic blocking agents, namely atropine, to increase heart rate.
   - Alpha and beta adrenergic drugs such as epinephrine and isoproterenol (Isuprel).
   - Beta adrenergic blocking agents such as propranolol (Inderal).

Electrical therapy

Restoration of normal cardiac rhythm may be accomplished by the use of drugs as well as by

- Defibrillation
- Cardiac pacemaker

Cardioversion. Cardioversion is used to terminate rapid cardiac arrhythmias such as atrial flutter, atrial fibrillation, and ventricular tachycardia, all of which decrease cardiac output to some degree. The electric current completely depolarizes the entire myocardium at one time so that the fastest normal pacemaker can regain control of the pacing function. Cardioversion avoids the time element and potential side effects encountered in the use of drug therapy.

In elective cardioversion there is time for the physician to explain the procedure to the patient and obtain his consent. Because the patient is generally anxious as a result of the tachycardia, explanation is limited to what he is able to comprehend. Where there is sufficient time, the physician may order an antiarrhythmic drug such as quinidine to be given orally several hours or a day prior to cardioversion so that a blood level of the drug will be achieved sufficient to maintain normal rhythm following cardioversion. Digitalis is usually withheld for a period prior to cardioversion because it is believed that its presence in myocardial cells increases the chance of the development of a fatal arrhythmia after the cardioversion procedure.

Defibrillation. The only treatment for venticular fibrillation is immediate defibrillation. Without it, the patient will die. Cardiorespiratory resuscitation is given immediately before and after defibrillation and should never be ceased for longer than 5 seconds, since blood flow and blood pressure can drop to zero. Usually a defibrillating shock of 400 watt seconds is delivered. Ventricular tachycardia which is accompanied by hypotension and loss of consciousness is likewise an extreme emergency; depending on the judgment of the physician, defibrillation may be used to restore normal sinus rhythm.

The patient with a pacemaker

A cardiac pacemaker (pulse generator) is used to maintain the ventricular rate at a minimum level for effective cardiac output. Formerly, an open-chest procedure was necessary to implant electrodes in the myocardium, so the use of a pacemaker was limited to "good risk" patients. Today, with the transvenous (or pervenous) technique, a permanent pacemaker

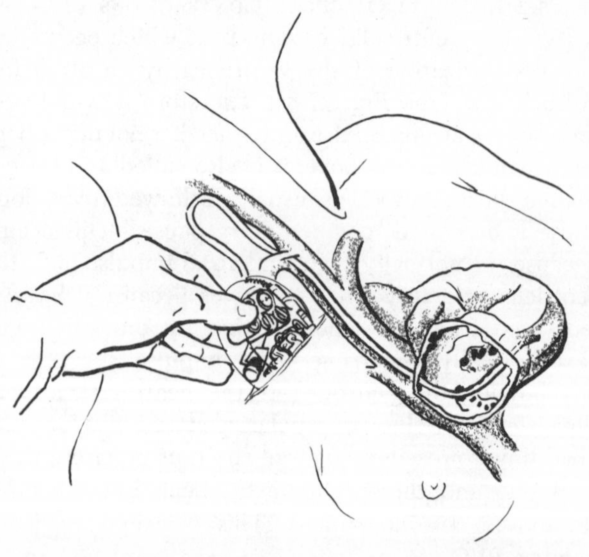

figure 47-9. An implanted cardiac pacemaker. The battery and circuitry that make up the pulse generator are placed under the skin below the collarbone. Attached to the pulse generator is an electrode consisting of two encapsulated wires running through a vein to the right ventricle through which the electrical stimulus is carried to the heart.

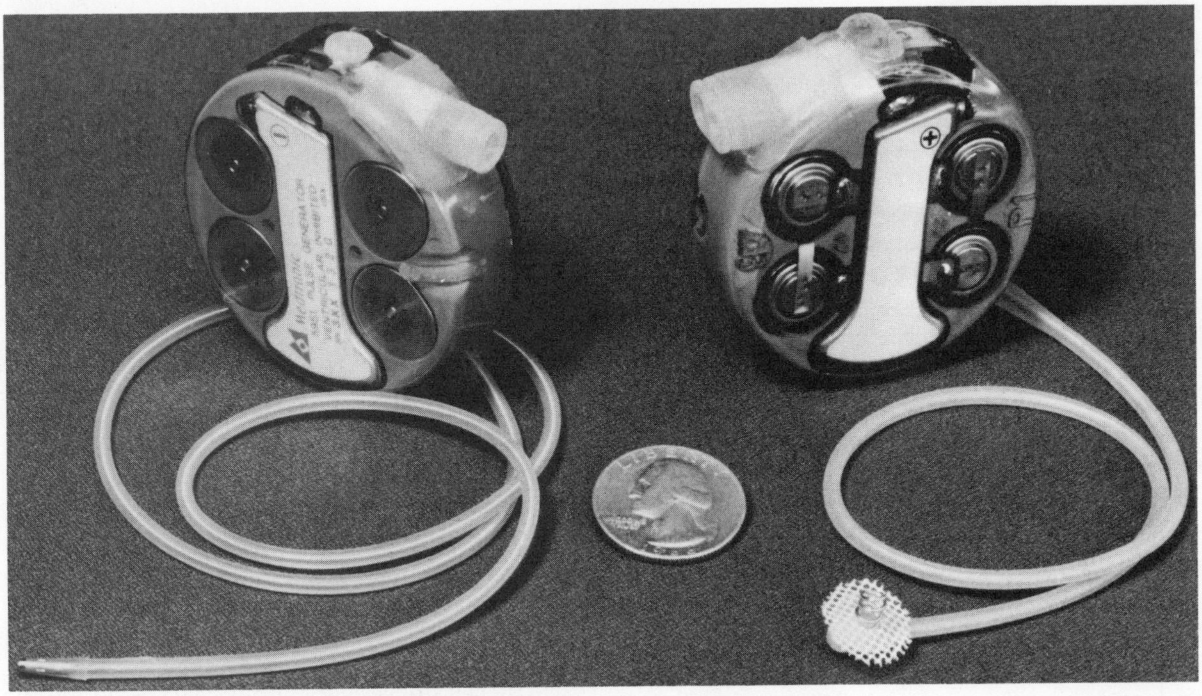

figure 47-10. The Medtronic implantable Xytron Pulse Generator with unipolar and bipolar leads. Note the size in comparison to a quarter. (Medtronic, Inc., Minneapolis, Minn.)

(Figs. 47-9 and 47-10) can be inserted quickly in most patients under local anesthesia with minimal surgical risk and discomfort.

The most frequent indication for permanent artificial pacing is to eliminate Stokes-Adams attacks associated with a variety of heart diseases, including coronary artery disease, rheumatic heart disease, and congenital malformations, or occurring as a direct complication of cardiac surgery.

Since pacing increases heart rate and therefore cardiac output, it may also be used to increase circulation in patients with slow heart rates and symptoms of right- or left-sided heart failure, angina, renal failure, or slow cerebration.

Temporary pacing is indicated in acute myocardial infarction complicated by heart block or other bradyarrhythmias, in digitalis toxicity with heart block, and in patients with slow heart rate and congestive failure who require digitalis. In most of these situations the pacemaker is removed when the normal sinus rhythm returns.

Some pacemakers are self-activating and are operational when the patient's pulse falls below a preset level. These are called "demand" pacemakers. Thus, if the physician sets this type of pacemaker at 72, the pacemaker unit is only operational when the patient's pulse falls below 72 per minute. Battery life is prolonged with the use of this type of pacemaker.

Another indication for temporary pacing is to suppress rapid arrhythmias such as recurrent ventricular tachycardia which does not respond to drugs or cardioversion.

Since there are many indications for pacing and several kinds of pacemakers, it is the responsibility of the nurse to know objectives of the pacing treatment, precautions to be taken, and observations to be made, and to be very familiar with the product literature which describes the individual pacing unit. The physician determines the rate of the heartbeat and the amplitude of the pacing stimulus.

Nursing management of the patient with bradycardia requiring a pacemaker

Patients who are subject to Stokes-Adams syndrome are often very apprehensive. Lightheadedness, fainting, and in some instances convulsions are symptoms of this syndrome. They do not know when the next attack will occur and then have only a few seconds to summon help before they become unconscious. It is not uncommon for patients to be admitted with acute physical injuries such as fractures or lacerations sustained while experiencing Stokes-Adams syndrome. Often attacks occur when the patient is away from his own community, and he may find himself admitted to a strange hospital under the care of a physician who is a stranger to him. Because Stokes-Adams attacks are a cardiac problem, the patient may be admitted to a coronary care unit.

When the physician decides that a pacemaker is to be inserted he explains this to the patient. A surgical consent is necessary. For most patients, the thought that their heart requires artificial electrical control is anxiety producing. They need time to talk about it and get used to the idea, but often there is very little time for this. The nurse should listen to the surgeon's explanation to the patient, and in her conversation with the patient review, clarify, and correct any misinterpretations that the patient or family might have. Language readily understood by the patient should be used.

For emergency temporary pacing, the catheter may be inserted into the right ventricle at the bedside, using electrocardiographic or fluoroscopic control. The implantation room is equipped with a cardiac monitor, a defibrillator and other equipment and drugs needed for cardiac arrest. Ventricular fibrillation can be provoked mechanically by the pacemaker lead tip as it enters the ventricle.

For permanent transvenous pacing, local anesthesia is usually used. The patient may find the procedure tedious and be uncomfortable after lying on a hard x-ray table. The patient hears what is going on though his eyes may be shielded. Strict surgical asepsis is essential. Contamination of the pacemaker lead or implantable pulse generator can result in infection and failure to pace properly. After the pacing lead is properly seated in the right ventricle the surgeon selects the correct pacing threshold and sets the voltage and rate. An amplitude of 6 mA. and rate of 70 is common.

Eventually the pacemaker lead becomes embedded in the right ventricular trabeculae. Immediately after insertion, the electrocardiographic display might show complexes with varying electrical potentials because the tip of the catheter might not touch the ventricle with the same force at first. PVC's are more frequent during the early postimplant period. The physician may order medication to suppress these. The patient spends several days in an environment where a defibrillator and other emergency equipment and drugs are available.

Table 47-1. Nursing management after insertion of a cardiac pacemaker

The patient is placed on a cardiac monitor. Check pulse and ECG pattern visually q15m for first 2 to 4 hours or as ordered.

Set Hi/Lo alarms on monitor as per physician's order or unit policy.

Measure patient's blood pressure and respirations q½-1h or as ordered.

Take patient's temperature q4h.

Run rhythm strips at ordered intervals and tape to patient's chart.

Measure intake and output.

If the pacemaker is external:

- Check site of insertion of lead(s) q1-2h.
- Report any bleeding around site of lead(s) insertion to the physician immediately.
- Report displacement or dislodging of the lead(s) to the physician immediately.
- Check the external pacemaker apparatus frequently to be sure it remains properly anchored to the patient's arm or chest.

Postimplantation Care (Table 47-1). Patients with newly implanted pacemakers are generally on an electrocardiographic monitor for an evaluation period after insertion. Each pacer has its own characteristic tracing. The electrical artifact or "blip" of the pacing stimulus should appear before the QRS of a ventricular pacer. It is usually identified on the oscilloscope as a thin, straight stroke. Absence of the artifact may mean faulty monitoring equipment, or more seriously, failure to pace due to malposition of the catheter, dislodgement of the catheter, catheter breakage, or rise of the pacing threshold due to tissue reaction to the catheter or to infection. The location of the artifact is particularly important. If the paced rhythm competes with the patient's spontaneous rhythm, the artifact can fall in the vulnerable period of the cardiac cycle.

To assist in determining that each pacing stimulus results in effective ventricular contraction, the patient's pulse should be taken simultaneously with observation of the cardiac monitor.

The small pulse generator of a temporary pacing system should be placed so that it is immovable and there is no tension on the wires. The patient should not be able to manipulate the controls. Only grounded electrical equipment should be used in the room and only one machine connected to a wall outlet should be used on the patient at one time.

Localized phlebitis and cellulitis can develop around the catheter exit site of a temporary pacemaker. The nurse will check the dressing for drainage and report discomfort to the physician.

If the patient develops singultus (hiccups), there can be current leakage across the diaphragm or perforation of the ventricle by the catheter. This symptom should be reported to the physician.

Nursing management depends on the condition of the patient. For example, if the patient developed heart block following acute myocardial infarction, he will continue to be on all coronary precautions. The physician will observe the patient after several days with the pacemaker off; if sustained normal sinus rhythm returns, the pacemaker will be removed.

The physician should be consulted regarding the initiation of exercise of the shoulder on the side of the catheter insertion. Unless this is mobilized early, the elderly patient is apt to develop "frozen" shoulder.

Discharge Planning. The patient's prognosis and activity depend on the adequacy of the myocardium. The pacemaker improves cardiac conduction, but cannot regenerate diseased myocardium. Some patients may needlessly restrict activities such as sexual intercourse because of unfounded fears. The patient and spouse need the opportunity to discuss activities with the physician and plan life realistically. Meeting a well-adjusted patient with a pacemaker may be a help.

If the patient has a permanent pacemaker, he may be taught to take his pulse for a full minute once or twice a day and is instructed to report rate changes and episodes of dizziness or unconsciousness.

All patients need continuing medical follow-up. The average life of a conventional battery pacemaker unit is about 2½ years, but this varies with the model. The average life of a nuclear-powered pacemaker is approximately 10 years. Battery failure is signalized by slight decrease in rate. Other components can fail, causing decrease or increase in rate, including the very rapid rate of a "runaway" pacemaker or absence of pacing. Symptoms of weakness or dizziness may be the patient's first clue that the pacemaker battery is becoming nonfunctional.

Some pacemakers are sensitive to outside electrical interference such as radiofrequency signals from diathermy and microwave ovens; proximity to these may interfere with the function of the pacemaker.

It is helpful for the patient with a pacemaker to wear a Medic Alert emblem or to carry a card indicating that he has a pacemaker in the event that he needs emergency medical care.

Cardiac arrest

Cardiac arrest is the sudden cessation of effective cardiac output. The electrical mechanism of cardiac arrest can be ventricular asystole or bradyarrhythmias, or ventricular tachyarrhythmias (ventricular tachycardia or ventricular fibrillation). An initially slow rhythm can induce myocardial hypoxia which can trigger ventricular fibrillation.

Care of the patient in cardiac arrest should encompass the following stages and maneuvers:

- If patient is on a cardiac monitor, respond to monitor alarm and check electrocardiographic patterns.
- Summon help.
- If necessary and possible, the patient should be defibrillated immediately. In a hospital intensive care unit this may be within 30 seconds.
- Observe the following steps (ABCDE's):

1. *Airway* should be established.
2. *Breathing,* using the mouth-to-mouth method or assistive device if available. Give three to four maximal insufflations before initiating circulation so that oxygenated blood will be pumped.
3. *Circulation* should be restored by closed chest cardiac compression. Check the pupils and carotid or femoral pulse.
4. *Definitive therapy* is ordered by the physician, depending on the cause and length of the period of arrest. Sodium bicarbonate, usually 44.0 mEq. for every 5 to 10 minutes in cardiac arrest, is given to treat the metabolic acidosis which results from the accumulation of lactic acid.
5. *Evaluation.* Dilation of the pupils starts 45 seconds after cardiac arrest and is complete in 1 to 2 minutes. Cerebral death begins in 30 to 90 seconds unless adequate cerebral oxygenation is restored. Since the pupil is the best index of brain oxygenation, pupillary response is the best indica-

tor of the effectiveness of heart-lung resuscitation. Adequate oxygenation and good blood flow to the brain are present if the pupil constricts on exposure to flashlight. Pulses should be present during cardiac compression and the patient's color should improve if he is responding.

Some additional important points about cardiopulmonary resuscitation are:

AIRWAY. A maximum backward tilt of the head is the easiest way to open an airway. Only an experienced person should attempt endotracheal intubation, since cardiac massage cannot be halted for more than 5 seconds. Endotracheal intubation is not essential for an adequate airway. Secretions need to be wiped out or suctioned from the pharynx. Establishment of an airway may be sufficient to permit spontaneous breathing to resume and to restore circulation.

BREATHING. Mouth-to-mouth breathing done effectively delivers about 18 percent oxygen to the patient. A self-inflating bag, such as the Ambu bag, used with a face mask or an endotracheal tube and oxygen, delivers about 50 percent oxygen only if used correctly. Three to four maximal insufflations should be given before compression is started so that oxygenated blood will be circulated. With two rescuers, one inflation should be interposed after each five compressions without any halting of compression (1:5 ratio or 12 breaths per minute). With one rescuer, two breaths are interposed after each fifteen compressions. The breather should see the chest rise and fall, feel the resistance of the lungs as they expand, and hear the noise of air escaping during exhalation.

Artificial ventilation may cause distention of the stomach. This can lead to regurgitation, reduced lung volume, or the initiation of vagal reflexes. The physician may exert moderate pressure between the umbilicus and the rib cage to expel the air. The patient's head should be lowered and turned to one side to avoid aspiration of gastric contents. Mouth-to-nose ventilation can be used if there is difficulty via the mouth-to-mouth route. Mechanical ventilators are also available when prolonged respiratory support is needed.

CARDIAC COMPRESSION. Rhythmic pressure applied over the lower half of the sternum results in compression of the heart and pulsatile arterial circulation.

The patient is placed on his back on a firm surface, such as the floor, the pavement, a bed board, or even a large tray slipped under the chest. (A soft mattress

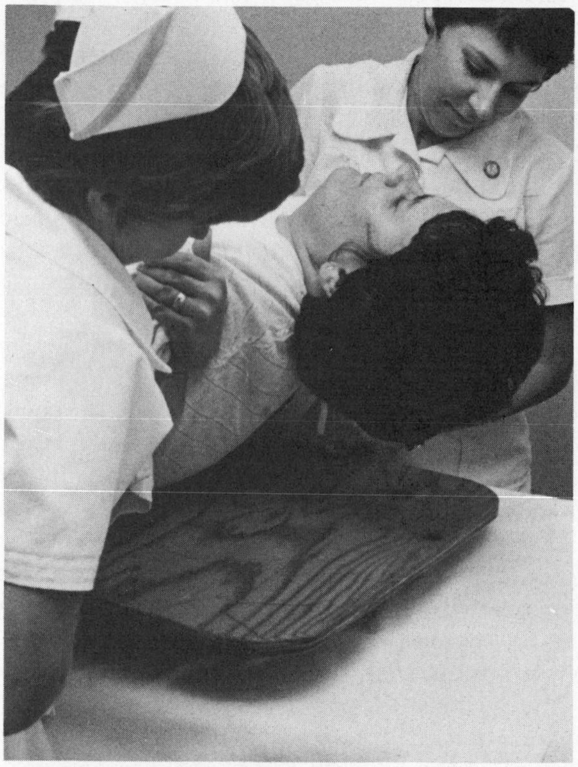

figure 47-11. A firm support, in this case a board, must be placed under the patient before cardiopulmonary resuscitation is initiated. (Photograph—D. Atkinson)

is depressed by pressure and would interfere with the massage.) As part of the emergency equipment, some hospitals keep a board that can be slipped between the patient and the bed (Fig. 47-11). It makes a hard surface from the waist to the shoulders.

The person kneels beside the patient, placing his hands at right angles on the lower sternum (Fig. 47-12). The hands, one on top of the other, are pressed vertically downward, pushing the sternum inward 1½ to 2 inches, thus compressing the heart between the sternum and the spine and forcing the blood out of the heart. Only the heels of the hands are used. The fingers are kept up, out of contact with the patient's ribs.

Manual pressure is released, allowing the heart to fill with blood, and then pressure is reapplied. The cycle is repeated approximately 60 to 80 times per minute with breathing interposed.

Closed cardiac massage is not without its dangers. Hands that are misplaced to one side may break ribs or rupture the liver or spleen.

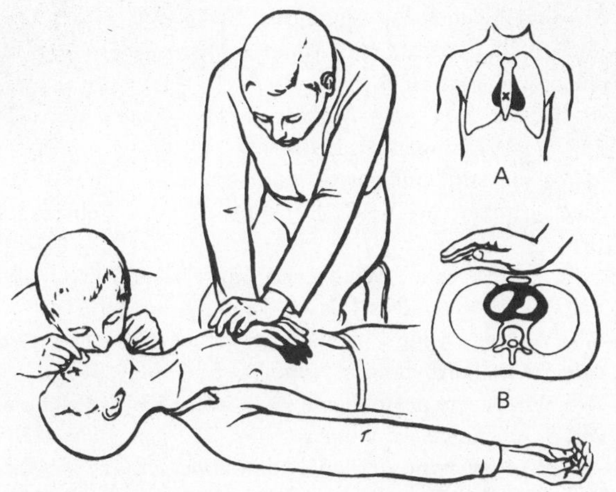

figure 47-12. Technique of closed chest cardiac massage. One rescuer gives mouth-to-mouth resuscitation. The other massages the heart by pressing downward on the patient's chest approximately 60 times a minute. (A) X indicates the area where pressure should be applied. (B) Manual pressure on the chest, compressing the heart and forcing blood out of it. (American Heart Association, Inc., New York, N.Y.; adapted from Kouwenhoven, W. B., *et al.*: Heart activation in cardiac arrest, *Modern Concepts of Cardiovascular Diseases* 30[2]:642)

When prolonged resuscitation or transportation of the patient is required, external cardiac compression machines are commercially available which are more consistent in the application of pressure than would be a number of different team members. The machine must be carefully and continually observed for correct placement and function.

During the resuscitation effort the physician may give an intracardiac injection of epinephrine and an intravenous injection of sodium bicarbonate to control acidosis. Calcium chloride to strengthen cardiac contractions also may be administered once heart action starts. Vasopressors may be given intravenously to maintain an adequate blood pressure. The nurse assists in the preparation and administration of drugs and by noting the patient's response.

External cardiac compression may be ineffective or contraindicated in such situations as crushing injuries of the chest and internal thoracic injuries, or in patients with advanced pulmonary emphysema with enlarged, fixed rib cages. The physician may elect to open the chest and do direct cardiac massage.

After successful cardiac resuscitation the patient needs to be observed closely. Vital signs are taken frequently; the patient will be attached to a monitoring device. Oxygen will be given to reduce the onset of arrhythmias due to hypoxemia. A nasogastric tube may be passed to prevent distention. Shock may have caused renal impairment. Other complications for which the nurse should observe include pneumothorax, hematoma of the liver, brain damage, fractured ribs or sternum, and fat embolism. To minimize the chance of cerebral damage, some physicians may use hypothermia for several days after cardiac arrest.

General pharmacological considerations

- Drug therapy for cardiac arrhythmias may include myocardial depressants (antiarrhythmics), cardiotonics, adrenergic drugs, cholinergic blocking agents, and electrolytes.
- Examples of myocardial depressants are quinidine, procainamide (Pronestyl), lidocaine, propranolol (Inderal), and phenytoin (Dilantin). When these drugs are used in the treatment of various cardiac arrhythmias, the patient's pulse rate and rhythm must be closely monitored. Patients receiving intravenous lidocaine or propranolol should be on a cardiac monitor during administration.
- Administration of lidocaine can result in serious side effects, including convulsions and cardiac arrest. An airway should be readily available. If hypotension or additional cardiac arrhythmias occur during administration, the intravenous infusion is adjusted to the slowest possible rate until the physician can examine the patient.
- The cardiotonics are digitalis and allied glycosides, including digoxin, digitoxin, and lanatoside-C. The apical-radial rate is taken before the drug is administered, especially during digitalization. Later, when the patient is fully digitalized, a radial rate may suffice.
- Signs of drug toxicity can occur even when normal doses of digitalis and allied glycosides are administered. Signs of toxicity include anorexia, nausea, vomiting, halos around dark objects, diarrhea, abdominal discomfort, disturbance of green/yellow vision, *cardiac arrhythmias* such as bradycardia, tachycardia, bigeminal pulse.
- The cholinergic blocking agent atropine may be used to treat the severe bradycardia of third degree heart block or digitalis intoxica-

tion. An emergency dose of 1 mg. (gr. 1/60) may be given intravenously. Isoproterenol (Isuprel), a beta adrenergic drug, may also be used to treat severe bradycardia. When either of these drugs is administered, the pulse must be closely monitored for drug response.

Bibliography

Andreoli, K. G. et al: *Comprehensive Cardiac Care,* ed. 3. St. Louis, Mosby, 1975.

Anthony, C. P.: *Structure and Function of the Body,* ed. 4. St. Louis, Mosby, 1972.

Conover, M. H.: *Cardiac Arrhythmias.* St. Louis, Mosby, 1974.

Pinneo, R.: Essentials of cardiac monitoring (pictorial). J. Prac. Nurs. 23:26, November, 1973.

Rodman, M. J. and Smith, D. W.: *Clinical Pharmacology in Nursing.* Philadelphia, Lippincott, 1974.

Scherer, J. C.: *Introductory Clinical Pharmacology.* Philadelphia, Lippincott, 1975.

Sharp, L. and Rabin, B.: *Nursing in the Coronary Care Unit.* Philadelphia, Lippincott, 1970.

Standards for cardiopulmonary resuscitation (CPR) and emergency cardiac care (ECC). JAMA 227:834, February 18, 1974.

Van Meter, M. et al: What every nurse should know about EKG's (pictorial). Part 1. Nurs. '75, 5:19, April, 1975.

———: What every nurse should know about EKG's (pictorial). Part 2. Atrial arrhythmias. Nurs. '75, 5:37, May, 1975.

———: What every nurse should know about EKG's (pictorial). Part 3. Junctional arrhythmias. Nurs. '75, 5:19, June, 1975.

———: What every nurse should know about EKG's (pictorial). Part 4. Ventricular arrhythmias. Nurs. '75, 5:31, July, 1975.

CHAPTER 48

The patient with acute myocardial infarction

On completion of this chapter the student will:

- List the symptoms of myocardial infarction.
- Define the functions of a coronary care unit.
- Describe the procedures for admitting a patient to a coronary care unit, including nursing measures instituted to make the patient comfortable and observations made during the admission period.
- Discuss the objectives and content of the admission patient history.
- Describe the methods used in the diagnosis of a myocardial infarction.
- Discuss the objectives of care of the patient with a myocardial infarction.
- List the complications of a myocardial infarction and their treatment.
- Formulate a nursing care plan for and participate in the nursing management of a patient with a myocardial infarction.
- Discuss the preparations made for the discharge of the patient from the coronary care unit.

In myocardial infarction the interference with the blood supply to a portion of the muscle of the heart is so severe that necrosis of a part of the heart results. This may be precipitated by the occlusion of a coronary artery from capillary hemorrhage within an atherosclerotic plaque or by the formation of a thrombus on one of the plaques. Myocardial infarction may occur without occlusion of an artery when there is a sudden reduction in the blood supply to the heart—for example, during shock or hemorrhage or during severe physical exertion—whenever, in fact, the need of the heart for blood is increased suddenly beyond that which the atherosclerotic arteries can deliver. Atherosclerosis is almost always the underlying cause of myocardial infarction. The narrowed, roughened vessels are very susceptible to obstruction.

Symptoms

The symptoms of myocardial infarction include sudden, severe pain in the chest, usually precordial or substernal, sometimes radiating to the shoulder and the arm, teeth, jaw, or throat, especially on the left side. The pain is more severe and of longer duration than that in angina pectoris, and it is not necessarily related to exertion. Patients sometimes describe it as "grinding" or "crushing" and so severe that every ounce of stamina is needed to endure it. Unlike that of angina pectoris, the pain of myocardial infarction is not relieved by rest or nitroglycerin. It may last several hours or as long as 1 or 2 days, and, finally, it becomes a soreness or an ache before it disappears entirely.

In some patients the pain is accompanied by symptoms of shock, pallor, sweating, faintness, a severe drop in blood pressure, and rapid, weak pulse brought about by sudden decrease in cardiac output.

It is not unusual for the patient to lose consciousness at the beginning of the attack and, as he regains consciousness, again to become aware of the excruciating pain in his chest. Sometimes the patient is more aware of feeling faint and weak than he is of chest pain. Nausea and vomiting may occur and lead the patient to believe that he has an attack of acute indigestion.

The suddenness and severity of symptoms of acute myocardial infarction have been described as being so stressful that primitive and virtually automatic responses to danger are aroused. Fear and restlessness almost invariably occur, unless shock is so profound that the patient is unable to respond emotionally to the situation. Most patients are well aware of the seriousness of chest pain, and they are immediately apprehensive. Symptoms of left-sided heart failure—dyspnea, cyanosis, and cough—may appear if the pumping of the left ventricle is sufficiently impaired.

The patient needs to be transferred as quickly as possible to a treatment facility where definitive measures such as defibrillation are available. The majority of deaths from acute myocardial infarction occur in the first hours after the onset of pain. Sudden death is attributed in most cases to ventricular fibrillation.

The coronary care unit

The emphasis in a CCU is on the prevention of the need for resuscitative measures by detecting early changes in the patient's condition. Thus all patients receive continuous close observation, including electrocardiographic monitoring, for several days. The nursing staff receives specialized education in the early recognition of cardiac arrhythmias and other complications. Prompt reporting of early warning signs enables the physician to institute treatment before complications become serious. Nursing care is directed toward the promotion of rest and healing, prevention of complications, support of the patient through the experience, and promotion of optimal rehabilitation.

Admitting the patient

The appearance of the patient on admission can vary widely. He may neither look nor feel very ill, or he may be in deep cardiogenic shock. He may have received pain medication in his doctor's office which gave relief, or he may be clutching his chest with muscle splinting of his shoulder and arm indicating severe pain. He may have a tachycardia, which may reflect a normal response to abruptly leaving one's place of work in an ambulance with flashing lights and siren, or which may mean the early onset of heart failure. A bradycardia does not mean that the patient is not excited. Rather this can be an ominous sign of involvement of the S-A or A-V node or marked vagal tone. A slow rate can lead to myocardial hypoxia which fosters lethal cardiac arrhythmias. Slowing of the rate can mean the patient is in heart block if the A-V node is ischemic from the episode. One patient may have a large area of muscle damaged; another, a relatively small area.

For each patient the admitting nurse has to determine priorities. The lifesaving activities always exert priority. Some other areas of nursing concern during the early admission period are:

▪ *Assisting the patient to bed* and undressing him with minimal expenditure of effort. A roller placed next to the patient on the stretcher can be used so that the patient does not have to be lifted.

▪ *Giving oxygen.* Equipment ready for immediate use is at the bedside. Adequate oxygenation contributes to the relief of pain and the prevention of arrhythmias. Physicians differ in opinion regarding routine oxygen administration. Patients who are dyspneic, tachycardic, or cyanotic are given oxygen as an emergency measure. The danger is that some emergency patients, unknown to the local physician and nursing staff, may have chronic obstructive lung disease. Giving oxygen routinely at high concentration may result in respiratory arrest by depriving the patient of the hypoxic stimulus to respiration. Asking the patient or family promptly on admission if he has lung disease is necessary. Unit policies should offer guidelines for action. For example, oxygen may be given at a lowered concentration and the physician promptly notified. The patient's response must be noted. If he becomes pink, but increasingly drowsy without drugs, this is an emergency sign!

▪ *Relieving pain.* It is imperative to relieve pain, which is often severe, crushing, and the source of great fear. Arrhythmias and shock can follow severe pain. Also, arrhythmias and hypotension can follow the administration of a drug such as morphine given to relieve pain.

The nurse will watch the patient's response to the pain-relieving drug. If pain is not relieved in an hour, the physician is called back. Often the pain is so severe that the narcotic does not completely relieve it, but makes it less intense and more bearable. Usually, the narcotic is given every 3 to 4 hours, as necessary, during the period when the pain is severe. It is important to note any depression of respiration, nausea, arrhythmias, and hypotension, particularly when morphine is given. The drug is given as often as it is required and permitted to control the pain. The period during which narcotics are needed usually lasts no more than 1 or 2 days; yet it is during this period that rest and the relief of apprehension are especially important. Oxygen should be given also.

▪ *Observation* of the patient is an ongoing process initiated when the nurse first greets the patient, who also observes the nurse. How the nurse confronts the patient during this period can influence the entire course of his illness. He can get a message of hope, warm caring, competence, and concern or one that is cold, impersonal, pessimistic, scolding, or panicky.

Using one's sensory apparatus skillfully can quickly give much data:

Eyes. What does the patient look like? What is his color? Is he splinting his shoulder muscles from pain? Is he working hard to breathe (dyspneic)? Does he have a calm or apprehensive look in his eyes? Is he alert or somnolent? Are his neck veins distended?

Ears. What do you hear? Are his respirations wheezing or stertorous? What does the patient have to say? Is he in pain? If talking does not distress him further, the nurse may ask what happened that brought him to the hospital. What questions does he have about the unit, the equipment, his condition?

Touch. Is the patient's skin cold and clammy? Warm and dry? Is there good skin turgor? What is the quality of his radial pulse? Full and bounding? Weak and thready? Is his abdomen or bladder distended?

Smell. What odors emanate from the patient? Does his breath smell like alcohol? Is there the sweet fruity odor of diabetic acidosis? Is there the odor of perspiration? Of excreta?

▪ *Placing chest electrodes* (Fig. 48-1) for cardiac monitoring.

The bedside cardiac monitor and a console at the nurses' station or a remote control monitoring system known as telemetry (Fig. 48-2) provide for a continuous display on an oscilloscope of 1 lead of the patient's ECG (Fig. 48-3).

The placement sites of electrodes are chosen so that the best cardiographic tracing appears on the oscilloscope. Care should be taken that electrodes and nonallergenic adhesive tape are so placed that they do not interfere with the taking of the chest leads of the 12-lead ECG or the placement of paddles for defibrillation.

Generally, high rate and low rate indicators are set on the cardiac monitor for each patient.

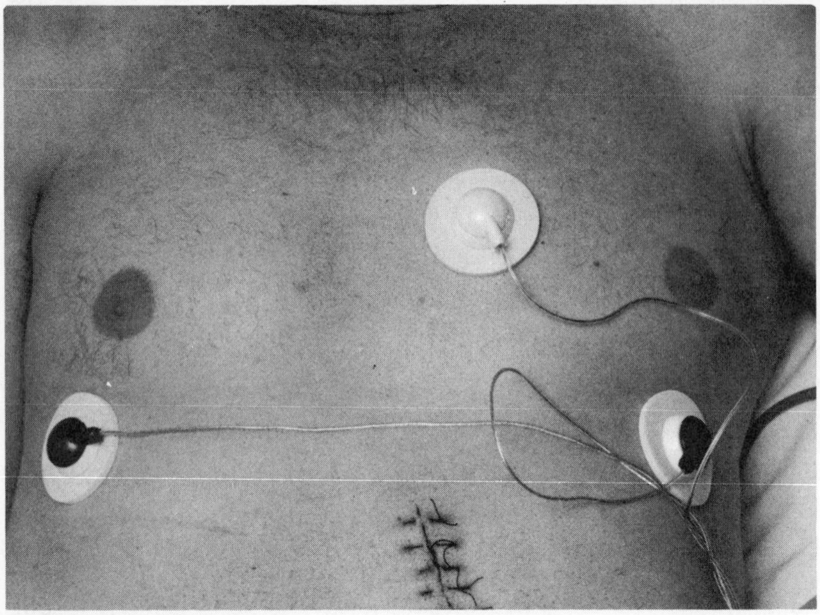

figure 48-1. Position of chest electrodes for cardiac monitoring. (Photograph—D. Atkinson)

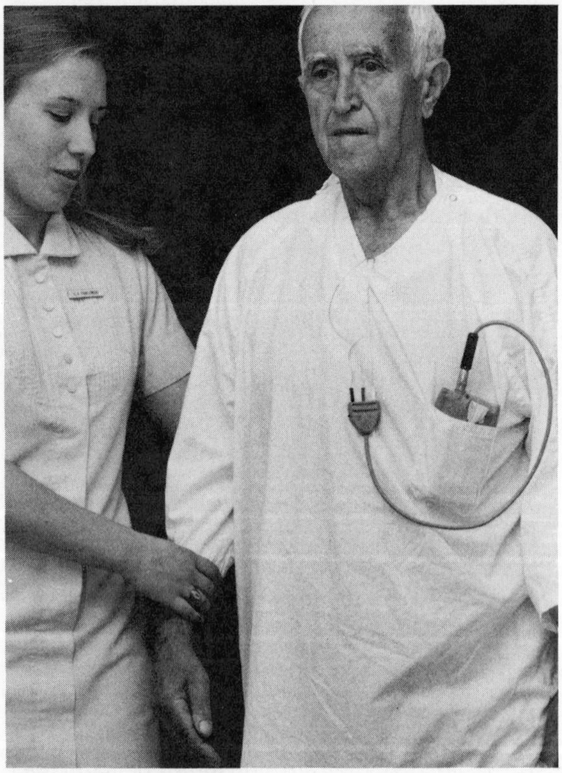

figure 48-2. The patient on remote telemetry can ambulate without being hindered by electronic hardware. A signal from the battery box carried in the patient's pocket is sent to the monitor/receiver at the nurses' station. (Photograph—D. Atkinson)

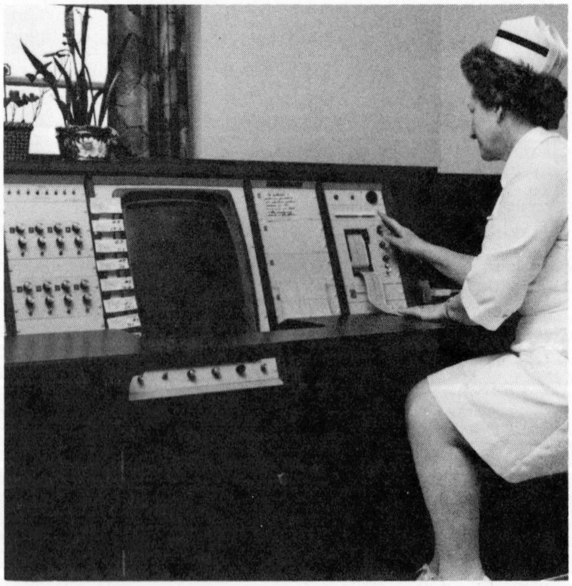

figure 48-3. Patients on remote telemetry can be monitored while carrying on various activities. This photograph shows the monitor in Phase II of the Coronary Care Unit at Sisters Hospital, Buffalo, New York. (Photograph—D. Atkinson)

Should the patient's pulse rate fall below or exceed these limits, an audiovisual alarm system is activated. On some machines, a writeout may be concurrent with that appearing on the oscilloscope or may be written out from a tape or memory-loop with a 10-second or longer delay. Hence, the cardiac rhythm immediately before the alarm situation can be identified. After the alarm, the nurse examines the cardiac tracing and observes the patient. Loosening of an electrode or excessive muscular activity can result in false alarms and an irregular monitor pattern. If an arrhythmia is the source of the alarm, the nurse makes a decision regarding nursing intervention.

The patient and family need to know that a cardiac monitor is not dangerous. Needless apprehension can be built up if the patient fantasizes about this piece of machinery that blinks, beeps, and causes people to jump and take note when an alarm goes off. False alarms frighten patients. Monitors are considered as aids to and not substitutes for nursing care and human contact with the patient.

Observation of the cardiac monitor rhythm must be accompanied by observation of the patient. The advantage of continuous cardiac monitoring of the hospitalized patient is that changes in rhythm or rate can be detected early and treated promptly, before the clinical condition of the patient deteriorates.

Because of subjective feelings such as palpitations, "jolting" sensations in the chest, or a fluttering feeling, patients are often aware of their arrhythmias. These abnormal sensations increase anxiety. Studies have shown that anxiety and other emotional states, in turn, contribute to the onset, severity, persistence, and recurrence of cardiac arrhythmias.

■ *Intravenous infusion.* Because cardiovascular collapse is an always present threat, an intravenous infusion is usually started to keep the vein opened. In an emergency, drugs can quickly be given and time is not wasted while the physician attempts to do a cut down on a collapsed vein.

■ *12-lead electrocardiogram.* This may be taken by the nurse on admission; though the results do not markedly influence nursing care at this point, the record serves as a basis for later comparison and immediate arrhythmia treatment.

■ *Spiritual care.* One role of the nurse is to expedite the availability of the patient's spiritual adviser. The suggestion of spiritual help from a clergyman of the patient's religion should be offered. The family can give information about religious affiliation and usual practices if the patient is too ill to be questioned. The clergyman can also be supportive of the family during this time of crisis.

■ *Diet.* Oral intake is restricted until specific orders are received. Because of the risk of cardiac arrest and aspiration, as well as the increased cardiac workload from digestion, intake for the critical period of the first 3 days is generally restricted to a full liquid diet. Iced water or iced beverages are contraindicated because they are vagal stimulants. Coffee and tea, which contain stimulants that may increase heart rate, may also be restricted. Carbonated beverages are not served because they promote gaseous distention.

■ *Admission interview.* Some specific questions that should be asked the patient or family are:

What allergies does the patient have? Is he allergic to *any* drugs? All allergies are reported to the physician; the specific substances and/or drugs to which the patient is allergic are listed on his Kardex and on the front of his chart.

Does the patient have any medical problems? Diseases and/or conditions might limit the use of some drugs or be relevant to the type of treatment instituted. For example, a patient with glaucoma would not be given atropine; a patient with severe spinal deformities might incur serious injury if closed chest cardiac massage is instituted.

Has the patient had any major surgery? The type of surgery should be ascertained, as well as when it was performed. Certain surgery, for example, cardiac surgery, could modify treatment.

Does the patient take *any* drugs, prescription or nonprescription? Insulin? Nitroglycerin? Cardiac drugs? Aspirin? Laxatives? If any drug is taken on a regular basis, when was the last dose taken?

What drugs has the patient been taking that shouldn't be stopped? Examples are steroids and phenytoin (Dilantin).

Obtaining answers to these questions is a

collaborative task of the physician and the nurse.

Diagnosis

A DISTINCTIVE HISTORY is a definite aid in diagnosis. Any symptoms experienced by the patient prior to admission are important and may aid in diagnosis. The patient may be acutely ill and the history may have to come from the family who may or may not be aware of the symptoms and/or problems the patient experienced prior to admission. The nurse will report any additional data which the patient discloses after the physician leaves him. If the patient is anxious, which is often the case, he may not recall or may distort events leading up to his admission.

PHYSICAL EXAMINATION includes nonauscultatory modes such as palpation as well as inspection of the chest. Auscultation of the heart and chest with the stethoscope can reveal heart murmurs, sounds of valve closure, changes in rhythm and rate, pericardial friction rub, and moist, crackling sounds in the lungs called rales, an early finding in left ventricular failure indicating pulmonary edema.

ELECTROCARDIOGRAM. Usually, it is ordered as soon as myocardial infarction is suspected, and it may be repeated several times (serial ECG's) in determining the diagnosis and in following the course of the illness.

LABORATORY STUDIES. Necrosis of myocardial tissue results in the release of intracellular enzymes into the circulation. These enzymes are not specific for myocardial tissue alone, but are useful as a diagnostic aid in this as well as other conditions involving tissue damage. The CPK (creatine phosphokinase), LDH (lactic acid dehydrogenase), and SGOT (serum glutamic oxalacetic transaminase) are especially used as indicators of the severity of tissue damage. Normal values vary according to laboratory methods.

An elevated erythrocyte sedimentation rate and white blood cell count are also evidence of tissue necrosis in myocardial infarction.

TEMPERATURE. Fever is common after a day or so. Usually, it is low or moderate, and lasts 4 or 5 days. Fever is one of the body's responses to necrosis of tissue. The oral thermometer is most often used. Rectal temperature is most accurate, but is not used in some cardiac units because of the potential harm from vagal stimuli. The use of a well-lubricated rectal thermometer inserted gently with the patient in a comfortable, safe position should prevent harmful vagal stimulation which could result in cardiac slowing and the appearance of arrhythmias.

Pathology

The site of a myocardial infarction is most frequently in the left ventricle. The area of a myocardial infarction heals by scar tissue. The size of the scar usually determines the amount of cardiac reserve that is lost. Thus, a large area of infarction decreases the pumping ability of the heart.

Necrosis can extend through the thickness of the myocardial wall to the subendocardium (transmural infarction), involve part of the myocardium, or may just involve the subendocardial area which is furthest from the blood supply. Different terms are used to describe the area of the heart which is affected. For example, in most people the right coronary artery and its branches supply the posterior wall of the ventricle. Occlusion of this artery results in what is called a posterior wall or diaphragmatic infarction. Heart block is more common with this type of infarction because a branch of the right coronary vessel supplies the A-V node. Another branch supplies the S-A node. Because it supplies these vital parts of the conduction system, the right coronary artery is thought to be the artery of sudden death.

The left coronary artery and its branches supply most of the anterior and apical portions of the left ventricle. Infarctions from occlusion of these branches are termed anterior wall, or anteroseptal.

The stages of healing can be correlated with the period of restriction of cardiac workload. From the onset until about the third day, there is acute tissue degeneration and the infarct area is soft, mushy and necrotic. It is dead tissue and therefore electrically inert. Dangerous arrhythmias are most apt to develop during this period, but they are thought to arise from the peri-infarction area which is ischemic and electrically unstable.

From the fourth to seventh days, softening of the infarcted area is greatest and there is danger of aneurysm formation. The weakened area in the ventricular wall may balloon out during systole. About the eighth to tenth day newly formed capillaries develop around the periphery of the infarct, but it is 2 to 3 weeks before there is a functionally significant collateral circulation.

Collagen begins to form about the twelfth day after the infarction. Rupture of the ventricle is likeliest from onset to the fourteenth day. It is 3 to 4 weeks before the scar begins to grow firm and 2 to 3 months before a scar of maximum strength is formed.

Objectives of care

Most of the time when the myocardial infarction patient arrives at the hospital, the heart damage has been done. The infarction can be extended, however, or other complications can develop. The objectives of care include the reduction of cardiac workload to prevent further damage and promote healing. This is accomplished through a program of optimal rest, which includes helping the patient and family to accept and adjust to the experience.

REST AND ACTIVITY. Optimal rest is a broad concept. Studies have shown that putting a patient to bed is not synonymous with putting him to rest. Prolonged bed rest favors the development of many complications which at worst can prove fatal, or at best prolong convalescence. A program of preventive measures—such as deep breathing and foot or leg exercises aimed specifically at reducing the hazards of immobility, and a bowel hygiene program—is essential if the chief treatment of infarction—rest—is not to become a liability.

Unlike a broken leg, which can be immobilized in plaster, the heart can never be immobilized. It works all the time, even when injured. It rests only during diastole. Therefore, the treatment of cardiac arrhythmias which adversely affect cardiac hemodynamics or the use of a drug such as digitalis to enhance cardiac systole and the diastolic or resting period of the cardiac cycle affords rest for the heart in the broad sense.

One of the hazards of bed rest is the Valsalva maneuver. This maneuver is accomplished with a forced expiration against a closed glottis. This can occur, for example, while straining to defecate or void, to lift oneself up in bed, during gagging, vomiting, or severe coughing. During the Valsalva maneuver, intrathoracic pressure is increased and blood is trapped in the great veins preventing it from entering the chest and right atrium. The heart actually gets smaller in size and, after an initial decrease in heart rate due to vagal stimulation, the rate accelerates. When the breath is released, blood gushes into the heart and rapidly distends it. This "overshoot" results in increased blood pressure and tachycardia which stimulate pressor receptors in the carotid sinus and aorta. A reflex bradycardia then ensues which can prove fatal for the patient with a damaged heart.

Since it is sometimes physically impossible to move patients precisely when they wish to be moved, patients should be instructed to avoid the Valsalva maneuver by exhaling rather than holding the breath when moving in bed.

Whenever caring for a patient with myocardial infarction, the nurse should find out specifically what the patient may and may not do. This information is shared with every member of the nursing staff caring for the patient by approximate notation on the nursing care plan so that one person does not let the patient feed himself at breakfast, and another insist that he be fed at lunch.

Certain principles apply to a program of rest, regardless of the exact program that has been prescribed:

- Do not allow the patient to exert himself. Straining at stool is one common example. Find out what the patient's usual bowel routine is and help him to maintain it in the hospital if it does not violate any physiological principles.

  Studies have shown that the use of the bedside commode often involves less energy expenditure than getting on and off and using the bedpan. The risk of inadvertently performing the Valsalva maneuver is minimized. The patient still requires assistance in cleansing himself after defecation.

  To avoid straining and bladder distention some physicians permit their male patients to stand at the side of the bed to void. Give the patient privacy, but stay close by to assist him to get back to bed.
- Place things within easy reach—the glass of water, the radio, the call bell—so that the patient does not have to use effort to reach them.
- If the patient strenuously objects to certain activity restrictions, discuss this with the physician, who may permit more flexibility, or who may be more effectively persuasive than the nurse. Refusal to accept activity restrictions is sometimes a manifestation of denial. Since this is an unconscious defense against anxiety, reasoning with the patient often does not help. Attempting to force restrictions can only increase the patient's anxiety and cardiac workload. The patient needs the nonjudgmental support of the nurse and family during this overwhelming adjustment period. Threatening or scolding increase his need for dangerous defense mechanisms. Supportive listening can

gradually assist the patient to begin to acknowledge what has happened.

Observe the patient as well as the cardiac monitor during changes of activity. Physical and emotional strain (such as from an upsetting visitor) can be reflected in cardiac arrhythmias as well as increased pain, pulse rate, dyspnea. The nurse then uses judgment in slowing down or eliminating the activity temporarily, then discussing it with the physician.

▪ If care is needed that may tire the patient, do it slowly, and allow for rest periods. Giving a bath and changing the bed may be fatiguing if they are undertaken all at once. In a well-staffed coronary unit, the bath can be given at any time of the day, according to the need and preference of the patient.

Many physicians believe that the safest, quickest, and most effective way of helping the patient to resume activity is to observe meticulously his reaction to slightly increased amounts of activity, and to be guided accordingly in allowing increases in activity. The patient is observed for arrhythmias on the cardiac monitor or irregularity of the pulse, chest pain, excessive fatigue, increased pulse and respiratory rates, and changes in the blood pressure. Such indices are being used increasingly in planning the patient's return to activity instead of regimens of bed rest for a stated number of weeks for every patient who has suffered myocardial infarction.

Sedation. Sedatives or tranquilizers are sometimes ordered after narcotics are no longer necessary for pain. These drugs should facilitate the patient's rest and relaxation, but should not make him so somnolent that he no longer initiates deep breathing, leg exercises, or moving in bed. Older patients, especially, may have paradoxical reactions to sedative drugs and become hyperactive.

Observation and accurate reporting are essential. Note carefully the location and the intensity of the chest pain, or whether there are any symptoms of dyspnea or cyanosis. Are physical or emotional activity associated with pain and/or arrhythmias? Absence of pain is not necessarily an indication that the patient is recovering. When the affected myocardial tissues die, the nerves in that portion of myocardium can no longer transmit impulses to the brain, and the pain ceases. Sometimes nurses are lulled into a false sense of security when the patient's pain abates or there is normal sinus rhythm. Do not relax vigilance; patients with myocardial infarction are disposed to sudden changes in their condition.

The patient's TPR and blood pressure are observed carefully. The temperature is usually taken every 4 hours. Note both the rate and the quality of the pulse. Blood pressure readings are usually ordered every 2 hours for the first several days. Intake and output are carefully noted for all patients for the first 3 days, or longer if the patient has symptoms of congestive heart failure or if shock has been severe.

Environment and Emotional Support. A well-managed coronary care unit is not a noisy, hectic place. The principle of the unit is to prevent the drama of resuscitation efforts by close observation and early treatment of complications. There is an element of heightened awareness and periods of sustained tension because changes can occur suddenly. Ideally the hospital area where coronary patients are admitted should be separate from but may be adjacent to the surgical or medical intensive care areas.

Though the patient may have a familiarity with the idea of a coronary care unit, coming upon it as he does abruptly and in the role of patient may make him more bewildered if he notices its difference compared with usual hospital units. He may ask specific or general questions but due to his anxiety answers may have to be repeated on other occasions. He may initially distort what is in his environment, and may show signs of disorientation and confusion.

The patient who suffers a myocardial infarction is beset by many fears. The two that predominate are the fear of death and the fear of living with impending death. The patient must cope with these as well as threats to his physical integrity, change in body image and self-concept, loss of status at work, reduction of income or even loss of job, loss of prestige in social life, restriction of favorite activities, loss of ability to care for family at least temporarily, and a potentially formidable barrier to the accomplishment of life goals.

Faced with many potential losses, small wonder that patients studied in a coronary care unit were found to experience many disturbing feelings—anxiety, anger, sorrow, depression, bitterness, clingingness, demandingness, and hopelessness. This last feeling, intermittent hopelessness, was found to be the most difficult for the patient and for the nursing staff to deal with. An appropriate response by the staff to this feeling was derived from the simple truth that we do not know that a situation is hopeless; all of our medical knowledge and skills are employed to help because there is some hope. It was thought that the major part of the struggle with hopelessness remained the patient's task to resolve. Helpful nursing action includes the capacity to confront the patient openly and humanly, to empathize with his situation, to think and feel about it and not turn away from him or rush to intervene in this painful circumstance over which the nurse has little control. Being able to say to a patient, "The other patient died," rather than "He was transferred," respects the patient's maturity and his capacity to employ defenses against facts which, temporarily, at least, are intolerable to him.

Inevitably some patients will die, many after a predictably downhill course. Assisting the patient to die with dignity is a formidable task in a coronary care unit where resuscitation attempt is a general rule. Visitors and other patients become aware when such an attempt is in progress—from the increase in activity, numbers of personnel, and characteristic sounds. It is well for one staff member to be assigned to visit these people, explain what is happening, discuss what needs to be discussed, and stay with visitors or find someone such as a clergyman to stay. Otherwise, a state of heightened anxiety pervades the environment with especially harmful physiological and psychological consequences on other patients.

Treatment of complications

Arrhythmias. Disturbances of Heart Rate, Rhythm, and Conduction. Many myocardial infarction patients have some type of arrhythmia during the acute phase. Over half of the deaths from myocardial infarction occur within 72 hours of admission to the hospital. Many of these deaths result from cardiac arrhythmias. Typically, the abnormal rhythm occurs suddenly within the first 3 days after the infarction, and it can be fatal within a few minutes. The arrhythmia can represent a transient abnormality in a heart that otherwise is capable of sustaining life and usual activity later. Consequently, prompt, effective treatment of arrhythmia assumes tremendous importance. If he can be helped to survive the episode of ectopic rhythm, he may not die from myocardial infarction.

Venous Thrombosis. This condition arises mostly in the veins of the lower extremities and pelvis. The exact cause is unknown. People who are ambulatory may also develop venous thrombosis. The use of Ace bandages, antiembolic stockings, positioning pillows, and foot and leg exercises on a regularly scheduled basis are measures employed to prevent thrombus formation.

Some physicians treat all patients who have myocardial infarcts, regardless of the severity, with anticoagulants. Others reserve this treatment for patients whose heart damage has been severe or who experience complications. Anticoagulants are given to decrease the likelihood of venous thrombosis and emboli and to prevent further increase in the size of a clot already formed.

Pulmonary Embolism. Most pulmonary emboli arise from venous clots in the lower extremities and pelvis. Many do not cause pulmonary infarction. A lung scan and angiocardiogram would be necessary if embolectomy were contemplated. For the patient with myocardial infarction, however, this is extremely risky. Anticoagulation and vena caval ligation would probably be considered.

Arterial Emboli. A clot can form in the left ventricular cavity overlying the infarcted area (mural thrombus). Part of it can break off and enter the systemic arterial circulation and cause occlusion of peripheral arteries, resulting in a mottled, cold, pulseless extremity, or of cerebral arteries, resulting in sudden stroke. The nurse should listen carefully to the patient's complaint of extremity pain and check for differences in temperature of the extremities. Arteriotomy and embolectomy may be necessary. The patient is also observed for severe pain in any part of the body, slurring of speech, change in level of consciousness, weakness, and paralysis, all of which are signs of an embolus.

Congestive Heart Failure. One complication of myocardial infarction is congestive heart failure. Onset may be sudden or the condition may develop over a period of hours or days. See Chapter 24 for the signs, symptoms, treatment, and nursing management of the patient with congestive heart failure and pulmonary edema.

Cardiogenic Shock. This is a dreaded complication because of the high mortality rate. Eighty percent of patients with this diagnosis die. The earlier shock is detected and treatment instituted, the better are the patient's chances of survival.

Because some believe that this mortality rate cannot be reduced further by conventional therapy, and because the size of the infarction is not always related to the extreme degree of shock, mechanical assistance devices for the failing ventricle following myocardial infarction have been successfully used in some patients.

Other complications include ventricular aneurysm and ventricular rupture.

Ventricular aneurysm decreases the pumping action of the heart, and angina or congestive failure may result. Some ventricular aneurysms can be surgically corrected. Those that cannot be corrected surgically may rupture at any time. Rupture of the aneurysm is fatal.

Cardiac rupture occurs when a soft necrotic area gives way. Hemopericardium, cardiac tamponade, and relatively sudden death ensue. There can also be rupture of the interventricular septum. Dyspnea, rapid right heart failure, and shock result; the prognosis is poor though survival is possible.

Preparation for transfer

Transfer from the coronary care unit generally means progress for the patient. He has survived one critical period and can go to an area of the hospital where the close observation of the CCU is unavailable but also unnecessary. "Can I get along without my monitor? What happens if I need a nurse right away? What about my chest pain—I still have angina? Can they help me if I have a cardiac arrest?" are questions which the patient probably poses to himself.

Ideally, patients with a myocardial infarction should be transferred to a postcoronary division where specially prepared staff can help the patient through the transition period. Remote control monitoring or telemetry may be available in such an area. This is not always possible. The staff who receives the patient, however, must be aware that despite the fact that the patient may look and feel well and has survived his CCU stay, he is still critically ill and subject to all of the complications of acute myocardial infarction.

The patient should have the opportunity in the CCU to discuss his thoughts and feelings about the transfer. A length of time in the CCU without a cardiac monitor and IV (weaning period) gives the patient confidence that he can, in fact, survive without them. A realistic projection of the length of stay in the CCU and visits from the staff of the transfer unit help the patient to make the adjustment when the time comes.

If possible, nursing visits from the CCU staff should continue after transfer. When all units where coronary patients are cared for are physically adjacent, staff can circulate among units and thus have the opportunity to care for the patient during the various phases of hospitalization. The clinical specialist may be able to follow patients through various hospital areas and stimulate and coordinate continuity of nursing care, including a patient-family education program.

Later management and rehabilitation

Of the approximately 80 percent of patients who survive their first myocardial infarction, some will be troubled by angina or congestive heart failure. Most patients, however, will look and feel well after their transfer from the CCU. They continue to need nursing care, but care at this point involves more of the counseling, teaching, and socializing aspects of the nursing role, rather than technical or mother-surrogate components.

This is the period when the patient begins to come to grips with some of the changes in life that the infarction has precipitated. This can be a long-term process with much of the "rethinking" coming after discharge. For many, this time has a profound philosophical dimension.

The nurse helps during this period by offering to be a listener as the patient attempts to work out his problems; by planning with the patient, family, or volunteer staff for appropriate diversion; and by reviewing with the patient and family those aspects of activity, drugs, diet, or other treatment such as a pacemaker which are part of the postdischarge medical plan.

A family member who might feel foolish or embarrassed to admit difficulty in coping with a situation may need to be encouraged to seek the care of a physician. Family members who themselves receive support are in a better position to offer support to the patient.

If the patient needs nursing or homemaker assistance at home, or a stay in an intermediate care facility, referrals are instituted early in the postdischarge period.

The nurse also contributes by assisting the patient to get answers to questions which may bother him, but which he may hesitate to ask. For example, it can be assumed that postcoronary patients will have questions about resumption of sex activity. Many are hesitant to ask questions about this. The nurse can detect clues that the patient may need help with this subject and can assist him and his spouse to formulate the questions and seek the physician's advice. When the limitations are reviewed and understood, the couple is in a better position to make their own decisions.

His arrival at home does not mean that the patient can resume his former activities. Usually, he is instructed to rest for at least 2 to 3 months, gradually increasing his activity as prescribed. Strenuous unprescribed physical exertion and emotional strain must be avoided. If all goes well, the patient may be permitted to return to work at the end of 2 to 3 months. The doctor may advise working part time, particularly at first. If the patient's work involves heavy responsibilities or considerable physical or emotional exertion, it may be necessary for him to find a less demanding type of work. There has been a trend in recent years toward a more scientific approach to the prescription of activity for patients after myocardial infarction and the enhancement of their physical fitness.

Prognosis

Although myocardial infarction is a serious event, constituting one of the major causes of death among older people, many patients not only survive the attack but also are able to return to work. Because the underlying condition of atherosclerosis is still present, the patient may have repeated attacks of myocardial infarction, or he may develop angina pectoris. Statistics concerning mortality apply to groups and not to specific individuals within groups. It is difficult to predict what the future holds for the individual patient. Some live comfortably and actively for many years afterward.

General nutritional considerations

- The patient admitted to the coronary care unit is usually allowed clear liquids (usually at room temperature); iced and hot fluids are omitted or allowed to come to room temperature. As food can be tolerated, the patient progresses to a full liquid diet and then to a soft and then a regular diet.
- Types of diets ordered for cardiac patients vary. Usual ones are the sodium-restricted diet (in which the amount of sodium allowed is expressed in milligrams), a low-cholesterol diet, a weight-reduction diet, and the cardiac prudent diet. Some physicians feel that special diets often cause anxiety, and therefore allow the patient to eat a house diet but omit adding salt to the food served.
- Once the patient is feeling better, any of the above-mentioned diets may prove unpalatable. If the patient complains about his food, this should be reported to his physician.

General pharmacological considerations

- Drugs administered to the patient in the coronary care unit are prescribed according to the symptoms presented and underlying disease processes. Drugs commonly used in a CCU include the following:

  Cardiotonic drugs such as digitalis and digoxin are used in management of congestive heart failure, atrial fibrillation, prevention of paroxysmal atrial or nodal tachycardia.

  Cardiac depressants such as quinidine, lidocaine, procainamide (Pronestyl), phenytoin (Dilantin), and propranolol (Inderal) are used in ventricular arrhythmias. Lidocaine and propranolol are used most often as emergency drugs for acute ventricular arrhythmias.

  Anticoagulants such as warfarin sodium (Coumadin), dicumarol, and phenindione (Hedulin) are usually used prophylactically to prevent development of venous thrombosis or atrial emboli.

  Narcotic analgesics such as meperidine (Demerol) and morphine are used to control severe chest pain.

  Tranquilizers such as chlorazepate (Tranxene), diazepam (Valium), and chlormezanone (Trancopal) are used in treatment of anxiety and as daytime sedatives.

  Sedatives/hypnotics such as secobarbital (Seconal), chloral hydrate, and flurazepam (Dalmane) are usually used in hypnotic doses (i.e., to produce sleep). The physician may also choose to order tranquilizers h.s. and not use a barbiturate or nonbarbiturate-type hypnotic.

  Diuretics such as mercaptomerin (Thiomerin), spironolactone (Aldactone), trichlormethiazide (Naqua), and furosemide (Lasix) are used in congestive heart failure and pulmonary edema.

  Electrolytes. Potassium (Kaochlor, Kay Ciel) is the usual electrolyte administered, especially when patients receive diuretics, to replace the potassium lost through massive diuresis.

- The nurse should consult appropriate references for the doses, precautions, contraindications, and side effects of drugs used to treat the patient with a myocardial infarction.

Bibliography

ALLENDORF, E. E. and KEEGAN, M. H.: Teaching patients about nitroglycerin. Am. J. Nurs. 75:1168, July, 1975.

ANDREOLI, K. G. et al: *Comprehensive Cardiac Care,* ed. 3. St. Louis, Mosby, 1975.

ARMINGTON, SISTER C. and CREIGHTON, H.: *Nursing of People with Cardiovascular Problems.* Boston, Little, Brown, 1971.

BATES, B.: *A Guide to Physical Examination.* Philadelphia, Lippincott, 1974.

BERGER, H.: Heart attack: Help the patient help himself. Consultant 114:132, March, 1974.

HOUSER, D.: Safer care for the M.I. patient. Nurs. '74, 4:42, July, 1974.

KÜBLER-ROSS, E.: *Questions and Answers on Death and Dying.* New York, Macmillan, 1974.

METHENY, N. M. and SNIVELY, W. D.: *Nurses' Handbook of Fluid Balance,* ed. 2. Philadelphia, Lippincott, 1974.

RIEHL, C. L.: *Coronary Nursing Care.* New York, Appleton-Century-Crofts, 1971.

RODMAN, T. et al: *The Physiologic and Pharmacologic Basis of Coronary Care Nursing.* St. Louis, Mosby, 1971.

ROMHILT, D. W. et al: Initial signs and early complications in acute myocardial infarction (pictorial). Hosp. Med. 10:8, November, 1974.

SANDERSON, R. G. et al: *The Cardiac Patient: A Comprehensive Approach.* Saunders Monographs in Nursing, No. 2. Philadelphia, Saunders, 1973.

SAYLOR, D. E.: Nursing response to behavioral changes in the cardiac patient. J. Prac. Nurs. 25:16, February, 1975.

SCHERER, J. C.: *Introductory Clinical Pharmacology.* Philadelphia, Lippincott, 1975.

SMITH, C. A.: Body image changes after myocardial infarction. Nurs. Clin. North Am. 7:663, December, 1972.

TYZENHOUSE, P. S.: Myocardial infarction: Its effect on the family. Am. J. Nurs. 73:1012, June, 1973.

What the EKG can tell about myocardial infarction (pictorial). Nurs. '75, 5:35, July, 1975.

WILLIAMS, S. R.: *Nutrition and Diet Therapy,* ed. 2. St. Louis, Mosby, 1973.

CHAPTER 49

Cardiac surgical nursing

On completion of this chapter the student will:

- **Discuss how surgery might improve cardiac function.**
- **Name some of the cardiac lesions requiring surgical correction.**
- **Describe the surgical correction employed for ischemic heart disease.**
- **Discuss the nursing management of a patient having cardiac surgery and describe nursing actions during the pre- and postoperative period.**
- **Formulate a nursing care plan for and participate in the nursing management of a patient with open-heart surgery.**

The patient who has decided to have surgery performed on his heart is taking a calculated risk for a longer and a more healthy life. Patients enter the hospital with varying degrees of emotional readiness to face the operation. The preoperative period can help them to feel secure in the hospital by demonstrating to them the competence and the concern of the physicians and the nurses. The patient's long illness, and, perhaps, a previous hospitalization that may have prevented his employment, as well as the high cost of past and present hospitalization with the necessary special equipment, drugs, and nursing management, may leave the patient drained physically, emotionally, and financially.

One important key to the nursing management of patients undergoing cardiac surgery is to remember that two physiological systems of the body have been affected, the cardiac and the respiratory. These systems are directly affected by anxiety and stress-producing situations. The nurse must take this phenomenon into consideration when she is noting physical characteristics and vital signs.

As she would with any patient, the nurse must be alert to the different forms that anxiety may take. She must allow the patient to express fear and anger, remembering that, in submitting to cardiac surgery, he is showing bravery in taking a calculated risk. The nurse refers medical questions to the physician, and helps the patient find answers to those questions which are answerable. Repeated experience has demonstrated that unanswered questions lead to increasing anxiety and lessened confidence in the staff.

Open-Heart Surgery or Intracardiac Surgery. A major breakthrough in cardiac surgery was due to understanding the hemodynamics of cardiopulmonary bypass. This information allowed engineers and biological technicians, as well as many others, to collaborate their efforts and develop the artificial heart-lung machine. The advent of this device provided a means by which the patient's circulation could be rerouted and supported during surgery. Certain drugs, such as concentrated solutions of potassium, can be used to stop the heartbeat temporarily. The surgeon can open the heart and correct the pathology under direct vision while working in a bloodless field.

Today we are in an era of development of a number of cardiovascular prostheses to repair many congenital and acquired defects.

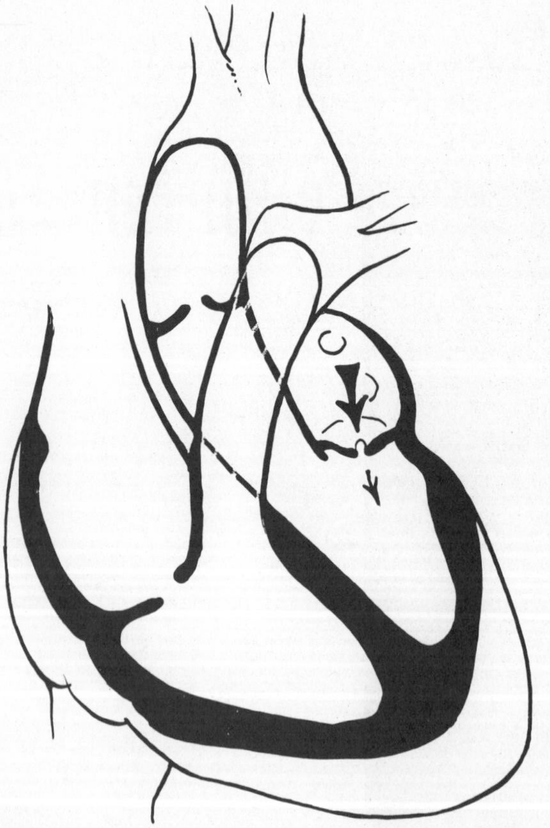

figure 49-1. Mitral stenosis. The narrowed valve does not permit blood to flow freely from the left atrium to the left ventricle.

Cardiac valve replacement

Severely damaged aortic, mitral, or tricuspid valves can be replaced by artificial valves. Some patients require multiple replacements and as many as two and three damaged valves have been successfully replaced. While artificial valves differ in design and in the materials from which they are constructed, they tend to share a number of common problems, one of which is the development of thrombi.

Cardiac lesions requiring corrective surgery

- Congenital heart lesions.
- Acquired heart lesions. Acquired heart disease includes pathological processes in the heart or great vessels that were not present at birth but have incurred since that time: acquired valvular disease due to an infectious process, ischemic heart disease, tumors of the heart, aneurysms of the heart, and traumatic injuries to the heart.

Acquired valvular diseases of the heart

Acquired lesions of the valves are most frequently of rheumatic origin. The initial process occurs early in life, usually between ages 5 and 15. Acquired valvular diseases may be caused by subacute or acute bacterial endocarditis which produces an inflammation of the lining of the heart including the lining of the valves. As an end result, heart valves, particularly the mitral and aortic valves, can become scarred and function improperly.

Undiagnosed and/or untreated cases of syphilis can also affect the aortic valve. Surgical reconstruction may be necessary for correction.

Pathologic valve processes

Stenosis (narrowing) of Cardiac Valves. The valve can become so tightened and narrowed that its lumen is reduced to pencil-point size (stenosis of valve) (Fig. 49-1). The scarred valve opens upon cardiac contraction, but the reduced size of the lumen limits the amount of blood that can flow through it.

Insufficient Valves. As a result of the processes of scarring, fusion of the valve leaflets, and eventual calcification, the valves are no longer capable of closing properly. Blood regurgitates backward, through the incompetent valve. A damaged heart valve may be stenotic or insufficient or both. Aortic insufficiency is the most serious of the valvular diseases.

Surgical repair of valvular heart disease

Closed Repair. The treatment of a stenotic valve used to be limited to closed repair (commissurotomy). The surgeon felt, rather than saw the abnormal valve, thus making this technique useful only to dilate fused valves. Open repair (see below) using cardiopulmonary bypass (heart-lung machine) is now the preferred method of valve repair.

Open Repair. Today the surgeon has the advantage of choosing to dilate, reconstruct (valvuloplasty), or replace diseased valves. The open-heart surgical technique is most frequently chosen.

Under direct vision, the surgeon can control the localization of the obstruction, prevent calcified tissue or an undetected atrial thrombus from dislodging to the bloodstream, and replace the damaged valve.

Mortality has been gradually decreasing. All patients do better if the valvular lesion is corrected before serious secondary involvement of the myocardium and lungs occur.

Ischemic heart disease

Atherosclerotic heart disease is the leading type of heart disease in the United States. Hence, extensive surgical research techniques have been established in an effort to increase the amount of blood reaching the heart muscle and to redirect blood to the ischemic myocardial muscle.

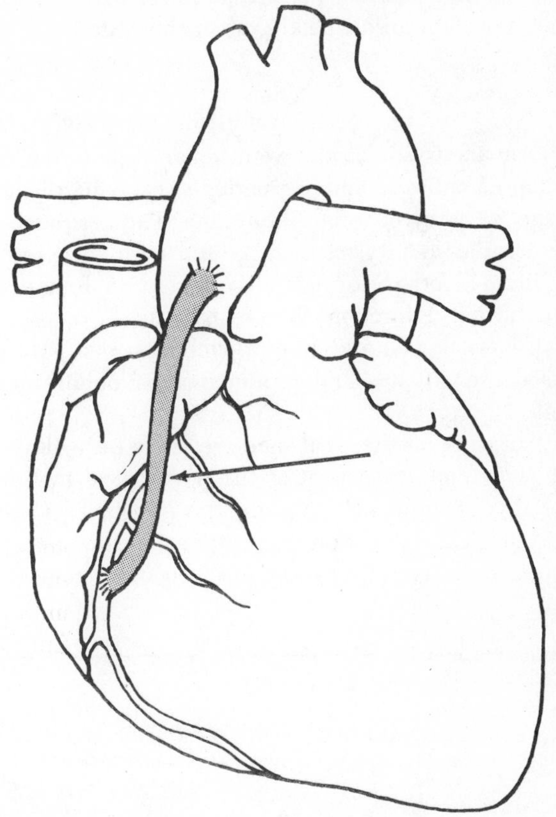

figure 49-2. Using a section of saphenous vein to bypass a coronary artery.

Coronary artery surgery

A widely used technique to increase the supply of blood to the myocardium is the saphenous vein revascularization procedure (Fig. 49-2). A section of saphenous vein is removed from the patient's leg and used to bypass the affected (blocked or narrowed) area of the coronary artery. In another type of coronary artery surgery, a branch of the internal mammary artery is used to bypass the affected area.

Direct open-heart approach

Atherosclerotic deposits or clots obstructing the coronary arteries are frequently confined to a relatively short section of artery. Arterial transplants of blood vessel graft, as well as artificial grafts, have been developed to correct this. The surgical approach is directed at opening the vessel, removing the plaque in the diseased intima (endarterectomy), or replacing the area with an artificial graft or homograft.

Ventricular aneurysm

An aneurysm of the ventricular wall is the most lethal complication among patients surviving the acute stage of a myocardial infarction. The frequency of ventricular aneurysms is increased with the presence of high blood pressure and overexertion following a myocardial infarction. The elasticity of the muscle wall is weakened and an outpouching occurs. The diseased area dilates and produces a ballooning of the wall.

Suturing off the weakened area may be required as an emergency treatment as the paradoxical motion of the myocardium may rupture the pouch. If possible, the surgical correction is postponed until after the acute stage. The damaged tissue becomes necrotic and cannot tolerate the correction until scar tissue appears. This may take 4 to 8 weeks.

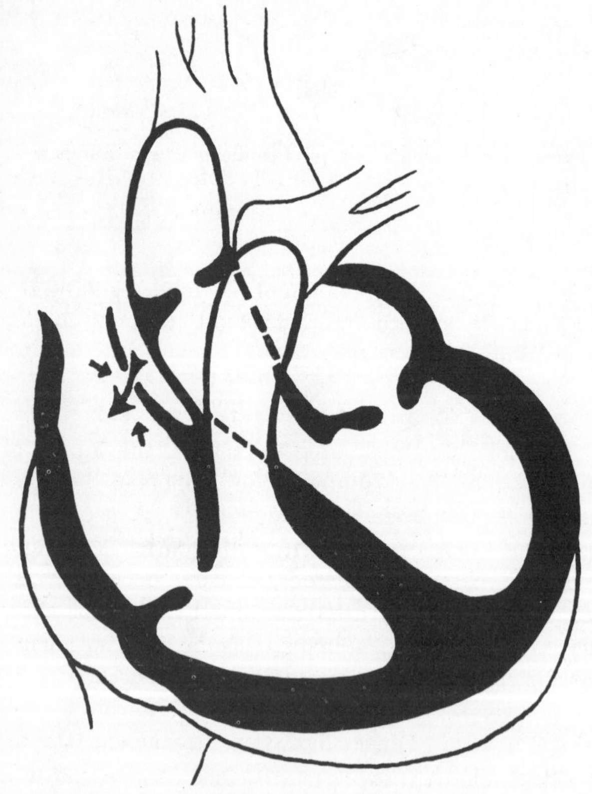

figure 49-3. Atrial-septal defect. The abnormal hole in the wall between the right and the left atria at first allows a left-to-right leakage of blood. Later, there may be a right-to-left shunting of blood.

Tumors of the heart

Primary tumors of the heart are rare. However, tumors may be benign or malignant. The clinical course usually depends upon the type of tumor and its location within the cardiac system, that is, if it occupies space within the chambers of the heart or is contained within the muscle. Large tumors located on the left side of the heart may produce signs of mitral valve disease.

Surgery, using cardiopulmonary bypass, may be undertaken as cardiac failure may occur, and the potential of embolization is often present. Benign tumors may stem from a base of a pedicle and their removal is usually uncomplicated. Malignant tumors are more difficult to remove, and the patient's prognosis is extremely poor.

Atrial-septal defect

An *atrial-septal defect* is a hole in the cardiac septum that separates the right and the left atria (Fig. 49-3).

Normally, the pressure within the heart is higher in the left atrium than in the right atrium; therefore, in a heart with an atrial-septal defect, blood flows from the left atrium through the hole to the right atrium. Because this blood has already been through the lungs, it is oxygenated. From the right atrium the blood goes to the right ventricle and back to the lungs. This inefficient functioning puts a strain on the right atrium, which enlarges in response to the extra load of blood. Over a period of time the right ventricle also enlarges, and, eventually, so does the pulmonary artery. If the condition is not corrected, pulmonary vessel resistance may increase, and right-sided pulmonary hypertension occurs. The right ventricle becomes unable fully to empty itself of blood during each contraction because of the increased resistance in the pulmonary vessels. As a result, blood is backed up into the right atrium. When the pressure in this chamber grows higher than the pressure in the left atrium, there will be a reversal of the direction of leakage of blood. Now it will go from the right to the left through the defect in the wall. But the blood that goes from the right to the left has *not* been through the lungs; nevertheless, it is sent on through the left atrium, the left ventricle and the aorta into the general circulation. Because the oxygen content of the blood being pumped from the left ventricle is lower than normal, the patient at this stage of the pathological process can develop cyanosis.

Symptoms of right-sided failure include venous distention, ascites, and peripheral edema as blood backs up through the venous system network. Patients also may experience bouts of palpitation and tachycardia fatigue and frequent respiratory infections.

Patients who have a small defect may be symptom-free. If the defect is repaired by surgery before a right-to-left shunt develops, there is an excellent chance of complete closure of the defect, followed by a lessening of the secondary pathological cardiac changes. Usually, open-heart surgery is the procedure of choice.

Traumatic heart lesions

A nonpenetrating injury of the chest may include bruising of the heart. For example, a patient who has been crushed against the steering wheel of a car may have some bleeding of the muscle of the heart. Because the heart is in a closed sac, blood will accumulate in the pericardial space and cause tamponade of the heart.

Most often the patient will need to have the fluid in the pericardial sac aspirated. The physician inserts a long needle into the pericardial sac (pericardial paracentesis). During this procedure the patient is usually placed at approximately a 45-degree angle. One aspiration is sufficient in many patients, but, if the bleeding continues, an open thoracotomy may be indicated to control the bleeding site.

The pulse is taken frequently of all patients with compressing chest injuries. There may be inhibition of the vagus nerve, with a slowing pulse, and perhaps cardiac standstill. Cardiac and respiratory resuscitation equipment is kept handy and ready for instant use. The pain from a bruised heart may be masked by the pain from other chest injuries.

Direct trauma to the myocardium, such as a stab wound, may also cause leakage of blood into the pericardium; the tear in the pericardium often seals with a clot, while the tear in the myocardium continues to bleed. If the wound is large enough to cause immediate shock from hemorrhage, the patient will be taken to the operating room from the ambulance.

A small wound of the myocardium may lose blood to the pericardium over a longer period of time. The nurse observes for shock and signs of cardiac compression, such as distention of the superficial veins of the neck, cyanosis, dyspnea, hypotension, and a paradoxical pulse. Relaxation of the anal sphincter, with fecal incontinence, is a serious sign not found in other types of chest injuries, and it should be reported to the physician immediately.

Sometimes traumatic tamponade of the heart is treated conservatively, with bed rest and careful observation of the patient. The increased pericardial pressure may serve to stop the leakage of blood and splint the wound. Larger tears will require suturing.

Preoperative nursing management of the cardiac surgical patient

The patient who is to have heart surgery may be hospitalized for 1 or 2 weeks prior to the day of operation and subjected to an extensive and exhausting medical evaluation. A thorough review of all body systems and a precise anatomic diagnosis of the lesion is desired. The patient undergoing surgery will be cared for by a large team of people, including surgeons, cardiologists, radiologists, nurses, dieticians, and technicians.

Diagnosis

During the preoperative period, the patient undergoes many diagnostic studies that determine the capacity of his vital systems. Cardiopulmonary evaluation may include tests and studies such as chest x-ray examinations, an electrocardiogram, pulmonary function studies, a phonocardiogram, laboratory blood studies, and cardioangiography.

The nurse has an obligation to prepare the patient for the test by explaining the importance of it and reviewing some aspects of it. Every effort should be made to ascertain the patient's understanding of the experience and correct any misgivings he may have.

When the procedure is completed the physician evaluates the data and discusses with the patient the findings and the recommended treatment. It is important for the nurse to know what the physician has explained to the patient. The nurse can learn this either by being present at the explanation or by discussing with the physician later what he told the patient.

Observations

There are many obvious symptoms that are associated with the pathology of cardiac disease. A patient's color and sitting position may indicate difficulty in breathing. Facial expression may be tense if chest pain exists. Signs of ankle edema may be noted if fluid retention occurs. Distention of the neck veins may indicate signs of increased venous pressure. Slurred speech, unsteady gait, facial paralysis may all be clues to previous embolic pathology. Clubbing of fingers can suggest congenital pathology.

The nurse observes the patient's symptoms when vital signs are taken. A weak, rapid, and/or irregular pulse beat may be felt and its effect on cardiac output reflected in the patient's color, level of alertness, degree of weakness, dyspnea, or chest pain. A blood pressure recording can denote hypertension or a reduced cardiac output. The rapid rate of respirations may indicate oxygen need or anxiety.

Vital signs, including rectal temperatures, are taken and recorded twice daily. They are important as their values serve as a baseline postoperatively. Observation during the preoperative period requires continuous assessment of the patient's physical and mental status. *Any* change in either is to be reported to the physician.

Environment

One advantage of the waiting period before surgery is to be more certain the patient is free from infection. Persons with cardiac disease and particularly those who have increased pulmonary pressure are prone to lung congestion and frequent upper respiratory tract infections. Patients should be kept away from other patients with contagious diseases. Family or friends with respiratory infections should be encouraged to telephone or send cards rather than visit. An antibiotic may be ordered preoperatively in an effort to prevent postoperative infections.

Preparation of surgical site

Careful preparation of the skin over the operative site is important. Bacteria are found on all levels of the skin. An infection introduced while performing a thoracotomy could be serious and can spread to the sternum, mediastinum, and into the circulatory system.

Usually a bacteriostatic soap is ordered for 1 or 2 days prior to surgery. The patient may assume responsibility for the scrub if he is able to shower himself. The nurse gives whatever assistance is required to those patients whose weakness prevents self-activity. The operative area (chest) is shaved the evening before surgery. Medications are usually discontinued 1 to 2 days prior to surgery; however, each patient is different and some may have medications continued until the night before surgery. A hypnotic is usually given the night before surgery to ensure the patient an adequate night's rest.

Fluid and electrolyte balance

Patients undergoing cardiac surgery are usually on a low-sodium diet during the preoperative period. The hospital prepared low-sodium diet may not be very palatable to the patient. As he becomes more preoccupied with the thought of surgery he may not feel like eating. Careful attention is given to the patient's nutrition so that he receives the necessary carbohydrates, proteins and fats. These play an essential part in the postoperative healing process.

There is a critical need for determining and maintaining fluid and electrolyte balance since most cardiacs have some fluid retention preoperatively and are placed on diuretic therapy and weighed daily. Change in weight indicates the daily fluid loss or gain and on the day of surgery serves as a baseline for calculating the volume of fluid needed in the heart-lung machine during surgery. Some diuretics tend to deplete the serum potassium level. Although they are usually discontinued prior to surgery, a supplement of potassium may be necessary.

Preoperative teaching

Preoperative preparation for surgery varies with each patient. The nurse begins by trying to ascertain what the patient already knows.

Preoperatively, the nurse should attempt to acquaint the patient and his family with the following:

- The purpose of the intensive care unit, that is, to provide a central, well-equipped and well-staffed facility to provide around-the-clock care. The time and length of visiting hours is explained to the family.
- The immediate physical preparation that takes place before the patient enters the operating room.
- The patient practices deep breathing and coughing which he will use later postoperatively.
- If it is anticipated that the patient will need oxygen administered by an intermittent positive-pressure breathing apparatus, preoperative practice with it is indicated until the patient is familiar with how it works and how it feels.
- Before the operation, the patient is taught the exercises that he will need to employ after-

ward. Both before and after surgery, the patient's condition may warrant only passive exercises.

- The patient is assured that analgesics are available for the control of postoperative pain.
- Most patients are placed on the serious list after surgery. This fact is explained to the patient and his family. The patient should also be allowed to see a member of the clergy if he so chooses.

How much information is given the patient and/or his family depends on the surgeon's evaluation of the patient and his family. Some patients are given a detailed explanation of the operative procedure and what will most likely occur during the postoperative period. The explanation may include a description of tubes, catheters, monitors, and so on, as well as a visit to the recovery room. Other surgeons feel that the patient should have the postoperative period explained, but that a detailed explanation or demonstration of equipment used only increases pre- and postoperative anxiety.

Postoperative nursing management

Although often lifesaving, all cardiac surgery is a severe insult to the body, and the patient requires expert care during the postoperative period. To make significant observations, the nurse needs to understand the nature of the condition, how the abnormality affected the patient's cardiac function, and how the surgery corrected it.

The operating room nurse and the anesthesiologist can briefly provide additional information about the patient's operative experience and the type of procedure done. Any problems during the operative course such as a prolonged time on the heart-lung machine, bleeding problems, or serious cardiac arrhythmias will alert the intensive care nurses to potential problem areas.

The nurse needs to learn as much as possible about the equipment used in connection with surgery—defibrillators, pacemakers, positive-pressure respirators—and know when, how, and why it is used.

After the patient is transferred to bed, the nurse notes the rate and quality of the apical and radial pulses and takes the blood pressure with an arm cuff, as ordered, to watch for signs of hypo- or hypertension. Postoperative observations can be accurate as they are constantly monitored on a cardiac monitor. Any change in the electrocardiogram can be noted immediately.

The patient may also have his arterial blood pressure recorded directly and continuously on another channel of the monitoring device. A small polyethylene catheter may have been left in place in the patient's femoral artery following the completion of the cardiopulmonary bypass. The pressure in this artery is transmitted via the tip of the catheter through rigid plastic tubing to a pressure-sensitive device called a transducer or strain gauge. The transducer converts the mechanical energy of pressure changes within the artery to electrical output. This is calibrated and equated to equivalent changes in millimeters of mercury which can be displayed on an oscilloscope or recorder. Small fluctuations in arterial blood pressure can be recorded and are obtainable at times when cuff blood pressures cannot be obtained. The arterial line also serves as a direct means by which blood for gas studies can be obtained.

A central venous pressure (CVP) reading is also done frequently. This line may also be used for drawing the venous blood samples that are necessary. The normal reading of the central venous pressure in or near the right atrium is estimated around 5 to 12 ml. of water. The numerical value is not as important as the occurrence of a change either increasing or decreasing. Because venous pressure is sensitive to an increased pressure in the respiratory system, the patient should be off the ventilator at the time of the recording.

An endotracheal tube or tracheotomy with mechanical ventilation, assisted or controlled, is used initially. A reduction in the patient's lung capacity may be due to the use of anesthetics or other drugs, a prolonged chronic disease process, pain or fear. The selection of the specific type of respirator to be used and the initial setting of the standard is the responsibility of the physician.

To evaluate the effectiveness of the breathing device and the patient's response, the nurse can use a respirometer. Blood gas studies are also done. The color of the patient's nailbeds and lips may be a clue to inadequate ventilation. Restlessness, flaring of the nares, and a poorly moving chest cage are causes for concern. The prepared nurse can listen to the patient's lungs and note the presence of congestion or diminished breathing sounds. The daily chest x-ray examination report is also valuable to the physician.

The type of intravenous solutions that are ordered will depend upon the patient's need for nourishment as well as laboratory reports of serum electrolytes. The surgeon prescribes the total amount that will effect fluid replacement without overloading the cardiovascular system and the approximate hourly rate. This may need to be adjusted because overloading the circulatory system would place an added strain on the vital organs at this time. The same serious state would occur if the amount of fluid volume were decreased as it may contribute to diminished tissue perfusion. Central venous pressure measurement is used as a guide to fluid replacement.

The major reason for the insertion of the Foley catheter is to allow observation of renal function, and especially to enable the early detection of renal shutdown—particularly if a problem with the kidneys is anticipated (for example, if there has been prolonged hypotension). An hourly output of 30 ml. is adequate; output below this should be reported to the physician. Urinary output upon arrival in the intensive care unit is often increased due to the osmotic diuretics used when the patient is on bypass. This situation corrects itself in a few hours. The patient may also have hemoglobinuria since lysis of blood cells can occur during prolonged cardiopulmonary bypass.

If the Foley catheter is irrigated to prevent clogging, the nurse must remember to deduct the irrigating solution from the total output. Specific gravity readings are taken for information about the patient's hydration and how well his kidneys are concentrating the urine. Drainage from the nasogastric tube also is recorded. Proper functioning of the tube is important as any abdominal distention may exert pressure upon the diaphragm and move it upward, restricting respiratory movement.

The nurse closely observes the chest tubes, making sure the tubes leading from the chest to the underwater seal bottles are not compressed, that there is no leak, and that the drainage flows through them. Unless the connecting tube lies lower than the wound, drainage will not take place. If drainage collects in the coils, the nurse changes the position of the tube so that the drainage flows into the collection bottle. Allowing drainage to remain stationary inside the tube may cause clotting and plugging of the tube. There is need for hourly observation of the amount of drainage. If the drainage is copious, it is recorded more frequently. The amount of blood replacement is determined by the loss of blood volume through the tube and the amount of blood drawn for specimens.

In mitral stenosis there is stasis of blood in the left atrium, and clots may have formed. Any clots observed during surgery are removed, but perhaps one escaped into the general circulation. There is no longer stasis of blood in the left atrium, and the free-flowing blood may push a clot along. The nurse observes for symptoms of emboli in the legs, especially after a commissurotomy. Embolization likewise is a danger after atrial fibrillation, which also allows blood to stay relatively still in the atrium, so that clots may form. After open-heart surgery there is danger of air emboli affecting the brain. Neurological symptoms, such as slurred speech, distortion of facial muscles or the tongue, and hemiparesis, may occur after air or a blood embolus to the brain. Dyspnea, cough, and expectoration of bloody sputum may indicate pulmonary embolism. An embolus to the spleen may cause sudden left flank pain, whereas an embolus to a kidney may result in hematuria and flank pain.

During the early postoperative period, the nurse is aware of the patient's color, his pulse and respirations, cardiac rhythm, his position, the state of his dressing, his blood pressure, the patency of the tubes leaving his body, and the steady drip of the infusions and transfusion. She must notice any changes immediately. A sudden but slight drop in blood pressure, central venous pressure, or hourly urine output may suggest a reduced cardiac output. A respiratory rate increase can result from an obstruction such as a mucous plug, improper positioning, splinting from incisional pain or circulatory insufficiency.

Psychological considerations

If the patient has been on the heart-lung machine (cardiopulmonary bypass or extracorporeal circulation), the lightest possible anesthesia was given, and because hypothermia facilitates anesthesia, the patient usually is conscious when he comes to the recovery unit.

As soon as possible, he should be told that the surgery is over. He may need to hear this several times. He may or may not be aware of the totality of the room, the people in it, and the whole situation. He is aware of his discomfort and the one person with whom he attempts to speak. If the patient complains of pain and the discomfort is not alleviated by positioning and other nursing measures, narcotics are given. The patient's vital signs and the cardiac monitor are checked before a drug is administered and periodically during the time of its effect. The dosage of narcotics given to patients who have had cardiac surgery is frequently less than average because of the danger of respiratory depression. Narcotics are given—only for pain as restlessness is often an indication of hypoxemia.

Some patients develop a psychoticlike reaction after cardiovascular surgery. They are disoriented and have hallucinations. These patients need protection with side rails and the reassurance of a human, caring presence. The cause of this reaction is not known. It may be related to some transient cerebral pathology induced by the surgery, the anesthesia, drug therapy, or the intensive care unit environment. The reaction is usually temporary.

Early mobility of patients is encouraged to prevent circulatory stasis and prevent the formation of thrombi. Active leg exercises are begun on the operative day when the patient's position is changed when possible.

General progression of patient care

As the patient's condition stabilizes the respirator is discontinued and the endotracheal tube is removed —usually in 24 to 48 hours. The patient may then be started on nasal oxygen and will be encouraged to use a Bennett or some other intermittent positive pressure respirator for deep breathing and coughing. The nasogastric tube is usually removed at the same time. The Foley catheter, one intravenous line, the central venous pressure line, and the arterial blood pressure line may be discontinued about a day later. The chest tubes may also be removed on the second or third postoperative day depending upon the amount of drainage that has been noted. If the patient has an artificial cardiac valve, he is started on anticoagulants at this time. They are not started earlier because additional bleeding from the chest may occur. Digitalis preparations may be restarted. Antibiotics are continued intravenously for another four or five days and then if needed are given orally.

The patient's vital signs are taken every 2 hours at this stage and he begins progressive ambulation. A restricted sodium liquid diet is ordered after the endotracheal tube is removed.

The patient who has had an endotracheal tube in place for a day or so will complain of a sore throat and excessive thirst for a few days after it is removed. If the patient is on restricted fluids he will need help in remembering and abiding by this regime. But, careful and consistent explanations from the physicians and nurse plus involving the patient in recording his intake and output gives the patient a chance to participate in his regime, distribute his allotment with some personal choice, and understand the reasons for it.

As the patient's course continues to progress, he begins to see signs of improvement (for example, ambulation) yet he is still feeling sick and remains in a potentially critical phase. While the need for constant observation and evaluation by the nurse is still important, the nurse must attempt to prepare him for his return to a general medical-surgical unit within the next few days.

The nurse begins to encourage him gradually to become more independent and let him begin to regain assurance in doing things for himself. Gentle encouragement accompanied by support as he tries each new activity can help the patient to pass through the period of extreme dependence on staff to greater independence.

Continuing care

While the patient is encouraged to progress at his own rate, careful assessment should be made of the patient's response to activity and his attitude towards it.

The expectation of what will happen after surgery can be important in the patient's postoperative adjustment. If he expected a complete cure and has had only partial relief of his symptoms, he may be resentful, and he may refuse to adhere to his low-sodium diet or to the restrictions on his activities.

These patient reactions are not unusual. Help the patient to identify what is troubling him and to express what he feels. His family may (or may not) be a comfort to him.

The amount of activity the patient can safely tolerate will be determined by the physician. It will be based upon the severity of his illness preoperatively as well as the nature of his operative procedure and the postoperative course.

It is important to collaborate with the physician in helping the family learn what activities the patient can safely assume after discharge. Often families who have experienced a lifetime of caring both physically and mentally for a patient will try to hold him back as they themselves cannot change their role from one which requires the patient to be dependent on them, or they may expect him to resume a full program of activities. He may or may not be able to do so.

If a patient needs domestic help at home arrangements can be sought with the help of social service. If health supervision and some nursing care are to be given a visiting nurse referral can be initiated several days prior to discharge so that there are no gaps in continuity of care.

Some patients are allowed to return to work 6 to 12 weeks postoperatively. Others have a more prolonged postoperative course. Many patients can, however, return to a more productive and satisfying way of life.

Bibliography

BROGAN, M. R.: Nursing care of the patient experiencing cardiac surgery for coronary artery disease. Nurs. Clin. North Am. 7:517, September, 1972.

BRUNNER, L. S. and SUDDARTH, D. S.: *Textbook of Medical-Surgical Nursing,* ed. 3. Philadelphia, Lippincott, 1975.

CALHOUN, P. L., et al: Postoperative care following coronary surgery. Heart Lung 3:912, November/December, 1974.

COLLINS, J. J., et al: Automated management of postoperative cardiac surgical care. Heart Lung 3:929, November/December, 1974.

ELLIS, R.: Unusual sensory and thought disturbances after cardiac surgery. Am. J. Nurs. 72:2021, November, 1972.

LE MAITRE, G. and FINNEGAN, J.: *The Patient in Surgery: A Guide for Nurses*. Philadelphia, Saunders, 1975.

NEVILLE, W. E.: *Care of the Surgical Cardiopulmonary Patient.* Chicago, Yearbook Medical Publishing Co., 1971.

PARSONS, M. C.: The surgical intensive care nurse and cardiac surgery. AORN J. 18:158, July, 1973.

CHAPTER—50

The patient in renal failure

On completion of this chapter the student will:

- **Discuss the etiology and prevention of renal disease.**
- **Discuss the symptoms, pathology, and diagnosis of renal insufficiency.**
- **Discuss the prognosis and objectives of treatment of renal disease.**
- **Formulate a nursing care plan for and participate in the nursing management of a patient with renal insufficiency.**
- **Describe the substitutes for kidney function—hemodialysis and peritoneal dialysis.**
- **Contrast hemodialysis and peritoneal dialysis as to the length of each procedure and the equipment required.**
- **Formulate a nursing care plan for and participate in the nursing management of a patient having hemodialysis and one having peritoneal dialysis.**

Renal failure, acute or chronic, is a serious inability of the kidneys to carry out the normal functions necessary to maintain fluid and electrolyte balance and to eliminate the end products of metabolism from the body. When kidney function is insufficient and such products as urea, other nonprotein nitrogens, creatinine, and uric acid accumulate in the blood, a state of *azotemia* is present. If unabated, the patient experiences the signs and symptoms of *uremia,* such as lethargy, irritability, and anorexia in the early stage, and progressively more ominous ones as uremia advances.

Etiology

Some conditions, such as shock or thrombosis of the arteries supplying the kidneys, markedly decrease the supply of blood to the kidneys. If the ischemia is not immediately remedied, renal failure and uremia can result.

The problem may be within the kidney itself as in acute renal tubular necrosis (lower nephron nephrosis) due, for example, to chemical poisoning from barbiturates, bichloride of mercury, or carbon tetrachloride or to transfusion with incompatible blood. In chronic glomerulonephritis and polycystic disease, progressively more nephrons are destroyed which can result in chronic renal insufficiency as well as acute shutdown.

Problems outside the kidney such as obstruction of the lower urinary tract can cause damage to the kidney parenchyma if not promptly treated.

Prevention

Renal failure occurs more frequently when body fluid reserves are depleted. Nurses contribute to its prevention by planning with hospitalized patients a system of oral fluid intake, particularly for those patients who may be too old, too weak, disinterested, or otherwise unable to reach for the water pitcher on the bedside stand.

Lowered cardiac output due to such conditions as cardiac arrhythmias, anaphylactic shock, or accidental blood loss compromises renal blood flow. Careful nursing observation of the patient and prompt reporting of lowered blood pressure to the physician assists him to initiate a course of action which minimizes the threat of renal damage.

The nurse in the teaching role can encourage patients with possible streptococcal infection to seek medical attention promptly to reduce the risk of glomerulonephritis. Alerting the public to the importance of keeping drugs where they cannot be accidentally ingested is important, as some drugs are nephrotoxic. Nurses and physicians, as well as ancillary personnel, must take utmost care to prevent the transfusion of incompatible blood.

Diagnosis, symptoms, and pathology

Although uremia sometimes has a sudden onset with pronounced initial symptoms, it usually starts so slowly that it is not recognized immediately. The early symptoms may be no more than headaches, fatigability, vague gastrointestinal complaints, irritability, and malaise. The patient just does not feel right, and active life becomes increasingly difficult.

Urine

Oliguria, or decrease in normal urinary output, may be present. However, the quantity of urine can be normal or even increased in volume when the kidneys are failing, but the specific gravity of the urine will be low since waste products appear in less than normal concentration.

Blood

Examination of the blood may show a gradual increase in the blood urea nitrogen (BUN) since the kidneys' ability to excrete urea, the end product of protein metabolism, is impaired. The BUN may become markedly elevated before any other symptoms are recognized. Mental clouding, confusion, and disorientation can accompany a rising BUN.

As the condition progresses, more and more products of metabolism—such as creatinine, uric acid, and sulfates—are retained in the blood, causing headaches and nausea. Acidosis appears. Nausea and vomiting, thirst, and air hunger are symptoms of acidosis. The deep and rapid respirations are indicative of a respiratory attempt to compensate for the metabolic acidosis.

So much sodium and water may be lost that the patient becomes dehydrated. Anorexia and vomiting intensify the losses. Muscular weakness, more anorexia, and overall debility characterize hyponatremia (deficient blood sodium). More rarely, depending on the original pathology causing the uremia, the patient is edematous instead of dehydrated.

In uremia, the blood level of calcium frequently is low because calcium is not reabsorbed in sufficient quantity from the glomerular filtrate. Early signs of calcium deficiency are numbness and tingling of the fingertips and toes, nose and ears. This can progress to symptoms of tetany, ranging from slight twitching to convulsions. Potassium retention is one of the most critical problems since potassium intoxication causes cardiac failure and pulmonary edema. The nurse observes the patient for excessive coughing, shortness of breath, respiratory wheezing or rales. Severe anemia is a common symptom of advancing renal failure.

BLOOD PRESSURE. Hypertension commonly accompanies renal failure. Dimness or blurring of vision and spots before the eyes may be the result of retinal hemorrhages caused by the hypertension.

APPEARANCE AND SKIN

The patient with renal insufficiency is usually pale and may have edema about the eyes and pitting edema of the ankles.

The patient may complain of torturous pruritus (itching of the skin). Since the skin also serves an excretory function, "uremic frost" (a white film composed of waste products excreted by the skin instead of by the kidneys) may become visible, especially in dark-skinned patients.

Halitosis is generally marked and ulceration of the oral mucosa due to increased capillary fragility is common. The patient may have a generalized body odor suggestive of urine.

THOUGHT PROCESS

Though some patients remain mentally alert for a long period of time considering their electrolyte imbalance, mental processes are progressively slowed. There may be dizziness and irritability. Behavior can be totally unpredictable and may even become psychotic. Cerebral edema can cause projectile vomiting, convulsions, and coma.

GASTROINTESTINAL

Ulceration and bleeding of the gastrointestinal tract is a fairly common component of renal failure. The mucous membranes of the mouth often bleed, and blood may be found in the feces. Hematemesis (vomiting of blood) is a frequent precursor of death in the patient with uremia. Relentless hiccoughing can also be present.

Prognosis and objectives of treatment

If the primary cause can be removed or quickly remedied, such as in acute renal tubular necrosis (lower nephron nephrosis) or urinary tract obstruction, renal failure is reversible in about 80 percent of such patients. The treatment objective is to keep the patient alive and free from complications during the 2 or 3 weeks required for regeneration of the damaged epithelium of the renal tubules. Kidney function may gradually return to normal over a period of several weeks.

Chronic renal diseases such as glomerular nephritis, nephrosis, pyelonephritis, and polycystic kidneys progress to deterioration of the nephron involving either the glomeruli or the tubules or both and may finally result in acute renal failure. The onset of oliguria or anuria is an ominous sign. Remissions can occur, however. One objective of treatment is to avoid conditions that increase the workload of the kidneys through control of diet, activity, and obesity and avoidance of infection. Another is to treat the various symptoms of the uremia itself.

A more aggressive approach is to prevent uremia in acute and chronic renal failure by substitution for kidney function through the use of such modes of therapy as ion exchange resins, hemodialysis (artificial kidney), or peritoneal dialysis.

Treatment and nursing management

GENERAL. Any decrease in urinary output below 500 ml. in a 24-hour period should be reported promptly. The nurse will remain alert for any symptoms that may indicate renal shutdown or beginning uremia. When the patient who is usually cheerful and pleasant becomes irritable and complains of a headache, it may not be because he has had a disagreeable visit with his family or has experienced some other unpleasant episode. The reverse may be true; his interpersonal relations may suffer because his BUN is elevated.

The patient with uremia is often very ill and may even be comatose. The episodes are long and taxing to both the patient and his family. Members of his family should be encouraged to participate in his care. (For instance, an unpalatable diet fed by a patient's wife or husband may not seem to be quite so depressing.) When the patient is irritable, the nurse can help the family to understand that his anger is not necessarily directed at them, but that it is rather the result of the accumulated chemicals in his bloodstream.

FLUID INTAKE. The physician determines how much fluid the patient can have based on exact measurements of intake and output via all routes.

In severe shutdown the patient may be limited to as little as 400 ml. intravenously (artfully regulated to last the 24 hours) and 100 ml. of oral fluid. Some days (depending on the output), tea, ginger ale, or water is given with as much sugar or Coca Cola syrup (to increase the caloric intake) as the patient can tolerate. Sucking glucose ice chips made by freezing

20 to 50 percent glucose in an ice tray can help alleviate thirst while providing needed calories. Ice chips can extend a small amount of fluid over 24 hours. To count intake accurately the nurse can measure in a graduate the same amount of ice which has been allowed to melt.

Unfortunately, most fruit juices contain potassium, and since the failing kidney cannot excrete excess potassium, they are not permitted.

DIET. In severe failure, the demand on the kidneys for the excretion of protein end products is limited by restricting protein foods. Feedings should be spaced so that there are no long periods of fasting. If the patient awakens during the night, for instance, he should be given a high carbohydrate snack or drink.

If the diet is limited to carbohydrate and fat, as for severe kidney shutdown, palatability becomes a problem. A well-chilled equal part mixture of Karo syrup and ginger ale with a drop or two of lemon juice provides a high carbohydrate intake which may be partially tolerated. The sodium intake of patients with edema is severely restricted.

If the patient with acute renal failure reaches the diuretic phase, nausea and vomiting subside after a few days and appetite returns. Urinary output can be quite large in volume because the patient loses surplus sodium and water previously present as edema. It may be necessary to compensate for excess sodium loss by encouraging the patient to eat salty foods. On the other hand, because sodium and water balance is unstable, sodium restriction is continued if edema is present. Daily body weight is used as a guide. Salt substitutes containing potassium for seasoning cannot be used. Rum, vinegar, mint, cloves, brown sugar, or cinnamon probably will be allowed. Diet is usually low in protein and high in calories until renal function returns to normal.

If the kidneys do not recover and the patient is in a state of chronic renal failure, fluids are forced provided that edema does not develop or urinary output decrease. Forced fluids are necessary because the kidneys are unable to concentrate solid wastes and more fluid is needed to excrete them. Some physicians recommend diets low in salt and protein to lessen the work of the kidneys. Others believe that the patient should have a liberal choice of foods that appeal to him with a basic balanced diet.

ACTIVITY. In the acute stage, metabolic demands are kept to a minimum by restricting activity to those measures necessary for preventing the hazards of bed rest. Chronic uremic patients in acute crises may have peripheral neuropathy and require considerable assistance from the nurse or physical therapist, to provide passive, then active, assistive exercise to maintain function. Rapid progressive ambulation with the preservation of patient safety is the goal.

ITCHING. Pruritus can occur with or without frost. Uremic frost can be removed with a weak solution of vinegar (2 tablespoons to a pint of water). The physician may order an anesthetic ointment to relieve the itching. Cleansing of the skin, without the use of soap, aids in the removal of accumulated uric acid crystals. Although the skin is not efficient for the disposal of such waste chemicals as uric acid, it is all that the body has available when the kidneys are not functioning, and a clean skin is always more efficient and more comfortable.

ANEMIA, secondary to hematopoietic depression, is common, and may be treated by blood transfusion to maintain the hematocrit in the normal range. The anemia contributes to the general weakness and lethargy of the chronic uremic patient.

PREVENTION OF INFECTION. Infectious processes increase protein catabolism and by increasing the workload of the kidneys hasten the onset or severity of uremia. Pulmonary complications are the most frequent cause of morbidity and mortality in acute renal failure. Those with upper respiratory infections—that is, visitors and nursing personnel—should avoid direct contact with the patient.

Frequent deep breathing, turning, and coughing are indicated, and may prevent complications such as atelectasis and pneumonia.

PATIENT AND FAMILY SUPPORT. Many patients with acute renal failure develop it as a complication after some major medical or surgical problem. Thus they have their initial problem plus a serious setback to deal with. Patients with chronic renal insufficiency who develop acute renal failure are often aware that they are approaching end-stage renal disease. For the patient and his close associates, fear of death is present. Added to this is the fear of losing control as the build-up of waste products in the blood affects the sensorium, causing the patient to become restless, confused, belligerent, disoriented, psychotic, or comatose. The nursing staff by their organization and manner can convey to the patient and his associates that they can be depended upon to keep the situation under control even though the patient may not be in control of himself.

Substitutes for kidney function

Renal dialysis (extracorporeal hemodialysis)

Hemodialysis is a process designed to bring blood into contact with a semipermeable membrane through which diffusion takes place. By "diffusion" is meant the spontaneous movement of solutes and solvent from areas of high concentration to areas of low concentration until a state of equilibrium is established. Substances which should be removed from the patient's blood, such as urea, creatinine, and dangerously high levels of potassium, are removed because these are all absent from the dialysate fluid. They move from the patient's blood through the semipermeable membrane to the dialysate fluid. Hemodialysis also permits the replacement of substances that may be low in the blood and present in the dialysate: for example, bicarbonate and calcium.

- In the many types of artificial kidneys (also called dialyzers) the basic components are cellophane tubing (coil) and dialysate fluid. The cellophane tubing acts as the semipermeable membrane. The dialysate fluid is similar to the electrolyte composition of normal *human plasma*. The composition is ordered by the physician and changed as needed. The patient's blood is removed from an artery, pumped through the coil, and returned to a vein. Water and ions are able to pass through the walls of the membrane, but protein and red blood cells cannot.
- Heparin is administered to prevent blood from clotting in the coil. To minimize the risk of systemic bleeding, regional heparinization may be used. This consists of infusing heparin into the blood as the blood passes from patient to coil and protamine sulfate as the blood returns to the patient, to neutralize the heparin. Clotting time tests are done frequently.
- Blood samples taken pre- and postdialysis for urea, creatinine, sodium, potassium, chlorides, CO_2, and hematocrit are indicators of the efficiency of dialysis.
- **External Arteriovenous Shunt.** When a patient is to be hemodialyzed, cannulas (the shunt) are placed surgically in an extremity where blood vessels are available. This allows for repeated treatments without having to cut down on vessels each time. Between treatments, the cannula ends are connected by an external Teflon joint and blood is shunted between the artery and the vein. To attach the patient to the artificial kidney the joint is opened and the arterial cannula is attached to the inflow tubing of the coil; the venous cannula is attached to the outflow tubing. When the treatment is finished, the joint is reconnected and blood flows through the shunt (Fig. 50-1).

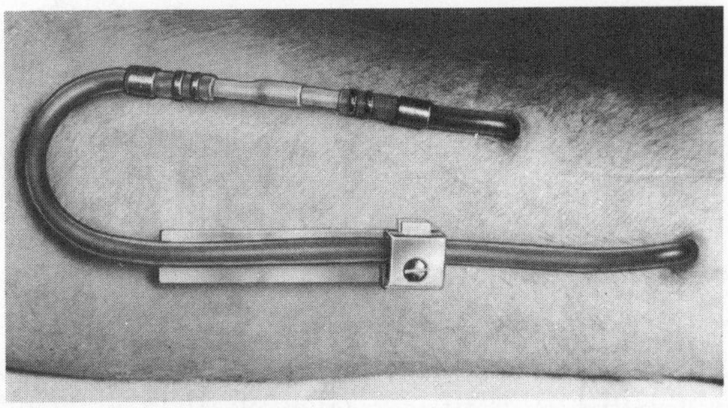

figure 50-1. Arteriovenous shunt between periods of use in hemodialysis. (Seattle Artificial Kidney Supply Company, Seattle, Wash.)

- Two cannula clamps (or rubber-tipped hemostats) should be close by at all times for use in the event that the cannulas disconnect at the Teflon joint.
- **Internal Arteriovenous Shunt.** Instead of an external shunt, some patients on permanent dialysis may have an arteriovenous fistula (internal shunt) formed by way of a surgical anastomosis of an artery and vein lying in close proximity. The vein enlarges and assumes the characteristics of an artery. Venipuncture is performed in a proximal site and is used for the outflow from the coil. A distal needle puncture is used for the inflow to the coil. When dialysis is completed, the needles are removed and pressure dressings applied for several hours. Blood pressures and blood samples should not be taken in the cannulated extremity.

Preparation of patient for hemodialysis

The confused, apprehensive, uremic patient can become more so when he encounters new faces, new surroundings, and new equipment. Because the seemingly unconscious patient may still be able to hear, attempts should be made to communicate with him.

If the situation is very critical, there may be little time afforded the patient to ask questions or otherwise review the explanation. The dialysis nurse should be informed regarding what explanation was given to the patient and his response so that she can more accurately assess the patient's need for continued support.

If the situation permits, the nurse's explanation can be enhanced by taking the patient to the dialysis room so that he can see the equipment the nurse describes and observe and talk to other patients as well.

The more the patient understands, the less bewildered he is; this reduces his feelings of helplessness. He recognizes that his well-being, his very life, depends upon the machinery, its correct operation, and the performance of the dialysis team.

The patient comes to the dialysis room in bed or ambulatory, depending on his clinical condition. He need not be fasting. In the dialysis room, emergency equipment and medications are readily available.

A pre- and postdialysis weight is important. A certain weight loss occurs with dialysis, depending upon blood flow rate and duration of dialysis. Fluid removal may be undesirable; a postdialysis weight enables the physician to order fluid replacement if necessary.

Nursing management during hemodialysis

Nursing requirements vary with each patient. The physical needs of chronic dialysis patients are minimal, but there is much opportunity for the professional nurse to function as a teacher or counselor. Nursing measures for acutely ill patients depend on the basic medical or surgical condition as well as the extent of renal failure, and may include frequent suctioning of airway to prevent aspiration; tracheostomy care; eye care; skin care for incontinence; cardiac and respiratory monitoring; gastric and chest drainage; intravenous feeding; and oxygen therapy.

Some important considerations for all patients are:

Support. During the procedure, especially if it is being done for the first time, a primary aspect of nursing is being there to explain, reassure, and respond to the patient.

Blood Pressure and Pulse. These are recorded predialysis, frequently at the start of dialysis, and depending on the clinical condition of the patient. Arrhythmias may result from potassium removal and low blood pressure from excess fluid removal.

Positioning. The patient's position should be changed frequently, as dialysis is a lengthy procedure. The length of the treatment depends on the condition of the patient as well as on the type of dialyzer and can vary from 4 to 8 hours two to three times per week. The patient may be turned, may sit up on the edge of the bed, may keep his head lowered or raised. A reclining chair can also be used. A drop in blood pressure may require a temporary flat position of the bed.

Prevention of Complications. Preventive measures and physical care are not interrupted because of dialysis. Diversion and socialization to the extent possible lessen boredom.

Thought Process. An unconscious patient may become aware and coherent during dialysis, or vice versa. Restlessness frequently occurs. Any change in the mental status of the patient should be reported to the physician.

Hemorrhage. Because of the administration of heparin, regionally or systemically, frequent observations should be made for bleeding, including inspection of dressings, stool specimens, and gastric drainage. Epistaxis and bleeding from gums are not uncommon.

Complications. Headache, muscle cramps, nausea and vomiting, fever, diaphoresis, anxiety, and/or chest pain occurring during hemodialysis may reflect serious complications.

Mechanical Problems. Membrane ruptures, clotting in coil or shunt, and reduced blood flow through the dialyzer may necessitate termination of hemodialysis. The nurse needs to be well prepared technically so that should problems arise, they can be promptly identified and steps taken to correct the situation.

Teaching and Counseling. A patient with end-stage renal disease anticipating chronic dialysis or renal transplant needs a nurse who recognizes that listening to his expression of thoughts and feelings as he contemplates his future is an important dimension of the nursing role. Some hospitals may utilize a home teaching team to prepare the patient and his family for home dialysis.

Nursing management after hemodialysis

Vital signs are taken frequently. The nurse continues to observe the patient for bleeding. No intramuscular injections are given for 2 to 4 hours postdialysis because, due to the administration of heparin, bleeding may occur at the injection site. Daily care is given to the external shunt and it is observed for patency.

Fluid and dietary restrictions are regulated according to the degree of recovery of renal function and the patient's clinical condition.

Chronic dialysis patients continue on fluid restrictions based on urinary output. The potassium and sodium content of the diet may be restricted. A normal protein diet may be allowed.

The long-term treatment of patients with end-stage renal disease by hemodialysis is not only a medical, nursing, and family problem. The large number of patients, the high monetary cost, and the limited number of specialized facilities and personnel make this a social and ethical problem for the community.

Peritoneal dialysis

The simplicity of peritoneal dialysis and the availability of the equipment for this procedure are in sharp contrast to the complexity of the technique and equipment used in hemodialysis. The latter is limited to hospitals that have the equipment and the personnel trained to use it, or to those who have been trained in the use of the equipment at home. Peritoneal dialysis can be performed in any hospital; however, it provides only a fraction of the plasma clearance that the artificial kidney can provide.

- In peritoneal dialysis, a bathing solution (dialysate) is made to flow into and out of the peritoneal cavity (Fig. 50-2). The peritoneum acts as the semipermeable membrane. The dialysate causes urea, electrolytes and dialyzable poisons to pass across the peritoneum and into the dialysate solution.
- The patient is weighed, the bladder is emptied, and a small incision is made in the midline of the abdomen. A catheter with many perforations is inserted by the physician so that the end lies free in the peritoneal cavity. The catheter is sutured in place and a dressing is applied. Blood pressure, pulse, and respirations are recorded.
- The bottles of dialysate are set up and the administration tubing (inflow tube) is attached to the catheter in the patient. The outflow tubing leading to a closed drainage system is clamped off.
- **Instillation Period.** Two liters of dialysate should run into the peritoneal cavity in 10 to 15 minutes by gravity. If the drip is slow, the physician may need to reposition the catheter. When the bottles are empty, but the tubing is still filled with dialysate to prevent entrance of air, the inflow tube should be clamped. The nurse records instillation time, the volume and type of dialysate, plus any medications added.
- **Equilibration Period.** The solution is left in the abdomen the length of time ordered by the physician (usually 30–45 minutes).
- **Drainage Period.** The outflow tube is unclamped and the dialysate drains into a closed sterile drainage system. Gravity drainage, facilitated by raising bed height or changing the patient's position, should take no longer than 10 to 15 minutes. If it does, the physician may need to irrigate the catheter to remove plugs, or he may need to reposition or replace the catheter.
- The time of the start and finish of the drainage period should be recorded. Note should be taken of the appearance of the fluid removed. It may be blood-tinged because of bleeding due to heparin, or cloudy from protein loss. The differences between the volume instilled and the volume removed is recorded. The physician should be notified of excessive fluid retained by or removed from the patient (±500 ml.).
- The number of exchanges performed in peritoneal dialysis is ordered by the physician. When dialysis is completed, the physician removes the catheter and applies a dry sterile dressing. A purse string suture may be necessary. A bacteriologic culture is obtained from the catheter tip as well as from the last dialysate drained. A postdialysis weight is obtained.

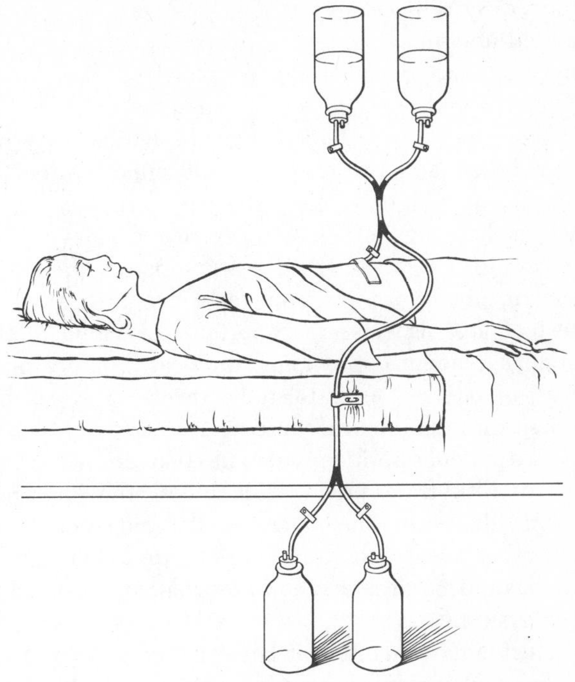

figure 50-2. Peritoneal dialysis. After the solution flows into the patient it is allowed to remain in situ for the period of time ordered by the physician. During this time, dialysis takes place. Then the clamps on the lower bottles are opened and the solution is drained off.

Observations

Blood pressure and pulse are taken frequently, usually at the end of each drainage period. A drop in blood pressure and increased pulse rate may occur when fluid removal is too rapid, especially when the dialysate has a high concentration of dextrose. If the patient is acutely ill, a bed scale is used for weight measurements. The physician may order the patient weighed as often as every 8 hours while the procedure is in progress.

Pain in the left shoulder may be due to diaphragmatic irritation caused by the high concentration of dextrose when present in the dialysate. Abdominal pain present at the end of the drainage period may be relieved by the next instillation. Pain accompanied by marked abdominal distention warrants contacting the physician and delaying the next dialysis cycle until the physician has examined the patient.

The procedure is tedious and the patient may become bored and restless. It is not sufficient for the nurse to appear only when she has some task to do such as hanging bottles or measuring drainage. This conveys to the patient that the equipment is the major concern, not him, though he may recognize too that the technical aspects are important. Listening to the patient's reactions, providing physical comfort measures, or offering some tolerable diversion assists the patient through the procedure.

The patient's position should be changed frequently; he can turn from side to side unless the physician orders otherwise. The patient undergoing peritoneal dialysis may eat and drink as permitted. His mental state should be observed and any changes reported to the physician.

Peritonitis (chemical or bacterial) is a major complication of peritoneal dialysis.

Renal transplantation

In some patients with chronic, progressive renal disease (end-stage renal disease) in whom kidney failure is a threat to life, a kidney transplant may be considered. This procedure is usually performed in hospitals with specialized transplant units.

General nutritional considerations

- As renal failure continues, dietary intervention becomes very important and will include restrictions to alleviate symptoms of uremia. The type of diet or dietary restriction usually depends on the degree of severity of renal disease.
- The diet may be restricted in sodium, potassium, protein, and fluids. Restrictions depend upon laboratory serum values, which show the kidneys' ability to eliminate specific waste products of metabolism.
- Anorexia and nausea may be present, also limiting dietary intake.
- Salt substitutes (some of which contain potassium) may *not* be used unless approved by the physician (by specific name-brand product).
- The patient will need detailed dietary instructions given by the dietitian and at times by the nurse. Patients and families should be informed of the availability of foods and recipes made especially for those with dietary restrictions.

General pharmacological considerations

- Drugs excreted from the body by the kidney are given with caution to the patient with renal disease. If the drug is deemed necessary, it may be given in lower than normal doses; the patient is closely observed for any changes in renal status if normal doses are necessary. The nurse should pay special attention to the patient's urinary output, as this is one method of determining a change in renal status.
- Drugs which are toxic to the kidney (nephrotoxic) are not given to the patient with renal disease unless the patient's life is in danger and no other therapeutic agent is of value.

Bibliography

Anger, D.: The psychologic stress of chronic renal failure and long-term hemodialysis. Nurs. Clin. North Am. 10:449, September, 1975.

Berne, T. V. et al: Hemodialysis for postoperative acute renal insufficiency. RN 35:ICU/CCU 5, March, 1972.

Desautels, R. E.: Managing the urinary catheter. Nurs. Dig. 3:30, September/October, 1975.

Dolan, P. O. et al: Renal failure and peritoneal dialysis (pictorial). Nurs. '75, 5:40, July, 1975.

Frye, C.: Toxic nephropathy. Canad. Nurs. 68:45, June, 1972.

Grant, M. M. and Kubo, W. M.: Assessing a patient's hydration status. Am. J. Nurs. 75:1306, August, 1975.

Guthrie, H. A.: *Introductory Nutrition,* ed. 3. St. Louis, Mosby, 1975.

Harrington, J. L. and Brener, E. R.: *Patient Care in Renal Failure.* Philadelphia, Saunders, 1973.

Hekelman, F. P. et al: Nursing approaches to conservative management of renal disease. Nurs. Clin. North Am. 10:431, September, 1975.

Hudak, C. M. et al: *Critical Care Nursing.* Philadelphia, Lippincott, 1973.

Levy, N. B.: *Living and Dying: Adaption to Hemodialysis.* Springfield, Thomas, 1974.

Prilook, M. E.: Renal failure: What to do when the kidneys shut down. Patient Care 5:40, December, 1971.

Robinson, C. H.: *Normal and Therapeutic Nutrition,* ed. 14. New York, Macmillan, 1972.

Stenzel, K. H. and Leonard, M. O.: End-stage kidney disease —current concepts in care. Part 2. Transplantation. J. Prac. Nurs. 26:16, March, 1976.

Topor, M. A.: Symposium on care of the patient with renal disease. Kidney transplantation. Nurs. Clin. North Am. 10:503, September, 1975.

Wiley, M.: Care of the patient with a kidney transplant. Nurs. Clin. North Am. 8:127, March, 1973.

CHAPTER 51

The burned patient

On completion of this chapter the student will:

- **Describe the two general classes of burns.**
- **Describe the "Rules of Nines" and how it is used to estimate the percentage of body surface covered by burns.**
- **Discuss the initial first aid treatment given the victim at the scene of the injury.**
- **Describe and discuss physiological changes that occur after a burn injury.**
- **Describe the initial hospital treatment and nursing management of the burned patient.**
- **Name the various methods of burn treatment and describe each.**
- **Name the different skin-grafting techniques and the advantages and rationale of each.**
- **Formulate a nursing care plan for and participate in the nursing management of the burned patient.**
- **List the complications of severe burns.**
- **Discuss the factors to be considered in the discharge planning of the burned patient.**

Suddenly a well person sustains serious burns, and is confronted with problems resulting from pain, mutilation, fear of death, disfigurement, separation, immobilization, helplessness, and possible abandonment. Together with his own injuries and problems he may be grieving over the death of others involved in the accident, such as spouse, children, or coworkers. He may experience guilt for having caused the accident or anger that this catastrophe should have happened to him. If he lives, he has a long battle with prevention of infection, continuing pain from dressing changes and surgery, scarring, malnutrition, financial need, social relationships, and many other problems.

Everything said about the severely burned patient in this chapter can apply also, with modification, to the patient with a milder or less extensive burn. A patient with a 1 percent burn is not likely to go into shock, but the basic pathology remains the same.

Classification of burns

Burns may be classified as *first-*, *second-*, *third-*, or *fourth-degree* burns. Another classification is *partial-thickness* or *full-thickness* burn. The relative depth of each is shown in Figure 51-1 and explained in Table 51-1.

Burns caused by *electricity* are characteristically deep, involving not only the skin, but also blood vessels, muscles, tendons, and bones.

Diagnosis of the depth of a burn is often difficult. There may be a combination of all degrees of burn. Both locally and systemically, the deeper the burn, the greater the damage.

The second measure of damage is the extent of the area: the larger the burn area, the greater the damage to the body. Severe sunburn (first-degree) over 85 percent of the body will cause a much greater disturbance of fluid and electrolyte regulation than a third-degree burn on the tip of a forefinger. Since physicians base their prescriptions for fluid replacement therapy on both the degree and the extent of the body surface injured, the diagnosis includes both these factors. The "Rule of Nines" (Fig. 51-2) is one method of estimating how much of the patient's skin surface is involved.

Prognosis

In recent years such large strides have been made in the treatment of burn shock that patients are saved today who would have died several years ago. This is especially true of patients who are not very young or very old, and who have no pre-existing disease. However, patients saved from dying in shock may later

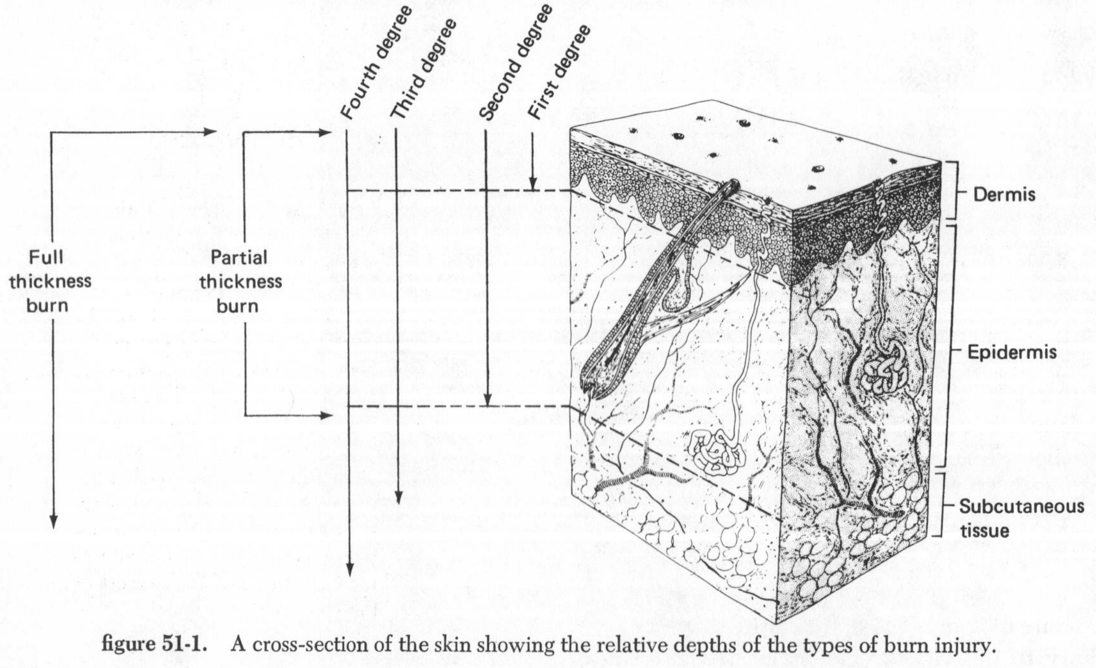

figure 51-1. A cross-section of the skin showing the relative depths of the types of burn injury.

Table 51-1.
Degree, depth, and characteristics of burn injuries

Degree of Burn	Depth	Characteristics
First-Degree (Partial-Thickness)	Epidermis	Red or pink in color; pain is present; edema may be present but subside quickly; no scarring occurs.
Second-Degree (Partial-Thickness)	Epidermis and dermis	Color may vary from mottled pink to red, white, dull white, tan (depending on depth); blistering, pain, some scarring occurs.
Third-Degree (Full-Thickness)	Epidermis, dermis, subcutaneous tissues	Color may vary: white, tan, black, brown, bright red; surface may be wet or dry; leathery covering (eschar is present); no pain; scarring occurs.
Fourth-Degree (Full-Thickness)	Epidermis, dermis, subcutaneous tissue; may include subcutaneous fat, fascia, muscle and bone	Surface is blackened, depressed; no pain; scarring occurs.

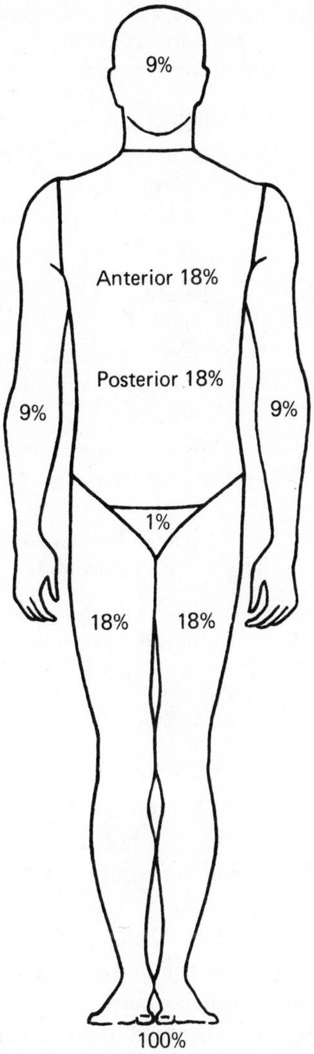

figure 51-2. The "Rule of Nines," a simplified method for estimating the percent of the body surface covered by burns. According to this method, the entire head is 9 percent of the body surface area; each entire arm is 9 percent; each entire leg is 18 percent; the genital region is 1 percent; the front torso is 18 percent; and the back torso is 18 percent. Physicians often sketch the area burned on a diagram such as this to facilitate the calculation of the percent of the body burned.

succumb to other complications, such as septicemia and renal failure. The prevention of infection, which has always been an important nursing consideration in the care of the burned patient, now assumes even more urgent proportions.

Initial first aid treatment

At the scene of a fire, the first priority is to prevent further injury to the victim. If the clothing is on fire, the victim should be *placed in a horizontal position*

Table 51-2.
Initial fluid, electrolyte, and blood disturbances in the burned patient

PROBLEM	RATIONALE
Fluid Loss (Dehydration)	Fluid moves toward the burned area resulting in localized edema.
	Fluid seeps from the burned area.
Electrolyte Disturbances	Potassium (K^+) levels are initially increased (hyperkalemia) as the ion moves *from* damaged cells *to* the bloodstream.
	Sodium (Na^+) levels may initially decrease (hyponatremia) as the ion leaves the body along with fluids lost from the wounds.
Anemia	Anemia is due to destruction of red blood cells at the site of the injury.

and rolled in a blanket to smother the fire. Laying the victim flat prevents the fire, hot air, and smoke from rising toward the head and entering the respiratory passages. The victim must be immediately taken to a hospital for examination. During transport, it is important that individuals who have been burned around the face and neck or who may have inhaled smoke, steam, or flames be observed *closely* for respiratory difficulty. When these substances are inhaled, the mucous membrane lining the respiratory passages may be damaged or extremely irritated. This can result in edema of the respiratory passages which decreases the amount of air reaching the lungs. In addition, there may be excessive mucous secretion, which also makes breathing difficult. The hospital should be made aware, if possible, that a burned patient will arrive shortly. Estimation of the extent of the burn and any problems the victim appears to have aids in mobilization and preparation of emergency room personnel.

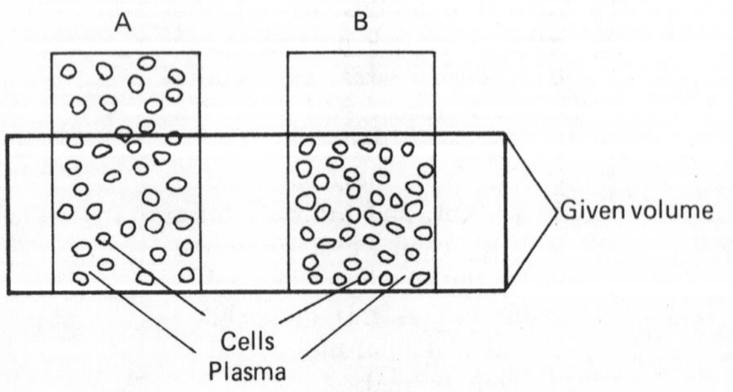

figure 51-3. (A) Normal plasma volume. (B) Loss of plasma volume.

Immediately upon the patient's arrival at the hospital, the physician assesses the extent of injury and the immediate problems and needs of the patient. Along with the burn, the patient may have incurred other body injuries—fractures, head injury, lacerations, and so on. The prime focus of the immediate treatment phase is to determine the respiratory status and then to meet the patient's fluid needs. Intravenous fluids are administered, including plasma expanders, for example, dextran (Gentran), if blood or excessive fluid is lost. A cutdown may be necessary and a central venous pressure (CVP) line may be inserted at this time or later to monitor the patient's fluid requirements. The patient is usually weighed with a bed scale to determine fluid gain and loss. Analgesics are also given, often intravenously, to relieve pain and apprehension.

Physiological changes after a burn injury

Many physiological changes occur almost immediately after a severe burn injury. Deep and widespread burns almost always result in a more drastic change (see Table 51-2) than do those that are less severe or widespread. It should also be noted that even small areas of injury can result in moderately severe to severe physiological changes in the very young and the very old.

The extent of physiological change is determined by laboratory studies—arterial blood gas studies and serum and urine electrolytes. After a burn, fluid from the body moves toward the burned area, accounting for the edema at the burn site. Some of the fluid is then trapped in this area, is unavailable for use by the body, and, therefore, becomes fluid "loss." Fluid is also lost from the burned area, often in extremely large amounts, in the form of water vapor and seepage.

Potassium levels increase as the ions move from the burned area into the bloodstream. Once diuresis begins, potassium levels decrease, but must be closely monitored because rapid diuresis will increase potassium loss. Potassium levels may decrease during profound diuresis. This condition is as serious as increased levels. Sodium levels may decrease initially as the ion leaves the body along with the fluid lost from the burned area. Protein is also lost.

Initial hemoglobin and hematocrit (the level of plasma volume to cell volume) levels may be reported as normal or above normal. Plasma, the liquid component of the blood, escapes from the bloodstream resulting in a *decrease* in the plasma volume (the total amount of plasma in all blood vessels). Figure 51-3 A and B illustrates normal plasma volume and reduced plasma volume. There are the same number of cells in B as in A, but the plasma in which the cells are suspended is less. When comparing, by means of the dotted lines, the number of cells in a *given amount* of fluid, there are more cells per milliliter of solution in B than in A. This is an illustration of *hemoconcentration.* The patient could be anemic, but because of plasma loss with resulting hemoconcentration, some blood studies may appear normal. Hemoconcentration presents another problem, namely, the sluggish flow of blood through blood vessels. This may result in inadequate nutrition of healthy body cells and organs; a fall in blood pressure usually follows. If physiological changes are not *immediately recognized* and *corrected,* irreversible shock can occur. These changes usually happen rapidly and may change from hour to hour, which is one reason why these patients require intensive care by skilled personnel.

Table 51-3.
Initial management of the burned patient

Establish and maintain an adequate airway.
Begin intravenous fluids. A cutdown may be necessary.
Administer intravenous analgesics for relief of pain.
Withhold oral fluids.
Insert Foley catheter.
Give tetanus and antibiotics if necessary.
Draw blood for laboratory studies.
Give burned areas initial care.

Initial hospital treatment

Once the patient is admitted, the medical team must work quickly to assess the extent of injury and formulate an immediate plan of care (see Table 51-3). Many hospital emergency rooms have set aside for immediate use materials necessary to manage the burned patient. There may also be a written procedure regarding initial management of the patient.

Personnel should observe clean technique (*clean* cap, gown, mask, gloves) during initial treatment, although some hospitals use sterile technique. If the patient has difficulty breathing, or if there is edema of the face and neck, an endotracheal tube may be inserted or a tracheostomy performed. A tracheostomy is rarely done if there are severe burns on the anterior neck. In this case, an endotracheal tube is inserted. It is *extremely important* that the respiratory rate be *closely* monitored and the patient observed for *any* sign of respiratory distress. Intravenous fluids are started immediately and the physician will determine which extremity will be used and what type of fluid will be administered. Blood samples are usually drawn at this time. A Foley catheter is inserted and attached to a closed drainage system as the urinary output will be closely observed during the first few days. The physician may order intravenous analgesics for pain, which in many cases is severe. Since pain can cause a drop in blood pressure, analgesics are very important at this time. Laboratory studies, such as serum electrolytes, may also be ordered. Blood pressure, pulse, and respirations are taken immediately and frequently thereafter. If both arms are burned, the blood pressure may be taken on the leg by wrapping the cuff around the thigh and placing the stethoscope over the popliteal artery behind the knee. This technique is not always possible in a busy and noisy emergency room as the systolic and diastolic sounds are often hard to hear because the popliteal artery is not close to the surface of the body. Tetanus shots and antibiotics may also be administered at this time or after the burned areas have been cleaned.

The first step in management of the burned area is removal of all clothing. As some pieces of clothing may have adhered to the injured area, care must be taken in separating clothing fibers from the wound. The body hair around the perimeter of the burn is usually shaved because hair is a source of bacterial wound contamination. When the head, neck, and upper chest are burned, singed eyebrows and eyelashes are clipped, head hair is shaved, the lips and mouth are cleansed, and the lips are lubricated. Eye ointments and/or irrigations are used to remove dirt and lubricate the lid margins.

The burned areas are cleansed to remove debris. This may be done in the emergency room or after the patient is transferred to the burn or general hospital unit. After cleansing, topical medications may be applied. Hospital procedures regarding initial management may vary, depending upon the extent of treatment given in the emergency room.

Burn treatment methods

When the emergency is over, the body must repair itself. The energy that was required to meet the emergency was greatly in excess of normal. Because large areas of fat deposits have been used, and the caloric intake over the past several days has been low, patients often are emaciated. As much as 20 pounds may be lost, even if the loss of edema is not considered. Debilitation is dangerous, because it reduces the patient's resistance to infection, delays the healing of the skin, and impedes the growth of new granulation tissue and the progress of new skin grafts. Accordingly, the nurse does everything possible to improve the patient's nutrition.

There is no one best method of treating burns; each method appears to have advantages and disadvantages.

The *open* or *exposure method* exposes the burned areas to air, allowing a formation of a hard crust on top of the burn. Over areas of a third-degree or full-thickness burn, a hard leathery crust (eschar) which is made up of dehydrated dead skin will form. The crust over a second-degree or partial-thickness burn forms in 2 or 3 days with a regrowth of skin (epithelialization) completed in approximately 2 to 3 weeks. At this time, the crust falls off. Eschar also forms in 2 to 3 days, gradually begins to loosen, and is cut away (debridement) or further loosened by whirlpool baths. A dressing may be used to cover the exposed areas as the eschar is removed. If the eschar constricts the area and impairs circulation, an escharotomy (an excision into the eschar) is done to relieve pressure on the affected area. New skin will not grow beneath eschar.

With the open method of treatment, the patient is placed in isolation, sterile linen is used, and personnel and visitors wear sterile gowns and masks. The skin of the burned patient is sensitive to drafts and temperature changes; therefore, a bed cradle or sheets may be placed over the patient for protection from drafts and temperature changes.

Occlusive dressings are mostly used when the arms, hands, feet, or legs are burned. Although there are variations, the burned area is covered with an ointment and gauze. Gauze impregnated with ointment is also used. Additional gauze, or a fluff dressing and gauze, is applied to cover the ointment/dressing adjacent to the skin. It is important that proper body alignment is attained: flexion of the foot is avoided to prevent footdrop, and the hand is curled in a relaxed position. The nurse checks the circulation of the extremity every 2 to 4 hours, noting color and skin temperature and asking the patient if numbness, tingling, or other sensations are experienced. If the entire extremity is wrapped, it is impossible to make these observations. Careful application of the dressing, making sure it is not constricting, may prevent circulation impairment.

Topical drugs

Various drugs are used in the treatment of burns: mafenide (Sulfamylon), silver nitrate ($AgNO_3$) 0.5 percent solution, povidone-iodine (Betadine), gentamicin (Garamycin) 0.1 percent cream, and silver sulfadiazine (Silvadene) 1 percent ointment. The solutions may be applied in the form of wet dressings or dabbed on the areas. The ointments are dabbed on the area or impregnated in gauze that is laid on the burn. Drugs have various advantages and disadvantages and no one preparation appears to be superior to another.

All drugs are applied by using sterile technique. Silver nitrate 0.5 percent is a solution applied by the continuous wet-dressing technique. The burned surface must be free of grease or oil film before gauze dressings are applied. The gauze is wet with the silver nitrate solution before application, anchored with stretch bandages, and kept continuously wet. Unusually thick dressings may have a catheter inserted in one of the middle layers to aid in the wetting of all layers of gauze. A blanket may be placed over the patient to slow down evaporation of the solution. One disadvantage in the use of silver nitrate is the loss of electrolytes—sodium and potassium—from body fluids. Silver nitrate is hypotonic and will draw fluid from a wound. Serum electrolyte levels must be monitored—usually 3 to 4 times a day—and oral or intravenous supplements given as needed. *Anything* coming in contact with the silver nitrate solution becomes stained dark brown/black, including bed linen, floors, metal, and skin. While skin stains will eventually wear off, stains on inanimate objects are usually permanent.

The dressings are changed 1 to 3 times a day, at which time a tub bath is usually given. Since dressing changes are painful, analgesics should be administered *20 to 30 minutes* before the procedure in order to be fully effective. One very important point to be remembered when using silver nitrate is that *the dressings must never be allowed to dry out,* as the silver nitrate solution becomes concentrated and can *harm* tissue.

Mafenide is a cream that is dabbed on the injured area, with the area left uncovered or covered with a single layer of fine mesh gauze. A generous amount of mafenide is applied by hand once or twice a day, using a sterile glove, or a sterile tongue blade. The cream is reapplied if rubbed off between applications. Tubbing—usually in a Hubbard tank—is used to remove previously applied cream.

Patients usually complain of a stinging or burning sensation when mafenide is first applied. They may require an analgesic 20 to 30 minutes before tubbing and application of the drug. Mafenide has carbonic anhydrase inhibitor properties and with continued use, acidosis can occur. Usually the respiratory system compensates for acidosis, but the physician may order oral sodium bicarbonate ($NaHCO_3$) to counteract this drug action, especially in patients who have had damage to the lining of the respiratory tract.

Silver sulfadiazine 1 percent is a water-soluble ointment applied in the same manner as mafenide. It does not sting when applied, nor does it disturb electrolyte or acid-base balances as do the previously mentioned drugs. This drug is particularly effective in controlling Pseudomonas infections, one of the most common burn wound infections. Other drugs are also applied using sterile techniques. As the manner of burn treatment varies, so too may the method or amount of drug applied vary.

Skin-grafting techniques

As stated before, first- and second-degree burns (partial-thickness burns) have the ability to heal without grafting; full-thickness burns require grafting because the skin layers capable of regeneration have been destroyed. Skin grafting is necessary during the management (or treatment) and rehabilitation stages of third-degree burns, and the management stage of most second-degree burns. Some second-degree burns may require grafting for cosmetic reasons. The purpose of a skin graft during the management stage is to lessen the possibility of infection, minimize fluid loss by evaporation, and prevent loss of function.

Bacteria present in the air, on the skin, and on objects in the environment cause no problem to others but *can* cause serious infections in burn wounds. The control of infection is of *prime* importance, because infection is one of the major causes of death in these patients. Body fluid lost by evaporation from the burned areas can be replaced with intravenous fluids, but there still remains the problem of *exact* replacement of fluids. Too much fluid results in overhydration, which places an added strain on the heart. Too little fluid results in dehydration, which is also serious. Fluid needs can be met, but the calculation of exact fluid requirements at any given moment is sometimes difficult. Unassisted healing, that is, not employing the use of temporary grafts, in second-degree burns can result in an overgrowth of granulation tissue. Good granulation tissue without excessive overgrowth is necessary for successful skin grafting during the rehabilitation stage. The purpose of skin grafting during the rehabilitation stage is the restoration of cosmetic appearance and function.

There are three sources of skin grafts: the patient's own body (autografts), skin from other living humans (homografts or allografts) or from cadavers, and the skin of animals (heterografts or xenografts). Heterografts are obtained from animals (pig or cow) or are made from synthetic materials. Only the patient's own skin or the skin from an identical twin can be used for permanent grafts, because other types of grafts are ultimately rejected by the body. Heterografts, which are temporary, are often used during the initial stages of treatment. Once healing has begun, the patient's own skin is used for final cosmetic reconstruction.

General nursing management of the burned patient

Patients who suffer severe burns require skilled management throughout hospitalization. Methods of treatment may vary; therefore, the nurse must be familiar with the policies and procedures outlined in the hospital procedure manual. Any order that seems unclear should be questioned and no procedure should be undertaken unless the nurse is thoroughly familiar with machinery, equipment, or methods of performance.

Patients admitted with severe burns are usually acutely ill. The extent or depth of burns is not always an accurate measurement of the patient's physical status. Elderly patients and children may show more intense physical symptoms than do young or middle-aged adults when only a small percentage of the body has been burned. Shock may be present in any patient, and this, along with other problems must be

Table 51-4.
Nursing management of the burned patient

Check blood pressure, pulse, respirations:
Hourly (or oftener) during the acute stage which may last 3 to 4 days.
Every 2 to 4 hours thereafter or according to the physician's order, unit policy, or nurse's judgment.
Check temperature every 1 to 4 hours or as ordered.
Record daily weights by use of a bed scale.
Monitor intake and output:
Urine output may be measured hourly during the acute phase.
Urine is tested for specific gravity, glucose, acetone, and protein hourly during the acute phase.
Output and other urine tests may be measured at less frequent intervals after the acute phase.
Nursing observations:
Describe burned areas with accuracy, noting any signs of crust or eschar formation, infection, cracking of crusts or eschar, oozing, bleeding.
Describe the patient's mental state: oriented, disoriented, confused, depressed, withdrawn, and so on.
Assure proper positioning of burned extremities which is important in preventing contractures.
Assist with active or passive exercises as ordered by the physician. The physical therapist may do some of the exercises with nursing personnel repeating the movements at specified intervals.

quickly and efficiently treated. Once emergency care is given, the following objectives of immediate and long-term management must be met:

1. Meeting the patient's needs now and in the future.
2. Keeping infection at a minimum.
3. Rehabilitation.

The patient's immediate needs are establishing an adequate airway, meeting fluid loss, relieving pain, observing sterile or clean techniques to prevent infection, and preventing or combating shock. Following emergency care, the patient will be transferred to the hospital unit (intensive care unit, burn treatment unit) or to another hospital with a specialized burn treatment center.

On arrival in the hospital unit, the patient may be placed on a regular bed, CircOlectric bed, or other type of turning frame. Sterile or clean linen will be used, depending on the method of treatment or hospital policy. Nonadherent absorbent pads are placed under the burned areas to absorb excess moisture. Personnel and visitors wear sterile or clean caps, gowns, and masks. Hospitals may use a special record sheet for recording nursing tasks and observations. If none is available, certain nursing tasks are to be included in a plan of care (see Table 51-4). These may be modified according to specific policies of the unit, the extent of burns, and the patient's condition.

Throughout the long hospitalization and rehabilitation period, the patient requires a great deal of emotional support. During the acute phase, mental changes may be due to electrolyte and fluid imbalances, lack of oxygen, or severe pain. Some burned victims may be alcoholics, drug addicts, or elderly persons who are senile. Withdrawal from alcohol or narcotics, or senility, can add to the behavior changes due to physiological problems, further compounding the problem of identifying the underlying cause(s) of the behavior disorder. Depression may occur after the acute phase has passed. The seriousness and the extent of the injury, pain and discomfort, the long recovery period, repeated surgery for skin grafts, the humdrum of hospital routine, financial needs, and concern about disfigurement can influence the patient's mental outlook. Coupled with this is the patient's previous emotional makeup and stability. The emotionally stable individual is more likely to cope with his problems than the unstable individual.

With little to occupy their minds except hospital routine, treatments, and their personal welfare, communication with the patient becomes an important and essential component in a plan of care. Television or radio is invaluable, but, if not available, nursing personnel must make an effort to provide contact with the outside world. Discussion of what is happening—the weather, sports, special news events, and so on—must be relayed to the patient, and visitors allowed if possible. Families also need emotional support for the seriousness of the injury and the long hospitalization will affect them as well as the patient. When possible, the methods of and reasons for treatment should be thoroughly explained to the patient and the family to help them adjust to this difficult situation. Thoughts uppermost in their minds will be disfigurement and what can be done to correct this problem, the costs of a long hospitalization and repeated surgeries, and the patient's future. Families need ample opportunity to discuss these problems with the physician. If it is noted that a particular problem is worrying the family or the patient, the nurse should report this to the physician. Team conferences are of great value in identifying the needs of the patient and his family.

Complications

Burns are frequently aggravated by complications. Although patients usually receive ample attention while they are in shock, it is harder to continue to give them the concentrated care that they need over a period of months.

Infection. Wound infection and septicemia are responsible for a large number of the deaths of burned patients who survive the shock period. Besides the overall lowered resistance of the burned patient, edema and thrombosis in the traumatized subcutaneous tissue obstruct bacterial-fighting mechanisms. There always is some infection in third-degree burns.

An increase in temperature may be the first indication of infection, and it characteristically mounts rapidly, rarely below 102° F. The pulse is rapid and yet regular. The odor or the appearance of the burn (if it is exposed) may change. The nurse should smell the burned area at least once a day. The odor of infection is different from that of burn exudate. On the other hand, a dry-appearing crust may harbor copious amounts of pus beneath its surface. By close and frequent contact with the patient the nurse is in an excellent position to be the first observer of infection, and should remain alert to its possible existence.

Treatment may include continuous saline soaks and antibiotics. The physician may order dressing changes every 4 hours with removal of the dead tissue loosened by the soaks. The saline should be warmed to normal body temperature before it is applied to the dressings.

Septicemia may result in oliguria, hypotension, tachypnea, paralytic ileus, disorientation (related to the degree of the fever), and cardiac failure. The patient may need oxygen, nasogastric suction, and blood; and intravenous fluid therapy may have to be resumed or increased.

Aspirin and sponging of the unburned areas may be ordered for the fever. Only those portions of the patient's body that are covered by unbroken skin should be sponged. If there is a high fever, the patient may be placed on a hypothermic blanket.

Kidney Failure. Oliguria or anuria are usual symptoms, but occasionally there is diuresis. If this complication is going to occur, it usually does so by the tenth to the twelfth day postburn.

Curling's Ulcer. For unknown reasons, burned patients sometimes develop a gastrointestinal ulcer. Ulcers are more common in patients with extensive burns, but may be seen in any burned patient. The symptom most suggestive of an ulcer is onset of, or increase in, anorexia, associated with abdominal distention due to gastric dilatation. As the patient recovers physiological balance from the widespread disturbances caused by the burn, his appetite should slowly improve. If there is reversal of this trend, it should be reported to the physician. The nurse also observes for blood in the stool and in the nasogastric tube or for hematemesis. Some patients have no symptoms until there is sudden gastrointestinal hemorrhage.

Gastrointestinal Disturbances. Dilatation of the stomach may occur, characterized by regurgitation of fluid, discomfort, anorexia, and nausea. The patient may be dyspneic, because the bloated stomach is pressing on the diaphragm, interfering with respiration. Also, fecal impaction may follow paralytic ileus.

Anemia. A number of factors contribute to the burned patient's anemia. Heat causes red blood cell destruction or makes the cells abnormally fragile which shortens their life. Red blood cells are trapped in dilated capillaries. Infection depresses the function of hematopoietic tissue. Blood is lost from granulating wounds at dressing changes. The treatment is blood transfusions, a high protein and iron-rich diet, with iron supplements.

Contractures. Due to the pull of tightening scar tissue, patients with third-degree burns may develop contractures that are both disfiguring and crippling. For example, a healed third-degree burn of the right side of the neck can twist and hold the head in a permanently fixed position. To minimize contractures, parts with third-degree burns sometimes can be held in extension during the period of immobilization with splints, sandbags, or casts. As soon as healing has advanced sufficiently so that movement will not crack the eschar, a program of physical therapy is started—perhaps whirlpool baths, and underwater and then dry exercises, both passive and active. If contractures develop, plastic surgery is indicated.

Decubitus Ulcers. Conditions are ripe for this complication as the patient has lost much body protein. He is immobilized for a time; therefore some areas of his body are compressed between the hard bed and an even harder bone. Frequent turning and good skin care to unburned areas help to prevent decubitus ulcers.

Respiratory Problems. Pneumonia also can follow immobilization and debilitation. A patient with burns of the chest finds it painful to cough up secretions, but he should be encouraged to do so anyway. Atelectasis may be caused by the aspiration of gastric contents following tube feedings or vomiting, as well as by mucus plugs retained in the respiratory passages.

Emotional considerations

Any questions that can be answered need answering. Some can be answered immediately, some may be referred to the physician, and the unknowns can be shared with a good listener.

Diversion may help the patient to keep from prolonged brooding. Can any of his special interests be tapped? The nurse should discuss this with him. A patient who is flat on his back and isolated in a tepee of sterile sheets may be able to watch television or the hall through a prism lens or by a strategically placed mirror. Initially, with mirrors, the patient may become frightened by his appearance. The patient's bed can be placed where he cannot easily see himself in the mirror until the edema phase is over, and until he has had a chance to see his chest or his arms start to heal. The patient's concept of his appearance can be a vital factor in restoring relations with his family and his friends. "How do I look?" and "Will people be repelled by my appearance?" may worry the patient. Also, he may worry about work in the future.

Discharge planning

Discharge planning should begin as soon as the acute phase is over. The scope of planning will depend on the patient, his family, the extent of burns, and the success of treatment. Patients with minimal injuries may require only basic discharge preparations whereas those with extensive injuries require thorough planning by means of a team approach. In addition to the physician, nurse, physical therapist, and social service worker, discharge planning may need to utilize community resources. The patient may require counseling (psychiatric, vocational), the supervision of a community health nurse, and financial assistance. There is no rigid guideline for long-range planning because each patient must be evaluated according to his specific needs. The points included in discharge planning will depend on the physician's orders, the patient's physical condition, and his or the family's ability to carry out these orders.

Long-range planning may need to include future surgery for cosmetic effects, for revision of scar tissue, or to restore function. Vocational rehabilitation may be necessary for patients who are unable to return to their previous work. As some patients incur severe functional limitation and disfigurement, discharge planning must be thorough, with *all* members of the health team making a concentrated effort to return the patient to as normal a life as possible.

General nutritional considerations

- The burned patient has lost massive amounts of fluid as well as serum proteins and electrolytes. Initially, these losses are replaced by intravenous or nasogastric feedings.
- Once food and fluid can be taken orally, the patient is usually given a diet high in calories and protein. Vitamin and protein supplements in the form of concentrates, such as multivitamin liquids (i.e., drugs), may be added to liquid supplemental feedings. Protein may be given as a liquid drink, for example, Sustagen, Lonalac, Meritine, and so on.
- Diet therapy for the burned patient must be focused on providing foods the patient will consume and providing foods that meet his nutritional requirements. If the patient does not eat an adequate diet, he may have to be tube fed, as a high-protein, high-caloric, high-vitamin and high-mineral diet is absolutely essential in the healing of burns.

General pharmacological considerations

- Various drugs are used in the treatment of burns with each product having advantages and disadvantages. Examples of products used in the treatment of burns are: mafenide (Sulfamylon), silver nitrate ($AgNO_3$) 0.5 percent solution, povidone-iodine (Betadine), gentamicin (Garamycin) 0.1 percent cream, silver sulfadiazine (Silvadene) 1 percent ointment.
- To be effective, each drug must be applied exactly as ordered by the physician.
- Silver nitrate soaks must be continuous and the dressings must not be allowed to dry out as a concentrated silver nitrate solution can harm tissue.
- Sterile technique is used in the application of all topical drugs used in the treatment of burns.

Bibliography

Anderson, L., et al: *Nutrition in Nursing*. Philadelphia, Lippincott, 1972.

Bowden, M. L. and Feller, I.: Family reaction to a severe burn. Am. J. Nurs. 73:317, February, 1973.

Calleia, P. and Boswick, J. A.: A home care nursing program for patients with burns. Am. J. Nurs. 72:1442, March, 1973.

Cosgriff, J. H. and Anderson, D. L.: *The Practice of Emergency Room Nursing*. Philadelphia, Lippincott, 1975.

Davidson, S. P.: Nursing management of emotional reactions of severely burned patients during the acute phase. Heart-Lung, 2:370, May/June, 1973.

Guthrie, H. A.: *Introductory Nutrition*, ed. 3. St. Louis, Mosby, 1975.

Hartford, C. E.: The early treatment of burns. Nurs. Clin. North Am. 8:447, September, 1973.

Jacoby, F. G.: *Nursing Care of the Patient with Burns*. St. Louis, Mosby, 1972.

Jelenko, C.: Emergency treatment of small deep burns (pictorial). Hosp. Med. 11:92, January, 1975.

Megan, B. J.: Initial care of the thermally injured (pictorial). AORN J 20:837, November, 1974.

Monafo, W. W.: *The Treatment of Burns: Principles and Practice*. St. Louis, Green, 1971.

Murphy, W. L.: Skin coverage for burn injury (pictorial). AORN J 20:794, November, 1974.

Polk, H. C. and Stone, H. H.: *Contemporary Burn Management*. Boston, Little, Brown, 1971.

Silverstein, P.: The development of porcine cutaneous xenograft as a biologic dressing (pictorial). Hosp. Care 4:4, March, 1973.

Stinson, V.: Porcine skin dressings for burns (pictorial). Am. J. Nurs. 74:111, January, 1974.

Wagner, M.: Positioning of burn patients. Nurs. Care 7:22, August, 1974.

CHAPTER—52

The patient with neurological disease

On completion of this chapter the student will:

- **Recognize the signs and symptoms of increased intracranial pressure.**
- **Discuss the nursing management of the patient who has or is in danger of developing increased intracranial pressure.**
- **Define the various types of brain injuries.**
- **Describe the observations made when the patient has or is suspected of having a brain injury.**
- **List the symptoms of a brain tumor.**
- **Describe the preoperative preparations of the patient having a craniotomy.**
- **Formulate a nursing care plan for and participate in the nursing management of a patient with a craniotomy.**

Increased intracranial pressure

The brain is enclosed in a sealed bony vault, the skull. Cerebrospinal fluid, produced in the ventricles, passes down into the spinal subarachnoid space, then up through the basilar cisterns and over the cerebral hemispheres to the region of the dural ve-

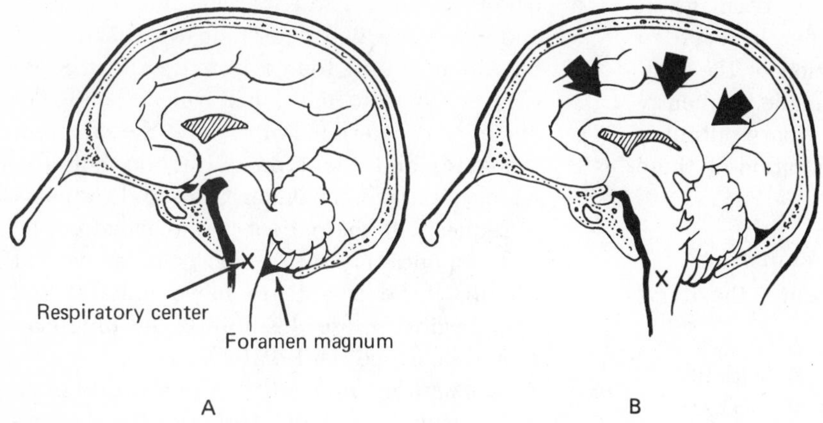

figure 52-1. (A) The normal brain. (B) Herniation of the lower portion of the brain stem (medulla) through the foramen magnum, caused by increased intracranial pressure. Note the position of the respiratory center.

Table 52-1.
Signs and symptoms of increased intracranial pressure

PULSE: may be increased initially, later becomes slow (40 to 60 per minute), full and bounding.

BLOOD PRESSURE: rises with a widening pulse pressure.

RESPIRATIONS: irregular, with Cheyne-Stokes or Kussmaul breathing.

PUPILS: may be unequal and may not react to light.

LEVEL OF CONSCIOUSNESS: progressive loss of consciousness; patient becomes comatose.

ADDITIONAL SIGNS: there may be vomiting which can be projectile and can occur without warning. Paralysis and headache may also be seen.

nous sinuses, where most of the absorption takes place. A tumor, a hematoma, or an abscess may increase intracranial pressure because of the added bulk within the rigid confines of the skull, as well as by obstruction of the cerebrospinal fluid pathways. A mass, such as a tumor, presses on and displaces the adjacent brain tissue, perhaps causing compression of the midbrain and displacement of the cerebellar tonsils through the foramen magnum, with compression of the medulla (Fig. 52-1).

The underlying pathology of increased intracranial pressure is basically constant, even though the etiology may vary. The most crucial pathological change is anoxia of the brain cells, or edema of white matter. Permanent brain damage may result.

Signs and symptoms

There are three cardinal signs and symptoms of increased intracranial pressure with an intracranial mass:

Headache. The pain is usually intermittent. Constant headache usually indicates that the patient's prognosis is grave. Anything that increases intracranial pressure, such as coughing, sneezing, or straining at stool, increases the headache. Lying quietly in bed—especially if the head of the bed is elevated—tends to reduce the intracranial pressure and thus helps to relieve the headache.

Vomiting. This usually occurs without the forewarning of nausea and without any relation to eating and it may be projectile.

Papilledema. This edema of the optic nerve at the point at which it enters the eyeball is caused by obstruction of venous drainage from the globe caused by the increased intracranial pressure.

The signs and symptoms of increased intracranial pressure are summarized in Table 52-1.

Treatment

The treatment may be medical or surgical, depending on the etiology. When possible, the underlying cause is removed: the infection is cured, the hematoma is drained, or the tumor is excised.

Cerebral edema may be treated with corticosteroids in high doses or with a hypertonic intravenous solution, such as mannitol or Urevert (intravenous urea).

Hypertonic solutions may be given by rectum as well as intravenously. When patients have been given mannitol or Urevert, the urinary output is recorded every 15 to 30 minutes, and observation of the vital signs and the level of consciousness is made frequently to assess the effects of the drug. The urinary output is expected to increase after the administration of these drugs.

Nursing management

In cases of increased cranial pressure, the nurse should:

- *Check vital signs q. 30 minutes.* As with all disease conditions, the vital signs tell a story to the observer. A rapid increase in the pulse rate usually occurs initially. The rate may vary as much as 10 to 20 beats from the original reading; then, there is usually a drop. If the pulse becomes less than 60 beats per minute and bounding, the physician should be notified immediately. Accompanying this change in pulse rate is an increase in the pulse pressure, and respirations may be variable. As the pressure on the cerebrum increases, there is likely to be an associated hypoxia. In order to compensate for this, the heart again beats faster.
- *Check the levels of consciousness and pupillary reaction.* The brain stem has a great deal to do with the maintenance of the conscious state. Any direct trauma or associated pressure on the brain stem will cause a change in the level of consciousness. If a person is hit on the back of the head, he is likely to lose consciousness much more quickly than if he is hit on the forehead; however, if there is edema, hemorrhage, or increased production of cerebrospinal fluid, the brain substance itself will press down on the pons and cause progressive stupor.

  If the temporal lobe is displaced medially by a mass, it may press on the third cranial (oculomotor) nerve, with the result that the muscles of the eye become paralyzed, and the corresponding pupil dilates and no longer reacts to a beam of light, such as that from a flashlight. Damage to the nuclei in the brain stem may result in constricted pupils, which are also unreactive.
- *Check for paralysis.* Loss of motor function is another valuable yardstick in ascertaining the amount of increased intracranial pressure. On admission of the patient, the physician and the nurse will determine whether or not he can move all four extremities. If the patient is asked to move his arm or hand, the nurse can determine not only the amount, the kind, and the type of motion but also whether the patient understands and responds to requests. If the patient is semicomatose, he will respond only to a pinch or other painful stimuli. If he is able to move initially and later begins to lose this ability, the physician should be called immediately.
- *Give nothing by mouth.* The previous three orders have been concerned with the recognition of increased intracranial pressure. This order is directed toward its prevention. If the patient is given food or fluid by mouth, he runs the risk of vomiting. Vomiting, sneezing, coughing, and hiccoughing cause an increase in pressure. This must be guarded against, since any sudden increase in the pressure may precipitate herniation of the brain through the foramen magnum, which results in compression of the medulla. The vital cardiopulmonary center is contained in the medulla. Pressure on this center will cause irregular respirations or apnea. An unconscious patient is never given fluids by mouth, because he may aspirate them.

  Although intake is prohibited by mouth, fluids are given intravenously. If the patient has been perspiring profusely, vomiting, or bleeding, additional fluid will be given. When there is marked increase in intracranial pressure, the fluid intake may be restricted. Overhydration or an infusion run too rapidly can increase intracranial pressure.
- *Elevate the head of the bed 30°, and maintain the patient's head to the side.* Patients with cerebral lesions are usually positioned with the head of the bed elevated to promote the return of venous drainage of blood and cerebrospinal fluid. The doctor orders the degree to which he wishes the bed elevated. Patients with basal skull fractures may be kept flat. In no instance should the patient's head be allowed to rest below the level of the rest of his body.

  Turning the patient on his side does not automatically result in a patent airway. He

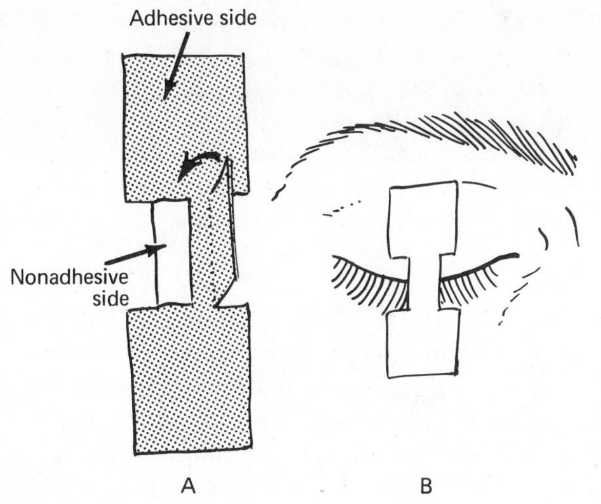

figure 52-4. A butterfly bandage to keep the eye closed. (A) Shows the side that goes on the patient. (B) Applied to the eye.

toms, such as vomiting, loss of consciousness, or cyanosis.

- Urinary output is important. A Foley catheter may be inserted if the patient has retention of urine. The amount voided by the patient who has had a pituitary tumor must be observed because damage to the gland may impair its manufacture of vasopressin, which regulates the amount of urine excreted. Postoperatively, the patient will usually be incontinent of urine and feces for one or two days, due to the depression of the voluntary cortical centers that control bladder and bowel habits.
- Edema may be present in the face, especially around the eyes. Ice compresses may be allowed. If the patient's face looks swollen and has ecchymotic areas, his family should be told before they see him that the swelling and the black-and-blue spots are both expected and temporary.
- The eyes should be observed. The patient may suffer a loss of the corneal reflex and keep his eyes open without blinking. Because blinking keeps the eye moist and free from specks of dust, the unblinking eye becomes dry and prone to corneal ulcers (Fig. 52-4).

Position. The neurosurgeon will prescribe the position in which the patient is to be placed postoperatively, depending on the surgery performed, the amount of cerebral edema, and his preference. In general, the heads of patients who have had craniotomies are kept elevated, often to 35° or 50°. If there is considerable edema, the physician may order that the head of the bed be kept at a 90° angle. Patients usually are not kept flat, because this position increases the blood supply to the brain and may start venous bleeding.

When the postoperative neurological patient is helpless, he is positioned as carefully as is any patient

Table 52-2.
Nursing management of the patient undergoing a craniotomy

Preoperative Preparation

Shaving of the scalp followed by a shampoo of the area. This may be done in the operating room after the administration of a general anesthetic.

Enemas or suppositories may be ordered to empty the bowel. Enemas are given with *great care*; straining by the patient must be avoided as this increases intracranial pressure.

An indwelling catheter is inserted.

Preoperative medications may be ordered and are usually limited to drugs that dry secretions (atropine, scopolamine).

Elastic stockings (antiembolitic stockings) may be applied to the legs.

Postoperative Management

Vital signs: blood pressure, pulse, respirations are checked as ordered.

Temperature is taken hourly or as ordered.

Fluids: nothing is given by mouth until ordered. Intravenous fluids may be ordered to infuse at a specific rate such as 20 drops per minute.

The patient's position is changed every 2 hours.

The patient's airway must be maintained. An oropharyngeal airway may be inserted until the patient is fully conscious.

Oral secretions are removed from the mouth by *gentle* suctioning.

Hourly evaluations are made of dressing, level of consciousness, motor activity, speech.

who cannot move himself. Special attention is given to placing the limbs in positions of function, so that even the patient whose prognosis is unfavorable will get as much use of his limbs as possible.

FLUID AND FOOD. After the patient has recovered from anesthesia, his intake is determined by his condition, which may necessitate intravenous feedings, gastric lavage, or a soft diet. Intravenous fluids should run at the rate ordered by the physician. Cerebral edema may cause the physician to order restricted fluids. Some postoperative patients who are otherwise able to eat may not be able to swallow well. They should be fed slowly and carefully to avoid aspiration of food or fluids, which may start a fatal pneumonia.

REHABILITATION. As soon as the patient returns from the operating room, his rehabilitation begins. Even the patient who is not expected to return to full activity should be given every chance and encouragement for as full a return of function as is possible. Proper positioning is the first step. Then passive exercises are done until the patient can move himself. At this point he is supervised in active exercises.

General pharmacological considerations

- Phenytoin (Dilantin) may be administered before and after cranial surgery as a prophylactic measure to prevent the convulsions which can occur in any patient undergoing this type of surgery.
- The use of narcotics, especially the opiate types, is avoided as these drugs tend to mask the signs of increased intracranial pressure. Some physicians may use codeine in low doses; this drug has minimal effect on the pupils, respiration, and level of consciousness when lower doses are given.
- Consistent use of aspirin or *products containing aspirin* for relief of pain is avoided. Aspirin can affect the blood clotting mechanism which in turn could cause increased bleeding during surgery.

Bibliography

AMERICAN CANCER SOCIETY: *A Cancer Source Book for Nurses.* New York, American Cancer Society, 1975.

BEESON, P. B. and MCDERMOTT, W., eds.: *Textbook of Medicine,* ed. 14. Philadelphia, Saunders, 1975.

BRUNNER, L. S. and SUDDARTH, D. S.: *Textbook of Medical-Surgical Nursing,* ed. 3. Philadelphia, Lippincott, 1975.

CARINI, E. and OWENS, G.: *Neurological and Neurosurgical Nursing,* ed. 6. St. Louis, Mosby, 1974.

COSGRIFF, J. H. and ANDERSON, D. L.: *The Practice of Emergency Nursing.* Philadelphia, Lippincott, 1975.

ERICKSON, R.: Cranial check: A basic neurological assessment. Nurs. '74, 8:67, August, 1974.

FREIDMAN, M.: *The Story of Josh.* New York, Ballantine Books, 1974.

GLASS, S. J.: Nursing care of the neurosurgical patient: head injuries. J. Neurosurg. Nurs. 5:49, December, 1973.

GREISHEIMER, E. M. and WIEDEMAN, M. P.: *Physiology and Anatomy,* ed. 9. Philadelphia, Lippincott, 1972.

HINKHOUSE, A.: Craniocerebral trauma. Am. J. Nurs. 73:1719, October, 1973.

HOLVEY, D. N., ed.: *Merck Manual of Diagnosis and Therapy,* ed. 12. Merck, Rahway, N.J., 1972.

JOHNSON, M. R.: Emergency management of head and spinal injuries. Nurs. Clin. North Am. 8:389, September, 1973.

KORTE, M. L.: Intensive care of the neurologic patient . . . meeting the challenge. Nurs. Clin. North Am. 7:335, June, 1972.

LE MAITRE, G. and FINNEGAN, J.: *The Patient in Surgery: A Guide for Nurses.* Philadelphia, Saunders, 1975.

MANDRILLO, M. P.: Brain scanning (pictorial). Nurs. Clin. North Am. 9:633, December, 1974.

PRESTON, D. N.: Diagnosed as glioma. Nurs. Times 67:1402, November 11, 1971.

LABORATORY VALUES

Laboratory Values

Abbreviations

cu.	cubic
cu. mm.	cubic millimeter
gm.	gram
hpf	high power field (refers to magnification power of microscope)
I.U.	international unit
L.	liter
lpf	low power field
kg.	kilogram
mcg.	microgram
mEq.	milliequivalent
mg.	milligram
mm.	millimeter
mm. Hg	millimeter of mercury
mU.	milliunit
ng.	nanogram

Abbreviations (*Continued*)

μ	micron
μg., mcg.	microgram
μl.	microliter
μU.	microunit

Blood Coagulation Tests (Normal Values)

bleeding time (Ivy or Duke)	up to 6 minutes
partial prothrombin time (PTT)	60-70 seconds
coagulation time (Lee-White)	6-17 minutes (glass tubes)
prothrombin time (one stage)	12-16 seconds; 70-100% of control

Hematology (Normal Values)

platelet count	150,000-400,000/cu. mm.

Hematology (Normal Values) (*Continued*)	
reticulocyte count	0.5-1.5%
sedimentation rate (ESR)	
male	0-15 mm./hr.
female	0-20 mm./hr.
complete blood count (CBC)	
hematocrit	
male	40-54%
female	38-47%
hemoglobin	
male	13-16 gm./100 ml.
female	12-14 gm./100 ml.
red cell count	
male	4,600,000-6,200,000/ cu. mm.
female	4,200,000-5,400,000/ cu. mm.
white cell count	4,500-11,000/cu. mm.
segmented neutrophils	56%
band neutrophils	3%
eosinophils	1-4%
basophils	0-0.5%
lymphocytes	20-30%
monocytes	2-6%
erythrocyte indices	
mean corpuscular volume (MCV)	82-98 (cu. microns)
mean corpuscular hemoglobin (MCH)	27-32 $\mu\mu$g. per cell
mean corpuscular hemoglobin concentration (MCHC)	32-36%
blood volume	
male	75 ml./kg. of body weight
female	67 ml./kg. of body weight
plasma volume	
male	39 ml./kg. of body weight
female	40 ml./kg. of body weight

Whole Blood, Serum, and Plasma Chemistries (Normal Values)	
ammonia	30-80 μg./100 ml. (enzymatic method)
amylase	80-150 Somogyi units/100 ml.
ascorbic acid	0.4-1.6 mg./100 ml.

Whole Blood, Serum, and Plasma Chemistries (Normal Values) (*Continued*)	
bilirubin, total	0.1-1.0 mg./100 ml.
direct	0.1-0.2 mg./100 ml.
indirect	0.1-0.8 mg./100 ml.
blood gases	
pH	7.35-7.45
$PaCO_2$	35-45 mm. Hg
PaO_2	80-100 mm. Hg
HCO_3 (bicarbonate)	22-26 mEq./L.
SaO_2	95% arterial blood 70-75% mixed venous blood
bromsulfophthalein (BSP)	5 mg./kg. of dye administered with less than 6% retention after 45 minutes
calcium	8.5-10.5 mg./100 ml.
carbon dioxide (CO_2 content)	24-32 mEq./L.
cephalin flocculation	negative to 1+
chloride (serum)	95-105 mEq./L.
cholesterol	150-300 mg./100 ml.
copper	65-170 μg/100 ml.
creatine phosphokinase (CPK)	0-20 I.U./L.
creatinine	0.7-1.5 mg./100 ml.
fibrinogin	200-400 mg./100 ml.
glucose (fasting)	65-110 mg./100 ml.
icterus index	1-6 units
insulin	4-24 μU./ml.
iodine, protein bound (PBI)	4.0-8.0 μg./100 ml.
iron, total	60-150 μg./100 ml.
iron-binding capacity	250-450 μg./100 ml.
iron saturation, percent	20-55%
ketone bodies	negative
17-ketosteroids	25-125 μg./100 ml.
lactate dehydrogenase (LDH)	80-200 mU./ml.
lipids (total)	400-1,000 mg./100 ml.
nonprotein nitrogen (NPN)	16-35 mg./100 ml.
phosphatase, acid	1.0-5.0 King-Armstrong units 0.5-2.0 Bodansky units
phosphatase, alkaline	5.0-13.0 King-Armstrong units 1.5-4.5 Bodansky units
proteins, total	6.0-8.0 gm./100 ml.
albumin	3.5-5.5 gm./100 ml.
globulin	1.5-3.0 gm./100 ml.
sodium	135-145 mEq./L.
T_3 uptake	25-35%

Whole Blood, Serum, and Plasma Chemistries (Normal Values) (*Continued*)	
thyroxine-binding globulin	10-26 μg./100 ml. thyroxine
thyroid-stimulating hormone (TSH)	up to 0.2 mU./ml.
transaminase	
SGOT	15-45 units/ml.
SGPT	5-36 units/ml.
triglycerides	10-190 mg./ml.
urea nitrogen (BUN)	8-20 mg./ml.
uric acid	2.5-8.0 mg./100 ml.

Urine	
acetoacetic acid	negative
acetone	negative
albumin (qualitative)	negative
aldosterone (24-hr. specimen)	2-26 μg./24 hr.
estrogens (24-hr. specimen)	
ovulation	28-100 μg./24 hr.
luteal peak	22-105 μg./24 hr.
at menses	4-25 μg./24 hr.
pregnancy	up to 45,000 μg./24 hr.
postmenopause	14-20 μg./24 hr.
male	5-18 μg./24 hr.
glucose	negative
17-hydroxycorticosteroids (24-hr. specimen)	
male	5.5-14.5 mg./24 hr.
female	4.9-12.9 mg./24 hr.
17-ketosteroids (24-hr. specimen)	
male	8.0-15.0 mg./24 hr.
female	6.0-11.5 mg./24 hr.
microscopic examination	up to 1-2 RBC, WBC, epithelial cells/hpf; occasional cast/lpf

Cerebrospinal Fluid	
cell count	0-8 cells/μl.
chloride	120-130 mEq./L.
colloidal gold curve	not more than 1 in any tube
glucose	45-80 mg./100 ml.
protein (total)	15-45 mg./100 ml.

Serology	
antistreptolysin-0 (ASLO)	less than 160 Todd units
cold agglutinins	less than 1:32
C-reactive protein (CRP)	0
fluorescent treponemal antibodies (HAA)	negative
herterophile antibodies	less than 1:56
latex fixation	negative
VDRL	nonreactive

Feces	
pH	7.0-7.5 (but may be acid)
RBC's	absent
WBC's	few
urobilinogen	40-280 mg./24 hr.
fat	less than 7 gm./24 hr.

Semen	
volume	more than 3 ml.
pH	7.2-8.0
count	more than 50 million/ml.

Drugs	
barbiturates: coma level	
phenobarbital	approximately 11 mg./100 ml.
most other barbiturates	2-4 mg./100 ml.
ethanol	0.3-0.4% marked intoxication 0.4-0.5% alcoholic stupor over 0.5% coma
salicylates	20-25 mg./100 ml. therapeutic range over 30 mg./100 ml. toxic range
cardiac drugs	
digitoxin	14-30 ng./ml. therapeutic range over 30 ng./ml. toxic range
digoxin	1.0-2.0 ng./ml. therapeutic range over 3.0 ng./ml. toxic range

Drugs (*Continued*)	
propranolol	20-50 ng./ml. therapeutic range
	over 50 ng./ml. toxic range
lidocaine	1.4-6.0 mcg./ml. therapeutic range
	over 6 mcg./ml. toxic range

Gastric	
free HCl	0-30 mEq./L.
total acidity	15-45 mEq./L.
combined acid	10-15 mEq./L.

NOTE: Laboratory values will vary somewhat when different references are consulted. Laboratory technique may also alter values.

GLOSSARY

abduction movement of the extremities away from the midline

abortion termination of pregnancy before the fetus is viable

abscess a localized collection of pus

accommodation the ability of the eye to focus at different distances

acetone bodies *see* ketone bodies

acetylcholine a neurohormone concerned with the transmission of nerve impulses

acidosis disturbance in acid-base balance with an accumulation of acid

ACTH adrenocorticotropic hormone, a hormone manufactured and secreted by the anterior pituitary gland

addiction a state of periodic or chronic intoxication produced by repeated consumption of a drug

adduction movement of the extremities toward the midline

adrenergic drugs drugs acting like or mimicking the action of the sympathetic nervous system

aerobic needing oxygen to live

albuminuria presence of albumin in the urine

alkalosis disturbance in acid-base balance with an accumulation of alkali

alkylating agent an antineoplastic drug that interferes with cell division

allergens substances that are inhaled, ingested, or come in contact with the skin and cause an allergy

alopecia abnormal loss of hair; baldness

amenorrhea absence of the menstrual flow

anabolism building up of body tissue; opposite of catabolism (adj., anabolic)

anaerobic unable to survive in the presence of oxygen

analgesic a drug relieving pain

anastomosis a joining, communication, or union (adj., anastomotic)

anemia a decrease in the number of red blood cells and a lower than normal hemoglobin (adj., anemic)

anesthesiologist a physician trained in the administration of anesthesia

aneurysm abnormal dilatation of a blood vessel due to a defect or weakness in the vessel wall
angina pectoris chest pain due to a decrease in blood supply to the myocardium
anorectal pertaining to the anus and rectum
anorexia loss of appetite (adj., anorectic)
anoxia lack of oxygen (adj., anoxic)
antibody protein substance manufactured by the body in response to the presence of a specific antigen
anticoagulant a drug interfering with the blood-clotting mechanism
antiemetic a drug used to treat or prevent nausea
antigen a substance which induces the manufacture of antibodies
antihistamine a drug that appears to compete with histamine receptor sites and is used in the treatment of allergy and motion sickness
antimetabolite an antineoplastic drug that interferes with cell growth by preventing use of necessary materials
antineoplastic a drug used in the treatment of neoplasms, more specifically malignant diseases
antipyretic a drug that lowers an elevated body temperature
antiseptic an agent that slows the multiplication of microorganisms
antitoxin a substance formed in the body after exposure to a toxin
antivenin a substance used to neutralize the venom of a poisonous animal
anuria suppression of urinary output
aphasia inability to use or understand spoken and written language
arrhythmia a deviation from the normal cardiac rhythm
arteriosclerosis loss of elasticity of an artery and thickening of the intima
arthrodesis surgical fusion of the joint surfaces
arthroplasty surgical repair of a joint
ascites fluid in the abdomen
asthma paroxysms of dyspnea, wheezing, and coughing, with production of thick tenacious sputum
astigmatism visual defect resulting from unequal curvature in the cornea or lens, usually correctable with glasses
atelectasis partial or total collapse of the lung
atheroma fatty plaque
atherosclerosis a deposit of fatty plaques in the intima of the artery causing the lumen to become narrowed
atrophy a wasting with a decrease in size
attenuate weaken
autograft a graft taken from one part of the body for another part of the body
aura in epilepsy, a warning preceding an epileptic seizure
axilla the armpit
azotemia an excess accumulation of nitrogens, creatinine, and uric acid in the blood

bacteremia bacteria in the bloodstream
bactericidal an agent that kills bacteria
bacteriostatic an agent that slows the duplication of bacteria
barbiturates a group of drugs used as sedatives, hypnotics, and anesthetic agents; these drugs have addiction potential
benign nonmalignant; also means not serious
biliary pertaining to bile, liver, gallbladder
biosynthesis manufacture of substances by living organisms
blanch to become pale
bleb a blister filled with fluid
BMR basal metabolic rate, a test for thyroid function
brachial plexus a group of nerves in the lower part of the neck and axilla
bradycardia slowing of the pulse
bronchiectasis chronic dilatation of bronchi and bronchioles in one or both lungs
bronchiolitis inflammation of the bronchioles
bronchitis inflammation of the bronchi
bronchodilator a drug that dilates the bronchi
bronchography x-ray visualization of the bronchi following injection of a radiopaque substance into the bronchi
bronchoscopy direct visual examination of the trachea, two major bronchi, and multiple smaller bronchi
bulla a bleb filled with fluid and sometimes air when located in the lung (pl., bullae)

cachexia a state of wasting, emaciation (adj., cachectic)
calculus stone (pl., calculi)
callus fibrous tissue formed at ends of fractured bone
cancellous bone the reticular tissue of bone
cannula a tube inserted into the body; the lumen of the cannula is obstructed with a trocar to facilitate insertion
carbuncle a large swollen lesion, surrounded by erythema, often located on the back of the neck
carcinogens agents capable of causing cancer (adj., carcinogenic)
carcinoma a malignant tumor (syn., cancer)
cardiogenic shock shock due to failure of the heart to act as an efficient pump
cardiopulmonary resuscitation emergency measures taken to restore heart-lung function (abbr., CPR)
cartilage fibrous connective tissue attached to articular surfaces of bone

catabolism breaking down of body tissue; opposite of anabolism (adj., catabolic)
cataract an opacity of the lens of the eye, reducing the amount of light reaching the retina
catecholamine organic compound normally found in the sympathetic nervous system, e.g., epinephrine
cathartic a drug producing bowel movements
catheterization insertion of a catheter
causalgia burning pain
cecostomy an opening made in the cecum for drainage of intestinal contents
cerebration mental activity, thinking
cerebrovascular accident lay term, "stroke"; bleeding in or loss of blood supply to a part of the brain (abbr., CVA)
cerumen waxlike secretion in the outer ear canal
cervicitis inflammation of the cervix
chancre a round, painless lesion on the genitalia
chemotherapy therapy by means of chemicals or drugs
Cheyne-Stokes respirations shallow, rapid breathing building in intensity and depth, then decreasing, followed by a period of apnea
cholecystectomy removal of the gallbladder
cholecystitis inflammation of the gallbladder
cholecystostomy surgical opening into the gallbladder
choledocholithiasis presence of stones anywhere in the ducts of the biliary system
choledochostomy surgical opening into the common bile duct
cholesterol a sterol contained in animal tissues
cholinergic blocking agent a drug inhibiting the action of acetylcholine, e.g., atropine
chordae tendineae cordlike structures attached to the atrioventricular valves
chronic disease a disease extending over a long period of time
cilia hairlike projections of some types of epithelial cells which propel mucus, dust, and other foreign particles out of a structure
cisternal puncture insertion of a needle between the cervical vertebrae into the cisterna at the base of the brain to withdraw cerebrospinal fluid
clonus alternate contraction and relaxation of muscles resulting in jerking movements and excessive thrashing of the arms and legs (adj., clonic)
colectomy removal of all or part of the colon
colic spasm causing pain; may be intestinal, uterine, renal, or biliary
collagen fibrous protein found in connective tissue
collateral circulation circulation in smaller blood vessels when a large vessel is occluded
colostomy an opening in the colon; usually one end of the colon is brought to the abdominal wall for the purpose of diverting the fecal stream
coma a deep, stuporous, unresponsive state
comedo blackhead (pl., comedones)
commissurotomy a surgical breaking or splitting of adherent tissue
concussion loss of consciousness caused by a blow to the head
congenital present at birth
connective tissue fibrous tissue supporting and connecting internal organs and bones
contracture an abnormal shortening of muscle(s) usually resulting in a deformity of the part and rendering the part resistant to movement
contusion an injury in which the skin is not broken; a bruise
convulsion involuntary muscle relaxation and contraction
COPD abbr. for chronic obstructive pulmonary disease
cordotomy surgical interruption of pain pathways in the spinal cord
cortex outer portion of an organ
corticosteroid any of the steroids manufactured by the cortex of the adrenal gland
crepitation a crackling or grating sensation or sound
cryosurgery use of extreme cold to produce cell destruction
cryptorchidism undescended testicle(s)
curettage scraping
cutaneous pertaining to the skin
cyanosis a bluish discoloration to the skin, nail beds, or mucous membranes due to oxygen deficiency
cyst a sac or capsule containing fluid or semisolid material
cystectomy surgical removal of a cyst or of the urinary bladder
cystitis inflammation of the bladder
cystocele herniation of the urinary bladder into the anterior vagina
cystoscopy visual examination of the inside of the bladder by use of a cystoscope

D and C dilatation and curettage
debridement removal of foreign material or dead tissue from a wound
decalcification loss of calcium from bone
decortication removal of the cortex or outer layer
decubitus a bedsore
decussate to cross
defibrillation to stop fibrillation of the heart through use of electrical current or drugs
defibrillator a machine delivering a specific amount of electrical current to the heart
dehiscence separation of wound edges without protrusion of organs
dehydration excessive loss of water from the body not compensated by intake

delirium a state of disorientation and confusion caused by interference with the metabolic processes of the brain
depolarization transfer of positive ions to the inside of the cell membrane
dermis the skin
desensitization subcutaneous administration of gradually increasing doses of antigen
dialysis removal of certain metabolic end products or other substances from the blood when the kidneys are nonfunctioning
diaphoresis profuse perspiration
diastole relaxation of the atria and ventricles (adj., diastolic)
digitalization rapid administration of relatively large doses of digitalis preparations to achieve a therapeutic blood level
diplopia double vision
distal farthest from a point of reference; opposite of proximal
diuresis secretion of large amounts of urine
diuretic a drug capable of causing diuresis
dyscrasias a large group of blood disorders
dysmenorrhea painful menstruation
dysphagia difficulty in swallowing
dyspnea difficult breathing; air hunger (adj., dyspneic)
dysuria difficult or painful urination

ecchymosis bleeding into skin or mucous membrane producing blue-black discolorations
ECG (also **EKG**) abbr. for electrocardiogram
ectopic out of place; not in correct position
eczema a skin rash characterized by swelling, oozing, itching, scaling of the skin
edentulous without teeth
electrocardiogram the electrical activity of the heart recorded on heat sensitive paper
electroencephalogram (EEG) a record of the electrical activity of the brain
electrolyte any compound that separates into charged particles (ions) when dissolved in water
embolectomy surgical removal of an embolus
embolism obstruction of a blood vessel with an embolus
embolus a mass present in a blood vessel
embryonal pertaining to an embryo
emollient skin softener
empyema collection of pus in the pleural cavity
emphysema specific morphologic changes in the lung characterized by overdistention of alveolar sacs, rupture of alveolar walls, and destruction of the alveolar capillary bed
encephalitis an infectious disease of the central nervous system
encephalopathy any dysfunction of the brain
endarterectomy removal of atherosclerotic plaques from the intima of an artery
endocardium a layer of endothelial tissue lining of the interior wall of the heart
endocrine gland a gland regulating body activity by the secretion of hormones released directly into the bloodstream
endogenous arising or coming from within
endometriosis a condition in which endometrial tissue is located outside the uterus and in various other structures of the pelvis or abdominal wall
endoscope a tube containing an optical system, often fiber optics, and a method of illumination whose diameter is small enough to allow insertion into a body cavity
endoscopy inspection of body cavities or organs by use of an endoscope
endotoxin a toxin present in a bacterial cell
endotracheal in the trachea
enema introduction of fluid into the rectum to remove fecal material
enterostomal therapist a nurse specifically trained in the care and teaching of ostomy patients
enzyme a complex substance that initiates and accelerates a chemical change
epidermis the outer layer of skin
epistaxis nosebleed
epithelium a type of cell covering internal and external body surfaces
erythema redness of the skin
erythrocyte a red blood cell
erythropoiesis the manufacture of red blood cells
eschar a hard leathery crust made up of dehydrated dead skin which forms over a full-thickness burn
esophagoscopy visualization of the esophagus with an endoscope
estrogen female sex hormone manufactured by the ovaries
etiology the science that studies the causes of disease
evisceration separation of wound edges with protrusion of organs
exacerbation an increase in intensity of symptoms or severity of a disease
excoriation an abrasion of the outer layer of the skin
exfoliated cells dead cells shed from the skin, mucous membrane or bone
exfoliative cytology study of dead cells shed from the skin or mucous membrane
exocrine gland a gland that secretes externally; opposite of endocrine gland
exogenous coming or arising from outside the organism
expectorant a drug that encourages raising of secretions from the lungs
extracorporeal outside of the body
extrasystole *see* premature ventricular contraction

exudate fluid usually containing pus, bacteria, dead cells

fibrillation a quivering of muscle fibers
fibroblast a cell from which connective tissue is developed
fibrosis formation of fibrous tissue
fibrous containing fibers
fissure a groove, crack, or slit
fistula a passageway or connection from one area to another
flaccid relaxed, weak
flatulence excessive intestinal gas
flatus gas in the intestinal tract
fluoroscopy visualization by use of x-rays and a fluorescent screen
footdrop inability to maintain the foot in a normal position; a dragging of the foot
furuncles whitish, raised painful lesions surrounded by erythema

gamma globulin a protein found in the blood and manufactured by lymphoid tissue and reticuloendothelial cells in response to infection
gamma rays one of three emissions from radioactive substances; similar to x-rays
ganglion a mass of nervous tissue
gangrene necrosis of tissue almost always due to a lack of blood supply to the affected part
gastrectomy surgical removal of the stomach; may be total (all) or subtotal (part)
gastritis inflammation of the stomach
gastroscopy visualization of the stomach by means of an endoscope
gastrostomy surgical opening into the stomach, usually for the purpose of feeding; usual reason for procedure is esophageal or gastric cancer
gingivitis inflammation of the gums
glaucoma a condition resulting from increased intraocular pressure due to a disturbance of the normal balance between the production and drainage of the aqueous humor that fills the anterior chamber
glomerulonephritis inflammation of the glomeruli; a form of nephritis
glomerulosclerosis hardening and degeneration of the glomeruli and the renal arterioles
glucagon manufactured by the pancreas; stimulates release of glucose by the liver
glucocorticoid one of the adrenal cortical hormones
glycogen a polysaccharide; starch
glycosuria presence of glucose in the urine
goiter enlargement of the thyroid gland
gonads sex glands; ovaries in the female, testes in the male
gram-positive a retention of the color of a Gram stain; opposite of gram-negative, which does not retain the Gram stain
granulation tissue tissue formed during the repair and healing of wounds
granulocyte a type of white blood cell
gumma a well-defined local lesion of tertiary syphilis

habituation a condition resulting from the repeated consumption of a drug
hallucination subjective sensory experiences that occur without stimulation from the environment
helminth a parasitic worm or wormlike organism
hematemesis vomiting of blood
hematocrit a measurement of the volume of red blood cells in a given amount of blood
hematogenic shock shock due to blood loss
hematoma a swelling containing blood
hematuria blood in the urine
hemianopsia vision in only one half of the normal visual field
hemiplegia paralysis of one side or one half of the body
hemodialysis the removal of chemical substances from the blood by passing the blood through a system of tubes surrounded by a dialysate
hemoglobin the red blood cell pigment containing iron
hemolysis destruction of red blood cells
hemoptysis spitting up of blood from the respiratory tract
hemostasis stopping of bleeding; stagnation of blood in one area
hepatitis inflammation of the liver
herniorrhaphy surgical repair of a hernia
heterogeneous unlike
heterogenous from another species
heterograft a graft taken from another individual
Homan's sign pain in the calf on dorsiflexion of the foot
homeostasis term used to describe a dynamic state of equilibrium of the body
homogeneous of uniform or like characteristics
homograft a graft taken from another person
hormone a chemical substance secreted by an endocrine gland and carried to another area by way of the bloodstream
hydrocele a collection of fluid in the testes
hydronephrosis swelling of the kidney pelvis with backflow of urine
hyperaldosteronism excess production of aldosterone, an adrenal hormone
hyperalimentation providing essential nutrients by the intravenous route by means of a catheter in the superior vena cava or an external arteriovenous fistula

hypercapnia excess carbon dioxide in the blood
hypercholesterolemia excessive amount of cholesterol in the blood
hyperextension extreme extension of a part
hyperglycemia excess glucose in the blood
hyperinsulinism excessive secretion of insulin
hyperkalemia excess potassium in the blood
hyperopia farsightedness
hyperparathyroidism overproduction of parathormone
hyperplasia extra growth of normal tissue
hypertension sustained elevation of arterial pressure
hyperthermia elevation of body temperature; fever
hyperthyroidism excessive secretion of thyroid hormone resulting in an increased rate of all metabolic processes
hypertonia increased tone of muscles or arteries (adj., hypertonic)
hypertonic solution a solution with a greater osmotic pressure than another solution
hypertrophy increase in size of an organ or structure (adj., hypertrophied)
hyperuricemia accumulation of uric acid in the blood
hypervolemia increased volume of circulating blood; opposite of hypovolemia (adj., hypervolemic)
hypnotic a drug used to produce sleep
hypocalcemia decrease in blood calcium below normal level
hypocapnia decrease in carbon dioxide in the blood
hypoglycemia decrease in blood glucose below normal level
hypokalemia decrease in potassium in the blood below normal level
hyponatremia decrease in sodium in the blood below normal level
hypoparathyroidism underproduction of parathormone
hypoproteinemia decrease in protein in the blood below normal level
hypostatic pneumonia pneumonia occurring from prolonged bed rest with failure to cough, move, and deep breathe
hypotension low blood pressure
hypothermia decrease in body temperature
hypothyroidism a deficiency of thyroid hormones causing a lowered rate of all metabolic processes
hypovolemia diminished volume of circulating blood; opposite of hypervolemia (adj., hypovolemic)
hypoxemia reduced oxygen in the blood
hypoxia diminished availability of oxygen to cells of the body (adj., hypoxic)
hysterectomy surgical removal of the uterus

illusion an inaccurate interpretation of stimuli within the environment
intracerebral within the brain
intractable pain pain which cannot be controlled by analgesic medications or good nursing management
intradermal an injection into the skin substance
intraocular within the eyeball
intrathecal injection into the subarachnoid space of the spinal cord; a lumbar puncture must be performed
intravenous injection or infusion into the vein
intrinsic factor a substance manufactured in the stomach, necessary for the assimilation of vitamin B_{12}; absence produces pernicious anemia
ion one or more atoms carrying a positive or negative electrical charge, e.g., Na^+, OH^-
ionization the breaking up of molecules into their constituent ions
IPPB abbr. for intermittent positive pressure breathing
iridectomy removal of a segment of the iris
iridencleisis surgical creation of a fistula in the iris for treatment of glaucoma
ischemia lack of blood to a part
isolated perfusion introduction of an antineoplastic drug to a tumor area after the blood supply is isolated from the rest of the circulation
isotonic having the same tone; also, a solution having the same osmotic pressure as the solution being compared to it
isotope any one of a series of chemical elements having the same atomic number but a different atomic weight

jaundice a yellowish color to the skin or sclera of eyes due to excess bile pigment

ketone bodies chemical intermediate products in the metabolism of fat; betahydroxybutyric acid, acetoacetic acid, acetone
ketonemia presence of ketone bodies in the blood
ketonuria presence of ketone bodies in the urine
ketosis an accumulation of ketone bodies in the body

laminectomy removal of the posterior arch of the vertebra to expose the spinal cord
laryngectomy removal of the larynx
laryngofissure removal of part of the larynx
latent hidden
lavage to wash out
lethargy sluggishness, stupor (adj., lethargic)
leukemia a malignant disease of the bone marrow characterized by an abnormal production of white blood cells
leukocyte a white blood cell
leukocytosis an increase in the number of leukocytes
leukopenia a decrease in the number of leukocytes

leukoplakia patches of white, thickened tissue in the mouth or mucous membrane often considered to be a forerunner of cancer
leukorrhea a white or yellow-white vaginal discharge
ligation tying off; application of a ligature to a part
lithiasis formation of stones
lobectomy removal of a lobe
lumbar puncture insertion of a needle into the subarachnoid space of the spinal cord in the lumbar region
lumen the inner space in a tube or tubular organ
lymphedema massive edema due to an obstruction of lymph channels
lymphadenitis inflammation of lymph glands
lymphocyte a type of white blood cell
lymphoid tissue lymph tissue; resembling lymph tissue
lymphoma a tumor of lymphoid tissue

malaise a feeling of discomfort or uneasiness
malignant harmful; capable of producing death
mastectomy removal of the breast
mastoiditis infection of the mastoid process
maximum breathing capacity the most air a person can voluntarily move in and out of the lungs within a period of one minute
medulla inner portion of a gland or organ; also a portion of the upper spinal cord
melena tarry stools
menarche the start of menstruation; usually occurs between ages of 10 and 14
meninges collectively the three coverings of the brain and spinal cord: pia mater, arachnoid membrane, dura mater
meningitis inflammation of the membranes that surround the brain and spinal cord
menopause the period of time when menstruation begins to wane and finally ceases
menorrhagia excessive bleeding at the time of normal menstruation
metabolism the sum total of the physical and chemical changes and reactions taking place in the body
metastasis spread; the spread of disease from one part of the body to another (adj., metastatic, verb, metastasize)
metrorrhagia bleeding at a time other than a menstrual period
mineralocorticoid hormone produced by the adrenal gland
miotic a drug that constricts the pupil
Monilia same as Candida, a genus of fungus
monocyte a type of white blood cell
morbidity sickness expressed as a rate in relation to population
mortality death rate
mucopurulent consisting of pus and mucus
mucus fluid secreted by mucous membrane
mydriatic a drug used to dilate the pupil; usually applied topically
myelogram an x-ray of the spinal cord using a radiopaque dye to outline the cord
myocardial infarction lay term "heart attack"; infarct of the muscle layer (myocardium) of the heart; (abbr., MI)
myocardium heart muscle
myopia nearsightedness
myringoplasty plastic surgery on the eardrum
myringotomy incision of the eardrum
myxedema hypothyroidism in the adult

narcotic a drug capable of producing stupor and sleep, usually used to relieve pain
nasogastric tube a tube passed through the nose into the stomach
nasopharynx the section of the pharynx above the soft palate
nebulizer an atomizer or sprayer producing a fine mist used for the delivery of medication to the upper respiratory passages
necrosis death of tissue (adj., necrotic)
neoplasm new growth (adj., neoplastic)
nephrectomy removal of the kidney
nephritis inflammation of the kidney
nephron the structural unit of the kidney
nephrosclerosis hardening of renal arteries and arterioles
nephrostomy an opening into the kidney
nephrotoxic toxic to the kidney
neuroma a tumor growing from a nerve
nocturia excessive urination during the night
nodule a small node
norepinephrine a neurohormone produced by the adrenal medulla, similar to epinephrine
normovolemia a normal blood volume (adj., normovolemic)
nuchal rigidity pain and stiffness of the neck
nystagmus involuntary eye movements

occlusion blockage of a passage
oculogyric crisis a rolling downward or upward of the eyes against the patient's will
olfactory pertaining to smell
oliguria decrease in the amount of urine secretion
oophorectomy removal of an ovary
opiate a drug obtained from opium; also, any drug that induces sleep
opisthotonos extreme hyperextension of the head and arching of the back
orchiectomy surgical removal of the testicle
orchitis inflammation of the testes
orifice entrance; opening

oropharyngeal airway an airway inserted in the mouth and extending as far as the oropharynx
orthopnea difficulty breathing when lying flat or almost flat
ossification formation of bone
osteoarthritis a chronic arthritic disease of the joints, especially the weight-bearing joints
osteoblast a cell concerned with the formation of bone
osteomyelitis infection of the bone
osteoporosis loss of density of bone; demineralization of bone
osteotomy artificial angling of the bone through a surgical fracture
ostomy a surgical opening, e.g., colostomy, ileostomy
OTC abbr. for over-the-counter or nonprescription drugs
otitis inflammation of the ear
otosclerosis hearing loss resulting from ankylosis of the stapes
ovulation release of an ovum (egg) from the mature graafian follicle of the ovary
oxidation the process of combining with oxygen

pacemaker the SA (sinoatrial) node; an artificial pacemaker is an electrical device which substitutes for the heart's own pacemaker
pain the sensation of physical and/or mental suffering or hurt that usually causes distress or agony to the one suffering it
palliative relieving symptoms without curing the disease
pancreatitis inflammation of the pancreas
panhysterectomy removal of the entire uterus
Papanicolaou smear (test) cytologic examination of exfoliated cells
papilledema swelling of the optic nerve at its point of entrance into the eye
paracentesis removal of fluid from a cavity
paradoxical pulse a pulse that weakens on deep inspiration
paralytic ileus paralysis of intestines and absence of peristalsis
paraplegia paralysis of both lower extremities
parathormone parathyroid hormone
parenchyma the essential parts of an organ (adj., parenchymal)
parenteral therapy the giving of food, fluids, or other substances by routes other than the alimentary canal
paroxysm a sudden spasm; a sudden recurrence of symptoms
patent open (n., patency)
pathogen an organism that produces harm (adj., pathogenic)
pathophysiology the physiology of disordered function
peptic ulcer an ulcer in the lower esophagus, stomach, or duodenum
percutaneous through the skin
perfusion a specialized method of giving a drug with administration of the maximum dose to an isolated part of the body
pericarditis inflammation of the pericardium
pericardium the covering of the myocardium
perineum the area between the vulva and anus of the female and the scrotum and anus of the male (adj., perineal)
periosteum the fibrous covering of bones
peripheral to the periphery or the outside edge
peristalsis wavelike movements of hollow organs such as the intestine, esophagus, ureter
petechiae tiny hemorrhagic spots on the skin (adj., petechial)
phlebothrombosis presence of clots in a vein with little or no inflammation
phlebotomy an opening into a vein
photocoagulation use of a laser beam for surgical coagulation
photophobia aversion to light
plasma the liquid part of blood
platelet a blood cell concerned with the clotting of blood; also called thrombocyte
plexus a network of blood vessels or nerves
pneumoencephalogram an air contrast study performed when there is a suspected abnormality in the brain
pneumonectomy removal of a lung
pneumothorax air in the thoracic cavity
polycythemia vera an abnormal increase in red blood cells
polydipsia drinking a great deal of water; excessive thirst
polyp a tumor or growth attached by a pedicle to a surface
polyphagia increasing the intake of food
polyuria excessive secretion of urine
postictal state the period of time following a convulsive seizure
postpartum after childbirth
postural hypotension a feeling of weakness, dizziness, or faintness when suddenly changing position
premature ventricular contraction a ventricular ectopic beat occurring before depolarization of the ventricles and followed by a long pause; the patient may complain of a fluttering sensation in the chest (abbr., PVC)
presbycusis loss of hearing as a result of aging
presbyopia loss of visual accommodation as a result of aging
proctoscopy visualization of the rectum and anus

prodromal phase the early stage of a disease
prognosis the outcome or prediction of the course of disease
prolapse a dropping of an organ out of its original place or position
prostate a gland surrounding the neck of the bladder and urethra in the male
prosthesis an artificial substitute for a part (pl., prostheses)
prosthetist an individual who makes and fits artificial limbs
prothrombin a chemical substance in the blood converted into thrombin during blood clotting
proximal nearest to a point of reference; opposite of distal
pruritus itching
psoriasis a dermatitis with dull red lesions surrounded by silver scales
psychosomatic symptoms bodily symptoms which are psychic or emotional in origin
ptosis drooping
purines end products of the digestion of certain proteins
purpura hemorrhage into the skin and mucous membrane
purulent containing pus
pustule a small elevation on the skin containing pus or lymph
PVC abbr. for premature ventricular contraction
pyelitis inflammation of the pelvis of the kidney
pyelogram an x-ray of the kidney and ureter
pyuria presence of pus in the urine

quadriplegia paralysis of all four extremities
quiescent inactive, dormant

radiation the emission or giving off of rays
radioactive isotope an isotope capable of giving off rays
radioactivity the ability of a substance to emit alpha, beta, and gamma rays
radioisotope an isotope that is radioactive
radiopaque not penetrable by x-rays
radiosensitive sensitive to radiation; easily affected by radiation
radiotherapy therapeutic application of ionizing radiation from x-ray machines or radioactive substances
refractory resistant to treatment
repolarization realignment of ions after depolarization
respirator a mechanical device substituting for or assisting with respirations
reticuloendothelial system cells throughout the body which ingest matter such as bacteria
rheumatic fever an inflammatory disease frequently followed by damage to the heart or kidney
rheumatoid arthritis an inflammatory disease of connective tissue characterized by chronicity, remissions and exacerbations
rhinitis a reaction of the nasal mucosa to various allergens commonly found in the environment
rhizotomy a sectioning of the posterior nerve root just before it enters the spinal cord for the relief of pain
rhythmicity rhythmic activity
roentgenogram x-ray
ROM abbr. for range of motion exercises

salicylism a set of symptoms resulting from excessive injestion of a salicylate
salpingectomy removal of a fallopian tube
saphenous vein a vein in the leg
sarcoma a malignant tumor arising from connective tissue
sclerectomy removal of a portion of the sclera
sedative an agent that exerts a calming effect
seizure another term for a convulsion or an epileptic attack
sensorineural hearing loss nerve deafness
septicemia the presence of infective organisms in the bloodstream
sigmoidoscopy visualization of the sigmoid colon, rectum, anus
specific gravity weight of a substance compared with water, which has a specific gravity of 1.000, measured with a hydrometer
sphincter a circular muscle around an opening
sphygmomanometer blood pressure cuff
splenectomy removal of the spleen
splenomegaly enlargement of the spleen
sputum fluid raised from the respiratory passage
stasis stagnation
stenosis constriction, narrowing
stertorous labored breathing producing a snoringlike sound
stoma opening; mouth; artificially created opening
stomatitis inflammation of the mouth
stool softener a drug which softens the stool thereby easing passage
stress incontinence incontinence of urine during sneezing or coughing
subcutaneous below or beneath the skin
supine lying on the back
suprapubic above the pubic bone
sympathectomy an excision of a portion of the sympathetic nervous system, usually of a nerve, ganglion, or plexus
syncope fainting
syndrome a group of signs and symptoms
synovectomy removal of a synovial membrane
synovial membrane the membrane lining the capsule of a joint

systole contraction of the atria and ventricles (adj., systolic)

tachycardia elevated pulse rate
tachypnea rapid respiratory rate
tamponade, cardiac fluid in the pericardial space that compresses the heart
tenacious clinging, adhesive
teratoma a congenital tumor containing embryonic elements
tetany tonic spasms
thoracotomy an opening into the thorax
thrombocytopenia decreased number of platelets
thrombophlebitis development of inflammation with the formation of clots within the vein
thrombus a clot obstructing the lumen of a blood vessel
thyroidectomy removal of the thyroid gland
thyrotoxicosis a toxic condition due to hyperactivity of the thyroid gland
tinnitus ringing in the ears
tonic characterized by rigid contraction of the muscles
toxin a poisonous substance
toxoid a weakened toxin
tracheostomy an opening into the trachea
tranquilizer a drug which calms the individual and reduces tension without interfering with normal mental activity
transcutaneous through the skin
transvenous through the vein
Trichomonas a parasitic protozoa
trochanter roll a roll placed parallel to the upper thigh
tuberculostatic drug a drug used in the treatment of tuberculosis

ulcer a depression or defect
ulcerative colitis inflammation and ulceration of the colon
ultraviolet light light beyond the violet end of the visible spectrum
urea the end product of protein metabolism
uremia accumulation of nitrogenous substances in the blood (adj., uremic)
ureter hollow tube transporting urine from the kidney to the bladder
urethra hollow tube transporting urine from the bladder to the outside
uricosuric drug a drug promoting the excretion of urates
urinalysis laboratory examination of the urine
urobilinogen "conjugated" bilirubin formed by the liver enters the bile ducts, reaches the intestine, and is changed into urobilinogen which is changed into urobilin, the brown pigment of the stool
urticaria hives

vaccine a specific infectious agent given for establishing resistance to an infectious disease
vaginitis inflammation of the vagina
vagotomy surgical interruption of the vagus nerve to terminate the transmission of impulses along the vagus nerve
vagus nerve tenth cranial nerve; innervates structures in the chest, abdomen, head, neck
Valsalva's maneuver pinching the nostrils while at the same time trying to blow air through the nose
vasoconstriction constriction or narrowing of a blood vessel
vasodilatation dilatation or enlargement of the diameter of a blood vessel
vasomotor nerves nerves having control over the size of blood vessels
vasopressor a drug capable of constricting blood vessels, particularly arteries and arterioles
venostasis the trapping of blood in an extremity by compression of a vein
ventilation the movement of air in and out of the lungs
vital capacity a measure of the amount of air a person can expire following maximal inspiration

wheal a raised lesion often accompanied by severe itching; a hive

INDEX